VOLUME 1

Imaging Children

*To our husband and wives who have
supported us throughout this project*

For Churchill Livingstone:

Commissioning Editor: Geoffrey Nuttall
Project Editor: Lowri Daniels
Copy Editor: Pat Croucher
Indexer: Monica Trigg
Production Controllers: Neil Dickson, Kay Hunston
Sales Promotion Executive: Douglas McNaughton

VOLUME 1

Imaging Children

Edited by

Helen Carty MB BCh FRCPI FRCR
Director of Radiology, Royal Liverpool Children's Hospital Trust,
Alder Hey Hospital; Lecturer in Radiodiagnosis, University of
Liverpool, Liverpool, UK

Francis Brunelle MD
Professor of Radiology, Hopital des Enfants Malades, Paris, France

Foreword by

Hans G. Ringertz MD PhD
Professor and Chairman, Department of Diagnostic Radiology,
Karolinska Hospital, Stockholm, Sweden

Donald Shaw MA MSc BM BCh DMRD FRCP
FRCR
Consultant Radiologist, Hospitals for Sick Children, Great Ormond
Street, London, UK

Brian Kendall FRCR FRCP FRCS
Director of Radiology, National Hospital for Neurology and
Neurosurgery, London; Neuroradiologist, Hospitals for Sick
Children, London, UK

CHURCHILL LIVINGSTONE
EDINBURGH LONDON MADRID MELBOURNE NEW YORK AND TOKYO 1994

CHURCHILL LIVINGSTONE
Medical Division of Longman Group Limited

Distributed in the United States of America by Churchill
Livingstone Inc., 650 Avenue of the Americas, New York,
N.Y. 10011, and by associated companies, branches and
representatives throughout the world.

First published 1994

ISBN 0 443 04260 8

British Library Cataloguing in Publication Data
A catalogue record for this book is available from the British Library.

Library of Congress Cataloging in Publication Data
A catalog record for this book is available from the Library of Congress.

The
publisher's
policy is to use
**paper manufactured
from sustainable forests**

Printed and bound in Great Britain by William Clowes Limited,
Beccles and London

Contents

VOLUME 2

Contributors

Laurence Abernethy MA MB ChB MRCP FRCR
Consultant Radiologist, Royal Liverpool Children's
Hospital Trust, Alder Hey, Liverpool, UK

Fred E. Avni MD PhD
Associate Professor, Department of Radiology,
University Clinics of Brussels, ULB Erasme Hospital,
Brussels, Belgium

Olivier Berges MD
Chef de Service Adjoint, Service d'Imagerie Médicale,
Fondation A. de Rothschild; Consultant
d'Echographie, Service d'Ophtalmologie, Paris, France

Francis Brunelle MD
Professor of Radiology, Hopital des Enfants Malades,
Paris, France

Helen Carty MB BCh FRCPI FRCR
Director of Radiology, Royal Liverpool Children's
Hospital Trust, Alder Hey Hospital; Lecturer in
Radiodiagnosis, University of Liverpool, Liverpool, UK

Philippe Demaerel MD
Staff Radiologist, Department of Radiology,
University Hospitals, Katholieke Universitat, Leuven,
Belgium

Claire Dicks-Mireaux BA MB BS DMRD MRCP
FRCR
Consultant Radiologist, The Hospitals for Sick
Children, Great Ormond Street, London, UK

Veronica Donoghue MB BCh BAO FRCR DMRD
(Lond)
Consultant Paediatric Radiologist, The Children's
Hospital, Dublin and The National Maternity
Hospital, Dublin, Eire

Josée Dubois MD FRCP
Assistant Professor, Department of Pediatric
Radiology, University of Montreal, St-Justine
Hospital, Montreal, Canada

J. Dubousset MD
Professor, Hopital St Vincent de Paul, Paris, France

Nadine Girard MD
Assistant Professor, Department of Radiology,
Hopital Nord, Marseille, France

Christine Hall MB BS DMRD FRCR
Consultant Paediatric Radiologist, Department of
Radiology, The Hospitals for Sick Children, Great
Ormond Street, London, UK

Anne S. Hollman MB ChB FRCR FRCP (Glas)
Consultant Paediatric Radiologist, Department of
Radiology, Royal Hospital for Sick Children, Yorkhill,
Glasgow, UK

G. Kalifa MD
Professor, Department of Radiology, Hopital St
Vincent de Paul, Paris

Brian Kendall FRCR FRCP FRCS
Director of Radiology, National Hospital for
Neurology and Neurosurgery, London;
Neuroradiologist, Hospitals for Sick Children,
London, UK

G. Lalande MD
Service de Radiologie, Hopital St Vincent de Paul,
Paris, France

Sylvia Neuenschwander MD
Head of Department of Radiology, Institut Curie,
Paris, France

Danièle Pariente MD
Practicien Hospitalier, Service de Radio-Pédiatrie,
Hopital Bicetre, Paris, France

Ethna Phelan MB BCh FRCR
Consultant Radiologist, Royal Children's Hospital,
Melbourne, Victoria, Australia

Peter D. Phelps MD FRCS FRCR
Consultant Radiologist, the Royal National Throat,
Nose and Ear Hospital, London and Walsgrave
Hospital, Coventry, UK

Charles Raybaud MD
Professor, Neuroradiologie, Hopital Nord, Marseille,
France

Peter Renton MB FRCR DMRD
Consultant Radiologist, Royal National Orthopaedic
Hospital, London and University College Hospital,
London; Honorary Senior Lecturer, University
College London, London, UK

CONTRIBUTORS

Michael B. Rubens MB BS DMRD FRCR
Consultant Radiologist, Royal Brompton National
Heart and Lung Hospital and London Chest Hospital;
Honorary Senior Lecturer, National Heart and Lung
Institute, University of London, London, UK

Steven W. Ryan MD MRCP
Senior Lecturer in Neonatal Medicine, University of
Liverpool; Honorary Consultant Neonatologist,
Liverpool Maternity Hospital, Liverpool;
Senior Lecturer in Neo-natal Medicine, Institute of
Child Health, R.L.C. National Health Trust, Alder
Hey, Liverpool, UK

Guy H. Sebag MD
Assistant Chef de Clinique, Service de Radiologie
Pédiatrique, Hopital des Enfants-Malades, Paris,
France

Donald Shaw MA MSc BM BCh DMRD FRCP FRCR
Consultant Radiologist, Hospitals for Sick Children,
Great Ormond Street, London, UK

John M. Stevens MB BS FRACR FRCR
Consultant Neuroradiologist, The National Hospitals
for Neurology and Neurosurgery, Maida Vale
Hospital, London, UK

Paul S. Thomas MB DMRD FRCR
Consultant Radiologist, Royal Belfast Hospital for
Sick Children, Belfast, UK

D. Van Gansbeke MD
Hopital Erasme, Radiology Department, Brussels,
Belgium

Ulrich Willi MD
Assistant Professor of Radiology, Head of Pediatric
Radiology, University Children's Hospital, Zurich,
Switzerland

Foreword

Paediatric radiology includes diseases that only occur in children, diseases that children have in common with adults but that are also affected by the growth of the child, and the normal development of all organ systems. This wide definition, combined with the recent development of numerous new radiological modalities, presents a challenging and stimulating background for a European textbook of paediatric radiology.

Imaging Children reflects the coming-of-age of the science of paediatric radiology in Europe. The book also parallels the co-operation in health care, education and science within and around the European Community. In my opinion, this book is the best thing that has happened in European paediatric radiology in the last few years. The members of the UK–French editorial team have taken an important initiative and

have been very successful in their endeavours. They, and their European contributors, have written a carefully structured text and the illustrations of pertinent cases and findings are of very high quality.

Paediatric radiology is practised in many forms, in specialized units by paediatric radiologists and in general radiology departments. In the same way, this book will be needed as an overview in the specialist unit and as a basic bench book in general departments of diagnostic radiology.

Whichever forum this book is used in, it will be very valuable. I congratulate the editors and authors on a successful joint effort.

Stockholm   Hans G. Ringertz

Preface

Children are precious — everywhere — representing the hope of continuity of our species and the promise of achievement over their forthcoming lifespan.

Children are different. They are not miniature adults. They suffer different illnesses and react in a different way from adults. Most illnesses are foreign to their nature, and happily children generally have great powers of recovery.

Children are frightening to doctors more familiar with adults and their diseases. Clinically this matters less because paediatricians have appropriate training. However, imaging children may be a marginal activity of a radiologist whose main interests and activities centre on adults.

There are already three splendid standard textbooks of paediatric radiology: Caffey, Swischuk and Kirk. All of these are American and reflect the generally excellent American medical culture. There is another culture of European Paediatric Radiology well reflected for some three decades by the European Society of Paediatric Radiology. While *Imaging Children* is in no way sponsored or underpinned by the ESPR it is the intention of the editors to make available in this textbook a summary of the challenges, agonies and delights of paediatric radiology from a European perspective.

It is a first throw in a keenly competitive game. We have done all we can to ensure that there will be second and subsequent throws. The decision rests with you, the readers.

We hope you enjoy it.

H.C.
D.S.
F.B.
B.K.

Acknowledgements

We would like to acknowledge our colleagues who helped us with advice and provided illustrations, our Secretaries and our Medical Illustration Departments. We would like, in particular, to thank Mrs Dorothy Turner, who performed the lion's share of the secretarial work associated with this book.

H.C.

Please note that Table 7.5.3 is based on information in Table 38–3 in *Caffey's Pediatric X-Ray Diagnosis 9E* (1992)

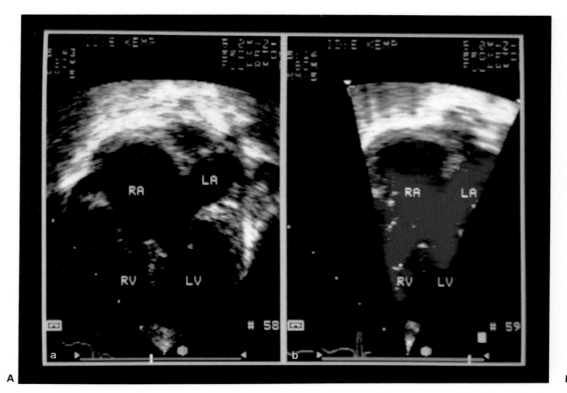

Fig. 2.1.16 A,B Colour-flow Doppler echocardiogram showing flow across a large primum ASD. RA = right atrium, LA = left atrium, RV = right ventricle, LV = left ventricle.

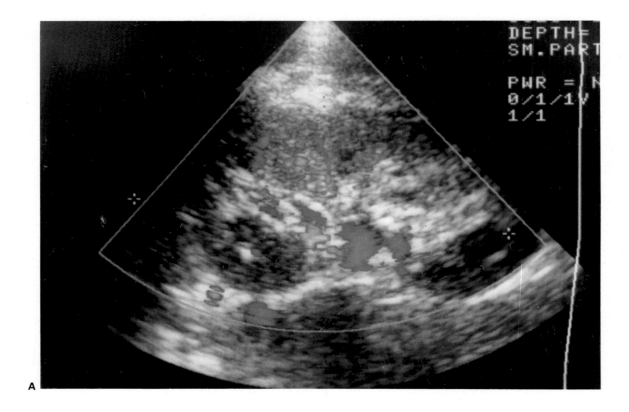

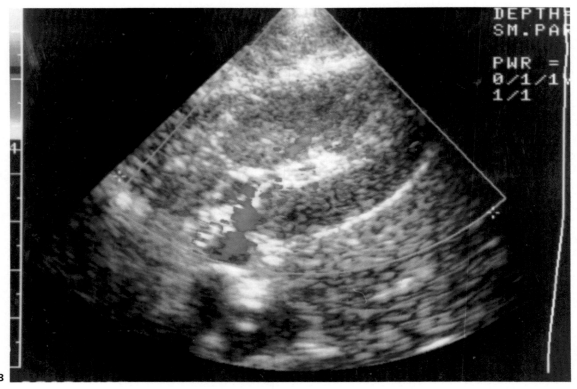

Fig. 5.1.14 Renal vascularization. Colour Doppler. Sagittal (A) transverse scans (B). Normal venous and arterial flow is displayed as far as the interlobar area.

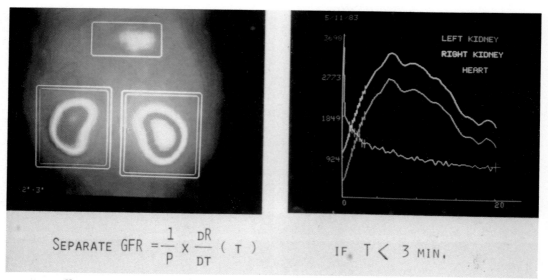

$$\text{SEPARATE GFR} = \frac{1}{P} \times \frac{DR}{DT} \; (T)$$

IF. T < 3 MIN.

Fig. 5.1.24 99mTc-DTPA isotope study. Glomerular filtration transit time, typical graph (right).

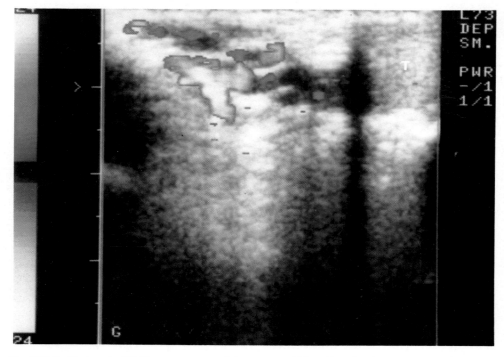

Fig. 5.12.7 Varicocele. US. Transverse scan of the scrotum. Colour Doppler demonstration of dilated vessels above and around the testis (T).

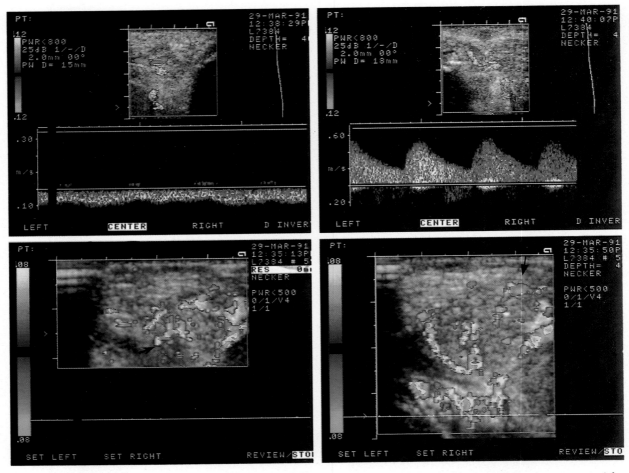

Fig. 9.2.1 Haemangioma of the nose. A Colour Doppler ultrasound. Hypervascular mass with feeding arteries forming an equatorial network at the periphery (arrow).

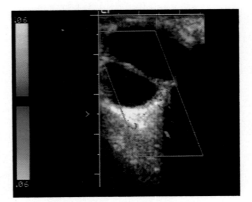

Fig. 11.4B Resistant hyperplastic primary vitreous. CDFI.

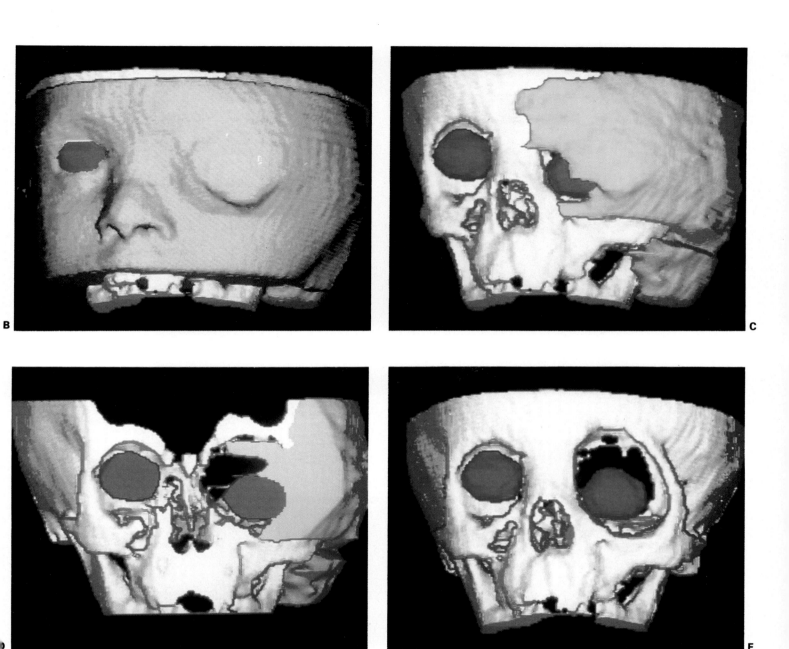

Fig. 11.5 Neurofibromatosis. **B – E** Three-dimensional reconstructions. These reconstructions help in understanding the different pathological conditions encountered in and around the orbit. **B** Anterolateral oblique view. The skin is coded in yellow, the eyes in dark blue, the left eye is hidden by a huge palpebral neurofibroma. **C** Same view after removal of the skin. The neurofibroma is coded in light blue. **D** After cutting of the superficial structures, it is easy to appreciate the infiltration of the superior part of the orbit by the neurofibroma. The eyeball is displaced downward. **E** After removal of the neurofibroma, the sphenoid bone dysplasia is obvious. The orbit is enlarged. There is no bone structure between the posterolateral orbit and mid-temporal fossa.

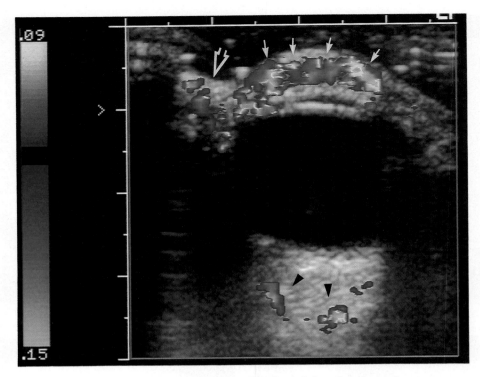

Fig. 11.12 Capillary haemangioma in a 1-year-old baby. A Colour Doppler section.

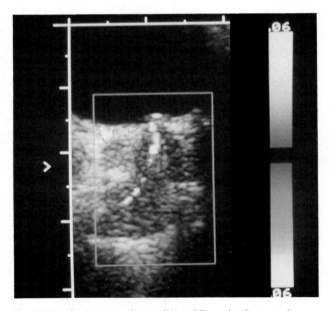

Fig. 11.16 Optic nerve glioma. **E** Axial B-mode ultrasound section with colour Doppler flow imaging.

1

The chest

D. Shaw

INTRODUCTION

THE DEVELOPMENT OF THE LUNG

At birth, lung development is far from complete. The bronchial tree is fully developed by 16 weeks' gestation. From 16 weeks to term, respiratory airways develop so that at birth primitive saccules, simple air spaces, are found in the lung periphery.

After birth, alveoli develop and from about 20 million primitive saccules present in the newborn, 300 million alveoli develop by the age of 8 years, following which there is an increase in size of the alveoli until thoracic growth ceases in adulthood.

In the extreme premature but viable infant there are many fewer primitive alveolar saccules than in the lungs of a term infant. A variety of conditions can inhibit the development of the non-respiratory airways before 16 weeks' gestation including congenital diaphragmatic hernia, renal malformation (in particular, agenesis), absent phrenic nerve associated with diaphragmatic amyoplasia, agenesis of the lungs and rhesus isoimmunization.

REFERENCES

Fawcitt J, Lind J, Wegelius C 1960 The first breath. Acta Paediatrica Scandinavica Supplement 123 49: 5–17
Inselman L S, Mellins R B 1981 Growth and development of the lung. Journal of Pediatrics 98: 1–15
Reid L 1977 The lung: its growth and remodeling in health and disease. American Journal of Roentgenology 129: 777–788
Reid L 1984 Lung growth in health and disease. British Journal of Diseases of the Chest 78: 113–134

RADIOGRAPHIC TECHNIQUE

Except in the neonate and very sick child, it is always desirable to radiograph the chest in the erect position. Whereas in the adult a PA projection is desirable, in practice in the younger child there is little difference between an AP and PA view. With a suitable chest stand, however, it is usually possible to achieve a satisfactory PA projection. Because the child's chest is more cylindrical than the adult, relatively small amounts of rotation will lead to asymmetry of the hemithoraces and this can lead to differing radiolucencies of the lung fields. An adequate inspiration is important as an expiratory film will lead to spurious impressions of cardiomegaly, abnormally prominent pulmonary vasculature and relative opacification of the lung fields, particularly in the bases (Fig. 1.0.1).

In a small child a poor inspiration is associated with buckling and deviation of the lower trachea to the right. If the aortic arch is on the right, the associated buckling is towards the left. These appearances should not be interpreted as a mediastinal tumour.

ARTEFACTUAL AND MISLEADING PSEUDOTUMOROUS APPEARANCES

The normal thymus in the small child and baby is a common pseudotumorous appearance. Fat in the mediastinum, particularly following steroid therapy, thymic haemorrhage and lymph node enlargement all at times lead to diagnostic difficulties. Superimposition of the scapulae and axillary folds in lateral films can simulate posterior mediastinal masses. The glenoid process of the scapula in lateral projection may cause apparent filling defects in the trachea, and if overlying the vertebral bodies give the false impression of vertebral collapse. In a thin child the anterior axillary folds overlying the lateral part of the upper thoracic cage can simulate a pneumothorax but the characteristic normal extension of a pneumothorax into the apex of the lungs is not seen (Fig. 1.0.2). Breast tissue in the pubertal girl at times casts confusing densities; in the presence of lipodystrophy, mammary tissue in the newborn can give marked rounded densities overlying the chest.

Encysted interlobar pleural effusions, which when seen side on give ovoid opacities, although commoner in adults, are well recognized in childhood particularly in association with congestive heart failure. Mucous impaction, rounded pseudotumorous pneumonia, rounded atelectasis and postinflammatory pseudotumours all occasionally give rise to confusing appearances. Normal pulmonary vasculature seen end on, particularly in the hilar regions, may be dense and the resulting rounded shadows may be misinterpreted either as hilar calcifications or as metastases. Usually on careful inspection vessels may be seen coursing peripherally in continuity with these shadows, thus indicating their true origins.

Long hair, particularly when plaited, causes a variety of bizarre yet sometimes misleading shadowing, particularly in the upper zones.

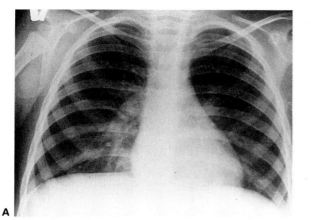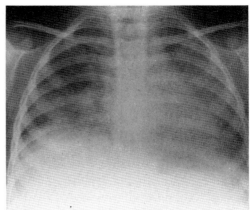

Fig. 1.0.1 Inspiratory (**A**) and expiratory (**B**) chest radiographs.

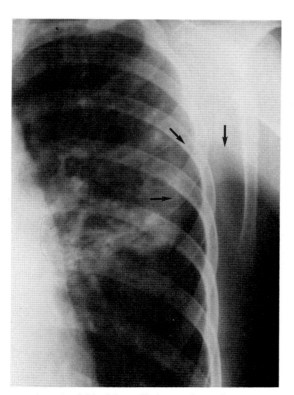

Fig. 1.0.2 Anterior fold of the axilla (arrows) simulating pneumothorax.

STERNAL OSSIFICATION CENTRES

Delayed ossification of the mesosternum in the small child is a useful but not absolute indicator of congenital heart disease. Defective ossification of the sternum may occur in Noonan's syndrome, campomelic dysplasia and de Lange's syndrome.

Premature sternal fusion and multiple manubrial ossification centres are described associations of congenital heart disease as is pectus carinatum, and are also seen in trisomy 18 and Noonan's syndrome.

The multiple sternal ossifications in childhood may cast misinterpreted shadows, particularly if frontal radiographs have been taken in a slightly oblique projection, and occasionally raise the spurious suggestion of inhaled foreign body if projected over a major airway.

Depressed sternum, pectus excavatum, is the displacement of the heart shadow to the left from its normal position of one-third of the heart shadow being to the right of the midline and two-thirds to the left (Fig. 1.0.3). The posterior ends of the ribs run a horizontal or even upward course and are steeply inclined inferiorly anteriorly. Increased shadowing may be seen medially in the right lower lung field. The lateral projection will confirm the degree of depression, for which surgery is sometimes undertaken.

REFERENCES

Fischer K C, White R I, Jordan C E, Dorse J P, Neill C A 1973 Sternal abnormalities in patients with congenital heart disease. American Journal of Roentgenology 119: 530–538

Kim O E, Gooding C A 1980–81 Delayed sternal ossification in infants with congenital heart disease. Pediatric Radiology 10: 219

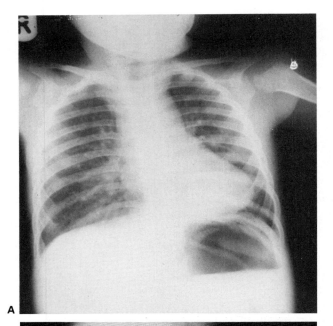

A

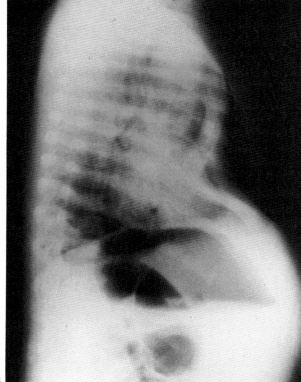

B

Fig. 1.0.3 **A,B** Depressed sternum. Note cardiac displacement to the left.

RIBS

Minor congenital anomalies of the ribs, especially bifid anterior ends, are common, as are mild hypoplasia and minor errors of segmentation; a possible association with childhood malignancy has been suggested.

Rib notching due to coarctation becomes more prominent in later childhood and is not a common feature in infancy. Asymmetrical or unilateral rib notching is a common consequence in the upper ribs following Blalock–Taussig shunts, and in the lower ribs in association with lower thoracic coarctation. Systemic collateral arterial supply to the lungs in congenital heart disease is also associated with rib notching (often unevenly distributed) as are lymphangiectasia, neurofibromatosis, sometimes following poliomyelitis and superior vena caval obstruction.

Widening of the anterior ends of the ribs may indicate rickets or a metaphyseal chondrodysplasia. Thickening of the ribs is seen in storage diseases such as the mucopolysaccharidoses, in haemoglobino-pathies (Fig. 1.0.4), and in infantile cortical hyperostosis in which rarely consequent rib fusion leads to a severe scoliosis, also seen following postoperative rib fusion after neonatal thoracic surgery.

Tumorous conditions of the ribs include the common osteochondroma seen in association with diaphyseal aclasis or in the margin of a radiation field, Langerhans' cell histiocytosis and a variety of rarer small round cell malignant tumours and neonatal mesenchymal hamartomas.

Hyperaemia in association with underlying pneumonia, often with pleural effusions but without frank empyema, may lead to development and subsequent organization of periosteal reactions along adjacent ribs, often a transitory appearance easily overlooked (Fig. 1.0.5). Haemothorax is described as a complication of costal cartilaginous exostoses.

Increased numbers of ribs and hypersegmentation of the vertebral column are associated with oesophageal atresia, tracheo-oesophageal fistula and anal atresia.

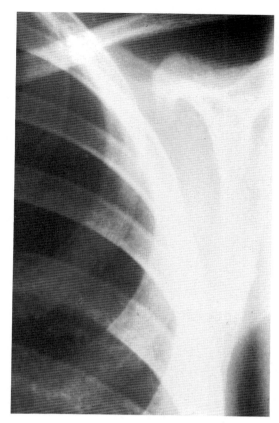

Fig. 1.0.4 Thalassaemia. Note the coarse rib trabecular pattern.

REFERENCE

Propfer R A, Young L W, Ward B P 1980 Haemothorax as a complication of costal cartilaginous exostoses. Pediatric Radiology 9: 135–137

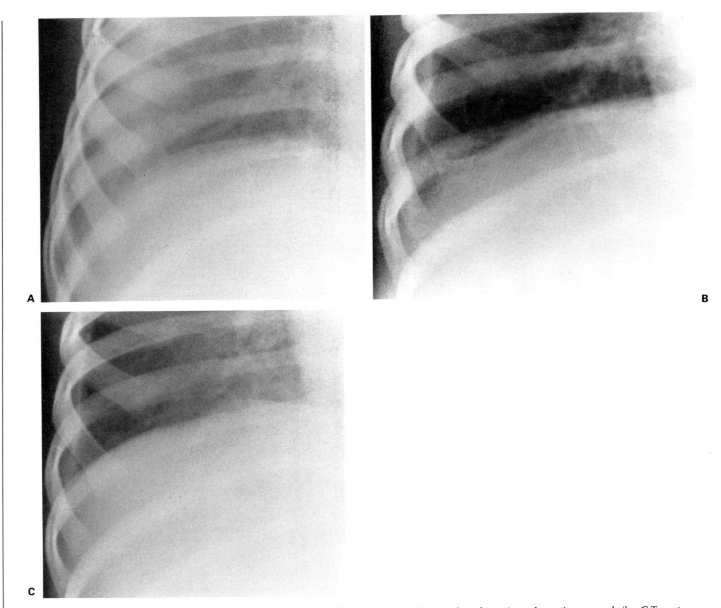

Fig. 1.0.5 Pleural effusion in bacterial pneumonia. **A** At presentation. **B** Ten days later with early periosteal reaction around ribs. **C** Twenty days, periosteal reaction consolidating with rib thickening now evident.

CERVICAL HERNIATION OF THE LUNG

Marked protrusions of the apices of the lungs are sometimes seen, extending into the root of the neck above the first rib, and can be unilateral or bilateral. Forced expiration or exertion can accentuate their prominence. The condition is of no significance other than cosmetic. Also in the root of the neck the suprasternal fossa may be deep enough to cast an ovoid, at times confusing, radiolucency.

REFERENCES

Hernandez R, Kubus L R, Holt J F 1978 The suprasternal fossa on chest radiographs in newborns. American Journal of Roentgenology 130: 745–746
Jones J G 1970 Cervical hernia of the lung. Journal of Pediatrics 76: 122–125
Palazzo W L, Garrett T A 1951 Cervical hernia of the lung. Radiology 56: 575–576

Respiratory difficulties are a feature of a variety of chest wall conditions. In osteogenesis imperfecta, multiple rib fractures and thoracic deformity in the severe forms are important predisposing causes towards often fatal pneumonia. Scoliosis whether idiopathic, paralytic or osteogenic, and restrictive conditions such as fibrodysplasia ossificans progressiva (Fig. 1.0.6) are also associated with restriction of thoracic movement and respiratory compromise.

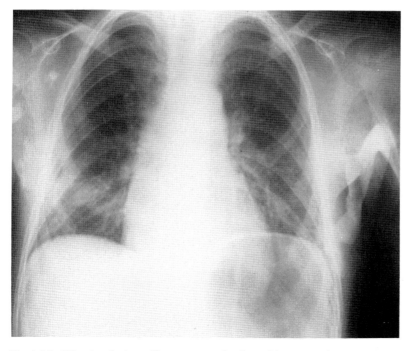

Fig. 1.0.6 Fibrodysplasia ossificans progressiva (myositis progressiva ossificans). Extensive abnormal ossification is seen in the soft tissues of the chest wall and this is associated with consolidation in the right lower zone.

THYMUS

The thymus in childhood is a relatively large organ occupying the anterior and superior mediastinum extending down into the diaphragm and up into the neck (Fig. 1.0.7). Rarely, thymic tissue occurs in the posterior mediastinum. Particularly on the right side the thymus may exhibit a characteristic sail-like shadow with a well-defined lateral and inferior margin. Noticeably on the left side the thymus moulds to the undulations of the inner thoracic wall caused by the ribs giving rise to a wavy lateral margin as seen in the frontal radiograph. Especially in the infant a prominent thymus can obscure the cardiac borders and differentiation of the cardiac shadow from the thymic shadow may be impossible. A radiographic determination of the cardiac size from a frontal radiograph in small children can be unreliable even in the absence of a large thymus, and echocardiography will allow a much better evaluation of cardiac morphology. Although thymic tissue may transiently disappear with illness in the small child the thymus is usually visible on chest radiographs for the first 3–4 years of life, whereafter it becomes relatively progressively smaller in relation to the size of the child, although reaching its largest absolute size around puberty.

Thymic hypoplasia is associated with a variety of diseases with immune deficiency although the value of this radiographic sign is not great, particularly with the frequent involution of the thymus with infection.

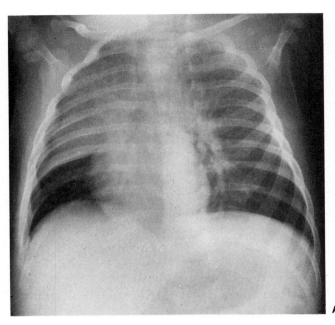

A

Fig. 1.0.7 Normal thymus. **A** The 'wave' shown to advantage due to some rotation. **B** 'Sail' sign. **C** 'Spinnaker' sign in the presence of pneumomediastinum.

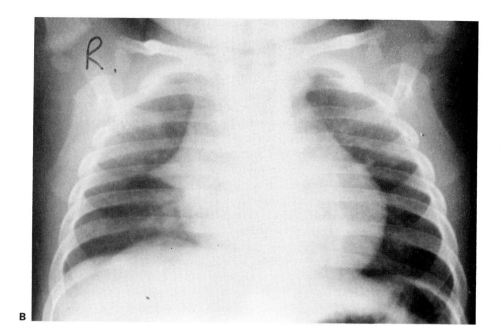

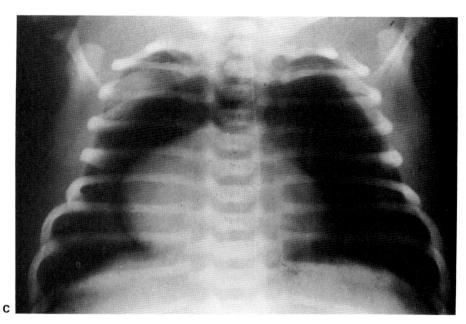

A similar difficulty occurs in the DiGeorge syndrome of congenital parathyroid dysfunction, aortic arch anomalies and malformation and maldevelopment of thymus, as chest radiographs in the first few days of life may show absence of thymic shadows for other causes and thus be of little use in the substantiation of diagnosis (Fig. 1.0.8).

Marked thymic enlargement can result from exogenous thyroid therapy, in addition to being described in other endocrine disorders such as thyrotoxicosis, acromegaly and Addison's disease. Considerable enlargement may occur as a rebound phenomenon after chemotherapy.

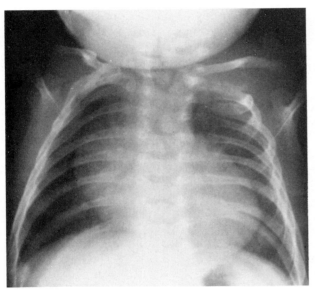

Fig. 1.0.8 DiGeorge's syndrome. Cardiomegaly, rib anomalies and narrow superior mediastinum.

Ectopic and accessory thymic tissue

The thymus is a confusing organ in the neonate and the normal prominence of the organ may simulate a tumour. Ultrasonography of the infant's chest is simple and the delineation of the normal thymic tissue with its uniform echogenicity and without evidence of displacement of the major thoracic vessels is a particularly useful technique (Fig. 1.0.9). Conventional computed tomographic examination of the anterior mediastinum in the very young is often relatively unrewarding, although ultrafast techniques provide better anatomical delineation.

Ectopic thymic tissue is present in about a fifth of the population, often occurring incidentally in the region of the thyroid, but less frequently as well-circumscribed nodules in the neck, measuring up to 1–2 cm diameter. Ectopic thymic cysts are usually larger. Accessory thymic tissue may occur in the anterior or posterior mediastinum (Fig. 1.0.10).

Although inconspicuous the thymus persists in the anterior mediastinum in the older and adolescent child with relatively clearly defined margins to its lobes particularly seen on CT. In early adulthood, fatty infiltration of the thymus can occur physiologically.

REFERENCES

Bar-Ziv J, Barki Y, Itzchak Y, Mares A J 1984 Posterior mediastinal accessory thymus. Pediatric Radiology 14: 165–167
Day D L, Gedgaudas E 1984 The thymus. Radiologic Clinics of North America. 22: 519–538
Harris V J, Ramilo J, White H 1980 The thymic mass as a mediastinal dilemma. Clinical Radiology 31: 263–269
Heiberg E, Wolverson M K, Sundaram M, Nouri S 1982 Normal thymus: CT characteristics in subjects under age 20. American Journal of Roentgenology 138: 491–494

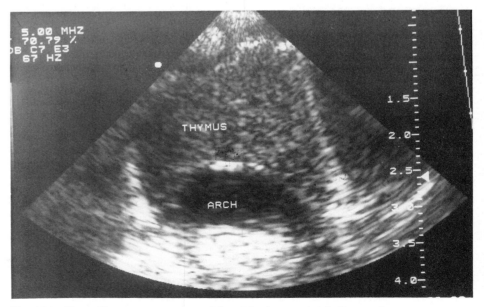

Fig. 1.0.9 Normal homogeneous echogenicity of the thymus. Axial ultrasound.

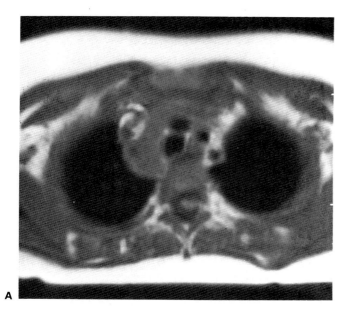

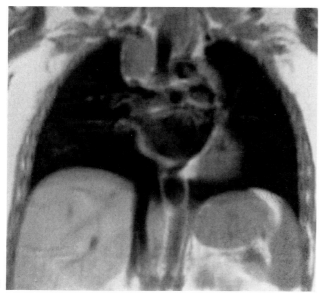

Fig. 1.0.10 Normal thymus. There is a posterior right-sided extension. **A** Axial T1. **B** Coronal T1.

Lanning P, Heikkinen E 1980 Thymus simulating left upper lobe atelectasis. Pediatric Radiology 9: 177–178

Moskowitz P S, Noon M A, McAlister W H, Mark B D J 1980 Thymic cyst hemorrhage: a cause of acute symptomatic mediastinal widening in children with aplastic anaemia. American Journal of Roentgenology 134: 832–836

Woodhead P J 1984 Thymic enlargement following chemotherapy. British Journal of Radiology 57: 932–934

POSITIVE CONTRAST BRONCHOGRAPHY

Positive contrast bronchography is a potentially dangerous investigation in the child. The indications for the investigation should be rigorously considered and it is important that the procedure be carried out in conjunction with a competent paediatric anaesthetist. Although in older children methods used in adults such as introduction of a catheter through the cricothyroid membrane by the Seldinger technique or direct installation through a locally anaesthetized larynx can be employed, in the young child endotracheal intubation under anaesthesia is a safer and more pleasant procedure. Preliminary physiotherapy and plain radiography should be undertaken; the place of atropinization is debatable and usually unnecessary. Installation of contrast medium through an endotracheal catheter passed through the endotracheal tube allows both general delineation of the bronchial tree or allows local specific examination of areas, for instance, of broncho- or tracheo-malacia.

It is prudent to investigate only one side of the bronchial tree unless satisfactory near-complete aspiration of contrast medium can be carried out. Bilateral bronchography in the child has led to unfortunate fatalities. Small volumes of non-ionic contrast medium are used following the withdrawal of Dionosil. The procedure should be carried out under fluoroscopic control so that the endobronchial volume of the contrast medium can be monitored and a dynamic appreciation of the airways made. Films may be taken fluorographically or following posturing in frontal, oblique and lateral views by conventional radiography. At the end of the procedure endotracheal and bronchial toilet should be performed, supplemented by physiotherapy on recovery of consciousness. If nursed in a lateral position, the examined side should be lower.

REFERENCES

Muller N L, Bergin C J, Ostrow D H 1984 Role of computed tomography in recognition of bronchiectasis. American Journal of Roentgenology 143: 971–976

Reid L 1950 Reduction of bronchial subdivision in bronchiectasis. Thorax 5: 233–247

Trapnell D H, Gregg I 1969 Some principles of interpretations of bronchograms. British Journal of Radiology 42: 125–131

COMPUTED TOMOGRAPHY (CT) OF THE PAEDIATRIC CHEST

This is now a well-established procedure in childhood and is of particular use in:

1. the detection and follow-up of pulmonary metastases
2. the evaluation of suspected tumours, particularly when involving the mediastinum
3. the evaluation of chest wall pathology, particularly tumour
4. when used with dynamic enhancement with intravenous contrast medium, clarification of the anatomy of the major thoracic vessels particularly when anomalous
5. indicating to some extent the pathology of mass lesions by identifying fat or calcification
6. particularly when used with high resolution and thin sections, the assessment of diffuse parenchymal infiltrates often underestimated on plain radiographs
7. the evaluation of the major airways and assessment of bronchiectasis.

There are certain problems in childhood which can lead to difficulties. Young children may need sedation, and babies and uncooperative children general anaesthesia. As a result, transient areas of collapse may be seen in dependent parts of the lung which can be confusing, particularly if metastases are to be excluded. Scanning the child prone instead of supine may help clarify these artefacts. The intrinsically small size of the infant can mean that image resolution may be suboptimal and even if respiration is controlled, this may be aggravated by tachycardia. The relatively small amount of fat means that tissue planes may not be so clearly identified as in older children and in adults. The normal thymus may be misinterpreted as pathological.

Needle biopsies of tumorous and parenchymal lesions can be guided by CT, but the radiation dose (in the order of 0.015 Gy) needs to be remembered. For sedation protocols for CT in childhood see Appendix.

Ultrafast CT by observing the normal variations of lung density during the respiratory cycle has been shown to be a non-invasive rapid method for evaluating pulmonary and particularly obstructive airways disease, both in the central and in the peripheral airways.

MAGNETIC RESONANCE IMAGING (MRI)

Although this technique is widely available in North America, access is relatively poor in Europe. There is a wide experience of paediatric neuroimaging but experience of body scanning with magnetic resonance is still relatively limited and applications are being constantly assessed and developed. The relatively slow acceptance of body imaging is partly related to difficulties with sedation and anaesthesia because of the length of the examination and an environment claustrophobic and frightening to a small child. Cardiac and respiratory motion degrades images and respiratory and cardiac gating are needed, although shorter sequences are being developed. Nevertheless, extensive evaluation of cardiac anatomy and function and of the thoracic great vessels has been achieved. In the thorax MRI is useful in evaluation of chest wall, soft tissue and spinal and paraspinal pathology. High soft tissue contrast is achieved but small areas of calcification are not adequately delineated. The technique is of particular use in the mediastinum and is perhaps the best technique for differentiating thymic pathology from a normal physiological enlargement. The relationship of the great vessels to the trachea is usually clearly defined and the ability to scan in any plane is particularly useful. Experience with the use of MRI in diffuse lung disorders is relatively small in the paediatric age group, but as with high definition thin slice CT, parenchymal lesions may be more striking than on plain radiographs. The place of dynamic changes and appearances with inspiration and expiration needs further evaluation but these are likely to prove fruitful in the evaluation of conditions such as Langerhans' cell histiocytosis, allergic alveolitis and the evaluation of pulmonary graft-versus-host disease.

DIGITAL RADIOGRAPHY

Digital radiography is being developed and evaluated and with its lower dose of radiation and facility to post-process images no doubt will be of increasing practical importance. It is as yet not widely available. CT scanners do provide a digital image with their localization facility and the opportunity to view at different windows. This finds practical application in airway evaluation (Fig. 1.0.11).

THIN SLICE HIGH RESOLUTION CT

This can replace positive contrast bronchography, especially if combined with ultrafast techniques, in many cases of bronchiectasis. If the lumen of the bronchus is wider than its associated vessel, giving rise to the 'signet ring' sign, bronchiectasis can be assumed (Fig. 1.0.12). In the small child and infant CT assessment of bronchiectasis may not be so satisfactory, but surgical intervention at this stage is also less likely. Assessment of the major airways in this age group, however, is feasible and can be supplemented by high kV filter techniques, fluoroscopy, aided sometimes by the instillation of small amounts of bronchographic contrast medium.

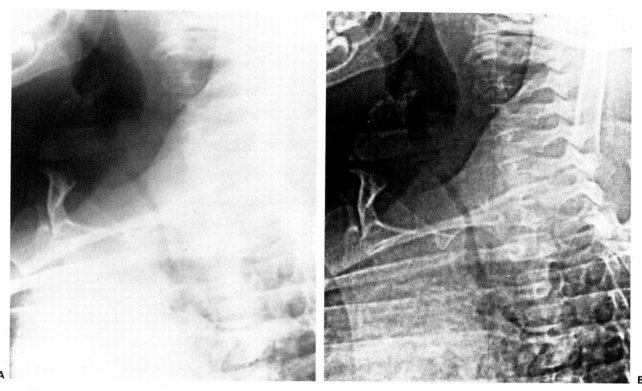

Fig. 1.0.11 Conventional radiograph (**A**) and digital radiograph (**B**), demonstrating good delineation of the airways with digital techniques.

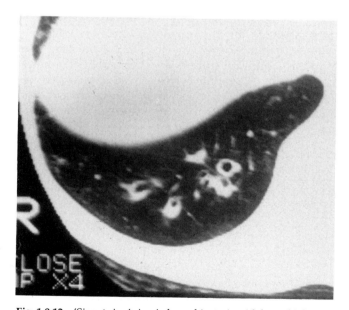

Fig. 1.0.12 'Signet ring' sign in bronchiectasis with bronchial lumen wider than accompanying vessel.

REFERENCES

Brody A S, Kuhn J P, Seidel F G, Brodsky L S 1991 Airway evaluation in children with use of ultrafast CT: pitfalls and recommendations. Radiology 178: 181–184
Mandell G, Harcke H T, Padman R, Brunson G, Delengowski R 1987 CT digital radiography. Pediatric Radiology 17: 505–508

RADIOLOGICAL ASSESSMENT OF THE OROPHARYNX AND LARYNGOPHARYNX

Nasal obstruction, noisy breathing and stridor are common clinical problems in children, especially in association with fever and ill health.

Lateral plain radiographs with air as a negative contrast medium allow satisfactory evaluation of the upper airways. In the newborn nasopharyngeal adenoidal lymphatic tissue is small, but by the age of 2 years the normal adenoidal pad will measure over 5 mm. In the older child, although the tonsils may be assessed by visual inspection, lateral films of the posterior nasal space allow evaluation of the size of the adenoids better than direct inspection and would allow estimation of the available airway between the adenoidal pad and the soft palate.

Difficulties are often experienced in the evaluation of the prevertebral soft tissues in young children. Radiographs should be obtained in deep inspiration and preferably with some extension of the neck. If a technically inadequate radiograph is obtained spurious thickening of the prevertebral tissues as seen on the lateral view, often associated with deviation of the upper trachea to the right on a frontal view, will give a false impression of prevertebral soft tissue pathology (Fig. 1.0.13).

CHOANAL ATRESIA

This is a congenital membranous or bony obstruction of the posterior nasal cavity. Bilateral atresia presents early with respiratory distress during feeding, but unilateral atresia may be later in presentation.

Plain radiographs are unhelpful. Instillation of a small amount of water-soluble contrast medium into the anterior nasal cavity with the child in the recumbent position will satisfactorily demonstrate obstruction. CT is more illuminating and is able to differentiate membranous from bony atresias.

REFERENCES

Slovis T L, Renfro B, Watts F B, Kuhns L R, Belenhy W, Spoylar J 1985 Choanal atresia: precise CT evaluation. Radiology 155: 345–348

Kleinman P, Winchester P 1975 Pseudotumour of the nasal fossa secondary to mucoid infection in choanal atresia. Pediatric Radiology 4: 47–48

CROUP

This is most often a viral infection of the upper airways, but can rarely result from bacterial infections, in particular staphylococcus and diphtheria. The radiographic findings of croup include a general lack of clarity of the laryngeal structures, as shown on a lateral plain radiograph, with often obliteration of the laryngeal sinus. Whereas the immediate subglottic area in a normal trachea is of much the same radiolucency as the body of the trachea, the side to side inflammatory reaction visible in an AP view is represented on a lateral view by a decrease in the radiolucency of the immediate subglottic trachea. Associated with this is frequent hypopharyngeal distension (Fig. 1.0.14).

Immediate subglottic narrowing is not entirely specific for croup and may be seen in the older child in allergic and angioneurotic responses.

EPIGLOTTITIS

Epiglottitis is usually due to *Haemophilus influenzae*. Clinical presentation is an acutely ill child with an open mouth, drooling and with an acutely inflamed oropharynx on visual inspection. The clinical signs are sufficiently suggestive of the diagnosis to warrant immediate admission to intensive care facilities. Radiographs should only be undertaken if facilities and personnel are available to maintain an airway, if necessary by endotracheal intubation. The plain radiographic findings are characteristic with gross swelling of the epiglottis and aryepiglottic folds with transformation of the normal leaf-like epiglottis into a rounded cherry-shaped mass (Fig. 1.0.15). There have been deaths recorded in children who have been sent inappropriately to X-ray departments rather than being admitted to intensive care.

REFERENCE

McCook T A, Kirks D R 1982 Epiglottic enlargement in infants and children: another radiologic look. Pediatric Radiology 12: 227–234

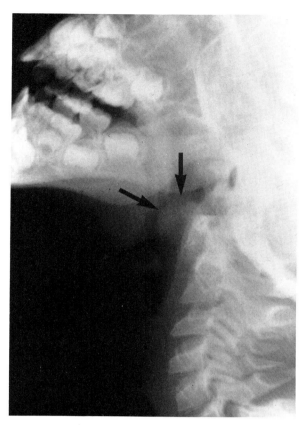

Fig. 1.0.13 Ear lobe (arrows) giving a false impression of pharyngeal soft tissue mass.

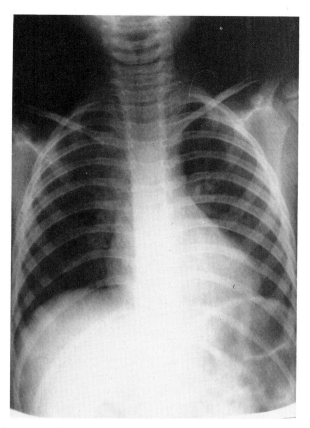

Fig. 1.0.14 Croup. Note extensive oedema of the trachea.

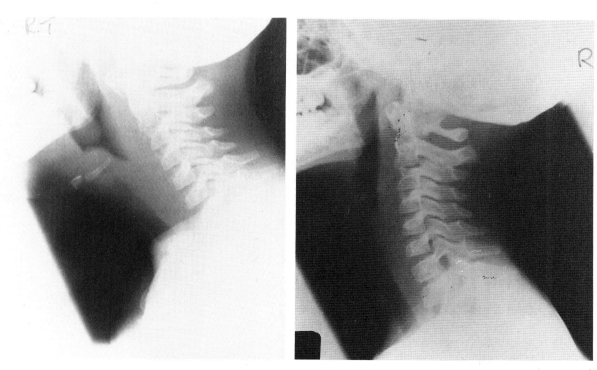

A

B

Fig. 1.0.15 Acute epiglottitis. (**A**) Rounded epiglottic shadow with some dilatation of the pharyngeal airway. (**B**) Following recovery, normal appearances.

15

OBSTRUCTIVE LESIONS OF THE LARYNX

Laryngomalacia

This functional flaccidity of the infant larynx is a common cause of stridor. The flaccidity of the laryngeal structures can be observed by fluoroscopy, but microlaryngobronchoscopy is a more appropriate method of investigation and will also reveal other local pathology such as laryngeal cysts and other tumours (Fig. 1.0.16), webs and stenoses (Fig. 1.0.17). Recently, delineation of pharyngeal anatomy and function has been performed using ultrasound and is proving a useful adjunct to endoscopy.

Subglottic stenosis

Congenital upper tracheal and subglottic stenosis is now less frequently encountered than the stenoses secondary to prolonged endotracheal intubation following respiratory support in the neonatal period. Although plain films, using air as contrast medium, will indicate narrowing (Fig. 1.0.18), evaluation is preferable by endoscopy, which will also reveal the presence of subglottic haemangioma or other tumorous conditions. In later childhood, lateral plain radiography of the trachea is useful for evaluation of the presence of tracheal granulomas (Fig. 1.0.19), especially in relation to tracheostomy sites and also to determine the correct positioning of fenestrations in tracheostomy tubes.

Retropharyngeal infections

Retropharyngeal infection with a true increase in the retropharyngeal space, as shown on a correctly exposed lateral radiograph, may arise from an extension of a quinsy from cervical adenitis, including that due to tuberculosis and in the young baby from iatrogenic perforation of the nasopharynx by feeding or suction tubes. Gas may be noted within the infection if abscesses are forming and careful inspection of the vertebral bodies for evidence of bony involvement should be carried out. Other mass lesions in this area can include cystic hygroma, haemorrhage following cervical injury, neurogenic tumours and lymphadenopathy due to lymphoma. All of these, however, are rare.

Lingual thyroid

Respiratory obstruction with enlargement of the tongue can be due to a variety of causes. Ectopic lingual thyroid or a thyro-glossal cyst are important causes. Haemangiomas, lymphangiomas and teratomas are well-described causes of mass lesions in this area. Generalized lingual enlargement is a

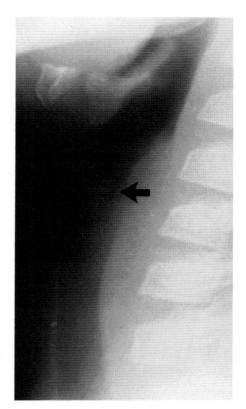

Fig. 1.0.16 Laryngeal papilloma (arrow).

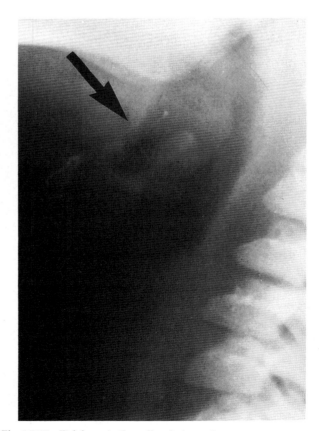

Fig. 1.0.17 Fish bone in the vallecula (arrow).

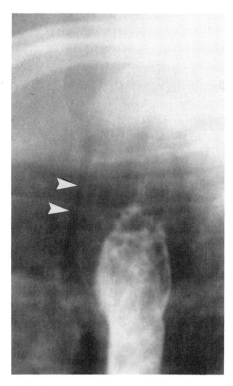

Fig. 1.0.18 Tracheomalacia (arrows) in a child who had oesophageal atresia.

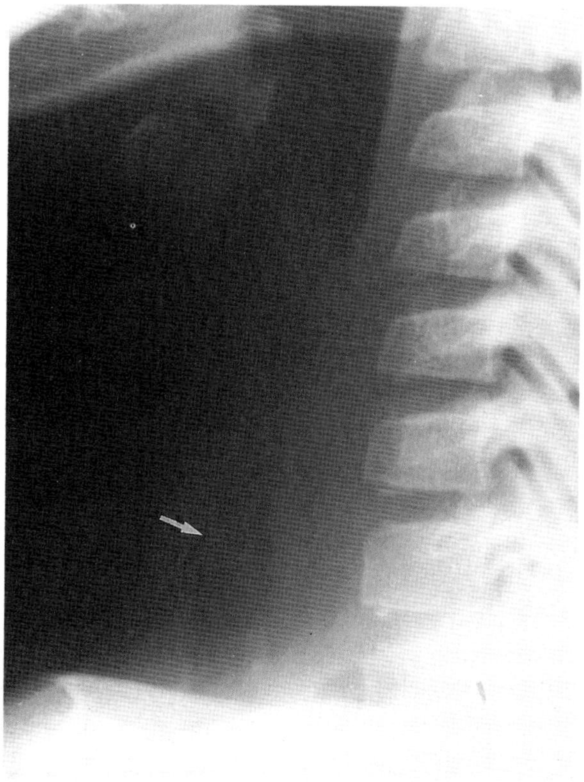

feature of congenital hypothyroidism, the Beckwith–Weidemann syndrome, and is a feature of mucopolysaccharidoses.

Tumours in the upper airways and soft tissues of the mouth and neck

Mass lesions which are causing respiratory distress in this region are best evaluated by a simple radiograph before endoscopic examination. After this, further simple evaluation can be performed by ultrasound by which means most cystic lesions will be identified. If the diagnosis remains unclear, more advanced cross-sectional imaging may then be appropriate. The evaluation of the lower face, lingual area and neck by CT in children is often unsatisfactory, particularly due to the high incidence of artefacts, some of which may be related to the endotracheal tubes and general anaesthesia. MRI is of particular value in this region. (Fig. 1.0.20).

Fig. 1.0.19 Post-tracheostomy granuloma (arrow).

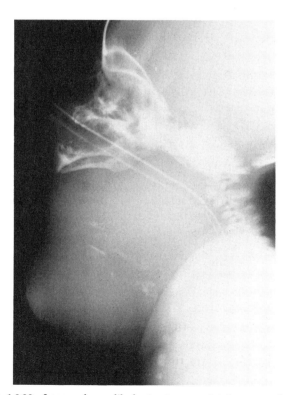

Fig. 1.0.20 Large submandibular teratoma containing areas of calcification. There is elevation and distortion of the mandible. Endotracheal tube.

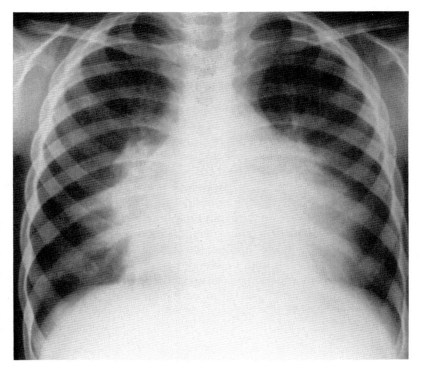

Fig. 1.0.21 Cardiomegaly and heart failure with patchy shadowing in the right middle lobe secondary to hyperventilation from enlarged adenoids in a negro child.

Sleep apnoea

This is a complication of upper airway obstruction, most commonly due to adenoidal hypertrophy but also seen in neuromuscular pharyngeal pareses. Hypoventilation may also be central as in trauma, encephalitis and the idiopathic Ondine's curse. Secondary pulmonary hypertension and cardiac failure may supervene (Fig. 1.0.21).

LARYNGEAL CLEFT

This failure of separation of the trachea from the oesophagus in prenatal development is commoner than the more severe manifestation of failure of separate canalization as shown by the oesophago-trachea. Clinical presentation is similar to H-type tracheo-oesophageal fistula with cough, intermittent cyanosis and aspiration pneumonia with additional features of abnormal phonation. The clinical presentation is likely to lead to a tube oesophagram for a suspected H-type fistula. Contrast typically will enter the upper trachea and radiologically it is very difficult to differentiate aspiration through a normal trachea from laryngeal cleft particularly if a minor deficit. The preferred investigation is microlaryngobronchoscopy. The condition might be suspected by abnormal sites of either endotracheal tubes or nasogastric tubes when they have traversed the deficit.

REFERENCE

Felman A H, Talbert J L 1972 Laryngotracheo-oesophageal cleft. Description of a combined laryngoscopic and roentgenographic diagnostic technique and report of two patients. Radiology 103: 641–644

1.1 NEONATAL DISORDERS

TECHNIQUE AND THE NEONATAL CHEST RADIOGRAPH

The normal neonate achieves good aeration of its lungs within the first few breaths of life. Variable degrees of residual lung fluid can, however, give some diffuse opacification, particularly in the first 4 hours of life. Careful radiographic technique is an essential prerequisite for correct evaluation of the neonate. In the child with respiratory distress any handling necessary for radiography should be reduced to the minimum, although care should be taken to remove as many extraneous leads as necessary and yet to include on the radiograph the position of the nasogastric and endotracheal tubes, vascular catheters and pleural drains.

Ideally, experienced radiographers should undertake such radiography and do so in collaboration with the nursing and medical staff so that films in adequate inspiration can be achieved, particularly in children with supportive ventilation. Fast film–screen combinations are preferable with careful collimation of the films. If possible thyroid shielding should be carried out with small pieces of lead or lead rubber, as should shielding of the gonads if abdominal films are also taken. The construction of modern incubators usually precludes macroradiography, which is now much less popular.

The newborn chest is virtually cylindrical. Small degrees of rotation, as shown by asymmetry of the anterior ribs, lead to considerable malprojections of the anterior ribs and sternum. The transverse diameter of the heart may be difficult to assess in the newborn because of superimposition of the thymic shadow. Cardiac enlargement may be better gauged from a lateral view but a baby with suspected cardiomegaly is better investigated by echocardiography. Normal diaphragmatic levels are usually about the 6th ribs anteriorly and the 8th ribs posteriorly. An air bronchogram can be seen in a normal child in the proximal airways, particularly behind the heart shadow, but if visible in the peripheral lung fields is abnormal indicating underaeration of the lung parenchyma.

NEONATAL RESPIRATORY DISTRESS

Causes of respiratory distress are tabulated in Section 1.9 and it is important to consider extrathoracic and cardiac causes, for which ultrasound is particularly helpful in evaluation. Appropriate haematological, microbiological and biochemical screens should be performed.

Transient tachypnoea of the newborn

Also known as transient respiratory distress of the newborn, wet lung disease, or neonatal retained fluid syndrome.

Retention of fluid normally present at birth in the lungs during the first few hours of life can give rise to variable degrees of respiratory distress. The condition is predisposed to by caesarean section, prematurity and some cases of maternal diabetes. Although mild cases may be asymptomatic, tachypnoea is associated with grunting and retraction of the chest wall and mild cyanosis. Symptoms are generally less severe than those of hyaline membrane disease and the temporal evolution of the condition, with resolution usually occurring in 48 hours, is quicker. The usual radiographic appearance is of diffuse patchy shadowing radiating from the perihilar regions, often associated with streaky shadowing. The generalized opacification of the lung fields can accentuate the air bronchogram. The condition is usually symmetrical but if asymmetrical the right lung is often more involved than the left. Patchy retained fluid can show a lobar distribution. By contrast with hyaline membrane disease, the lungs may show mild to moderate overaeration. Sometimes a small amount of pleural fluid can be noted extending into the lung fissures. The heart size is essentially normal. Although the radiographic signs may be non-specific the relatively mild symptoms and the usual resolution of clinical and radiographic signs in the first 2 days of life is characteristic and helps differentiate the condition from hyaline membrane disease, neonatal pneumonia, aspiration and congestive heart failure.

REFERENCES

Kuhn J P, Fletcher B D, Delemon R A 1969 Roentgen findings in transient tachypnea of the newborn. Radiology 92: 751–757
Rimmer S, Fawcitt J 1982 Delayed clearance of pulmonary fluid in the neonate. Archives of Disease in Childhood 57: 63–67
Wesenberg R L, Graven S N, McCabe E B 1971 Radiological findings in wet-lung diasease. Radiology 98: 67–74

The respiratory distress syndrome, hyaline membrane disease

This important and common cause of neonatal morbidity and mortality is due to a deficiency of pulmonary surfactant contributing to alveolar atelectasis and associated with dilatation of the terminal bronchioles. Prematurity, perinatal asphyxia, caesarean section, being the second of twins or an infant of a diabetic mother are predisposing conditions. Clinically, tachypnoea and retraction of the chest wall with expiratory grunting are associated with cyanosis starting within the first few hours of life and with progressive respiratory compromise.

The chest radiograph will usually be abnormal by 6 hours. Mild hyaline membrane disease shows symmetrical fine reticular shadowing throughout both lung fields with accentuation of the air bronchogram. As the condition becomes more severe, the reticulogranular shadowing becomes more confluent and hypoaeration of the lungs which are typically small leads to progressive loss of clarity of the diaphragmatic and cardiac contours (Figs 1.1.1–1.1.3). The air bronchogram becomes more easily visible throughout the lung fields and the diameter of the major airways is often increased. In the most severe cases, the lung fields become virtually opaque (Fig. 1.1.4). Uncomplicated hyaline membrane disease is a bilaterally symmetrical disease, although there may be some gradation in radiographic opacification from the upper zones to the lower zones. Asymmetrical changes may be seen when some areas have been differentially aerated by, for instance, misplaced endotracheal tubes or in the presence of localized pathology such as interstitial emphysema.

Hyperechogenicity in the lower lung fields demonstrated by abdominal ultrasound in the retrohepatic or retrosplenic area has been described as a specific pattern of hyaline membrane disease. This hyperechogenicity of the lung fields may be due to sonographic summation of the peripherally aerated bronchioles and alveolar ducts surrounded by collapsed alveoli.

REFERENCE

Avni E F, Braude P, Pardou A, Matos C 1990 Hyaline membrane disease in the newborn: diagnosis by ultrasound. Pediatric Radiology 20: 143–146

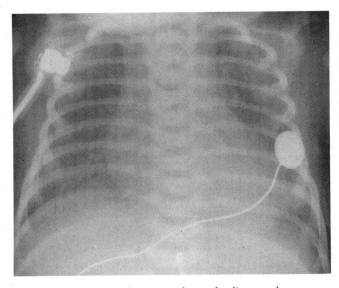

Fig. 1.1.1 Respiratory distress syndrome: hyaline membrane disease. Premature baby (with endotracheal tube), second day of life; generalized granularity in the lung fields.

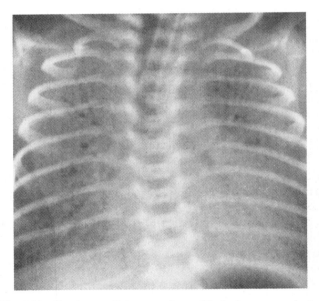

Fig. 1.1.2 Respiratory distress syndrome. Marked even granularity of lung fields with an air bronchogram.

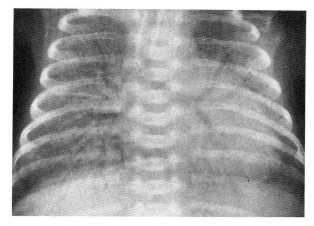

Fig. 1.1.3 Respiratory distress syndrome. Marked granularity with prominent and relatively wide airways.

COMPLICATIONS OF NEONATAL INTENSIVE CARE

Assisted ventilation and other advances in neonatal intensive care have dramatically improved the prognosis for low birthweight infants and for those with neonatal respiratory distress. Ventilatory support can be effected through endotracheal intubation and mechanical ventilation or the use of head boxes or facial masks to provide a continuous positive airway pressure.

Pulmonary interstitial emphysema, pneumothorax, pneumomediastinum and other air leak complications

The considerably improved survival rate following intermittent positive pressure respiration, in the respiratory distress syndrome in particular, has been associated with a variety of clinical complications due to air leak following alveolar rupture.

Pulmonary interstitial emphysema

Alveolar dehiscence allows gas to pass from the bronchial tree into the interstitial tissues of the lung and also into the lymphatics. This initially may be quite localized but usually quickly spreads throughout the affected lung to give a characteristic radiographic appearance of numerous small radiolucencies (Fig. 1.1.5). Less frequently, larger air cysts either within the lung parenchyma or in a subpleural situation may be visible. The volume of the affected lung is consequentially increased leading to contralat-

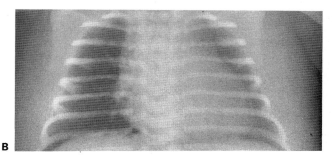

Fig. 1.1.4 **A** Hyaline membrane disease. Note gross general opacification, aortic oxygen electrode and endotracheal tube. **B** Pancuronium oedema. Gross oedema of the soft tissues. Mild streakiness in the lung fields.

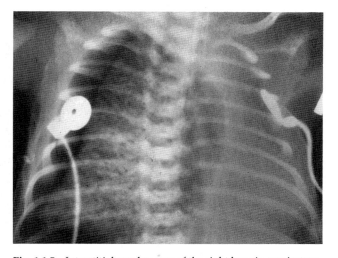

Fig. 1.1.5 Interstitial emphysema of the right lung in respiratory distress syndrome. Note right pneumothorax and reticular shadowing present in the right lung fields with deviation of the mediastinum to the left.

eral deviation of the mediastinum. If both lungs are involved the compressive effect can lead to restriction of the return of venous blood to the heart and compromise the circulation.

Pneumomediastinum

Interstitial air may track along the peribronchial fascia through the hilar structures and into the mediastinum, most frequently collecting anteriorly. A central radiolucency is apparent delineated by the parietal pleura and usually extends superiorly above the heart shadow (Fig. 1.1.6). In the anterior and superior mediastinum, gas surrounding the thymus makes it more clearly visible than usual and when lifted up gives rise to a sail-shaped shadow (Fig. 1.1.7). Extensive pneumomediastinum can extend behind the heart or project laterally when loculated in the inferior pulmonary ligaments extending down from the hilar regions towards the diaphragm. Radiological interpretation of mediastinal gas shadows at times can be difficult and a horizontal ray lateral radiograph of the chest can be helpful (Fig. 1.1.8). This is particularly so in posterior collections when it may be still difficult to differentiate a loculated medial pneumothorax from mediastinal collections, particularly in the pulmonary ligaments or when there is a small anterior predominantly unilateral pneumomediastinum. Gas in the lower mediastinum inferior to the heart shadow gives rise to the 'continuous diaphragm' sign.

Venous air embolism

A rare but often fatal complication of interstitial pulmonary emphysema, pneumomediastinum and pneumothorax is the entrance of gas into the circulation. If massive, this is usually fatal and air is seen within the cardiac chambers and to a variable extent in the vascular tree.

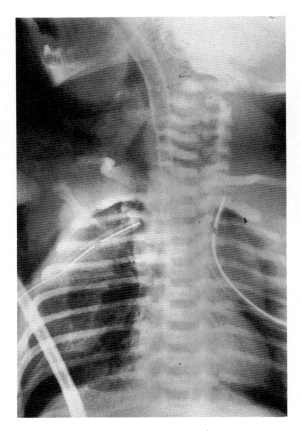

Fig. 1.1.6 Pneumothoraces and pneumomediastinum are present in a neonate being ventilated for hyaline membrane disease. The left lobe of the thymus is easily seen. Note subcutaneous emphysema.

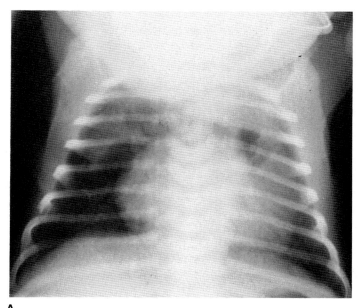
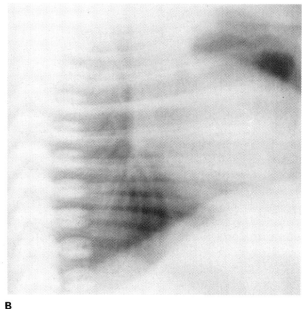

A   **B**

Fig. 1.1.7 AP (**A**) and lateral (**B**) view of pneumomediastinum with elevation of the thymic shadow and anterior mediastinal radiolucency on the lateral view.

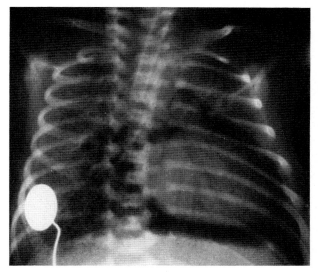

Fig. 1.1.8 Pneumomediastinum and pneumopericardium in respiratory distress syndrome.

REFERENCES

Bowen A III, Quattromani F L 1980 Infraazygos pneumomediastinum in the newborn. American Journal of Roentgenology 135: 1017–1021

Campbell R E 1970 Intrapulmonary interstitial emphysema: a complication of hyaline membrane disease. American Journal of Roentgenology 110: 449–456

Donald I, Steiner R E 1953 Radiography in the diagnosis of hyaline membrane disease. Lancet ii: 846–849

Giedion A, Haefliger H, Dangel P 1973 Acute pulmonary x-ray changes in hyaline membrane disease treated with artificial ventilation and positive end-expiratory pressure (PEP). Pediatric Radiology 1: 145–152

Greenough A, Dixon A K, Roberton N R 1984 Pulmonary interstitial emphysema. Archives of Disease in Childhood 59: 1046–1051

Hall R T, Rhodes PG 1975 Pneumothorax and pneumomediastinum in infants with idiopathic respiratory distress syndrome receiving continuous positive airway pressure. Pediatrics 55: 493–496

Johnson J F, Dean B L 1982 The expiratory film in hyaline membrane disease: preliminary observations. American Journal of Roentgenology 139: 31–34

Reilly BJ 1975 Regional distribution of atelectasis and fluid in the neonate with respiratory distress. Radiologic Clinics of North America 13: 225–250

Shook D R, Cram K B, Williams H J 1975. Pulmonary venous air embolism in hyaline membrane disease. American Journal of Roentgenology 125: 538–542

Swischuk L E 1976 Two lesser known but useful signs of neonatal pneumothorax. American Journal of Roentgenology 127: 623–627

Bronchopulmonary dysplasia

This was the term used by Northway, Rosan and Porter in 1967 to describe the lung changes occurring in hyaline membrane disease treated by artificial ventilation and increased inspired oxygen tensions, the pathological changes of which consist of alveolar cell hyperplasia, bronchial hyperplasia and interstitial fibrosis leading to areas of localized emphysema, dilated lymphatics and vascular changes of pulmonary hypertension. These changes follow a variety of iatrogenic insults to the lung including the mechanical effects of artificial ventilation, increased oxygen tensions, following meconium aspiration, interstitial pulmonary emphysema, neonatal pneumonia and in congenital heart disease. Radiographically (Figs 1.1.9–1.1.11) the condition is usually realized by failure of normal resolution of predominant changes of hyaline membrane disease or some other precipitating condition. Characteristic findings are areas of emphysema separated by linear streaky shadowing, representing poorly aerated parenchyma. The common pattern shown on the chest radiograph has changed with increasing expertise and knowledge of desirable pressure cycles in artificial ventilation, and the grossly coarse reticular patterns associated with larger pseudocystic lesions in the lung fields are now less commonly seen. A finer reticular pattern with varying degrees of pulmonary opacification associated with scattered areas of compensatory emphysema is more usually seen. In less severe cases the radiographic pattern may stabilize and improvement in the lung fields be seen but pulmonary compromise can be progressive and fatal with compromised gas exchange and cor pulmonale.

As with uncomplicated hyaline membrane disease, attempts have been made to score the radiographic changes, but in both these conditions the prognostic usefulness is dubious and clinical evaluation is superior. Nevertheless, gross radiographic changes are likely to be associated with a poorer outcome.

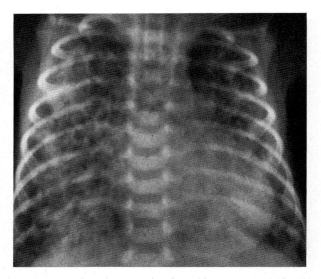

Fig. 1.1.9 Bronchopulmonary dysplasia. Note coarse reticular shadowing which is confluent in some areas.

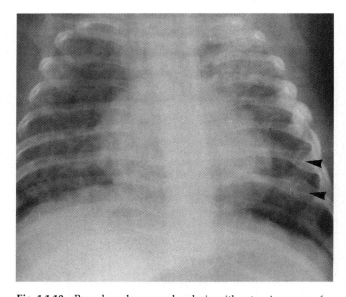

Fig. 1.1.10 Bronchopulmonary dysplasia with extensive areas of fibrosis. Note rib fractures (arrows).

REFERENCES

Heneghan M A, Sosulski R, Baquero J M 1986 Persistent pulmonary abnormalities in newborns: the changing picture of bronchopulmonary dysplasia. Pediatric Radiology 16: 180–184

Miller K E, Edwards D K, Hilton S, Collins D, Lynch F, Williams R 1981 Acquired lobar emphysema in premature infants with bronchopulmonary dysplasia: an iatrogenic disease? Radiology 138: 589–592

Northway W H Jr, Rosan R C 1968 The radiographic features of pulmonary oxygen toxicity in the newborn: bronchopulmonary dysplasia. Radiology 91: 49–58

Oppermann H C, Willie L, Bleyl U, Obladen M 1977 Bronchopulmonary dysplasia in premature infants. A radiological and pathological correlation. Pediatric Radiology 5: 137–141

Sickler E A, Gooding C A 1976 Asymmetric lung involvement in bronchopulmonary dysplasia. Radiolody 118: 379–383

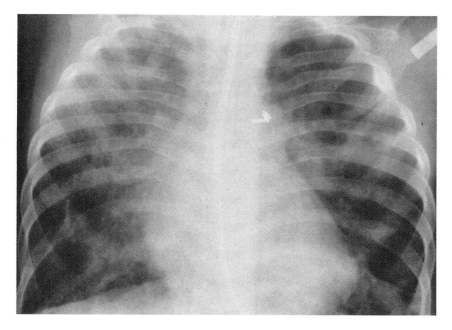

Fig. 1.1.11 Bronchopulmonary dysplasia. The ductus arteriosus has been closed with metallic clips.

Spontaneous localized pulmonary interstitial emphysema

Rarely, persistent apparently spontaneous interstitial pulmonary emphysema occurs as a localized cystic area, usually unilateral and involving only one part of the lung. Histological examination shows interstitial air and dilated air-containing lymphatics. Initially, parenchymal densities in the newborn can progress to overinflated cystic spaces without obvious precipitating cause (Fig. 1.1.12).

REFERENCE

Smith T H, Currarino G, Rutledge J C 1984 Spontaneous occurrence of localised pulmonary interstitial and endolymphatic emphysema in infancy. Pediatric Radiology 14: 142–145

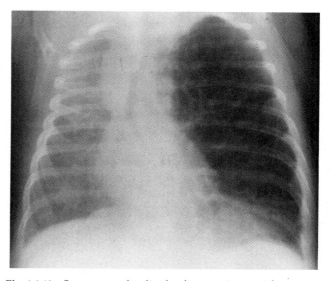

Fig. 1.1.12 Spontaneous localized pulmonary interstitial emphysema.

Idiopathic subpleural cysts in the newborn

Rare reports of cystic subpleural collections of gas, typically basal, in full-term newborn babies without evidence of coexistent disease has been recorded. No clear aetiology have been suggested for these and spontaneous regression may occur, encouraging an expectant management policy.

REFERENCE

Sag F, Marco A, Martinez A, Lopez J A, Vita M J, Paramo C, Larrea F 1985 Transient idiopathic subpleural cysts in the newborn. Pediatric Radiology 15: 249–250

Radiographic changes after surfactant therapy

In premature neonates with respiratory distress syndrome, artificial surfactant instilled into the bronchial system results in a rapid improvement in clinical and biochemical state although the radiographic findings show a slower change with improvement being seen up to 24 hours. The incidence of pneumothoraces and lobar atelectasis is less in treated infants, but no difference has been reported between the treated and a control group in complications such as intracranial haemorrhage, bronchopulmonary dysplasia and significant ductus arteriosis.

REFERENCE

Clarke E A, Siegle R L, Gong A K 1989 Findings on chest radiographs after prophylactic pulmonary surfactant treatment of premature infants. American Journal of Roentgenology 153: 799–802

Pulmonary haemorrhage

This serious complication of neonatal respiratory distress is notably seen in severe hyaline membrane disease treated with artificial ventilation, although may be seen in other conditions such as neonatal pneumonia, aspiration and bronchopulmonary dysplasia, where there may also be severe hypoxia. If the haemorrhage is relatively mild the radiographic features may not be prominent and the associated patchy parenchymal shadowing difficult to differentiate from the appearances of the underlying condition.

In those babies more severely affected, deterioration in the clinical state with blood-stained fluid in the airways is reflected by widespread opacification of the lung fields which in its most severe form shows as virtual complete opacification, 'white-out' (Fig. 1.1.13). Such severe and fulminating haemorrhages are a frequent terminal event; lesser degrees of pulmonary haemorrhage will resolve quite rapidly in survivors.

Haemorrhagic disease of the newborn due to vitamin K deficiency is only very rarely seen now but may, together with congenital coagulation factor deficiencies and thrombocytopenia, present as neonatal pulmonary haemorrhage. Disseminated intravascular coagulation is a much more frequent aetiology in perinatal haemorrhage.

REFERENCES

Bomsel F, Couchard M, Larroche J C, Magder L 1975 Radiologic diagnosis of massive pulmonary haemorrhage of the newborn. Annales de Radiologie 18: 419–430
Trompeter R, Yu V Y H, Aynsley-Green A, Roberton N R C 1975 Massive pulmonary haemorrhage in the newborn infant. Archives of Disease in Childhood 50: 123–127

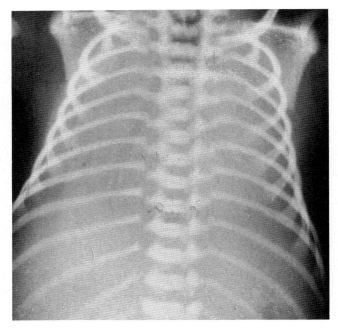

Fig. 1.1.13 Pulmonary haemorrhage in a neonate. Opacification of both lung fields.

Bilateral pulmonary hypoplasia

Bilateral pulmonary hypoplasia is a relatively common and an important cause of respiratory compromise.

Potter's syndrome, in which renal agenesis and oligohydramnios are associated with a compressive inhibition of normal pulmonary growth, is well known. Oligohydramnios may be associated with other renal disease such as obstructive uropathy and cystic disease of the kidneys but may occur due to amniotic fluid loss. Abnormal development of the thoracic cage may be either due to skeletal dysplasias or myopathies. Intrathoracic masses, frequently diaphragmatic hernias, abdominal distension either from masses, ascites or distended gut can all compromise normal pulmonary development. Such lungs are lighter than normal and show poor development of the bronchovascular tree and a decrease in alveolar numbers. Air-leak problems such as pneumomediastinum and pneumothorax may be spontaneous but are often due to resuscitative attempts to attain adequate ventilation.

REFERENCE

Langes R, Kaufmann H J 1986 Primary (isolated) bilateral pulmonary hypoplasia: a comparative study of radiologic findings and autopsy results. Pediatric Radiology 16: 175–179

Extracorporeal membrane oxygenation

Facilities for this form of cardiorespiratory support vary from country to country with the greatest experience in North America, especially in cases of diaphragmatic hernia. During extracorporeal oxygenization, the ventilatory pressures on the lungs are reduced and this is accompanied by diffuse dense pulmonary opacification as a consequence, which is not necessarily of poor prognostic significance. Catheters are placed in the right atrium from the jugular vein and aortic arch from the right carotid artery. Radiographic monitoring of tube positions is vital.

REFERENCES

Schlesinger A, Cornish J D, Null D M 1986 Dense pulmonary opacification in neonates treated with extra-corporeal membrane oxygenation. Pediatric Radiology 16: 448–451

Gross G W, Cullen J, Kornhouser M S, Wolfson P J 1992 Thoracic complications of extracorporeal membrane oxygenation. American Journal of Roentgenology 158: 353–358

Taylor G A, Lotze A, Kapur S, Short B L 1986 Diffuse pulmonary opacification in infants undergoing extracorporeal membrane oxygenation. Clinical and pathologic correlation. Radiology 161: 347–350

NEONATAL ASPIRATION

Aspiration of a small amount of amniotic fluid, meconium or blood into the lungs appears to be relatively innocuous, particularly if limited to the major tracheobronchial divisions and prompt post-natal toilet of the airways is performed (Fig. 1.1.14). In the presence of fetal distress, however, especially in the postmature baby, aspiration of meconium can lead to neonatal distress (Fig. 1.1.15). In mild cases where probably relatively small amounts of meconium in relation to fluid are aspirated, the chest radiograph may remain normal or show transitory patchy nodular shadowing clearing within a few hours. In more severe cases tachypnoea, cyanosis with chest retraction and grunting is associated with extensive air trapping and overaeration of the lung fields due to peripheral meconium impaction. Pneumothorax and pneumomediastinum are frequent complications which can result in hypoxia and lead to pulmonary artery vasoconstriction, hypertension and right-to-left shunting across the ductus arteriosus, the persistent fetal circulation. Recovery from meconium aspiration is typically slow and overaeration, nodular patchy infiltrates and reticular shadowing can persist for many days or even weeks. In the most severe cases secondary changes of bronchopulmonary dysplasia may supervene.

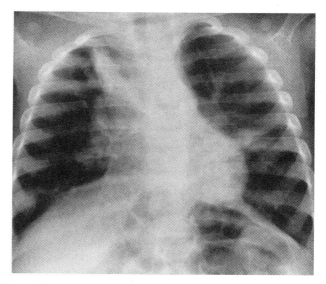

Fig. 1.1.14 Aspiration pneumonia. Extensive collapse in right upper lobe with other areas of collapse in right middle lobes.

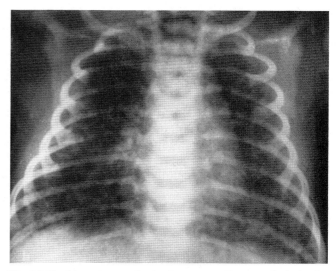

Fig. 1.1.15 Meconium aspiration in neonate. Coarse reticulation is present and persisted for several days.

REFERENCES

Gooding C A, Gregory G A 1971 Roentgenographic analysis of meconium aspiration of newborn. Radiology 100: 131–135

Hoffman R R Jr, Campbell R E, Decker J P 1974 Fetal aspiration syndrome: clinical roentgenologic and pathologic features. American Journal of Roentgenology 122: 90–96

Neonatal aspiration of vernix caseosa

Postmature babies shed vernix into the amniotic fluid and such contamination may give rise to an aspiration pneumonia similar to that associated with the aspiration of meconium.

REFERENCE

Ohlsson A, Cunning W A, Najjar H 1985 Neonatal aspiration syndrome due to vernix caseosa. Pediatric Radiology 15: 193–195

WILSON–MIKITY SYNDROME

There has been considerable speculation about the true aetiology of this condition. It is characteristically seen in premature babies, often male, who usually do not show respiratory symptoms for the first day or two of life. Transient cyanosis, tachypnoea and chest retraction start in the first 1–4 weeks after birth. The lung fields are initially well aerated but a coarse reticular pattern with areas of hyperinflation develops with the onset of respiratory distress. This leads to a characteristically coarse honeycomb pattern throughout the lung fields representing areas of alveolar atelectasis and hyperaeration (Fig. 1.1.16). Cellular infiltration and fibrosis are not common and if seen probably represent the onset of dysplastic change. If the infant survives the compromise of alveolar gas exchange and does not develop intracranial pathology, such as intraventricular haemorrhage, progressive recovery of the radiographic features occurs which may, however, take many months before the alternating areas of collapse and overaeration disappear.

REFERENCE

Wilson M G, Mikity V G 1960 A new form of respiratory disease in premature infants. American Journal of Diseases of Children 99: 489–499

PERSISTENT PULMONARY HYPERTENSION OF THE NEWBORN; PERSISTENT FETAL CIRCULATION

This is usually associated with such conditions as central nervous abnormalities leading to depression of ventilation, infections, polycythaemia, upper airway obstruction due to conditions such as micrognathia, pulmonary aspiration or some congenital heart defects (Fig. 1.1.17). Although reopening and persistence of the ductus arteriosus is an important complication in the sick premature neonate, infants with idiopathic persistent pulmonary hypertension are usually term babies. Unless the condition is due to pulmonary parenchymal abnormalities such as meconium aspiration, the lung fields are usually well aerated but the right to left shunt manifests as oligaemia of the lung fields. Occasionally, however, pulmonary oedema may be noted secondary to cardiac valvular incompetence.

REFERENCES

Merten D F, Goetzman B W, Wennberg R P 1977 Persistent fetal circulation; an evolving clinical and radiographic concept of pulmonary hypertension of the newborn. Pediatric Radiology 6: 74–80
Nielson H C, Riemenschneider T A, Jaffe R B 1976 Persistent transitional circulation. Roentgenographic findings in thirteen infants. Radiology 120: 649–652

THE IMMATURE LUNG

In small premature babies with a birthweight often well below 1500 g, the radiograph may show a diffuse fine granularity in the lung fields but without accentuation of the air bronchogram. The clinical features of the respiratory distress syndrome such as grunting, tachypnoea and desaturation are not in evidence and there is no biochemical evidence of inadequate pulmonary surfactant activity. The immaturity of such small premature babies may be associated with episodes of apnoea and persistent patency of the ductus arteriosus. However, the outcome in such babies is usually determined by serious pathology in other systems such as intracranial haemorrhage, necrotizing enterocolitis or the development of bronchopulmonary dysplasia secondary to ventilatory support for recurrent apnoea.

In the extremely immature infant histological studies show the radiographic pattern of linear densities and patchy consolidation is related to pulmonary haemorrhage, interstitial and air space oedema and occasionally underexpansion. Radiographic features in the extremely young premature baby are usually non-specific and could also reflect surfactant deficiency and associated hyaline membrane disease.

REFERENCE

Wood B P, Davitt M A, Metlay L A 1989 Lung disease in the very immature neonate: radiographic and microscopic correlation. Pediatric Radiology 20: 33–40

NEONATAL ATELECTASIS

The sick neonate is at risk of collapse of the lung due to the small diameter of the airways, general debilitation, extrinsic pressure from tumour or enlarged heart or from wrongly positioned endotracheal tubes. Although collapse of lobes or lungs may be associated with mediastinal shift, this is by no means universal and major airway obstruction may be accompanied by filling of the peripheral airways and alveoli by fluid

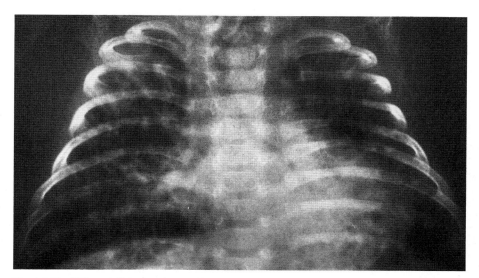

Fig. 1.1.16 Wilson–Mikity syndrome. Note coarse reticulation with some areas of more marked opacification.

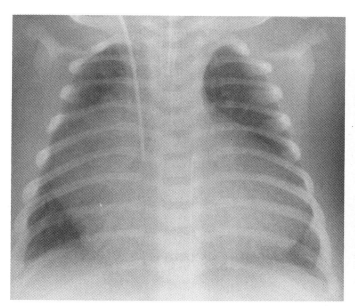

Fig. 1.1.17 Persistent fetal circulation.

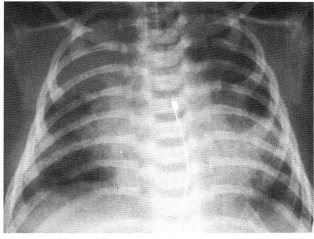

Fig. 1.1.18 Consolidation of right upper lobe due to pneumonia and retained secretions. Patchy consolidation is present medially in the lower zones.

(Fig. 1.1.18). Endobronchial toilet with suction aspiration of mucosal plugs and repositioning of endotracheal tubes with appropriate physiotherapy will usually lead to reaeration of the collapsed lung. Postextubation atelectasis is more common in the right lung, particularly the upper lobe, but may affect other lobes, often sequentially.

REFERENCES

Finer N N, Moriartey R R, Boyd J, Phillips H J, Stewart A R, Vlan O 1979 Post-extubation atelectasis: a retrospective review and a prospective controlled study. Journal of Pediatrics 94: 110–113

Wyman M L, Kuhns L R 1977 Lobar opacification of the lung after tracheal extubation in neonates. Journal of Pediatrics 91: 109–111

BRONCHIAL COMPRESSION BY AN ENLARGED LEFT ATRIUM IN INFANTS

An enlarged left atrium may compress the left main bronchus and occasionally produce hypovascularity of the left lung but without the usual signs of obstructive hyperinflation with mediastinal shift, depressed hemidiaphragm and a hyperlucent lung field. Hypoxic vasoconstriction has been hypothesized as the cause.

REFERENCE

Corr L, McCarthy P A, Lavender J B, Hallidie-Smith K A 1988 Bronchial compression by an enlarged left atrium in infants; a cause of hypovascularity of the left lung. Pediatric Radiology 18: 459–463

CENTRAL VENOUS CATHETERS

These are frequently used for nutritional support and their tip should ideally be in the right atrium. It is possible for them to pass through the right heart and into the pulmonary arteries where, if situated peripherally, infusions of nutritional substances such as triglycerides for instance may cause localized pulmonary damage (Fig. 1.1.19, 1.1.20).

REFERENCE

Landry B A, Melhem R E 1989 Pulmonary nodules secondary to total parenteral alimentation. Pediatric Radiology 19: 456–457

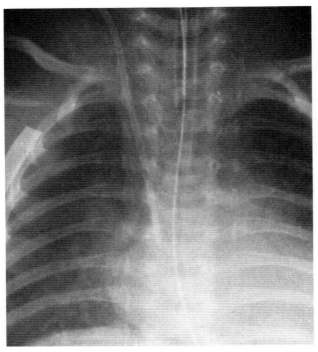

Fig. 1.1.19 Calcification in soft tissues of right side of the neck in association with central venous catheter.

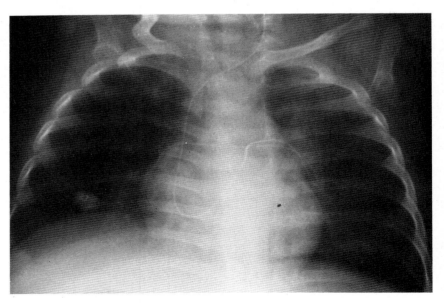

Fig. 1.1.20 The intravenous catheter has passed through the heart into the lung as shown by contrast medium.

CHYLOTHORAX

Chylothorax is an uncommon cause of respiratory distress in neonates. The aetiology is uncertain but is probably related to trauma during birth. Respiratory distress is apparent soon after birth although onset of symptoms may be delayed.

Chylothorax is more common on the right (Fig. 1.1.21) but effusions on the left or bilaterally are by no means rare (Fig. 1.1.22). Opacification of the affected hemithorax may be complete or the appearances of pleural effusion may be more obvious. The presence of fluid in the chest can be shown by ultrasound and the diagnosis confirmed by pleural aspiration. In the child who has not been fed the pleural fluid may be straw coloured but once feeding has been established the fluid becomes chylous and fat can be shown on microscopic examination. Treatment is relatively simple and dependent upon removal of the fluid which may be affected by multiple aspirations or by the insertion of a chest drain.

Chylothorax is a complication of major heart surgery and chest trauma and can be secondary to thoracic duct obstruction from a tumour. In such cases, lymphangiography, either using conventional contrast media or radioactive isotopes, is far from universally successful in showing the site of the leak.

HAEMOTHORAX

This is an uncommon cause of respiratory distress in the neonatal period which may arise secondary to haemorrhagic disease of the newborn or to birth or neonatal trauma. The condition can arise spontaneously.

REFERENCES

Gates G F, Dore E K, Kanchanopoom V 1972 Thoracic duct leakage in neonatal chylothorax visualized by [198]Au lymphangiography. Radiology 105: 619–620
Kramer S S, Taylor G A, Garfinkel D, Simmons M A 1981 Lethal chylothoraces due to superior vena caval thrombosis in infants. American Journal of Radiology 137: 559–563
Oppermann H C, Wille L 1980 Hemothorax in the newborn. Pediatric Radiology 9: 129–134
Willich E, Kundert J G 1971 Chylothorax in the newborn. Radiological features. Annales de Radiologie 14: 155–160

INFANTILE POLYCYTHAEMIA

Although this may be a primary phenomenon it can occur following twin to twin transfusion. Pulmonary oedema, prominent pulmonary vasculature and enlarged heart shadow are radiological features which are not however shown by all affected babies.

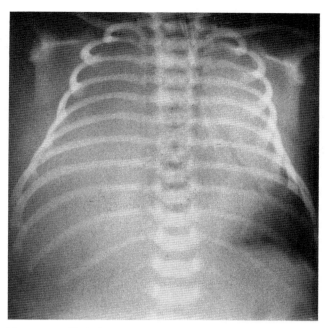

Fig. 1.1.21 Chylothorax. Large right pleural effusion with oedema of the right chest wall.

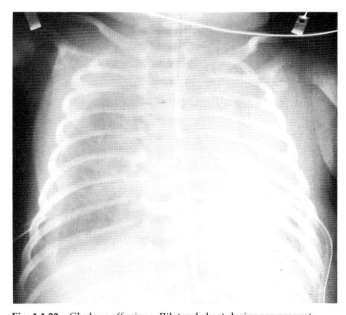

Fig. 1.1.22 Chylous effusions. Bilateral chest drains are present.

REFERENCES

Saigal S, Wilson R, Usher R 1977 Radiological findings in symptomatic neonatal plethora resulting from placental transfusion. Radiology 125: 185–188
Wesenberg R L, Rumack C M, Lubchenco L O, Wirth F H, McGuinness G A, Tomlinson A L 1977 Thick blood syndrome. Radiology 125: 181–183

NEONATAL SEPTICAEMIC CONDITIONS

The incidence and type of those organisms causing neonatal septicaemia has changed over the past decades. Of current importance are Group B strepto-cocci, *Escherichia coli*, *Staphylococcus aureus*, *Listeria monocytogenes*, klebsiella, enterobacter and pseudo-monas (Fig. 1.1.23). Group B haemolytic streptococci infections (Fig. 1.1.24) have variable manifestations on the chest radiograph including widespread streaky or more confluent shadowing, but an important manifes-tation is an even granularity which can mimic the appearances of the idiopathic respiratory distress syndrome, although the clinical picture is usually different. Often associated with disseminated intravascular coagulation the lung findings may in part be due to a neonatal manifestation of a secondary adult respiratory distress syndrome for which there is some histological evidence in fatal cases. Pneumatocoele formation in the neonate is uncommon but may be seen in association with *E. coli*, *Haemophilus influenzae* and now less frequently *S. aureus*. Viral infections may show marked inflammatory oedema-tous changes (Fig. 1.1.25). Congenital infections may be septicaemic but are often the result of prolonged rupture of the membranes.

Pneumocystis carinii

This protozoan organism is now more commonly encountered in immune compromised patients, yet epidemics have occurred particularly in premature debilitated infants. The parenchymal lung infiltration radiates from the hilar region typically without lymph node enlargement. Air-leak phenomena such as pulmonary interstitial emphysema, pneumomedi-astinum and pneumothorax are relatively common with occasional pneumatocoele formation.

REFERENCES

Bier S, Halton K, Krivisky B, Leonidas J 1986 *Pneumocystis carinii* pneumonia presenting as a single pulmonary nodule. Pediatric Radiology 16: 59–60

Vessal K, Post C, Dutz W, Bandarizadeh B 1974 Roentgenologic changes in infantile pneumocystis carinii pneumonia. American Journal of Roentgenology 120: 254–260

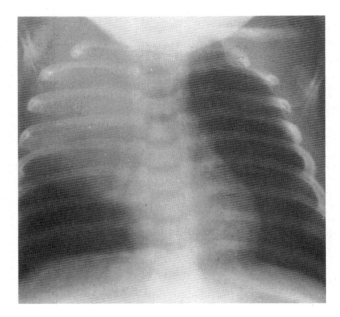

Fig. 1.1.23 Suppurative pneumonia in the right upper lobe.

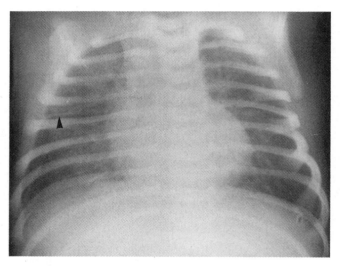

Fig. 1.1.24 Group B haemolytic streptococcal infection. Widespread streaky shadowing, fine granularity, small right pleural effusion and accentuation of the fissures in the right lung (arrowhead).

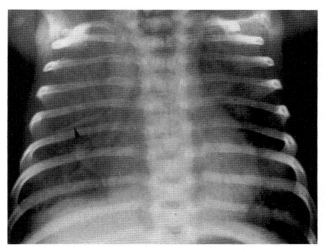

Fig. 1.1.25 Adenovirus. Oedematous consolidations with pleural fluid in lesser fissure (arrowhead).

Rubella

Although the bony lesions and cardiovascular lesions are more prominent in the congenital rubella syndrome, pulmonary parenchymal infiltration is seen particularly in infections occurring in late pregnancy and aplasia of the diaphragm and thymic hypoplasia have also been recorded.

REFERENCE

Phelan P, Campbell P 1969 Pulmonary complications of rubella embryopathy. Journal of Pediatrics 75: 202–212

Cytomegalovirus

Central nervous system manifestations and occasional irregularities in the metaphyses of the long bones are the more common manifestations of this condition, but eventration of the diaphragm has also been noted (Fig. 1.1.26).

REFERENCES

Hayes K, Gibas I I 1971 Placental cytomegalovirus infection without fetal involvement following primary infection in pregnancy. Journal of Pediatrics 79: 401–405
Merten D F, Gooding C A 1970 Skeletal manifestations of cytomegalic inclusion disease. Radiology 95: 333–334
Whitley R J, Brassfield D, Reynolds D W et al 1976 Protracted pneumonitis in young infants associated with perinatally acquired cytomegaloviral infection. Journal of Pediatrics 89: 16–22

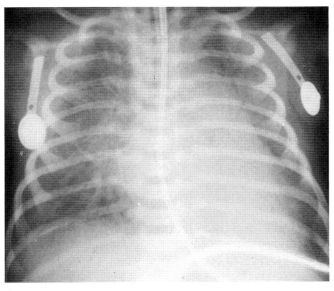

Fig. 1.1.26 Cytomegalovirus pneumonia.

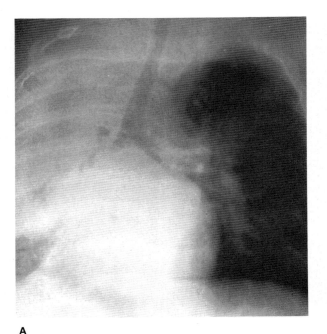

A

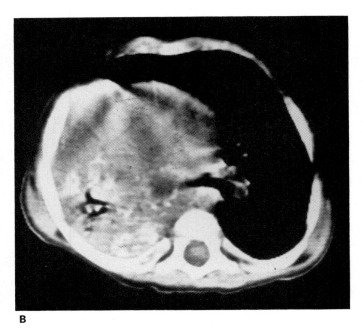

B

Fig. 1.1.27 Congenital tuberculosis. **A** Plain radiograph with right pleural effusion and collapse and consolidation in right lower lobe. **B** CT.

Congenital tuberculosis

Transplacental congenital tuberculosis infection is rare. The primary complex is usually in the liver or abdominal lymph nodes and lung findings, although often present at birth, may be delayed in onset. Widespread lung shadowing may be relatively discrete or miliary in nature (Fig. 1.1.27).

REFERENCES

Bate T W P, Sinclair R E, Robinson M J 1986 Neonatal tuberculosis. Archives of Disease in Childhood 61: 512–514
Polansky S M, Frank A, Ablow R C, Effmann E L 1978 Congenital tuberculosis. American Journal of Roentgenology 130: 994–996

Candida

Although a frequent commensal in the adult, *Candida albicans* is an important pathogen particularly in the immunocompromised or in the sick neonate. The chest radiographic features are non-specific and consist of variable consolidation but typically without hilar lymph node enlargement or cavitation. In the neonate candida lung infections are frequently associated with widely disseminated infection of which candida pyelonephritis with obstructive fungus balls, cardiovascular and central nervous system involvement are serious complications.

REFERENCE

Kassner E G, Kaufman S L, Yoon J J 1981 Pulmonary candidiasis in infants. Clinical, radiological and pathological features. American Journal of Roentgenology 137: 707–716

Chlamydial pneumonia

Chlamydial pneumonia has recently been appreciated as an important infection starting after the neonatal period and during the first 6 months of life, often acquired from the 5–10% of women who harbour chlamydia in the genital tract. Clinical presentation is of a respiratory infection with tachypnoea and paroxysmal coughing. Often there is no fever but eosinophilia is common. The radiological signs (Fig. 1.1.28) are similar to those seen in viral infections with streaky perihilar infiltrates with areas of atelectasis, often with hyperinflation.

REFERENCES

Attenburrow A A, Barker C M 1985 Chlamydial pneumonia in the low birthweight neonate. Archives of Disease in Childhood 60: 1169–1172
Radkowski M A, Kranzier J K, Beem M O, Tipple M A 1981 Chlamydia pneumonia in infants: radiography in 125 cases. American Journal of Roentgenology 137: 703–706

Listeria

Listeria monocytogenes is a vaginal organism causing septicaemia, meningitis and bilateral patchy pulmonary infiltrates, an infection predisposed by prolonged rupture of the membranes.

PULMONARY LYMPHANGIECTASIA

This pathological dilatation of the pulmonary lymphatics is very uncommon.

Lymphangiectasia can occur as an isolated defect in the lungs without any obvious obstructive lesion. Commoner in males, the presentation is of severe immediate respiratory distress and cyanosis with usually a quickly fatal outcome. Radiographic features are of a fine reticular pattern throughout the lung fields.

In a second group obstruction to pulmonary venous return is associated with a dilatation of the lymphatics. This is particularly associated with total anomalous pulmonary venous drainage, either supradiaphragmatic or infradiaphragmatic, and also with the hypoplastic left heart syndrome. The prognosis is usually poor. A third group of patients have generalized lymphangiectasia which may affect the limbs, alimentary tract and bones, and may be unilateral and asymmetrical. Pulmonary involvement in this group is less likely to compromise respiratory function and disability is usually related to severity of involvement of other systems. In the thorax, involvement of the chest wall can lead to destruction and deformity of the ribs with which pleural effusions may be associated. Rarely, gross pulmonary and pleural involvement is lethal in later childhood.

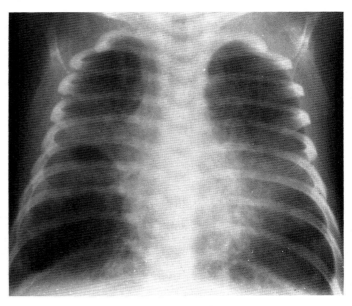

Fig. 1.1.28 Chlamydial pneumonia. Eight-day-old neonate.

LATER SEQUELAE OF NEONATAL LUNG DISEASE

In survivors of uncomplicated prematurity and respiratory distress syndrome, radiographic findings in later childhood are uncommon and usually consist of mild linear shadowing representing fibrosis or deep pleural fissuring. To some extent parallelling the lack of improvement in pulmonary function in middle and later childhood, about three-quarters of survivors of neonatal bronchopulmonary dysplasia will show abnormal radiographic findings. Most frequently, linear shadows representing strands of fibrosis or pleural fissuring are seen with, less commonly, areas of irregular aeration and distortion of the bronchovascular architecture (Fig. 1.1.29). The plain radiographic abnormalities decrease with age. The AP dimension of the chest in survivors of neonatal bronchopulmonary dysplasia is decreased in childhood but in adolescence, probably due to increased airways resistance secondary to bronchial lability, an increase in AP diameter is common.

REFERENCE

Griscom N T, Wheeler W B, Seveezey N B, Kim Y C, Lindsey J C, Wohl M E B 1989 Bronchopulmonary dysplasia: radiographic appearance in middle childhood. Radiology 171: 811–814

ECHO PLANAR IMAGING

MRI using the technique of echo planar imaging in which each image may be achieved within 100 milliseconds has been used to estimate lung volumes in infants. Other uses of this technique include evaluation of the heart and proximal pulmonary vessels in which the inherently poor resolution is of not such great importance.

REFERENCE

Chapman B, O'Callaghan C, Coxen R, Glover P, Jaroszkiewicz G, Houseman A, Mansfield P, Small P, Milner A D, Coupland R E 1990 Estimation of lung volume in infants by echo planar imaging and total body plethysmography. Archives of Disease in Childhood 65: 168–170

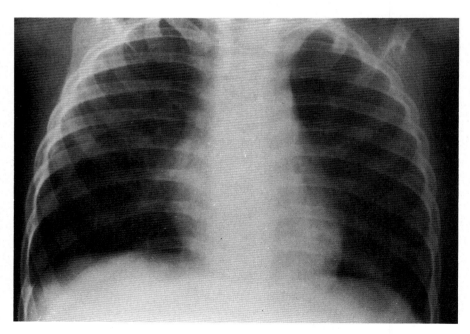

Fig. 1.1.29 Late sequelae of bronchopulmonary dysplasia. Streaky parenchymal and pleural shadowing in a 2 year old.

1.2 CONGENITAL ABNORMALITIES (EARLY PRESENTATION)

TRACHEAL AGENESIS

This is usually found in association with other congenital defects, particularly the VATER association, and death is inevitable in early infancy. Three types have been described. In type I the proximal trachea is deficient with distal direct communication with the oesophagus. In type II, accounting for about two-thirds of all cases, virtually the whole of the trachea is absent with a distal tracheo-oesophageal fistula. In type III the bifurcation of the trachea is absent and both the right and left main bronchus open directly from the oesophagus. Ventilation of the lungs is possible by intubation of the oesophagus.

REFERENCES

Milstein J M, Lau M, Bickers R F 1985 Tracheal agenesis in infants with VATER association. American Journal of Diseases of Children 139: 77–80

Rovira J, Morales L, Rottermann M, Julia V, Llaurado F, Perez del Pulgar J 1989 Agenesis of the trachea. Journal of Pediatric Surgery 24: 1126–1127

Statz T, Lynch J, Ortmann M, Roth P 1989 Tracheal agenesis: case report. European Journal of Paediatrics 149: 203–204

CONGENITAL TRACHEAL STENOSIS

In this condition the trachea is intrinsically narrowed. The tracheal cartilages are smaller than normal, more ridid and the posterior membranous tracheal structures are missing. As a result the trachea is rigid and the term 'stove-pipe' trachea has been applied to the anomaly.

Presentation is usually in the first year with respiratory distress, stridor and wheeze. Stenosis of the bronchi, hypoplasia or agenesis of the lung, tracheal bronchus, anomalous origin of the left pulmonary artery from the right pulmonary artery and H-type tracheo-oesophageal fistula are associated conditions. Although plain radiography, high kV films and microlaryngobronchoscopy have been used to evaluate the condition, CT has several advantages. In particular, evaluation of the distal extent of the lesion can be made, the narrowing of the trachea can be compared with the conus elasticus in the immediate subglottic region where tracheal cartilaginous rings are absent and is thus usually of normal calibre, and extrinsic compression of the trachea by mediastinal masses can be excluded.

Fluoroscopy of the major airways has a place in differentiating the rigid narrowing of this condition from the variable narrowing of tracheomalacia related to respiratory phase. This can be supplemented by positive contrast evaluation of the trachea and proximal bronchi with small volumes of bronchographic contrast medium.

REFERENCE

Hernandez R J, Tucher G F 1987 Congenital tracheal stenosis. Pediatric Radiology 17: 192–196

OESOPHAGEAL LUNG

Rare anomalies of the bronchial tree include origin of a right main bronchus from the distal oesophagus, the so-called oesophageal lung and the bridging bronchus in which a bronchus to the right lower lobe arises from the left bronchial tree across the mediastinum, often associated with a sling left pulmonary artery (Fig. 1.2.1).

REFERENCES

Starshak R J, Sty J R, Woods G, Kreitzer F V 1981 Bridging bronchus: a rare airway anomaly. Radiology 140: 95–96

Wells T R, Stanley P, Padua E M, Landing B H, Warburton D 1990 Serial reconstruction of anomalous tracheobronchial branching patterns from CT scan images. Bridging bronchus associated with sling left pulmonary artery. Pediatric Radiology 20: 444–446

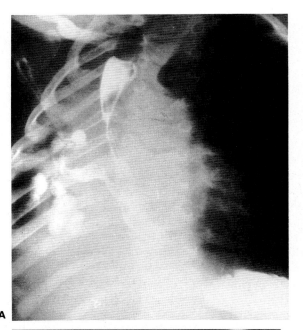

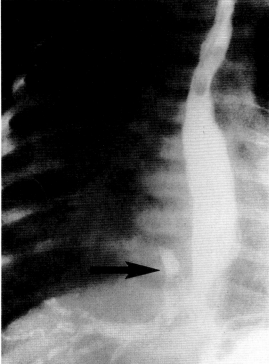

Fig. 1.2.1　Two examples of oesophageal lung. **A** Associated marked right pulmonary hypoplasia.
B Arrow points to bronchus running upwards which connected with hilar bronchial tree.

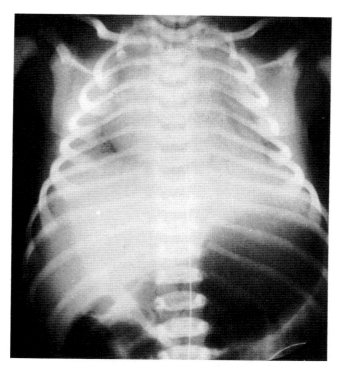

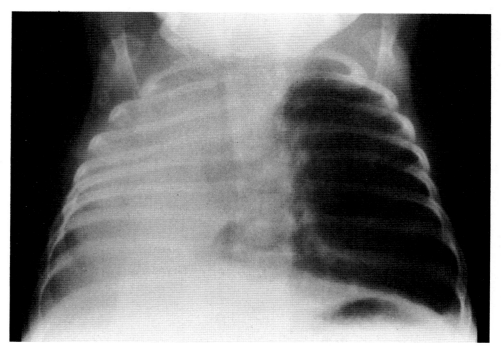

PULMONARY AGENESIS, HYPOPLASIA

Unilateral pulmonary agenesis is associated with a high incidence of congenital anomalies in other organs, particularly the cardiovascular system, the alimentary tract with anal and oesophageal atresia, tracheo-oesophageal fistula and with renal agenesis. Skeletal anomalies involve the ribs and vertebra but particularly ipsilateral hypoplasia of the thumb with varying metacarpal and radial anomalies.

A single mediastinal unilobar lung has been described as a possible form of subtotal pulmonary agenesis (Figs 1.2.2, 1.2.3).

REFERENCE

Osborne J, Masel J 1989 A spectrum of skeletal anomalies associated with pulmonary agenesis: possible neural crest injuries. Pediatric Radiology 19: 425–432

Fig. 1.2.2 Severe neonatal pulmonary hypoplasia with a small bell-shaped thorax and apparent cardiomegaly.

Fig. 1.2.3 Congenital gross hypoplasia of the right lung. The right ribs are crowded.

UNILATERAL PULMONARY HYPOPLASIA

Congenital unilateral hypoplasia may result from failure of normal lung development secondary to some other anomaly such as a large diaphragmatic hernia or may be a primary embryological defect, a group which may be divided into five types.

1. Simple hypoplasia

In these sometimes asymptomatic patients the heart is displaced towards the hypoplastic side and in some cases a retrosternal density representing extrapleural areolar connective tissue is seen. The plain radiograph reveals decreased vascularity of the small lung which can typically be confirmed by pulmonary angiography, or radioisotope perfusion scans. The pulmonary venous pattern is similar to the arterial tree (Fig. 1.2.4).

Fluoroscopy and radiographs taken in expiration and inspiration typically do not reveal the paradoxical movement of significant major air trapping.

Bronchography similarly will show a pattern usually corresponding with the pulmonary artery branching.

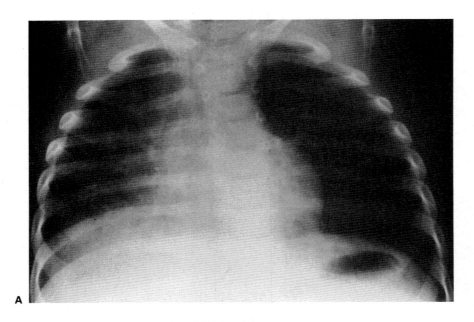

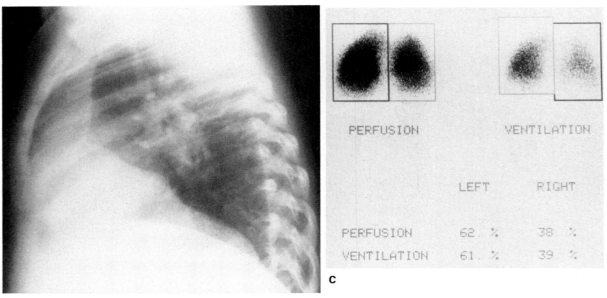

Fig. 1.2.4 Right pulmonary hypoplasia. **A** Frontal radiograph. **B** Lateral view with retrosternal density from alveolar tissue. **C** Ventilation-perfusion scan, posterior images.

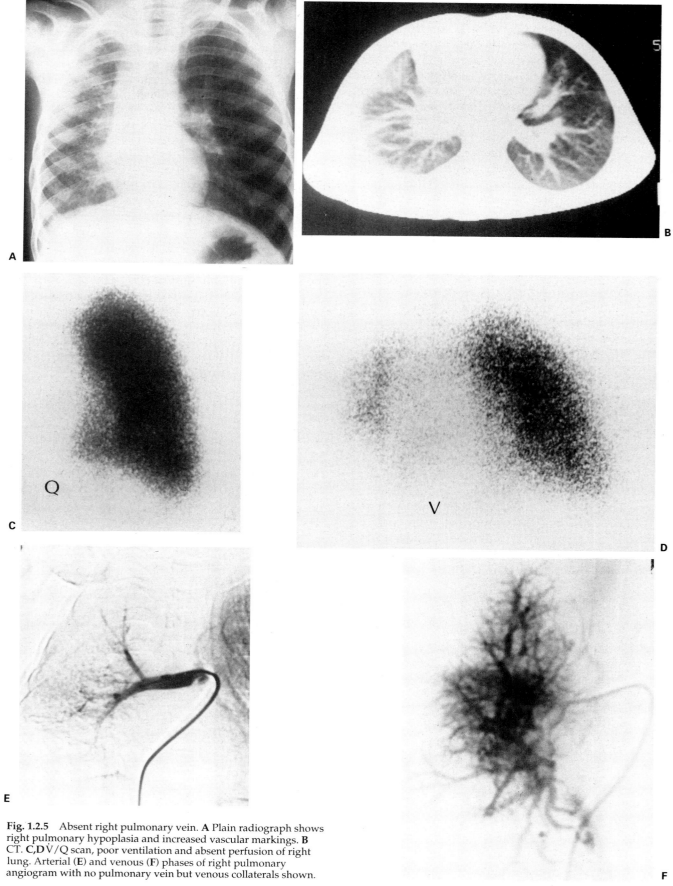

Fig. 1.2.5 Absent right pulmonary vein. **A** Plain radiograph shows right pulmonary hypoplasia and increased vascular markings. **B** CT. **C,D** V̇/Q scan, poor ventilation and absent perfusion of right lung. Arterial (**E**) and venous (**F**) phases of right pulmonary angiogram with no pulmonary vein but venous collaterals shown.

2. Absence of a pulmonary artery

This is more common on the right. Absence of the left pulmonary artery is associated with a right aortic arch. A small lung is associated with decreased vascularity and displacement of the heart ipsilaterally. The cardiac and superior mediastinal borders are usually clearly defined although a retrosternal density may be noted. At angiography the pulmonary artery cannot be identified although a systemic arterial supply and bronchial collaterals may be seen. The bronchial tree may be normal at bronchography or there may be varying degrees of bronchial tree deficit. Absent pulmonary veins are associated with hypoplasia (Fig. 1.2.5).

3. Anomalous venous return: scimitar syndrome

Pulmonary hypoplasia is also a feature of a malformation complex involving often severe congenital heart lesions but with anomalous pulmonary venous return into the inferior vena cava, right atrium, coronary sinus or the hepatic or portal veins. The right lung is small with mediastinal shift and the anomalous veins create the eponymous 'scimitar sign' as they run inferiorly. The right pulmonary artery is typically small although abnormal systemic arteries may perfuse the affected lung. The right heart border is often poorly defined.

Horseshoe lung, in addition to some features of the scimitar syndrome, is a condition in which the lungs are fused behind the heart. The posterior mediastinal pleural reflections may be absent and fluoroscopy reveals lung tissue between the lower oesophagus and the heart shadow. Left bronchial isomerism is described. The diagnosis is established by demonstrating angiographically continuity of the pulmonary artery vasculature in the isthmus of the lung behind the heart.

4. Accessory diaphragm

This is usually associated with pulmonary hypoplasia and particularly occurs on the right. A partial duplication of the right hemidiaphragm extends upwards and backwards separating a greater or lesser amount of the right lower lobe from the hemidiaphragm.

Typically the right cardiac border lacks clarity and there is deviation of the mediastinum to the right reflecting the associated lung hypoplasia with a retrosternal density due to anterior areolar tissue. These radiographic signs are much more frequently elicited than the considerably rarer observation of the obliquely and posteriorly inclined true accessory diaphragm above the normally situated hemidiaphragm. There is, in addition to the usual right-sided hypoplasia, a variety of other associated abnormalities including vascular anomalies of the lungs, congenital heart disease and diaphragmatic hernia.

5. Pulmonary sequestration

Pulmonary hypoplasia may be associated with pulmonary sequestration. In this category, a spectrum of abnormalities involving systemic arterial supply to a varying proportion of a small lung is associated with variable deficiencies in the bronchial tree. Defects in the right hemidiaphragm occur with this form of hypoplasia. Pulmonary sequestration, however, is typically not associated with significant hypoplasia of the affected lung in which the radiographic features suggesting the diagnosis are usually repeated localized episodes of pneumonia in lungs otherwise not radiographically grossly abnormal.

REFERENCES

Boyden E A 1972 The structure of compressed lungs in congenital diaphragmatic hernia. American Journal of Anatomy 134: 497–508

Currarino G, Williams B 1985 Causes of congenital unilateral pulmonary hypoplasia: a study of 33 cases. Pediatric Radiology 15: 15–24

Hislop A, Hey E, Reid L 1979 The lungs in congenital bilateral renal agenesis and dysplasia. Archives of Disease in Childhood 54: 32–38

Langer R, Kaufmann H J 1986 Primary isolated bilateral pulmonary hypoplasia: a comparative study of radiologic findings and autopsy results. Pediatric Radiology 16: 175–179

Orjan F, Angelum P, Ogliecti J, Leachman R D, Coxley D A 1977 Horseshoe lung: report of two cases. American Heart Journal 93: 501–505

Perlman M, Levin M 1974 Fetal pulmonary hypoplasia, anuria, and oligohydramnios: clinicopathologic observations and review of the literature. American Journal of Obstetrics and Gynecology 118: 1119–1123

Renert W A, Berdon W E, Baker D H, Rose J S 1972 Obstructive urologic malformations of the fetus and infant: relation to neonatal pneumomediastinum and pneumothorax (air block). Radiology 105: 97–105

Swischuk L E, Richardson C J, Nichols M M, Ingman M J 1979 Bilateral pulmonary hypoplasia in the neonate (a classification). American Journal of Roentgenology 233: 1057–1063

CONGENITAL DIAPHRAGMATIC HERNIA

Occurring in about 1 in 2500 live births, congenital diaphragmatic hernia is an important neonatal surgical emergency. The most common site of herniation lies posteriorly and lateral to the spine to which the inaccurate but established term of the Bochdalek foramen hernia is applied. The incidence of left-sided hernias is several times that of right sided. Other sites of herniation are anterior, through or adjacent to the foramina of Morgagni, and rarer sites include those associated with hemidiaphragmatic duplication cysts, through the crura of the diaphragm and midline defects arising anteriorly either retrosternally or into the pericardial sac. Antenatal ultrasound examination is an increasingly important and common method of recognition, but progressive and early respiratory distress in the newborn is the usual clinical presentation.

Typical radiographic findings (Figs 1.2.6, 1.2.7) in the commoner left congenital diaphragmatic hernia may initially show an opaque left hemithorax with deviation of the mediastinum to the right as shown by the course of a nasogastric tube or endotracheal tube. Once the alimentary tract begins to fill with air, radiolucencies due to the stomach and the small bowel in particular will be seen in the left hemithorax and there may be progressive contralateral deviation of the mediastinum. In addition to the upper alimentary tract, parts of the colon, spleen and kidney and pancreas can herniate and their position can be identified by ultrasound examination. Loops of bowel may be seen running in an unusually vertical pattern towards the herniation sac and the abdomen may show a paucity of intestinal gas. Malrotation and malfixation of the small bowel are associated problems.

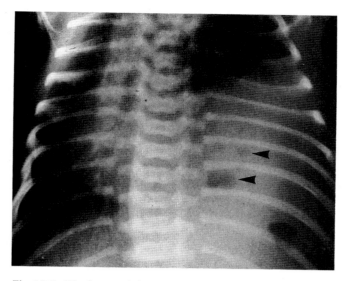

Fig. 1.2.6 Diaphragmatic hernia. The mediastinum is displaced to the right and bowel occupies the lower left chest (arrows). The left lung is hypoplastic.

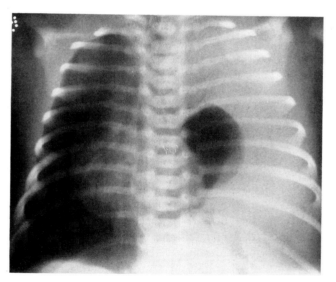

Fig. 1.2.7 Diaphragmatic hernia. The stomach is in the thorax indicating a poor prognosis. The left lung is hypoplastic and there is a right pneumothorax.

In the less common right-sided hernia the liver and intestine may be seen in the right hemithorax, in which case the right upper abdomen lacks the normal hepatic shadow (Fig. 1.2.8). Delineation of the site of the liver has previously been determined by contrast medium studies of the umbilical vein, but this has been superseded by ultrasound; the use of radionuclide liver scans in this context is generally inappropriate.

Urgent surgical repair is the treatment, although increasingly the neonate may undergo a period of stabilization and assisted ventilation for 24 hours before correction of the defect. Extracorporeal membrane oxygenation has proved a successful supportive technique. Following repair of the hernia a balanced induced pneumothorax is frequently left by the surgeon to counteract the usually small lung on the involved side and to maintain the mediastinal structures central. A few days later this pneumothorax may be replaced by pleural fluid, both of which resorb as the lung expands.

Pulmonary hypoplasia is a most important complication. In extreme cases underdevelopment of the lungs will not support extrauterine life. The degree of hypoplasia may be indicated by the site of the stomach on the postnatal film. The compromise of pulmonary development is early in fetal development. If the stomach can be identified in the thorax this usually indicates an early herniation in utero and is associated with a significantly poorer prognosis. In the neonate pulmonary hypoplasia can be associated with re-establishment and persistence of the fetal circulation. In survivors the affected lung may remain small and relatively radiolucent with a paucity of pulmonary vessels. Radionuclide studies confirm a diminished predominantly ipsilateral pulmonary artery perfusion although ventilation is reasonable.

Other anomalies are associated with congenital diaphragmatic hernia, although commonly the defect is isolated. Congenital heart disease, limb deformities, extra pairs of ribs, pleural effusions, particularly on the right, and extralobar sequestrations have been described (Fig. 1.2.9).

The radiographic differential diagnosis includes congenital adenomatoid malformation and pneumatocoele formation secondary to staphylococcal or enteropathic bacterial infection. In reality, evaluation of the plain abdominal and chest radiographs supplemented by ultrasound should allow correct diagnosis.

Diaphragmatic palsy

Neonatal diaphragmatic palsy may result from birth trauma affecting the phrenic nerve and is usually associated with an ipsilateral brachial plexus palsy. Strongly associated with breech delivery, the right hemidiaphragm is more frequently involved. Bilateral diaphragmatic paralysis is rare and usually lethal.

Less common factors are viral infections, damage from positioning vascular catheters and drainage tubes and damage to the cervical spinal cord. Diaphragmatic palsy may follow cerebrovascular catastrophes. Clinical features include respiratory distress, tachypnoea usually but not necessarily of immediate onset. A left diaphragmatic paralysis may be associated with feeding difficulties due to distortion of the oesophagogastric junction and pyloric region. Recovery is usual but may be slow during which period there is an increased risk of pneumonia, lung collapse and recurrent aspiration. Diaphragmatic movement and the detection of paradoxical movement can be demonstrated by carefully timed double exposed plain radiographs, one in expiration and one in inspiration, by rapid fluoroscopy or by ultrasound with which technique simultaneous evaluation of both hemidiaphragms is only achieved with two scanners.

Occasionally, elevation of the affected leaf of the diaphragm may be delayed for a few days. Complete congenital eventration of the hemidiaphragm where there is muscular deficiency can mimic diaphragmatic palsy and be very difficult to differentiate. However, persisting diaphragmatic elevation in both these conditions is similarly treated by surgical plication, making distinction less important.

Eventration of the diaphragm

A relative weakness of the diaphragm which may be bilateral or unilateral is sometimes associated with severe neonatal respiratory distress and the clinical features are essentially those of true congenital diaphragmatic hernia. Frequently the clinical symptoms are not marked and the radiographic findings are of a localized bulge on the diaphragm. Anterior bulges on the right hemidiaphragm are not infrequent and fluoroscopy will show good movement of the diaphragm and liver at this site. Such children could be treated conservatively.

Aplasia and hypoplasia of the diaphragm

This rare but often autosomal recessive condition may be bilateral or unilateral, in which case the appearances are similar to the more common congenital diaphragmatic hernia.

REFERENCES

Ambler R, Gruenewald S, John E 1985 Ultrasound monitoring of diaphragm activity in bilateral diaphragmatic paralysis. Archives of Disease in Childhood 60: 170–172

Moccia W A, Kaude J V, Felman A H 1981 Congenital eventration of the diaphragm. Diagnosis by ultrasound. Pediatric Radiology 10: 197–200

Wexler H A, Poole C A 1976 Neonatal diaphragmatic dysfunction. American Journal of Roentgenology 127: 617–622

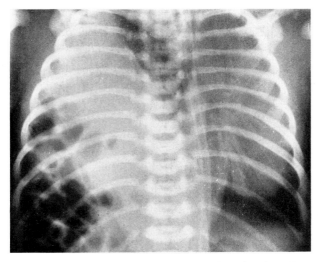

Fig. 1.2.8 Diaphragmatic hernia. Liver and bowel in the right hemithorax.

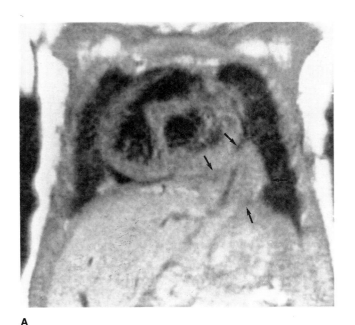

A

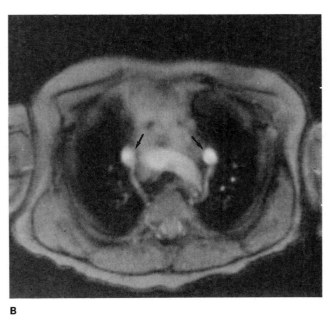

B

Fig. 1.2.9 Localized herniation of the liver through the diaphragm. **A** MR coronal T1 (arrows). **B** Incidental finding of bilateral superior vena cavas (arrows). FISP.

LOBAR EMPHYSEMA

This is an important cause of respiratory distress in infancy. Overdistension of lung tissue compromises gas exchange and can deviate the mediastinum in a contralateral fashion. The upper lobes are most frequently involved, more commonly the left, although middle lobe emphysma is frequent. Involvement of the lower lobes or of both lungs is rare.

The radiographic signs include gross overinflation of the affected lobe with compression of the remaining lobes of the lung (Fig. 1.2.10). The mediastinum is shifted contralaterally. Immediately after birth, the overdistended lobe may sometimes be opaque but will gradually become hyperlucent as the lung fluid clears (Fig. 1.2.11). The embarrassment to respiration is frequently so severe that urgent lobectomy has to be carried out, but in some cases of congenital lobar emphysema where surgery has been refused on religious grounds, spontaneous resolution has occurred. A trial of conservative management is often merited. Aetiology has not been clearly defined but several different mechanisms such as a developmental alveolar abnormality, lobar bronchial obstruction, possibly from inspissated secretion, alveolar damage from infection, bronchomalacia from poorly developed or absent bronchial cartilage or the condition of polyalveolar lobe may be involved.

A persistent patent ductus arteriosus can give rise to a similar appearance of overdistension of the left upper lobe as a result of secondary compression of the bronchial tree. In such cases, however, the degree of compression of the lingula and left lower lobe is typically less marked than in true congenital lobar emphysema. If the origin of the left pulmonary artery is aberrant arising from the right pulmonary artery, the left main bronchus may be compressed by the artery as it passes backwards into the lung.

There is a well-established association between congenital heart disease and infantile lobar emphysema, in particular, ventricular septal defects and persistent ductus arteriosus, but also with tetralogy of Fallot, especially in the presence of aneurysmal dilatation of the pulmonary arteries or absence of the pulmonary valve. Such lobar emphysema generally needs to be surgically treated before corrective cardiac surgery is attempted.

REFERENCES

Cremin B J, Movsowitz H 1971 Lobar emphysema in infants. British Journal of Radiology 44: 692–696

Fagan C J, Swischuk L E 1972 The opaque lung in lobar emphysema. American Journal of Roentgenology 114: 300–304

Pierce W S, DeParedes C G, Friedman S, Waldhausen J A 1970 Concomitant congenital heart disease and lobar emphysema in infants; incidence, diagnosis, and operative management. Annals of Surgery 172: 951–956

Tapper D, Schuster S, McBridge J, Eraklis A, Wohl M E, Williams A, Reid L 1980 Polyalveolar lobe: anatomic and physiologic parameters and their relationship to congenital lobar emphysema. Journal of Pediatric Surgery 15: 931–937

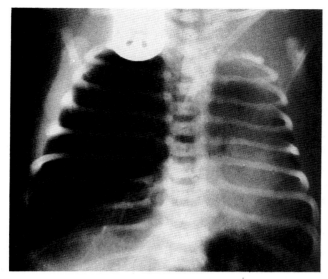

Fig. 1.2.10 Congenital lobar emphysema of the right middle lobe compressing the remaining right lung and displacing the mediastinum to the left.

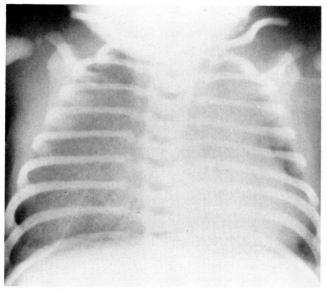

A

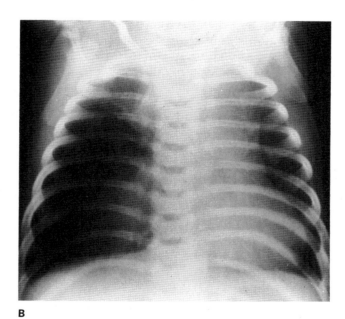

B

Fig. 1.2.11 Congenital lobar emphysema of the right middle lobe. **A** Pulmonary opacification after birth. **B** Overdistension of affected lobe at 1 week.

CYSTIC ADENOMATOID MALFORMATION OF THE LUNG

This is a rare congenital abnormality in which there is abnormal proliferation of the distal bronchial and terminal respiratory structures with varying sizes of communicating cysts which are lined with a pseudo-stratified or ciliated columnar epithelium. The mucosa becomes polypoid and there are increased amounts of elastic tissue in the walls of the cystic parts of the lesion. Three types have been described. Type 1, the most common, shows obvious cystic spaces within the malformation. Occasionally one large cyst is surrounded by smaller cysts. In type 2 lesions, multiple smaller cysts are evenly distributed throughout the lesion, while type 3 malformations appear homogeneous with no macroscopic cysts and a histological appearance similar to the lung in its earlier stages of development.

Type 1 lesions present usually with respiratory symptoms within the first few months of life, although later presentation with a history of chronic or recurrent pneumonia may occur. The cystic areas are filled with fluid after birth and present a space-occupying lesion within an expanded lobe or lung. As the cysts usually communicate with the airway the fluid is replaced by gas and a coarse reticular cystic pattern replaces the previous opacities. In such cases the circular radiolucencies can mimic the pneumatocoeles of staphylococcal pneumonia or a congenital diaphragmatic hernia. In congenital diaphragmatic hernia, the abdomen often appears scaphoid with a relative paucity of gas shadows. The lesions occur with equal frequency in either lung and usually involve one lobe with a slightly increased incidence in the upper lobes. Although usually affecting only one lobe, multiple lobes can be involved. The vascular supply and drainage are typically normal.

Cystic adenomatoid malformations are increasingly detected by obstetric ultrasound; type 1 lesions are characterized by their larger fluid-filled cystic appearance, while type 2 and 3 lesions show a finer cystic appearance or a homogeneous echo pattern. Type 2 lesions are often associated with severe congenital abnormalities, particularly with renal agenesis, and type 3 abnormalities, although very rare, carry an equally poor prognosis. Maternal hydramnios and fetal hydrops are associations. In type 1 lesions the prognosis is generally good following excision of the space-occupying mass in infancy or of lesions presenting in later life as recurrent pneumonia (Figs 1.2.12–1.2.14).

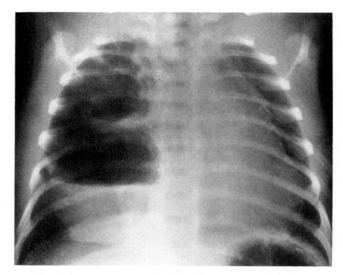

Fig. 1.2.12 Congenital cystic adenomatoid malformation. Multiple air-filled cysts with fluid levels.

REFERENCES

Cave A P D, Adam A E 1984 Cystic adenomatoid malformation of the lung found on antenatal ultrasound examination. British Journal of Radiology 57: 176–178

Gaisie G, Oh K S 1983 Spontaneous pneumothorax in cystic adenomatoid malformation. Pediatric Radiology 13: 281–283

Hulnick D H, Naidich D P, McCauley D I, Feiner H D, Avitabile A M, Greco M A, Genieser N B 1984 Late presentation of congenital cystic adenomatoid malformation of the lung. Radiology 151: 569–574

Madewell J E, Stocker J T, Korsower J M 1975 Cystic adenomatoid malformation of the lung: morphologic analysis. American Journal of Roentgenology 124: 346–448

Tucker T T, Smith W L, Smith J A 1977 Fluid-filled cystic adenomatoid malformation. American Journal of Roentgenology 129: 323–325

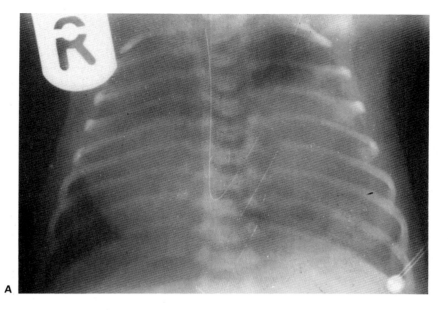

A

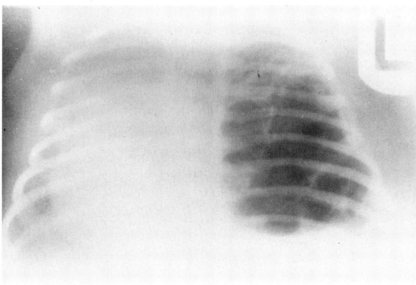

B

Fig. 1.2.13 Congenital cystic adenomatoid malformation. Initially opaque left lower lobe lesion (**A**), develops gas-filled cysts (**B**).

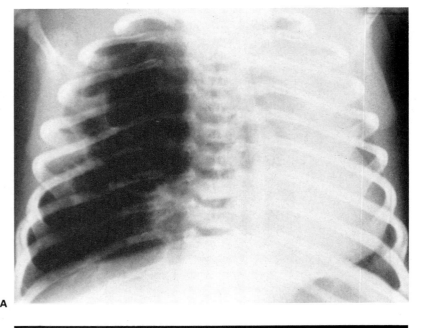

A

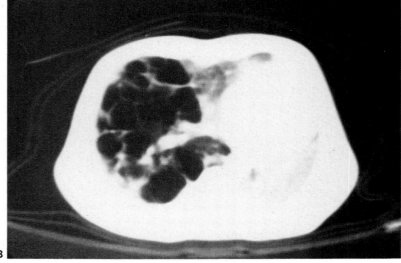

B

Fig. 1.2.14 Cystic adenomatoid malformation. **A** Plain radiograph. **B** CT scan with multiple cysts deviating the mediastinum.

TRACHEOBRONCHOMALACIA

The lumen of the major airways is dependent upon the cartilaginous structures in the walls. Structural deficiencies in these may arise as part of an intrinsic congenital malformation or associated with external causes of which compression by the dilated oesophagus proximal to oesophageal atresia and aberrant vessels are important causes (Figs 1.2.15, 1.2.16). Local infection, foreign body or extrinsic mass may also compromise the airway lumen. Evaluation of the airways is best performed by fluoroscopy and observing inappropriate movement of the tracheobronchial walls and attenuation of the lumen. Detection of local bronchomalacia may be less satisfactory with conventional fluoroscopy but can be supplemented by local positive bronchography with selective catheterization of suspected parts of the bronchial tree. Such procedures will usually involve general anaesthesia and careful endotracheal intubation. Ultrafast CT is a valuable investigation if available.

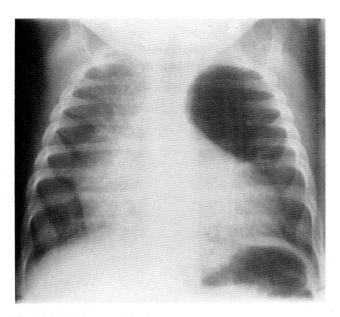

Fig. 1.2.15 Left upper lobe distension. At surgery, the left upper lobe showed severe localized bronchomalacia.

REFERENCES

Cook R C M, Bush G H 1978 Tracheal compressions as a cause of respiratory symptoms after repair of oesophageal atresia. Archives of Disease in Childhood 53: 246–248

Wittenberg M H, Gyepes M T, Crocker D 1967 Tracheal dynamics in infants with respiratory distress, stridor, and collapsing trachea. Radiology 88: 653–662

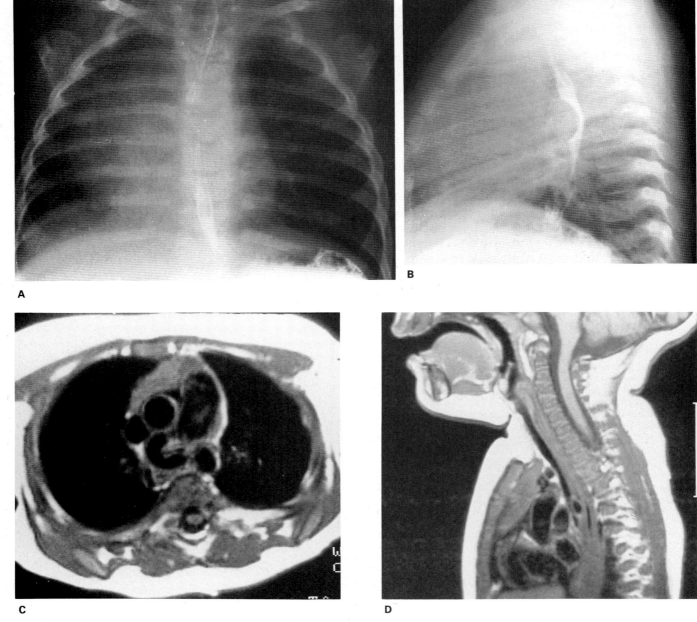

Fig. 1.2.16 Aberrant left pulmonary artery (pulmonary sling). **A** Radiograph with dextroversion of the heart. **B** Lateral view with barium in oesophagus, indenting it anteriorly and pushing forward tracheal bifurcation. **C** MR showing aberrant left pulmonary artery passing (**D**) between carina and oesophagus.

BRONCHO-BILIARY FISTULA

This rare congenital condition consists of a fistula from the right main stem bronchus to the left hepatic duct system. Diagnosis can be confirmed by localized bronchography at bronchoscopy.

REFERENCE

Chang C C, Giulian B B 1985 Congenital bronchobiliary fistula. Radiology 156: 82

TRACHEOBRONCHOMEGALY

The Mounier–Kuhn syndrome was described in 1932 as dilatation of the tracheobronchial tree associated with recurring respiratory tract infections. Progressive dilatation of the trachea and main bronchial tree begins in childhood and becomes more marked in adult life, although onset in infancy has been described. In addition to the generalized dilatation associated with more peripheral cylindrical or saccular bronchiectasis, localized saccular recesses occur particularly in the central tracheobronchial tree.

The aetiology of this condition is not clear but tracheobronchomegaly may be seen in patients with connective tissue abnormalities such as cutis laxa and the Ehlers–Danlos syndrome.

The Williams–Campbell syndrome is associated with deficiency of the bronchial cartilages involving the fourth and more peripheral generations of divisions. Persistent cough and wheeze, which may start in the first year of life, is associated with overinflation of the lung fields and bronchial dilatation which is accentuated on inspiration, with collapse on expiration.

Dilatation of the trachea and proximal bronchi is also associated with immune deficiency states including severe combined immune deficiency and ataxia telangiectasia. Plain film and CT data of tracheal dimensions are available.

REFERENCE

Griscom N T, Wohl M E B, Fenton T 1989 Dimensions of the trachea to age 6 years related to height. Pediatric Pulmonology 6: 186–190

VARIOUS SKELETAL LESIONS

Poland's syndrome

Partial or complete absence of the pectoral muscles leads to increased radiolucency of the ipsilateral hemithorax. Syndactyly and hypoplasia of the ipsilateral arm and hand are associated and there may occasionally be rib deformities, lung herniation and sternal anomalies (Fig. 1.2.17).

Cerebrocostomandibular syndrome

In this condition deficiency of the ribs posteriorly with irregular ossification and malformation of the costovertebral joints is associated with micrognathia and severe brain defects (Fig. 1.2.18).

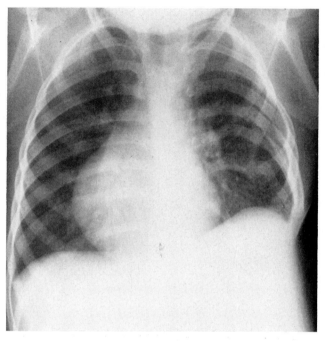

Fig. 1.2.17 Poland's syndrome. Absence of left pectoral muscles with multiple rib anomalies.

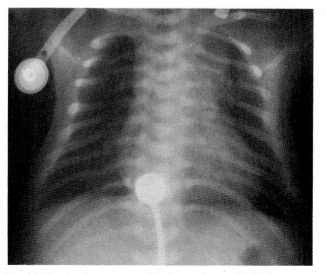

Fig. 1.2.18 Cerebrocostomandibular syndrome. Multiple posterior rib defects.

REFERENCES

Burton E M, Oestreich A E 1988 Cerebro-costo-mandibular syndrome with stippled epiphysis and cystic fibrosis. Pediatric Radiology 18: 365–367
Clark E A, Nguyen V D 1985 Cerebro-costo-mandibular syndrome with consanguinity. Pediatric Radiology 15: 264–266

Many skeletal dysplasias are associated with narrow chests (see Chapter XX); asphyxiating thoracic dystrophy (Jeune's syndrome) (Fig. 1.2.19) and achondroplasia (Fig. 1.2.20) are two relatively common diseases. Spinal dysraphism is often associated with rib cage deformity (Fig. 1.2.21). The ribs are particularly narrow in trisomy 18 (Edward's syndrome) (Fig. 1.2.22) and are a useful radiographic marker of this condition with a very poor prognosis.

Common mass lesions in the newborn are cystic hygroma (Fig. 1.2.23), teratoma (Fig. 1.2.24) and foregut duplication cysts.

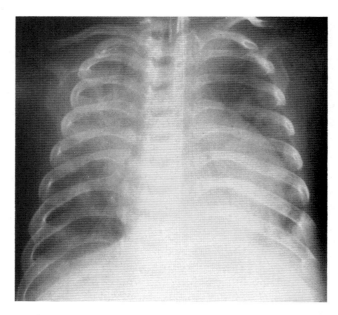

Fig. 1.2.19 Asphyxiating thoracic dystrophy. The thorax is narrow with short ribs; the clavicles are projected above the first ribs.

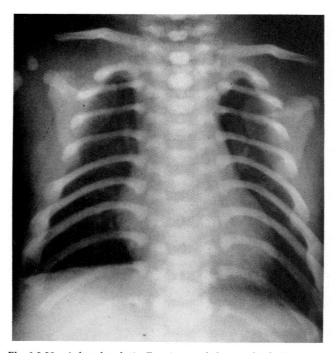

Fig. 1.2.20 Achondroplasia. Respiratory failure and infection.

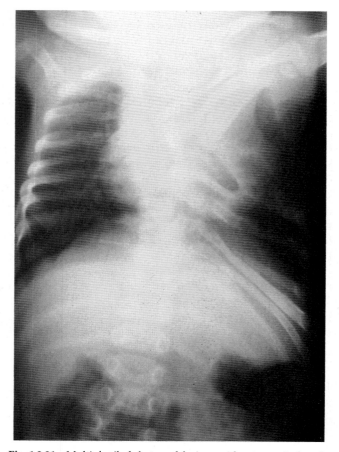

Fig. 1.2.21 Multiple rib defects and fusions with osteogenic dorsal scoliosis.

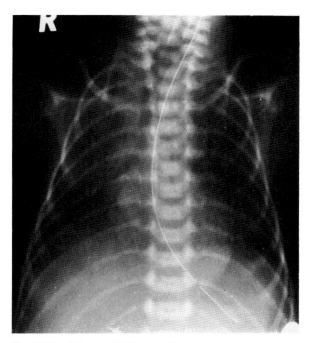

Fig. 1.2.22   Trisomy 18. Narrow ribs.

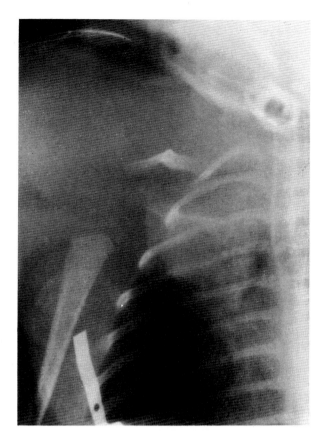

Fig. 1.2.23   Cystic hygroma extending into chest.

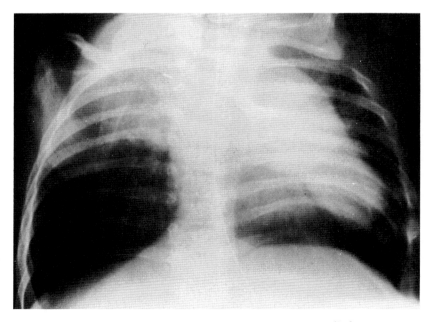

Fig. 1.2.24   Teratomatous twinning with anterior thoracic accessory limbs.

1.3 INFECTIONS

GENERAL CONSIDERATIONS

The lungs of small children differ from those of adults in that the peripheral airways are relatively smaller in size and that small amounts of oedema or intraluminal mucus or pus have a proportionately larger obstructing effect giving rise to air trapping or areas of collapse. The collateral airways of ventilation consisting of the pores of Kohn and the canals of Lambert are less efficient in childhood. There are relatively more mucous glands in the airways of young infants and the trachea and major bronchi appear more collapsible.

As a consequence of these factors inflammatory exudates in the central airways of the lung in the small child are likely to lead to areas of air trapping with local or generalized overinflation associated with irregular areas of localized atelectasis. True lobar consolidations and localized lobar collapse also appear in infancy but are a less common response to lower respiratory tract infection.

Acute inflammatory disease of the airways is often associated with peribronchial infiltration and oedema and radiographically presents as thickened ring shadows of bronchi seen end on or parallel line shadows ('tram-lines or railroad shadows') in those seen from the side. Such peribronchial thickening is usually transitory in pulmonary infections but is persistent in mucoviscidosis and young asthmatics.

BACTERIAL PNEUMONIA

The common bacterial infections encountered in childhood are due to pneumococcus, streptococcus, haemophilus, staphylococcus and less commonly, except in immune-compromised children, pseudomonas and klebsiella. Infective lung pathogens rarely produce absolutely characteristic radiographic patterns but lobar or segmental pulmonary consolidation, often with an air bronchogram giving the characteristic appearance of pulmonary consolidation, is a commoner feature of bacterial than of viral pneumonias which in many Western societies are probably now more common (Figs 1.3.1–1.3.3). Necrosis and cavitation are generally uncommon but pneumatocoele formation is an important complication of staphylococcal pneumonia (Figs 1.3.4, 1.3.5). These pneumatocoeles may rapidly enlarge, cause mediastinal displacement and perforate into the pleural space giving a pyopneumothorax (Fig. 1.3.6). Thin-walled residual cysts may be observed for several months following a staphylococcal pneumonia. In the newborn or young baby, haemophilus has been associated with pneumatocoele formation as has a variety of enteric organisms. Pleural effusions (Fig. 1.3.7) are frequently seen in association with bacterial pneumonias and are usually small and transitory. If they become significantly infected an empyema results. Some of these spontaneously reabsorb but if persistent

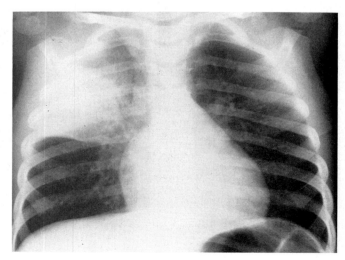

Fig. 1.3.1 Right upper lobe consolidation. Pneumococcus.

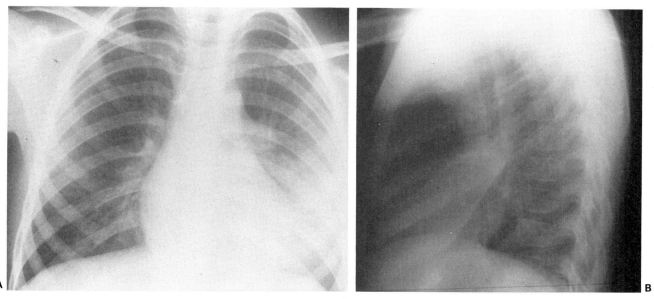

Fig. 1.3.2 **A** and **B** Lingular consolidation demonstrating well the 'silhouette sign' with loss of the left heart border.

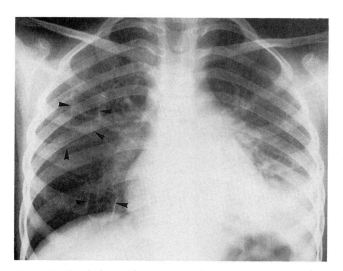

Fig. 1.3.3 Staphylococcal pneumonia. Extensive pneumatocoeles (arrows) in addition to areas of pneumonic consolidation.

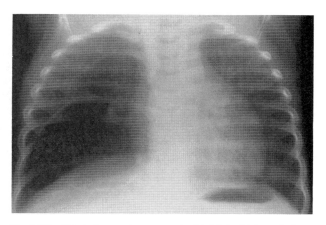

Fig. 1.3.5 Staphylococcal pneumonia. Multiple thick-walled pneumatocoeles.

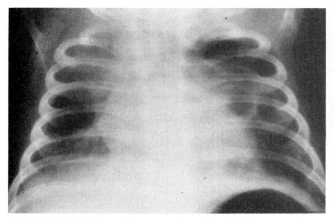

Fig. 1.3.4 Staphylococcal pneumonia with multiple areas of cavitation.

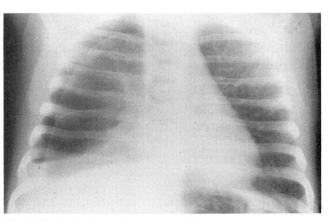

Fig. 1.3.6 Staphylococcal pneumonia. Pyopneumothorax.

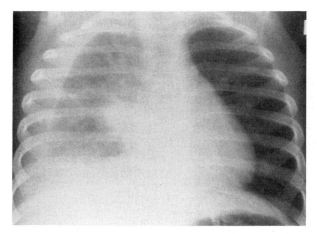

Fig. 1.3.7 Pleural effusion. Staphylococcal pneumonia.

and loculated, ultrasound can demonstrate loculation, the thickness of the rind and indicate satisfactory sites for aspiration (Fig. 1.3.8). Should the empyema become chronic and undergo organization, CT especially if decortication of the lung is considered, will allow good delineation of the parietal and visceral rind (Figs 1.3.9, 1.3.10).

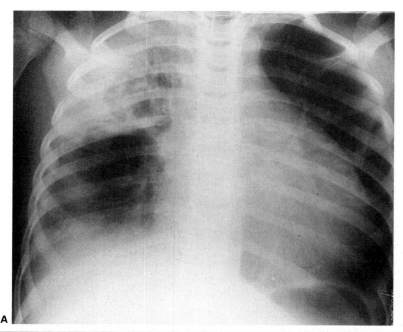

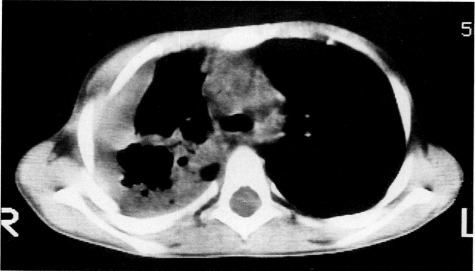

Fig. 1.3.8 **A** Radiograph of cavitated right upper lobe. Pneumococcal pneumonia with pleural effusion. **B** CT at the level of the carina.

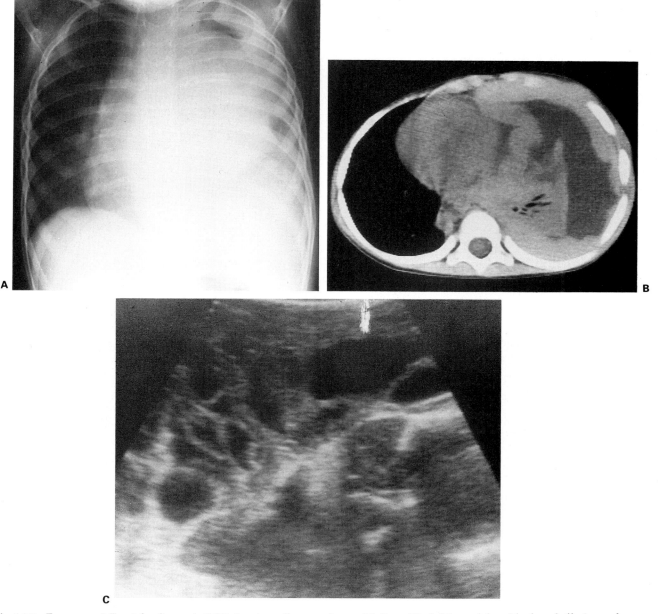

Fig. 1.3.9 Empyema. **A** Frontal radiograph. **B** CT showing collapse and consolidation of the left lower lobe with pleural effusion and parietal and visceral rind. **C** Ultrasound showing loculation.

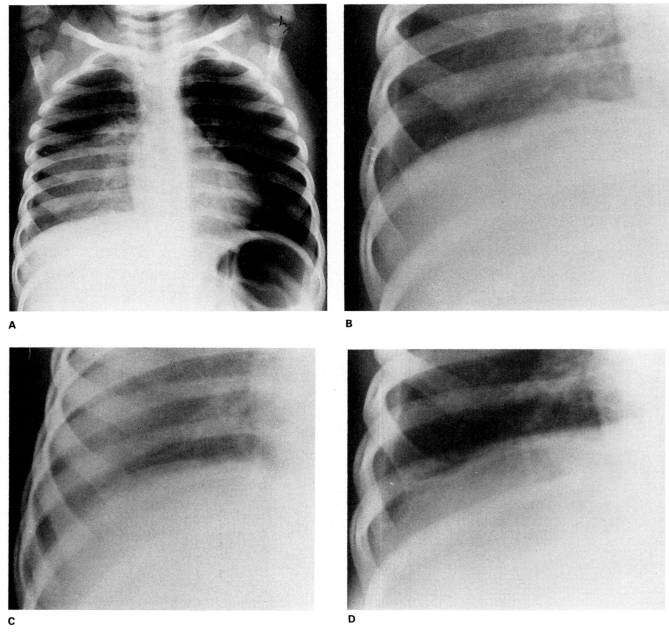

A

B

C

D

Fig. 1.3.10 Subtle periosteal reaction of the ribs in a child with right lower lobe haemophilus pneumonia. **A** At presentation showing extensive right lower lobe consolidation with a small pleural reaction. **B** Localized view of the right costaphrenic angle. **C**. Ten days later showing fine periosteal reaction around the anterior ends of the ribs. **D** Three weeks later the periosteal reaction has consolidated leading to some thickening of the ribs.

ROUNDED OR PSEUDOTUMOROUS PNEUMONIA

Pneumonic consolidation, usually bacterial and frequently pneumococcal in origin, gives rise to confusing and at times alarming radiographic images. An acute lower respiratory tract infection is associated initially with a sharply defined rounded lung opacity (Fig. 1.3.11). The opacity is usually situated in the posterior part of the lung and more frequently the lower lobes. An air bronchogram may be visible within the area of consolidation which is usually unilobar but may affect two adjacent lobes.

The clinical features are usually characteristic of an infective process, with cough, fever and leucocytosis. However, the remarkable clarity of the margins of these lesions in their early evolution can mimic posterior mediastinal masses and neuroblastoma is a frequently entertained incorrect diagnosis.

HILAR LYMPHADENOPATHY IN THE CHILD

Hilar lymph node enlargement is frequently seen as a response to parenchymal pulmonary infection. Simple pneumonias and viral infections of the lung are much more commonly associated with enlargement of the ipsilateral hilar lymph nodes in childhood than in the adult. Although it is always important to consider tuberculosis as a cause of hilar lymphadenopathy in childhood, it should also be appreciated that the lymphadenopathy can result from infections running a more benign and shorter course. Mediastinal lymph node enlargement from infections, particularly tuberculosis, can significantly narrow the major airways in childhood, and at times the mass effect of infective lymphadenopathy is difficult to differentiate from that associated with the malignant lymphomas (Fig. 1.3.12).

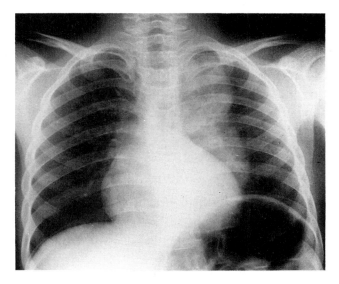

Fig. 1.3.11 Pseudotumorous pneumonia. Involvement of two lobes is uncommon.

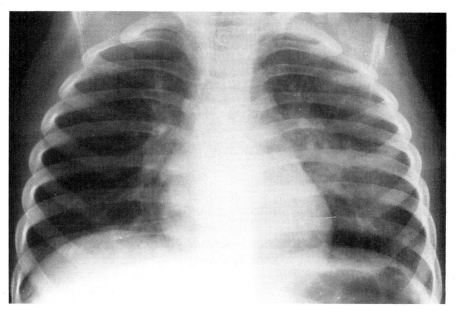

Fig. 1.3.12 Left hilar lymph node enlargement, simple bacterial pneumonia of left lower lobe.

THE ANATOMICAL LOCALIZATION OF LOBAR PATHOLOGY

It is possible to localize most lobar consolidations by recourse to the 'silhouette sign'.

The right upper lobe is adjacent to the right superior mediastinal structures and loss of clarity of these indicates lack of aeration in the right upper lobe. Similarly, lack of clarity of the lower right border arises from collapse or consolidation in the middle lobe of the right lung; and of the superior contour of the right hemidiaphragm from right lower lobe consolidation. The corresponding findings in the left lung are obscuring of the left upper mediastinum from left upper lobe consolidation or collapse, of the lower left heart border by lingular pathology, and of the left dome of the diaphragm by loss of aeration in the left lower lobe. Such evaluation can limit the need for lateral radiographs, particularly in simple pneumonias, with subsequent radiation reduction. The 'silhouette sign' is generally reliable but in complete collapse of the right middle lobe, there may be an entirely normal frontal radiograph. Peripheral segmental lesions and subsegmental lesions may be difficult to localize on a frontal radiograph.

PLEURAL EFFUSION, OPACIFICATION OF ONE HEMITHORAX

A common cause of opacification of one hemithorax is pleural effusion. Small pleural effusions separate the lung from the chest wall and are easily recognized by plain radiography. In small children and infants because of small distances and consequently less hydrostatic pressure changes, pleural fluid often surrounds the lung completely without the concave blunting of the costo-phrenic angles seen in the adult. However, as in the adult subpulmonary effusions occur and can be suspected from apparent elevation of the hemidiaphragm or abnormal separation of the lung and gastric air bubble.

Large effusions lead to opacification of the hemithorax. If the underlying lung is aerated or there is an associated mass, the mediastinum, and trachea in particular, will be deviated contralaterally. If the lung is collapsed, the mediastinum can remain central.

If plain radiographs supplemented by decubitus views are insufficient for evaluation, ultrasound of the chest will confirm the presence, site and loculation of pleural fluid facilitating aspiration and drainage. The character of the pleural fluid (bloody, purulent, clear, proteinacous, chylous) will indicate possible diagnoses. If an intrathoracic mass is suspected with an associated pleural effusion causing major opacification of the hemithorax, CT or MRI can supplement ultrasonography.

PNEUMOTHORAX

Spontaneous pneumothorax in the young child is uncommon but is not infrequent in adolescence. Presenting with pleuritic pain, respiratory embarrassment is typically not great, but occasionally tension pneumothoraces are seen. Pneumothorax is a relatively common complication of cystic fibrosis and may occur in association with the more common pneumomediastinum of the asthmatic child. Iatrogenic causes of pneumothorax, particularly following cardiac surgery and diaphragmatic repair for congenital diaphragmatic hernia, are commoner than those associated with chest trauma, particularly if there are rib fractures.

Detection of pneumothoraces with separation of the lung margin from the chest wall is usually easy on an upright frontal radiograph. Although an expiratory film will facilitate the diagnosis, small pneumothoraces are typically inconsequential and such a procedure may not be deemed worthwhile. Care must be taken to differentiate the anterior axillary fold from a loculated pneumothorax and in the supine position, small pneumothoraces are difficult to detect, but may be identified in the anterior cardiophrenic angles. Horizontal beam radiographs are more informative to exclude small pneumothoraces in sick children nursed supine if it is clinically important to detect them. Decubitus views with horizontal beams are a supplementary technique as they are in the detection and assessment of fluidity of small pleural effusions. The principal use of radiography is in management and the assessment of the correct position of intercostal drains.

SECONDARY COLLAPSE AND CONSOLIDATION

Glandular enlargement and neoplasms particularly affecting the mediastinum and hilar regions may compromise airway patency. Oesophageal dilatation, cardiac enlargement (Fig. 1.3.13) and the spine in scoliotics can also cause significant bronchial compression.

PERSISTENT RIGHT MIDDLE LOBE COLLAPSE AND CONSOLIDATION

Recurrent and often persisting collapse and consolidation in the right middle lobe is a frequent feature of the asthmatic child and may also be seen in association with tuberculosis where extrinsic compression of the middle lobe bronchus by hilar lymphadenopathy leads to persistent collapse. Medical treatment with antibiotics, bronchodilators and physiotherapy should be diligently tried before too hasty radiographic investigation of these children. Should the collapse and consolidation be refractory, bronchoscopy and often

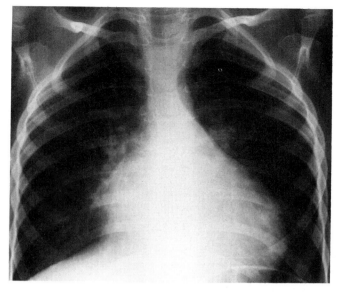

Fig. 1.3.13 Right middle lobe consolidation, ventricular septal defect.

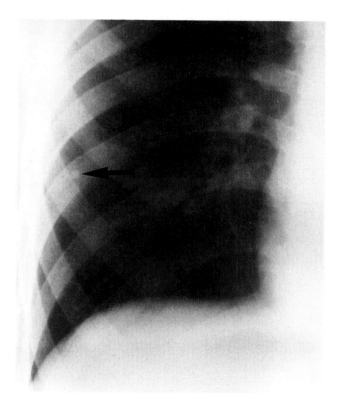

Fig. 1.3.14 Calcification in primary Ghon focus (arrow).

bronchial lavage may be combined with broncho-graphic evaluation of the bronchial tree in this region to exclude mural pathology or distal bronchiectasis.

REFERENCES

Rose R W, Ward B H 1973 Spherical pneumonias in children simulating pulmonary and mediastinal masses. Radiology 106: 179–182
Talner L B 1967 Pulmonary pseudotumors in childhood. American Journal of Roentgenology 100: 208–213

TUBERCULOSIS

Mycobacterium tuberculosis usually gains entrance to the child by air-borne inhalation. The site of initial infection in the lungs is most frequently under the visceral pleura. Growth of organisms here leads to development of the primary tuberculous focus. Polymorphs, histiocytes and lymphocytes are present within the lesion and caseation quickly follows. The regional lymph nodes associated with the focus enlarge and together with the focus form the primary complex. With the development of tuberculin sensitivity, the primary focus heals with or without calcification which usually takes a year or so to develop (Fig. 1.3.14). The peripheral primary focus is manifest on the chest radiograph as a small parenchymal lesion a few millimetres in diameter and more commonly in the right lung. In many patients the primary tuberculous focus may not be radiographically visible, yet the hilar nodes of the primary complex enlarge. The paratracheal nodes may also be involved.

The enlarged mediastinal and hilar lymph nodes can lead to incomplete bronchial obstruction with distal hyperinflation. If the compression effect is sufficiently great, distal collapse of lobes or segments may occur (Figs 1.3.15–1.3.18). Erosion of the bronchial wall by caseating hilar nodes can lead to endobronchial occlusion with collapse or consolidation. This may result in widespread tuberculous bronchopneumonia (Fig. 1.3.19). Usually, however, the segmental lesions clear both radiologically and clinically. Some residual bronchostenosis may persist and calcified tuberculous lymph nodes may be clearly seen in close relation to a narrowed area of the bronchus and occasionally may ulcerate into the bronchus as a broncholith.

Cylindrical bronchiectasis may be a late complication in areas in which there has been previous tuberculous collapse.

The development of the primary complex may be associated with pleural effusion and very occasionally can progress to tuberculous empyema. Although usually ipsilateral to the primary complex, effusions may occur contralaterally.

A serious complication of mediastinal lymphadenopathy is involvement of the pericardium with subsequent pericarditis and pericardial effusion. Compression of the oesophagus may occasionally be seen and fistula may develop into the oesophagus. Traction diverticula, especially in the region of the tracheal bifurcation, are a well-recognized complication of adhesive mediastinal lymphadenopathy.

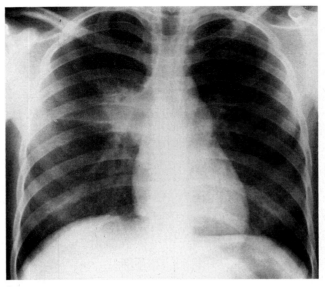

A

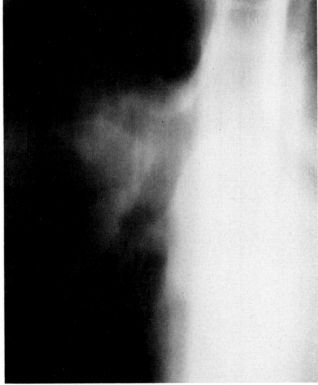

B

Fig. 1.3.15 Tuberculous adenopathy. **A** Plain radiograph **B** Conventional tomogram.

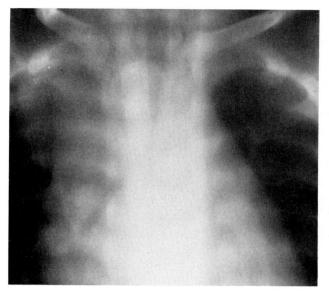

Fig. 1.3.16 Tuberculosis. Massive mediastinal lymphadenopathy is significantly narrowing the trachea.

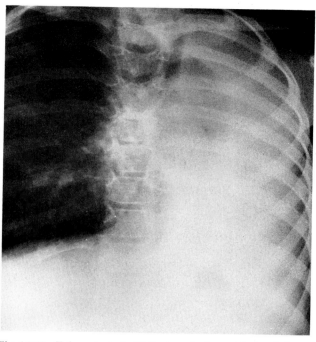

Fig. 1.3.17 Tuberculosis. Left hilar lymphadenopathy has led to bronchostenosis and collapse in the left lung.

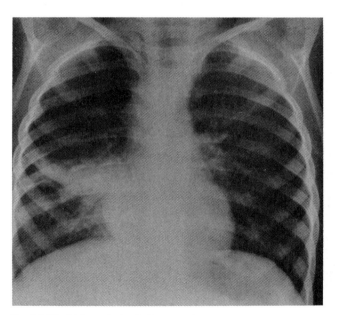

Fig. 1.3.18 Tuberculosis. Collapse and consolidation in the right middle lobe with right hilar and mediastinal lymphadenopathy.

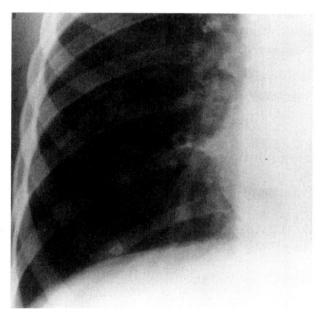

Fig. 1.3.19 Calcification in the lung as a consequence of previous tuberculous bronchopneumonia.

Miliary tuberculosis

Miliary tuberculosis usually develops within a year of an untreated primary tuberculosis lesion. In the early phase of haematogenous dissemination, the lung lesions are very small and inconspicuous, particularly in the first 2 or 3 weeks. As they develop multiple small shadows appear evenly distributed throughout both lung fields giving a characteristic fine even nodularity (Fig. 1.3.20). Although hilar lymph node enlargement may be seen, this is an uncommon finding.

With treatment the finely nodular shadows of miliary tuberculosis usually disappear without persisting change or calcification. However, calcification may be seen in the granulomas in the liver and spleen on chest radiographs. The former are usually well-circumscribed small calcific lesions while the latter may be larger and more amorphous.

Sites affected

The predilection of tuberculosis to affect the apices of both upper and lower lobes as in adult secondary disease is uncommon in the child. Parenchymal lesions involving the right upper lobe and middle lobes are half as common again as those occurring in the left upper lobe and lingula. Bronchographic studies have revealed that the residual bronchial deformities are more frequent in the upper lobes, the right middle lobe and lingula, with sparing generally of the lower lobes. Tuberculosis can arise in a rib or in the soft tissues of the thoracic cage and then may spread to involve either the ribs or the sternum when the resulting soft tissue mass may be a presenting symptom. There is, however, usually evidence elsewhere of tuberculous infection such as parenchymal lung disease or mediastinal lymphadenopathy.

REFERENCE

Lamont A C, Cremin B J, Pelteret R M 1986 Radiological patterns of pulmonary tuberculosis in the paediatric age group. Pediatric Radiology 16: 2–7

BCG VACCINATIONS

Reports of lung involvement in disseminated BCG are rare. The recorded appearances are essentially similar to those usually found with ordinary *Mycobacterium tuberculosis*. A nodular pattern can occur and these may in time calcify. In immune-compromised children a progressive and fatal tuberculosis infection of the lungs with adenopathy and widespread consolidation and cavitating lesions may occur.

PERTUSSIS (WHOOPING COUGH)

The radiographic appearances of this disease have changed over the past few decades with the advent of antibiotics and vaccination. Older studies suggest that collapse was the commonest pulmonary complication and that bronchiectasis was a significant sequel. More recent studies of children admitted to hospital with acute whooping cough show that radiographic abnor-

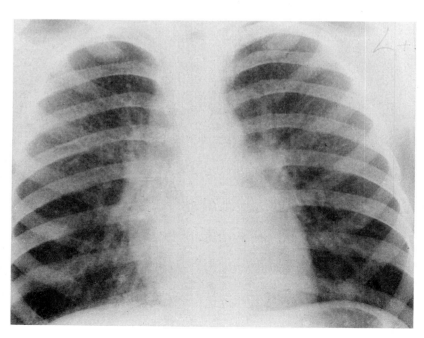

Fig. 1.3.20 Miliary tuberculosis.

malities in the chest are seen in about a quarter of the patients. Of these, pulmonary consolidation was much more frequent than collapse and lymphadenopathy occurred in about a third. Collapse is usually peribronchial in character and both collapse and consolidation were commoner on the right, particularly involving the lower and middle lobes. Current follow-up studies indicate that significant radiographic persisting abnormalities are most unlikely.

REFERENCE

Bellamy E A, Johnston I D A, Wilson A G 1987 The chest radiograph in whooping cough. Clinical Radiology 38: 39–43

EMPYEMA

Empyema is often due to staphylococcal pneumonia. Ultrasound of the pleural space with change in posture helps delineate the size and loculation of these infected effusions, assisting aspiration or the insertion of a drain. CT also allows delineation of an empyema and by doing prone and supine scans will indicate if the effusion is mobile. The degree of loculation and the thickness of the pleural reaction can also be assessed.

REFERENCE

Highman J H 1969 Staphylococcal pneumonia and empyema in childhood. American Journal of Roentgenology 106: 103–108

PRIMARY ATYPICAL PNEUMONIA

The term primary atypical pneumonia was introduced some 50 years ago to characterize lower respiratory tract infections other than those due to the common pneumococcal pneumonia. A feature was that the clinical state was of a moderate illness with chest radiographs demonstrating quite florid widespread changes. The term has now been broadened to include pneumonia due to viruses, rickettsia, chlamydia and *Mycoplasma pneumoniae*. With the relative decine in the incidence of bacterial pneumonia such agents constitute the majority of lower respiratory tract infections in children.

Mycoplasma pneumoniae

An important cause of primary atypical pneumonia in teenagers, mycoplasma pneumonia, or Eaton agent pneumonia also affects younger patients. Although the young child is frequently less ill than the adolescent, the condition can lead to severe toxicity. Infection is more common in autumn and winter and epidemics vary from year to year. Initial symptoms are of upper respiratory tract infection, otitis media and bronchitis with an incubation period of 2–3 weeks. Radiological features are varied. Three different patterns have been described. Peribronchial and perivascular interstitial infiltrates occur bilaterally. Of equal incidence are patchy non-homogeneous consolidations and thirdly homogeneous ground-glass consolidations are seen. The mid and lower lung fields are more frequently affected. The disease can be predominantly unilateral and may rarely be associated with pleural effusions. Enlargement of the hilar nodes is common but mediastinal lymphadenopathy is not usually apparent. A unilobar reticular shadowing, sometimes associated with an added nodularity, is highly suggestive of this condition (Fig. 1.3.21).

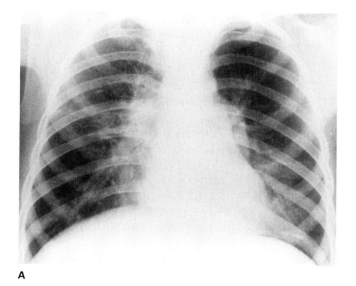

A

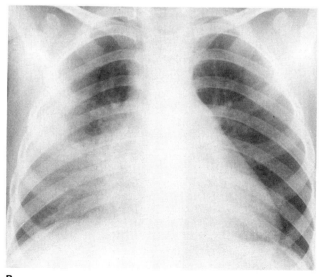

B

Fig. 1.3.21 Mycoplasma pneumonia. Two different cases. **A** There is hilar lymphadenopathy. **B** Extensive parenchymal consolidation.

Severe pulmonary manifestations are frequently seen in children with sickle cell disease with multiple infiltrates and pleural effusions.

Although most infections with *Mycoplasma pneumoniae* are benign, unresolved lobar pneumonia, pneumatocoeles and lung abscesses have all been described as complications. An unusual complication is obliterative bronchiolitis which can progress to a MacLeod or Swyer–James syndrome; persistent functional abnormalities of small airway function have also been recorded.

REFERENCES

Mok J Y, Waugh P R, Simpson H 1979 Mycoplasma infection: a follow up study of 50 children with respiratory illness. Archives of Disease in Childhood 54: 506–511
Vales A F, Masel J, O'Duffy J 1987 Obliterative bronchiolitis due to *Mycoplasma pneumoniae* infection in a child. Pediatric Radiology 17: 109–111
Guikel C, Benz-Bohm G, Widemann B 1989 Mycoplasmal pneumonias in childhood. Pediatric Radiology 19: 499–503

LEGIONELLA PNEUMONIA

Infection with this organism in children usually affects those who are debilitated by other systemic disease or those who suffer from some immune compromise. Both the clinical and radiographic features are non-specific but in addition to pneumonic consolidation, hilar lymphadenopathy and pleural effusions and occasional abscess formation may be noted. Parenchymal lesions may progress following the institution of antibacterial therapy and both clinical and radiographic resolution may be slow.

SYPHILIS

Radiological manifestations of this are usually observed as typical osseous changes of metaphyseal lucencies and periostitis. Syphilitic involvement of the lungs leads to the morbid anatomical appearance of pneumonia alba. Radiographically the appearances are however non-specific and consist of patchy shadowing throughout the lungs, associated clinically with respiratory distress.

REFERENCE

Macias E G, Eller J J, Huber T W, Abraham G, Diserens H W, Crawford S T 1974 Immunofluorescence of tracheal secretions in neonatal syphilis. Pediatrics 53: 947–949

NECROTIZING PNEUMONIA DUE TO *FUSOBACTERIUM NECROPHORUM*

Fusobacterium, a gram-negative anaerobe, is a normal oral commensal. Local infections such as severe pharyngitis, cervical abscesses and ear infections may be associated with severe pulmonary involvement. In contradistinction to adults where infection with this bacterium is usually associated with debilitation or alcoholism, affected children are usually normal. Diffuse interstitial disease with septal lines and nodular shadows which cavitate are seen as may be more confluent areas of consolidation especially in the lower lobes. Central lymphadenopathy and pleural effusions may occur.

REFERENCES

Kleinman P K, Flowers R A 1984 Necrotising pneumonia after pharyngitis due to *Fusobacterium necrophorum*. Pediatric Radiology 14: 49–51
Landay M J, Christensen E E, Bynum L J, Goodman C 1980 Anaerobic pleural and pulmonary infections. American Journal of Roentgenology 134: 233–240

ADENOVIRUS INFECTION, BRONCHIOLITIS OBLITERANS

Bronchiolitis obliterans with chronic obstructive airways disease can be due to a variety of causes, but in childhood lower respiratory tract infections with adenovirus, particularly types 3, 7 and 21, are important causes. Although these agents affect children of all ages, the complication of bronchiolitis obliterans is most common following initial infection below the age of 2 years (Figs 1.3.22, 1.3.23).

The initial disease starts as a severe necrotizing pneumonia and is indistinguishable from other forms of viral pneumonia. However, the destruction of the smaller airways and consequent poor perfusion are associated with persisting signs of obstructive lung disease. Radiographically the lungs are hyperinflated with diminution in the pulmonary vascular tree. Although very rarely indicated, bronchography will reveal failure of the positive contrast agent to reach the peripheral airways of the bronchial tree, giving rise to the so-called 'broken bough' appearance.

If the condition is mostly unilateral, an ipsilateral small hyperlucent lung may result, the MacLeod or Swyer–James syndrome. Plain radiographs show a small lung with increased radiolucency while fluoroscopy demonstrates air trapping with contralateral deviation of the mediastinum on expiration. Ventilation/perfusion scans show diminution in ventilation and perfusion. Although some defective lobes or lungs may improve, severe involvement is associated with significant diminution in growth of the affected rib cage and a persisting small relatively hyperinflated and poorly perfused lung with poor gas exchange.

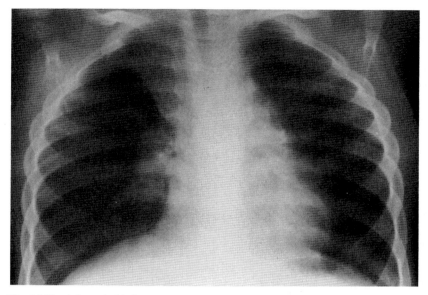

Fig. 1.3.22 Adenoviral infection. Widespread patchy shadowing with right upper lobe collapse and consolidation with air bronchogram.

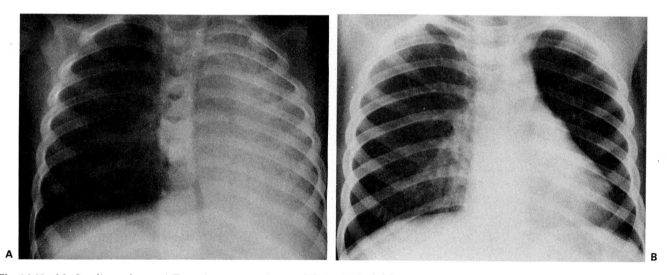

A

B

Fig. 1.3.23 MacLeod's syndrome. **A** Extensive pneumonic consolidation in the left lung associated with severe adenoviral infection. **B** Seven years later, the left hemithorax is smaller with diminished vascularity and hypertranslucency.

RESPIRATORY SYNCYTIAL VIRUS

Although the appearance of respiratory syncytial virus pneumonia is predominantly one of over-inflation with peribronchial and perihilar streaky shadowing, lobar collapse has been described with an incidence varying from some 7% to 25%. Some series have shown a preponderance of collapse and consolidation in the right upper lobe (Fig. 1.3.24).

REFERENCES

Eriksson J, Nordshus T, Carlsen K H, Orstadvik I, Westrik J, Eng J 1986 Radiological findings in children with respiratory syncytial virus infection. Pediatric Radiology 16: 120–122

Osborne D 1978 Radiologic appearance of viral disease of the lower respiratory tract in infants and children. American Journal of Roentgenology 130: 29–33

Quinn S F, Erickson S, Osborne D, Hayden F 1985 Lobar collapse with respiratory syncytial virus pneumonitis. Pediatric Radiology 15: 229–230

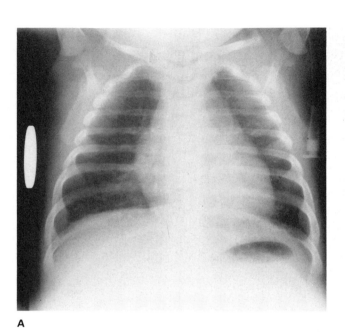

A

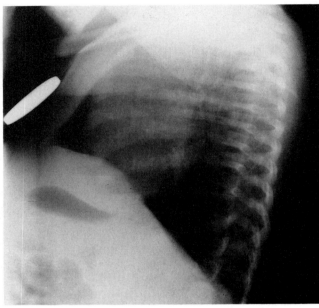

B

Fig. 1.3.24 Respiratory syncytial virus. **A** There is overdistension of the lung fields with a marked retrosternal and retrocardiac lucency visible on the lateral view. **B** The metallic opacity is a coin used to assess magnification.

ATYPICAL MEASLES AFTER MEASLES IMMUNIZATION

Killed measles vaccine provides only partial protection as it does not induce respiratory antibodies. Live vaccines may not be very effective in the first year of life. Consequently an atypical measles may occur in such children. In the acute phase of the disease paratracheal and hilar lymphadenopathy with patchy sometimes nodular lung shadowing may occur. Pleural effusions are common in extensive lung involvement. Persisting nodular lesions have been described in pneumonia of atypical measles and have been mistakenly thought to be metastases (Figs 1.3.25, 1.3.26).

CHICKENPOX PNEUMONIA

In childhood, varicella pneumonia is usually a complication of immune deficiency, malignancy, nephrotic syndrome or occurs in the neonate. The radiographic features in the lungs, consisting of widespread ill-defined patchy shadowing which may at times be confluent, are often in excess of the clinical state. Resolution of the lung changes is usually complete. In adult varicella pneumonia, a rare finding is secondary small punctate calcifications but these are not a typical feature of the disease in childhood.

REFERENCES

James A G, Lang W R, Liang A Y et al 1979 Adenovirus type 21 bronchopneumonia in infants and young children. Journal of Pediatrics 95: 530–533

Epler G R, Colby T V 1983 The spectrum of bronchiolitis obliterans. Chest 83: 161

Margolin F R, Gandy T K 1979 Pneumonia of atypical measles. Radiology 131: 653–655

Nemir R L 1977 Varicella pneumonia in: Kendig E L Jr, Chernick V (eds) Disorders of the respiratory tract in children, 3d edn. W B Saunders, Philadelphia, p 955

Ruuskanen O, Meurman O, Sarkkinen H 1985 Adenoviral diseases in children: a study of 105 hospital cases. Pediatrics 76: 79–83

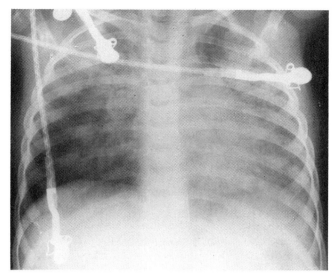

Fig. 1.3.25 Measles pneumonia in immune compromise.

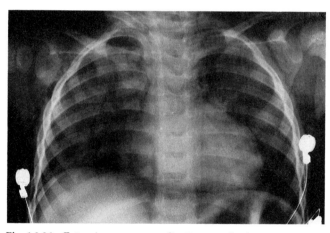

Fig. 1.3.26 Extensive pneumomediastinum and subcutaneous emphysema in measles in an African child.

AIDS

Children with the acquired immune deficiency syndrome suffer from pneumonia due to agents such as *Pneumocystis carinii* and cytomegalovirus in a similar way to adult patients (Fig. 1.3.27). A second group of children show abnormal chest radiographs and respiratory distress but have no obvious laboratory or biopsy evidence of infectious agents. The radiographs in such patients are non-specific and show diffuse reticulonodular shadowing with variable perihilar shadowing and central lymphadenopathy (Fig. 1.3.28). The histological lesions corresponding to this radiographic appearance include lymphocytic interstitial pneumonia (LIP), chronic interstitial pneumonia, bronchus associated lymphoid tissues (BALT) and immunoblastic lymphosarcoma. The relatively large amount of lymphoid tissue in the lungs of children is the probable reason why this reticulonodular non-specific appearance is seen in childhood although most uncommon in adult AIDS patients.

The widespread variability and the non-specificity of the radiographic appearances in children with AIDS either due to opportunistic infection or those lymphoid associated or interstitial pneumonias may mean lung biopsy is needed for adequate differentiation, particularly as the therapy of the lymphoid disorders differs from opportunist infections.

Hilar and mediastinal lymph node enlargement may also be due to coincident infection with mycobacteria including atypical forms, cytomegalovirus, lymphoma, Kaposi's sarcoma and fungal infections. Enlargement of the heart with sudden onset of acute congestive heart failure can result from a non-specific cardiomyopathy with myocardial lymphocytic infiltration.

REFERENCES

Rubinstein A, Morecki R, Silverman B, Charytan M, Krieger BZ, Andiman W, Ziprkowski M N, Goldman H 1986 Pulmonary disease in children with acquired immune deficiency syndrome and AIDS-related complex. Journal of Pediatrics 108: 498–503

Zimmerman D L, Haller J O, Price A P, Thelmo W L, Fikrig S 1987 Children with AIDS. Is pathologic diagnosis possible based on chest radiographs? Pediatric Radiology 17: 303–307

ACTINOMYCOSIS

Thoracic actinomycosis is rare in childhood. Immuno-compromise and mental retardation predispose. The radiological features include chronic pulmonary consolidation, pleural effusion and associated rib periostitis (Fig. 1.3.29).

REFERENCES

Thompson A J, Carty H 1979 Pulmonary actinomycosis in children. Pediatric Radiology 8: 7–9

Wilson D C, Redmond A O B 1990 An unusual cause of thoracic mass. Archives of Disease in Childhood 65: 991–992

COCCIDIOIDOMYCOSIS

This fungal disease, sometimes known as San Joaquin Valley Disease, occurs frequently in the arid regions of the south west of the USA. The infection is frequently asymptomatic but can clinically present as pneumonia with parenchymal consolidation and associated regional hilar lymph node enlargement. Calcification of the peripheral primary lung lesion and hilar lymph nodes occurs. Pleural reaction is usually minimal but at times significant. As in several fungal diseases,

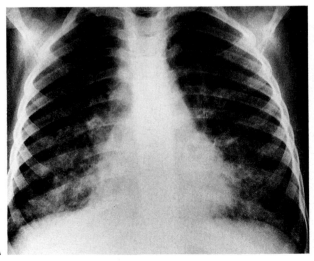
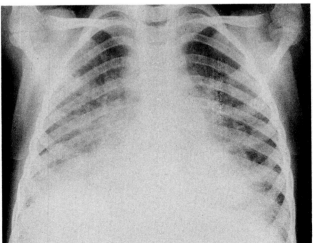

Fig. 1.3.27 Immune compromise. **A** Cytomegalovirus pneumonia. **B** *Pneumocystis carinii.*

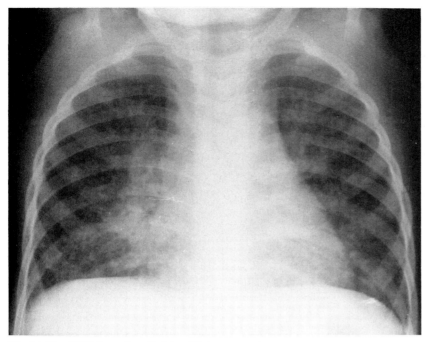

Fig. 1.3.28 AIDS. Lymphocytic interstitial pneumonia.

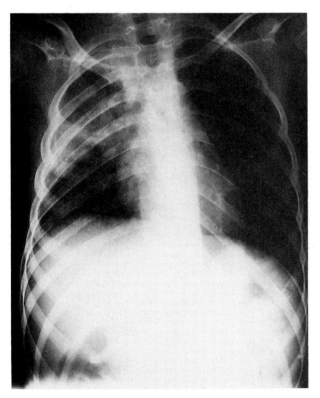

Fig. 1.3.29 Pulmonary actinomycosis.

thin-walled cavitation occurs and may lead to pneumothorax.

In addition to a cutaneous granuloma from direct infection, a serious disseminated form of the condition is described which is often fatal.

BLASTOMYCOSIS

So called North American Blastomycosis due to *Blastomyces dermatitidis* is geographically widespread. Peripheral lung lesions with hilar lymph node enlargement, sometimes with cavitation or a miliary pattern are features.

MUCORMYCOSIS

This serious fungal infection, particularly common in leukaemia and lymphoma, also occurs in children who are leucopenic, immune compromised or taking steroids or cytotoxic drugs. The radiographic appearances are non-specific with irregular areas of consolidation in which cavitation may occasionally be seen. Pleural effusion is a rare association but discrete lesions and mycetomas have been described.

CRYPTOCOCCOSIS

Peripheral areas of consolidation in this condition which are often subpleural are associated with hilar lymphadenopathy. Cavitation and pleural effusions are uncommon.

NOCARDIASIS

Often associated with immune compromise pulmonary infection with this organism leads to extensive areas of pulmonary consolidation, often rounded, associated with hilar and mediastinal lymphadenopathy (Fig. 1.3.30).

PULMONARY HISTOPLASMOSIS

Histoplasma capsulatum, an important disease in many parts of the USA, the Middle East and sub-Saharan Africa, has many pathological similarities to primary tuberculosis. The primary complexes are usually multiple. Healing is associated with widespread calcifications. Disseminated histoplasmosis, often in immune compromise, shows a similar pulmonary miliary pattern to that seen in miliary tuberculosis. As with tuberculosis, it can cause a fibrosing mediastinitis.

ECHINOCOCCOSIS

Hydatid cysts are common in those parts of the world where the dog tapeworm is endemic, although ease of worldwide travel and sporadic infestations mean that the diagnosis should be considered in any child with clearly defined rounded lesions in the lung fields.

Lung involvement, although not as frequent as that of the liver, is common. Distribution of the characteristically rounded or ovoid opacities is at random throughout the lung fields and may be multiple, unilateral and show considerable variation in size (Fig. 1.3.31). Less commonly, pericardial or cardiac involvement is present. Chest symptoms are unimpressive. Breakdown of the cysts can lead to crescentic air shadows or air-fluid levels within which a clump of endocyst may be seen. Rupture into pleural space can produce pneumothorax with effusion.

REFERENCE

Grunebaum M 1975 Radiological manifestations of lung echinococcus in children. Pediatric Radiology 3: 65–69

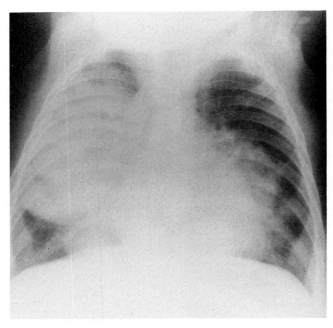

Fig. 1.3.30 Nocardiasis. Note the extensive rounded consolidation.

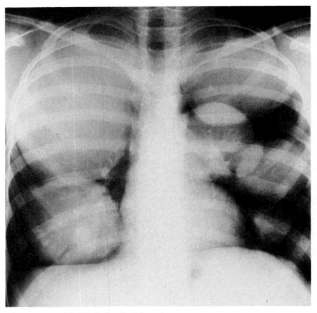

Fig. 1.3.31 Multiple hydatid cysts.

PARAGONIMIASIS

In the Far East and South East Asia, infestation with the lung fluke *Paragonimus westermanii* in many ways mimics pulmonary tuberculosis with haemoptysis and multiple calcified foci throughout the lungs and hilar regions.

REFERENCES

Fischer G, McGrew G L 1980 Pulmonary paragonimiasis in childhood. Journal of the American Medical Association 243: 1360–1362
Ogakwa M, Nwokolo C 1973 Radiologic findings in pulmonary paragonimiasis as seen in Nigeria: a review based on 100 cases. British Journal of Radiology 46: 699–705

TROPICAL EOSINOPHILIA (WEINGARTEN'S SYNDROME)

Tropical eosinophilia is associated with the presence of microfilariae in pulmonary eosinophilic granulomas in the absence of circulatory adult filarial worms. Pulmonary eosinophilia in temperate climates is more likely to be due to asthma (often with allergic aspergillosis), polyarteritis and rarely eosinophilic leukaemia (Fig. 1.3.32).

IMMUNE DEFICIENCY

IgA deficiency

This is the most common primary immune deficiency and occurs in about 1 in 700 of the population. Although associated with autoimmune and allergic disorders, recurrent respiratory infections involving the lungs, paranasal sinuses and ears are common and occur in about 40% of affected individuals. Recurrent croup is an association. Bronchiectasis is a rare complication as the respiratory manifestations of IgA deficiency are less marked than in some other deficiencies.

X-linked agammaglobulinaemia

This condition is associated with depression of the serum antibody levels of IgM, IgG and IgA. The thymus is morphologically normal but lymphatic tissue is hypoplastic. Maxillary and ethmoid sinusitis, chronic bronchitis and widespread bacterial pneumonias are common. Bronchiectasis affecting the lower lobes is an important complication and may be severe. Lung abscesses and chronic areas of collapse with associated pleural effusions are also features (Fig. 1.3.33).

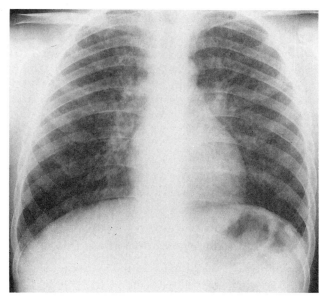

Fig. 1.3.32 Tropical eosinophilia.

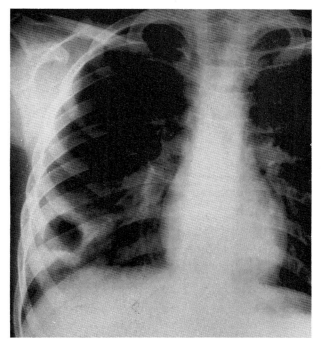

Fig. 1.3.33 Lung abscess. An air-fluid level is present in the thick-walled cavity.

Common variable immunodeficiency

All immunoglobulin classes are reduced and T-cell function is variable. Recurrent pneumonias are very common and progress to bronchiectasis in a high proportion of the patients. Radiographs will reveal widespread air trapping with pleural reactions and bullae, particularly in the lower lobes.

IgG subclass deficiency

Recurrent pneumonias and asthma are well-described complications of these conditions. Despite a subclass deficiency, the total IgG levels may be normal.

Transitory hypogammaglobulinaemia of infancy

This condition is usually self-limiting by the age of 1 or 2 years and can be associated with recurrent bronchitis and upper respiratory tract infections.

Severe combined immune deficiency

This is a heterogeneous group in which cell-mediated immunodeficiency is associated with recurrent infections and particularly by opportunistic organisms. Pneumocystis and viral infections are common. Unless successful bone marrow transplantation can be carried out, the condition is usually fatal. The type of combined immune deficiency associated with adenosine-deaminase deficiency may sometimes show abnormalities of the costochondral junctions on the chest radiograph.

DiGeorge's syndrome

This dysmorphic syndrome has many manifestations. Defective development of the third and fourth pharyngeal pouches leads to hypoparathyroidism, absent thymus and vascular lesions, especially interrupted aortic arch and truncal abnormalities. The chest radiograph will reveal a narrow superior mediastinum, due to absence of the thymus and parenchymal consolidation, which can result from a variety of opportunistic infections, particularly pseudomonas and viral infections.

Ataxia telangiectasia

Cerebellar ataxia, telangiectasia and immune deficiencies are associated in this condition. There is a moderate increase in the incidence of pulmonary infections. There is an exceptional sensitivity to the effects of radiation therapy in these children and marked tissue damage can follow small doses of ionizing radiation. There is an increased incidence of lymphoma and of acquired tracheobronchomegaly (Fig. 1.3.34).

Wiskott–Aldrich syndrome

Thrombocytopenia, eczema and recurrent infections are a feature of this X-linked recessive disease. There is a high incidence of pneumonia and of upper respiratory tract infection, usually bacterial but also from pneumocystis and viruses such as herpes.

Complement deficiencies

The two pathways, classical and alternative, can be associated with a variety of specific deficiencies. These may manifest as vascular conditions such as lupus erythematosis or glomerulonephritis and as repeated infections. An important deficiency is that of C1 esterase inhibitor. This deficiency is not associated with increased incidence of infections but can be associated with severe angioneurotic oedema which can lead to fatal laryngeal obstruction.

Phagocytic defects, chronic granulomatous disease

This multisystemic, usually X-linked recessive disorder of phagocytosis is associated with widespread granulomatous pyogenic infections (Fig. 1.3.35). Chemotaxis and phagocytosis are normal but intracellular organisms are not killed. Presenting usually in the first 2 years of life, chronic infection involves most organs, particularly the skin, alimentary tract, bones and genitourinary tract. Pulmonary disorders are very common and most patients suffer from recurrent pneumonia, with hilar lymphadenopathy, empyema and pulmonary abscesses. Common organisms are staphylococcus, *E. coli* and klebsiella. Fungal infections, particularly with aspergillus and candida, occur and are sometimes associated with spread from the lungs into the chest wall with rib osteomyelitis.

Extensive lung infections can lead to widespread consolidation progressing later to extensive fibrosis with honeycomb formation in the lung. Extension from the lung into the mediastinum or mediastinitis secondary to infections in the alimentary tract are often fatal.

Diagnosis is by the nitroblue tetrazolium (NBT) test which measures the ability of the phagocytes to reduce NBT to an intracytoplasmic dye.

Chediak–Higashi syndrome

This rare lysosomal storage disorder is associated with oculocutaneous albinism, hypersplenism, a lymphoma-like condition with coagulation defects, and recurrent pyogenic infections of the paranasal air sinuses and lungs. Important pathogens include *Staphylococcus aureus*, *Haemophilus influenzae* and haemolytic streptococci.

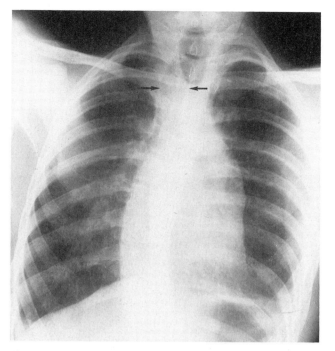

Fig. 1.3.34 Ataxia telangiectasia. The trachea (arrows) is wide, a recognized feature of diseases with immune compromise.

Hyper IgE syndrome

Although originally described as Job's syndrome in red-headed females, this condition, affecting both sexes, is associated with recurrent staphylococcal abscesses, skin infections and recurrent chest infections. Markedly elevated IgE levels in the serum are found. Pulmonary manifestations are usually apparent in the first year of life with chronic cough and bronchitis. Recurrent pneumonia, abscesses and empyema are associated with pneumatocoeles and cyst formation. The lung cysts may resolve spontaneously or can become infected with thickening of their walls. They often persist and may need to be removed surgically. Whereas bronchopleural fistula with persisting pneumothorax are important complications, bronchiectasis is not very common. Upper respiratory tract involvement includes chronic sinusitis and recurrent ear infections.

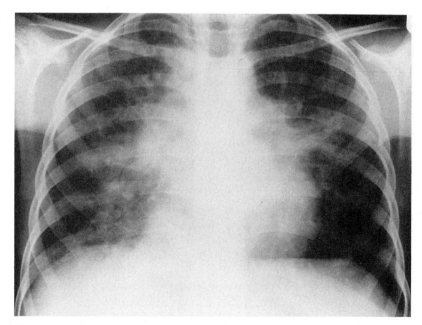

Fig. 1.3.35 Chronic granulomatous disease. Widespread parenchymal shadowing, particularly marked in the perihilar regions.

In the immune-compromised child, including those with AIDS and undergoing chemotherapy for malignant disease, parenchymal lung opacification associated with fever is often due to opportunistic infection. Of particular importance is pneumocystis, cytomegalovirus and *Mycobacterium tuberculosis*. Pneumocystis often gives a ground-glass appearance throughout the lung fields, with accentuation of the air bronchogram and elevation of the diaphragm reflecting the reduced compliance of the lungs. Bronchial lavage and transbronchial biopsies may identify the infecting agents. Percutaneous lung biopsy is practised in some centres, but many prefer open biopsy as a safer technique, since pneumothorax complicating needle biopsy of the lung in such sick children may seriously compromise pulmonary ventilation. Occasionally immune compromise is associated with calcification in the aorta (Figs 1.3.36, 1.3.37).

REFERENCES

Imoke E, Dudgeon D L, Colombari P et al 1983 Open lung biopsy in the immunocompromised pediatric patients. Journal of Pediatric Surgery 18: 816–821
Prober C G, Whyte H, Smith C R 1984 Open lung biopsy in immunocompromised children with pulmonary infiltrates. American Journal of Diseases of Children 138: 60–63
Sotomayor J L, Douglas S D, Wilmott R W 1989 Pulmonary manifestations of immune deficiency diseases. Pediatric Pulmonology 6: 275–292

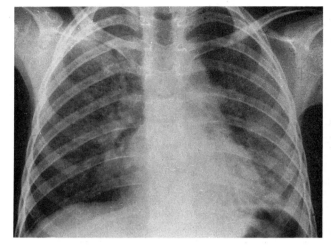

Fig. 1.3.36 Pneumocystis pneumonia in leukaemia. Widespread parenchymal shadowing with more marked left lower lobe consolidation.

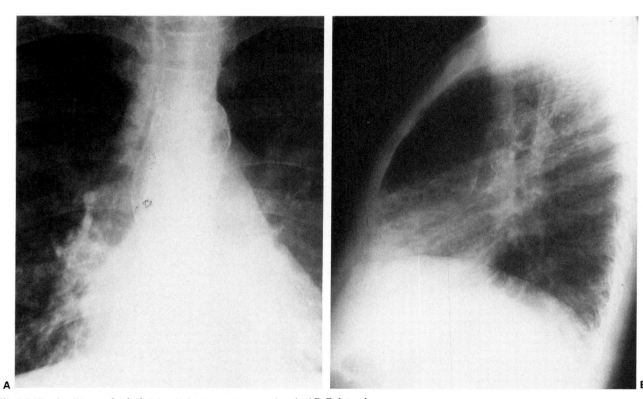

Fig. 1.3.37 Aortic mural calcification in immune compromise. **A**, AP; **B**, lateral.

CILIARY DYSKINESIA

Primary ciliary dyskinesia is a condition in which there is a deficiency of the dynein arms in cilia and spermatozoa and the consequent reduction in ciliary ATPase activity results in uncoordinated ciliary function and sperm immotility. The condition is heterogeneous with a variety of electron micrographic appearances, although the clinical symptoms are essentially similar. Inheritance is autosomal recessive with an incidence of about 1 in 30 000.

Mucociliary transport is grossly inefficient with consequent recurring respiratory tract infections beginning in early childhood. Chronic rhinorrhoea, sinusitis and otitis media are associated with chronic bronchitis resulting in bronchiectasis in most patients by early adulthood. Kartagener's syndrome consists of a triad of sinusitis, bronchiectasis and situs inversus and represents a subgroup of the condition. Male patients are infertile.

Recurrent paranasal air sinus infections are a distressing feature and may be complicated by direct extension beyond the sinuses resulting in osteomyelitis and intracranial disease. Radiographic features in the lungs include peribronchial thickening and variable areas of collapse and consolidation with a generalized overinflation. Bronchiectasis usually involves the lower lobes, lingula and middle lobe. Metastatic brain abscess is a recognized complication. The diagnosis can be established by microscopic examination of the ciliary activity in epithelial cells obtained by brushing the nasal mucosa. The saccharin test analyses the time of recognition of a sweet taste when a drop of saccharin is placed on the anterior turbinate bones, the time being elongated in affected patients. Delayed transport from the anterior nose to the nasopharynx of a small amount of radioactive material can also be recorded using a gamma camera.

REFERENCES

Faure C, Verderi D, Schmit P, Sirinelli D 1985 Chest x-ray findings in children with congenital ciliary abnormalities. Pediatric Radiology 15: 269
Nadel H R, Stringer D A, Levison H, Turner J A P, Sturgess J M 1985 The immotile cilia syndrome: radiological manifestations. Radiology 154: 651–656
Reyes De La Rocha S, Pysher T J, Leonard J C 1987 Dyskinetic cilia syndrome. Pediatric Radiology 17: 97–103
Rossman C M, Newhouse M T 1988 Primary ciliary dyskinesia. Pediatric Pulmonology 5: 36–50
Schidlow D V, Moriber S, Turtz M G, Donner R M, Capasso S 1982 Polysplenia and Kartagener syndromes in a sibship: association with abnormal respiratory cilia. Journal of Pediatrics 100: 401–403

MEDIASTINITIS

Suppurative mediastinitis is now infrequently encountered secondary to surgery with consequent infection, but can be due to perforation of the oesophagus or pharynx, extension from infections in the neck and from suppurating lymph nodes. It may also be a persistent and frequently fatal complication of immune-compromised patients, particularly those with chronic granulomatous disease (Fig. 1.3.38).

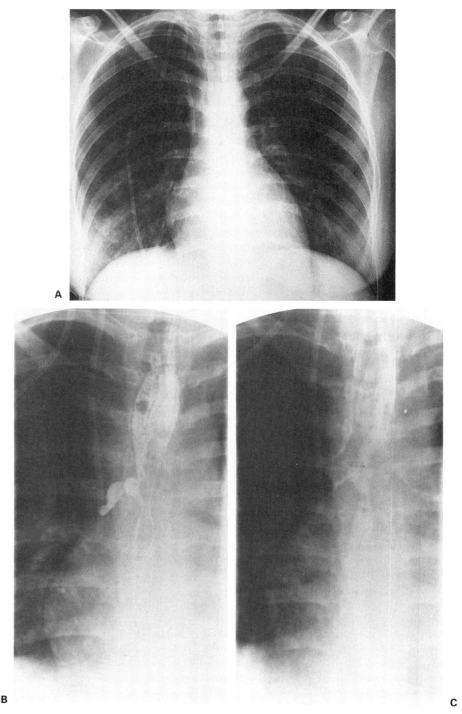

Fig. 1.3.38 Broncho-oesophageal fistula following candidiasis in immune compromise. **A** Frontal radiograph. **B** Contrast medium is extravasating from the oesophagus and entering the tracheobronchial tree (**C**).

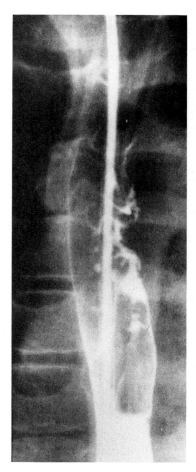

Fig. 1.3.39 Mediastinal tuberculosis involving the oesophagus in an Asian child.

Mediastinal fibrosis

This can result from infection with *Histoplasma capsulatum* or *Mycobacterium tuberculosis*, but most commonly is of unknown aetiology (Fig. 1.3.39). Presenting radiographically as widening of the mediastinal shadow with hilar or paratracheal masses, bronchial obstruction and compression of the vena cava and pulmonary veins are clinical findings, although the condition may be asymptomatic in its early presentation. Although usually widespread the fibrotic mass may be well circumscribed and sometimes calcified. Histologically there are many similarities with retroperitoneal fibrosis and orbital pseudotumour (Fig. 1.3.40).

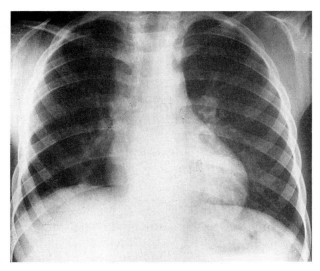

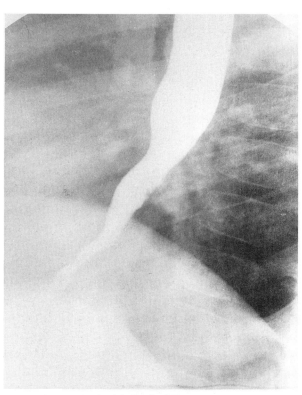

Fig. 1.3.40 Mediastinal fibrosis, inflammatory pseudotumour. There is widening of the lower posterior mediastinum. The lower oesophagus is compressed and narrowed. **A** Plain radiograph. **B** Barium swallow. **C** CT.

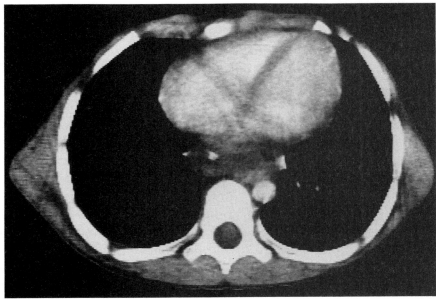

SICKLE CELL DISEASE

Hypoxaemia is a prominent feature of this condition. Pulmonary infarction is considered to be the cause of much acute or chronic lung disease, but pneumonia is many times more common in sickle cell disease than in the general population. The differentiation of pneumonia from pulmonary infarction is not clear cut: pulmonary infarction is more likely in later childhood; if positive (only about 10%) blood cultures favour infection; infarction is commoner in lower lobes; $\dot{V}/Q$ scans are unreliable but a negative gallium scan favours infarction; jaundice suggests infarction (Figs 1.3.41, 1.3.42).

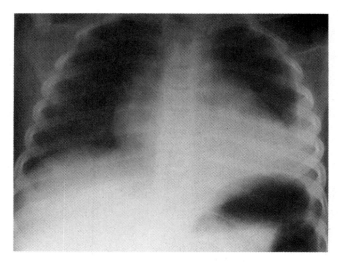

Fig. 1.3.41 Sickle cell disease. There is a left pleural effusion and cardiomegaly.

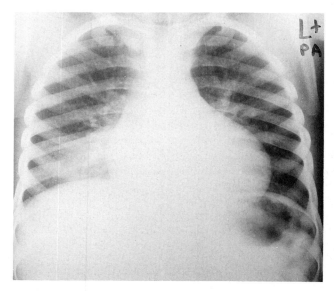

Fig. 1.3.42 Sickle cell disease. Consolidation in this condition may be due to infective pneumonia, pulmonary infarction or both. The heart shadow is enlarged.

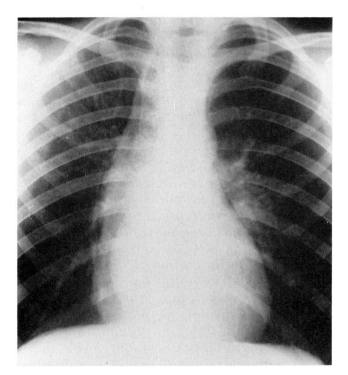

Fig. 1.3.43 Achalasia of the oesophagus.
The dilated oesophagus is seen running parallel to the right cardiac border.

MISCELLANEOUS MEDIASTINAL PATHOLOGY

Achalasia of the cardia is an important cause of repeated infection and although uncommon in the young, is well recorded. The dilatation of the oesophagus can be identified with air-fluid levels and enlargement of the mediastinal structures, particularly to the right. The gastric fundal air bubble may be insignificant, but in childhood is often present (Fig. 1.3.43). A rare manifestation of pancreatitis is extension of a pancreatic pseudocyst into the mediastinum, or even more rarely, into the pericardium. Although plain radiographs and ultrasound may adequately delineate such pancreatic pathology, CT is more definitive (Fig. 1.3.44).

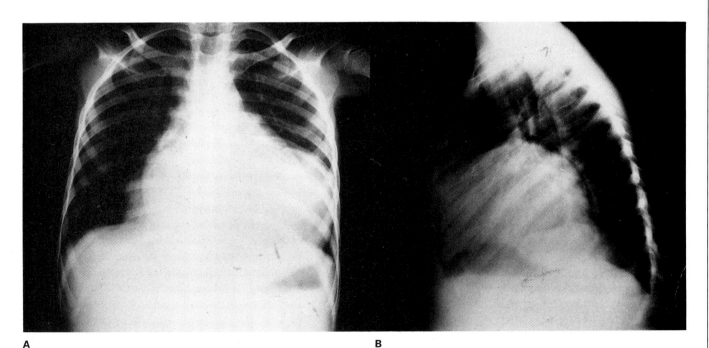

A   **B**

Fig. 1.3.44 There is an extensive retrocardiac mass which is a mediastinal extension of a pancreatic pseudocyst. **A**, AP view. **B**, Lateral view.

1.4   CYSTIC DISEASE OF THE LUNG

CYSTIC FIBROSIS OF THE PANCREAS (MUCOVISCIDOSIS)

Cystic fibrosis is inherited as an autosomal recessive disease with many organ systems affected; chronic suppurative lung disease and pancreatic insufficiency are the major features. There is some variation in the frequency of the disease. In European populations, the heterozygote carrier rate is about 1 in 25, but the disease is much less common in negroes. The gene locus has been determined on chromosome 7, allowing prenatal and definitive diagnosis, and possibly in years to come permitting gene therapy. However, recent earlier diagnosis and better treatment have led to a dramatic increase in life expectancy from death in early childhood to increasing survival to the fourth and fifth decades, although there is a high mortality still in teenage and early adult life.

The lungs appear normal at birth but abnormal mucociliary clearance soon leads to obstruction, particularly of the smaller bronchi. Infections predominantly with *Staphylococcus aureus*, pseudomonas, Escherichia and fungi quickly supervene. In infancy overinflation of the lungs or of individual segments due to mucous plugs in the bronchi leads to flattening of the diaphragm and bulging of the chest wall with sternal bowing and kyphosis. Accentuation of the bronchial wall pattern is shown as ring shadows or parallel line shadows and, although also seen in asthma and chronic bronchitis, in cystic fibrosis is usually more obvious and persistent becoming more prominent during exacerbations of infections (Fig. 1.4.1). Histologically, the bronchial wall is infiltrated by lymphocytes and plasma cells and the alveoli adjacent to the bronchi show collapse and epithelialization. There is cellular infiltration of the adjacent interalveolar septa. In 1962 Hodson and France correlating radiological and pathological findings found that small discrete opacities occurring either singly or in groups peripherally in the lung fields, seen first at about 4 years of age, resulted from peripheral abscesses, usually limited by interlobular septa and due to lobular consolidation with subsequent suppuration. The terminal bronchiole is often completely destroyed as a result and drainage from such abscesses is typically directly into the bronchus. Thin-walled air spaces persist following drainage of the mucopus.

The bronchiectasis may be of two types. Segmental bronchiectasis affects major pulmonary segments resulting in segmental collapse or consolidation and is similar to classical bronchiectasis, although the upper

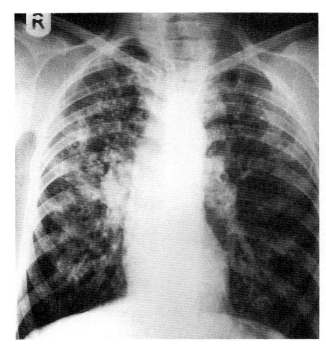

Fig. 1.4.1 Fibrocystic disease. Patchy and reticular shadowing throughout all zones with prominent hilar shadowing and generalized hyperinflation.

lobes may be involved more frequently than usual (Fig. 1.4.2). A more specific form of bronchiectasis arises from peribronchial abscesses which lie close to the medium-sized bronchi and give rise to a characteristic 'blob bronchiectasis' with widespread, irregular distribution throughout the lung fields. Enlargement of the hilar shadows is another feature. This is frequently due to hilar lymph node enlargement associated with acute infective exacerbations (Fig. 1.4.3) and will often dramatically decrease with adequate treatment of the precipitating infection. The hilar shadows may also be enlarged when pulmonary hypertension supervenes. This is usually irreversible and is associated with a poor prognosis. The heart shadow is usually rather narrow associated with the typical general overinflation of the lung fields, but may show an increase in diameter as a sign of cor pulmonale and an ultimately poor prognosis. Bronchial obstruction may give rise to segmental collapse which may persist and not respond to physiotherapy. In such cases, the alveoli become lined by cuboidal epithelium and show thick interalveolar septa with mononuclear and plasma cell infiltration.

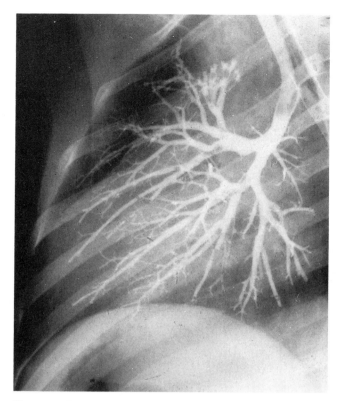

Fig. 1.4.2 Cystic fibrosis. Right upper lobe bronchiectasis.

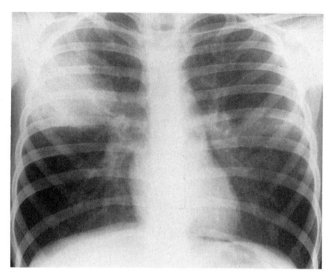

Fig. 1.4.3 Cystic fibrosis. Bacterial consolidation in right upper lobe and left mid zone.

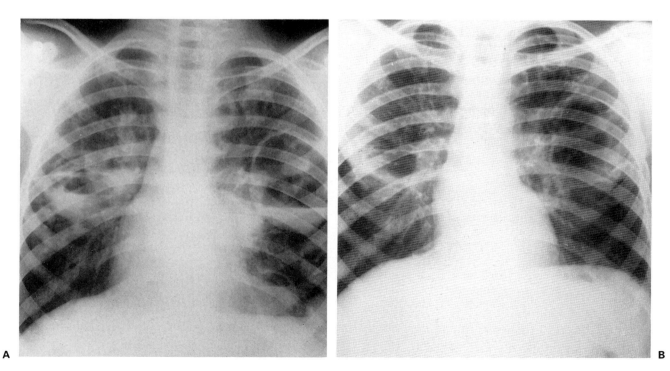

A

B

Fig. 1.4.4A, B Cystic fibrosis. Multiple large pneumatocoeles secondary to acute bacterial infection.

Occasionally thin-walled air-containing cavities may be seen in areas where there has been acute consolidation, often due to staphylococcus, representing lobular abscesses which have drained. Such large pneumatocoeles are typically seen in lungs relatively previously spared as gross widespread involvement with fibrosis and scarring will usually inhibit the development of larger thin-walled cysts (Fig. 1.4.4). Pneumothorax is a well-recognized complication and can lead to an acute deterioration in already compromised lungs (Figs 1.4.5, 1.4.6).

Coexistent bronchopulmonary aspergillosis is an important complication with often large areas of consolidation which may rapidly appear and clear. Extensive parenchymal destruction is a serious result in some cases (Fig. 1.4.7).

The paranasal air sinuses are virtually always opaque and clear sinuses is a reasonably certain exclusive sign of mucoviscidosis. Nasal polyposis leads to expansion of the nasal cavity (Fig. 1.4.8).

Electrocoagulation with alternating current and a bipolar electrode has been used in addition to embolization in the management of severe bronchial artery haemorrhage arising from bronchial suppuration and inflammation.

Radiographic scoring methods in cystic fibrosis

Several scoring methods for evaluating chest radiographs in mucoviscidosis have been devised. Such features as bronchial line shadows, mottled and ring shadows, larger shadows, air trapping, etc., form the basis of these methods, none of which shows a statistical superiority above the others. Standard errors of measurement are large and all methods suffer from the criticism that by the time radiographic features are well established major damage to the lungs has already occurred and the scoring methods are in fact evaluating the radiographic appearances of complications which may not necessarily correlate with the true parenchymal involvement.

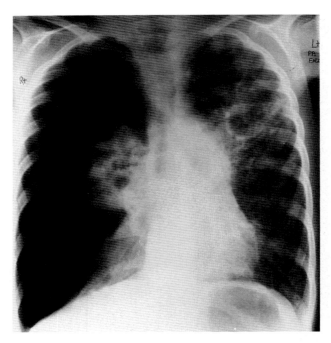

Fig. 1.4.5 Cystic fibrosis (mucoviscidosis). Advanced parenchymal changes complicated by right pneumothorax.

REFERENCES

Brunelle F, Ford F, Beacher D, Clairmont P 1985 Successful electrocoagulation of an internal mammary artery in a child. Pediatric Radiology 15: 251–252

Hodson C J, France N E 1962 Pulmonary changes in cystic fibrosis of the pancreas. Clinical Radiology 13: 54–61

Holsclaw D S, Grand R J, Shwachman H 1970 Massive hemoptysis in cystic fibrosis. Journal of Pediatrics 76: 829–838

Lloyd-Still J D, Khaw K T, Shwachman H 1974 Severe respiratory disease in infants with cystic fibrosis. Pediatrics 53: 678–682

Nathanson I, Riddlesberger M M 1980 Pulmonary hypertrophic osteoarthropathy in cystic fibrosis. Radiology 135: 649–651

Reinig J W, Sanchez F W, Thomason D M, Gobien R T 1985 The distinctly visible right upper lobe bronchus on the lateral chest: a clue to adolescent cystic fibrosis. Pediatric Radiology 15: 22–224

Te Meerman G J, Dankert-Ruelse J, Martijn A, van Woerden H H 1985 A comparison of the Shwachman, Crispen–Norman and Brassfield methods for scoring the chest radiographs of patients with cystic fibrosis. Pediatric Radiology 15: 98–101

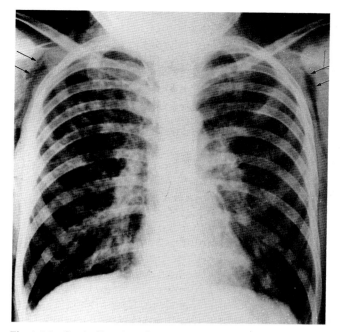

Fig. 1.4.6 Cystic fibrosis with pneumomediastinum and subcutaneous emphysema (arrows).

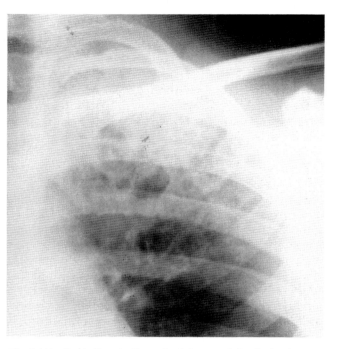

Fig. 1.4.7 Cystic fibrosis. Extensive left upper lobe shadowing from aspergillus.

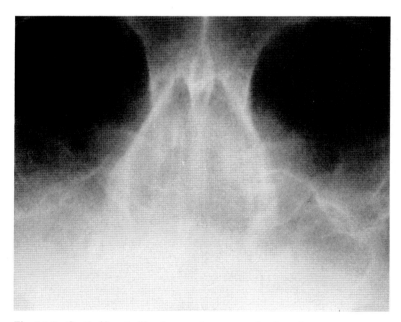

Fig. 1.4.8 Cystic fibrosis. Nasal expansion, mucosal polyposis.

BRONCHIECTASIS

Chronic dilatation of the bronchial tree is now much less common with reduction in pulmonary sepsis, particularly as a result of a lower incidence of tuberculosis, prophylactic measures against measles and whooping cough, and with better antibiotic treatment and physiotherapy for acute pneumonias. However, diseases such as cystic fibrosis, acute infections, particularly viral, endoluminal bronchial obstruction, ciliary dyskinesia and immune compromise remain as predisposing causes.

Although most bronchiectasis is acquired, congenital forms are seen rarely, especially in relation to pulmonary sequestrations and other maldevelopments of the bronchial tree.

A pathological classification has been made into cylindrical bronchiectasis with smooth dilatation of the affected parts of the bronchial tree, varicose where variable degrees of luminal irregularity are superimposed on a generally cylindrical dilatation, and thirdly saccular bronchiectasis with which is associated more severe purulent expectoration.

Early cylindrical bronchiectasis may show minimal radiographic signs. As the disease progresses crowding of the bronchi, accentuation of the peribronchial tissues giving roughly parallel lines, and varying degrees of lobar loss of volume, particularly in the lung bases, will be accompanied by compensatory emphysema in the upper zones with distortion downwards of the main pulmonary vasculature emanating from the hilar regions. Advanced bronchiectasis with saccular changes will show ring shadows within which air-fluid levels may be seen, with visualization of secretion or pus-filled bronchi as opaque tubular structures.

Postinfective bronchiectasis has an essentially basal distribution (Fig. 1.4.9). Localized upper lobe bronchiectasis is highly suggestive of mucoviscidosis in particular or some immune or ciliary dysfunction which need to be excluded as predisposing causes in any unusual or very extensive case of bronchiectasis.

Surgical resection of bronchiectatic segments is considerably less commonly practised than in the past. This is a consequence of better medical management, more effective antibiotics and in particular good physiotherapy and the realization that localized areas of bronchiectatic change typically in the lower lung fields are often multilobar and more extensive, albeit often mildly so, than previously appreciated. Surgical excision, however, is useful for severely affected areas of the lung, particularly for symptomatic relief, and may be curative for local areas of bronchiectasis following, for instance, endobronchial occlusion or where the rest of the lungs can be shown to be virtually normal.

Plain radiographs are an insensitive indicator of mild bronchiectasis. Ventilation/perfusion scans are a relatively non-invasive and effective screening technique for bronchiectasis. A normal scan virtually precludes any form of bronchiectasis for which surgery would be deemed currently appropriate.

Thin slice high resolution CT can demonstrate bronchiectasis well, will define sacalar changes, show associated lobar or segmental collapse and will in practice replace positive contrast medium bronchography. The normal bronchus is not larger than its associated accompanying vessel and bronchiectasis and dilatation of the bronchi leads to the 'signet ring' sign.

Bronchography remains a method of delineating the bronchial tree, particularly in the evaluation of bronchiectasis before surgery to reassure normality in presumed unaffected parts of the lung. It is also an important technique in the evaluation of localized bronchostenosis and bronchomalacia, particularly in the major divisions beyond the carina where fluoroscopic and high kilovoltage examination of the airways is less efficient.

REFERENCES

Gamsu G, Klein J S 1989 High resolution computed tomography of diffuse lung disease. Clinical Radiology 40: 554–556

Muller N L, Bergin C J, Ostrow D H, Nichols D M 1984 Role of computed tomography in recognition of bronchiectasis. American Journal of Roentgenology 143: 971–976

Reid L 1950 Reduction of bronchial subdivision in bronchiectasis. Thorax 5: 233–237

Swensen S J, Aughenbaugh G L, Douglas W W, Myers J L 1992 High-resolution CT of the lungs: findings in various pulmonary diseases. American Journal of Roentgenology 158: 971–979

Trapnell D H, Gregg I 1969 Some principles of interpretations of bronchograms. British Journal of Radiology 42: 125–131

Vandevivere J, Spehl M, Dab J, Baran D, Piepsz A 1980 Bronchiectasis in childhood. Comparison of chest roentgenograms, bronchography and lung scintigraphy. Pediatric Radiology 9: 193–198

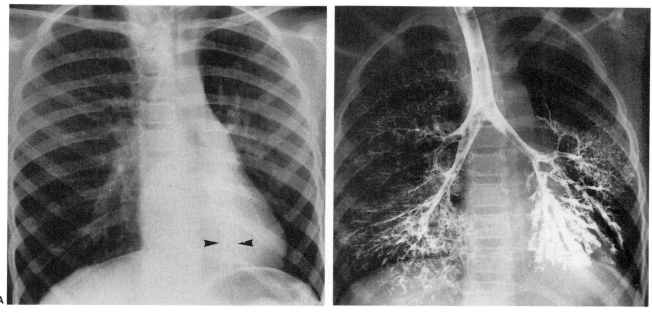

Fig. 1.4.9 Postinfective bronchiectasis. **A** Plain radiograph. **B** Bronchogram.

YELLOW NAIL SYNDROME

Bronchiectasis, hypoplasia of the lymphatic system and recurrent pleural effusions and chylothorax are associated in the yellow nail syndrome, the onset of which is usually in adult life but rarely described in childhood.

PROTEUS SYNDROME

Lung cysts have been described as a feature of the Proteus syndrome, a constellation of abnormalities with partial gigantism of extremities, hemihypertrophy, subcutaneous tumours, and macrocephaly as part of a wide spectrum of mesodermal malformations.

REFERENCE

Azouz E M, Costa T, Fitch N 1987 Radiologic findings in the Proteus syndrome. Pediatric Radiology 17: 481–485

ASTHMA

Recurrent episodes of wheezing or dyspnoea with a significant increase in resistance to air flow defines asthma which may be extrinsic, intrinsic, mixed or exercise induced. In childhood the type most commonly seen is extrinsic representing a Type I immediate hypersensitivity to various allergens such as pollens, housedust, animal dander, drugs (particularly aspirin) and foodstuffs.

The chest radiograph in asthma can be normal but the typical radiographic feature is generalized overinflation of the lungs leading to a low, flat diaphragm which, when longstanding, will lead to widening of the thoracic cage and intercostal spaces with accentuation of the muscle attachments of the diaphragm to the ribs. The AP diameter of the chest is typically increased accompanied by sternal bowing and a consequent increase in the radiolucency of the retrosternal space. Peribronchial thickening due to eosinophilic infiltration leads to ring shadows and parallel line shadows ('tramlines or rail-roads') in the perihilar regions in particular, but not extending as far peripherally as may be seen, for instance, in mucoviscidosis. Mucous plugs cause variable degrees of collapse and in particular the middle lobe is frequently involved.

Pneumomediastinum (Fig. 1.4.10) is a well-recognized complication of asthma in childhood, often with subcutaneous emphysema in the neck and occasionally associated with pneumothorax. Extensive mucous impaction in the bronchial tree shown as branching shadows (the 'gloved hand' appearance) may be rarely seen in uncomplicated asthma. It is, however, more commonly found in association with allergic bronchopulmonary aspergillosis which is relatively uncommon in childhood (Fig. 1.4.11).

The frequency of radiographs in the management of asthma in childhood has been the subject of considerable debate. It is important not to overlook persistent lobar collapse and a normal radiograph between acute attacks is reassuring. Unnecessary radiographs in the acute phase should be avoided. Overinflation in particular, if localized, or any focal lesion should be followed to its resolution.

PULMONARY EOSINOPHILIA

Eosinophilia in the blood is seen in many patients with asthma and this may be associated with areas of pulmonary consolidation, usually transitory, with poorly defined homogeneous peripheral opacities. Characteristically these shadows flit from one part of the lung field to another and they last from several days to months. Although such infiltrations may be seen with helminthic infestation, filariasis and drug reactions, allergic aspergillosis is the common cause. Precipitins to *Aspergillus fumigatus* are usually found with both Type I and Type III skin responses. The IgE levels are elevated in the blood.

Repeated inflammatory changes in the bronchi can lead to permanent fibrosis with bronchiectasis particularly occurring in the upper and middle parts of the lungs. Peribronchial thickening with parallel line and ring shadows are seen and mucoid impaction can give rise to branching shadows in the lung fields like fingers of a glove. Bronchography, although rarely indicated, shows a characteristic proximal bronchial dilatation with a more normal peripheral bronchial tree. Longstanding bronchopulmonary aspergillosis leads to extensive upper lobe honeycomb shadowing which may be confused with tuberculosis.

MYCETOMA

The formation of intracavitatory fungus balls in childhood is uncommon but immune-compromised patients and those undergoing chemotherapy are candidates for this complication which is typically seen in the upper lobes. Adjacent pleural thickening and a periosteal reaction along adjacent ribs are other radiological features.

In childhood a more common finding is invasive aspergillosis, again particularly in the debilitated or immune-compromised child. This is usually part of a widespread colonization of multiple organs. Initial radiographic findings in the lung may be insignificant, but with progression usually bilateral infiltrations with confluent rounded densities develop. Areas of low parenchymal density ringing areas of pulmonary consolidation are a characteristic late radiographic finding in invasive aspergillosis which are not related to air in cavities but are probably a thrombotic or infarctive lesion.

REFERENCES

Brooks I J, Cloutier M M, Afshani E 1982 Significance of roentgenographic abnormalities in children hospitalized for asthma. Chest 82: 315–318
Hodson C J, Trickey S E 1960 Bronchial wall thickening in asthma. Clinical Radiology 11: 183–191

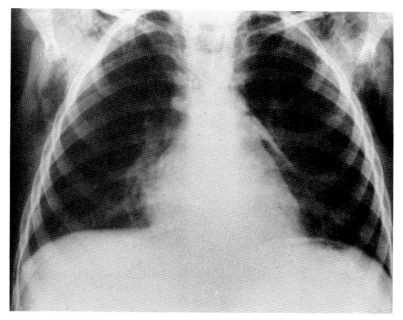

Fig. 1.4.10 Asthma with pneumomediastinum and subcutaneous emphysema in the neck.

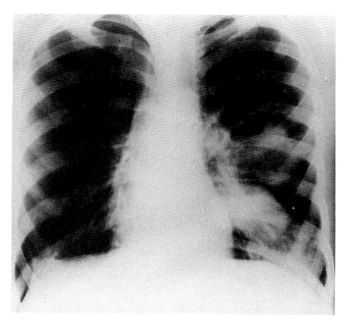

Fig. 1.4.11 Asthma. Widespread shadowing from allergic bronchopulmonary aspergillosis.

1.5   CONGENITAL ABNORMALITIES (LATER PRESENTATION)

PULMONARY SEQUESTRATIONS

These are usually divided into two broad groups, extralobar and intralobar sequestrations.

Extralobar sequestrations are less common and can be considered as a form of accessory lung arising from abnormal differentiation of an additional lung bud. The characteristic abnormal bronchial development and usually absent connection with the normal bronchial tree, common features of sequestration, are typically associated with a lesion showing separate pleural covering with a very high left-sided preponderance situated posteriorly in a supradiaphragmatic position and sometimes associated with diaphragmatic hernia or eventration. Usually the arterial supply is from the systemic circulation (but not exclusively so) whilst venous drainage is usually into the systemic azygous systems but occasionally into pulmonary venous channels. Clinically, there is a high male preponderance. The lesions are frequently found in infancy and may be discovered incidentally at autopsy in children with other severe developmental abnormalities.

Intralobar sequestrations are of more clinical importance. By contrast with the extralobar type, the lesion is contained within the pleura of the affected lung. There is a high incidence in the posterior lung bases with a left-sided preponderance but less marked than with the extralobar type. Typically, the arterial supply is from the systemic circulation, often from the aorta and via large vessels, while venous drainage is usually into the pulmonary veins.

Clinical presentation is commonly with recurrent attacks of pneumonia in a posterior basal segment of the lung and the diagnosis is usually established in later childhood. Some authors have suggested that intralobar sequestrations are acquired lesions with secondary enlargement of systemic arteries supplying an area in which chronic or recurrent infection occurs. However, intralobar sequestrations can occur in the very young baby and can be associated with contralateral sequestrations, extralobar sequestrations and with an increased incidence of other congenital malformations, and an as yet undetermined proportion of sequestrations are highly likely to be congenital in origin.

The plain radiographic findings of intralobar sequestrations are initially recurrent areas of pneumonia usually in the posterior basal regions of the lung fields, although intralobar sequestrations have been recorded in the upper lobes. Initial infections may be transient with clearing of the parenchymal shadowing but progressive change leads to cavitation with air-fluid levels and persisting shadows. Occasionally a sequestration may present as an opacity without gas within it which is believed to pass there by collateral air drift. A parenchymal opacity is a common presentation of the extralobar type of sequestration. Although not usually indicated, bronchography will confirm the isolation of the bronchial tree of the sequestration with normal bronchi being draped around the affected segment. Occasionally contrast medium can enter a sequestration through, it is believed, fistulous connections, probably resulting from the infections to which the lesions are predisposed (Fig. 1.5.1).

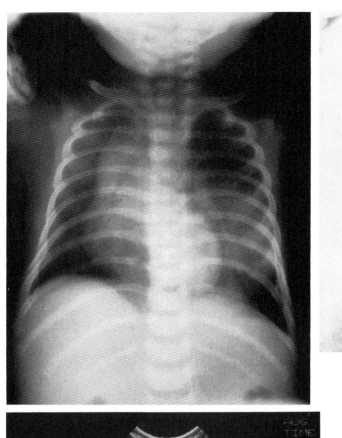

A

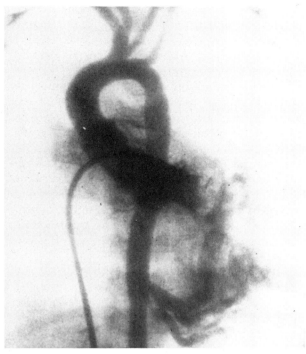

C

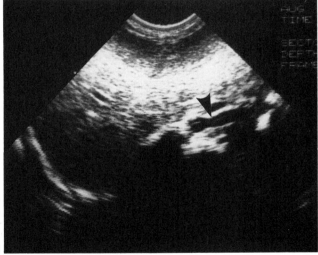

B

Fig. 1.5.1 Intrapulmonary sequestration. **A** Plain radiograph showing left lower zone opacity. **B** Ultrasound showing large feeding vessel (arrowed). **C** Aortogram showing large feeding vessels.

Arteriography, by digital vascular imaging preferably, delineates the arterial supply. The systemic arteries supplying the lesion are often large and can lead to significant shunting. Although the vessels usually arise from the thoracic aorta, blood supply is often from the abdominal aorta or from some of its major branches (Fig. 1.5.2). Although, practically, delineation of the arterial supply is of more consequence to the surgeon, evaluation of the venous drainage into the pulmonary veins will typically confirm an intralobar sequestration and into the azygous system an extralobar sequestration. Contrast medium enhanced CT scans may show anomalous arterial supply to the usually clearly defined lung parenchymal abnormality. Ultrasound, particularly with Doppler techniques, can identify the feeding systemic artery and establish the diagnosis noninvasively.

Ventilation/perfusion scans will show an area of absent perfusion and of absent ventilation, although slow gas exchange by collateral gas drift can be demonstrated by radionuclide ventilation scans. This technique is useful particularly in the early evaluation of an intralobar sequestration where, in particular, there has been recurrent pneumonia in the basal regions with intermittent good radiographic resolution.

Bronchopulmonary sequestration, spontaneous haemothorax

Haemothorax is a very rare complication of bronchopulmonary sequestration. Multiple aneurysms in the supplying artery have been described with a localized fibrinoid necrosis and aneurysm formation similar to the postcardiomyotomy syndrome.

REFERENCES

Clements B J, Warner J O 1987 Pulmonary sequestration and related congenital broncho-pulmonary-vascular malformations Thorax 42: 404–408

Clements B J, Warner J O, Shinebourne E A 1987 Congenital bronchopulmonary vascular malformations. Thorax 42: 409–416

Felker R E, Tonkin I L D 1990 Imaging of pulmonary sequestration. American Journal of Roentgenology 154: 241–249.

Holden P D, Langston C 1986 Intralobar pulmonary sequestration (a nonentity?) Pediatric Pulmonology 2: 147–153.

Ikegoe J, Murayama S, Godwin J D, Done S L, Verschahelm J A 1990 Bronchopulmonary sequestration. CT assessment. Radiology 176: 375–379

Kaude J V, Laurin S 1984 Ultrasonographic demonstration of systemic artery feeding extrapulmonary sequestration. Pediatric Radiology 14: 226–227

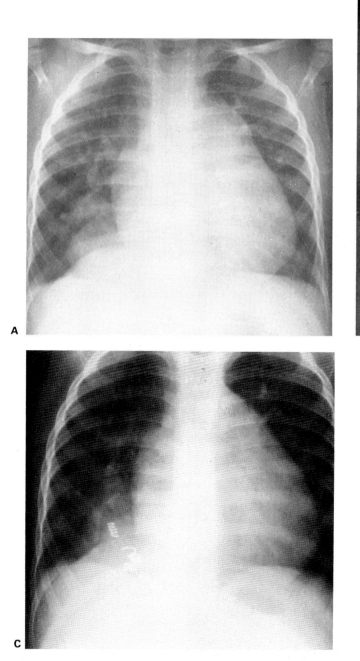

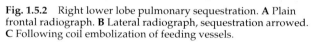

Fig. 1.5.2 Right lower lobe pulmonary sequestration. **A** Plain frontal radiograph. **B** Lateral radiograph, sequestration arrowed. **C** Following coil embolization of feeding vessels.

BRONCHIAL ATRESIA

This is a rare congenital abnormality particularly affecting a single bronchus. The upper lobes are more fequently involved, particularly the left upper lobe. The lung distal to the atretic bronchus is characteristically overdistended by collateral air drift. The bronchus distal to the atresia may fill with mucus and present as an ovoid opacity, sometimes containing an air-fluid level. Bronchography reveals absence of filling of the associated bronchus and some compression of the remaining lung by the overdistended affected segment or lobe. Initial presentation is usually in childhood or early adulthood, most commonly due to pneumonia in the affected lung (Fig. 1.5.3).

REFERENCES

Oh K S, Dorst J P, White J J, Haller J A Jr, Johnson B A, Byrne W D 1976 Syndrome of bronchial atresia or stenosis with mucocele and focal hyperinflation of the lung. Johns Hopkins Medical Journal 138: 48–53

Schuster S R, Harris G B C, Williams A, Kirkpatrick J, Reid L 1978 Bronchial atresia: a recognizable entity in the pediatric age group. Journal of Pediatric Surgery 13: 682–689

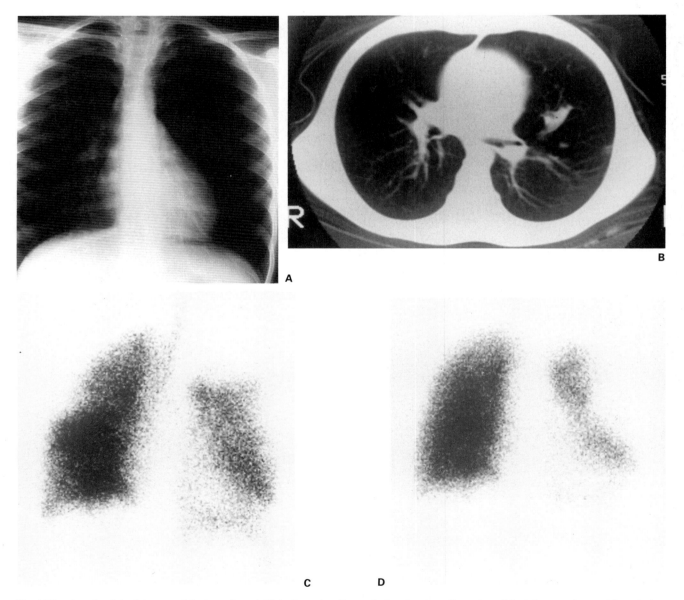

Fig. 1.5.3 Atresia of the left upper lobe bronchus. **A** Plain frontal radiograph showing overdistension of the left upper lung with central opacity. **B** CT showing mucocoele peripheral to the atretic bronchus. **C** The ventilation scan with radioactive krypton technetium perfusion; scan **D** showing decreased perfusion and ventilation in the left lung.

TRACHEAL BRONCHUS

Although a normal feature in many domesticated animals, this is a relatively rare variant in which the apical segment right upper lobe bronchus enters the trachea directly (Fig. 1.5.4).

REFERENCES

Iannaccone G, Capocaccia P, Colloridi V, Roggini M 1983 Double right tracheal bronchus. Pediatric Radiology 13: 156–158
Siegel M J, Shackelford G D, Francis R J, McAlister W H 1979 Tracheal bronchus. Radiology 130: 353–355

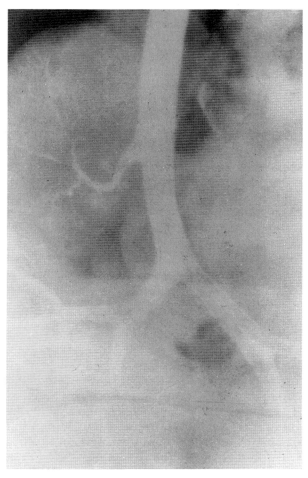

Fig. 1.5.4 Post-mortem bronchogram showing right tracheal bronchus.

PULMONARY ARTERIOVENOUS MALFORMATION

Arteriovenous malformations allow the passage of unsaturated blood directly into the pulmonary venous system and into the systemic circulation, bypassing the pulmonary capillary bed. This shunting may lead to cyanosis, decrease of exercise tolerance, shortness of breath, finger clubbing and polycythaemia. It can also cause paradoxical embolism. However, many cases are asymptomatic and may be discovered as abnormalities on routine chest radiographs, particularly in early adult life. Clinical presentation in the very young is rare.

About half the lesions are solitary but a more prominent single lesion may be associated with scattered arteriovenous malformations throughout the lungs or there may be more diffusely distributed lesions. Many patients suffer from hereditary haemorrhagic telangiectasia (Osler–Rendu–Weber syndrome), a dominant trait with widespread angiodysplasias.

The larger lesions show a peripheral, often poorly defined radiopacity in which the associated enlarged vessels may be seen coursing serpiginously towards the hilum of the lung. In the presence of a large shunt, secondary signs of high output failure and cardiac enlargement can be seen. Shunting can be evaluated using radiolabelled albumin microspheres.

The lesions can be demonstrated on CT and MRI, but pulmonary angiography especially using digital vascular techniques is the best method of delineation with which can be combined embolization with coils or balloons for the larger lesions. Should surgical excision be considered, careful examination of both lungs should be undertaken to assess the incidence and size of any other associated arteriovenous malformations (Fig. 1.5.5).

The Hughes–Stovin syndrome is the rare association of multiple pulmonary aneurysms and peripheral venous thromboses. Pulmonary varix, a local venous dilatation, is a rare cause of an intrapulmonary mass.

REFERENCES

Higgins C B, Wexler L 1976 Clinical and angiographic features of pulmonary arteriovenous fistulas in children. Radiology 119: 171–175
Taylor G A 1983 Pulmonary arteriovenous malformation: an uncommon cause for cyanosis in the newborn. Pediatric Radiology 13: 339–341

LATE PRESENTATION OF DIAPHRAGMATIC HERNIA

Small congenital diaphragmatic deficiencies and those associated with infantile pneumonias, often streptococcal, may present in later childhood. Because of the often small diaphragmatic deficit, herniated loops of bowel may strangulate and clinical presentation is of a pleural effusion. The presence of an air-fluid level in the strangulated bowel can mimic an intrathoracic abscess. Obstruction of the bowel, particularly associated with markedly compromised herniated bowel, can mimic the paralytic ileus of pneumonia and compound the clinical confusion.

REFERENCES

McCue J, Ball A, Brereton R J, Wright V M, Shaw D G 1985 Congenital diaphragmatic hernia in older children. Journal of the Royal College of Surgeons of Edinburgh 30: 305–310
Newman B M, Afshani E, Karp M P, Jewett T C, Cooney D R 1986 Presentation of congenital diaphragmatic hernia past the neonatal period. Archives of Surgery 121: 813–816

α-I ANTITRYPSIN DEFICIENCY

The chronic obstructive airways and emphysema associated with this is rarely seen in childhood but the diagnosis should be considered in a child who has cough and wheezing with a chest radiograph showing hyperinflation.

REFERENCE

Talamo R C, Levison H, Lynch M J, Hercz A, Hyslop N E Jr, Bain H W 1971 Symptomatic pulmonary emphysema in childhood associated with hereditary α-1 antitrypsin, antitrypsin and elastase inhibitor deficiency. Journal of Pediatrics 79: 20–26

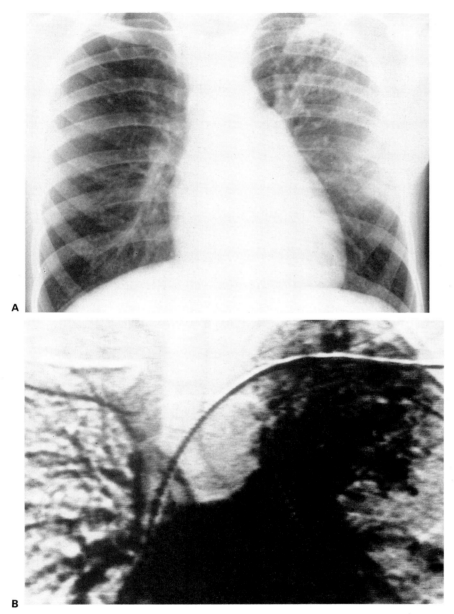

Fig. 1.5.5 Pulmonary arteriovenous malformation. Linear branching shadow in the left upper lobe (**A**) with digital arteriogram showing the arteriovenous malformation (**B**).

MARFAN'S SYNDROME

Although musculoskeletal manifestations with arachnodactyly and joint laxity, cardiovascular disease with valvular abnormalities and aortic aneurysm and ectopia lentis and myopia are the most characteristic features of this disease, pulmonary disorders are an important but less common feature. The connective tissue disorder with abnormal collagen formation is reflected in an increased incidence of spontaneous pneumothorax, pulmonary emphysema, pulmonary cystic disease and an increased susceptibility to lower respiratory tract infections.

Similar connective tissue diseases such as Ehlers–Danlos syndrome, pseudoxanthoma elasticum, cutis laxa and Beal's congenital contractual arachnodactyly are conditions which should be considered with Marfan's syndrome in the differential diagnosis of unusual emphysematous change and spontaneous pneumothorax. Artificial and assisted ventilation in these conditions can be associated with an exaggerated barotraumatic response.

REFERENCES

Day D L, Burke B A 1986 Pulmonary emphysema in a neonate with Marfan syndrome. Paediatric Radiology 16: 518–521
Travis R C, Shaw D G 1985 Congenital contractural arachnodactyly. British Journal of Radiology 58: 1115–1117

SARCOIDOSIS

As in adults, pulmonary involvement with this systemic granulomatous disease is an important manifestation. The incidence in childhood has probably been underestimated. Asymptomatic expression with hilar lymphadenopathy, sometimes with parenchymal lung lesions, has been discovered in countries such as Hungary and Japan where mass chest radiographic screening has been carried out. The disease appears to be more common in the negro population. In childhood, the symptoms are of cough, wheezing, variable dyspnoea and sometimes pleuritic pain. In the very young child, in whom sarcoid is much rarer, abnormalities on the chest radiograph are often absent, with preponderant clinical features of rash, uveitis and arthritis.

There are differences between radiological features of pulmonary sarcoidosis in the child and those seen in later life. At the time of diagnosis thoracic lymphadenopathy is seen in virtually all children while absent in about one-sixth of adults. Bilateral paratracheal lymph node enlargement is very much more common in childhood than in the adult. Enlargement of subcarinal, anterior and posterior mediastinal lymph nodes is also more frequently seen in childhood. Involvement of the lung parenchyma in childhood has an incidence similar to that in adults (Figs 1.6.1–1.6.3).

The common radiographic features are small reticulonodular shadows scattered throughout both lung fields. This may uncommonly be associated with some streaky shadowing and softer peripheral lung opacities. Pleural granulomas can lead to spontaneous pneumothorax and mediastinal emphysema. Pleural effusions are an uncommon association. Pulmonary involvement with sarcoid as in adults can be asymptomatic and discovered incidentally. Generally in childhood the disease appears benign with eventual resolution. However, fibrosis and emphysematous changes with bullae and secondary pulmonary hypertension together with uveitis and nephrocalcinosis are important complications of the disease in childhood.

Although the diagnosis can be indicated by the Kveim test, serum levels of angiotension-converting enzyme and immunological responses, in practice, it is often one of exclusion. Transbronchial or open lung biopsy or lymph node excision allow a more definitive histological diagnosis.

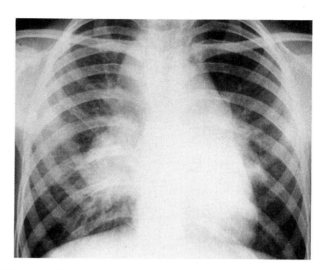

Fig. 1.6.1 Sarcoid. Bilateral hilar and paratracheal lymphadenopathy.

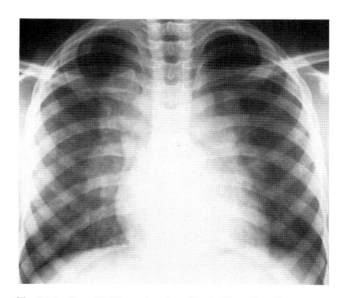

Fig. 1.6.2 Sarcoid. Bilateral and mediastinal lymph node enlargement. Diffuse parenchymal nodular shadowing.

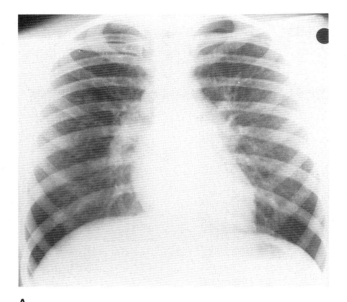

A

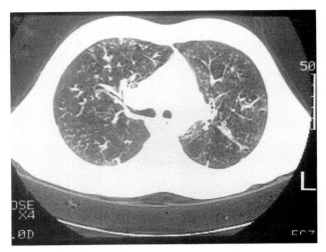

B

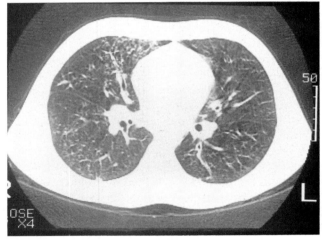

C

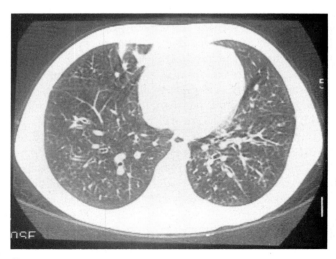

D

Fig. 1.6.3 Sarcoid. Chest radiograph (**A**) and high resolution CT scans (**B–D**).

REFERENCES

Harris R O, Spock A 1978 Childhood sarcoidosis: pulmonary infiltrates as an early sign in a very young child. Clinical Pediatrics 17: 119–121

Hetherington S 1982 Sarcoidosis in young children. American Journal of Diseases of Children 136: 13–15

Kirks D R, McCormick V D, Greenspan R H 1973 Pulmonary sarcoidosis: roentgenologic analysis of 150 patients. American Journal of Roentgenology 177: 777–786

Merten D F, Kirks D R, Grossman H 1980 Pulmonary sarcoidosis in childhood. American Journal of Roentgenology 135: 673–679

Toomey F , Bautista A 1970 Rare manifestations of sarcoidosis in children. Radiology 94: 569–573

HISTIOCYTOSIS X (LANGERHANS' CELL HISTIOCYTOSIS)

This frequently generalized disease is also known as Letterer–Siwe disease, Hand–Schüller–Christian disease and eosinophilic granuloma. Lung disease may be seen as part of systemic involvement or as a primary condition, in which case there is high preponderance in young male adults. In childhood it seems some quarter of the patients will have lung involvement again with a high male preponderance. Histiocytic involvement of the lung gives rise to a reticular or reticulonodular pattern with areas of peribronchial thickening. Pleural reactions are uncommon. Hilar and mediastinal adenopathy are variable in incidence. Pneumothorax can be an early complication and may indeed be a presentation (Fig. 1.6.4). With evolution of the disease a coarse honeycombing may develop, as may multiple pulmonary cysts, which are believed to be due to necrotic areas at the site of histiocytic infiltration or where there has been previous bronchial infiltration and consequent obstruction. These changes are accompanied by fibrosis which can contribute to retraction of lung tissue and the cyst formation. The cystic areas in the lung parenchyma may communicate with the bronchial tree directly (Fig. 1.6.5).

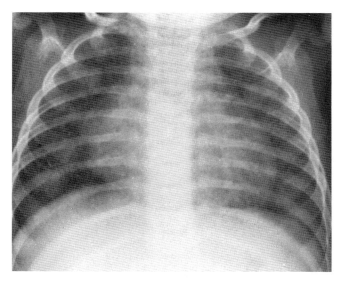

Fig. 1.6.4 Histiocytosis X (Langerhans' cell histiocytosis). Diffuse reticular nodular shadowing.

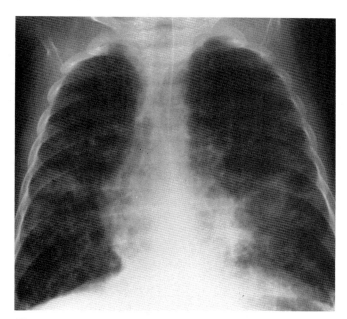

Fig. 1.6.5 Later evolution of histiocytosis with honeycomb formation.

103

In young children anterior mediastinal masses have been infrequently reported. During resolution these anterior mediastinal masses which may be partly due to thymic infiltration can undergo cavitation with marked cyst formation. This cavitation has been suggested as being due either to necrosis within histiocytic masses or to fibrosis and adhesion to adjacent lung and pleural tissue with communication from the peripheral lung tissue into the mediastinal cysts (Fig. 1.6.6).

The plain radiographic manifestations of lung histiocytosis may be absent or extremely subtle, and in such cases lung function tests show deficient diffusion capacity and restrictive lung volumes. Similarly, ^{67}Ga-citrate may show an enhanced uptake in the lungs of patients with early clinical symptoms but equivocal or normal chest radiographs. Involvement of the thoracic skeleton may be incidentally observed.

REFERENCES

Abramson S J, Berdon W E , Reilly B J , Kuhn J P 1987 Cavitation of anterior mediastinal masses in children with histiocytosis X. Pediatric Radiology 17: 10–14
Basset F , Corrin B , Spenser H 1978 Pulmonary histiocytosis X. American Review of Respiratory Disease 118: 811
Carlson R A , Hattery R H , O'Connell E J , Fontana R S 1976 Pulmonary involvement by histiocytosis X in the pediatric age group. Mayo Clinic Proceedings 51: 542–547

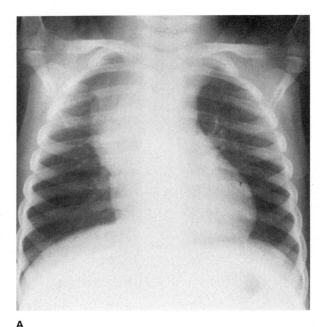

A

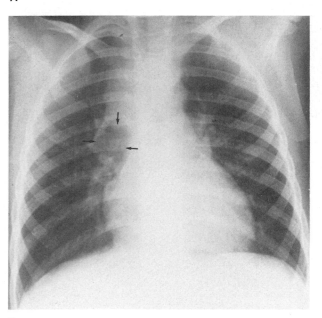

B

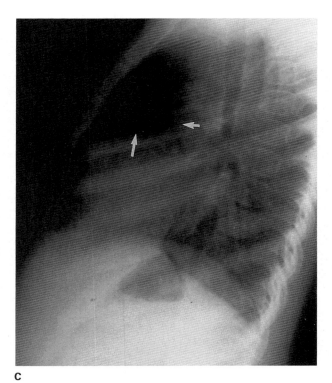

C

Fig. 1.6.6 Histiocytosis. Anterior mediastinal mass (**A**), frontal (**B**) and lateral (**C**) views showing gas containing a cyst (arrows) at the site of the previous mass.

IDIOPATHIC INTERSTITIAL PNEUMONIA

Clinically this group of conditions is associated with respiratory distress and hypoxaemia, often more marked than the plain chest radiograph would indicate, variably progressive yet sometimes quickly with a fatal outcome. The hypoxaemia is associated with clubbing of the fingers.

The characteristic radiograph (Figs 1.6.7–1.6.10) shows fine bilateral infiltrates radiating from the hilar regions, particularly towards the lung bases. Radiographic changes may be minimal in the presence of severe respiratory embarrassment. Progressive fibrosis leads to a honeycomb lung appearance.

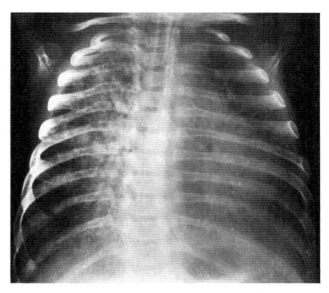

Fig. 1.6.7 Desquamative interstitial pneumonia. Fine reticulogranular shadowing throughout both lungs.

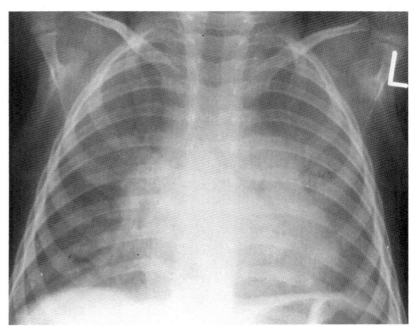

Fig. 1.6.8 Desquamatous interstitial pneumonitis. Widespread pulmonary opacification.

Histological classification into usual interstitial pneumonia, desquamatous interstitial pneumonia, lymphocytic interstitial pneumonia and giant cell interstitial pneumonia can be established following lung biopsy which may be performed by a percutaneous needle technique or, more satisfactorily and particularly with the good tolerance of thoracotomy in childhood, by open lung biopsy. CT in idiopathic pulmonary interstitial pneumonitis and fibrosis demonstrates that the subpleural opacities are more commonly seen in the inferior and posterior parts of the lung. The bullous changes are well demonstrated, particularly in the later stages of the development of the honeycomb lung. Spontaneous pneumothorax is uncommon, as are mediastinal lymphadenopathy and pleural effusion.

^{67}Ga-citrate uptake by the lungs reflects the alveolitis and is particularly useful in those cases where cough, dyspnoea and hypoxia are out of proportion to incipient and mild early radiographic changes. Pulmonary fibrosis has been recorded in some families with neurofibromatosis. Pulmonary infiltrates are seen in rheumatoid disease (Fig. 1.6.11).

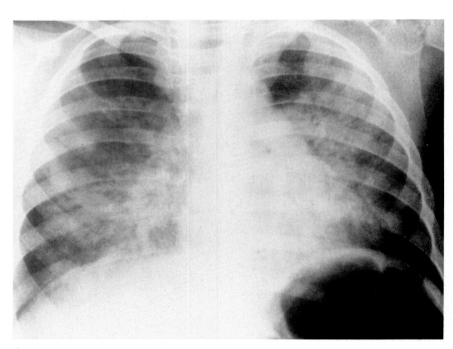

Fig. 1.6.9 Interstitial pneumonitis.

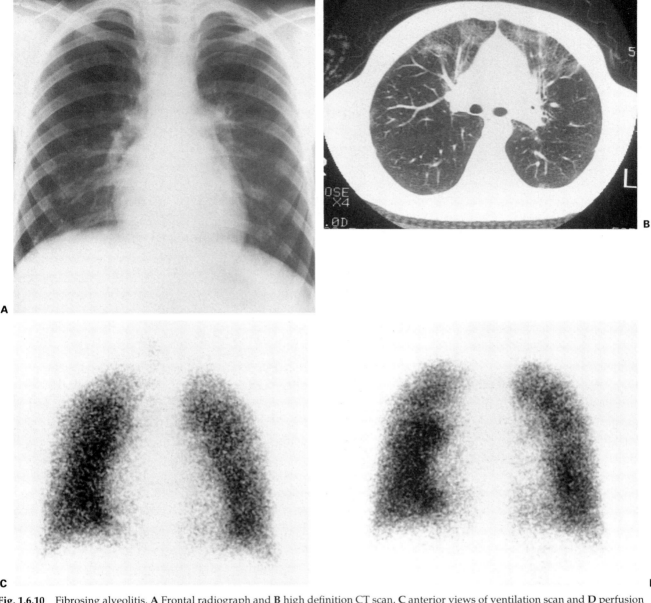

Fig. 1.6.10 Fibrosing alveolitis. **A** Frontal radiograph and **B** high definition CT scan, **C** anterior views of ventilation scan and **D** perfusion scan showing some mild irregularity of perfusion in the upper zones and demonstrating the usefulness of high resolution computed lung tomography.

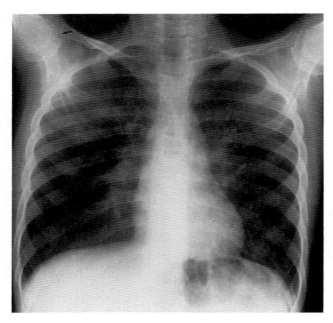

Fig. 1.6.11 Rheumatoid disease. Pulmonary infiltration with periarticular erosions (arrow).

^{99}Tc^{m}-DTPA aerosol lung clearance in interstitial pneumonias

Accelerated clearance of ^{99m}Tc-DTPA aerosol from the lungs is a simple rapid sensitive method for the investigation of interstitial pneumonia and the changes of chronic graft-versus-host disease and can indicate pathology before the chest radiograph becomes abnormal. Response to therapy for interstitial pneumonia can also be assessed and followed by serial studies.

REFERENCES

Hewitt C J, Hull D, Keeling J W 1977 Fibrosing alveolitis in infancy and childhood. Archives of Disease in Childhood 52: 22–37
Nezelof C, Brieu A, Beal G, Meyer B, Paupe J, Vialatte J 1974 Familial pulmonary fibrosis; two cases. Annales de Pediatrie 21: 135–144
Webb W R, Goodman P C 1977 Fibrosing alveolitis in patients with neurofibromatosis. Radiology 122: 289–293

EXTRINSIC ALLERGIC ALVEOLITIS

Associated with a large number of occupations in adults, this hypersensitivity disease is more likely to be seen as a result of contact with birds, particularly pigeons and budgerigars, or to a variety of allergens in children in rural communities. Asthma is unusual since the subject is usually not atopic. Although shortness of breath and respiratory distress may be episodic following contact with the antigen, respiratory symptoms may be progressively insidious in prolonged exposure such as to housedust. Radiological findings include a fine ground-glass hazy loss of radiolucency over part or all of the lung fields. Although more obvious at the bases, the whole lung can be involved. Fine micronodules may be seen, but more common are mottled shadows some 2–3 mm in size, predominantly prominent in the upper zones. Widespread patchy consolidation with poorly defined margins found anywhere throughout the lung fields are a common manifestation. The end stages of gross pulmonary fibrosis seen in adults following prolonged exposure with the formation of bullae and bronchiectasis are rarer in childhood. Enlargement of the mediastinal lymph nodes and pleural effusions are not typical features.

REFERENCES

Eisenberg J D, Montaneu A, Lee R G 1992 Hypersensitivity pneumonitis in an infant. Pulmonology 12: 186–190
Pierce J W, Kerr I H 1978 Immunologic diseases and the lung. Radiologic Clinics of North America 16: 389–406

IDIOPATHIC PULMONARY HAEMOSIDEROSIS (CEELEN'S DISEASE)

This is an uncommon condition essentially affecting infants and children. It is rare after 20 years of age. Episodic bleeding into the lung gives rise to breathlessness, coughing, wheeze, fever, haemoptysis and anaemia. Finger clubbing may occur. Haemosiderin-laden macrophages are present in the sputum and gastric washings and tests for faecal occult blood may be positive. Intravenous injection of radioactive-labelled erythrocytes will show increased radioactivity in the lungs. The serum bilirubin may rise. Pulmonary diffusion and compliance may be reduced.

The intermittent pulmonary haemorrhages give rise to transitory widespread patchy shadowing which resolves when the bleeding stops (Fig. 1.6.12). Initially, during remission, the lung fields will appear normal. Repeated haemorrhage, however, leads to the development of a fine granularity and as a consequence interstitial fibrosis becomes more marked. Later in the disease, fine linear and reticular shadows develop. Pleural effusions are very rare and pneumothorax is not a feature. The prognosis is poor, with death frequently occurring in an acute episode of bleeding.

The aetiology of the condition remains obscure and no real evidence of an autoimmune process has been advanced. Some response to corticosteroids and immunosuppressive agents has been recorded, although it is possible, however, that in some of these particular children the pulmonary haemorrhage is an early sign of glomerulonephritis or a collagen vascular disease, especially if associated with pancreatitis or myocarditis.

Secondary pulmonary haemosiderosis has been described in mitral stenosis with elevated pulmonary venous pressures, in association with collagen vascular disease and with certain haemorrhagic states such as anaphylactoid purpura, microangiopathic haemolytic anaemia and pulmonary lymphangio-leiomyomas.

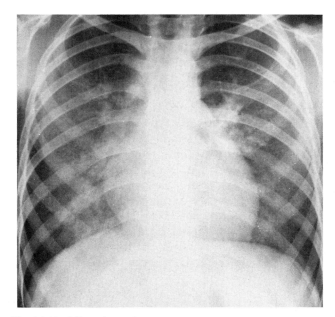

Fig. 1.6.12 Idiopathic pulmonary haemosiderosis. Widespread shadowing associated with haemoptysis.

REFERENCE

Levy J, Wilmott R W 1986 Pulmonary hemosiderosis. Pediatric Pulmonology 2: 384–391

PULMONARY CALCIFICATION AND OSSIFICATION

Metastatic pulmonary calcification is most usually associated with chronic renal failure and primary hyperparathyroidism, especially if there is extensive bone destruction. It may also be noted following vitamin D intoxication and administration of calcium salts. Pulmonary calcification is rarely detected on premortem radiographs although histologically may be quite extensive. The chest radiographs can be essentially normal or can mimic pulmonary oedema or pneumonia. An increased uptake of $^{99}Tc^m$-labelled phosphates has been recorded. Massive pulmonary calcification has been described in infants with congenital cardiac lesions but which was not clearly associated with the underlying cardiac abnormality.

Other causes of pulmonary calcification include chronic pulmonary venous hypertension, granulomatous infections and chronic granulomatous disease. Idiopathic disseminated pulmonary ossification consisting of branching linear densities is usually seen in the lower zones. Pulmonary ossification metaplasia in mitral stenosis is rare in children.

REFERENCES

Beerman P J, Crowe J E, Sumner T E, Lorentz W, Young L W 1983 Radiological case of the month – metastatic pulmonary calcification from chronic renal failure. American Journal of Diseases in Children 137: 1119–1120

Chinn D H, Gamsu G, Webb W R, Godwin J D 1981 Calcified pulmonary nodules in chronic renal failure. American Journal of Roentgenology 137: 402–405

Mani T M, Lallemand D, Corone S, Mauriat P 1990 Metastatic pulmonary calcifications after cardiac surgery in children. Radiology 174: 463–467

Phelan M S, Lewis P 1983 Massive pulmonary calcification in two infants with congenital cardiac lesions. Clinical Radiology 34: 381–384

LEIOMYOMATOSIS

Pulmonary leiomyomatosis is a rare condition affecting females with onset in late teenage. A generalized reticular nodular pattern of shadowing throughout the lung fields progresses to a honeycomb appearance which may be associated with pleural effusions and with spontaneous pneumothorax. Hamartomatous overgrowth of smooth muscle cells in multiple cysts throughout the lungs with similar changes in the pleural septa and vascular structures is seen histologically. Similar radiographic changes are seen in the rare pulmonary manifestations of tuberose sclerosis (Fig. 1.6.13).

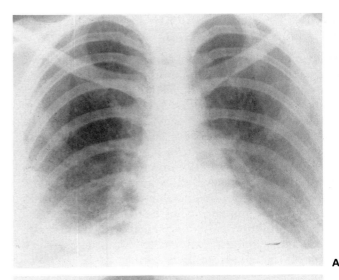

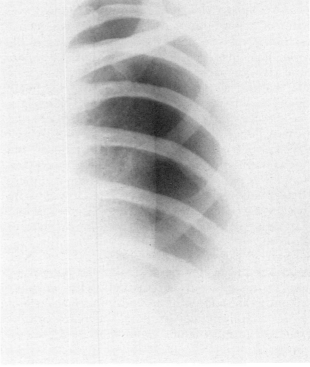

Fig. 1.6.13 Pulmonary leiomyomatosis (**A**) with complicating pneumothorax (**B**).

REFERENCE

Aberle D R, Hansell D M, Brown K, Tashkin D P 1990 Lymphangiomyomatosis: CT chest radiographic and functional correlations. Radiology 176: 381–387

GAUCHER'S DISEASE AND NIEMANN–PICK DISEASE

These are lipid storage diseases in which, due to enzymic defects, glucocerebroside accumulates in Gaucher's disease and sphingomyelin accumulates in Niemann–Pick disease. Lung involvement has been described in both type A and type B Niemann–Pick disease and in type I Gaucher's disease. Pulmonary infiltration with storage cells gives rise to a diffusely reticular nodular or miliary pattern affecting both lungs. The resulting respiratory insufficiency can be fatal (Fig. 1.6.14).

REFERENCE

Wolson A H 1975 Pulmonary findings in Gaucher's disease. American Journal of Roentgenology 123: 712–715

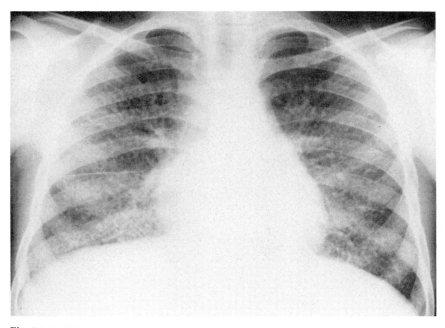

Fig. 1.6.14   Niemann–Pick disease.

MUCOPOLYSACCHARIDOSES; STORAGE DISEASES

Storage diseases, in particular the mucopolysaccharidoses (MPS), may be associated with reduced tracheal calibre, potentially of considerable significance in patients undergoing general anaesthesia.

Patients with MPS 1H and MPS 2 have a high incidence of often fatal pneumonia, in which limitation of chest wall movement is a contributory factor. Large tongues, infiltration of the soft tissues of the oropharynx and bony deformity of the face also contribute to respiratory embarrassment. Post-mortem examination in fatal cases has shown infiltration of the airways and laryngopharyngeal structures with the relevant mucopolysaccarides and mucolipids (Fig. 1.6.15).

REFERENCE

Peters M E, Arya J, Langen L O, Gilbert E F, Carlson R, Adkins W 1985 Narrow trachea in mucopolysaccharidoses. Pediatric Radiology 15: 225–228

PULMONARY ALVEOLAR MICROLITHIASIS

This exceedingly rare disease of unknown aetiology has a highly characteristic radiographic appearance. Tiny calculi are present in the alveoli which leads to a fine sand-like calcific micronodular pattern throughout the lung fields with a denser fine rim outlining the visceral pleura not only against the chest wall but also against the mediastinal structures. The interlobar fissures are prominent. $^{99}Tc^m$-DTPA accumulates in the pulmonary parenchyma. The disease can occur in the newborn and be familial (Fig. 1.6.16).

REFERENCE

Valle E, Kaufmann H J 1987 Pulmonary alveolar microlithiasis. Pediatric Radiology 17: 439–442

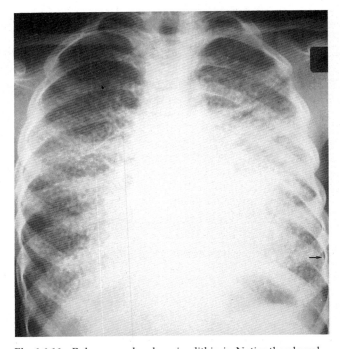

Fig. 1.6.16 Pulmonary alveolar microlithiasis. Notice the pleural opacification accentuation (arrow).

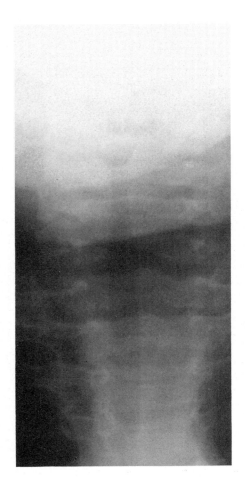

Fig. 1.6.15 Hurler's disease. The trachea is frequently narrowed in the mucopolysaccharidoses.

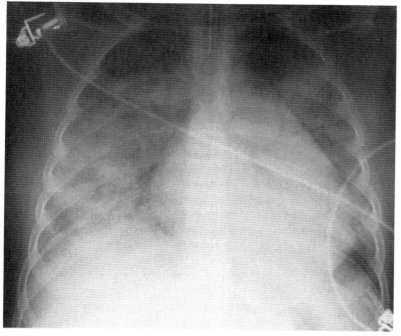

Fig. 1.6.17 Systemic lupus erythematosis. Widespread alveolar oedematous opacification with accentuation of the air bronchogram.

WEGENER'S GRANULOMATOSIS

In this condition necrotizing granuloma in both the upper and lower respiratory tract are associated with a necrotizing vasculitis and glomerulitis. It is commoner in adulthood, but rarely encountered in the child.

Opacification of the paranasal air sinuses can be seen with destruction of bone and nasal cartilage with septal perforation. In the lungs, single or multiple poorly or relatively well-defined shadows may be noted which can become confluent. Occasionally much more prominent widespread infiltrations may occur, which may be transient but can cavitate in an irregular fashion with usually thick walls. Vasculitis and pulmonary infiltrates, often oedematous, are features of systemic lupus erythematosis and Henoch–Schönlein purpura (Figs 1.6.17, 1.6.18).

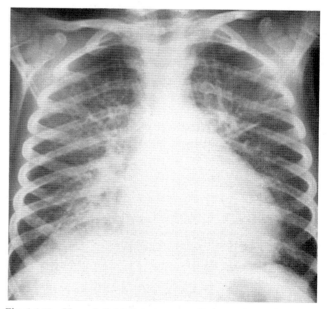

Fig. 1.6.18 Henoch–Schönlein purpura. Perivascular and deep lymphatic lines are seen radiating from the hilar regions.

REFERENCE

Singer J, Suchet J, Horwitz T 1990 Paediatric Wegener's granulomatosis. Two case histories and a review of the literature. Clinical Radiology 42: 50–51

ALLERGIC GRANULOMATOUS ANGIITIS

Asthma, fever and eosinophilia with vasculitis in abdominal organs was described by Churg and Strauss. Lung involvement consists of widespread patchy shadowing but also with streaky shadowing related to infiltration, particularly eosinophilic, of the lung septa.

REFERENCE

Churg J, Strauss L 1951 Allergic granulomatous allergic angiitis and periarteritis nodosa. American Journal of Pathology 27: 277

PULMONARY VENO-OCCLUSIVE DISEASE

This is a rare condition in which pulmonary hypertension arises from progressive obliteration of the pulmonary veins. Shortness of breath on exertion is a common symptom, although haemoptysis and fever are also presenting features. Sex distribution is equal and the age range is from infancy to middle age with half the cases being children. This disease is of unknown aetiology, although there have been some associations with Hodgkin's disease, chemotherapy and bone marrow transplantation. The radiographic features show prominent main pulmonary arteries and fine linear shadows, especially basally. Pulmonary oedema and septal lines are prominent, and the fissures are accentuated. The appearances may be predominantly unilateral. The condition, however, is usually progressive with a fatal outcome. Congenital stenosis of the pulmonary veins and obstructive lesions of the left atrium such as myxoma and cor triatriatum can be differentiated by echocardiography and cardioangiography (Fig. 1.6.19).

REFERENCE

Shackelford G D, Sacks E J, Mullin J D et al 1977 Pulmonary veno-occlusive disease: case report and review of the literature. American Journal of Roentgenology 128: 643–648

HEPATOGENIC PULMONARY ANGIODYSPLASIA

In this condition hepatic cirrhosis is associated with arterial desaturation caused by right to left shunting through small pulmonary arteries which show dilatation and peripheral arteriovenous shunting. Radiographically, a fine reticular diffuse interstitial pattern is distributed throughout the lungs, often more obvious in the bases. Central cyanosis and finger clubbing are clinical correlates.

Portopulmonary venous anastomosis is a rare association with portal hypertension.

REFERENCE

Sang O K, Bender T M, Bowen A, Zelesma-Media J 1983 Plain radiographic, nuclear medicine and angiographic observations of hepatogenic pulmonary angiolyoplasia. Pediatric Radiology 13: 111–115

KAWASAKI'S DISEASE

A particular granular pattern with occasional peribronchial cuffing, pleural effusion and atelectasis may be noted on the chest radiographs of children with Kawasaki's disease, often without signs of heart failure. It is likely that these radiographic findings are due to associated lower respiratory tract inflammation or pulmonary arteritis. Cardiac features are discussed elsewhere.

REFERENCE

Umejawa T, Saji T, Matsuo N, Odagin K 1989 Chest X-ray findings in the acute phase of Kawasaki disease. Pediatric Radiology 20: 48–51

PULMONARY ALVEOLAR PROTEINOSIS

Once considered essentially a disease of adults, the rare incidence of this condition in infancy and childhood has recently been appreciated. Presentation is often through failure to thrive, vomiting and diarrhoea and sometimes pyogenic infections. There is an association with lymphopenia, immune deficiency, haematological neoplasia and lymphoproliferative disease. Degeneration of enlarged alveolar pneumatocytes leads to accumulation of proteinaceous material which stains characteristically red with periodic acid-Schiff stain.

The chest radiograph usually shows bilaterally symmetrical fine nodular perihilar shadows which spread outwards from the hilar regions and can coalesce to give marked central opacification with some relative peripheral sparing (Fig. 1.6.20). Appearances can mimic pulmonary oedema and in the very young hyaline membrane disease. The heart size is normal and other signs of pulmonary venous hypertension such as pleural effusions and septal lines are not seen. Respiratory embarrassment can be fatal but lung lavage by which the diagnosis can be made is also therapeutic. Similar radiographic and histological appearances can be seen in *Pneumocystis carinii* pneumonia.

REFERENCES

McCook T A, Kirks D R, Merten D F, Osborne D R, Spock A, Pratt P C 1981 Pulmonary alveolar proteinosis in children. American Journal of Roentgenology 137: 1023–1027

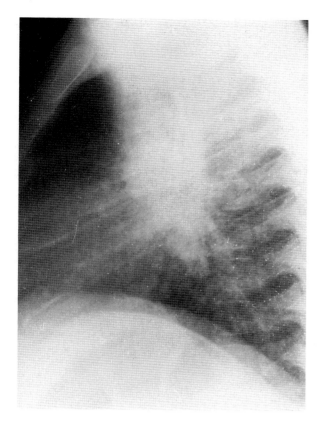

Fig. 1.6.19 Pulmonary veno-occlusive disease. Right lateral radiograph showing prominent pulmonary artery and septal lines.

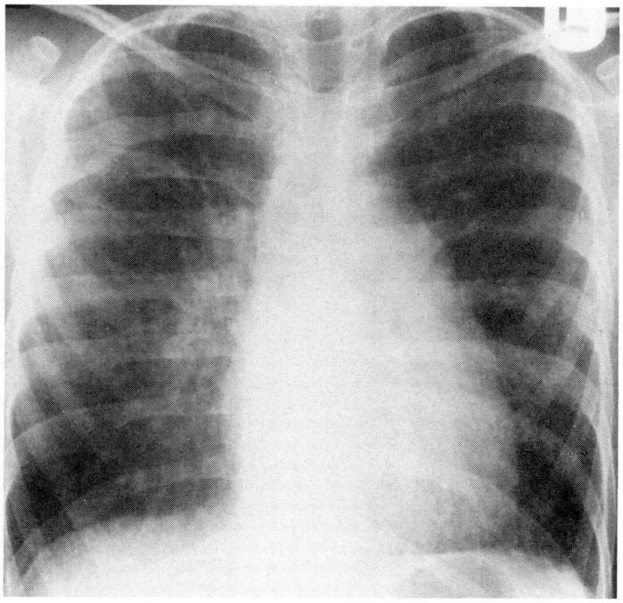

Webster J R Jr, Batttifora H, Furey C, Harrison R A, Shapiro B 1980 Pulmonary alveolar proteinosis in two siblings with decreased immunoglobulin. American Journal of Medicine 69: 786–789

LYMPHOMATOID GRANULOMATOSIS

This is a rare condition characterized by multiple pulmonary nodules in the lower lung fields, unilateral or bilateral, and frequently rapidly cavitating. Clinical symptoms include fever, cough or weight loss. A lymphoproliferative granulomatous reaction with vasculitis is the underlying pathology and there may be involvement of other systems, particularly the central nervous system, skin and kidneys. Some patients progress to frank lymphoma. Acquired immune deficiency, secondary to infection with Epstein–Barr, virus is the underlying pathology in some cases.

REFERENCES

Bridges R A, Aerendes H, Good R A 1959 A fatal granulomatosis disease of childhood: the clinical, pathological and laboratory features of a new syndrome. American Journal of Diseases of Children 97: 387–408

Glickstein M, Kornstein M J, Pietragg et al 1986 Non-lymphomatous lymphoid disorders of the lung. American Journal of Roentgenology 147: 227–237

Fig. 1.6.20 Pulmonary alveolar proteinosis, proved by open biopsy of right lung.

HEART–LUNG TRANSPLANTATION

For patients with end-stage lung disease such as mucoviscidosis or with irreversible pulmonary arterial hypertension, combined heart–lung transplantation has become a reasonable therapy. In the early post-operative period complications include infection, haemorrhage, breakdown of the tracheal anastomosis and acute rejection.

The radiographic features of rejection of bilateral lung and heart–lung transplantation are similar and the diagnosis of acute rejection is essentially imprecise and clinical. Radiographic changes consist usually of mid-zone and basal consolidation but may not be associated with obvious plain radiographic changes. It has been suggested that the combination of septal lines and developing pleural effusions is suggestive of acute rejection.

The response of non-cardiogenic pulmonary oedema from ischaemia and damage to nerves and lymphatic vessels is more marked in lung transplantation than in heart–lung transplantation and the usual radiographic findings of patchy bilateral perihilar basal consolidation usually reaches a maximum by 4 days, after which a deteriorating chest radiograph is unlikely to be due to this reimplantation response. In the assessment of the integrity of tracheal and bronchial anastomoses and evaluation of their patency CT is considerably more accurate than plain chest radiography.

The development of bronchiolitis obliterans in long-term survivors is an important complication. In such patients the chest radiograph shows a variable mixture of nodular and linear or diffuse alveolar opacities which are essentially non-specific and indistinguishable from other infectious and non-infectious conditions in the transplanted lung. Central bronchiectasis has however been described and may prove to be a distinctive feature not seen in the bronchiolitis obliterans of other patients without transplants.

Although the main cause of obliterative bronchiolitis after heart–lung transplantation is immunological, the aetiology is probably multifactorial. Cytomegalovirus infection may be an initiating cause and in some patients bronchiectasis, chronic cough, gastro-oesophageal reflux and slow gastric emptying have been ascribed to vagal injury at surgery (Figs 1.6.21, 1.6.22).

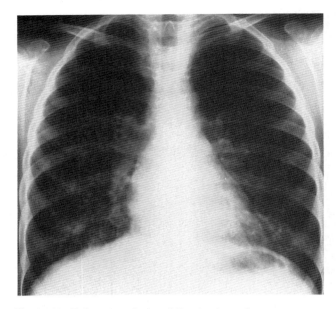

Fig. 1.6.21 Pulmonary changes following heart–lung transplantation. There is peribronchial shadowing and scattered basal opacities.

REFERENCES

Bergin C J, Castillino R A, Blank N, Berry G J, Sibley R K, Staines V A 1990 Acute lung rejection after heart–lung transplantation. American Journal of Roentgenology 155: 23–27

Sheens J L, Fuhrman C R, Yousem S A 1989 Bronchiolitis obliterans in heart–lung transplantation patients. American Journal of Roentgenology 153: 253–256

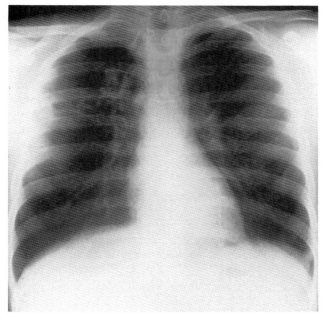

A

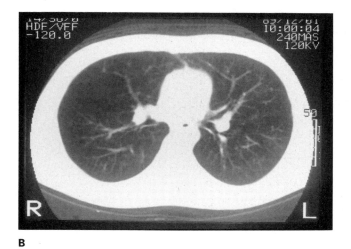

B

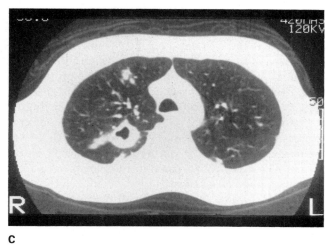

C

Fig. 1.6.22 Obliterative bronchiolitis with cavitating lesions in the right upper lobe following heart–lung transplant. **A** Chest radiograph. **B** CT showing marked attenuation of the pulmonary vasculature. **C** CT showing cavitating thick-walled lesion in the right upper lobe.

LUNG DISEASE FOLLOWING ALLOGENIC MARROW TRANSPLANTATION

Bone marrow transplantation is increasingly used in the treatment of leukaemia, other malignancies and aplastic anaemia. Following high dose cytotoxic drugs often with total body irradiation, 'rescue' is affected with marrow from a histocompatible donor. The principal complications are infection, graft-versus-host disease and, less commonly, graft rejection.

During the first 3–4 weeks following marrow transplantation, profound neutropenia may be complicated by lung infection, usually bacterial, but sometimes fungal.

The establishment of marrow engraftment and subsequent improvement in neutropenia can, however, be associated with the onset of graft-versus-host disease affecting skin, gut, liver and the lungs. Interstitial pneumonias are common and may be due to cytomegalovirus, herpes simplex, adenovirus or other viruses or pneumocystis but often without any established pathogen. Clinical features of cough, shortness of breath and fever are accompanied radiographically by scattered pulmonary infiltrates.

An important later complication of marrow transplantation is the development of chronic obstructive lung disease. Symptoms include cough and increasing dyspnoea which may progress to severe pulmonary compromise. The chest radiograph is usually clear by comparison with the diffuse or patchy shadowing of interstitial pneumonia. Open lung biopsy demonstrates an obliterative bronchiolitis similar to that seen following adenovirus or influenzal pneumonia in the young. The airways obstruction is often progressive, carrying a poor prognosis.

Calcified small peripheral ill-defined nodular lesions in the lower lung fields on CT examination of the chest have been observed following bone marrow transplantation. It has been suggested that these are thromboembolic in origin, although possibly also due to endothelial injury from pretransplant irradiation with associated thrombosis and dystrophic calcification.

REFERENCE

Allen B T, Day D L, Dehner L P 1987 CT demonstration of asymptomatic pulmonary emboli after bone marrow transplantation. Pediatric Radiology 17: 65–67

PULMONARY EMBOLISM

Pulmonary embolism is much less common at autopsy than in adults. In the neonatal period pulmonary embolism often associated with cerebral and hepatic venous occlusion are unlikely to have manifestations on a chest radiograph. In older children, pulmonary embolism is an important complication of the nephrotic syndrome, sickle cell disease and also of ventriculo-venous shunts for hydrocephalus. Mismatched defects on ventilation/perfusion radioisotope scans are more diagnostic than localized pulmonary parenchymal shadows.

REFERENCES

Arnold J, O'Brodovich H, Whyte R, Coates G 1985 Pulmonary thromboemboli after neonatal asphyxia. Journal of Pediatrics 106: 806–809
Buck J R, Connors R H, Coon W W, Weintraub W H, Wesley J R, Coran A G 1981 Pulmonary embolism in children. Journal of Pediatric Surgery 16: 385–392

1.7 TUMOURS

JUVENILE LARYNGEAL PAPILLOMATOSIS

The most common laryngeal tumour of the young child is the benign, usually multiple, epithelial papilloma. These can extend down into the trachea and occasionally into the bronchi. Parenchymal spread is well recognized but uncommon. Multiple small parenchymal nodules gradually cavitate and slowly enlarge (Fig. 1.7.1). Typically they do not fill with bronchographic contrast medium but may show air-fluid levels sometimes in association with infection.

CT has shown that these lesions are more frequent in the posterior parts of the lung which may be consistent with one theory that the lung nodules are seedlings from endoscopic procedures coming to rest in dependent parts of the lung. Whereas juvenile laryngeal papillomas often regress in later adolescence, such regression in the lung lesions is not a feature and there is a significant risk of development of carcinoma in parenchymal lesions, perhaps related to radiotherapy.

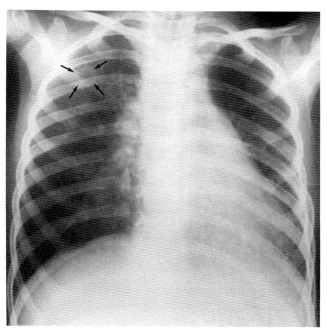

Fig. 1.7.1 Laryngotracheal papillomatosis. Cavitating lesion in the right upper lobe (arrows). A tracheostomy has been performed.

REFERENCES

Clements R, Graville I H 1986 Laryngeal papillomatosis. Clinical Radiology 37: 547–550
Dallimon N S 1985 Squamous bronchial carcinoma arising in a case of multiple juvenile papillomatosis. Thorax 40: 797–798
Kawanami T, Bowen A 1985 Juvenile laryngeal papillomatosis with pulmonary parenchymal spread. Paediatric Radiology 15: 102–104
Reaner S S, Wehunt W D, Stocker J T, Kashima H 1985 Pulmonary manifestations of juvenile laryngotracheal papillomatosis. American Journal of Roentgenology 144: 687–694
Smith L, Gossling C A 1974 Pulmonary involvement in laryngeal papillomatisis. Pediatric Radiology 2: 161–166

GRANULAR CELL MYOBLASTOMA

This arises from Schwann cells, particularly in skin but also in the tongue and upper respiratory tract. Radiographic features are of a progressive endotracheal lesion, symptomatic by virtue of airways obstruction. The lesion is typically slow growing and surgical extirpation is usually curative.

BRONCHIAL ADENOMA

Bronchial adenoma, although the most common primary lung tumour in children, is rare. The most common histological type is carcinoid which accounts for about two-thirds of the tumours and derives from argentaffin cells which can become endocrinologically active. Presentation is typically as a polypoidal endobronchial mass producing segmental bronchial obstruction or predominantly extrabronchial extension which displaces rather than infiltrates the lung tissue.

Mucoepidermoid tumours account for about a quarter of the lesions arising from the glandular tissue. Cylindromas are rare and arise in the mucus-producing glands. In childhood, there is a greater preponderance of mucoepidermoid and a lesser preponderance of carcinoid tumours by comparison with the incidence in adults. Most tumours occur in the main bronchi and are unusual in the trachea. Males are affected twice as commonly as females. Recurrent pneumonia and areas of collapse with a chronic cough reflect the consequent local obstruction caused by the tumour. Although in adulthood cylindromas and carcinoids can infiltrate and expand into the lung parenchyma and metastasize, in childhood the incidence of malignancy in these tumours is considerably less. In a small percentage of children dying from metastases increased 5-hydroxy-indole-acetic acid levels are present.

CT can assess extrabronchial spread in particular and assess mediastinal lymphadenopathy which is more frequently due to reactive change from infection than from metastasis. In view of the low incidence of malignancy, conservative therapy such as endoscopic excision or sleeve resection is preferable to lobectomy or pneumonectomy.

REFERENCE

Wildeburger R, Hoolworth M E 1989 Bronchoadenoma in childhood. Paediatric Surgery International 4: 373–380

MESENCHYMAL AND EMBRYONIC BLASTEMAS

These form a rare and small group of potentially malignant tumours of the lung. Histological types include fibrosarcoma (Fig. 1.7.2), leiomyosarcoma and rhabdomyosarcoma (Fig. 1.7.3), all of which usually present as often large intrathoracic and radiographically non-specific masses.

PRIMARY LEIOMYOSARCOMA OF THE LUNG

This rare tumour arises from smooth muscle in the bronchi and blood vessels. Metastasis is haematogenous and not through lymphatics. The characteristic clinical course is of fever, cough and worsening dyspnoea and a chest radiograph showing the presence of a mass of variable size with usually well-defined borders or with atelectasis as a consequence of bronchial obstruction.

REFERENCE

Beluffi G, Bertolotti P, Mietta A, Manara G, Luisetti M 1986 Primary leiomyosarcoma of the lung in a girl. Pediatric Radiology 16: 240–244

PULMONARY HAMARTOMA

These lesions are usually detected in adult life but are seen in paediatric practice. The lesions are small and clearly defined, usually single and may show characteristic curvilinear and speckled calcification, although this is more commonly seen in the older age group. If no calcification is present the diagnosis is unlikely to be made radiographically and biopsy, either by surgical excision or percutaneous needle biopsy, will be required.

REFERENCES

Hedlund G L, Bisset G S, Bove K E 1989 Malignant neoplasms arising in cystic hamartomas of the lung in childhood. Radiology 173: 77–79
Weinberg A G, Currarino G, Moore G C, Vatteler T P 1980 Mesenchymal neoplasia and congenital pulmonary cysts. Pediatric Radiology 9: 179–182

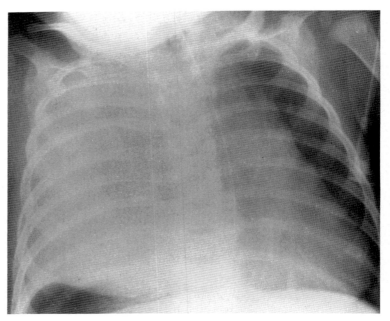

Fig. 1.7.2 Fibrosarcoma occupying most of right hemithorax.

BRONCHOGENIC CARCINOMA

Bronchogenic carcinoma in childhood is rare. It is usually very aggressive with early metastases; most tumours are undifferentiated adenocarcinomas. Squamous cell tumours form only a small proportion. The majority of the lesions are circumscribed, peripheral masses, but perihilar and central lesions have been described.

REFERENCE

Shelley B E, Lorenzo R L 1983 Primary squamous cell carcinoma of the lung in childhood. Pediatric Radiology 13: 92–94

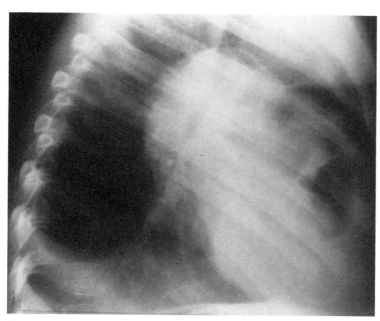

A

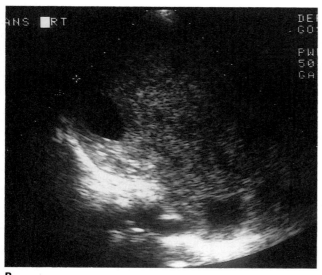

B

Fig. 1.7.3 A Lateral view of right-sided rhabdomyosarcoma occupying middle and anterior mediastinum. Gas containing necrotic areas anteriorly. **B** Ultrasound showing necrotic area in mass.

SECONDARY SMOKING

Exposure of infants to tobacco smoke results in an increased incidence of pneumonia and bronchiolitis. Although cigarette smoking is too common among teenagers, consequent development of bronchogenic carcinomas is likely to be delayed until early adult life.

CONGENITAL PULMONARY CYSTS AND MESENCHYMAL NEOPLASIA

A rare association of congenital pulmonary cysts is the development of embryonal tumours, including rhabdomyosarcomas, cystic pulmonary blastomas and malignant mesenchymomas. These tumours are associated with and seen to arise in predominantly unilocular peripheral cysts of bronchiolar origin. This defined risk of development of malignancy in a truly congenital cyst is an indication, in addition to respiratory distress and secondary infection, for surgical removal.

PULMONARY METASTASES

Secondary haematogenous dissemination to the lungs is the commonest cause of lung malignancy. Tumours particularly metastasizing to the lungs are Wilms' tumours, rhabdomyosarcomas and skeletal malignancies. CT is more sensitive than plain radiography for detection of lung deposits. A frontal plain radiograph should be supplemented by a lateral view in elucidation of possible lung metastases, a practice which in the general evaluation of the pulmonary parenchyma is not indicated. Response to chemotherapy can be followed particularly by CT and a successful response will be accompanied by disappearance of the typically rounded shadows. The exclusion of micrometastases, however, is not possible. In certain parts of the world, granulomatous infections of the lung can cause confusion with malignant deposits, especially if the granulomas do not show calcification. In childhood, cavitation of pulmonary metastases is rare but has been recorded before, and also following, chemotherapy and therapeutic radiation and in osteogenic sarcoma. Although not widely practised, percutaneous biopsy of pulmonary parenchymal lesions, especially if situated in the peripheral lung fields, is a practical proposition which can be facilitated by the use of CT or fluoroscopy for accurate localization. Although osteogenic sarcoma usually metastasizes to the lung fields, involvement of the mediastinal lymph nodes is a very uncommon metastatic site causing dysphagia and bronchial erosion and compression (Fig. 1.7.4).

THYMUS

Pure thymic cysts are rare, and may be uni- or multi-locular. Though calcification may be seen in adult thymic cysts it is very rare in childhood.

THYMOMA

Thymomas usually occur in later childhood and are often found as incidental anterior mediastinal masses on plain radiographs. Respiratory distress from local obstruction and displacement is a common symptom, but myasthenia gravis is not a typical feature in childhood. Linear calcification, either capsular or in the walls of associated cystic components, may be more easily demonstrated by CT than plain radiographs. Malignant thymomas are rare in childhood, but pleural metastases occur often as in adults.

THYMOLIPOMA

This rare fatty benign tumour of the thymus is less common than a non-thymic mediastinal lipoma. Although the patients are usually asymptomatic, cough, dyspnoea and chest pain may be presenting signs, and the condition is associated with Graves' disease, aplastic anaemia, hypogammaglobulinaemia and myasthenia gravis. Sometimes lipomas are seen in other adjacent organs such as the thyroid and the pharynx. Plain radiographs are often incorrectly interpreted as demonstrating a large heart shadow. The tumours can be very large and associated with pleural effusions. Ultrasound may show increased echogenicity from the fatty components. CT shows thymic tissue interspersed between whorls of low density fatty tissue, although such appearances may also be seen in thymic hyperplasia.

REFERENCE

Faerber E N, Balsain R K, Schidlow D D, Marron L M, Zaen N 1990 Thymolipoma: computed tomographic appearances. Pediatric Radiology 20: 196–197

THYMIC CYSTS

Congenital pure thymic cysts are very rare lesions arising from a persistent thymopharyngeal duct. They can be uni- or multi-locular. Though calcification may be seen in adult thymic cysts, it is very rare in childhood. Thymic cysts may occur in Hodgkin's disease, probably from intrinsic involvement rather than as a result of therapy. Persistence of such cystic lesions may falsely indicate persistent or recurrent lymphoma.

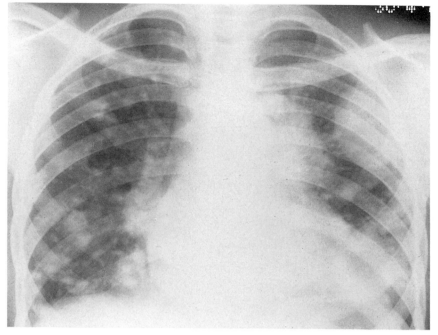

A

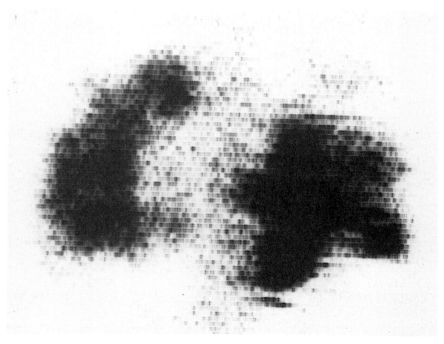

B

Fig. 1.7.4 Metastatic osteogenic sarcoma. **A** Chest radiograph. **B** Uptake by radioactive diphosphonates.

CYSTIC HYGROMA

These soft tissue multicystic lymphoid and haemangiomatous lesions most commonly occur in the neck (Fig. 1.7.5). Some 10%, however, extend into the superior mediastinum anteriorly and, very rarely, they occur exclusively in the mediastinum. Smaller cystic hygromas may produce few symptoms other than their presenting mass, but larger lesions can distort both the airways and adjacent bony structures, although cystic hygromas have less propensity to infiltrate than histologically more simple lymphangiomas. Pleural effusions can be a serious complication.

Plain radiographic assessment of size is usually adequate but CT gives a better delineation of extension into the thorax. The diagnosis may be suggested by the characteristic multiple sonolucent cysts demonstrated by ultrasound.

Evaluation of anterior mediastinal masses, particularly those based in and around the thymus, is a common problem in paediatric practice. MRI is of particular value and signal characteristics are indicated in Table 1.7.1.

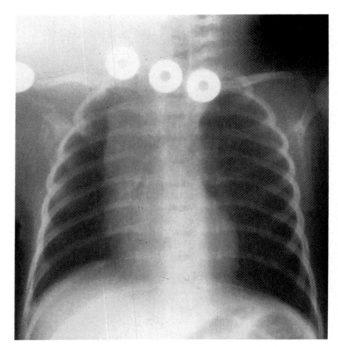

Fig. 1.7.5 Cystic hygroma extending from right side of neck into superior mediastinum.

REFERENCES

Cohen M D, Weber T R, Sequeira F W 1983 The diagnostic dilemma of the posterior mediastinal thymus: CT manifestations. Radiology 146: 691–692

Day D L, Gedgaudas E 1984 Symposium on non-pulmonary aspects in chest radiology. The thymus. Radiologic Clinics of North America 22: 519–538

Fonkalsrud E W, Herrmann C Jr, Mulder D G 1970 Thymectomy for myasthenia gravis in children. Journal of Pediatric Surgery 5: 157–165

Francis I R, Glazer G M, Bookstein F L et al 1985 The thymus: re-examination of age-related changes in size and shape. American Journal of Roentgenology 145: 249–254

Rose J S, Lam C 1982 Thymic enlargement in association with hyperthyroidism. Pediatric Radiology 12: 37–38

Table 1.7.1 Thymic typical MR characteristics		
Lesion	T1 weighted	T2 weighted
Normal	Low, slightly more than muscle	High
Thymic cyst	Low	High
Thymic cyst + haemorrhage	Increased	High
Lymphoma	Low	High (may be low)
Post-therapy fibrosis	Low	Low
Leukaemia	Low	High
Thymolipoma	High	High
Germ cell	Variable depending upon fat and calcification	
Lymphangioma, Cystic hygroma	Occasionally high from fat	High

GERM CELL TUMOURS

Some 8% of germ cell tumours occur in the anterior mediastinum in childhood and comprise about 10% of mediastinal masses. Sex incidence is usually equal in teratomas but there is male preponderance in the malignant forms. Klinefelter's syndrome may be associated with an increased risk of development of malignant mediastinal germ cell tumours. Clinical presentation can be of respiratory distress, chest pain, obstructive emphysema or superior vena caval obstruction. Rare presentations are rupture of cystic components into the pleura or pericardium or even into the trachea. Ectopic pancreatic or gastric tissue may secrete digestive enzymes and ectopic hormone production, such as in hyperinsulinaemia, is a rare complication. Malignant teratomas can be clinically monitored by elevated blood levels of alphafetoprotein and gonadotrophins.

Plain radiographs (Fig. 1.7.6) may show a surprisingly large anterior mediastinal mass displacing and obstructing the lung or heart. Calcification is present in about a third of teratomas and can represent bone, calcified cartilage or teeth. The cystic components of teratomas (Fig. 1.7.7) may be well demonstrated by CT and poor definition of the capsule with areas suggestive of haemorrhage and necrosis in partially cystic masses may be indicative of malignant neoplasia. Such tissue differentiation would be more easily demonstrated by nuclear magnetic resonance imaging than by conventional CT. These tumours are often large and situated in the anterior mediastinum, and it is often possible to evaluate them by ultrasound, in which case the cystic and calcific components may be well demonstrated.

Germinomas or seminomas are rare in childhood and need to be differentiated both histologically and radiographically from malignant lymphoma. The tumours are often large, lobulated but without demonstrable calcification.

Endodermal sinus tumours (yolk sac carcinoma) are rare in childhood, with a male preponderance, and are usually solid but may show partial necrosis. Choriocarcinoma is an agressive lesion of young females, with a poor prognosis.

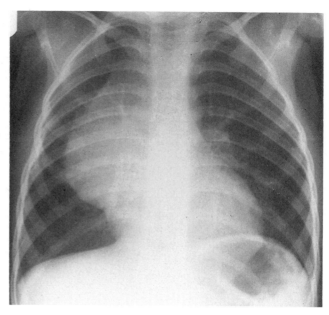

Fig. 1.7.6   Anterior mediastinal teratoma.

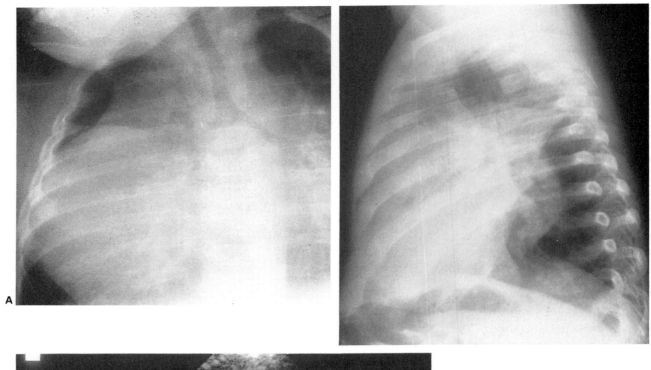

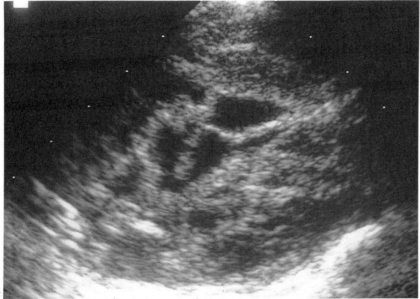

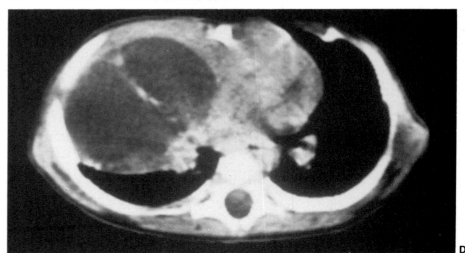

Fig. 1.7.7 Teratoma. Frontal (**A**) and lateral (**B**) radiographs showing anterior mediastinal mass. Ultrasound (**C**) and CT (**D**) showing cystic components.

MALIGNANT LYMPHOMAS

Both Hodgkin's and non-Hodgkin's lymphomas are common malignancies involving the chest (Figs 1.7.8, 1.7.9). Acute lymphoblastic leukaemia may also lead to thymic and mediastinal lymph node enlargement and at times differentiation from lymphoblastic lymphoma may not be clear and depend upon bone marrow findings. The nodular sclerosing type of Hodgkin's disease has a high incidence of mediastinal involvement usually affecting adolescent girls. In younger children there is a predominance of boys and the more common lymphocytic predominant Hodgkin's disease at this earlier age is less frequently associated with mediastinal widening. Involvement of the lung parenchyma in Hodgkin's disease is relatively infrequent and is associated with mediastinal disease. Parenchymal lung lesions in continuity with hilar and mediastinal structures do not alter the staging of the disease but peripheral discrete lesions, if indeed due to lymphoma, indicate Stage IV disease.

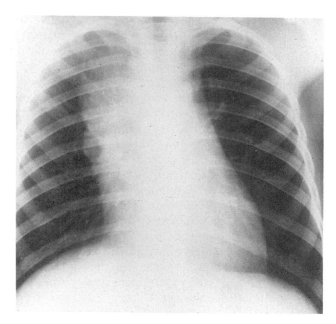

Fig. 1.7.8 Lymphoma with right paratracheal and hilar mass.

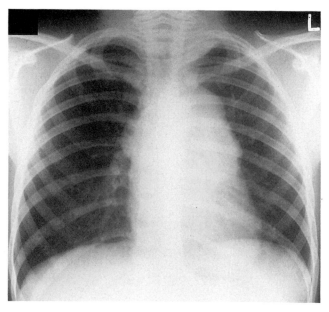

Fig. 1.7.9 Lymphoma. The hilar and left mediastinal lymph nodes are enlarged. There is lymphadenopathy in the left side of the neck overlying the apex of the left lung.

Non-Hodgkin's lymphoma (Figs 1.7.10, 1.7.11) of the small convoluted cell type shows a mediastinal mass in about half of the cases. These lymphoblastic lymphomas may grow very rapidly and present with superior vena caval obstruction, often associated with severe respiratory distress from tracheal compression. Non-Hodgkin's lymphoma is associated with a much greater incidence of pleural effusions, pericardial effusions and parenchymal lung involvement than Hodgkin's disease.

Radiography does not contribute significantly to the cellular diagnosis of lymphomas and usually plain films are adequate to monitor clinical progress either to chemotherapy or radiotherapy. The differentiation of thymic enlargement due to lymphomatous infiltration from enlarged mediastinal lymph nodes is difficult and usually of little clinical significance. However, CT and MRI relying particularly upon the change in tissue character and irregularity of shape of the thymus in the lymphomas may allow some differentiation.

PULMONARY LEUKAEMIA

Leukaemic involvement of the lungs usually gives rise to a diffuse interstitial pattern but very occasionally a nodular leukaemic infiltration may be observed, the precise pathology of which is unclear. Peribronchial connective tissue infiltration, thrombotic or leukaemic pulmonary infarcts have been suggested as causes.

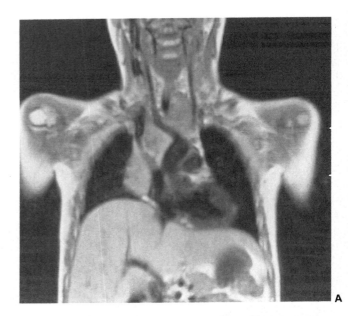

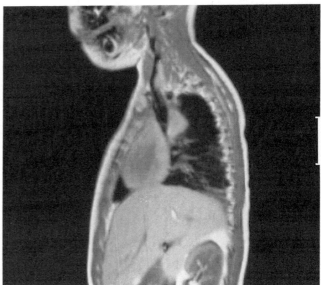

Fig. 1.7.10 Non-Hodgkin's lymphoma with superior vena caval obstruction. **A** Coronal and **B** sagittal T1-weighted images.

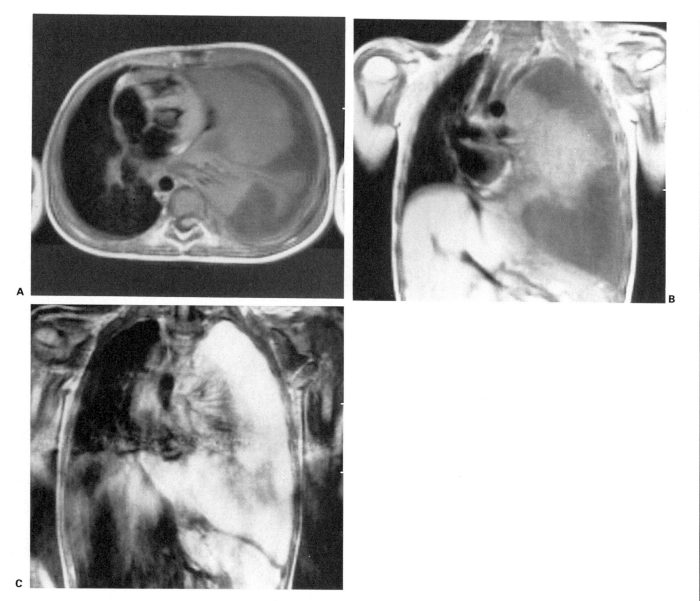

Fig. 1.7.11 T-cell non-Hodgkin's lymphoma with left-sided pleural effusion. **A** Axial T1-weighted image. **B** Coronal T1-weighted image. **C** Coronal T2-weighted image.

CALCIFIED MEDIASTINAL LYMPH NODES IN HODGKIN'S DISEASE AND NON-HODGKIN'S LYMPHOMA

Following radiotherapy and sometimes chemotherapy calcification of mediastinal lymph nodes affected by Hodgkin's disease is well documented in children, although occurring less frequently than in adults. Calcification in lymphoma before treatment is extremely rare. Intrathoracic opacities may result from lymphangiography (Fig. 1.7.12).

LYMPHOPROLIFERATIVE DISEASE SECONDARY TO CYCLOSPORIN

A complication arising several months after exhibition of cyclosporin in transplant patients is the development of a lymphoproliferative condition with pulmonary masses, single or multiple, with hilar and mediastinal lymph node enlargement, most probably due to uninhibited B-cell proliferation due to Epstein–Barr virus.

CYSTS

About 10–15% of mediastinal masses are cystic and predominantly found in the middle or posterior mediastinum. Although usually congenital broncho-pulmonary foregut malformations, Hodgkin's disease, germ cell tumours and thymoma may be predominantly cystic and as such are more typically found in the anterior mediastinum.

Duplication cysts

Primitive foregut duplication cysts are properly divided into enteric duplication and bronchogenic cysts (Fig. 1.7.13). About 3% of mediastinal masses in childhood are due to bronchogenic cysts. Usually presenting in the first 2 years of life with recurrent pneumonia and respiratory distress, the cysts are typically in the region of the carina but can present in the paratracheal, paraoesophageal, and the hilar regions. They may also present with scoliosis due to associated vertebral abnormalities. Although the common sites are the middle and posterior mediastinum (Figs 1.7.14, 1.7.15), bronchogenic duplication cysts may also occur in the neck. Air-fluid levels may be seen when communication develops with the bronchial tree, particularly in the presence of infection.

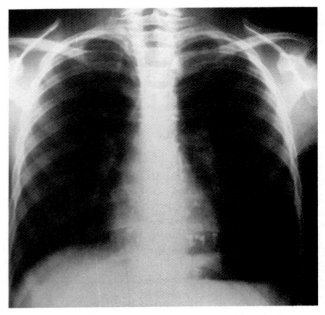

Fig. 1.7.12 Intrathoracic densities following lymphography.

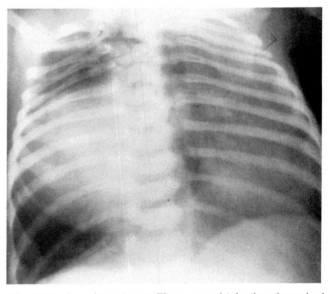

Fig. 1.7.13 Bronchogenic cyst. There are multiple rib and vertebral deformities and displacement of the heart to the left.

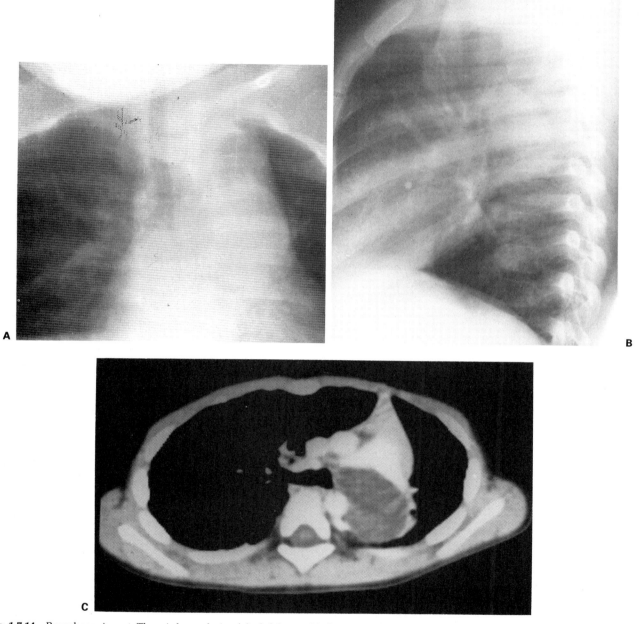

Fig. 1.7.14 Bronchogenic cyst. There is hypoplasia of the left lung with deviation of the mediastinum to the left and hypovascularity of the left lung from the cyst lying in the left posterior hilar region. **A** and **B** are plain radiographs. **C** is a CT scan.

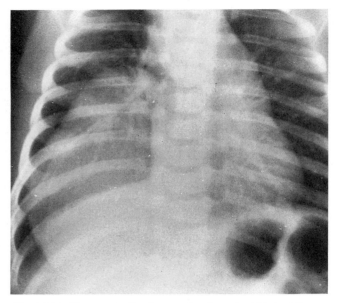

Fig. 1.7.15 Foregut duplication cyst in a 3-week-old baby. The rounded mass lies posteriorly. The lower lobe vessels can be seen superimposed on the mass.

Enteric duplication cysts are typically juxtaposed to the oesophagus. Occasionally, duplication cysts may connect through the diaphragm to the jejunum (Fig. 1.7.16). The variable incidence of gastric mucosa within them may lead to inflammation, necrosis and superinfection but may also facilitate diagnosis by the uptake of radioactive pertechnetate. Some enteric cysts are associated with vertebral anomalies and a defect in the neurospinal axis, the split notochord syndrome, presenting as posterior mediastinal masses (Figs 1.7.17, 1.7.18).

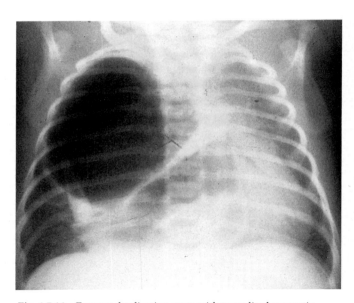

Fig. 1.7.16 Foregut duplication cysts with transdiaphragmatic connection to the jejunum.

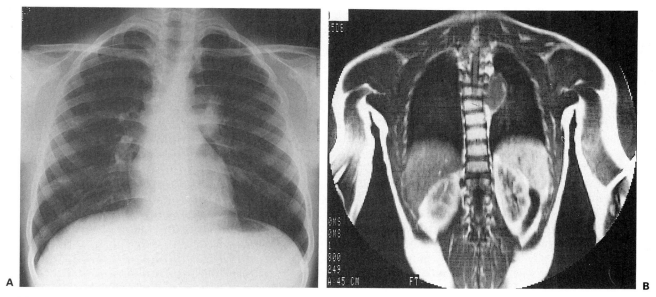

Fig. 1.7.17 Neurenteric cyst. **A** Plain radiograph. **B** Coronal MR.

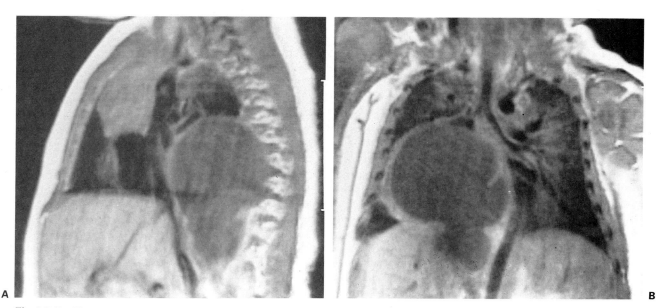

Fig. 1.7.18 Neuroenteric cyst. **A** Sagittal T1-weighted image. **B** Coronal T1-weighted image.

NEUROGENIC TUMOURS

Neurogenic tumours in childhood are a common cause of mediastinal mass, particularly posteriorly. Neuroblastoma (Figs 1.7.19, 1.7.20) and ganglioneuroblastoma occur in the younger child whereas ganglioneuroma, a benign lesion, is more frequent in later childhood. Some tumours show decreasing malignant features with age. Benign lesions may be discovered incidentally on chest radiography. Symptoms with benign lesions are usually those of pressure due to size or neurogenic pain from nerve involvement. Malignant lesions may present with the full range of clinical features associated with neuroblastoma, including pain, neurological deficit and endocrine manifestations. High thoracic and cervical neuroblastoma may present with Horner's syndrome. The radiographic appearances are usually of a well-defined posterior paravertebral mass which may show some lobulation. Although predominantly unilateral, the mass can extend across the midline displacing the heart and other mediastinal structures. Erosion and separation of the ribs posteriorly is an important diagnostic and characteristic finding. Extension into the spinal canal is common and spinal cord compression is one of the presenting features of the disease. Erosions of vertebral bodies and pedicles may be appreciated on plain radiographs but is better demonstrated on CT or MRI. Fine calcification in the lesion is highly suggestive of a neurogenic origin, although thoracic tumours show less calcification than those in the abdomen.

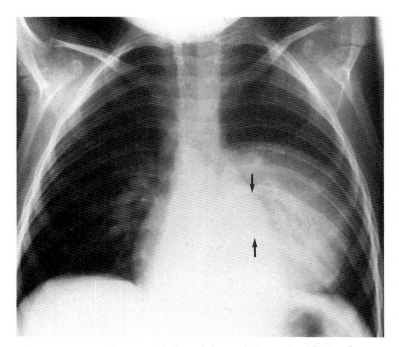

Fig. 1.7.19 Neuroblastoma. The large left rounded mass is widening the intercostal space (arrows).

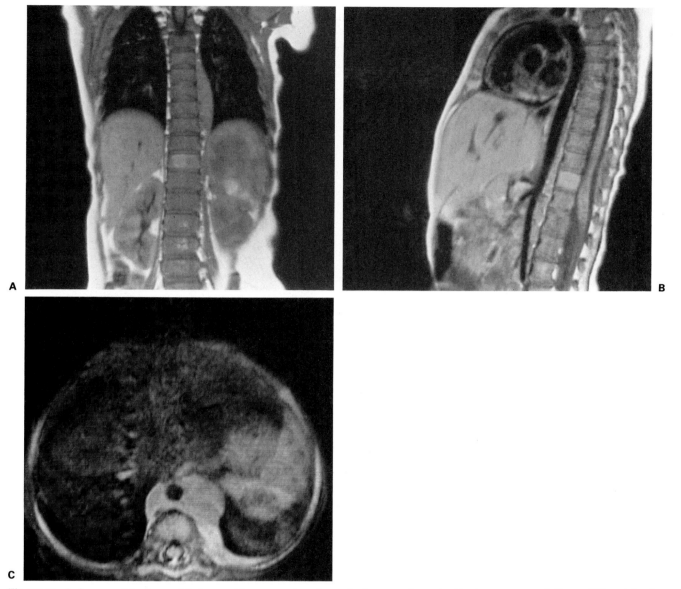

Fig. 1.7.20 Left paravertebral neuroblastoma with para-aortic and vertebral mass and vertebral body metastases. **A** Coronal T1-weighted image. **B** Sagittal T1-weighted image. **C** Axial T2-weighted image.

Ganglioneuromas (Fig. 1.7.21) represent the benign end of the spectrum of sympathetic nervous system tumours and present as paravertebral posterior mediastinal tumours, often with extension into the spinal canal. They show similar radiographic features to neuroblastoma from which differentiation is essentially histological and biochemical. Nerve sheath tumours include neurofibroma, neurilemmoma and malignant Schwann cell tumours. These are often associated with generalized neurofibromatosis and although these tumours are well documented in childhood, radiographic and clinical manifestations are more common in adult life. The common site for neurofibromatous lesions is in the posterior part of the mediastinum closely applied to the vertebral column where pressure erosion of the adjacent vertebra is a frequent finding. Scalloping of the vertebral bodies in neurofibromatosis may be due to dural ectasia in addition to localized tumour involvement. Although typically occurring posteriorly, nerve sheath tumours may affect central mediastinal structures, particularly when arising from the vagus nerve, and can arise anteriorly from an intercostal nerve.

The site and extent, especially intraspinal, of neurogenic tumours is usually adequately demonstrated by plain radiography supplemented by cross-sectional imaging using CT or MRI. MIBG radioactive scanning is widely used in the assessment of neuroblastoma but more so for metastatic involvement than delineation of the primary lesion, in which uptake of the isotope is further confirmation of a neurogenic origin.

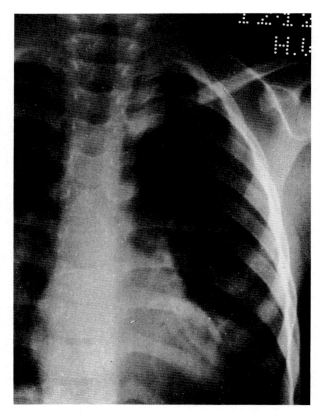

Fig. 1.7.21 Ganglioneuroma in the left upper paravertebral region (arrowheads).

AORTO-SYMPATHETIC PARAGANGLIOMA

About a third of intrathoracic paragangliomas occur in children and may present as masses in either the anterior or posterior mediastinum. Although usually benign, about one-fifth of patients will show metastases, either regional or distant.

PRIMITIVE NEUROECTODERMAL TUMOUR

In many ways resembling neuroblastoma, but typically without elevation of catecholamines, this neurogenic tumour of the mediastinum may occur either in a paravertebral area or more centrally in the mediastinum, and also in the chest wall, as Askin's tumour. Diagnosis is histological.

MENINGOCELES

Intrathoracic meningoceles are cystic lesions occurring in the posterior mediastinum, sometimes in association with neurofibromatosis but more frequently with other spinal dysraphisms.

PERICARDIAL CYSTS

These are probably acquired lesions accounting for their typical discovery in later life. An opacity of relatively low radiographic density is seen adjacent to the heart shadow, usually in the right cardiophrenic angle.

REFERENCES

Bergstrom J R, Yost R V, Ford K T, List R M 1973 Unusual roentgen manifestations of bronchogenic cysts. Radiology 107: 49–54

Blair T C, McElvein R B 1963 Hamartoma of the lung. A clinical study of 25 cases. Diseases of the Chest 44: 296–302

Castellino R A, Parker B R 1977 Non-Hodgkin's lymphoma. In: Parker B R, Castellino R A (eds): Pediatric oncologic radiology. St Louis: Mosby, p. 183

Chalmers A H, Armstrong P 1977 Plexiform mediastinal neurofibromas. A report of two cases. British Journal of Radiology 591: 215–217

Cohen M, Slabaugh R, Smith J A 1982 Unusual non-metastatic nodules in the lungs of children with cancer. Clinical Radiology 33: 57–59

Cohen M, Smith W L, Weetman R et al 1981 Pulmonary pseudometastases in children with malignant tumors. Radiology 141: 371–374

Dumontier C, Grauiss E R, Siberstein M J, McAllister W H 1985 Bronchogenic cysts in children. Clinical Radiology 36: 431–436

Ekloff O, Gooding C A 1967 Intrathoracic neuroblastoma. American Journal of Roentgenology 100: 202–207

Fermaglich D R 1975 Pulmonary involvement in infectious mononucleosis. Journal of Pediatrics 86: 93–95

Hurt R, Bates M 1984 Carcinoid tumours of the bronchus: a 33 year experience. Thorax 39: 617–623

Kantrowitz L R, Pais M J, Burnett K, Choi B, Pritz M B 1986 Intraspinal neurenteric cyst containing gastric mucosa: CT and MRI findings. Pediatric Radiology 16: 324–327

Karl S R, Dunn J 1985 Posterior mediastinal teratomas. Journal of Pediatric Surgery 20: 508–510

Kolygin B A, Vesnin A G 1976 Hodgkin's disease in children: clinicoroentgenologic features of the lesion in the chest. Pediatric Radiology 4: 144–148

McCall I W, Woo-Ming M 1978 The radiological appearance of plasma cell granuloma of the lung. Clinical Radiology 29: 145–150

McLatchie G R, Young D G 1980 Presenting features of thoracic neuroblastoma. Archives of Disease in Childhood 55: 958–962

Niitu Y, Kubota H, Hasegawa S et al 1974 Lung cancer (squamous cell carcinoma) in adolescence. American Journal of Diseases of Children 127: 108–111

Pike M G, Wood A J, Corrin B, Warner J O 1984 Intrathoracic extramediastinal cystic hygroma. Archives of Disease in Childhood 59: 75–77

Resjo M, Harwood-Nash D C, Fitz C R, Chuang S 1979 CT metrizamide myelography for intraspinal and paraspinal neoplasms in infants and children. American Journal of Roentgenology 132: 367–372

Rivero H, Gaisie G, Bender T M, Oh K S 1984 Calcified mediastinal lymph nodes in Hodgkin's disease. Pediatric Radiology 14: 11–13

Shackelford G D, McAlister W H 1976 Mediastinal teratoma confused with loculated pleural fluid. Pediatric Radiology 5: 118–119

Sinner W N 1982 Fine-needle biopsy of hamartomas of the lung. American Journal of Roentgenology 138: 65–69

Solomon A, Rubistei Z J, Rogoff M et al 1982 Pulmonary blastoma. Pediatric Radiology 12: 148–149

Wellons H A, Eggleston P, Golden G T et al 1976 Bronchial adenoma in childhood. Two case reports and review of the literature. American Journal of Diseases of Children 130: 301–304

INTRATHORACIC KIDNEY

This rare site of renal ectopia predominantly affects the left side, with a high male preponderance. The condition may be secondary to neonatal diaphragmatic hernia but can occur in the presence of an intact diaphragm. Presentation may be delayed and the entity should be considered as a rare cause of a left posterior lower zone chest mass or of renovascular arterial hypertension due to renal artery stenosis secondary to distortion and stretching of the renal vessels.

CHEST WALL TUMOURS

Ewing's sarcoma of the thorax and soft tissues, together with Askin's malignant small cell tumour, are the important small round cell neoplasms. The soft tissue component of these tumours is often large and the destructive lesion of the involved rib, usually with a periosteal reaction, may be inconspicuous and easily overlooked. Large pleural effusions are often associated (Fig. 1.7.22).

The differentiation of Askin's tumour from Ewing's sarcoma cannot be made radiologically, and is based on the presence of intracellular neurosecretory granules on electron microscopy and neurone-specific enolase indicating they are peripheral primitive neuroectodermal tumours. Askin's tumours are three or four times more common in girls. Other chest wall tumours with similar radiological features include rhabdomyosarcoma, malignant lymphoma and, much more rarely, osteosarcoma, histiocytoma, fibrosarcoma and synovial sarcomas. Osteochondromas arising in ribs can extend into the vertebra and spinal canal (Fig. 1.7.23).

REFERENCES

Askin F B, Rosai J, Sibley R K, Dehner L P, McAlister W H 1979 Malignant small cell tumour of the thoracopulmonary region in childhood. A distinctive clinicopathological entity of uncertain histogenesis. Cancer 43: 2438–2451

O'Keefe F, Lorigan J G, Wallace S 1990 Radiological features of extraskeletal Ewing's sarcoma. British Journal of Radiology 63: 456–460

Shamberger R C, Grier H E, Weinstein H J, Perez-Atayde A R, Tarbell N J 1989 Chest wall tumours in infancy and childhood. Cancer 63: 774–785

Shuman L S, Libshitz H I 1984 Solid pleural manifestations of lymphoma. American Journal of Roentgenology 142: 269–273

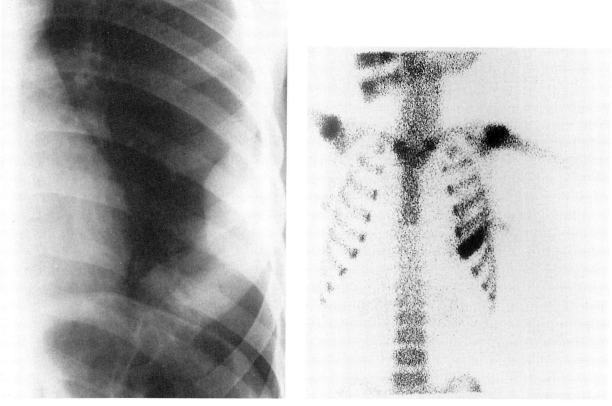

Fig. 1.7.22 Askin's tumour of left rib with soft tissue mass (**A**) and increased uptake on bone scan (**B**). The soft tissue mass is often much larger and associated with pleural effusion.

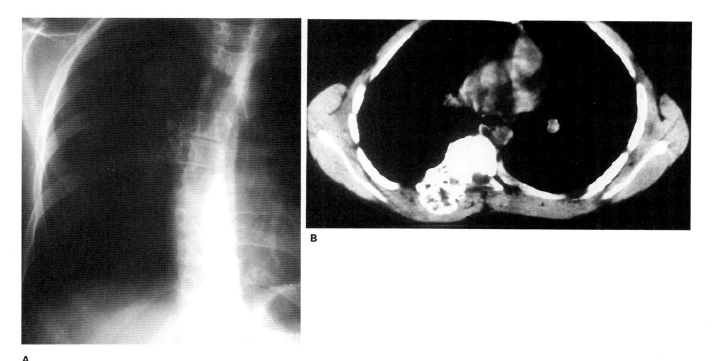

Fig. 1.7.23 Osteochondroma arising from the posterior end of the sixth right rib is deforming the adjacent rib (**A**) and the adjacent vertebra (**B**, CT).

LIPOMA

These are rare lesions in childhood which may occur in the mediastinum or in the chest wall. Mediastinal tumours may show deviation of normal structures. The characteristic low attenuation of fatty tumours usually visible on CT may not be evident on plain radiographs. Chest wall or subpleural lipomas can directly erode, enlarge and deform adjacent ribs. Lymphangiomas and haemangiomas may involve the chest wall (Figs 1.7.24, 1.7.25) and diaphragm (Figs 1.7.26, 1.7.27).

REFERENCE

Whyte A M, Powell N 1990 Case report: mediastinal lipoblastoma of infancy. Clinical Radiology 42: 205–206

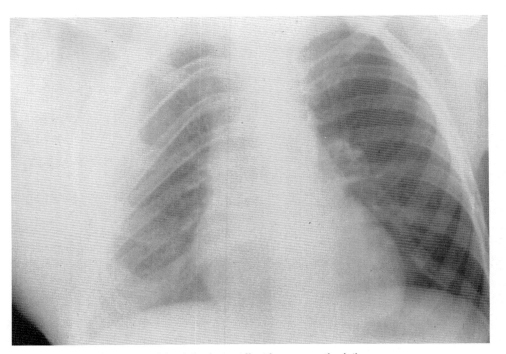

Fig. 1.7.24 Lymphangioma of the right chest wall with overgrowth of ribs.

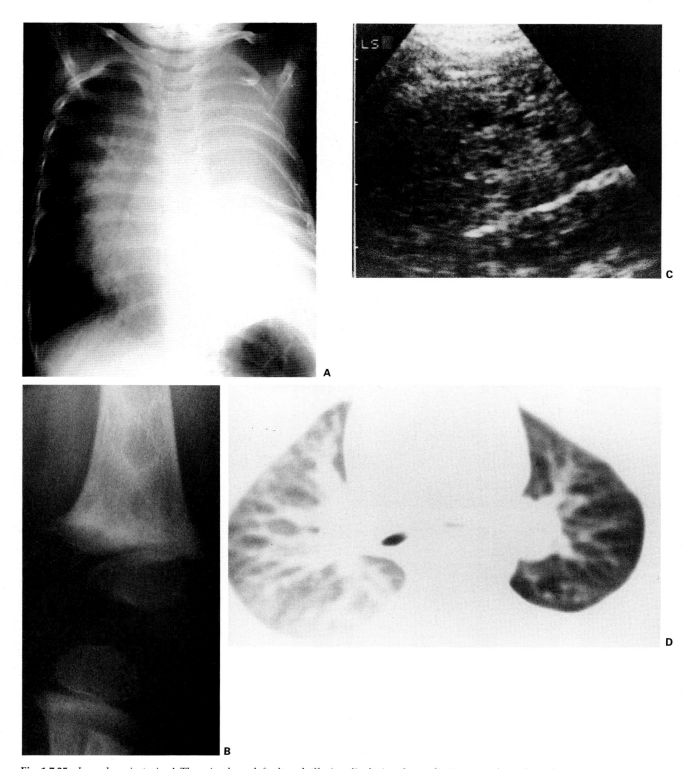

Fig. 1.7.25 Lymphangiectasia. **A** There is a large left pleural effusion displacing the mediastinum to the right with multiple rib erosions. **B** Metaphyseal radiolucencies from intraosseous lymphangioma. **C** Longitudinal ultrasound scan of the spleen showing echolucent lymphangiomatous lesions. **D** CT scan of the chest before development of the left pleural effusion and multiple left rib lesions showing lymphangiomatous involvement of the right lung.

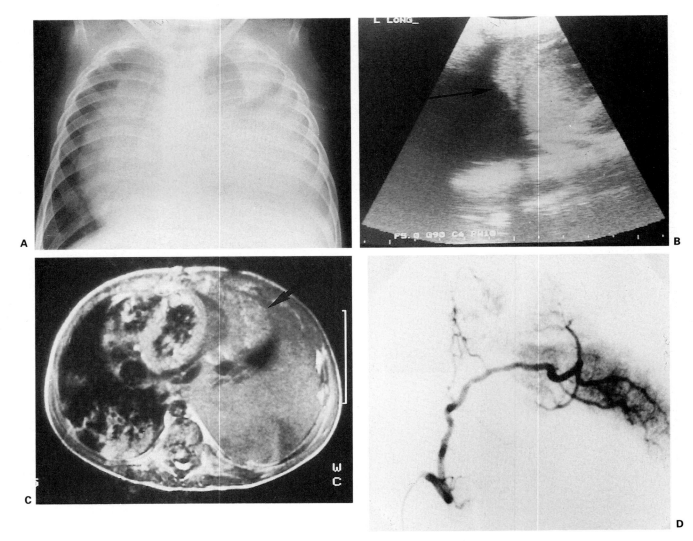

Fig. 1.7.26 Hemangioma of the left hemidiaphragm with consumptive coagulopathy. **A** Left haemorrhagic pleural effusion. **B** Echogenic mass (arrow) on left hemidiaphragm. **C** Anterior diaphragmatic mass (arrow). T1-weighted MRI. **D** Selective angiography of the mass.

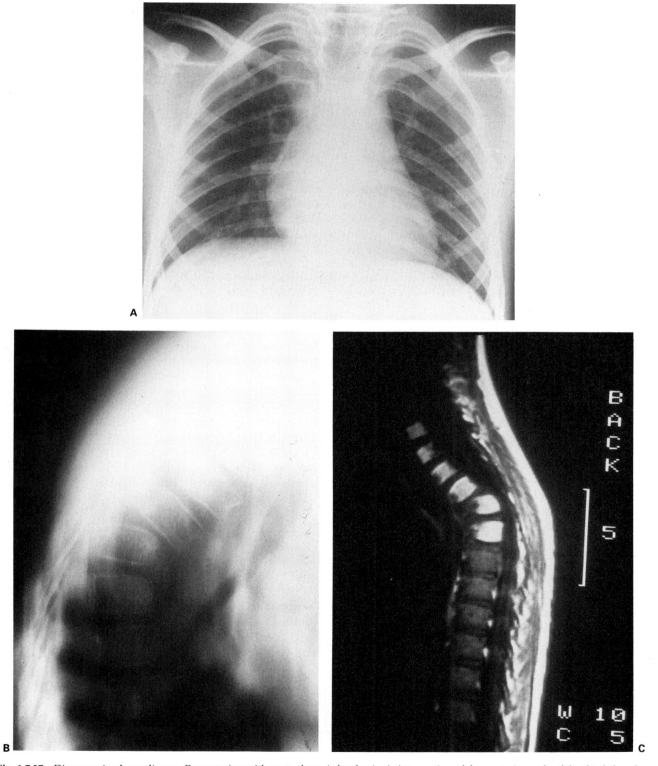

Fig. 1.7.27 Disappearing bone disease. Presentation with acute thoracic kyphosis. **A** Attenuation of the posterior ends of the third, fourth and fifth ribs, in particular. **B** Conventional tomography showing subluxation of the dorsal vertebral bodies. **C** T1-weighted MRI with high signal from affected vertebral bodies. The posterior laminae in the affected area are deficient.

BENIGN MESENCHYMOMA OF THE CHEST WALL

This very rare tumour presents shortly after birth or in infancy. Discovery may be incidental or due to the effect of lung compression. A chest wall mass (Fig. 1.7.28), mild respiratory distress or scoliosis are more frequent presentations. An extrapleural mass arises from one or two ribs, usually away from the axial skeleton. Irregular calcification and ossification can be seen within the mass and the peripheral nature of bone within the lesion can be well shown on CT. Histologically, mesenchymal cells are seen forming both cartilage and mature bone. Aneurysmal bone cyst formation has been described as an association. Although often markedly hypercellular, the lesions are benign, and rarely spontaneous regression has been seen.

REFERENCE

Oakley R H, Carty H, Cudmore R E 1985 Multiple benign mesenchymomata of the chest wall. Pediatric Radiology 15: 58–60

PANCREATIC PSEUDOCYSTS

Extension of pancreatic pseudocysts into the chest can present as pleural or pericardial effusion or as lower mediastinal masses. Ultrasonic demonstration of pericardial and pleural fluid in a child with upper abdominal pain is suggestive of this rare complication of pancreatitis in which CT will allow delineation of the thoracic disease and assessment of the pancreas and upper abdomen.

REFERENCE

Mallard R E, Stilwell C A, O'Neill J A Jr, Karzon D T 1977 Mediastinal pancreatic pseudocyst in infancy. Journal of Pediatrics 91: 445–447

FIBROMATOSIS

These desmoid tumours of the mediastinum are very rare in childhood, sometimes associated with Gardner's syndrome and present as mediastinal masses which can show extension into the chest wall and diaphragm. Mediastinal masses with predominantly fibrous histology can be the presentation of nodular sclerosing Hodgkin's disease in which a representative histological section has not been obtained.

REFERENCES

Campbell A N, Chan H S L, Daneman A, Martin D J 1983 Aggressive fibromatosis in childhood. Computed Tomography 7: 109–113
Krause L M, Schey W L, Bassak A, Shrock P 1985 Intrathoracic desmoid tumours in a child. Paediatric Radiology 15: 131–133

EXTRAMEDULLARY HAEMOPOIESIS

Thalassaemia is an important cause of extramedullary haemopoiesis of which the thoracic manifestations are more frequently seen in later childhood. Paravertebral soft tissue masses with rib expansion and occasional extension into the vertebral canal with spinal cord compromise is the usual manifestation, but in severe cases rib expansion, particularly of the anterior ends with extensive soft tissue rounded masses, may also be noted.

CASTLEMAN'S DISEASE, GIANT LYMPH NODE HYPERPLASIA

Seen in later childhood and in early to middle adult life, this essentially benign condition has a high incidence of mediastinal lymph node involvement, particularly affecting the anterior mediastinum. Occasional posterior mediastinal nodes and nodal calcification may be seen, as can occasional bony involvement. Iron-deficiency anaemia, a polyclonal hypergammaglobulinaemia and poor growth may accompany the plasma cell variant of this condition. Considerable improvement in systemic symptoms may follow resection of the nodal mass. The hyaline vascular type of the condition can show enhancement with intravenous contrast media on CT.

INFECTIOUS MONONUCLEOSIS

The widespread peripheral adenopathy associated with Epstein–Barr virus infection may also be accompanied by mediastinal lymph node enlargement which may radiographically suggest a more sinister differential diagnosis. Parenchymal lung involvement may be seen although sometimes due to associated non-viral pneumonia.

PLASMA CELL GRANULOMA; INFLAMMATORY PSEUDOTUMOUR

Also known as fibroxanthoma, xanthogranuloma or histiocytoma. This is a benign tumour-like aggregation of plasma and reticuloendothelial cells, occurring in early adulthood and in childhood. Although likely to be a postinflammatory lesion, the lesions are usually asymptomatic and found fortuitously. The radiographic presentation is typically of a single well-defined rounded pulmonary mass which can grow to a large size and may occasionally show cavitation or calcification without a pleural reaction.

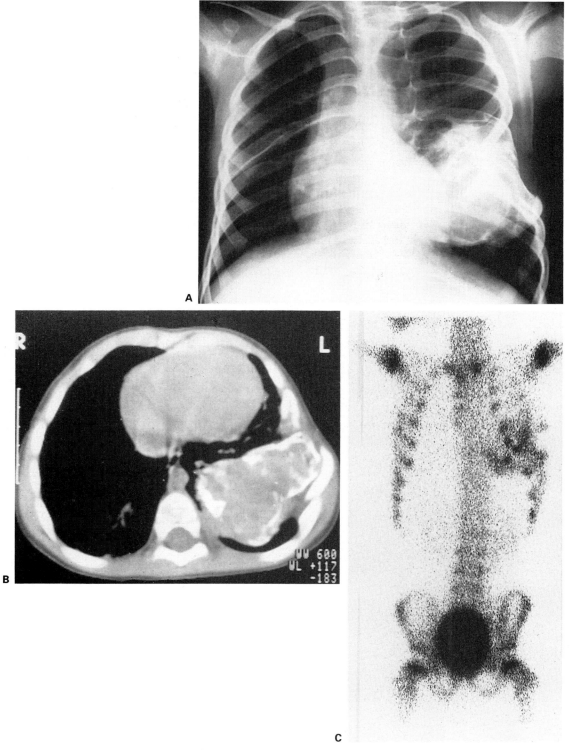

Fig. 1.7.28 Mesenchymoma of the chest wall. **A** Plain radiograph. **B** CT scan. **C** Bone scan showing extensive uptake in the mass.

Although usually parenchymal in origin, lesions may occur within the bronchial tree or the mediastinum and thereby cause areas of local pulmonary collapse. Fibrous histiocytomas can closely mimic these lesions.

SINUS HISTIOCYTOSIS (ROSAI–DORFMAN DISEASE)

This disease, of unknown aetiology, occurring predominantly in childhood, typically presents with peripheral lymphadenopathy, particularly involving the neck. Extranodal manifestations are common in the head and neck but skeletal manifestations, central nervous system involvement and visceral involvement are well recorded. Mediastinal and hilar lymph node enlargement, either unilateral or bilateral, is present in about a third of patients. Involvement of the lung is by direct extension of the hilar regions along the vessels producing accentuated interstitial shadowing. Nodular infiltration, although described, is most unusual.

REFERENCE

McAlister W H, Herman T, Dehner L P 1990 Sinus histiocytosis with massive lymphadenopathy (Rosai–Dorfman disease). Pediatric Radiology 20: 425–432

PLEURAL FIBROMA

Histologically very similar to desmoid fibromatosis of the mediastinum, these pleural-based well-circumscribed masses may present with a pneumothorax.

1.8 PHYSICAL AGENTS

FOREIGN BODIES

Sudden choking and cough with subsequent respiratory distress are highly suggestive of inhalation of a foreign body. A significant number of deaths result from this. Although clinical presentation may be immediate with severe respiratory distress, presentation may be significantly delayed and the clinical signs may then consist of cough, haemoptysis and pneumonia. Most foreign bodies are non-opaque and frequently vegetable matter, of which peanuts and other nuts are common.

The majority of foreign bodies are found in the main bronchi (Fig. 1.8.1). Some studies have shown a preponderance for the right main bronchus but this is not a universal finding. A foreign body in a major bronchus with partial obstruction of the airway typically leads to overdistension of the lung distal to the obstruction with deviation of the mediastinum contralaterally, a low hemidiaphragm and widening of the rib spaces (Figs 1.8.2, 1.8.3). Gross changes are easily discerned on conventional plain radiographs supplemented by a high kV filter view for evaluation of the airways. Lesser changes can be confirmed by an expiratory film in a cooperative child, showing the obstructive emphysema, or by quick fluoroscopy. More complete obstruction of the airway leads to distal lung collapse (Fig. 1.8.4). In smaller children in particular, acute occlusion of the airway can be associated with alveolar oedema in which collapse is not so prominent. Very occasionally a localized pneumothorax may develop peripheral to a collapsed lobe. Some foreign bodies are mobile in the bronchial tree giving rise to changing patterns of obstructive emphysema or of collapse.

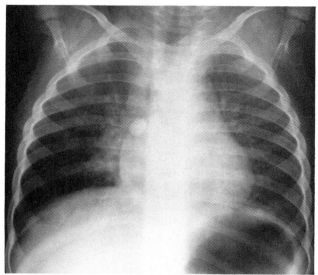

A

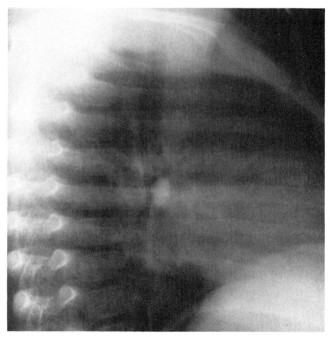

B

Fig. 1.8.1 Dense foreign body in right main bronchus. **A** AP view. **B** Lateral view.

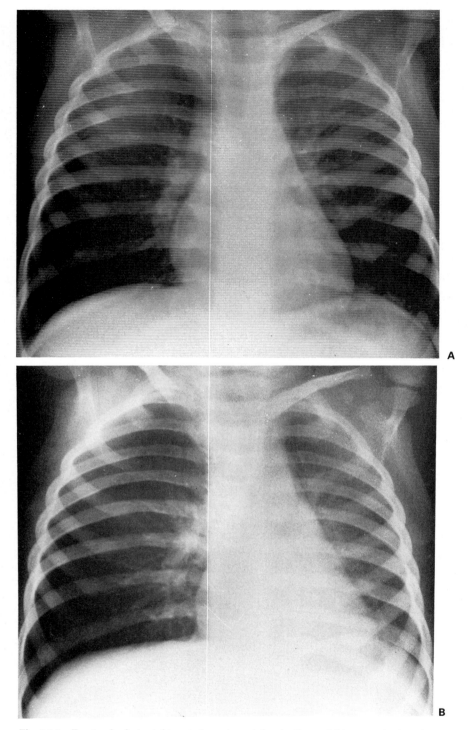

Fig. 1.8.2 Foreign body in right main bronchus. **A** Inspiration: mild increase in size of right lung with splaying of ribs. **B** Expiration: air trapping in the right lung with mediastinal contralateral swing.

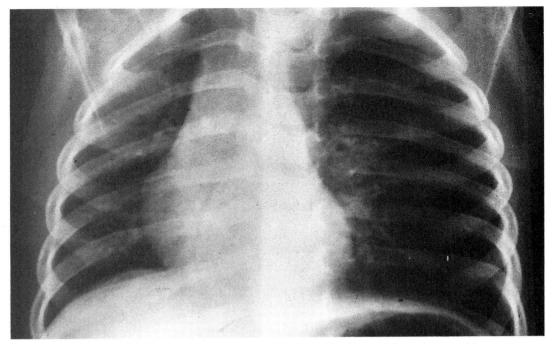

Fig. 1.8.3 Foreign body in the right main bronchus is causing partial collapse of the right lung with hyperinflation of the left lung (inspiration film).

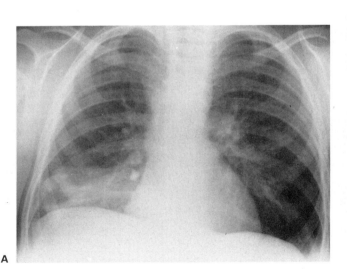

A

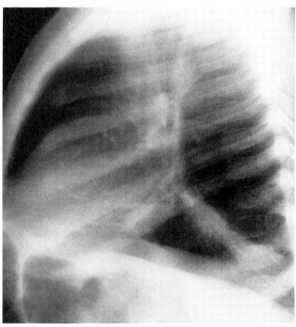

B

Fig. 1.8.4 **A,B** Dense foreign body in a right lower lobe bronchus with associated collapse and consolidation of the obstructed segment of lung.

Undiagnosed aspiration of foreign bodies is an important cause of chronic pneumonia often with the development of bronchiectasis (Fig. 1.8.5). Bronchial damage can be potentiated by vegetable oils, particularly in peanuts, and longstanding endobronchial obstructions can ulcerate and subsequently be partially epithelialized.

In all cases clinical evaluation should be paramount and apparently normal radiographic findings either on plain films or fluoroscopy should not lead to the exclusion of a potentially fatal diagnosis. Late sequelae of foreign body inhalation have been evaluated by scintigraphy. Many children have persistent matched defects of perfusion and ventilation 6 or more months after the removal of the foreign body, even when plain chest radiographs were considered normal. The time interval between inhalation and removal of the foreign body appears an important factor and most children will have scintigraphic abnormalities if the foreign body was present for more than 6 weeks. If the initial plain radiograph showed parenchymal abnormalities other than changes in aeration, persisting scintigraphic abnormalites were also much more common.

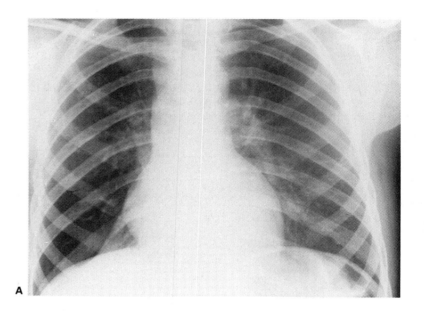

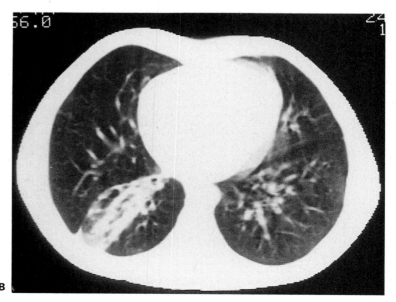

Fig. 1.8.5 A–D Bronchiectasis in the right lower lobe with matched defect in the right base on V/Q scan (p. 151) following aspiration of foreign body (posterior view).

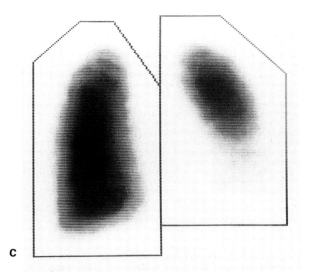

C

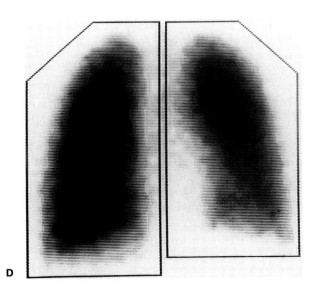

D

Pneumomediastinum is a well-recognized complication of the inhalation of foreign bodies and in one series was seen in over 10% of children under 2 years of age following peanut aspiration, but is more often seen following oesophageal perforation (Fig. 1.8.6).

REFERENCES

Berdon W E, Dee G J, Abramson S J, Altman R P, Wung J T 1984 Localized pneumothorax adjacent to a collapsed lobe: a sign of bronchial obstruction. Radiology 150: 691–694
Blazer S, Naveh Y, Friedman A 1980 Foreign body in the airway: review of 200 cases. American Journal of Diseases of Children 134: 68–71
Burton E M, Pizzo W, Kaufmann R A, Houston C S 1984 Pneumomediastinum caused by foreign body aspiration in children. Pediatric Radiology 20: 45–47
Piepsz A 1988 Late sequelae of foreign body inhalation. European Journal of Nuclear Medicine 13: 578–581
Swedstrom E, Pukakka H, Kero P 1989 How accurate is chest radiography in the diagnosis of tracheobronchial foreign bodies in children? Pediatric Radiology 19: 520–522

ASPIRATION

Pulmonary aspiration and gastro-oesophageal reflux

Occasionally during a fluoroscopic examination severe gastro-oesophageal reflux is seen to be accompanied by aspiration of the contrast medium into the trachea and bronchial tree (Fig. 1.8.7). Because the radiation dose with radionuclides is significantly less and monitoring can be performed over a longer period, milk scans with $^{99}Tc^m$-sulphur colloid have been used to identify pulmonary aspiration. A typical dose of 7.4×10^6 Bq of $^{99}Tc^m$ gives a whole body dose of 6.5×10^{-6} C/kg. There has been considerable variation in the reported incidence of pulmonary aspiration using radioactive milk scans in the investigation of gastro-oesophageal reflux in infancy. There has been some indication that placing the child in the prone position may lead to more pulmonary aspiration and that giving a second dose of radioisotope-labelled milk at midnight may also increase the detection rate of pulmonary aspiration. Other reports, however, indicate a very low detection rate of pulmonary aspiration and the place of radioactive isotope scans is as yet undetermined.

REFERENCES

Fawcett H D, Hayden C K, Adams J C, Swischuk L E 1988 How useful is gastro oesophageal reflux scintigraphy in suspected childhood aspiration? Pediatric Radiology 18: 311–313
Itani Y 1988 Upper GI examinations in older prem infants with persistent apnoea: correlation with imaging. Pediatric Radiology 18: 464–467
McVeagh P, Howman-Giles R, Kemp A 1987. Pulmonary aspiration studied by radionuclide milk scanning and barium swallow roentgenography. American Journal of Diseases of Children 141: 917–921
Willich E 1986 Gastrooesophageal reflux: radiological aspects. Pediatric Surgery International 1: 144–160

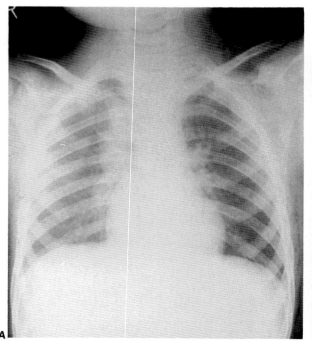

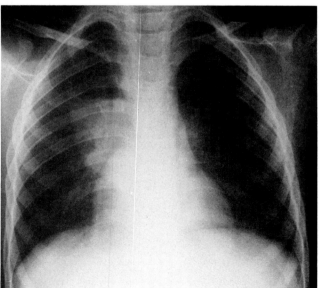

Fig. 1.8.6 A Perforation of trachea (postinstrumentation) with mediastinal widening and subcutaneous emphysema in neck, lateral view. **B** Later development of mediastinal abscess with air-fluid level.

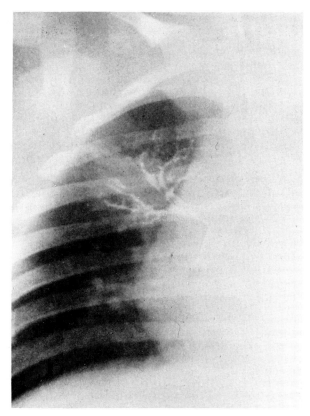

Riley–Day syndrome, familial dysautonomia

This is an autosomal recessive condition usually affecting Ashkenazi Jews. Swallowing is frequently incoordinated with resulting tracheal aspiration and recurring pneumonia. Distribution of the pulmonary lesions is irregular but may involve complete lobar collapse and consolidation. In addition to defective lacrimation, poor pain sense, emotional instability and irregular hypertension, scoliosis is a frequent concurrence (Fig. 1.8.8). Poor coordination between oesophageal peristalsis and the oesophagogastric sphincter can aggravate episodes of tracheal aspiration.

Fig. 1.8.7 Infant presenting with right upper lobe consolidation and subsequent image during barium swallow showing aspiration from gastro-oesophageal reflux.

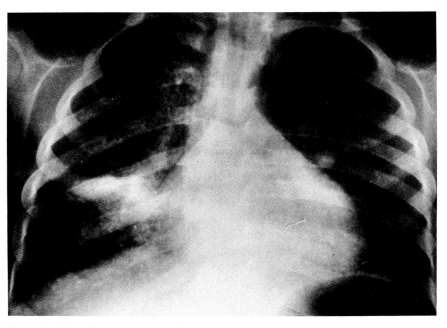

Fig. 1.8.8 Riley–Day syndrome. Widespread densities due to aspiration with right middle lobe consolidation. Note the scoliosis.

Lipid aspiration pneumonia

First described at necropsy in a child given mineral oil nose drops, aspiration of oils, often with gastro-oesophageal reflux, has been associated with shadowing in the perihilar regions and posterior parts of the lung, more frequently on the right. These non-specific radiographic features have been complemented by looking for lipid-laden macrophages following bronchial lavage. Medium chain triglycerides have been used for parenteral feeding and pneumonia associated with this has shown typical appearances of aspiration pneumonia. There have, however, been reports of an unusual progression of lipid aspiration pneumonia secondary to gastro-oesophageal reflux in the presence of nasogastric feeding where perihilar streaky infiltrates in hyperinflated lungs have progressed to diffuse parenchyma alveolar opacities which rapidly became confluent.

REFERENCE

Wolfson B J, Allen J C, Paritch H B, Karmajin N 1984 Lipid aspiration pneumonia due to gastroesophageal reflux. Pediatric Radiology 19: 545–547

Inhalation of talc

Inhalation of baby talcum powder can lead to acute or chronic respiratory distress and compromise. Massive inhalation can be fatal. Chest radiographs will show initial general hyperinflation followed by widespread patchy consolidation.

REFERENCES

Hughes W T, Kalmer T 1966 Massive talc aspiration – successful treatment with Dexamethazone. American Journal of Diseases of Children 111: 653–654
Motomatsu K, Adachi H, Uno T 1979 Infant deaths after inhaling baby powder. Chest 75: 448–450

SMOKE INHALATION

Although inhalation of toxic substances and carbon monoxide can be quickly fatal, survivors of fires may show acute damage to the upper airways from direct heat but more frequently inflammatory response in the alveolae and smaller airways, with oedema, haemorrhage or obliterative bronchiolitis. The radiographic appearances are variable and dependent upon the extent to which pulmonary oedema, sometimes haemorrhagic, contributes to variable patchy and sometimes confluent parenchymal shadowing.

REFERENCE

Zec M J, O'Connell D J 1988 The plain chest radiograph after acute smoke inhalation. Clinical Radiology 39: 33–37

NEAR-DROWNING

Abnormal radiographs are found in many victims of near-drowning. Although the chest radiograph may be normal, usually widespread patchy shadowing due to oedema which may be haemorrhagic is noted, and there may also be scattered areas of lung collapse (Fig. 1.8.9). Initial abnormal radiographs often deteriorate over a period of days, although delayed onset of radiographic abnormalities is well substantiated. Resolution of lung changes should begin within 3 or 4 days and usually be complete after a week.

Persisting abnormalities may be due to superimposed pneumonia or adult respiratory distress syndrome. Grossly contaminated water in the bronchial tree can lead to pulmonary necrosis and abscess formation.

The prognostic value of the chest radiograph on admission varies in differing reports. Although the importance of late onset of radiographic abnormalities is an important consideration, a normal chest radiograph on admission is generally a good prognostic sign. The clinical outcome is much more dependent upon central nervous system damage for which length of submersion, age and water temperature are important. Cold water has a better prognostic significance whereas salinity does not appear of great importance.

Central nervous system damage can be assessed by CT where low densities in the basal ganglia, cerebral oedema and atrophy are important signs. Central nervous system damage is almost certainly an important cause of secondary pulmonary parenchymal problems due to neurogenic oedema.

REFERENCES

Hunter T B, Whitehouse W M 1974 Fresh-water near-drowning: radiological aspects. Radiology 112: 51–56
Rapprecht E, Weinderlick P, Treffty F, Thomsen H, Burkhardt J 1985 Chest radiographs of near drowned children. Paediatric Radiology 15: 297–299
Taylor S B, Quencer R M, Holzman H H et al 1985 Central nervous system anoxic-ischemic insult in children due to near-drowning. Radiology 156: 641–646

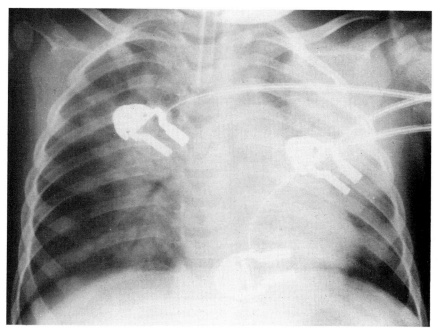

Fig. 1.8.9 Near-drowning. Widespread pulmonary opacification.

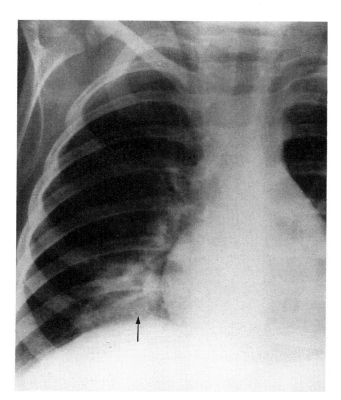

Fig. 1.8.10 Hydrocarbon inhalation. Right basal shadowing is present. This film shows developing pneumatocoele formation (arrow).

HYDROCARBON PNEUMONIA

Accidental ingestion of hydrocarbons, particularly paraffin and petroleum products, all too frequently stored domestically in old soft drink bottles, remains an important but largely avoidable hazard. The caustic effect of these liquids in the pharynx is the major cause of pulmonary aspiration. The consequent radiographic changes are usually seen in the lower lobes and although changes may be seen quickly, parenchymal shadowing may be delayed for a day or two. The typical scattered patchy opacities may increase and pneumatocoele formation may occur towards the end of the first week. Such changes are usually a direct result of the chemical pneumonitis, although secondary bacterial infection is a recognized complication. Resolution may be slow and take several months (Fig. 1.8.10).

REFERENCES

Harris V J, Brown R 1975 Pneumatoceles as a complication of chemical pneumonia after hydrocarbon ingestion. American Journal of Roentgenology 125: 531–537
Stones D K, Van Niekerk C H, Gilliers C 1987 Computerised tomography in pneumatocoeles after paraffin ingestion. Pediatric Radiology 17: 443–446

TRACHEOBRONCHIAL RUPTURE

Intrathoracic tracheobronchial rupture is a rare condition in life as associated trauma, usually acquired in an automobile accident, is often fatal. However, localized AP compression of the chest, particularly if there is an associated reflex closure of the glottis, can lead to bronchial rupture, the majority of which occur close to the carina. The increased relative elasticity of the chest wall in the child may account for the higher incidence of these injuries in the young. Parenchymal or hilar vascular damage is not usually associated. Similarly, contusion of the lung parenchyma is not a common association. Fractures of the thoracic cage may be noted but are by no means an obligatory association. Persistent leakage of air into the mediastinum or pleura, persistent atelectasis of a segment of the lung or of the entire lung and the presence of cervical emphysema should arouse suspicion of a ruptured bronchus. The rare 'fallen lung' sign in which the lung with the transected bronchus falls away from the mediastinum in the presence of a pneumothorax may be seen. Diagnosis, often delayed, is by bronchoscopy with which bronchography is rarely needed. The rare condition of post-traumatic torsion of the lung can be diagnosed by plain radiographs in which the normal distribution of the pulmonary vasculature is inverted. As with bronchial rupture, fractured ribs in such cases are by no means necessarily associated.

REFERENCE

Mahbouli S, O'Hara A E 1981. Bronchial rupture in children following blunt chest trauma. Pediatric Radiology 10: 133–138

LUNG CONTUSION

The radiographic changes in the lung following blunt chest trauma are variable, ranging from patchy, irregular shadowing to extensive confluent widespread consolidation (Figs 1.8.11, 1.8.12). Onset of these changes quickly follows trauma in contradistinction to the later radiographic findings in pulmonary fat embolism following extensive limb trauma seen usually in an older child. Cavitation in the lung fields may result in the acute phases from parenchymal tearing or as a later manifestation of more localized haematomas in which air-fluid levels can develop. Slow and gradual resolution of cavitating haematomas is usual although clinical and radiographic deterioration indicate superadded infection (Fig. 1.8.13). Traumatic pneumatocoeles may rupture into the pleural space and cause a pneumothorax.

REFERENCES

Fagan C J, Swischuk L E 1976 Traumatic lung and paramediastinal pneumatoceles. Radiology 120: 11–18
Mills S A, Johnston F R, Hudspeth A S et al 1982 Clinical spectrum of blunt tracheobronchial disruption illustrated by seven cases. Journal of Cardiovascular Surgery 84: 49–58
Sivit C J, Taylor C A, Eichelberger M R 1989 Chest injury in children with blunt abdominal trauma: evaluation with CT. Radiology 171: 815–818
Sorsdahl O A, Powell J W 1965. Cavitary pulmonary lesions following non-penetrating chest trauma in children. American Journal of Roentgenology 95: 118–124

COMPLICATIONS OF TREATMENT OF CHILDHOOD CANCER

Radiation pneumonitis

Damage to the lung is dose related. Less than 20 Gy rarely causes symptoms whereas 35 Gy or more is likely to induce radiation pneumonitis. Drugs such as bleomycin, cyclophosphamide and some other chemotherapeutic agents can potentiate the effects of radiation.

The evolution of the pneumonitis in childhood seems to have a time-course essentially similar to that seen in adults with initial radiation damage being noted at about 3 months with progressive evolution up to 2 years. Early changes include diffuse opacification in the irradiated part of the lung, often sharply demarcated corresponding to the incident field. During this phase pleural reaction is uncommon. As pulmonary fibrosis occurs in the damaged areas there is associated loss of volume and attenuation of the blood vessels which can give rise to extensive streaky shadowing. Pericardial effusion is now a very rare complication of mediastinal radiation. Although the incidence of pneumothorax in pulmonary metastasis is well established this does not appear to be related to radiation therapy.

Osteochondromas are a relatively common response to radiation therapy and may be noted on chest radiographs in the ribs, clavicle and scapula. Radiation-induced malignant bone tumours are a rare complication. Interference with normal growth and development of the spine and of the sternum can lead to kyphoscoliosis and consequent chest deformity.

The lung and antineoplastic drugs

Lung changes in children receiving chemotherapy for malignant disease may be due to a variety of causes. The primary disease may progress if the tumour is unresponsive. Opportunistic infections precipitated by neutropenia and decreased immune responses may be bacterial, viral or due to pneumocystis. The radiographic appearances are often non-specific.

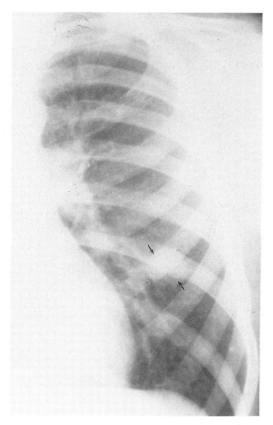

Fig. 1.8.11   Pulmonary contusion following blunt trauma (arrows).

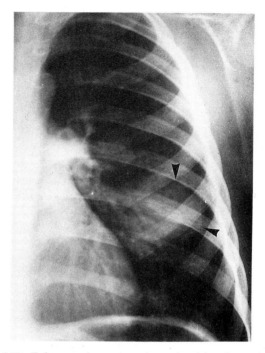

Fig. 1.8.12   Pulmonary haematoma (arrowheads) without rib fracture following a fall.

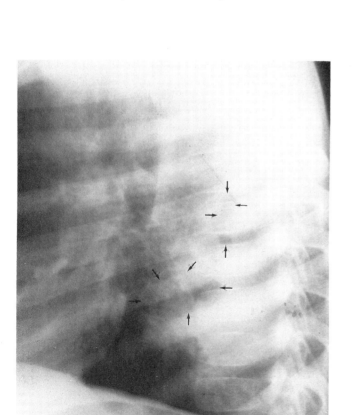

Fig. 1.8.13   Cavitating post-traumatic haematomas (arrows).

Cardiac failure from adriamycin and cyclophosphamide can be reflected in pulmonary oedema which is also caused by cytarabine. Rounded and nodular shadows in the lung fields are likely to be metastases but granulomatous conditions such as histoplasmosis, small areas of pseudotumorous rounded pneumonia, inflammatory pseudotumours and lymphoid granulomatosis are among other causes. Differentiation from metastases may depend upon percutaneous or open biopsy.

A wide variety of cytotoxic drugs can produce interstitial pneumonia and fibrosis. In particular bleomycin and methotrexate are associated with lung damage. Radiological appearances can be variable with a variety of linear, nodular and patchy shadowing more common at the bases. Though plain radiographs may be relatively unremarkable in methotrexate toxicity, changes are usually present in symptomatic patients treated with bleomycin. Lung CT demonstrates more extensive parenchymal shadowing than would be suggested from a plain radiograph. The nitrosureas and alkylating agents are also causes of pneumonitis. Although the parenchymal changes associated with pulmonary toxicity from therapeutic agents are usually reasonably symmetrical, the rarer associated pleural effusions, particularly with methotrexate, may be unilateral.

REFERENCE

Athanasion A, Leonidas J C, Hungerwider J E 1985 Iatrogenic Disorders of the Fetus, Infant and Child, vol I. 1985. Springer, Berlin, pp 339–379

DRUGS

Nitrofurantoin

Reactions to this drug can be acute or chronic. Fevers, respiratory distress and eosinophilia, which can mimic an asthmatic attack, characterize the acute response beginning within hours or up to 10 days following exposure to the drug. The radiographic features are diffuse alveolar opacification sometimes with added interstitial streaky shadowing. Pleural effusions may occur. Resolution of the changes usually follows in a day or two of stopping treatment. Chronic reaction is uncommon in children and is considerably more insidious, starting months to years after beginning treatment with the drug. The radiographic features are usually of a diffuse streaky interstitial involvement of the lungs typically without pleural effusion.

Phenytoin

Mediastinal lymphadenopathy and patchy shadowing in the lung periphery have been described in association with fever, eosinophilia and splenomegaly as a result of this drug.

Intal

This is widely used in the treatment of asthma. Occasional hypersensitivity to this drug arises. A few adult patients with eosinophilia associated with hypersensitivity have shown parenchymal patchy shadowing which disappeared following withdrawal of the drug.

Other drugs

A wide variety of medications including aspirin, penicillin, *para*-aminosalicylic acid and sulphonamides have been associated with lung infiltrates. Warfarin causes tracheal and bronchial cartilage calcification (Fig. 1.8.14).

REFERENCE

Holmberg L, Boman G, Bottiger L et al 1980 Adverse reactions to nitrofurantoin. Analysis of 921 reports. American Journal of Medicine 69: 733–738

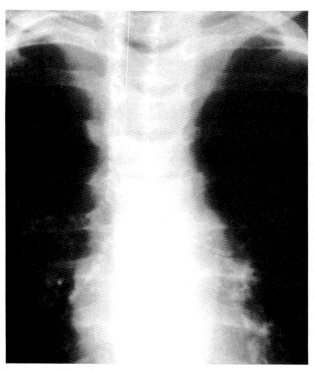

Fig. 1.8.14 Calcification of tracheobronchial cartilages due to warfarin following mitral valve replacement.

POST-PNEUMONECTOMY CHANGES

Following pneumonectomy in children the remaining lung usually shows relatively mild compensatory overinflation with a generally good clinical course, although pulmonary hypertension may occur during exercise. However the rotation and mediastinal displacement after pneumonectomy can lead to airways obstruction.

1.9 GAMUTS

Pseudotumours (Figs 1.9.1–1.9.8)

- Buckling of the trachea due to poor inspiration
- False widening of prevertebral tissues in expiration
- Ear lobes
- Posterior part of the inferior turbinate bones
- Vascular causes – ectasia of the jugular vein, high aortic arch
- Mediastinal haemorrhage associated with catheter placement
- Normal thymus
- Mediastinal fat (steroids, Cushing's syndrome)
- Prominent ductus arteriosus (hump) in newborn
- Pseudocoarctation of the aorta
- Left superior intercostal vein (aortic nipple)
- Pseudotumorous rounded pneumonia; post-inflammatory pseudotumour
- Rounded atelectasis
- Interlobar pleural effusion.

Artefactual appearances arise from catheters, endotracheal and feeding tubes, monitoring apparatus, etc.

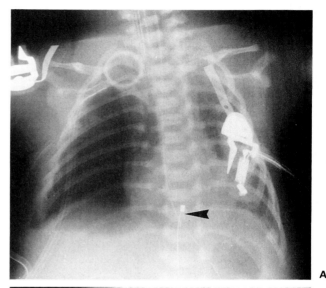

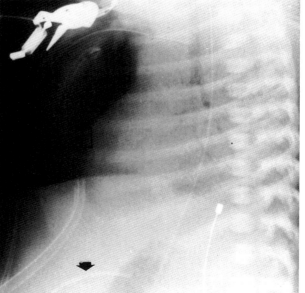

B

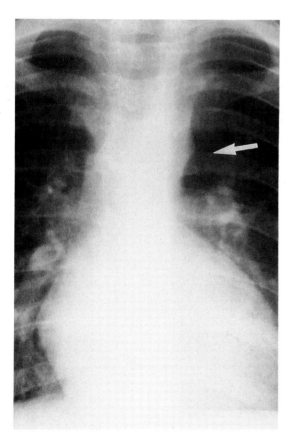

Fig. 1.9.1 Aortic nipple (arrow). This is caused by the left superior intercostal vein coursing over the aortic arch.

Fig. 1.9.2 A, B Neonate with respiratory distress undergoing intensive care. Note the numerous support aids. There is a right pneumothorax with pleural drain (open arrow). The lateral view is a horizontal decubitus view showing the anterior position of the pneumothorax. There is a nasogastric tube and endotracheal tube. An aortic oxygen electrode tip overlies the 11th dorsal vertebra (arrowhead). There is an umbilical venous catheter curved into a right hepatic vein (small arrow). Electrode monitors can be seen over the left chest and over the region of the right clavicle medially and the right upper arm.

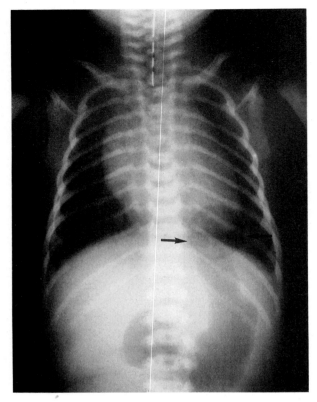

Fig. 1.9.3 Rounded radiolucency (arrow) due to a hole in the incubator. This child had oesophageal atresia and duodenal atresia.

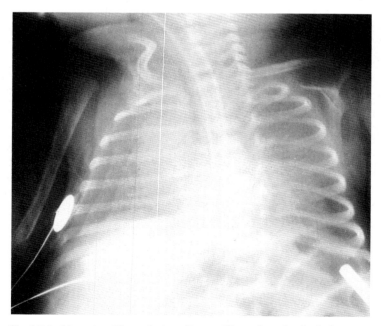

Fig. 1.9.4 Neonate with respiratory distress. The endotracheal tube lies in the oesophagus.

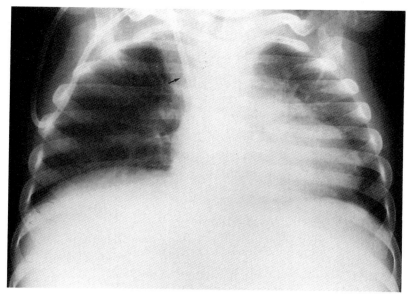

Fig. 1.9.5 Right upper mediastinal widening associated with haemorrhage induced by central venous catheter (arrow).

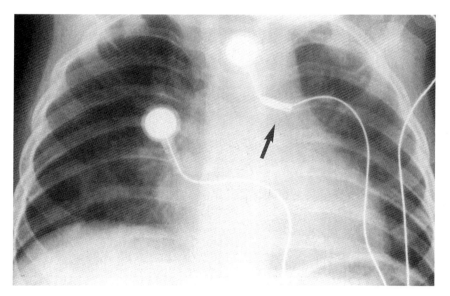

Fig. 1.9.6 A surgical clip has been put on the patent ductus arteriosus (arrow). Note monitoring electrodes.

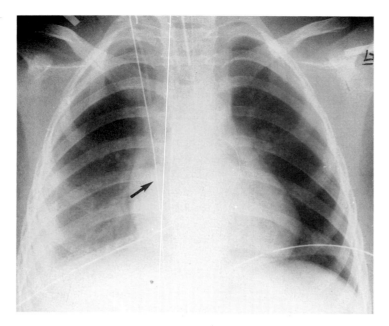

Fig. 1.9.7 Retained guide-wire following femoral venous catheterization (arrow).

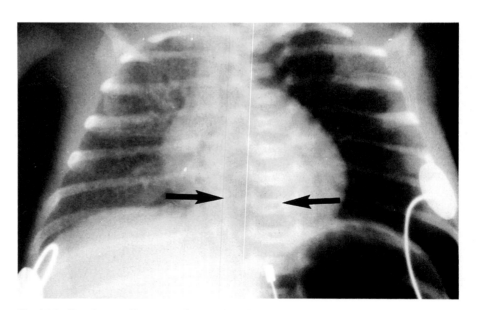

Fig. 1.9.8 Respiratory distress syndrome. Note the capacious lower oesophagus (arrows). The difference in radiolucency of the lung fields is due to rotation of the child.

Neonatal respiratory distress

- Pulmonary
— Transient tachypnoea, wet lung
— Immature lung of the extreme premature
— Hyaline membrane disease, and complications
   i.   interstitial emphysema
   ii. pneumomediastinum
   iii. pneumothorax
   iv. air embolism
   v.   pulmonary haemorrhage
   vi. bronchopulmonary dysplasia
— Wilson–Mikity syndrome
— Aspiration
— Neonatal pneumonia
— Lobar emphysema
— Atelectasia
— Lymphangiectasia
— Diaphragmatic hernia, eventration
— Diaphragmatic paresis
— Tracheobronchomalacia
- Alimentary and abdominal
— Tracheo-oesophageal fistula
— Oesophageal atresia
— Pharyngeal incoordination
— Gastro-oesophageal reflux
— Abdominal mass
— Intestinal obstruction, perforation
— Ascites
- Nasopharynx and larynx
— Haemangioma
— Micrognathia
— Cystic hygroma
— Cleft larynx
— Conradi's syndrome
— Laryngomalacia
- Skeletal
— Asphyxiating thoracic dystrophy
— Achondroplasia
— Osteogenesis imperfecta
— Myopathies
— Hypophosphatasia
— Thanatophoric dysplasia
- Tumour
— Bronchogenic cyst
— Cystic adenomatoid malformation
— Neurenteric cyst
— Teratoma, dermoid
— Neuroblastoma
- Nervous system
— Intracranial haemorrhage
— Tumour
— Meningitis
- Metabolic, etc.
— Septicaemia
— Acidosis
— Renal failure
— Anaemia, polycythaemia
— Hypoglycaemia
- Pleura
— Chylous effusion
— Empyema
— Haemothorax
- Cardiac and vascular
— Pulmonary sling
— Pulmonary hypoplasia syndromes
— Persistent fetal circulation.

Thymus

- Prominent
— Physiological
— Haemorrhage
— Lymphoma, leukaemia
— Thymoma, cyst
— Rebound following chemotherapy
- Small
— DiGeorge syndrome
      Absent parathyroids
— Immune deficiency
   i.   Thymic alymphoplasia
   ii. Wiskott–Aldrich
   iii. Agammaglobulinaemia
— Chemotherapy and other drugs, e.g. steroids
— Radiation
— Intercurrent disease
   i.   Infection
   ii. Malnutrition
   iii. Abuse
   iv. Cardiac and other debilitating disease.

Pneumomediastinum

- Postoperative
- Asthma
- Inhaled foreign body
- Perforation of oesophagus
- Rupture of trachea, bronchus, trauma
- Post-resuscitation
- Pneumoperitoneum
- Measles.

Mass between trachea and oesophagus

- Duplication cyst: bronchogenic or foregut
- Anomalous left pulmonary artery sling
- Lymph nodes
- Leiomyomatosis of oesophagus
- Hydatid cyst.

Reticular shadowing

- Pulmonary oedema
- Interstitial pneumonia
- Bronchopulmonary dysplasia
- Tuberose sclerosis, leiomyomatosis
- Lymphangiectasia: local or generalized with heart lesions
- Histiocytosis (Langerhans' cell)
- Lipoid storage disease
- Haemosiderosis, haemorrhage
- Allergic alveolitis
- Drug induced
- Lymphangitis carcinomatosa.

Intrapulmonary rounded lesion

- Tumour
— Metastasis: osteogenic and Ewing's sarcoma, Wilms' tumour, rhabdomyosarcoma
— Adenoma
— Hamartoma
— Parenchymal lymph node
- Infective
— Abscess
— Rounded pseudotumorous pneumonia
— Atelectasis
— Tuberculosis
— Fungi
— Hydatid
— Plasma cell granuloma
- Encysted pleural effusions
- Arteriovenous malformations, pulmonary varix
- Pulmonary haematoma
- Pseudotumours
— Chest wall lesions, buttons, hair
- Fluid-filled cyst
— Bronchogenic, congenital
- Parenteral alimentation
— Lipid emboli.

Cystic disease

- Congenital diaphragmatic hernia
- Late-presenting diaphragmatic hernia
- Pneumatocoele
- Lung abscess
- Cystic adenomatoid malformation
- Congenital cysts
- Bronchogenic and duplication cysts
- Bronchiectasis
- Necrotizing pneumonia
- Necrotic malignant tumour
- Sequestration
- Hydrocarbon pneumonia
- Loculated hydropneumothorax

- Hydatid cyst
- Histiocytosis (Langerhans' cell)
- Bullae
- Artefacts: e.g. hair plaits, bifid ribs.

Chest wall masses

- Lipoma
- Cystic hygroma
- Lymphangioma, haemangioma
- Rhabdomyosarcoma
- Osteochondroma
- Neurofibroma
- Mesenchymoma
- Histiocytosis
- Askin's tumour, Ewings' sarcoma
- Metastasis
— Neuroblastoma, rhabdomyosarcoma
- Leukaemia
- Haematoma
- Abscess.

Pleural effusion

- Congestive heart failure; pulmonary venous hypertension
- Hypoproteinaemia
- Nephrotic syndrome
- Chylothorax
— Pulmonary, lymphangiectasia, post-thoracotomy, congenital
- Neoplastic
— Metastasis
— Local
  i.   Lung
  ii. Chest wall
  iii. Lymphoma, leukaemia
  iv. Mediastinal mass
- Infection
— Usually bacterial
— Rarely viral
- Trauma
— Postoperative
— Lung or chest wall, rib fractures, haemothorax
- Mediastinitis, oesophageal perforation
- Vasculitis, SLE, rheumatoid
- Subphrenic abscess
- Ascites
- Pancreatitis.

Anterior mediastinal mass

- Teratoma, dermoid cyst
- Thymus, both physiological and pathological
- Lymphoma, benign lymph node enlargement
- Pericardiac and cardiac tumours

- Diaphragmatic hernia, 'morgagni'
- Mesenchymal and embryonal cell tumours
- Thyroid and parathyroid tumour
- Lipomatosis, lipoma
- Postoperative collections.

Middle mediastinal mass

- Lymph node enlargement
- Bronchogenic cyst, duplication cyst, foregut malformations
- Oesophageal dilatation
- Vascular anomalies, aneurysm
- Hiatus hernia
- Abscess
- Cystic hygroma
- Mesenchymal tumour
- Pericardial cysts.

Posterior mediastinal mass

- Neurogenic tumour
- Dural ectasia
- Neurenteric cyst
- Foregut malformations, bronchogenic cyst, duplication cyst
- Vertebral infection
- Mesenchymal tumours
- Diaphragmatic hernia
- Extramedullary haematopoiesis
- Intrathoracic kidney
- Aortic aneurysm, dilated veins (azygos systems)
- Local abscess.

Bronchiolitis obliterans

- Adenoviruses especially 3, 7 and 21
- Influenza virus
- Pertussis
- Measles
- Toxic inhalation
- Foreign bodies
- Graft-versus-host disease
- Post heart–lung transplant.

2

The heart and great vessels

M. Rubens

INTRODUCTION

INCIDENCE OF CARDIOVASCULAR DISEASE IN CHILDREN

Acquired heart disease is unusual in children under 5 years old, and is very rare under 2 years of age. Therefore, most cardiac disease in the paediatric age group is congenital. Congenital heart disease (CHD) occurs in approximately 0.75% of live births, and in approximately 25% of these cases the cardiac abnormality will be fatal within 1 year. Early diagnosis and treatment of CHD is, therefore, vital.

Most cases of CHD are due to simple malformations. Isolated ventricular septal defect (VSD) accounts for 30% of cases and patent ductus arteriosus (PDA) for 10%. Approximately two-thirds of cases of CHD seen in a paediatric cardiology clinic are due to VSD, PDA, pulmonary stenosis, ASD, coarctation of the aorta, aortic stenosis or tetralogy of Fallot. The commonest complex malformations are complete transposition of the great arteries, atrioventricular septal defect and hypoplastic left heart syndrome, which each account for 3–5% of cases.

AETIOLOGY OF CHD

Most cases of CHD occur sporadically, and are probably the result of both environmental and genetic factors. In a minority of cases definite aetiological factors may be identified. These include inherited, chromosomal and environmental factors.

Examples of CHD which behave as autosomal dominant traits include hypertrophic obstructive cardiomyopathy, supravalvar aortic stenosis, mitral valve prolapse and some cases of ASD. Marfan's syndrome, Holt–Oram syndrome and Noonan's syndrome may all exhibit cardiac defects, and also show autosomal dominant inheritance.

CHD is particularly common in Down's syndrome, trisomy 13, trisomy 18 and Turner's syndrome. Table 2.0.1 lists some inherited syndromes which may involve the cardiovascular system.

Environmental factors that predispose to CHD in the developing fetus include maternal drug taking, rubella and diabetes mellitus. The most commonly implicated drugs are alcohol, amphetamines, phenytoin, lithium, oestrogens and progestogens.

If one parent has CHD the chances of a child having CHD is 1–4%. There is also an increased incidence of CHD in children born to mothers over 40 years old.

CLINICAL PRESENTATION OF HEART DISEASE

Most cases of heart disease in infancy and childhood present as a manifestation of congestive heart failure or cyanosis or both. Cardiac failure in this age group may present as dyspnoea, tachypnoea, poor feeding, failure to thrive, abnormal weight gain despite poor feeding and cyanosis. Examination of the patient may reveal hepatomegaly and pulmonary crepitations. Cardiac murmurs may or may not be present, and the differentiation between primary cardiac or respiratory disease may, therefore, be difficult.

Conditions associated with decreased pulmonary flow usually present with cyanosis and are rarely complicated by heart failure, whereas conditions with increased flow may exhibit both cyanosis and signs of heart failure.

The age at which a lesion manifests may be of diagnostic value. The commonest congenital cardiac problems presenting in the first week of life are hypoplasia of the left heart, transposition of the great arteries, coarctation of the aorta with VSD and/or PDA and multiple complex cardiac defects.

Table 2.0.1 Inherited syndromes with associated cardiovascular abnormalities

1. Trisomy syndromes	
a. 21 (Down's syndrome)	— VSD, atrioventricular septal defect, tetralogy of Fallot
b. 18 (Edward's syndrome)	— ASD, VSD, PDA
c. 13–15 (Patau's syndrome)	— ASD, VSD, PDA
2. Turner's syndrome	— coarctation of aorta, aortic stenosis
3. Noonan's syndrome	— pulmonary valve stenosis, HOCM
4. Mucopolysaccharidoses	— cardiomyopathy, mitral regurgitation
5. Ellis–Van Creveld syndrome	— single atrium
6. Marfan's syndrome	— aortic aneurysm and dissection, aortic regurgitation, mitral regurgitation
7. Homocystinuria	— thrombosis of medium-sized arteries and veins
8. Holt–Oram syndrome	— ASD, VSD
9. Alkaptonuria	— atheroma, aortic stenosis
10. Osteogenesis imperfecta	— aortic regurgitation, mitral regurgitation

Heart failure as the presenting problem in the first week of life is likely to be due to hypoplasia of the left heart, coarctation of the aorta syndrome, severe aortic stenosis, a large arteriovenous fistula or total anomalous pulmonary venous connection with obstruction. From 1 week to 1 month heart failure indicates transposition of the great arteries, cardiomyopathy, anomalous origin of the left coronary artery or a large left-to-right shunt; and from 1 month to a year a left-to-right shunt, truncus arteriosus, total anomalous pulmonary venous connection without obstruction or cor triatriatum.

Cyanosis as the presenting sign in the first week of life is likely to be due to transposition of the great arteries, hypoplasia of the left heart, pulmonary atresia, Ebstein's anomaly, tricuspid atresia or total anomalous pulmonary venous return. From 1 week to 1 month cyanosis indicates tetralogy of Fallot, tricuspid atresia or truncus arteriosus, and older than 1 month tetralogy of Fallot or an Eisenmenger shunt.

PERINATAL HAEMODYNAMICS

Pulmonary vascular resistance in the fetus is high and the pulmonary arterial and aortic pressures are equal. In the normal fetal circulation blood shunts from right atrium to left atrium across the foramen ovale, and from pulmonary artery to descending aorta through the ductus arteriosus. The pulmonary blood flow is, therefore, very low.

At birth, as the lungs expand with air there is a dramatic fall in pulmonary vascular resistance and this leads to a massive increase in pulmonary blood flow. The pulmonary artery pressure normally falls to adult levels within 2 weeks. The foramen ovale is functionally closed at birth, and by 10–15 hours the ductus arteriosus is also functionally closed, although complete closure of the duct usually takes 2–3 weeks. The resistance of the placental circulation is low and its removal at birth causes systemic resistance to rise. Thus, soon after birth the pressures in the right side of the heart are significantly lower than those in the left side.

If, after birth, a communication persists between the two sides of the heart (and there is no obstruction to flow through the right side of the heart) then a left-to-right shunt will occur. The effects of this shunt will depend upon its site and its size. If the shunt is at atrial level the right ventricle will usually accommodate increased flow by increasing its volume and contraction, and its pressure may be normal or only mildly increased. This situation may be tolerated well for many years, until the chronically increased flow through the lungs causes pulmonary arterial hypertension and eventual elevation of right heart pressures to similar or higher levels than left heart pressure. On the other hand, a large VSD will create similar pressures in the two ventricles, and there will be both high pressure and high flow in the lungs. This situation, if untreated, is likely to lead to early irreversible pulmonary arterial hypertension. When right-sided pressure exceeds left-sided pressure the shunt reverses (i.e. becomes right-to-left), desaturated blood bypasses the lungs and cyanosis develops. This is known as Eisenmenger's syndrome, and the timing of its development depends upon the size and site of the underlying abnormality.

A SEQUENTIAL APPROACH TO CHD

Most cases of CHD are due to a single, easily described abnormality, e.g. secundum ASD or pulmonary valve stenosis. However, many cases of complex CHD do not fall into a simple category, e.g. the term tricuspid atresia does not describe if a rudimentary right ventricle is present, how the great vessels arise from the heart, or whether or not there is any obstruction to pulmonary flow. With the advent of modern surgical techniques such details are vital in planning appropriate treatment. In terms of function the relationship between the cardiac chambers and great vessels is not as important as their connections. However, relationships may have some bearing on surgical strategy. A widely accepted sequential approach to CHD has been developed (Table 2.0.2). This approach is based on defining the connections between the cardiac chambers and great vessels, then describing their relationships and finally listing any additional lesions. Before attempting to describe connections it is necessary to determine situs and to be able to recognize the morphological features of the atria and ventricles.

Table 2.0.2	Sequential segmental analysis

Atrial situs
        Solitus (or usual)
        Inversus (or mirror-image)
        Ambiguous: Right isomerism
                Left isomerism
Atrioventricular connection:
        Concordant
        Discordant
        Ambiguous (implies atrial isomerism)
        Univentricular: Absence of one AV valve
                Double inlet ventricle
Ventriculo-arterial connection
        Concordant
        Discordant
        Double outlet ventricle
        Single outlet ventricle

Situs solitus or normal situs

Normally the thoracic and abdominal viscera are asymmetrical. The liver and inferior vena cava lie to the right and the heart and spleen lie to the left. The left main bronchus is normally at least 1.5 times the length of the right main bronchus (Fig. 2.0.1). The normal right lung has three lobes and a horizontal fissure, but the left lung comprises two lobes only and no horizontal fissure. The right atrium almost always receives the inferior vena cava, and atrial situs almost always corresponds to bronchial situs.

Situs inversus

In complete situs inversus the thoracic and abdominal viscera are situated as the mirror image of normal (Fig. 2.0.2). This condition is not usually associated with serious CHD. However, if the thoracic viscera are inverted and the abdominal viscera are not, then there is a high incidence of complex CHD. This situation may be termed isolated dextrocardia. The mirror image of isolated dextrocardia is abdominal situs inversus with isolated laevocardia (Fig. 2.0.3), and is also associated with a high incidence of CHD.

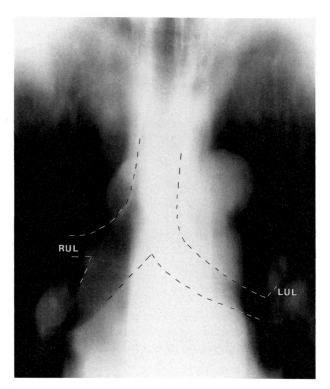

Fig. 2.0.1 Bronchial situs solitus. A tomogram of normal trachea and bronchi shows the left main bronchus to be at least 1.5 times the length of the right main bronchus. (RUL, right upper lobe; LUL, left upper lobe.)

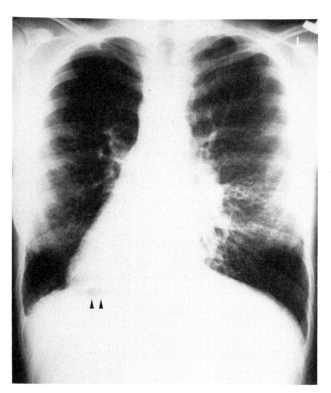

Fig. 2.0.2 Complete situs inversus. The cardiac apex, aortic knuckle and stomach (arrowheads) are all right-sided. Patient with Kartagener's syndrome – note signs of middle lobe bronchiectasis in left lung.

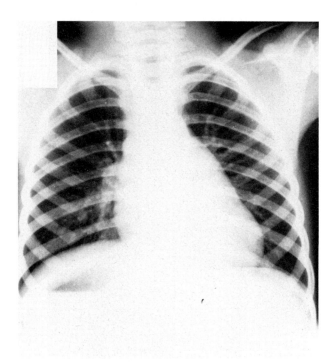

Fig. 2.0.3 Abdominal situs inversus and isolated laevocardia. Note stomach on right. Patient with polysplenia, interrupted inferior vena cava and ASD.

Situs ambiguous

In some cases thoracic or abdominal situs may not be definitely solitus or inverted, and such cases may then be described as situs ambiguous. The possible variations are bilateral right-sidedness, bilateral left-sidedness or indeterminate situs.

In bilateral right-sidedness (or right isomerism) both atria have right atrial morphology. The main bronchi are symmetrical, both having right bronchial morphology, and both are eparterial. The stomach and liver are usually midline and the spleen is usually absent (Fig. 2.0.4). Bilateral right-sidedness is often associated with transposition of the great arteries, total anomalous pulmonary venous return and pulmonary stenosis or atresia. Other cardiac defects are common. This condition, therefore, almost always presents in early infancy and long-term survival is rare. In bilateral left-sidedness (or left isomerism) both atria have left atrial morphology. The main bronchi are symmetrical, both having left bronchial morphology, and both are hyparterial (Fig. 2.0.5). The liver is often midline and there are usually multiple spleens. Bilateral left-sidedness is usually associated with interruption of the hepatic segment of the inferior vena cava. CHD is often present, but is less frequent and is of less severity than in bilateral right-sidedness.

Morphology of the cardiac chambers and great vessels

Right atrium (Fig. 2.0.6)

The morphological hallmark of the right atrium is the presence of the limbus of the fossa ovalis on its septal aspect. The right atrium is more heavily trabeculated than the left, and its appendage has a broader base. It usually receives the inferior vena cava.

Left atrium (Fig. 2.0.7)

The morphological hallmark of the left atrium is the absence of the limbus of the fossa ovalis. It is smooth walled and its appendage typically narrow based.

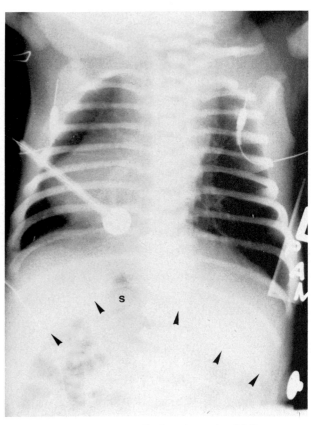

Fig. 2.0.4 Right isomerism. The liver (arrowheads) lies symmetrically across the midline. The stomach (s) is to the right of the midline. The cardiac apex is on right. Bilateral horizontal fissures were visible on the original film. Patient with asplenia.

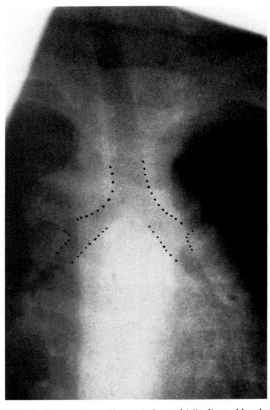

Fig. 2.0.5 Left isomerism. The main bronchi (indicated by dots) are symmetrical with left bronchial morphology.

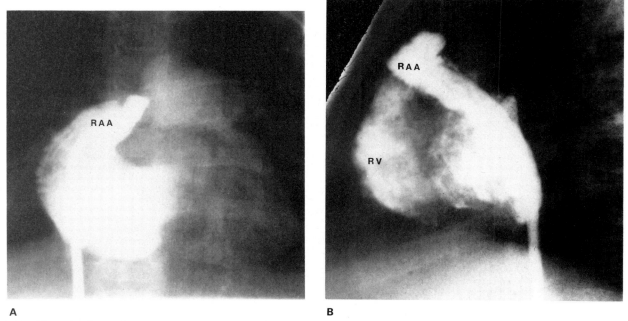

Fig. 2.0.6 Normal right atrial angiogram. AP (**A**) and lateral projections (**B**). Catheter in inferior vena cava. Note broad-based right atrial appendage (RAA). RV = right ventricle.

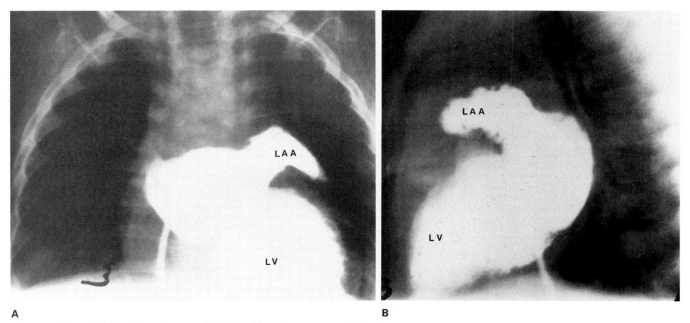

Fig. 2.0.7 Normal left atrial angiogram. AP (**A**) and lateral projections (**B**). Catheter passing from inferior vena cava into right atrium and through foramen ovale into left atrium. LAA = left atrial appendage, LV = left ventricle.

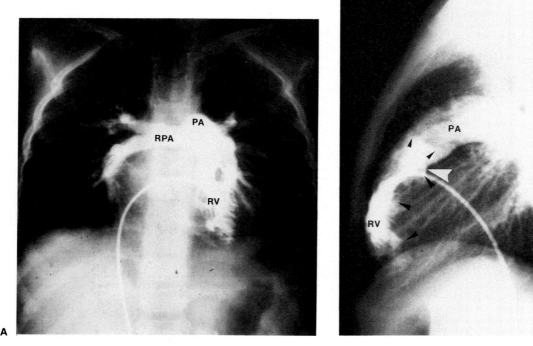

Fig. 2.0.8 Normal right ventriculogram. AP (**A**) and lateral projections (**B**). Note that in **B**, inlet and outlet valves (black arrowheads) are separated by muscular conus (white arrowhead). RV = right ventricle, PA = main pulmonary artery, RPA = right pulmonary artery.

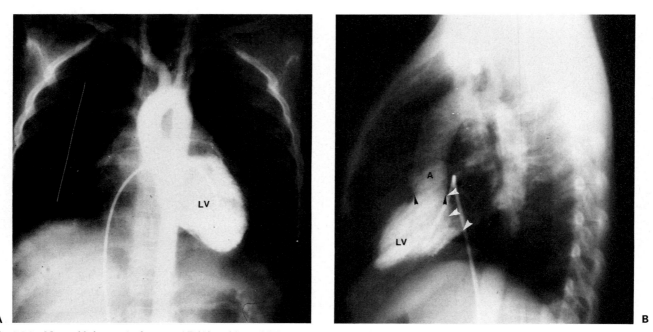

Fig. 2.0.9 Normal left ventriculogram. AP (**A**) and lateral (**B**) projections. Note that inlet and outlet valves (arrowheads) are in continuity with one another. LV = left ventricle, A = ascending aorta.

Right ventricle (Fig. 2.0.8)

The morphological hallmark of the right ventricle is separation of its inlet and outlet valves by a muscular conus or infundibulum. The septal aspect is heavily trabeculated and part of the inlet valve is attached directly to the septum by chordae tendinae of the papillary muscle.

Left ventricle (Fig. 2.0.9)

The morphological hallmark of the left ventricle is fibrous continuity between its inlet and outlet valves. The septal aspect is smooth and there is no attachment of its inlet valve to the septum.

Connections (Fig. 2.0.10)

Following identification of situs and atrial and ventricular morphology it is then necessary to determine how the central vessels and cardiac chambers are connected. Henceforth the terms right and left, when applied to a cardiac chamber, refer to morphology and not position.

The normal arrangement of the right atrium connecting to right ventricle, and left atrium connecting to left ventricle is termed atrioventricular concordance. Similarly, pulmonary artery arising from right ventricle and aorta from left ventricle is ventriculo-arterial concordance. Where the atrioventricular or ventriculo-arterial connections are the reverse of normal the connections are discordant. Thus, in transposition of the great arteries there is atrioventricular concordance, but ventriculo-arterial discordance.

When there is atrial isomerism and each atrium connects with a ventricle, one of the atria must be inappropriately connected. In this situation there is an ambiguous atrioventricular connection.

In some cases the atria connect to only one ventricle. This may be due to absence of the right atrioventricular valve (as in tricuspid atresia), absence of the left ventricular valve, or both atrioventricular valves may connect to the same ventricle, as in double inlet ventricle. These are all examples of a univentricular atrioventricular connection.

Double outlet ventricle occurs when both great arteries arise from the same ventricle. By convention, each artery is considered to arise from whichever ventricle it overrides by at least half of its diameter. Thus, in classical tetralogy of Fallot the aorta overrides the ventricular septum by less than 50%, whereas in a double outlet right ventricle the aorta overrides by more than 50%.

A single outlet heart occurs when a single artery arises from the heart as in truncus arteriosus, pulmonary atresia or aortic atresia.

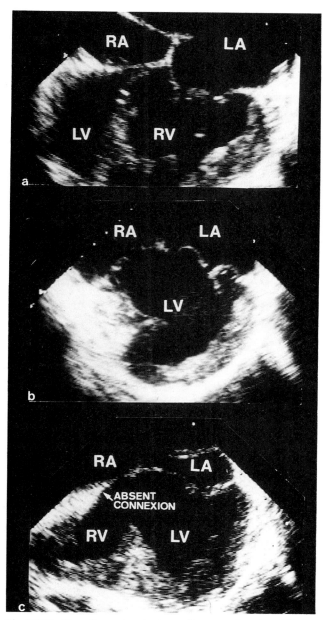

Fig. 2.0.10 Two-dimensional echocardiograms showing different types of atrioventricular connections. **A** Discordant. Patient with corrected transposition of the great arteries. The right atrium (RA) connects to the left ventricle (LV), and the left atrium (LA) connects to the right ventricle (RV). **B** Univentricular. Both atria connect with the left ventricle in double inlet left ventricle. **C** Univentricular. Absent right atrioventricular connection in tricuspid atresia. (Courtesy of Dr. A. N. Redington.)

Having described the connections it is necessary to describe the valves at atrioventricular and ventriculo-arterial level in more detail. At the atrioventricular connections there may be one or two valves. If there is only one valve the possibilities are that either one valve is absent or a common valve is present. Each valve should be assessed further to determine whether it is normal, imperforate, stenotic, prolasping, or straddling or overriding the septum. At the ventriculo-arterial connection there may be one or two valves. Aortic and pulmonary valves, if present, may be normal, imperforate, stenotic, prolapsing or overriding.

REFERENCES

Hoffman J I E, Christianson R 1978 Congenital heart disease in a cohort of 19 502 births with long-term follow-up. American Journal of Cardiology 42: 641–647

Burn J 1987 Aetiology of congenital heart disease. In: Anderson R H, Macartney F J, Shinebourne E A, Tynan M (eds) Paediatric cardiology, vol 1. Churchill Livingstone, Edinburgh, pp 15–63

Rudolph A M 1970 The changes in the circulation after birth. Circulation 41: 343–359

Shinebourne E A, Macartney F J, Anderson R H 1976 Sequential chamber localisation – logical approach to diagnosis in congenital heart disease. British Heart Journal 38: 327–340

2.1 METHODS OF INVESTIGATION

The last decade has seen remarkable changes in the investigation of cardiac disease. Formerly the chest radiograph and cardiac angiography were the main methods of imaging. However, non-invasive methods have now developed to a stage where many cases of CHD can be comprehensively diagnosed without the need for angiography.

THE CHEST RADIOGRAPH

The chest radiograph is widely available, relatively easy and cheap to perform, and if properly analysed may provide considerable diagnostic information. Consequently it remains a procedure performed in virtually all cases of suspected heart disease. A 'full cardiac series' comprising frontal, lateral and both oblique views with barium in the oesophagus is no longer current practice. A frontal film alone is usually sufficient, unless cardiomegaly is suspected, in which case a lateral film is necessary to obtain an accurate impression of cardiac volume. A barium swallow may be useful in assessing vascular anomalies, but has been superseded by echocardiography in assessing left atrial size.

Technique

In infants and young children a straight, erect AP film at end inspiration using fast screens and 60–70 kV is ideal. It may be better to take the film supine if the baby is very small or sick. A PA film should be obtained with older children.

Analysis

Technical considerations

On an overexposed film the lungs are blacker than normal and may mimic pulmonary oligaemia. Conversely, the lungs on an underexposed film may appear plethoric. On a rotated film some structures may appear abnormally prominent, and others abnormally small.

The bones

Analysis of the bony thorax may give hints about possible or likely cardiovascular disease and evidence of previous surgery (Figs 2.1.1, 2.1.10). Several of the syndromes in Table 2.0.1 may have characteristic skeletal abnormalities visible on the chest radiograph, e.g. in Down's syndrome there may be only 11 pairs of ribs (Fig. 2.1.7). In addition certain skeletal deformities may be associated with or secondary to particular cardiovascular abnormalities (Table 2.1.1).

Deformity of the thoracic cage, such as depressed sternum, may alter the appearances of the mediastinum and suggest the presence of heart disease when the heart is intrinsically normal.

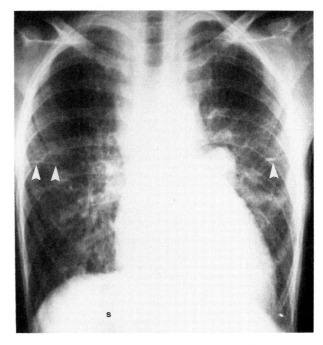

Fig. 2.1.1 Right isomerism. Bilateral rib notching relates to previous bilateral Blalock shunts. Bilateral horizontal fissures (arrowheads) and stomach (s) in midline suggest right isomerism. Patient with asplenia, pulmonary atresia and total anomalous pulmonary venous return.

Table 2.1.1

A. Skeletal abnormalities associated with cardiovascular disease:	
1. Scoliosis	— ASD, VSD, PDA, tetralogy of Fallot, pulmonary atresia
2. Straight back	— mitral valve prolapse, ASD
3. Sternal depression	— mitral valve prolapse, ASD
4. Premature sternal fusion	— ASD, VSD
5. Absent sternum	— various cardiac anomalies
6. Klippel–Feil syndrome	— VSD, coarctation of aorta
B. Skeletal abnormalities secondary to cardiovascular disease:	
1. Surgical changes in ribs or sternum	
2. Rib-notching	— coarctation of aorta, Blalock–Taussig shunt pulmonary atresia, vena caval obstruction
3. Sternal bowing	— VSD

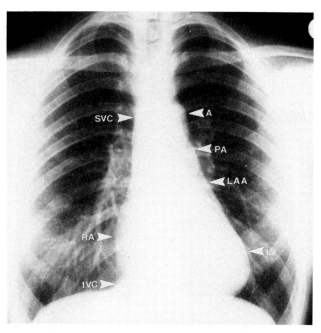

Fig. 2.1.2 Normal adolescent chest radiograph. Note symmetrical pulmonary vasculature, and lower zone vessels larger than upper zone vessels. The right side of the cardiovascular silhouette is formed by the superior vena cava (SVC), right atrium (RA) and inferior vena cava (IVC). The left side comprises aortic knuckle (A), main pulmonary artery (PA), left atrial appendage (LAA) and left ventricle (LV).

Situs

Atrial situs may be assessed by looking at the anatomy of the main bronchi (Figs. 2.0.1, 2.0.5). This may be easier on a penetrated film or a film taken with added filtration. A horizontal fissure indicates a morphological right lung (Fig. 2.1.1). The upper abdomen should be examined to assess the position of the liver, stomach and spleen (if present) (Figs. 2.0.2–2.0.4, 2.1.1). In left isomerism the azygos vein may be visibly enlarged.

The lungs

The pulmonary vasculature pattern may provide important insight into cardiovascular physiology. The pulmonary vascular pattern may be normal, increased, decreased or uneven. In normal vascularity (Fig. 2.1.2) the main pulmonary arteries are similar in diameter to the trachea, and a few vessels are visible in the peripheral thirds of the lungs. If the film is taken erect then the lower zone vessels are larger than the upper zone vessels. A normal vascular pattern is reassuring, but does not exclude a small intracardiac shunt or mild valvular disease. Moreover, in the neonate, if pulmonary vascular resistance is high, a lesion that would usually cause pulmonary plethora may not be apparent.

There are four distinct patterns of increased pulmonary vascularity:

1. Pulmonary venous hypertension (Fig. 2.1.3)
2. Pulmonary arterial hypertension (Fig. 2.1.4)
3. Pulmonary overcirculation or plethora (Fig. 2.1.5)
4. Systemic supply to the lungs (Fig. 2.1.6)

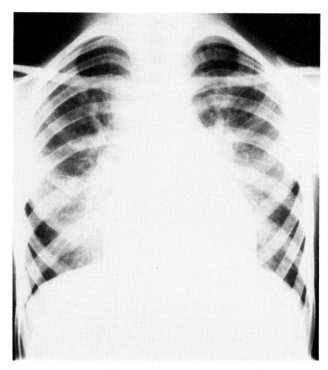

Fig. 2.1.3 Pulmonary venous hypertension. The upper zone vessels are distended and the lower zone vessels and hila are indistinct. Patient with cor triatriatum.

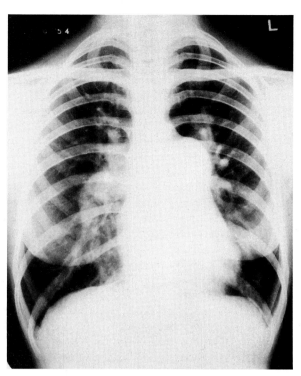

Fig. 2.1.4 Pulmonary arterial hypertension. The central pulmonary arteries are very large, and the peripheral arteries are pruned. Patient with Eisenmenger ASD.

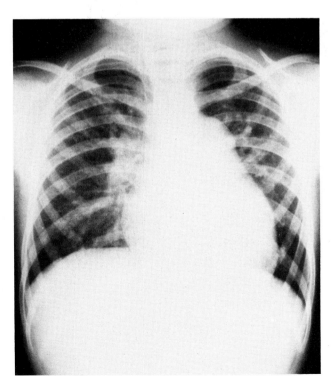

Fig. 2.1.5 Pulmonary plethora. There is enlargement of both central and peripheral pulmonary vessels. Patient with VSD and 3 : 1 left-to right shunt.

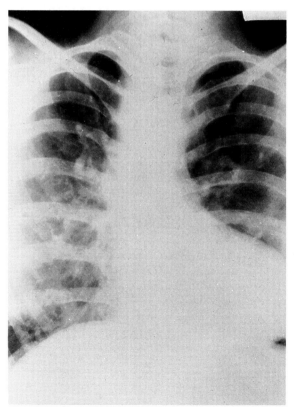

Fig. 2.1.6 Systemic supply to lungs. The main pulmonary arteries are not visible. Several large, disorganized vessels are seen at the hila. Patient with pulmonary atresia. The aortic arch is right-sided.

Pulmonary venous hypertension may be due to left ventricular failure, mitral valve disease, aortic valve disease or pulmonary venous obstruction. On an erect film there is redistribution of blood flow such that the lower zone vessels constrict and the upper zone vessels enlarge. With further increase in pulmonary venous pressure fluid accumulates in the interstitial spaces of the lung producing septal lines, peribronchial cuffing and lack of clarity of the hilar and more peripheral vessels. Subpleural fluid may cause thickening of the interlobar fissures. Further elevation of pulmonary venous pressure leads to fluid accumulating in the alveolar spaces causing alveolar oedema.

Pulmonary arterial hypertension may be secondary to pulmonary venous hypertension, lung disease, pulmonary embolism or left-to-right shunts. Occasionally it is idiopathic. The typical radiological appearance of enlargement of the central pulmonary arteries and pruning of the peripheral arteries is unusual below the age of 5 years.

Pulmonary overcirculation or plethora indicates increased flow through the lungs, and may be caused by a left-to-right shunt, a bidirectional shunt or increased cardiac output. The central pulmonary arteries are enlarged and pulmonary vessels are easily visible in the outer third of the lungs. These changes usually indicate a pulmonary-to-systemic flow ratio of at least 2:1. It is often difficult to differentiate pulmonary plethora from pulmonary venous hypertension. In plethora the lungs are often hyperinflated and vessels are usually visible projected over the diaphragm. Conversely with pulmonary venous hypertension the lungs are stiff and tend to be of smaller volume, and the lower zone vessels are constricted.

Systemic supply to the lungs occurs in severe right ventricular outflow obstruction. The pulmonary trunk is either small or absent. The peripheral vessels are disorganized with an abnormal branching pattern that may produce a reticular or nodular pattern.

Pulmonary oligaemia (Fig. 2.1.7) indicates decreased blood flow in the lungs, and is usually due to right ventricular outflow obstruction associated with a right-to-left shunt. The pulmonary trunk may be small or inapparent and the peripheral vessels are smaller and fewer than normal.

Uneven pulmonary vascularity is most often due to lung disease, but important cardiovascular causes are pulmonary embolism, previous shunt operations for CHD, pulmonary artery stenosis and pulmonary arteriovenous malformation.

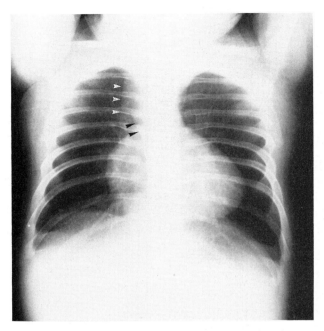

Fig. 2.1.7 Pulmonary oligaemia. The pulmonary trunk and peripheral vessels are small. Patient with tetralogy of Fallot and Down's syndrome. Only 11 pairs of ribs are present. The aortic arch (black arrowheads) is right-sided displacing the superior vena cava (white arrowheads) laterally.

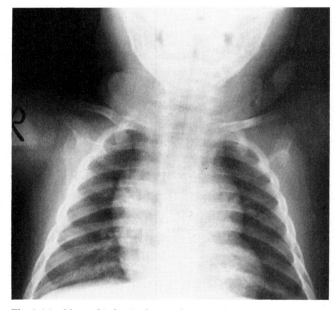

Fig. 2.1.8 Normal infant's chest radiograph. The thymus widens the superior mediastinum and obscures the superior part of the cardiovascular silhoutte.

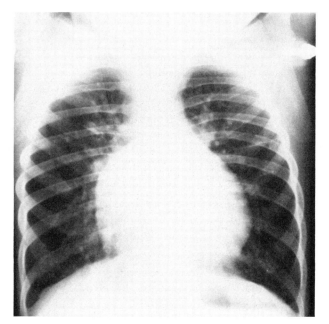

Fig. 2.1.9 Right atrial enlargement. The right heart border is more prominent than normal. The lungs are plethoric. Patient with primum ASD.

The mediastinum

The right side of the cardiovascular silhouette comprises (Fig. 2.1.2), from above downward, superior vena cava, body of right atrium and inferior vena cava. The left side comprises aortic knuckle, pulmonary trunk, left atrial appendage and left ventricle. In infancy the thymus often widens the upper mediastinum (Fig. 2.1.8).

The heart size may be assessed by using the cardiothoracic ratio, i.e. the ratio of transverse cardiac diameter to maximum internal diameter of the thorax. The normal cardiothoracic ratio in infants is up to 60%, on an AP film; by the second year, on a PA film, the ratio does not normally exceed 50%. Cardiomegaly usually indicates dilatation of one or more cardiac chambers, or pericardial effusion.

Right atrial enlargement usually occurs in association with right ventricular enlargement, with prominence of the right side of the heart shadow (Fig. 2.1.9).

Right ventricular enlargement displaces the left ventricle laterally causing elevation of the cardiac apex (Fig. 2.1.10). On the lateral view there is greater than usual contact between the anterior aspect of the heart and the sternum.

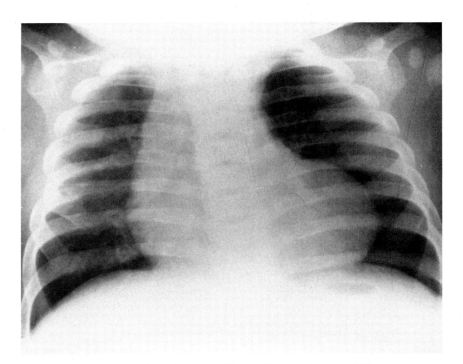

Fig. 2.1.10 Right ventricular enlargement. The cardiac apex is elevated. The pulmonary artery is not visible and there is surgical deformity of the right fifth rib. Patient with tetralogy of Fallot and right Blalock shunt.

Left atrial enlargement (Fig. 2.1.11) may displace the left main bronchus superiorly and posteriorly, and it may create an extra density over the right heart border. If barium is present in the oesophagus, it may be seen to be displaced posteriorly. Enlargement of the left atrial appendage may cause straightening or bulging of the upper left heart border. The normal confluence of the pulmonary veins may create a laterally rounded density behind the right side of the heart shadow and should not be confused with atrial enlargement.

Left ventricular enlargement causes displacement of the cardiac apex downward and to the left (Fig. 2.1.11A). On the lateral film an enlarged left ventricle may be seen to extend posteriorly.

In general, the plain radiographic signs of left atrial enlargement are more reliable than the signs for the other chambers.

The aortic arch is normally left-sided, i.e. it arches over the left bronchus. A right-sided aortic arch is often seen in association with CHD, and may be recognized by absence of a normal left arch, indentation of the right side of the trachea by the right arch and lateral displacement of the superior vena cava (Fig. 2.1.7).

ECHOCARDIOGRAPHY

Ultrasound examination has become the most important diagnostic investigation in suspected or known paediatric cardiac disease. It can provide detailed and accurate data on both anatomy and function of the heart and great vessels, and is painless, harmless and relatively inexpensive. It is more operator dependent than other imaging methods used in cardiology. A complete examination may involve cross-sectional, M-mode and Doppler scans.

Cross-sectional (or two-dimensional) echocardiography

Cross-sectional echocardiography provides a two-dimensional view of the heart. By scanning in different planes the anatomy of the heart and great vessels is seen, and their connections can be elucidated. Real-time scanning allows assessment of function of the cardiac chambers and valves, and facilitates M-mode and Doppler examinations.

The heart is scanned in three orthogonal planes:

1. The long axis view (Fig. 2.1.12) is usually achieved by placing the transducer over the 4th left

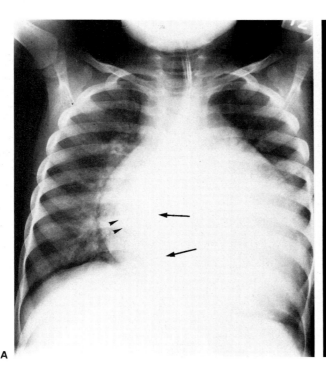

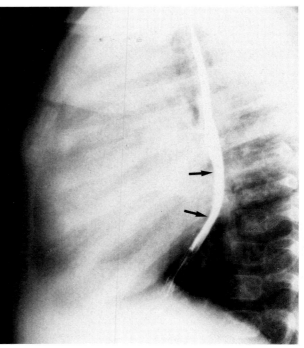

A **B**

Fig. 2.1.11 Left atrial enlargement. **A** There is generalized cardiomegaly, but in particular an extra density is visible over the right heart border (arrowheads), and the barium-filled oesophagus is displaced to the right (arrows). The lungs show signs of pulmonary venous hypertension. Patient with congestive cardiomyopathy. **B** Lateral film of patient with VSD shows posterior displacement of barium-filled oesophagus by enlarged left atrium (arrows).

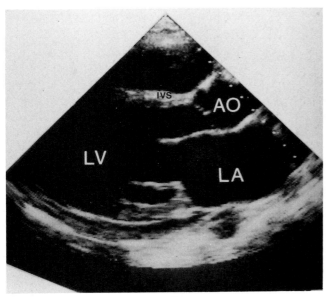

Fig. 2.1.12 Normal parasternal long axis two-dimensional echocardiogram. AO = aortic root, LA = left atrium, LV = left ventricle, IVS = interventricular septum. (Courtesy of Dr M. St. J. Sutton.)

intercostal space immediately lateral to the sternum, and aligning the sector between cardiac apex and aortic root. It provides visualization of the left ventricle, part of the right ventricle, the interventricular septum, left atrium and aortic and mitral valves.

2. The short axis view may be achieved by placing the transducer over the 4th left intercostal space, as for the long axis view, and then rotating it 90°. In this plane the ventricles are seen in cross-section, and by angulating the transducer the heart may be viewed at the level of the aortic valve, the mitral valve or the papillary muscles. At the level of the aortic valve, the right ventricular outflow is seen anteriorly and the atria and interatrial septum are seen posterior to the aorta (Fig. 2.1.13).

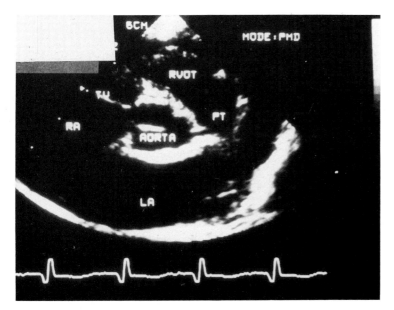

Fig. 2.1.13 Normal parasternal short axis two-dimensional echocardiogram at level of aortic valve. RVOT = right ventricular outflow tract, PT = pulmonary trunk, LA = left atrium, RA = right atrium, TV = tricuspid valve. (Courtesy of Dr A. N. Redington.)

3. The four-chamber view may be obtained by placing the transducer over the cardiac apex or by scanning from the subcostal position. It demonstrates both ventricles, both atria, the interventricular and interatrial septa and the tricuspid and mitral valves (Fig. 2.1.14).

The standard views are merely a guide, and in any individual patient it may be necessary to alter the transducer position and angulation depending on the findings and the information that is required.

The suprasternal view is used to visualize the aortic arch and its branches (Fig. 2.1.15).

Transoesophageal echocardiography is not used routinely in paediatric practice, but it allows particularly good visualization of the atria, the atrial septum, the atrioventricular valves, pulmonary veins and the aorta.

M-mode echocardiography

M-mode scanning has been largely superseded by two-dimensional scanning, but is still used to assess left ventricular function and movement of the valves.

Doppler echocardiography

Doppler scanning allows the detection of blood flow within the heart and great vessels. It is possible to determine accurately the site of blood flow, its direction and velocity and whether or not the flow is turbulent. Valvular stenosis and regurgitation can be measured and intracardiac shunting may be identified and assessed.

Pulsed Doppler allows accurate sampling of small volumes at precise locations within the heart, provided the velocity is not high. Continuous wave Doppler allows measurement of high velocities along its path but depth resolution is poor. Colour flow mapping combines pulsed Doppler and two-dimensional scans, superimposing the Doppler information on the two dimensional image (Fig. 2.1.16), with different colours representing flow towards and away from the transducer.

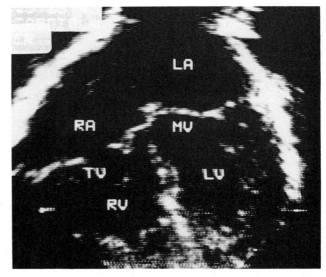

Fig. 2.1.14 Normal apical four-chamber two-dimensional echocardiogram. RA = right atrium, TV = tricuspid valve, RV = right ventricle, LA = left atrium, MV = mitral valve, LV = left ventricle. (Courtesy of Dr A. N. Redington.)

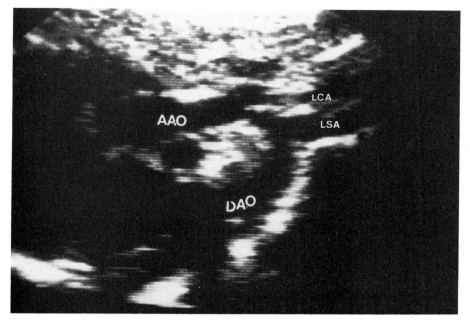

Fig. 2.1.15 Normal suprasternal two-dimensional echocardiogram of aortic arch. AAO = ascending aorta, DAO = descending aorta, LCA = left common carotid artery, LSA = left subclavian artery. (Courtesy of Dr A. N. Redington.)

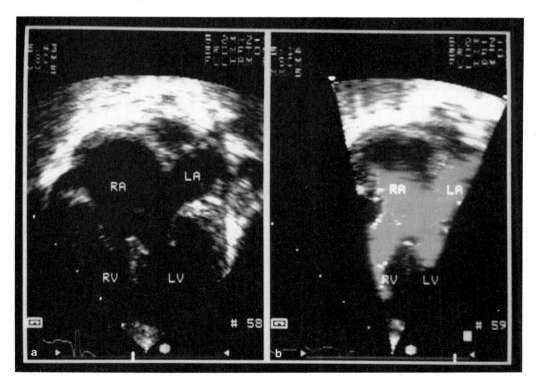

Fig. 2.1.16 **A,B** Colour-flow Doppler echocardiogram showing flow across a large primum ASD. RA = right atrium, LA = left atrium, RV = right ventricle, LV = left ventricle.

CARDIAC MAGNETIC RESONANCE IMAGING (MRI)

MRI can provide detailed anatomical and haemodynamic data which is in many respects similar to that obtained by echocardiography. Sectional images through the heart and great vessels may be displayed in any plane (Fig. 2.1.17). Ventricular function may be accurately assessed (Fig. 2.1.18). Flowing blood is easily identified, and its velocity and direction can be measured. There is natural contrast between the soft tissues and blood so that contrast media are not required. Data are degraded by movement, but ECG-gating enables data to be collected over several cardiac cycles. Therefore, it is necessary to sedate restless patients. Unlike with echocardiography the surrounding lungs do not prevent imaging the entire mediastinum, so that MRI is useful for assessing subjects in whom ultrasound results are technically poor.

The main disadvantages of MRI are its expense and the time required to perform the examination, often about 1 hour. Some patients become claustrophobic in the scanner. An irregular heart rate is a relative contraindication to MRI. An implanted pacemaker is an absolute contraindication, but most implanted surgical clips are non-ferromagnetic and do not present a problem.

MRI is an excellent method of defining cardiac anatomy and connections. Its ability to image the entire aorta may be used to show vascular rings.

Surgically created shunts may be assessed for patency non-invasively. MRI is also an excellent method of assessing the extent and severity of heart muscle disease, intracardiac masses and pericardial disease, although it cannot detect calcification. Functionally, MRI can identify and quantify flow across intracardiac shunts and regurgitation through valves.

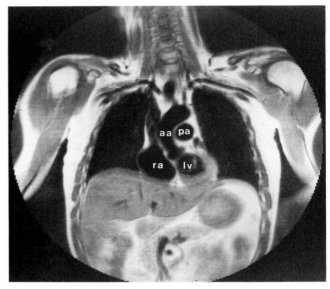

Fig. 2.1.17 Normal coronal MRI scan. ra = right atrium, aa = ascending aorta, pa = main pulmonary artery, lv = left ventricle.

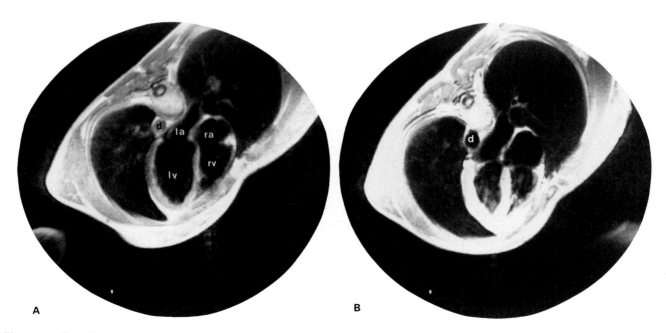

Fig. 2.1.18 Four-chamber MRI scan. **A** Ventricular diastole. **B** Ventricular systole. Note change in signal in descending aorta. la = left atrium, lv = left ventricle, ra = right atrium, rv = right ventricle, d = descending aorta.

CARDIAC COMPUTED TOMOGRAPHY (CT)

CT is an excellent method of assessing the pericardium (Fig. 2.1.19). To assess the heart and great vessels, however, it is necessary to use intravenous contrast medium. Cross-sectional images and reconstruction in other planes are both helpful. Where MRI is unavailable, CT is useful for assessing the aorta, vascular rings and myocardial disease.

Ultrafast-CT scanners now available have many advantages over conventional CT scanners. Scanning time is significantly shorter, e.g. two sections may be scanned in 50 milliseconds, or in the ciné mode, two levels may be scanned simultaneously at 17 frames per second (Fig. 2.1.20). In addition the scanner table may be slewed so that long or short axis sections through the heart may be scanned. The scanning time is so fast that sedation is only rarely necessary. The ciné mode gives functional data that cannot be obtained on conventional CT scanners.

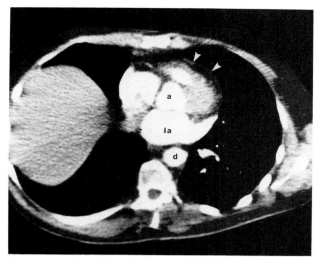

Fig. 2.1.19 Contrast-enhanced ciné CT scan. Part of the pericardium is seen (arrowheads) over the right ventricular outflow tract. a = aortic root, la = left atrium, d = descending aorta.

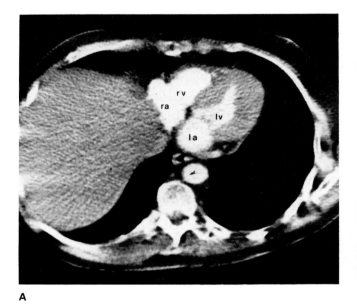

A

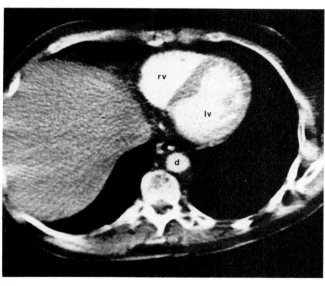

B

Fig. 2.1.20 Contrast-enhanced coné CT scans through ventricles during systole (**A**) and diastole (**B**). ra = right atrium, rv = right ventricle, la = left atrium, d = descending aorta.

CARDIAC CATHETERIZATION

The majority of paediatric cardiac abnormalities can be accurately assessed non-invasively, on the basis of the history, clinical examination, electrocardiogram, chest radiograph and echocardiogram. Cardiac catheterization is now performed to resolve specific questions concerning anatomy or physiology which have not been answered non-invasively, or as part of a therapeutic procedure. The operability of many cardiac lesions depends upon the level of pulmonary vascular resistance, and this can only be determined accurately by catheterization. Coronary artery anatomy can be completely assessed only by angiography, and it is also the most reliable method of assessing the pulmonary blood supply in most cases of pulmonary atresia. If angiography is being performed to demonstrate an anatomical point, it is important that the most appropriate projection is used, e.g. if it is required to demonstrate a defect or defects in the muscular interventricular septum, then a long axial oblique projection should be used, since this profiles the septum.

Angiography provides excellent spatial and temporal resolution, but is associated with significant morbity and mortality in sick infants. Low osmolarity contrast media should be used. The use of digital subtraction angiography enables production of diagnostic images with smaller amounts of contrast medium, although the temporal and spatial resolution is inferior to ciné film.

Percutaneous therapeutic procedures are being increasingly used in paediatric heart disease. Balloon atrial septostomy for palliation of transposition of the great arteries has been performed since 1966. Balloon valvuloplasty is now regarded as the treatment of choice for isolated pulmonary valve stenosis, and may also be used to dilate other valves. Other sites where balloon angioplasty may be used are coarctation of the aorta (both unoperated and recurrent), superior and inferior vena caval obstruction following Mustard's operation for transposition of the great vessels, pulmonary artery stenoses and stenosed Blalock–Taussig shunts. Detachable balloons, umbrellas and coils may be used to close PDA, ASD, systemic collaterals to the lungs and arteriovenous malformations.

NUCLEAR ANGIOGRAPHY

The main use of radionuclide scanning in paediatric heart disease is to assess intracardiac shunting. This is usually achieved by a first-pass study using $^{99}Tc^m$-labelled pertechnetate or DTPA. Following a rapid intravenous injection of a bolus of radionuclide, the sequence in which activity appears in the various cardiac chambers and great vessels will show whether or not intracardiac shunting exists; and the amount of shunting, if present, may be quantified.

By labelling erythrocytes with technetium-99m, multigated equilibrium (MUGA) studies may be performed for assessment of ventricular function, particularly in cardiomyopathy and after cardiotoxic drugs such as adriamycin.

REFERENCES

Bank E R, Hernandez R J 1988 CT and MR of congenital heart disease. Radiologic Clinics of North America 26: 241–262

Elliott L P, Bargeron L M, Soto B et al 1980 Axial cineangiography in congenital heart disease. Radiologic Clinics of North America 18: 515

Elliot L P, Schiebler G L 1979 The X-ray dignosis of congenital heart disease in infants, children and adults, 2nd edn. Charles C Thomas, Springfield, Illinois

Freedom R M, Culham J A G, Moes C A F 1984 Angiocardiography of congenital heart disease. Macmillan, New York

Leung M P, Mok C K, Lau K C et al 1986 The role of cross sectional echocardiography and pulsed Doppler ultrasound in the management of neonates in whom congenital heart disease is suspected. British Heart Journal 56: 73–82

Rees S 1990 The George Simon Lecture: magnetic resonance studies of the heart. Clinical Radiology 42: 302–316

Silverman N H, Snider A R 1982 Two dimensional echocardiography in congenital heart disease. Appleton-Century-Crofts, Norwalk

Steiner R, Flicker S, Eldredge J et al 1986 The functional and anatomic evaluation of the cardiovascular system with rapid acquisition computed tomography (cine CT). Radiologic Clinics of North America 24: 503

Verel D, Grainger R G 1978. Cardiac catheterisation and angiocardiography, 3rd edn. Churchill Livingstone, Edinburgh

2.2 PULMONARY PLETHORA WITHOUT CYANOSIS

Pulmonary plethora in a non-cyanosed patient indicates left-to-right intracardiac shunting. This may be due to a shunt at atrial level, ventricular level, great vessel level or at more than one level.

ATRIAL LEVEL SHUNTS

Approximately 10% of cases of CHD are accounted for by ASDs, of which most are ostium secundum defects, and the remainder are ostium primum, sinus venosus and coronary sinus defects. Ostium primum defects are part of the spectrum of ASDs and are discussed under that heading.

Ostium secundum ASD

This defect is caused by a deficiency in the fossa ovale due to failure of the septum secundum to obliterate the ostium secundum. The septum primum lies between the defect and the atrioventricular valves (Fig. 2.2.1).

In early infancy the compliance, and therefore filling pressures, of the right and left ventricles are similar. At this time, therefore, no significant shunting occurs across an ASD. However, as pulmonary vascular resistance falls, right ventricular pressure decreases leading to a decrease in right atrial pressure and left-to-right shunting across the atrial septum. The size of the shunt depends upon the size of the defect and the right atrial pressure.

It is unusual for an isolated ASD to present in infancy or childhood, unless the defect is large. A large defect may cause tiredness, exertional dyspnoea and frequent chest infections. A more usual presentation in childhood or adolescence is the incidental discovery of a murmur on routine examination. In later life an untreated ASD may present with atrial dysrhythmia, right heart failure or pulmonary arterial hypertension. There is an association between secundum ASD and mitral valve prolapse, and in approximately 15% of cases there is partial anomalous pulmonary venous return.

The chest radiograph may be normal if the shunt is small. Larger shunts will show pulmonary plethora and signs of right atrial and ventricular enlargement (Fig. 2.2.2). In adulthood signs of pulmonary arterial hypertension may develop (Fig. 2.1.4).

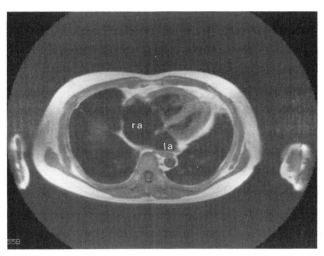

Fig. 2.2.1 Ostium secundum ASD. MRI scan shows the defect above the intact septum primum. ra = right atrium, la = left atrium.

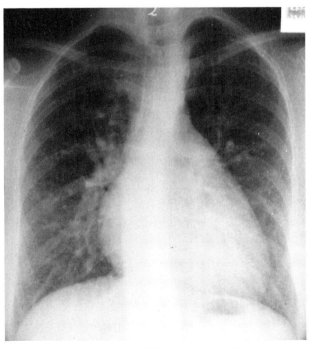

Fig. 2.2.2 Ostium secundum ASD in adolescent. There is pulmonary plethora, a prominent pulmonary trunk and mild cardiomegaly. The shape of the heart is consistent with right heart enlargement. There is also a mild dorsal scoliosis.

Cross-sectional echocardiography in the four-chamber view (Fig. 2.2.3) will differentiate the various ASDs from one another, and the shunt may be demonstrated by Doppler. Similar information may be obtained by MRI (Fig. 2.2.1), or nuclear angiography.

Cardiac catheterization is rarely necessary, but will show a rise in oxygen saturation in the right atrium and similar atrial pressures.

Sinus venosus ASD

This defect is in the superior, posterior portion of the atrial septum close to the insertion of the superior vena cava. It is usually associated with anomalous drainage of the right upper lobe pulmonary vein into the right atrium. The anomalous vein may be visible on the plain film.

Coronary sinus defect

This rare anomaly occurs when a defect in the roof of the coronary sinus causes communication between the coronary sinus and the left atrium.

Partial anomalous pulmonary venous return

Approximately 50% of cases of partial anomalous pulmonary venous return are associated with CHD. This is usually an ASD. In secundum defects the anomalous veins usually drain the lower part of the right lung to the inferior vena cave or right atrium (Fig. 2.2.4). The anomalous pulmonary venous return in sinus venosus defects is described above.

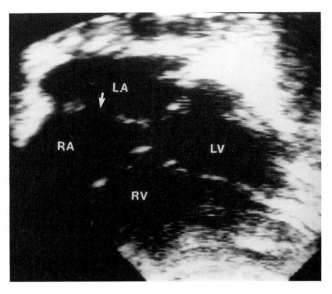

Fig. 2.2.3 Ostium secundum ASD (arrow). Two-dimensional echocardiogram, four-chamber view. RA = right atrium, LA = left atrium, RV = right ventricle, LV = left ventricle. (Courtesy of Dr A. N. Redington.)

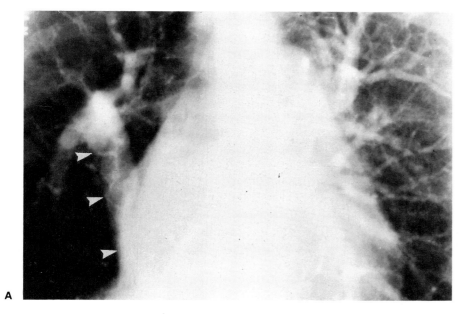

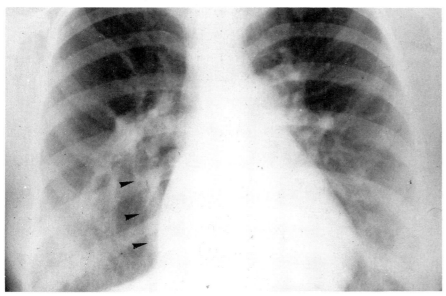

Fig. 2.2.4 Ostium secundum ASD with partial anomalous pulmonary venous return. **A** The chest radiograph shows pulmonary plethora and a vertical band shadow (arrowheads) to the right of the heart. **B** The venous phase of the pulmonary arteriogram shows that the band shadow is an anomalous pulmonary vein (arrowheads) draining to the junction of the inferior vena cava and right atrium.

When partial anomalous venous return occurs as an isolated lesion it again usually involves the right lung, and the anomalous vein may connect with the superior or inferior vena cava, the right atrium, or more rarely with the coronary sinus or azygos vein. Connection with the inferior vena cava may be by a large scimitar-shaped vein that descends through the right lower thorax (Fig. 2.2.5). This may be associated with hypoplasia of the right lung and abnormal systemic arterial supply to the right lung.

Although partial anomalous pulmonary venous return causes a left-to-right shunt, it is rarely of haemodynamic significance. However, the presence of anomalous vessels, and their site of drainage may be of importance when surgical repair of an associated cardiac defect is planned.

With the exception of the scimitar shadow, anomalous veins are difficult to see on the chest radiograph. Anomalous veins may be identified by echocardiography or MRI, but if there is doubt about identifying all of the pulmonary veins then angiography may be necessary.

ATRIOVENTRICULAR SEPTAL DEFECT

The inferior part of the interatrial septum is derived from the septum primum. It is continuous with the base of the interventricular septum. Absence of this part of the atrioventricular septum may occur with or without developmental defects of the atrioventricular valves. The various malformations that may occur are currently known as atrioventricular defects and were previously known as endocardial cushion or atrioventricular canal defects. They may be classified as partial, intermediate or complete atrioventricular septal defects:

• A partial atrioventricular defect comprises a defect in the septum primum, and is often termed an ostium primum ASD (Fig. 2.1.16). It is almost always associated with a cleft in the anterior leaflet of the mitral valve.

• A complete atrioventricular defect comprises defects in the septum primum and upper interventricular septum with a common atrioventricular valve (Fig. 2.2.6). This was formerly known as a complete atrioventricular canal.

• In the intermediate form tethering of valve tissue to the crest of the ventricular septum limits the size of the interventricular defect (Fig. 2.2.7).

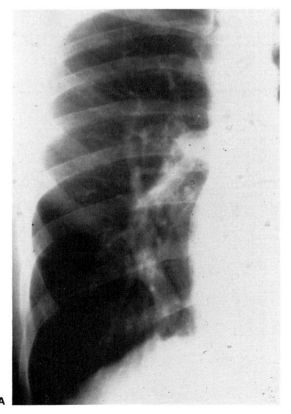

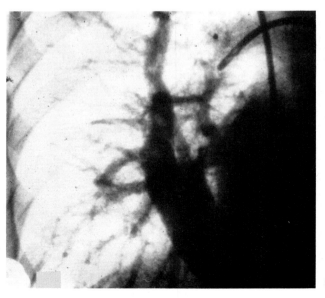

Fig. 2.2.5   Isolated partial anomalous pulmonary venous drainage. **A** The chest radiograph shows a scimitar shadow in the right lower zone. **B** The venous phase of a pulmonary arteriogram shows that the scimitar shadow is due to an anomalous pulmonary vein draining to the inferior vena cava.

Partial atrioventricular septal defect or ostium primum defect

Approximately 20% of ASDs involve the ostium primum. The defect is situated immediately above the atrioventricular valves (Fig. 2.1.16). There is almost always a cleft in the anterior leaflet of the mitral valve, which may cause mitral regurgitation, the degree of which varies from trivial to severe. Regurgitant blood may pass directly from the left ventricle into the right atrium via the septal defect. Occasionally there is a cleft in the tricuspid valve.

The presentation of a partial atrioventricular septal defect depends upon the degree of mitral regurgitation. If the mitral valve is competent the clinical picture is similar to that of an ostium secundum ASD, except that the electrocardiogram will usually show left axis deviation. When there is significant mitral regurgitation, symptoms may occur in childhood and include fatigue, dyspnoea, frequent chest infections and congestive cardiac failure.

The chest radiograph may be similar to a secundum defect, but if the mitral valve is incompetent the signs of pulmonary plethora and right heart enlargment may be more severe (Fig. 2.1.9), and there may also be evidence of left ventricular enlargement and heart failure. Untreated cases develop signs of pulmonary arterial hypertension.

The defect is best demonstrated by two-dimensional echocardiography in the four-chamber view (Fig. 2.1.16). This will show the ASD immediately above the atrioventricular valves, and will demonstrate any abnormality of the atrioventricular valves.

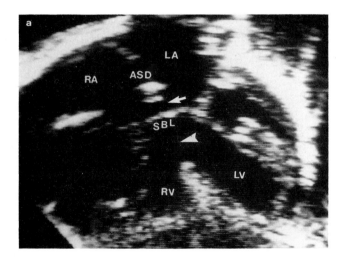

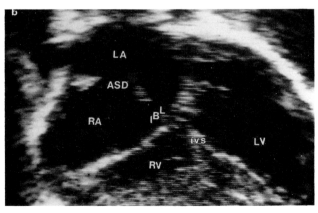

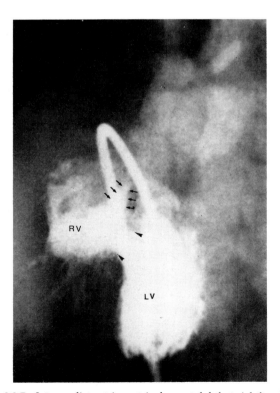

Fig. 2.2.6 Complete atrioventricular septal defect. This patient also has a secundum ASD. Four-chamber two-dimensional echocardiograms. **A** The interatrial component of the defect (arrow) lies above the superior bridging leaflet (SBL) of the common atrioventricular valve, and the interventricular component of the defect (arrowhead) lies below this leaflet. **B** The inferior bridging leaflet (IBL) of the common valve is attached to the crest of the interventricular septum (IVS). RA = right atrium, RV = right ventricle, LA = left atrium, LV = left ventricle. (Courtesy of Dr A. N. Redington.)

Fig. 2.2.7 Intermediate atrioventricular septal defect. A left ventriculogram in the four-chamber projection shows a small interventricular defect (arrowheads). Contrast medium is seen trapped (arrows) by chordae which tether bridging leaflet tissue to the interventricular septum. RV = right ventricle, LV = left ventricle.

The atrioventricular valves are attached to the crest of the interventricular septum, and occasionally a small ventricular septal defect is seen. The right atrium and ventricle are enlarged. Doppler studies may be used to identify and quantify the left-to-right shunting and mitral regurgitation.

Angiocardiography is not usually necessary but the defect can be demonstrated by injecting contrast medium into the right upper pulmonary vein and recording images in the four-chamber view. A left ventriculogram may be used to assess accurately the mitral regurgitation.

Complete atrioventricular septal defect

Approximately 30% of patients with complete atrioventricular septal defect have Down's syndrome. Complete atrioventricular septal defect usually presents in early infancy with symptoms due to congestive heart failure. There is left-to-right shunting at atrial and ventricular levels and the atrioventricular valves are almost always incompetent. Pulmonary arterial hypertension frequently occurs. As pulmonary vascular resistance increases pulmonary flow decreases and cyanosis develops.

The appearance of the chest radiograph depends upon the degree of intracardiac shunting and the severity of valvular regurgitation. Usually there is pulmonary plethora, often with superimposed signs of pulmonary venous hypertension, and generalized cardiomegaly.

Two-dimensional echocardiography in the four-chamber view (Fig. 2.2.6) demonstrates the interatrial and interventricular septal defects, and also the atrioventricular valve morphology.

Cardiac catheterization is necessary to assess pulmonary vascular resistance if surgery is contemplated. Cardiac angiography is unnecessary but a left ventriculogram in the four-chamber projection will show the septal defects and atrioventricular valve morphology. An AP left ventriculogram will show the typical 'goose-neck' appearance of the left ventricular outflow tract.

VENTRICULAR LEVEL SHUNTS

Ventricular septal defect (VSD) may occur in isolation, or in association with other congenital cardiac defects (such as ASD, pulmonary valve stenosis and coarctation of the aorta), or as an integral part of a more complex malformation (such as tetralogy of Fallot, double outlet ventricle, or truncus arteriosus). This section describes isolated VSD.

The currently favoured classification of isolated VSD requires some knowledge of the anatomy of the interventricular septum. The septum comprises a small membranous portion and a much larger muscular portion. The muscular septum comprises inlet, trabecular and outlet portions, which respectively separate the inlet, apical and outflow portions of the two ventricles. The three components of the muscular septum fan out from the membranous septum, which is situated where the tricuspid, mitral and aortic valves are in fibrous continuity. VSDs are classified as follows.

Perimembranous defects

Most VSDs occur in the membranous septum (Fig. 2.2.8). They almost always extend beyond the membranous septum and into the muscular septum and therefore are best called perimembranous. Posterior extension into the inlet septum produces an inlet defect (Fig. 2.2.9), anterior extension below the aortic root produces an outlet defect, and extension into the trabecular septum produces a trabecular defect. A confluent perimembranous defect involves all three parts of the muscular septum.

Muscular defects

Muscular defects are surrounded entirely by muscle (Fig. 2.2.10). They may occur in any part of the muscular septum and are termed inlet, trabecular or outlet defects. Muscular defects may be single or multiple.

Doubly committed subarterial defects

These defects, also known as supracristal defects, are situated directly beneath the aortic and pulmonary valves.

A left ventricle-to-right atrial communication

This is known as a Gerbode defect, and develops if there is a defect in that part of the septum which separates the left ventricle and right atrium close to the tricuspid valve (Fig. 2.2.11).

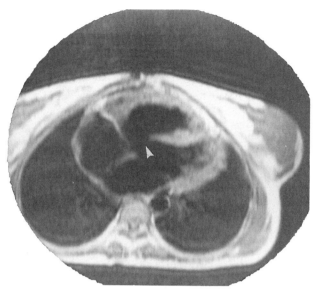

Fig. 2.2.8 Perimembranous ventricular septal defect. MRI scan shows the defect (arrowhead) just below the tricuspid valve.

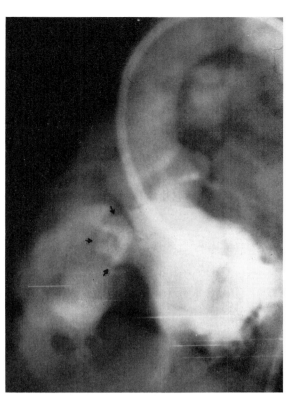

Fig. 2.2.9 Perimembranous ventricular septal defect. Left ventriculogram in left anterior oblique projection shows an inlet defect which has partly closed, producing an 'aneurysm' (arrows) of the interventricular septum.

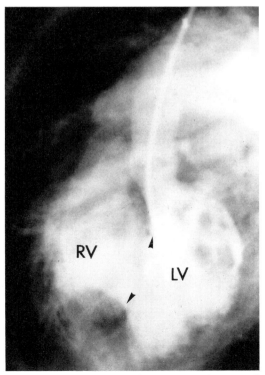

Fig. 2.2.10 Muscular ventricular septal defect. Left ventriculogram in left anterior oblique projection shows a large trabecular defect (arrowheads). RV = right ventricle, LV = left ventricle.

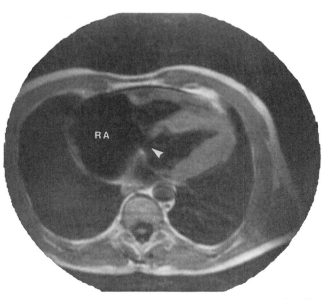

Fig. 2.2.11 Gerbode defect. MRI scan shows a defect (arrowhead) allowing direct communication between the left ventricle and right atrium (RA), which is enlarged.

The natural history of a VSD depends upon its size and location. Inlet perimembranous VSDs often close spontaneously, usually by adhesion of tricuspid valve tissue to the margin of the defect. This may create a so-called aneurysm of the interventricular septum (Fig. 2.2.9). Muscular VSDs may close spontaneously by hypertrophy of the adjacent myocardium.

Subarterial defects and outlet muscular defects may be associated with prolapse of the right coronary cusp of the aortic valve and cause aortic regurgitation.

The clinical presentation depends upon the size of the defect and the pulmonary vascular resistance. Small defects are often asymptomatic, and are discovered as a pansystolic murmur on routine examination. Larger defects do not usually cause symptoms until a month or so after birth, when pulmonary vascular resistance has fallen, allowing significant left-to-right shunting to occur. At this time the patient may develop feeding difficulties, breathlessness, chest infections and heart failure. Very large defects may cause heart failure within 2 or 3 weeks of birth.

Approximately 70% of VSDs will close spontaneously. When a large defect does not close, infundibular stenosis may develop, but more usually pulmonary arterial hypertension. Either of these will, in the first instance, limit pulmonary blood flow and improve symptoms. However, if pulmonary hypertensive changes become irreversible, then an Eisenmenger complex will eventually develop. In a small minority of patients with large VSDs pulmonary vascular resistance does not fall after birth. These patients may be asymptomatic until late childhood, when they present with cyanosis.

The chest radiograph of patients with small VSDs is usually normal. In approximately 3% of cases of isolated VSD the aortic arch is right-sided. Pulmonary plethora is usually visible when the ratio of pulmonary to systemic flow is greater than 2 : 1 (Fig. 2.2.12). With larger shunts there may be evidence of heart failure and enlargement of the left atrium and both ventricles. If pulmonary arterial hypertension has developed the peripheral pulmonary vascular pattern is attenuated.

Echocardiography is used to assess VSDs. Two-dimensional scanning will identify most defects and any associated abnormalities (Fig. 2.2.13). Small or multiple defects may be missed on two-dimensional scanning, but can usually be detected by Doppler scanning and colour flow mapping. With small- and medium-sized defects a gradient is detectable between the ventricles, but with large defects there is no gradient. The flow across the defect is left to right unless an Eisenmenger complex has developed. MRI may give similar information as echocardiography (Fig. 2.2.8).

Cardiac catheterization is necessary if surgery is contemplated and pulmonary vascular resistance needs to be determined.

Angiography may also be performed if there is doubt about the site or number of defects. The long axis projection is used to image the outlet septum, and the four-chamber projection is used for the inlet septum.

GREAT VESSEL LEVEL SHUNTS

Communication between the aorta and pulmonary artery via the ductus arteriosus is part of the normal fetal circulation. Persistent patency of the ductus arteriosus, after birth, is the commonest cause of a great vessel level shunt. Rarer causes include aorto-pulmonary window, coronary artery fistula and ruptured aneurysm of sinus of Valsalva.

Patent ductus arteriosus (PDA)

Normal closure of the ductus arteriosus depends upon specialized contractile tissue, which does not usually develop until the last trimester of fetal development. PDA is, therefore, commoner in premature babies. Hypoxaemia is a stimulus to continued patency of the ductus, so that respiratory distress syndrome may be an additional factor. It may also be due to maternal rubella during the first trimester, and is occasionally familial. Approximately 15% of cases of PDA are associated with other congenital heart defects. In some cases the patient's survival may depend upon continued patency of the duct, e.g. in hypoplastic left heart syndrome where the duct supplies the aorta, or in pulmonary atresia where the duct may be the main pulmonary supply. This section deals with isolated PDA.

The ductus arteriosus is usually situated on the left and extends from the bifurcation of the main pulmonary artery to the inferior surface of the aortic arch opposite the origin of the left subclavian artery (Fig. 2.2.14). The direction of blood flow in a PDA depends upon pulmonary vascular resistance, and the amount of shunting depends upon both the pulmonary vascular resistance and the calibre of the duct. In premature babies a PDA may close spontaneously up to 3 months after birth, but in full-term babies spontaneous closure is unlikely after 2 weeks.

Patency of the ductus in utero is maintained by prostaglandins which prevent contraction of its muscular wall. Indomethacin, which is a prostaglandin synthetase inhibitor, may be administered to close a PDA. Conversely, in situations where continued duct patency is desirable, prostaglandins may be given; these may cause periosteal reactions.

A small PDA does not cause any symptoms and is

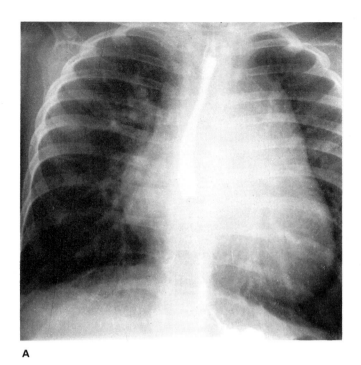

A

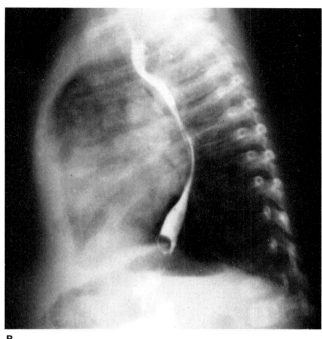

B

Fig. 2.2.12 Ventricular septal defect. **A** The lungs are plethoric. **B** The lateral view shows posterior displacement of the barium-filled oesophagus by an enlarged left atrium. A posterior impression on the upper oesophagus is caused by an incidentally present aberrant subclavian artery.

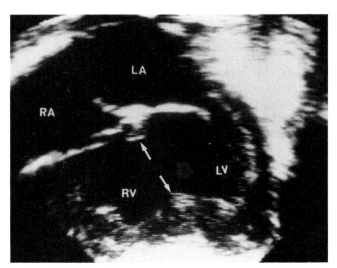

Fig. 2.2.13 Large ventricular septal defect. Four-chamber two-dimensional echocardiogram shows a large confluent perimembranous defect (arrows). LA = left atrium, LV = left ventricle, RA = right ventricle, RV = right ventricle. (Courtesy of Dr A. N. Redington.)

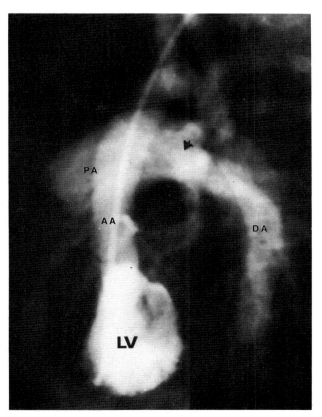

Fig. 2.2.14 Patent ductus arteriosus. Left ventriculogram in left anterior oblique projection shows a patent ductus (arrow) connecting the aorta and pulmonary artery (PA). AA = ascending aorta, DA = descending aorta, LV = left ventriculogram.

usually detected as a continuous murmur in the pulmonary area on routine examination. A moderate duct may present between 2 and 5 months of age with slow feeding, chest infections or tachypnoea. A large duct may present earlier with signs and symptoms of heart failure. If pulmonary vascular resistance does not fall after birth or rises in response to a large left-to-right shunt an Eisenmenger situation may develop, and the shunt will reverse. This may result in cyanosis of the lower half of the body. The chest radiograph with a small PDA is likely to be normal. A larger shunt may produce pulmonary plethora, and evidence of biventricular and left atrial enlargment. A small bulge may be visible on the distal aortic knuckle corresponding to the origin of the ductus (Fig. 2.2.15). In older patients the aortic knuckle may be prominent, and occasionally a PDA will calcify: if an Eisenmenger situation develops there will be evidence of pulmonary arterial hypertension.

The diagnosis is usually confirmed by two-dimensional echocardiography scanning from the suprasternal notch. It is usual to visualize the duct, and with Doppler it is possible to determine the size and direction of the shunt. In a moderate or large shunt the left atrium and ventricles will be enlarged. Echocardiography will also detect any other cardiac abnormalities. MRI may be used to provide this information, if echocardiography proves difficult.

Cardiac catheterization is rarely necessary to diagnose PDA. It may be performed if there is doubt about the diagnosis or to assess additional abnormalities. A right heart catheter may pass from the pulmonary artery into the descending aorta via a PDA (Fig. 2.2.16). The duct may be opacified by left ventricular or aortic injection of contrast medium, and is best visualized in the left anterior oblique projection. It may be possible to close a PDA by catheter placement of a collapsible umbrella in the duct.

Aortopulmonary window

Aortopulmonary window is a rare anomaly caused by incomplete partition of the truncus arteriosus, which leaves a communication between the aorta and pulmonary trunk (Fig. 2.2.17). The defect lies above the aortic and pulmonary valves, both of which are normal. It may be associated with other congenital cardiac anomalies.

The presentation depends upon the size of the defect and the pulmonary vascular resistance. When pulmonary vascular resistance is low there is left-to-right shunting. With a large defect pulmonary arterial pressure will rise and eventually pulmonary vascular resistance will increase.

Large shunts usually present in infancy with signs and symptoms of heart failure, but small shunts may be asymptomatic.

Depending on the size of the shunt the chest radiograph may show pulmonary plethora, cardiomegaly and evidence of left atrial enlargement. Signs of pulmonary arterial hypertension may also be evident. Two-dimensional and Doppler echocardiography make the diagnosis by demonstrating the defect and shunt above normal aortic and pulmonary valves. Echocardiography will also demonstrate or exclude any other lesions. MRI may provide the same information.

Angiography is rarely necessary, but aortography may be used to demonstrate the defect.

Coronary artery fistula

Coronary artery fistulas are rare. The commonest communication is right coronary artery to right atrium, but the right coronary artery may develop a fistula into either ventricle. These right coronary to right heart fistulas are left-to-right shunts. They are usually asymptomatic unless the shunt is large, when heart failure may develop. Physical examination may reveal a continuous murmur similar to that of a PDA.

The chest radiograph may show pulmonary plethora. If the fistula is associated with particularly large or tortuous vessels, these may produce an unusual bulge on the cardiovascular silhouette.

Echocardiography may demonstrate these fistulas, but aortography or coronary angiography are usually necessary to define the precise anatomy. Anomalous origin of the left coronary artery from the pulmonary trunk usually causes left heart failure, and is discussed in Topic 2.6.

Ruptured aneurysm of sinus of Valsalva

Aneurysm of a sinus of Valsalva is due to a localized congenital weakness. It is a rare abnormality which may rupture into an adjacent structure and thus create a fistula. The commonest fistula of this type is from the right sinus to the right ventricular outflow tract, but other fistulas that have been reported are non-coronary sinus to right atrium, and left sinus to pulmonary artery or left atrium.

Fistulas of this sort at birth are clinically very similar to PDA, but rupture of a sinus aneurysm later in life may cause chest pain and heart failure.

The chest radiograph may show plethora, depending on the size of the shunt and pulmonary vascular resistance. Echocardiography and angiography will demonstrate the lesion.

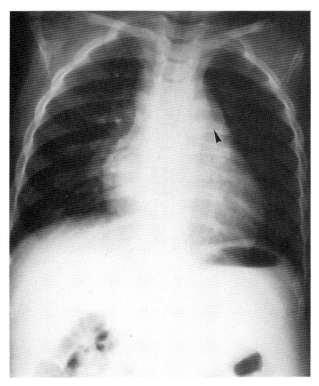

Fig. 2.2.15 Patent ductus arteriosus. A ductus 'bump' (arrowhead) is visible on the distal aortic arch.

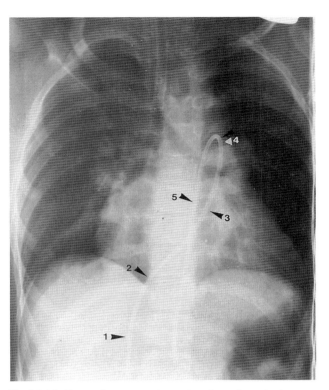

Fig. 2.2.16 Patent ductus arteriosus. A catheter from the femoral vein passes through the inferior vena cava (1), into the right atrium (2), across the tricuspid valve and into right ventricle (3), and then across the patent ductus (4), into the descending aorta (5).

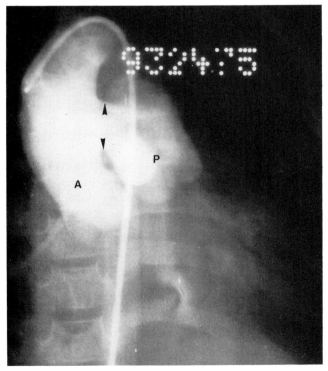

Fig. 2.2.17 Aortopulmonary window. Root aortogram shows communication (arrowheads) between the ascending aorta (A) and main pulmonary artery (P) above normally formed aortic and pulmonary valves.

REFERENCES

Bargeron L M, Elliott L P, Soto B et al 1977 Axial cineangiography in congenital heart disease: section 1. Concept, technical and anatomic considerations. Circulation 56: 1075–1083

Bierman F Z, Williams R G 1979 Sub xyphoid two dimensional imaging of the interatrial septum in infants and neonates with congenital heart disease. Circulation 60: 80–90

Elliott L P, Bargeron L M, Bream P R et al 1977 Axial cineangiography in congenital heart disease: section II. Specific lesions. Circulation 56: 1084–1093

Rashkind W J, Mullins C E, Hellenbrand W E, Tait M A 1987 Non-surgical closure of patent ductus arteriosus: clinical application of the Rashkind P.D.A. occluder system. Circulation 75: 583–592

Smallhorn J F, Anderson R H, Macartney F J 1982 Two-dimensional echocardiographic assessment of communications between ascending aorta and pulmonary trunk or individual pulmonary arteries. British Heart Journal 47: 563–572

Sutherland G R, Godman M J 1986 The natural history of ventricular septal defects. A long-term prospective cross-sectional echocardiographic study. In: Hunter A S, Hall R J C (eds) Clinical echocardiography. Castle House, Tunbridge Wells, Ch 16

Suzuki Y, Kambara H, Kadota K et al (1985) Detection of intracardiac shunt flow in atrial septal defect using a real-time two-dimensional color-coded Doppler flow imaging system and comparison with contrast two-dimensional echocardiography. American Journal of Cardiology 56: 347–350

Tobin R B, Schwartz D C 1981 Endocardial cushion defects, embryology, anatomy and angiography. American Journal of Radiology 136: 157

2.3 PULMONARY PLETHORA WITH CYANOSIS

Pulmonary plethora on the chest radiograph is due to increased flow of blood through the lungs, and indicates the presence of a left-to-right shunt. If, in addition, the patient is cyanosed then desaturated blood is bypassing the lungs and reaching the systemic circulation, i.e. the shunt is bidirectional.

COMPLETE TRANSPOSITION OF THE GREAT ARTERIES

Complete transposition implies that the atrioventricular connections are concordant and the ventriculo-arterial connections are discordant, i.e. the right atrium connects with the right ventricle which connects with the aorta, and the left atrium connects with the left ventricle which connects with the pulmonary trunk. This should be distinguished from congenitally corrected transposition where atrioventricular and ventriculo-arterial connections are all discordant. Complete transposition may be described as simple, or complex, if there are associated cardiac anomalies.

Complete transposition with intact ventricular septum

Simple transposition is compatible with life only if the foramen ovale or ductus arteriosus remain patent after birth, and allow mixing of the systemic and pulmonary circulations. Balloon atrial septostomy is often performed to create an ASD and improve mixing. Following such palliation more definitive surgery may be performed.

The anatomy of the great vessels in transposition is variable, but usually the aortic valve lies anterior and to the right of the pulmonary valve, and the aorta and pulmonary trunk ascend parallel to one another (Fig. 2.3.1). This contrasts with the normal heart, where the right ventricular outflow tract and pulmonary trunk twist around the left ventricular outflow tract and aorta.

Simple transposition usually presents in the first few days of life with increasing cyanosis which is usually precipitated by closure of the ductus arteriosus. Without treatment there is progressive metabolic acidosis and breathlessness.

The chest radiograph may not show plethora for several days, until pulmonary vascular resistance has fallen. The heart is usually moderately enlarged, and, since the pulmonary trunk lies posterior to the aorta, the vascular pedicle of the heart is narrow (Fig. 2.3.2).

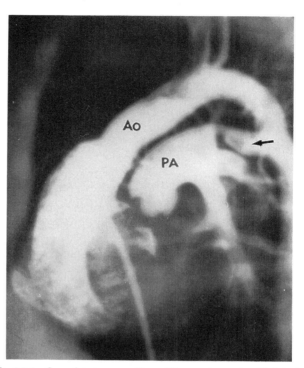

Fig. 2.3.1 Complete transposition of the great vessels with intact ventricular septum. Right ventriculogram, lateral projection, shows the aorta (AO) arising from the right ventricle. The aorta lies anteriorly and ascends parallel to the main pulmonary artery (PA). The pulmonary artery is filling via a patent ductus arteriosus (arrow).

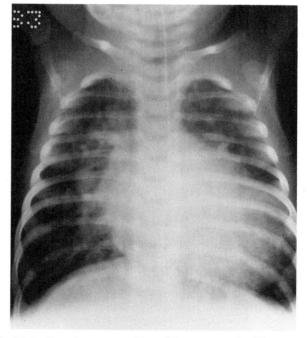

Fig. 2.3.2 Complete transposition of the great arteries. Neonate with cyanosis. The lungs are plethoric. The heart is enlarged. The pulmonary trunk is not visible.

Two-dimensional echocardiography or MRI will demonstrate normal intracardiac anatomy. The aorta and pulmonary artery will be seen to arise from the inappropriate ventricles, and then to ascend in parallel (Fig. 2.3.3). It is usually possible to demonstrate that the anterior great vessel becomes aortic arch, and that the posterior vessel divides into left and right pulmonary arteries.

Cardiac catheterization is not usually required for diagnosis, but is often undertaken in order to perform balloon atrial septostomy. A balloon catheter is passed across the foramen ovale, from right atrium to left atrium. The balloon is than inflated and pulled back across the septum, rupturing it and creating an ASD.

Complete transposition with VSD

Approximately 20% of cases of complete transposition have a VSD, 7% have a VSD and pulmonary stenosis and 7% have a VSD and coarctation of the aorta.

Complete transposition with VSD usually causes mild cyanosis at birth. Over the subsequent 3 or 4 weeks there is progressive heart failure. The chest radiograph shows gross cardiomegaly and a narrow vascular pedicle (Fig. 2.3.4). Echocardiography shows enlargement of the cardiac chambers, VSD (which is usually subarterial) and arterioventricular discordance (Fig. 2.3.5).

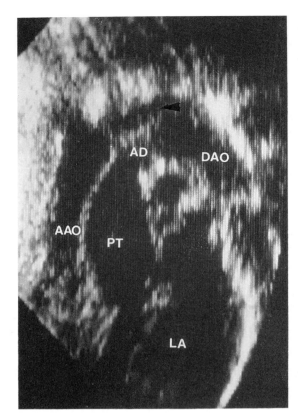

Fig. 2.3.3 Complete transposition of the great arteries. Parasternal long axis two-dimensional echocardiogram shows ascending aorta (AAO) anteriorly and parallel to main pulmonary artery (PT). The ductus arteriosus (AD) is patent. DAO = descending aorta, LA = left atrium. (Courtesy of Dr A. N. Redington.)

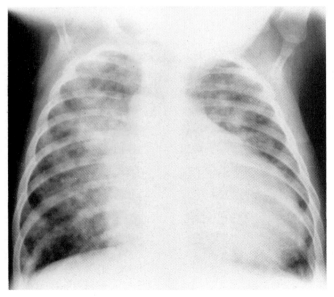

Fig. 2.3.4 Complete transposition of the great arteries with ventricular septal defect. The lungs are markedly plethoric and the heart is grossly enlarged.

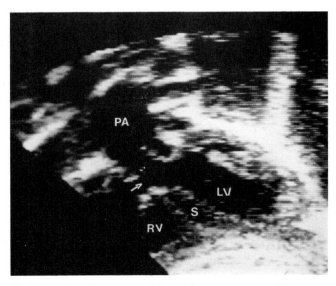

Fig. 2.3.5 Complete transposition of the great arteries with ventricular septal defect. Two-dimensional echocardiogram shows the pulmonary artery (PA) arising from the morphological left ventricle. A defect (arrow) is present in the interventricular septum (S). RV = right ventricle, LV = left ventricle. (Courtesy of Dr A. N. Redington.)

Complete transposition with VSD and pulmonary stenosis usually presents with cyanosis in the first few days of life. If the pulmonary stenosis is mild, cyanosis is usually mild but heart failure is likely to develop. With severe pulmonary stenosis cyanosis is more severe. The chest radiograph may show normal or plethoric lungs, but echocardiography is required to make the diagnosis.

Complete transposition with VSD and coarctation typically causes heart failure within the first few days of life. Echocardiography usually gives the complete diagnosis.

SINGLE VENTRICLE OR UNIVENTRICULAR HEART

A normal ventricle comprises three parts: inlet, trabecular and outlet portions. Without an inlet portion a ventricle becomes an outlet chamber, and absence of both inlet and outlet portions creates a trabecular pouch. These are examples of rudimentary chambers. In single ventricle one 'complete' ventricle is present; it receives either one or two atrioventricular valves. In the former instance there is either tricuspid or mitral atresia, and in the latter case there is a double inlet ventricle. The other ventricle, if identifiable, is represented as a rudimentary chamber.

Double inlet ventricle

In the majority of cases of double inlet ventricle the atria connect with a morphological left ventricle (Fig. 2.0.10B), a VSD is present, and the right ventricle is represented by an outlet chamber which is situated anterosuperiorly. The ventriculoarterial connections are usually discordant so that the aorta arises from the outlet chamber, i.e. transposition. If the VSD is small it will cause subaortic obstruction. Less often the ventriculo-arterial connections are concordant, in which cases a small VSD will restrict pulmonary blood flow. Approximately 40% of cases of double inlet left ventricle are associated with aortic coarctation, and 30% with pulmonary stenosis.

In cases of double inlet right ventricle a rudimentary left ventricle is usually found posteriorly and to the left. Occasionally, double inlet ventricle is of indeterminate morphology, and in some cases the atrioventricular connection may be via a common valve.

The clinical presentation depends upon the degree of pulmonary stenosis and the presence or absence of other lesions. Patients with severe pulmonary stenosis or atresia are cyanosed at birth or soon after. Patients without pulmonary stenosis are not severely cyanosed, but develop breathlessness and heart failure within a few weeks secondary to high pulmonary flow.

The chest radiograph in double inlet ventricle reflects the clinical picture. In the absence of pulmonary stenosis the lungs are plethoric, but with pulmonary stenosis the lungs may appear oligaemic. In the presence of heart failure there is usually cardiomegaly.

Echocardiography and MRI are the best methods of diagnosing double inlet ventricle and any additional lesions. The four-chamber view enables assessment of the atrioventricular connection (Fig. 2.0.10B), and a parasternal long axis view will show an anterior rudimentary chamber in double inlet left ventricle and a posterior rudimentary chamber in double inlet right ventricle. The presence or absence of any subarterial obstruction should be determined, and then the ventriculo-arterial connections. Finally, other associated anomalies should be looked for.

Cardiac catheterization is usually not necessary, although appropriately angled projections may give a full anatomical assessment. However, before surgical correction it is usual to measure pulmonary vascular resistance.

Tricuspid atresia

Tricuspid atresia may be described as single ventricle with absent right atrioventricular connection. The tricuspid valve is absent and the right atrium empties into the left atrium via a defect in the atrial septum (Fig. 2.3.6). The left atrium empties through the mitral valve into a morphological left ventricle. The right ventricle is usually represented by an outlet chamber situated anterosuperiorly. The ventriculo-arterial

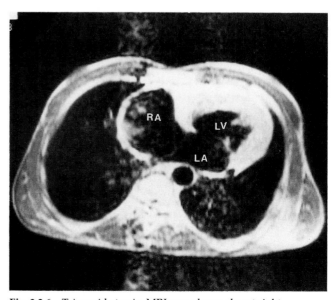

Fig. 2.3.6 Tricuspid atresia. MRI scan shows absent right atrioventricular connection. The right atrium (RA) connects with the left atrium (LA) via an ASD. LV = left ventricle.

connection is usually concordant with the pulmonary artery arising from the outlet chamber and the aorta arising from the main ventricle. Less often the ventriculo-arterial connection is discordant, i.e. transposed, and rarely there is some other ventriculo-arterial connection. When there is ventriculo-arterial concordance pulmonary blood flow is often restricted by the small VSD or by subpulmonary stenosis. When there is ventriculo-arterial discordance subpulmonary stenosis is unusual, but aortic flow is often restricted by the size of the VSD or by coarctation of the aorta.

Most cases of tricuspid atresia present in the first few days of life with cyanosis. The degree of cyanosis is dependent upon the severity of obstruction of pulmonary flow. Cases in which pulmonary flow is high may present at 1 or 2 months with heart failure.

Radiographic appearance depends upon the pulmonary blood flow. Where pulmonary flow is not obstructed the lungs appear plethoric and the heart is enlarged. Where pulmonary flow is restricted the lungs appear normal or oligaemic and the heart size is normal (Fig. 2.3.7).

Echocardiography in the four-chamber projection will demonstrate an absent right atrioventricular connection. The only atrioventricular valve enters a dominant left ventricle (Fig. 2.3.8). Further examination will demonstrate the VSD (Fig. 2.0.10C), the ventriculo-arterial connections and any other malformations. MRI will provide similar information.

Angiography in the appropriate projections will show the anatomy and connections but is not usually necessary unless corrective surgery is planned, when it may be necessary to delineate the pulmonary arteries and measure pulmonary vascular resistance.

DOUBLE OUTLET RIGHT VENTRICLE (DORV)

The term 'double outlet ventricle' implies that more than one and a half great vessels arise from the same ventricle. In the large majority of cases the great vessels arise from a morphological right ventricle. Double outlet left ventricle, and double outlet from a single, indeterminate ventricle are very rare and will not be discussed further. DORV is usually associated with a normally developed left ventricle and a VSD (Fig. 2.3.9). Both great vessels usually have their own outflow tract or infundibulum and, therefore, in contrast to tetralogy of Fallot, neither semilunar valve is in fibrous continuity with the mitral valve.

The clinical presentation depends on the site of the VSD, its relationship to the great vessels, the presence or absence of infundibular stenosis, and any additional lesions. DORV with a large subaortic VSD and no infundibular stenosis mimics an isolated VSD, whereas if the VSD is subpulmonary (the so-called Taussig–Bing malformation) the presentation is similar to complete transposition of the great arteries with a VSD. If infundibular pulmonary stenosis is present the haemodynamics and clinical presentation are similar to tetralogy of Fallot. Pulmonary stenosis is often present when the VSD is subaortic. Infundibular aortic stenosis and coarctation of the aorta may be associated with DORV and subpulmonary VSD. If the VSD is small or becomes small there is left ventricular outflow obstruction, which presents as dyspnoea and pulmonary oedema.

The chest radiograph reflects the haemodynamic situation. If there is a large VSD and no pulmonary stenosis the lungs are plethoric, and the heart enlarged, whereas with pulmonary stenosis the lungs are usually oligaemic and the heart size normal. If there is a restrictive VSD then the chest film shows signs of pulmonary venous hypertension.

In most cases echocardiography is able to demonstrate the ventriculo-arterial connections and the site and size of the VSD, and MRI is likely to be able to provide similar data. Both of these techniques should also demonstrate any other lesions.

Angiography may be necessary if there is any doubt about the relationship of the VSD to the great arteries. Right and left ventriculography in the long axis projection will usually suffice. The pulmonary vascular resistance may also be measured at the time of angiography.

The surgical treatment is particularly dependent upon the position of the VSD. If the VSD is subaortic, patching the VSD so that the left ventricle drains to the aorta is possible. However, simple patching of a subpulmonary VSD creates the same connections as in transposition of the great arteries. Therefore, surgical correction in this situation requires an arterial switch operation.

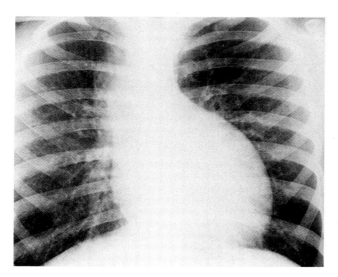

Fig. 2.3.7 Tricuspid atresia. Mild pulmonary plethora and cardiomegaly.

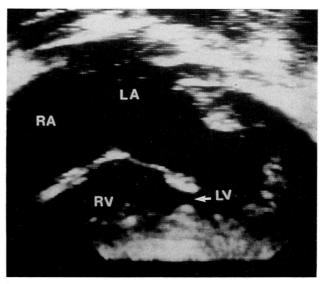

Fig. 2.3.8 Tricuspid atresia. Two-dimensional echocardiogram shows absent connection between right atrium (RA) and right ventricle (RV). There is a large ASD and a small ventricular septal defect (arrow). LA = left atrium, LV = left ventricle. (Courtesy of Dr A. N. Redington.)

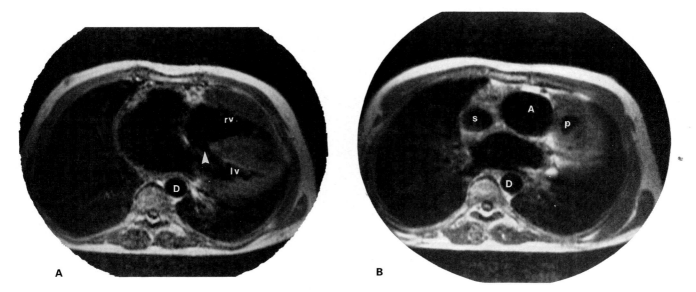

Fig. 2.3.9 Double outlet right ventricle. MRI scans shows: **A** ventricular septal defect (arrowhead) and **B** aortic root (A) to the right of the pulmonary trunk (P). Both great arteries arise from the right ventricle (rv). lv = left ventricle, s = superior vena cava, D = descending aorta.

TOTAL ANOMALOUS PULMONARY VENOUS RETURN (TAPVR)

In TAPVR none of the pulmonary veins connect with the left atrium and pulmonary venous return is into a systemic vein or veins. The site of TAPVR may be supracardiac, cardiac, infracardiac or mixed.

Supracardiac TAPVR is the commonest form. The pulmonary veins usually all drain into a vertical vein (or left superior vena cava), which drains into the brachiocephalic vein, the right superior vena cava and then the right atrium (Fig. 2.3.10). Less often the pulmonary veins drain into the azygos vein and then into the right superior vena cava. In TAPVR at the cardiac level the pulmonary veins usually drain into the coronary sinus, but sometimes directly into the right atrium. In the infracardiac type the pulmonary veins drain into a common vein which descends vertically, and passes through the diaphragm to terminate in the portal vein (Fig. 2.3.11), or rarely into the inferior vena cava. In all forms of TAPVR an ASD is present.

In most cases of supracardiac and cardiac TAPVR the pulmonary venous return is not obstructed and pulmonary blood flow is increased. However, in virtually all cases of infracardiac TAPVR there is some obstruction to pulmonary venous return. This may occur where the common pulmonary vein passes through the diaphragm or where it enters the portal vein, or be due to the resistance of the portal venous system. Obstruction in supracardiac TAPVR is usually due to kinking of the vertical vein at its junction with the brachiocephalic vein or compression by the left main bronchus. In the obstructed cases pulmonary blood flow is not greatly increased but there is pulmonary venous hypertension.

Babies with non-obstructed TAPVR are not usually symptomatic until 2 or 3 months and sometimes not for a year or more. They present with tachypnoea, chest infections and mild cyanosis. Obstructed cases present much earlier, usually within a day or two of birth, with severe cyanosis, dyspnoea and heart failure. Approximately 40% of cases of TAPVR have other congenital cardiac malformations.

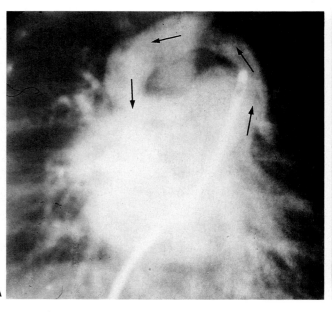 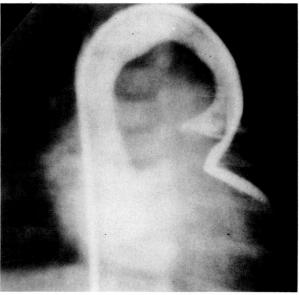

Fig. 2.3.10 Supracardiac total anomalous pulmonary venous return. **A** The venous phase of a pulmonary arteriogram shows that all the pulmonary veins converge to a vertical vein on the left, which drains into the right atrium via the brachiocephalic vein and superior vena cava. The arrows indicate the direction of flow. **B** Retrograde injection into vertical vein.

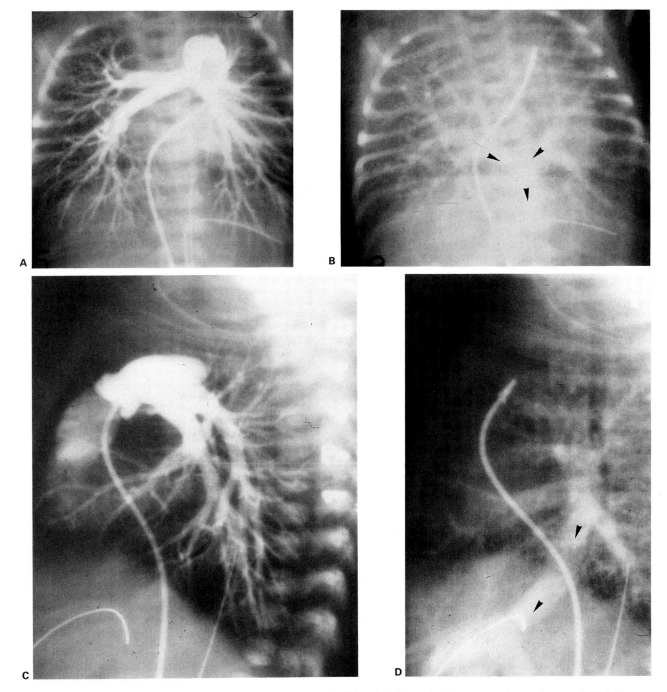

Fig. 2.3.11 Infracardiac total anomalous pulmonary venous return. **A, C** Arterial phase of pulmonary angiogram is normal. **B, D** Venous phase shows all the pulmonary veins draining into a retrocardiac venous confluence, and then into a common vein which traverses the diaphragm to reach the portal vein. Arrowheads show the direction of flow.

Chest radiographic findings depend in large part on whether or not the pulmonary venous return is obstructed. In unobstructed cases the lungs are plethoric (Fig. 2.3.12), and in obstructed cases the lungs show signs of pulmonary oedema. In the neonate this is often a diffuse reticular or nodular pattern, which may be similar in appearance to diffuse lung disease. There is usually obvious cardiomegaly, due to right heart enlargement in unobstructed cases, but a normal heart size is typical in obstructed cases. In unobstructed cases the vein or veins that receive the anomalous pulmonary venous return enlarge. Thus, in typical cases of supracardiac TAPVR the upper mediastinum widens bilaterally, but the classical 'cottage loaf', 'snowman' or 'figure of eight' appearance does not usually develop until the patient is at least a few months old.

Two-dimensional echocardiography will usually identify the common pulmonary vein behind the left atrium, and show that it does not connect with that atrium (Fig. 2.3.13). Doppler and colour flow scanning are useful in demonstrating the direction of flow in anomalous veins and identifying areas of obstruction. The ASD and any other cardiac lesions may also be identified.

Angiography may be necessary if there is doubt whether the anomalous venous return is total or partial. The pattern of pulmonary venous return may be shown by pulmonary arteriography or by direct injection into the anomalous veins.

TRUNCUS ARTERIOSUS

Failure of the embryonic truncus arteriosus to divide into aorta and pulmonary trunk leaves a common arterial trunk arising from the ventricular mass. The truncus almost always overrides a large VSD, but rarely it may arise from one ventricle. The truncal valve usually has three or four leaflets, but there may be two or five. The valve is often incompetent and sometimes stenosed.

In approximately 70% of cases (Type I) a short main pulmonary artery arises from the left side of the truncus (Fig. 2.3.14), in 25% of cases (Type II) the left and right pulmonary arteries arise close together on the posterior aspect of the truncus, and in the remaining cases (Type III) the pulmonary arteries arise from opposite sides of the truncus.

The patient may be asymptomatic at birth, but as pulmonary vascular resistance falls the pulmonary blood flow increases dramatically causing congestive cardiac failure, usually within the first 2 or 3 months. These babies are only mildly cyanosed. However, if the pulmonary vascular resistance remains high, heart failure is unusual but cyanosis is severe. When the truncal valve is incompetent presentation is earlier.

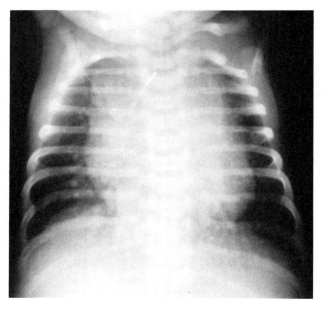

Fig. 2.3.12 Supracardiac total anomalous pulmonary venous return. The lungs are plethoric. The superior mediastinum is widened by dilated systemic veins.

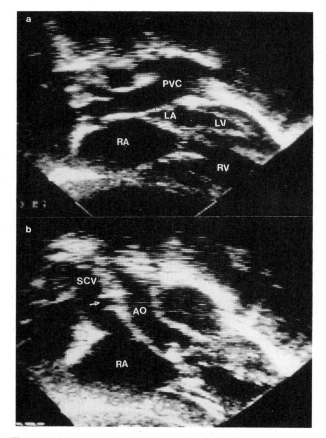

Fig. 2.3.13 Supracardiac total anomalous pulmonary venous return. Two-dimensional echocardiography shows **A** the pulmonary venous confluence (PVC) posterior to the left atrium (LA) receiving all four pulmonary veins. **B** This scan shows the brachiocephalic vein (arrow) entering the superior caval vein (SCV). RA = right atrium, RV = right ventricle, LV = left ventricle, AO = ascending aorta. (Courtesy of Dr A. N. Redington.)

A radiograph usually shows pulmonary plethora. The heart may be enlarged and there may be signs of heart failure. In 30–40% of cases the aortic arch is right-sided (Fig. 2.3.15).

Two-dimensional echocardiography will almost always demonstrate the large truncal root overiding a large VSD (Fig. 2.3.16). The truncal valve anatomy may be visualized, and Doppler scanning is useful to determine the presence and severity of valvar regurgitation and stenosis, and shunting across the VSD Echocardiography will also usually identify any other associated anomalies such as interruption of the aortic arch. MRI is also able to provide the same morphological and haemodynamic data.

Cardiac catheterization may be performed to measure pulmonary vascular resistance. If angiography is required a left ventricular injection in the long axis projection will demonstrate the VSD and a truncal injection in the four-chamber projection will usually demonstrate the type of truncus and any truncal valve incompetence.

COMMON ATRIUM

Common or single atrium is due to almost complete absence of the atrial septum. It is often associated with a cleft in the anterior leaflet of the mitral valve. The clinical presentation and the radiological features are, therefore, similar to a large complete atrioventricular septal defect. It is rarely found as an isolated defect, and is often seen in right isomerism. The diagnosis is usually readily apparent with two-dimensional echocardiography.

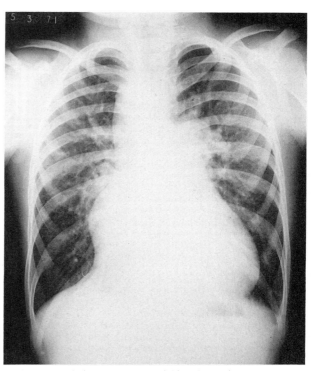

Fig. 2.3.15 Truncus arteriosus. There is pulmonary plethora, the heart is enlarged and the aortic arch is on the right.

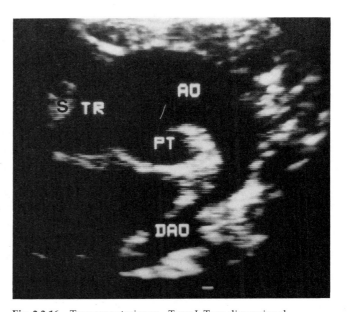

Fig. 2.3.16 Truncus arteriosus – Type I. Two-dimensional echocardiogram shows a persistent truncus (TR) overriding the ventricular septum (S) and dividing into ascending aorta (AO) and pulmonary trunk (PT). DAO = descending aorta.

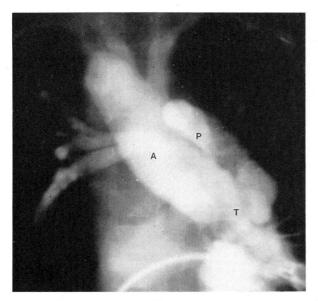

Fig. 2.3.14 Truncus arteriosus – Type I. Left ventriculogram shows a persistent truncus (T) overriding a ventricular septal defect. The truncus divides into aorta (A) and pulmonary trunk (P). The aortic arch is right-sided.

REFERENCES

Daskalopoulos D A, Edwards W D, Driscoll D J, Seward J B, Tajik A J Hagler D J 1983 Correlation of two-dimensional echocardiographic and autopsy findings in complete transposition of the great arteries. Journal of the American College of Cardiologists 2: 1151–1157

DeLisle G, Ando M, Calder A L, Zuberbuhler J R, Rochemacher S, Alday L E, Mangino O, Van Praagh S, Van Praagh R 1976, Total anomalous pulmonary venous connection: report of 93 autopsied cases with emphasis on diagnostic and surgical considerations. American Heart Journal 91: 99–122

Hagler D J, Tajik A J, Seward J B, Mair D D, Ritter D G 1980 Wide-angle two-dimensional echocardiographic profiles of conotruncal abnormalities. Mayo Clinic Proceedings 55: 73–82

Huhta J C, Gutgesell H P, Nihill M R 1985 Cross sectional echocardiographic diagnosis of total anomalous pulmonary venous connection. British Heart Journal 53: 525–534

Macartney F J, Rigby M L, Anderson R H et al 1984 Double outlet right ventricle: cross sectional echocardiographic findings, their anatomical explanation, and surgical relevance. British Heart Journal 52: 164

Rashkind W J, Miller W W 1966 Creation of an atrial septal defect without thoracotomy. A palliative approach to complete transposition of the great arteries. Journal of the American Medical Association 196: 991–992

Rigby M L, Anderson R H, Gibson D, Jones O D H, Joseph M C, Shinebourne E A 1981 Two-dimensional echocardiographic categorisation of the univentricular heart. Ventricular morphology, type and mode of atrioventricular connection. British Heart Journal 46: 603–612

Sutherland G R, Godman M J, Anderson R H, Hunter S 1981 The spectrum of atrioventricular valve atresia: a two-dimensional echocardiographic/pathological correlation. In: Rijsterborgh H (ed) Echocardiology. Martinus Nijhoff, The Hague, pp 345–353

2.4 PULMONARY OLIGAEMIA WITH CYANOSIS

Pulmonary oligaemia indicates a severe obstruction to pulmonary blood flow; the associated presence of cyanosis indicates right-to-left shunting, which may occur at either atrial or ventricular level.

TETRALOGY OF FALLOT

Tetralology of Fallot is the commonest congenital cyanotic heart disease. It comprises infundibular pulmonary stenosis, a VSD, overriding of the aorta and right ventricular hypertrophy (Fig. 2.4.1). The basic defect is anterior displacement of the infundibular septum. This creates the infundibular stenosis and a large subaortic VSD; the right ventricular hypertrophy develops as a consequence of the right ventricular outflow obstruction and the VSD. If the aorta overrides the septum by over 50% the ventriculo-arterial connection is DORV. The degree of the infundibular stenosis varies from mild to severe. Frequently there is also pulmonary valve stenosis, stenosis of the pulmonary trunk or one of the main pulmonary arteries, or peripheral pulmonary artery stenosis (Fig. 2.4.2). Other associations include complete atrioventricular septal defect, absence of the pulmonary valve, absence of one of the pulmonary arteries and secundum ASD. In cases

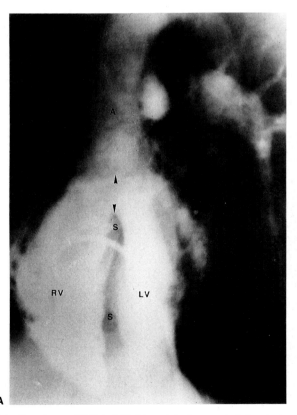
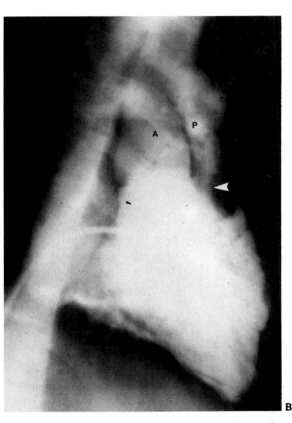

Fig. 2.4.1 Tetralogy of Fallot. **A** Right ventriculogram in left anterior oblique projection shows right ventricular hypertrophy, a subaortic ventricular septal defect (arrowheads) and the aorta (A) overriding the ventricular septum (S). **B** The right anterior oblique projection shows infundibular stenosis (arrowhead). RV = right ventricle, LV = left ventricle, P = pulmonary trunk.

with severe pulmonary stenosis systemic arteries from the descending aorta may provide collateral flow to the pulmonary circulation, as in pulmonary atresia.

Coronary artery anomalies are common in tetralogy of Fallot. Of importance to the surgeon contemplating right ventriculotomy are the origin of the anterior descending artery from the right coronary artery and enlargement of the conus branch of the right coronary artery.

The clinical presentation depends upon the severity of the pulmonary stenosis. Since the VSD is always large the right ventricle is at systemic pressure. With severe pulmonary stenosis blood shunts across the VSD from right to left causing severe cyanosis. With mild pulmonary stenosis shunting may be mostly left to right and the presentation is similar to a simple VSD.

The most severe cases present within a few days of birth with increasing cyanosis as the ductus arteriosus closes. Most cases, however, do not develop cyanosis until 3 or 4 months, as infundibular stenosis increases; they may present with fainting spells due to infundibular spasm.

The pulmonary vasculature radiographically usually appears normal or oligaemic, but in the few cases where there is only mild pulmonary stenosis the lungs may appear plethoric. The pulmonary trunk is usually small. The heart size is usually normal, but the cardiac apex is often elevated due to right ventricular hypertrophy (Fig. 2.1.7). If the heart is enlarged the possibility of an associated lesion, such as atrioventric-ular septal defect, should be considered. The ascending aorta is often prominent and the aortic arch is seen to be right-sided in about 25% of cases.

Two-dimensional echocardiography using a combination of parasternal long axis, parasternal short axis and apical or four-chamber views will demonstrate an enlarged aortic root overriding a large VSD, infundibular stenosis and right ventricular hypertrophy (Fig. 2.4.3). It should also be possible to determine the size of the pulmonary annulus, whether or not the pulmonary valve is dysplastic, and the presence or absence of stenoses in the central pulmonary arteries. Other lesions such as atrioventricular septal defect should be looked for. The side of the aortic arch can be confirmed on the suprasternal view. Doppler scanning is useful to assess the size and direction of shunting across the VSD, and the gradient across the right ventricular outflow tract. Similar data may be obtained by MRI (Fig. 2.4.4).

Angiocardiography may be necessary before surgery if non-invasive examination has not assessed the pulmonary arteries adequately. A pulmonary arteriogram performed in the 'sitting up position' (i.e. AP projection with 45° cranial tilt of the image intensifier) usually demonstrates the bifurcation of the main pulmonary artery (Fig. 2.4.5). The other features of tetralogy of Fallot may be demonstrated by biplane right ventriculography in the long axial oblique projection. Some surgeons require preoperative coronary arteriography to show any anomalous vessels crossing the infundibulum.

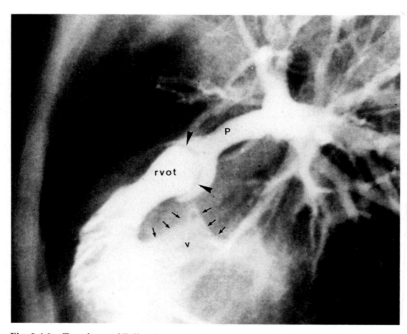

Fig. 2.4.2 Tetralogy of Fallot. Lateral right ventriculogram in systole shows a doming, stenosed pulmonary valve (arrowheads) and a hypoplastic pulmonary trunk (P). rvot = right ventricular outflow tract. Contrast medium in the subaortic ventricular septal defect (v) outlines the cusps of the aortic valve (arrows).

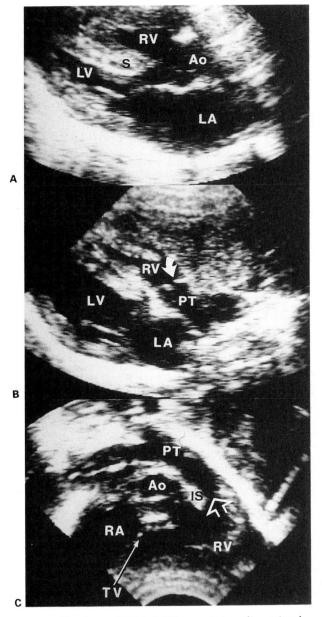

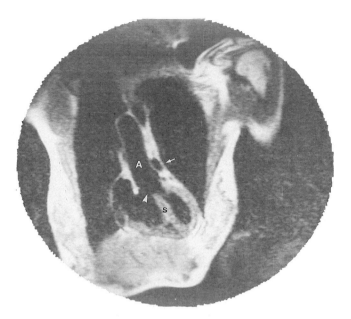

Fig. 2.4.4 Tetralogy of Fallot, MRI scan, coronal section, shows a subaortic ventricular septal defect (arrowhead). The aortic arch is right-sided. The pulmonary trunk (arrow) is hypoplastic. A = aorta, S = septum.

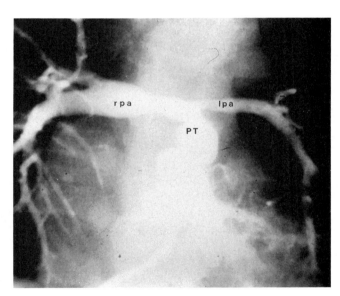

Fig. 2.4.3 Tetralogy of Fallot. **A, B** Long axis two-dimensional echocardiograms show a hypertrophied right ventricle (RV), a large aortic root (Ao) which overrides the interventricular septum (s), a subaortic interventricular septal defect and thickened pulmonary valve leaflets (arrow). **C** A short axis echocardiogram shows infundibular stenosis (open arrow) due to anterior displacement of the infundibular septum (IS). LV = left ventricle, LA = left atrium, PT = pulmonary trunk, TV = tricuspid valve. (Courtesy of Dr A. N. Redington.)

Fig. 2.4.5 Tetralogy of Fallot. Pulmonary arteriogram 'sitting up' projection, shows hypoplastic left pulmonary artery (lpa) and stenosis of origin of right pulmonary artery (rpa). PT = pulmonary trunk.

PULMONARY ATRESIA

Pulmonary atresia may occur with a VSD, or the ventricular septum may be intact.

Pulmonary atresia with VSD

This may be regarded as an extreme form of tetralogy of Fallot in which the infundibulum is completely obstructed. The development of the central pulmonary arteries is variable. They are almost always small, the right and left pulmonary arteries may or may not be confluent, and one or both may be absent. The aorta overrides a large VSD. The right and left ventricular pressures are similar and the right ventricle becomes hypertrophied. The entire output of both ventricles is to the aorta. Pulmonary blood flow must, therefore, be derived from a ductus arteriosus, from bronchial collateral vessels or from aortopulmonary collateral vessels (Fig. 2.4.6). There are often significant stenoses where these collaterals join lobar or segmental pulmonary arteries.

Clinical presentation is usually within a few days of birth with severe cyanosis. This may be precipitated by closure of the ductus arteriosus. If pulmonary blood flow is via well-developed systemic collaterals presentation may be later.

The lungs on a chest radiograph appear oligaemic or the pulmonary vasculature may have a disorganized pattern due to systemic supply to the lungs (Fig. 2.1.16). The pulmonary trunk is usually inapparent. The heart size is normal or mildly enlarged, and its apex may be elevated. The ascending aorta is often prominent and in approximately 30% of cases the aortic arch is right-sided.

Two-dimensional and Doppler echocardiography will usually demonstrate the large VSD and overriding aorta, the absent pulmonary valve and possibly the central pulmonary arteries and the origins of any aortopulmonary collateral vessels. The same data may be obtained by MRI, which is likely to be a more reliable method of assessing the systemic collateral flow to the lungs.

Surgical treatment is most successful when true central pulmonary arteries are present, and the right and left pulmonary arteries are confluent. In many cases this information may only be obtained by aortography, selective injection of aortopulmonary collaterals or by pulmonary venous wedge angiography (Fig. 2.4.7).

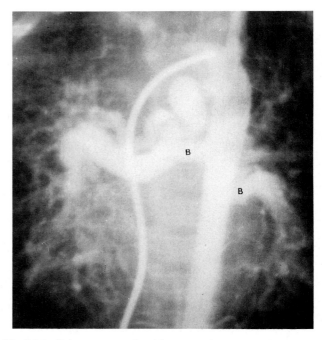

Fig. 2.4.6 Pulmonary atresia with ventricular septal defect. Descending aortogram shows large systemic, bronchial collateral arteries (B) supplying the pulmonary circulation.

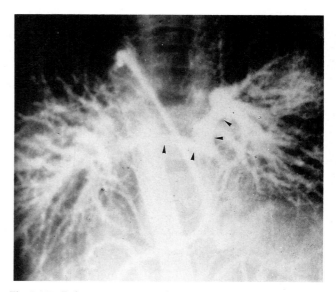

Fig. 2.4.7 Pulmonary atresia with ventricular septal defect. Descending aortogram has opacified confluent, hypoplastic right and left pulmonary arteries (arrowheads). The aortic arch is right-sided.

Pulmonary atresia with intact ventricular septum

In all cases of pulmonary atresia the pulmonary valve is imperforate. In pulmonary atresia with intact ventricular septum the main pulmonary artery is usually well developed and perfused by the ductus arteriosus (Fig. 2.4.8).

In most cases the tricuspid valve is small and reasonably competent, and the right ventricular cavity is very small. In some of these cases there are intramyocardial sinusoids which connect the right ventricular cavity and the coronary circulation. If right ventricular pressure is suprasystemic, right-to-left shunting through these sinusoids may cause myocardial ischaemia.

In the remaining cases the tricuspid valve is a good size, but is usually incompetent, so blood may flow to and fro into the right ventricle. In these cases the right ventricle, although hypoplastic, may reach a fair size. In all cases of pulmonary atresia with intact ventricular septum there is right-to-left shunting across an ASD.

Cyanosis in the first day or two of life is the usual presentation, with rapid, severe deterioration as the ductus closes. Congestive heart failure secondary to tricuspid incompetence may also be present.

Usually the lungs are oligaemic and there is cardiomegaly due to right atrial and left ventricular enlargement.

Two-dimensional echocardiography in the parasternal long axis and subcostal and apical four-chamber views will show the atretic pulmonary valve, the size of the atria and ventricles, the ASD and the state of the tricuspid valve. Suprasternal views will demonstrate the pulmonary arteries and the ductus. Doppler interrogation of the right ventricular outflow tract will differentiate pulmonary atresia from severe pulmonary stenosis.

Cardiac catheterization is not necessary to make the diagnosis. However, if corrective surgery is planned it is important to demonstrate any myocardial sinusoids, and this is best achieved by right ventriculography.

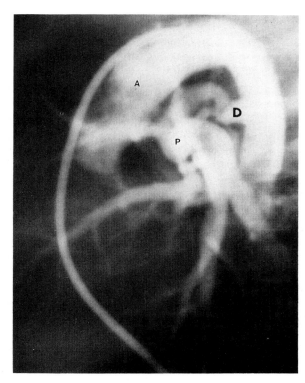

Fig. 2.4.8 Pulmonary atresia with intact ventricular septum. Arch aortogram, lateral projection, shows a large patent ductus arteriosus (D) supplying a well-developed main pulmonary artery (P). A = aorta.

EBSTEIN'S ANOMALY OF THE TRICUSPID VALVE

Ebstein's anomaly is an abnormality of the right atrioventricular valve. The valve annulus is in its normal position, but the valve leaflets are not attached to it as usual (Fig. 2.4.9). Instead, they are displaced into the right ventricular cavity and arise from the right ventricular wall. The portion of the ventricle between the annulus and the valve is functionally part of the right atrium. The size of the 'atrialized' part of the right ventricle and that of the remainder of the ventricle are inversely related, depending upon the degree of displacement of the valve. The leaflets are usually dysplastic and often redundant. The valve is typically incompetent, sometimes stenotic and occasionally both. The right atrium and ventricle enlarge secondary to tricuspid regurgitation, and there is usually right-to-left shunting across a patent foramen ovale or atrial septal defect.

Ebstein's anomaly may be associated with maternal lithium ingestion during pregnancy. It is rarely an isolated malformation being most frequently associated with an ASD, but also with VSD, pulmonary stenosis, pulmonary atresia with intact ventricular septum, corrected transposition of the great vessels and Wolff–Parkinson–White syndrome.

Presentation may be with cyanosis, dyspnoea, congestive heart failure or a tachyarrhythmia. In the severest cases this may occur in the first few weeks of life, but milder cases may not present until adulthood.

The chest radiograph shows normal or decreased pulmonary vascularity. The heart size may be normal, but it is usually increased and it may be massive (Fig. 2.4.9), with its shape suggesting right heart enlargement. Dilatation of the right ventricular outflow tract may cause a bulge high on the left heart border, and a dilated inferior vena cava may be visible (Fig. 2.4.10).

Two-dimensional echocardiography in a four-chamber view will demonstrate the displaced tricuspid valve leaflets and show if they are dysplastic or redundant. Echocardiography will also show the size of the right atrium and ventricle, and detect any associated malformations. Doppler scanning is useful in assessing the severity of any tricuspid regurgitation and shunting across the atrial septum.

Angiocardiography rarely adds to an adequate echographic study, but the anomaly may be demonstrated by right ventriculography in which the tricuspid valve deformity may make catheterization difficult.

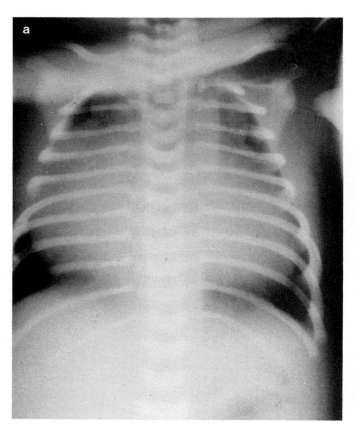

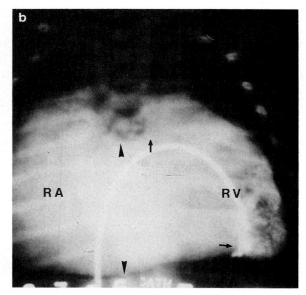

Fig. 2.4.9 Ebstein's anomaly. **A** The chest radiograph shows gross cardiomegaly and pulmonary oligaemia. **B** Right ventriculogram shows massive enlargement of the right atrium (RA) and right ventricle (RV). 'Atrialized' right ventricle lies between the tricuspid valve ring (arrowheads) and the attachments of the displaced tricuspid valve leaflets (arrows).

REFERENCES

Anderson R H, Macartney F J, Shinebourne E A, Tynan M 1987 Fallot's tetralogy. In: Paediatric cardiology, vol 2. Churchill Livingtone, Edinburgh, pp 765–798

Rees R S O, Somerville J, Underwood S R, Wright J, Firmin D N, Klipstein R H et al 1987 Magnetic resonance imaging of pulmonary arteries and their systemic connections in pulmonary atresia: comparison with angiographic and surgical findings. British Heart Journal 58: 621–626

Silverman N H, Birk E 1988 Ebstein's malformation of the tricuspid valve: cross-sectional echocardiography and Doppler. In: Anderson R H, Neches W H, Park S C, Zuberbuhler J R (eds) Perspectives in pediatric cardiology, vol 1. Futura, Mount Kisco, New York, pp 113–125

Soto B, Pacifico A D, Ceballos R, Bargeron L M 1981 Tetralogy of Fallot: an angiographic–pathologic correlative study. Circulation 64: 558–566

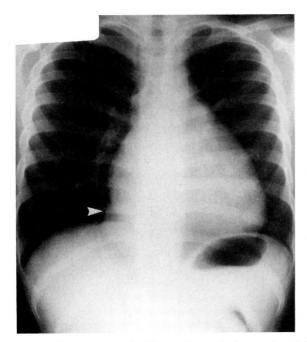

Fig. 2.4.10 Ebstein's anomaly. Chest radiograph shows only mild cardiomegaly. Prominence of the upper left heart border is due to dilated right ventricular outflow tract. The inferior vena cava (arrowhead) is dilated. The lungs are oligaemic.

2.5 NORMAL PULMONARY VASCULATURE WITHOUT CYANOSIS

PULMONARY STENOSIS

Obstruction of the right ventricular outflow tract may occur proximal to the pulmonary valve, at the level of the valve or distal to the valve. It may be an isolated abnormality or part of a more complex malformation.

Pulmonary valve stenosis

Isolated pulmonary valve stenosis accounts for 8–10% of all cases of CHD. The valve leaflets are usually thickened and may be partially fused. In those cases associated with Noonan's syndrome the valve is dysplastic and its annulus is small. The valve is unable to open fully, and in systole it becomes dome shaped with a small opening at the apex of the dome (Fig. 2.5.1). If the valve is significantly obstructed the right ventricle hypertrophies, and this may cause infundibular stenosis, which may be more severe in systole. Increased right ventricular filling pressure causes elevation of right atrial pressure, and this may lead to right-to-left shunting across the atrial septum via a patent foramen ovale or an ASD if present. In extreme cases the right ventricle may fail. The jet of blood that emerges through the stenosed valve strikes the anterior wall of the pulmonary trunk and can cause post stenotic dilatation. Turbulence in the pulmonary trunk is transmitted to the left pulmonary artery, which also enlarges.

The clinical presentation depends upon the severity of the stenosis. Most cases are asymptomatic and come to light in infancy, childhood or adulthood as an incidentally discovered murmur. Some cases present with fatigue and dyspnoea on exercise, and more severe cases develop overt heart failure. If there is right-to-left shunting across the atrial septum the patient may be cyanosed.

In most cases the chest radiograph shows normal pulmonary vasculature, normal heart size and enlargement of the pulmonary trunk and left pulmonary artery (Fig. 2.5.2). In severe cases with heart failure the lungs may appear oligaemic and there may be gross cardiomegaly.

Two-dimensional echocardiography will demonstrate thickened, restricted pulmonary valve leaflets, and may also show post stenotic dilatation of the pulmonary trunk and left pulmonary artery. Interrogation of the valve with Doppler echocardiography enables assessment of the gradient across the valve.

Cardiac catheterization is rarely necessary for diagnosis, but a right ventriculogram in the lateral projection usually demonstrates the abnormality. However, angiography may be a prelude to balloon dilatation of a stenosed valve.

Subvalvar pulmonary stenosis

Obstruction of the right ventricular outflow tract proximal to the pulmonary valve is usually due to narrowing of the infundibulum by fibrosis or muscle hypertrophy (Fig. 2.5.3). Isolated infundibular stenosis is rare, and is usually seen secondary to pulmonary valve stenosis or as part of a more complex malformation such as tetralogy of Fallot. A much rarer form of subvalvar stenosis is due to a ring of muscular hypertrophy between the inlet and outlet portions of the right ventricle, producing a so-called 'two-chambered right ventricle'.

The clinical presentation of isolated infundibular stenosis is similar to that of pulmonary valve stenosis. The chest radiograph shows a normal pulmonary vascular pattern, unless an ASD is present, in which case there may be oligaemia. However, in contrast to pulmonary valve stenosis, post stenotic dilatation of the pulmonary artery does not occur unless the valve is also abnormal. The diagnosis is usually confirmed by two-dimensional echocardiography.

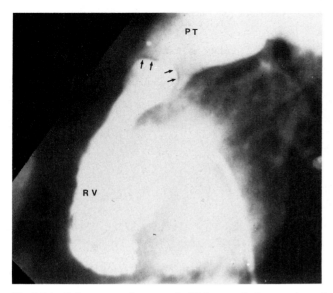

Fig. 2.5.1 Pulmonary valve stenosis. Right ventriculogram, lateral projection in systole, shows thickened, doming pulmonary valve leaflets (arrows). The pulmonary trunk (PT) is dilated. RV = right ventricle.

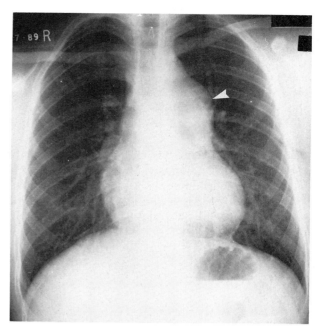

Fig. 2.5.2 Pulmonary valve stenosis. The pulmonary trunk and left pulmonary artery (arrowhead) are dilated. The right pulmonary artery, peripheral pulmonary vessels and heart size are normal.

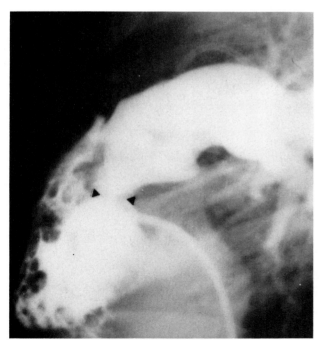

Fig. 2.5.3 Subvalvar pulmonary stenosis. Right ventriculogram, lateral projection, shows discrete narrowing of the infundibulum (arrowheads). The right ventricle is hypertrophied.

Pulmonary artery stenosis

Significant narrowing of the central pulmonary arteries occurs in approximately 40% of cases of tetralogy of Fallot, the origin of the left pulmonary artery being most commonly involved. Peripheral pulmonary stenoses may be due to maternal rubella, and are also associated with William's syndrome (Fig. 2.5.4).

The chest radiograph may show oligaemia distal to a pulmonary artery stenosis. These stenoses are best demonstrated by pulmonary arteriography. Stenoses of the origins of the right and left pulmonary arteries are often seen only in the 'sitting-up' projection (Fig. 2.4.5).

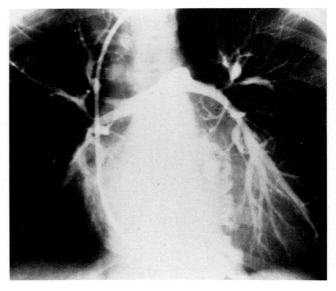

Fig. 2.5.4 Peripheral pulmonary artery stenoses. Pulmonary arteriogram William's syndrome.

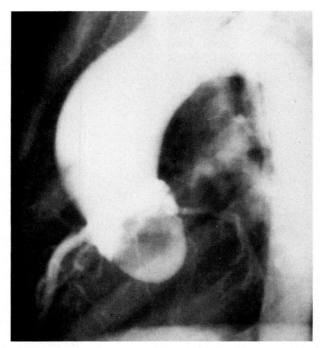

Fig. 2.5.5 Aortic valve stenosis. Root aortogram shows a bicuspid aortic valve and mild poststenotic dilatation of the ascending aorta.

AORTIC STENOSIS

Congenital aortic stenosis most commonly occurs at the level of the valve, but it may be sub- or supra-valvar.

Aortic valve stenosis

Approximately 85% of cases of congenital aortic stenosis, and 7% of all cases of CHD are due to aortic valve stenosis. Isolated aortic valve stenosis affects boys four times more commonly than girls, and may occur in association with Turner's syndrome. In most cases the valve is bicuspid (Fig. 2.5.5). A bicuspid valve is rarely symptomatic during childhood.

Narrowing of the valve orifice is due to partial fusion of one or both commissures. With the passage of time the cusps become fibrotic and calcified, and most cases present between 15 and 65 years of age. Cases that present in the neonatal period and infancy usually have a unicuspid valve with a small central orifice (Fig. 2.5.6) or a single commissure. In approximately 10% of cases the valve is incompetent (Fig. 2.5.7).

Clinical presentation depends upon the severity of the stenosis. Most cases discovered in childhood and adolescence are asymptomatic and have an incidentally heard murmur. These cases may develop left ventricular hypertrophy and eventually left heart failure, but this is unusual in childhood. The cases that present in infancy have critical stenosis and develop congestive heart failure, sometimes in the first few days of life.

The chest radiograph appearance depends upon the presentation. Neonates and infants with critical stenosis show signs of pulmonary venous hypertension and have cardiomegaly due to left ventricular dilatation. In older children, with milder stenosis, the lungs appear normal. The heart is not usually enlarged, but its shape may suggest left ventricular stress. Eccentric, turbulent flow through the valve may cause post stenotic dilatation of the ascending aorta, but calcification in the valve is rarely visible before adulthood.

Two-dimensional echocardiography in the parasternal long and short axis projections will show the number of aortic valve cusps, their thickness and mobility, and the size and position of the valve orifice in systole. It is also possible to assess the size of the left ventricular cavity and its wall thickness and contractility. Doppler interrogation allows assessment of the gradient across the valve, and will also detect any regurgitation. The gradient is usually too high for assessment by pulsed Doppler, and, therefore, the continuous wave mode is required. The gradient assessed by Doppler echography is the maximum instantaneous gradient in a usually unsedated patient,

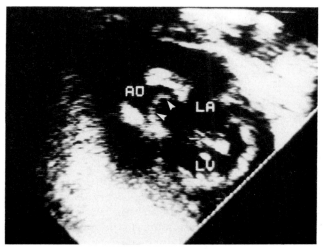

Fig. 2.5.6 Aortic valve stenosis. Critical stenosis in a neonate. Two-dimensional echocardiogram shows a thickened, doming aortic valve (arrowheads). AO = aortic root, LA = left atrium, LV = left ventricle. (Courtesy of Dr A. N. Redington.)

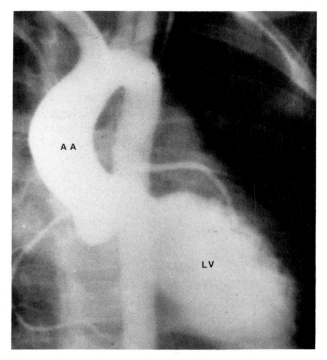

Fig. 2.5.7 Aortic valve stenosis and incompetence. Root aortogram, AP projection, shows severe aortic regurgitation filling the left ventricle (LV). There is mild poststenosis dilatation of the ascending aorta (AA).

and, therefore, is often higher than the gradient measured at cardiac catheterization.

MRI is able to demonstrate the morphological abnormalities of aortic valve stenosis, and with ciné MRI the severity of aortic stenosis can be graded.

Cardiac catheterization is usually only necessary if there is a conflict between the clinical and echocardiographic evaluations of the patient.

Subaortic stenosis

Subaortic stenosis may be dynamic or fixed. Dynamic subaortic stenosis is due to overgrowth of the muscular part of the ventricular septum and occurs in hypertrophic cardiomyopathy, discussed below. Fixed subaortic stenosis is usually caused by a fibrous ring just below the valve (Fig. 2.5.8), but in some cases a more diffuse fibromuscular overgrowth creates a tubular subaortic narrowing. Approximately 30% of patients with subaortic stenosis also have aortic valve stenosis, and some cases are associated with VSD.

Presentation is usually similar to that of moderate or mild aortic valve stenosis, with many patients having a symptomless murmur. Most patients remain asymptomatic until middle or late childhood when left ventricular hypertrophy may cause chest pain and breathlessness.

The lungs appear normal on the chest radiograph, unless heart failure has developed. The heart size is normal, but the shape suggests left ventricular stress. In contrast to stenosis at valvar level, there is no poststenotic dilatation of the ascending aorta.

Two-dimensional echocardiography in the long axis projection defines the subaortic abnormality, and as in valvar stenosis the gradient may be estimated by Doppler scanning. Angiography is seldom necessary.

Supravalvar aortic stenosis

Supravalvar aortic stenosis may be due to a discrete stricture immediately above the aortic sinuses, or it may take the form of a more diffuse hypoplasia of the proximal aorta (Fig. 2.5.9). Together with mental retardation, hypercalcaemia and 'elfin facies' it forms William's syndrome, which may be associated with peripheral pulmonary artery stenoses and coarctation of the aorta. Supravalvar aortic stenosis causes left ventricular hypertrophy and the clinical presentation is similar to subvalvar aortic stenosis.

Two-dimensional echocardiography demonstrates the lesion, and the gradient can usually be measured by Doppler scanning.

Angiography is not usually necessary but is useful to demonstrate extensive hypoplasia of the aortic arch and its branches.

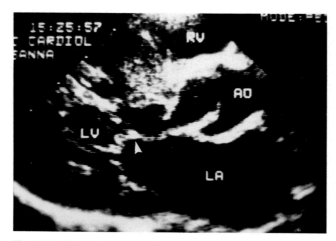

Fig. 2.5.8 Subaortic stenosis. Long axis two-dimensional echocardiogram shows a discrete fibrous ring (arrowhead) below a thickened aortic valve. AO = aortic root, RV = right ventricle, LV = left ventricle, LA = left atrium. (Courtesy of Dr A. N. Redington.)

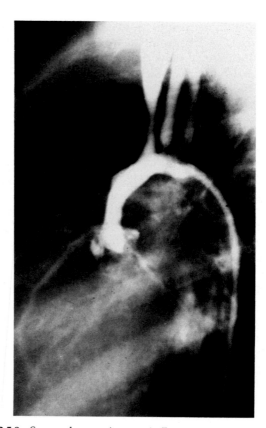

Fig. 2.5.9 Supravalvar aortic stenosis. Root aortogram shows a hypoplastic ascending aorta and strictures at the origins of the brachiocephalic and left common carotid and subclavian arteries. Patient with William's syndrome.

COARCTATION OF THE AORTA

Coarctation of the aorta accounts for approximately 10% of cases of CHD; in about half of these cases there is an additional congenital cardiovascular defect. The commonest associations are bicuspid aortic valve, PDA, VSD and complete transposition of the great arteries. It is a stricture in the aorta related to its junction with the ductus arteriosus or its remnant, the ligamentum arteriosum. The obstruction in the aorta is often due to a discrete shelf of tissue on its posterior wall (Fig. 2.5.10), but there may also be tubular hypoplasia of the aortic arch immediately proximal to the ductus (Fig. 2.5.11).

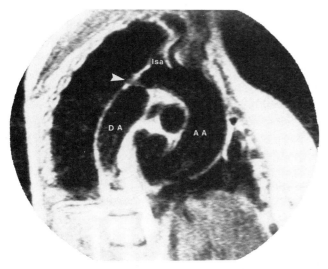

Fig. 2.5.10 Coarctation of aorta. MRI scan through aortic arch shows ascending aorta (AA), descending aorta (DA) and discrete shelf of tissue (arrowhead) distal to origin of left subclavian artery (lsa).

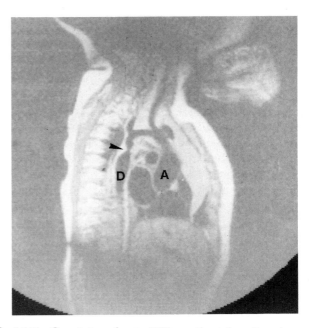

Fig. 2.5.11 Coarctation of aorta. MRI scan through aortic arch shows severe coarctation (arrowhead) distal to origin to left subclavian artery, and also hypoplasia of the whole transverse aorta. A = ascending aorta, D = descending aorta.

If the aortic obstruction is severe, perfusion of the descending aorta and its branches depends upon adequate right ventricular function and patency of the ductus arteriosus. In this situation presentation is often in the first few days or weeks of life and is precipitated by closure of the ductus or heart failure.

In milder cases long-term survival, usually without symptoms, is the rule. The aortic obstruction is bypassed by the development of collateral arterial channels which are derived from branches of the subclavian arteries. This collateral circulation causes enlargement of the internal mammary, intercostal and scapular arteries. These cases may be discovered incidentally with systemic hypertension in the arms, weak or delayed femoral pulses or an abnormal chest radiograph (Fig. 2.5.12).

The chest radiograph of a symptomatic neonate or infant will usually show signs of pulmonary venous hypertension and cardiomegaly. However, in older patients the pulmonary vasculature and heart size are usually normal, although the shape of the heart may suggest left ventricular stress. In these patients there may be rib notching, which typically involves the fourth to eighth ribs posteriorly, and is caused by enlargement of the intercostal arteries. Rib notching is unusual before 10 years of age and is very rare before 5 years. The appearance of the aortic knuckle is almost always abnormal, with loss of its normal smooth contour which may be more or less prominent than usual.

Two-dimensional echocardiography in the suprasternal projection will usually demonstrate the site and extent of the coarctation, as well as the size of the aortic arch, the position of the left subclavian artery and the state of the ductus arteriosus (Fig. 2.5.13). Other views may be useful to confirm or exclude associated abnormalities. Doppler interrogation enables assessment of the gradient across the coarctation. MRI is able to provide similar information, and in older children and adults it will consistently show the entire aorta, which is not always possible with echocardiography.

Angiography is only required if after non-invasive investigation there is some doubt about the precise anatomy of the coarctation or associated anomalies. A left ventriculogram or root aortogram in the left anterior oblique or lateral projection show the region of the coarctation (Fig. 2.5.14). Primary balloon angioplasty is not yet routinely used to treat coarctation, but is widely used to treat re-stenosis after surgical correction.

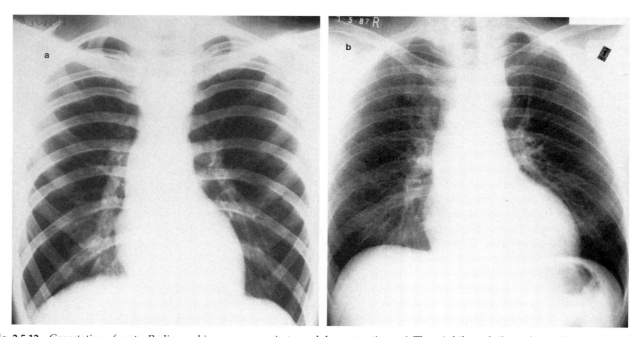

Fig. 2.5.12 Coarctation of aorta. Radiographic appearances in two adolescent patients. **A** There is bilateral rib notching. The aortic knuckle is flatter than normal. **B** There is mild, bilateral rib notching. The shape of the heart suggests left ventricular stress. The aortic knuckle is deformed; the left subclavian artery is prominent creating a double density over the aortic knuckle. The ascending aorta is prominent secondary to a bicuspid aortic valve.

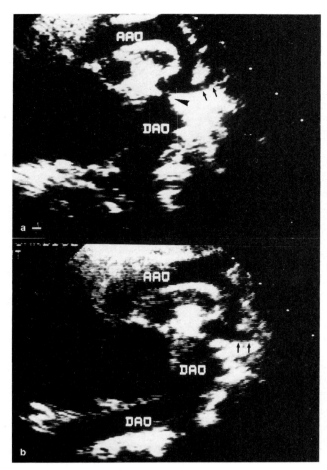

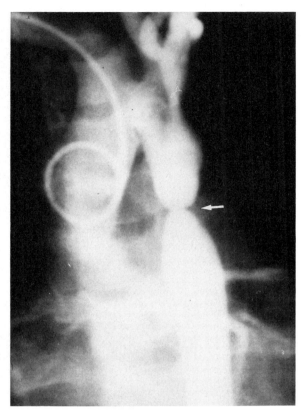

Fig. 2.5.13 Coarctation of aorta (**A**, **B**). Suprasternal two-dimensional echocardiograms show discrete narrowing of the aorta (arrowhead) distal to origin of left subclavian artery (arrows). AAO = ascending aorta, DAO = descending aorta. (Courtesy of Dr A. N. Redington.)

Fig. 2.5.14 Coarctation of aorta. Root aortogram shows discrete narrowing of aorta (arrow) distal to origin of left subclavian artery.

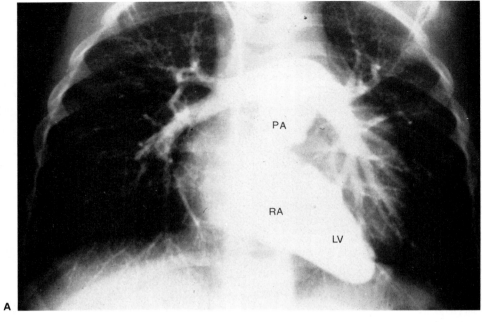

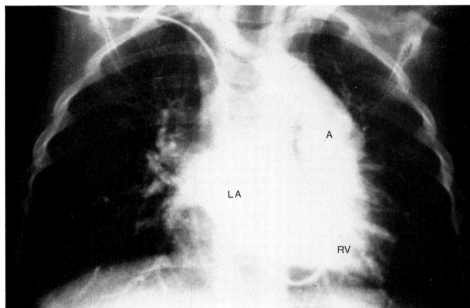

Fig. 2.5.15 Corrected transposition of the great arteries. Cardiac angiography shows: **A** right atrium (RA) connecting with morphological left ventricle (LV) from which the pulmonary artery (PA) arises, and **B** the left atrium (LA) connecting with the morphological right ventricle (RV) from which the aorta (A) arises. Note that the upper part of the left cardiovascular silhouette is formed by the ascending aorta.

CONGENITALLY CORRECTED TRANSPOSITION OF THE GREAT ARTERIES

In this condition there is both atrioventricular discordance and ventriculo-arterial discordance (Fig. 2.5.15). The right atrium connects via the mitral valve to the morphological left ventricle from which the pulmonary artery arises, and the left atrium connects via the tricuspid valve to the morphological right ventricle from which the aorta arises. Therefore, in the absence of any other abnormality, deoxygenated blood flows to the lungs and oxygenated blood flows into the aorta, and the patient is likely to be asymptomatic. However, most cases are complicated by an associated anomaly, most commonly VSD, pulmonary stenosis, dysplasia of the tricuspid valve and heart block.

Clinical presentation depends upon the associated anomalies. The combination of VSD and pulmonary stenosis may mimic tetralogy of Fallot, and regurgitation across the tricuspid valve mimics mitral regurgitation.

On the chest radiograph the upper part of the left heart border is often prominent (Fig. 2.5.16) due to the ascending aorta lying on the left side. The pulmonary vasculature may be normal, plethoric or oligaemic, depending on associated abnormalities.

Two-dimensional echocardiography will usually provide the diagnosis (Fig. 2.0.10A) and detect any associated anomalies. In most cases the morphological right ventricle lies to the left, the morphological left ventricle lies to the right, and the aorta lies to the left of the main pulmonary artery. A parasternal view typically shows the pulmonary valve more posterior than usual and in continuity with its atrioventricular valve. The aortic valve, however, is seen to be separated from its atrioventricular valve. Doppler investigation is useful to assess intracardiac shunting or valve regurgitation or stenosis, if present. MRI is also able to provide the same data. Cardiac catheterization is rarely necessary to make the diagnosis but may be performed preoperatively if non-invasive studies are inconclusive.

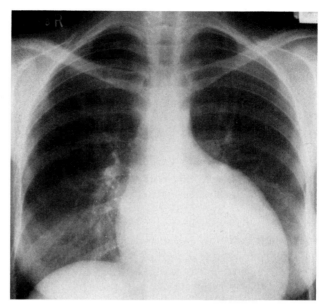

Fig. 2.5.16 Corrected transposition of the great arteries. The left heart border is prominent due to the abnormal position of the ascending aorta – see Fig. 2.5.15

REFERENCES

Gomes A S 1989 MR imaging of congenital anomalies of the thoracic aorta and pulmonary arteries. Radiologic Clinics of North America 27: 1171–1181

Huhta J C, Gutgesell H P, Latson L A, Huffines F D 1984 Two-dimensional echocardiographic assessment of aorta in infants and children with congenital heart disease. Circulation 70: 417–424

Kan J S, White R I, Mitchell S E, Gardener T J 1982 Percutaneous balloon valvuloplasty: a new method for treating congenital pulmonary valve stenosis. New England Journal of Medicine 307: 540–542

Sutherland G R, Smallhorn J F, Anderson R H, Rigby M L, Hunter S 1983 Atrioventricular discordance. Cross-sectional echocardiographic–morphological correlative study. British Heart Journal 50: 8–20

2.6 PULMONARY VENOUS HYPERTENSION

HYPOPLASTIC LEFT HEART SYNDROME

Hypoplasia of the left ventricle, aortic atresia and severe stenosis or atresia of the mitral valve constitute the hypoplastic left heart syndrome. In this situation blood can only leave the heart via the pulmonary artery. The systemic circulation, therefore, depends upon the ductus arteriosus remaining open and perfusing the aorta. Moreover, since the ascending aorta is not directly connected to the heart, the direction of the blood flow in the aortic arch and ascending aorta is the reverse of normal (Fig. 2.6.1). Blood entering the left atrium is obliged to cross the atrial septum into the right atrium and then into the right ventricle. The right ventricle is responsible for maintaining both the pulmonary and systemic circulation.

Hypoplastic left heart syndrome is the commonest cause of heart failure and death from heart disease in the first 2 or 3 days of life, both are precipitated by closure of the ductus arteriosus.

The chest radiograph usually shows cardiomegaly, which is due to right heart failure, and signs of pulmonary venous hypertension. Before the ductus closes the pulmonary blood flow may be greater than normal and the lungs may, therefore, be plethoric (Fig. 2.6.2).

Two-dimensional echocardiography is usually diagnostic. The left ventricle and aortic root are seen to be very small and there is enlargement of the right heart and pulmonary artery.

Cardiac catheterization is rarely necessary, but angiography will demonstrate the retrograde flow in the aortic arch and ascending aorta.

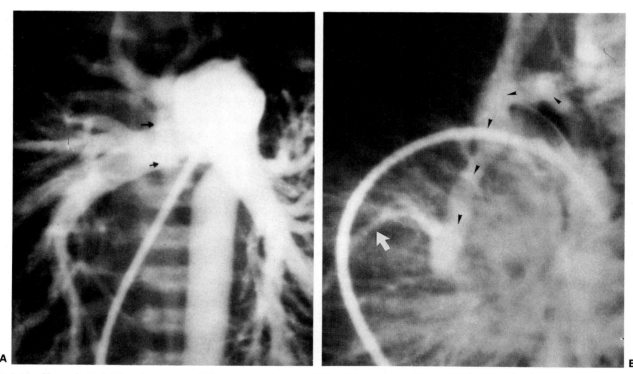

Fig. 2.6.1 Hypoplastic left heart syndrome. Pulmonary angiogram. **A** The AP projection shows well-developed pulmonary arteries and a hypoplastic ascending aorta (arrows) which has filled via the patent ductus arteriosus. **B** The lateral projection show the hypoplastic aortic arch. The arrowheads indicate the direction of flow in the aorta – it is the reverse of normal. The right coronary artery is arrowed.

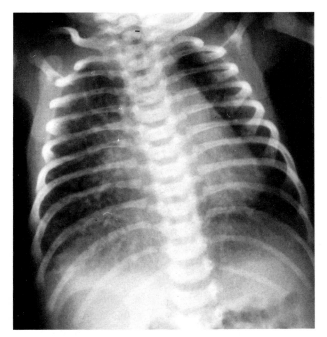

Fig. 2.6.2 Hypoplastic left heart syndrome. Radiograph in a neonate shows pulmonary plethora, before the ductus arteriosus has closed.

COR TRIATRIATUM

Cor triatriatum is caused by a perforated membrane dividing the left atrium into two compartments (Fig. 2.6.3). The upper compartment usually receives the pulmonary veins and the lower one connects with the atrial appendage and the mitral valve. The hole in the membrane is generally small enough to cause pulmonary venous obstruction.

Presentation is usually in the first 2 years with cough, dyspnoea and tachypnoea.

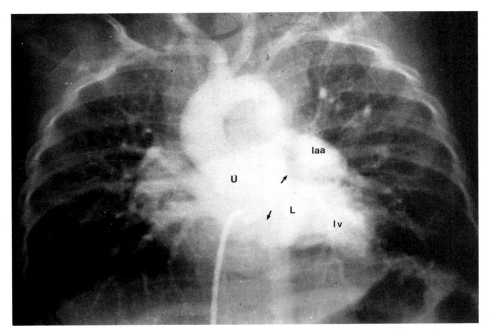

Fig. 2.6.3 Cor triatriatum. Angiogram shows left atrium divided by a membrane (arrows) into upper (U) and lower (L) compartments. The pulmonary veins enter the upper compartment and the left atrial appendage (laa) is connected to the lower compartment. lv = left ventricle.

The chest radiograph typically shows signs of pulmonary venous hypertension, often with alveolar oedema (Fig. 2.1.3). There may be signs of right heart enlargement, but in contrast to mitral valve disease, the left atrium does not appear enlarged. Two-dimensional echocardiography usually demonstrates the membrane dividing the left atrium (Fig. 2.6.4). This may also be seen on MRI. Cardiac catheterization is rarely necessary but will show elevated pulmonary artery and wedge pressures, and the laevophase of a pulmonary arteriogram may show the membrane.

ANOMALOUS ORIGIN OF THE LEFT CORONARY ARTERY

If the left coronary artery arises from the pulmonary trunk its perfusion pressure is lower than normal, and this may cause left ventricular ischaemia. Moreover, if there are well-developed collateral vessels between the normal right coronary and the anomalous left coronary, then flow in the left coronary may be reversed so that blood shunts left to right from right coronary to pulmonary artery (Fig. 2.6.5), and this may cause severe left ventricular ischaemia.

Presentation occurs when pulmonary vascular resistance has fallen and is unusual before 1 or 2 months. Milder cases may present later in childhood. Symptoms are due to myocardial ischaemia and include bouts of screaming related to exertion, pallor and sweating. There may also be signs of heart failure and mitral regurgitation.

The chest radiograph shows signs of pulmonary venous hypertension and cardiomegaly. Two-dimensional echography may identify the anomalous origin of the left coronary artery. The left ventricular size and wall motion may be assessed, and Doppler interrogation may show mitral regurgitation. Thallium scanning may demonstrate areas of ischaemia or infarction. Aortography or coronary angiography will also show the anomaly.

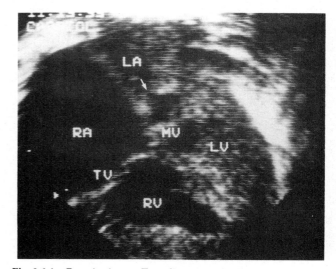

Fig. 2.6.4 Cor triatriatum. Two-dimensional echocardiogram shows a membrane (arrow) dividing the left atrium (LA) into two compartments. MV = mitral valve, LV = left ventricle, RA = right atrium, TV = tricuspid valve, RV = right ventricle. (Courtesy of Dr A. N. Redington.)

REFERENCE

Greenberg M A, Fish B G, Spindola-Franco H 1989 Congenital anomalies of the coronary arteries. Classification and significance. Radiologic Clinics of North America 27: 1127–1146

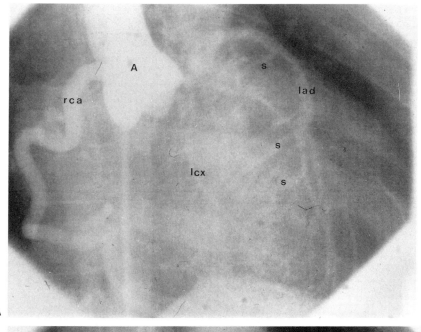

A

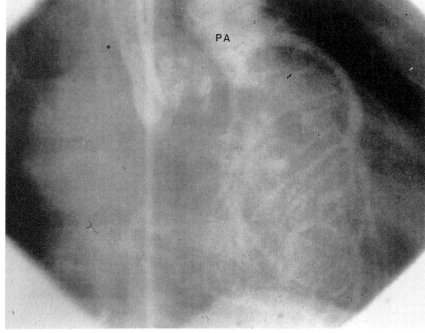

B

Fig. 2.6.5 Anomalous origin of left coronary artery. **A** Root aortogram shows normal origin of right coronary artery (rca). However, the left circumflex (lcx) and left anterior descending (lad) arteries are filling via septal collaterals (s) and the left main coronary artery does not appear to arise from the aorta. **B** A later frame shows that the left coronary artery arises from the main pulmonary artery (PA) which has now opacified. There is, therefore, a left-to-right shunt.

2.7 SURGERY FOR CONGENITAL HEART DISEASE

Approximately two-thirds of patients with CHD will undergo surgical treatment. Ideally surgery will restore the anatomy and physiology to as close to normal as possible. The sooner that this is achieved the greater is the opportunity for the heart and lungs to develop normally. If corrective surgery is not possible, then a palliative procedure may be performed. Many palliative procedures are performed with a view to corrective surgery at some later time.

PALLIATION

Systemic to pulmonary artery shunts are created to increase pulmonary blood flow in cases of cyanotic heart disease due to inadequate pulmonary flow, e.g. tetralogy of Fallot, pulmonary atresia and any malformation associated with severe right ventricular outflow obstruction. A classical Blalock–Taussig shunt involves transection of the subclavian artery which is then anastamosed to the ipsilateral pulmonary artery (Fig. 2.7.1). A modified Blalock–Taussig shunt involves insertion of a Gore-Tex conduit between the subclavian artery and ipsilateral pulmonary artery. Waterston–Cooley shunts (between ascending aorta and right pulmonary artery) and Pott's shunts (between descending aorta and left pulmonary artery) are now performed rarely. The chest radiograph of patients who have undergone right Blalock or Waterston shunts may show signs of a right thoracotomy, and those with left Blalock or Pott's shunts may have signs of a left thoracotomy. Following a classical Blalock shunt rib notching may develop on the side of the operation (Fig. 2.7.2).

A Glenn shunt, between superior vena cava and right pulmonary artery, for treatment of tricuspid atresia with severe pulmonary stenosis or atresia, is now rarely performed.

Banding of the pulmonary trunk is performed to restrict pulmonary flow in cases where there is severe pulmonary arterial hypertension due to left-to-right shunting and a corrective procedure is inadvisable in the first instance. This includes multiple VSDs and single ventricle without pulmonary stenosis. It is performed via a left thoracotomy.

The Blalock–Hanlon procedure via a right thoracotomy, which involves surgical creation of an ASD, has been replaced by Rashkind balloon septostomy in the palliation of complete transposition of the great arteries.

RADICAL PALLIATION

These procedures are intended to restore near normal physiology despite anatomical correction being difficult or impossible. They are performed via a sternotomy and are often associated with long-term survival and well-being.

The Mustard and Senning procedures for complete transposition involve surgery to the atrial septum and creation of an intra-atrial baffle that directs systemic venous blood to the left ventricle and pulmonary venous blood to the right ventricle. Complications of these procedures include both systemic and pulmonary venous obstruction.

The Rastelli procedure may be used to treat complete transposition with a VSD and pulmonary stenosis, DORV with pulmonary stenosis, pulmonary atresia with VSD and truncus arteriosus types I and II. The operation involves patching the VSD so that left ventricular blood enters the aorta and inserting a valved conduit between right ventricle and pulmonary artery.

The Fontan procedure involves insertion of a conduit between the right atrium and pulmonary trunk. It is usually performed to treat tricuspid atresia, but may also be appropriate for some cases of pulmonary atresia and single ventricle. Homograft valves in conduits frequently calcify (Fig. 2.7.3), but this process usually spares the cusps.

CORRECTIVE PROCEDURES

The most commonly performed extracardiac corrective procedures are ligation of a PDA and repair of coarctation of the aorta. These are performed via a left thoracotomy. Correction of coarctation of the aorta is now usually done with a subclavian flap. Use of prosthetic patches to repair coarctation of the aorta has been abandoned due to aneurysm formation being a late complication. Development of this complication is best screened for by MRI (Fig. 2.7.4).

Virtually all other corrective procedures are intracardiac and performed via a sternotomy. The more frequent operations include patching ASDs and VSDs and total correction of tetralogy of Fallot (i.e. closure of the VSD and relief of infundibular stenosis).

Transposition of the great arteries may now be treated by an arterial switch operation. This involves transection of both the pulmonary artery and aorta, which are then anastomosed to their appropriate ventricles, with implantation of the coronary arteries into the aorta.

In general, valve replacement is avoided in children since prosthetic valves have a limited life expectancy and do not keep up with the growth of the child. Wherever possible attempts are made to repair incompetent valves and dilate stenosed valves.

The ultimate corrective operations are heart transplantation and heart–lung transplantation if there is irreversible pulmonary disease.

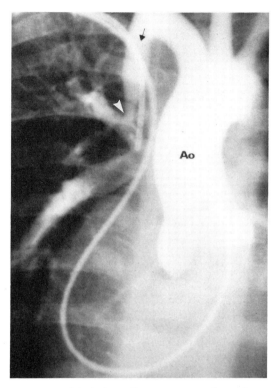

Fig. 2.7.1 Right Blalock shunt. Root aortogram shows that the right subclavian artery (arrow) has been transected and anastamosed to the right pulmonary artery (arrowhead). Ao = ascending aorta.

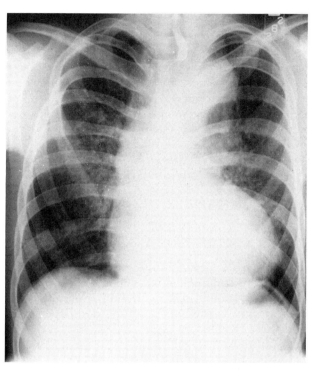

Fig. 2.7.2 Right Blalock shunt. Patient with pulmonary atresia. Surgical deformity of right fourth rib and notching of right third to fifth ribs.

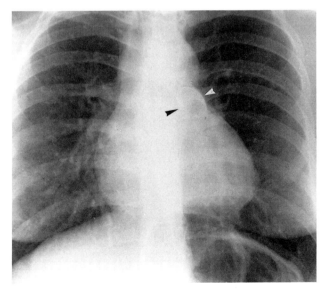

Fig. 2.7.3 Calcified homograft. Patient with pulmonary atresia. A valved homograft (arrowheads) between right ventricle and pulmonary trunk has calcified.

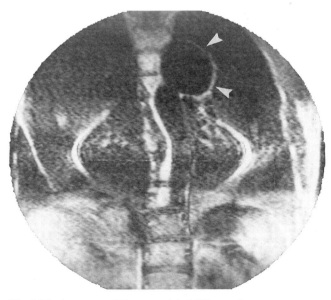

Fig. 2.7.4 Aneurysmal Dacron patch. MRI scan shows an aneurysm (arrowheads) at the site of previous repair of coarctation of the aorta.

2.8 ANOMALIES OF THE AORTIC ARCH AND VASCULAR RINGS

There are many possible anomalies of the aortic arch and its branches. They are frequently asymptomatic, but they may cause symptoms if they are part of a vascular ring, and they may be associated with congenital cardiac defects. In some cases, such as anomalous origin of the left subclavian artery associated with coarctation of the aorta, they may be of considerable importance to the surgeon.

A vascular ring occurs when the oesophagus and trachea are completely encircled by vascular structures. This may cause stridor or dysphagia.

The development of the normal aortic arch and all of its anomalies is explicable on the basis of the hypothetical double aortic arch system (Fig. 2.8.1) first described by Edwards.

THE LEFT AORTIC ARCH

The normal left aortic arch is formed by regression of the right fourth branchial arch between the origin of the right subclavian aorta and the descending thoracic aorta. In approximately 0.5% of the population a left aortic arch is formed by regression of the right fourth branchial arch between the right subclavian and common carotid arteries. This creates anomalous origin of the right subclavian artery, which arises as the fourth branch of the aortic arch, and passes from left to right posterior to the oesophagus. This condition is rarely symptomatic, and is usually discovered incidentally during a barium study, when a posterior impression on the oesophagus is seen. Occasionally, however, it presents with dysphagia. In cases of coarctation of the aorta proximal to the origin of an anomalous right subclavian artery, the blood pressure measured in the right arm is lower than in the left, and if rib notching develops it will be confined to the left side. Other anomalies of the brachiocephalic vessels in association with a left aortic arch are rare.

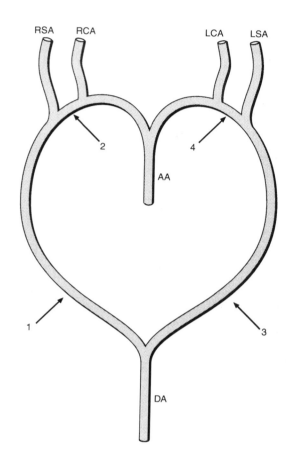

Fig. 2.8.1 Hypothetical double aortic arch. Regression of segment (1) creates a normal left aortic arch. Regression of segment (2) creates a left aortic arch with anomalous origin of the right subclavian artery. Regression of segment (3) creates a right aortic arch with branching that is the mirror image of normal. Regression of segment (4) creates a right aortic arch with anomalous origin of the right subclavian artery. AA = ascending aorta, DA = descending aorta, RSA = right subclavian artery, RCA = right common carotid artery, LCA = left common carotid artery, LSA = left subclavian artery.

THE RIGHT AORTIC ARCH

Regression of the left fourth branchial arch between the origin of the left subclavian artery and the descending aorta creates a right aortic arch with branches that are the mirror image of normal. The ductus arteriosus is almost always left-sided, so that a vascular ring is rarely present. Right aortic arch with mirror-image branching is usually associated with CHD (Figs 2.1.6, 2.1.7, 2.4.4). The commonest associations are tetralogy of Fallot, pulmonary atresia with VSD and truncus arteriosus. Other associations are VSD, complete transposition of the great arteries and tricuspid atresia.

Right aortic arch with aberrant left subclavian artery is created by regression of the fourth left branchial arch between the origins of the left common carotid and subclavian arteries. It is the mirror image of a left arch with aberrant right subclavian artery. It is uncommonly associated with heart disease and is usually asymptomatic. Rarely right aortic arch is associated with aberrant left innominate artery and isolation of a subclavian artery.

The chest radiographic signs of right aortic arch have already been described. The distinction between cases with mirror-image branching and aberrant left subclavian artery can be made by barium swallow (Fig. 2.8.2). In cases with mirror-image branching the swallow is either normal or only shows a right-sided indentation, but in the presence of an aberrant left subclavian artery there is a posterior oesophageal indentation. The precise vascular anatomy may be demonstrated by angiography, MRI or CT.

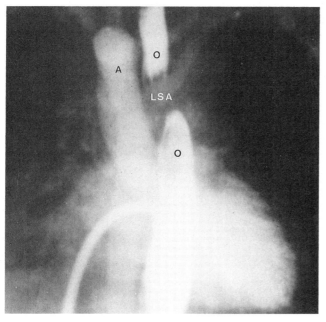

Fig. 2.8.2 Right aortic arch with aberrant left subclavian artery. Angiogram combined with barium swallow shows right aortic arch (A) and diagonal compression of oesophagus (o) by aberrant left subclavian artery (LSA), which arises as the fourth branch of the arch.

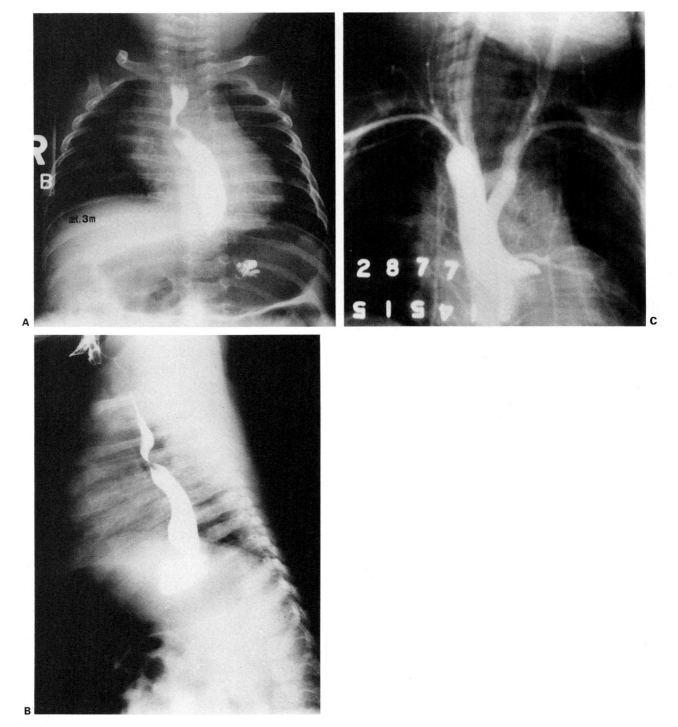

Fig. 2.8.3 Double aortic arch. **A** Frontal radiograph with barium in oesophagus shows compression of both sides of the oesophagus. **B** The lateral view shows posterior compression of the oesophagus. **C** The aortogram shows persistent double arch. The right arch is larger and more cephalad.

DOUBLE AORTIC ARCH

Double aortic arch occurs when neither side of the hypothetical double arch regresses. It is a rare anomaly, which is isolated in 80% of cases, but associations include VSD and Tetralogy of Fallot.

The double arch is usually asymmetrical, the left side often being hypoplastic. A complete vascular ring surrounds the trachea and oesophagus, and presentation is usually during infancy with stridor or dysphagia.

The chest radiograph is rarely diagnostic in infants, but in older children bilateral indentation of the trachea may be visible. The right component is usually more prominent than the left. Posterior indentation of the trachea may be visible on the lateral film. Barium swallow is often diagnostic (Fig. 2.8.3), showing bilateral and posterior indentation of the upper oesophagus. The right indentation is usually larger and more cephalad than the left. The precise vascular anatomy may be demonstrated by angiography, echocardiography, MRI or CT.

CERVICAL AORTIC ARCH

Cervical aortic arch is a rare condition in which the transverse aorta is situated more cephalad than normal. In most cases it is right-sided, and it may be associated with CHD, and present as a pulsatile supraclavicular mass, or with symptoms of airway compression.

The superior mediastinum is widened on the side of the arch. The diagnosis may be confirmed by two-dimensional echography, MRI, CT or angiography.

INTERRUPTED AORTIC ARCH

Interrupted aortic arch is a rare anomaly in which the ascending and descending aorta are disconnected. The arch may be interrupted between the left subclavian artery and the isthmus, between the left common carotid and subclavian arteries (Fig. 2.8.4), or most rarely between the innominate and left common carotid arteries. As in severe coarctation of the aorta the circulation to the descending aorta and its branches depends upon the ductus arteriosus remaining patent. Other cardiac malformations are often present, and include VSD, subaortic stenosis, hypoplastic left heart syndrome and complete transposition.

Clinical presentation is often in the first few days of life and is usually precipitated by closure of the ductus. Interruption of the aortic arch in association with hypoplasia or aplasia of the thymus and parathyroid glands is the DiGeorge syndrome.

The chest radiograph may show pulmonary

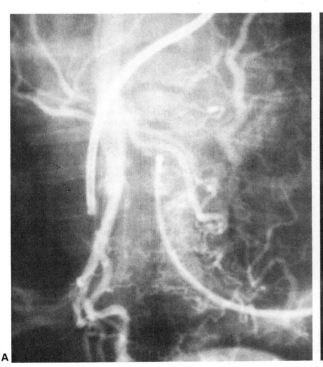
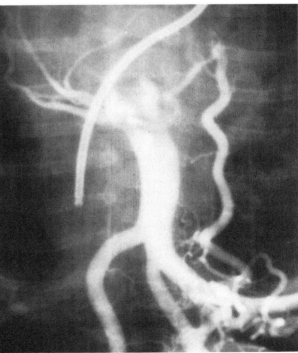

Fig. 2.8.4 Interrupted aortic arch. **A** Root aortogram shows that the aortic arch is interrupted immediately distal to the origin of the left common carotid artery. **B** A later frame shows retrograde flow in the left vertebral artery filling the left subclavian artery and descending aorta.

plethora or pulmonary venous hypertension, and cardiomegaly due to right heart enlargement.

Two-dimensional echocardiography may demonstrate the interruption, and will diagnose any associated anomalies. Angiography, however, may be necessary to show the precise vascular anatomy.

ANOMALOUS ORIGIN OF THE LEFT PULMONARY ARTERY FROM THE RIGHT PULMONARY ARTERY

This is a rare anomaly in which the left pulmonary artery arises from the right pulmonary artery and passes between the oesophagus and trachea to reach the left hilum, sometimes called pulmonary artery sling. The main pulmonary artery in this condition may cause anterior compression of the trachea, and the aberrant left pulmonary artery may cause posterior tracheal compression and also compression of the right bronchus. Approximately 50% of cases of pulmonary sling have additional cardiovascular abnormalities, and approximately 50% have congeni-

tal anomalies of the trachea or bronchi. Most cases present before 6 months of age with stridor.

The chest radiograph may show indentation of the right bronchus or distal trachea, and there may be areas of collapse, consolidation or hyperinflation in the lungs (Fig. 2.8.5). The anomalous pulmonary artery may be visible on the lateral film between the trachea and oesophagus. A barium swallow will demonstrate an anterior indentation on the mid-oesophagus. The abnormality is best demonstrated by a pulmonary angiogram in the 'sitting up' projection, or by MRI.

HEMITRUNCUS

This is a rare anomaly in which one of the pulmonary arteries arises from the ascending aorta. In most cases the right pulmonary artery arises anomalously, and there is frequently an associated cardiac malformation, such as as VSD, PDA or tetralogy of Fallot.

Cardiomegaly and plethora of the lung on the abnormal side are seen on the chest radiograph. The definitive diagnosis may require angiography.

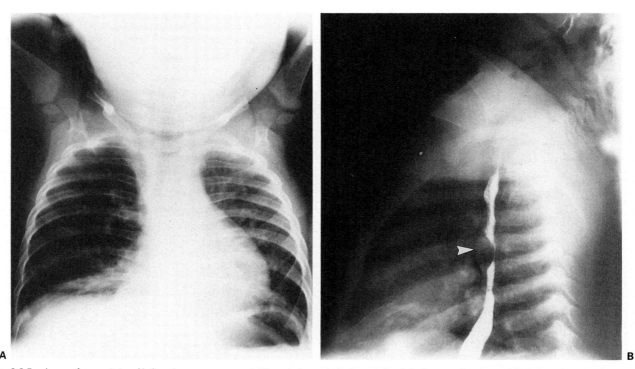

A **B**

Fig. 2.8.5 Anomalous origin of left pulmonary artery. **A** There is hyperinflation of the right lung and right middle lobe collapse and consolidation. **B** Lateral film with barium in oesophagus shows the anomalous left pulmonary artery as an oval density (arrowhead) which is compressing the oesophagus behind, and the trachea in front.

2.9   RHEUMATIC FEVER

Rheumatic fever is now uncommon in Western Europe and North America, but remains the most important worldwide cause of valvular heart disease.

Acute rheumatic fever is rare before 3 years of age, and most cases occur between 5 and 15 years. The major criteria for the diagnosis of rheumatic fever are carditis, polyarthritis, chorea, erythema marginatum and subcutaneous nodules. Carditis occurs in approximately 55% of patients and it may involve any part of the heart: pericarditis may cause pericardial effusion, myocarditis may cause heart failure, endocarditis may cause valvar regurgitation, and involvement of the conducting tissues may cause heart block. In the chronic phase the heart valves may become thickened and fibrous, leading to stenosis and/or regurgitation.

In acute rheumatic fever the chest radiograph may be normal. However, mitral regurgitation and heart failure may give rise to signs of pulmonary venous hypertension. Enlargement of the cardiac shadow may be due to myocarditis or pericardial effusion. Echocardiography may demonstrate mitral valve prolapse secondary to stretching of the chordae tendineae, enlargement of the cardiac chambers and pericardial effusion.

2.10 PERICARDIAL DISEASE

PERICARDITIS

There are many causes of acute pericarditis in infancy and childhood. Pyogenic pericarditis, usually due to staphylococcus, may be secondary to pulmonary infection or septicaemia. In older children and adolescents most cases of acute pericarditis are viral. Other important causes are tuberculosis and rheumatic fever, and less common causes in childhood include rheumatoid disease, other connective tissue disorders, leukaemia and postpericardiotomy syndrome.

The clinical presentation depends upon the cause, but in general, in addition to signs and symptoms of any underlying cause, there may be fever, malaise and chest pain. A pericardial effusion is invariably present and may cause tamponade.

Constrictive pericarditis is rare in childhood and is most often due to tuberculosis, but any acute pericarditis or haemothorax may lead to pericardial thickening and constriction. Clinical features may include lassitude, abdominal pain and swelling, hepatomegaly and ascites.

PERICARDIAL EFFUSION

Pericardial effusion is invariably present in acute pericarditis and is often present in heart failure. Most effusions in childhood do not compromise cardiac function, but rapid accumulation of a large amount of fluid may cause dyspnoea, raised central venous pressure and hepatic enlargement. A chronic pericardial effusion may present with ascites.

PERICARDIAL CYST

Pericardial cysts are fluid-filled sacs that lie adjacent to the heart. They rarely communicate with the pericardium, but their contents are similar to pericardial fluid. The majority are situated in one or other cardiophrenic angle, more often on the right.

PNEUMOPERICARDIUM

Pneumopericardium may be a complication of assisted ventilation or be related to trauma or surgery.

PERICARDIAL DEFECTS

Congenital absence of all or part of the parietal pericardium over the left side of the heart is a rare, usually benign, congenital abnormality. In complete absence the heart shifts toward the left hemithorax. The left atrial appendage may herniate through a partial defect. Ventral diaphragmatic defects are associated with pericardial and lower sternal defects, deficiency of the upper abdominal wall and intracardiac anomalies in the pentalogy of Cantrell.

PERICARDIAL TUMOURS

Primary pericardial tumours are very rare, and in infants and children are usually teratomas, although lipomas, fibromas and angiomas may occur. The pericardium may be involved in leukaemia, lymphoma and metastatic disease when pericardial thickening and effusion may occur.

IMAGING THE PERICARDIUM

The typical appearance of pericardial effusion on the chest radiograph is symmetrical enlargement of the cardiac shadow in association with normal pulmonary vasculature. If tamponade develops the systemic veins may enlarge and the lungs may appear oligaemic. It is very unusual for pericardial calcification to develop in childhood.

Pericardial cysts usually appear as well-defined round soft tissue opacities, contiguous with the heart, in one or other cardiophrenic angle. A partial pericardial defect may cause a prominent bulge on the left heart border, due to herniation of the left atrial appendage. A complete defect may result in the heart being shifted into the left hemithorax, and a radiolucent band may be visible between its inferior surface and the left hemidiaphragm.

Echocardiography is the most widely used method of assessing the pericardium (Fig. 2.10.1). It is able to detect pericardial effusion, thickening, cysts and tumours, and also provide information about cardiac function. Two dimensional scanning is superior to M-mode for defining the amount and extent of pericardial fluid. The parietal pericardium is seen to be separated from the myocardium by a relatively echo-free space of at least 2 mm thickness. The fluid may be echogenic if it is haemorrhagic or purulent. In patients with cardiac tamponade collapse of the free wall of the right ventricle during diastole is seen. In the presence of both pericardial and pleural effusion accurate measurement of the thickness of the pericardium may not be possible. Echography enables differentiation between pericardial cysts (which are completely echo free) and other paracardiac masses. Since echography provides real-time data it is often used for guidance during percutaneous drainage of pericardial fluid.

CT or MRI is useful in differentiating paracardiac fat from other paracardiac masses or collections. Pericardial effusion and pericardial thickening may also be assessed. If an effusion appears radiodense it may be haemorrhagic, and if it is of low radiodensity it may be due to chyle. MRI also has the potential to characterize the nature of pericardial fluid. Both MRI and CT may be useful to assess the amount and distribution of pericardial fluid if echography is unsatisfactory. In addition, MRI and ciné CT may provide functional data on the cardiac chambers.

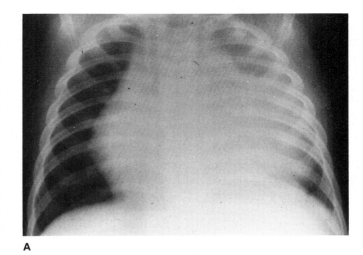

A

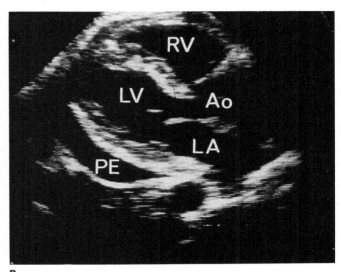

B

Fig. 2.10.1 Pericardial effusion. **A** Chest radiograph, characteristic cardiac contour. **B** Long axis two-dimensional echocardiogram shows an echo-free fluid collection (PE) posterior to the heart. RV = right ventricle, LV = left ventricle, Ao = aorta, LA = left atrium. (Courtesy of Dr M. St. J. Sutton.)

2.11   INFECTIVE ENDOCARDITIS

Infective endocarditis is uncommon under the age of 10 years and rare before the age of 2 years. In this younger age group it often involves previously normal heart valves, but in older children CHD is an important factor. The malformations that most commonly predispose to infective endocarditis are VSD, PDA, bicuspid aortic valve, tetralogy of Fallot and coarctation of the aorta. In older patients rheumatic heart disease is an important predisposing factor.

The chest radiograph may show evidence of heart failure superimposed on the signs of any underlying abnormality. Right-sided endocarditis may give rise to pulmonary infection. Two-dimensional echocardiography is useful in identifying vegetations, which appear as echogenic masses attached to valves or the endocardium. Echography, CT or MRI may also identify mycotic aneurysms associated with PDA and coarctation of the aorta (Fig. 2.11.1).

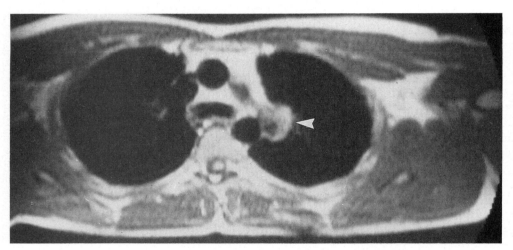

Fig. 2.11.1   Mycotic aneurysm (arrowhead) following repair of coarctation of aorta demonstrated by MRI scan.

2.12   CARDIAC TUMOURS

Cardiac tumours are rare in paediatric practice. The clinical presentation depends upon the location of the tumour.

MYXOMAS

Myxomas may arise in any of the cardiac chambers, but are most commonly seen in the left atrium, attached to the atrial septum by a pedicle. They may produce a syndrome of malaise, fever and weight loss, and may also cause systemic emboli or mimic mitral valve disease.

RHABDOMYOMAS

Rhabdomyomas of the myocardium are often multiple and associated with tuberous sclerosis. Depending on their location they may cause obstruction to the inflow or outflow of either ventricle. Spontaneous resolution can occur.

FIBROMAS

Fibromas in the myocardium are usually solitary. They may present with ventricular outflow obstruction.

IMAGING CARDIAC TUMOURS

The chest radiography may show generalized cardiomegaly or a discrete bulge may be visible. Fibromas and myxomas may be partly calcified. Left atrial myxoma may cause signs of pulmonary venous hypertension and left atrial enlargement.

The presence of a cardiac tumour can usually be identified on two-dimensional echocardiography, but CT or MRI may also be useful (Fig. 2.12.1). Angiography is rarely necessary.

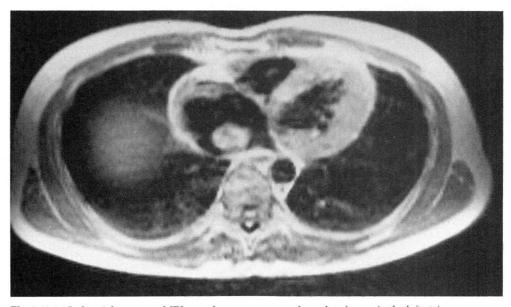

Fig. 2.12.1   Left atrial myxoma. MRI scan demonstrates a pedunculated mass in the left atrium.

2.13 CORONARY ARTERY DISEASE

Myocardial ischaemia in childhood is rare. Causes include anomalous origin of the left coronary artery from the pulmonary artery (discussed above), mucocutaneous lymph node syndrome (MCLS), idiopathic arterial calcification of infancy (Fig. 2.13.1) and familial hypercholesterolaemia.

MCLS or Kawasaki's syndrome comprises a number of symptoms including fever, conjunctivitis, dry and red mucous membranes, fissured lips, generalized erythematous rash, oedema and induration of the hands and feet, and cervical lymph node enlargement.

The cause is not known, and approximately 20% of cases develop cardiac involvement. The most important cardiac complication is a coronary arteritis leading to coronary artery aneurysms which may rupture or thrombose. When coronary aneurysms develop they almost always involve the origins of the arteries, and are, therefore, usually visible on echocardiography. However, coronary angiography may be required to show the full extent of coronary involvement.

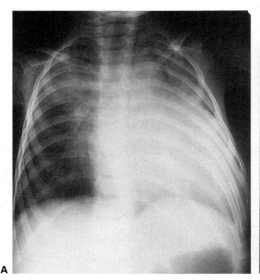
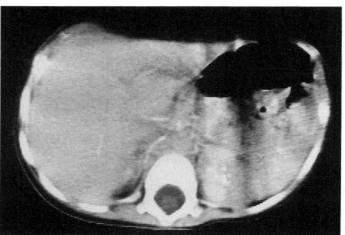

Fig. 2.13.1 Idiopathic infantile arterial calcification. **A** Cardiac failure and enlargement. **B** CT showing arterial calcification.

2.14 HEART MUSCLE DISEASE

ACUTE MYOCARDITIS

Acute myocarditis is usually due to a viral infection, often a Coxsackie B virus. Following a viral illness symptoms and signs of heart failure develop, the severity of which depends upon the amount of left ventricular damage. Of patients presenting with severe heart failure approximately 35% die within 1 year, 15% survive with some degree of permanent left ventricular impairment, and about 50% recover completely.

The chest radiograph shows cardiomegaly and signs of pulmonary venous hypertension. The severity of these changes depends upon the amount of left ventricular dysfunction.

Two-dimensional echocardiography may show enlargement of all cardiac chambers, but particularly the left ventricle. There is decreased contractility of the left ventricle and reduction of its ejection fraction. Doppler scanning may demonstrate mitral regurgitation.

The diagnosis may be confirmed by endomyocardial biopsy.

ENDOCARDIAL FIBROELASTOSIS

Isolated endocardial fibroelastosis is characterized by a severely dilated left ventricle which contracts poorly (Fig. 2.14.1), and a layer of fibrous tissue lining its endocardium. Most cases are probably due to a previous viral myocarditis, and present in the first year of life with symptoms and signs of heart failure. Fibrous thickening of the endocardium is often found in association with CHD, especially when there is left heart obstruction (e.g. in aortic stenosis, coarctation of the aorta and hypoplastic left heart syndrome). In these cases the signs and symptoms are those of the basic abnormality.

In isolated endocardial fibroelastosis the chest radiograph typically shows severe cardiomegaly and pulmonary venous hypertension. Two-dimensional echocardiography shows a severely dilated, globally hypokinetic left ventricle with a markedly reduced ejection fraction. The thickened, fibrotic endocardium is highly echogenic. Doppler scanning may demonstrate mitral regurgitation.

CONGESTIVE CARDIOMYOPATHY (Fig. 2.1.11A)

Congestive cardiomyopathy is similar in most respects to endocardial fibroelastosis, and the two entities may well be different parts of the spectrum of the same disease. The main point of distinction is the absence of endocardial fibrosis in congestive cardiomyopathy.

ENDOMYOCARDIAL FIBROSIS (EMF)

Endomyocardial fibrosis is relatively common in Central and East Africa and parts of South America and India, but is rare elsewhere. Following an acute eosinophilic myocarditis, the endocardium becomes fibrotic and lined by thrombus. Progressive fibrosis and thrombosis cause obliteration of the ventricular cavities, and distortion of the atrioventricular valves.

In the acute phase there may be fever and eosinophilia. In the chronic phase there may be right or left heart failure.

Radiographic appearances are variable. Right heart involvement may be associated with cardiomegaly, and left heart involvement with signs of pulmonary venous hypertension.

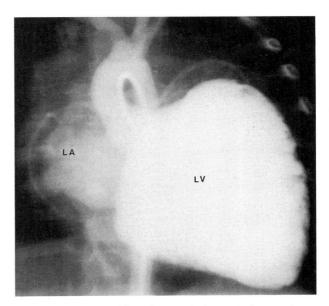

Fig. 2.14.1 Endocardial fibroelastosis. Left ventriculogram shows a severely dilated left ventricle (LV). Opacification of the left atrium (LA) indicates mitral regurgitation.

Two-dimensional echocardiography shows enlargement of the atria and obliteration of the ventricular cavities. The ventricles may be seen to be lined by echogenic masses (thrombi), particularly toward the apices. The atrioventricular valves may appear deformed, and Doppler scanning may detect regurgitation.

Endocardial biopsy may provide definitive histology, but is potentially hazardous due to the possibility of dislodging emboli.

HYPERTROPHIC CARDIOMYOPATHY (HCM)

Hypertrophic cardiomyopathy is a genetic disorder characterized by hypertrophy of one or both ventricles, but usually the left, in the absence of any predisposing cause. The myocardial hypertrophy is often asymmetrical and particularly involves the septum. Left ventricular hypertrophy may cause obstruction of the left ventricular outflow, and distortion of the mitral valve may cause regurgitation.

Many cases in childhood are discovered by screening the siblings and children of known patients with HCM. Other cases present as symptomless murmurs, chest pain, dyspnoea and sudden death.

The chest radiograph may be normal. The heart may appear bulky, but is not usually enlarged, except late in the disease. Signs of left atrial enlargement and pulmonary venous hypertension may be visible.

Two-dimensional echocardiography is usually diagnostic. Important signs are thickening of the left ventricular wall, especially involving the septum, obliteration of the left ventricular cavity at end-systole, systolic anterior movement of the anterior leaflet of the mitral valve, and premature systolic closure of the aortic valve. The gradient across the left ventricular outflow tract and any mitral regurgitation may be assessed by Doppler scanning.

CT and MRI can demonstrate the amount and distribution of the ventricular hypertrophy (Fig. 2.14.2), and most of the echographic features of the disease may also be demonstrated by angiography.

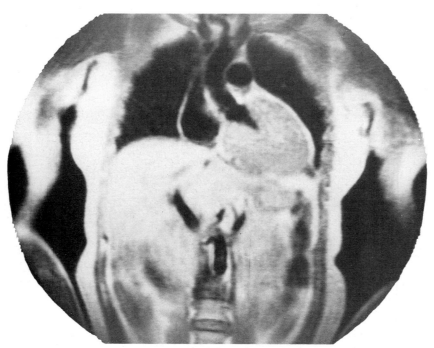

Fig. 2.14.2 Hypertrophic cardiomyopathy. MRI scan shows diffuse, severe hypertrophy of the left ventricle, and a small cavity.

2.15   VALVULAR HEART DISEASE

TRICUSPID VALVE DISEASE

Tricuspid stenosis in children and infants is almost always associated with Ebstein's anomaly or pulmonary atresia with intact ventricular septum. Tricuspid regurgitation is usually due to Ebstein's anomaly or less often endomyocardial fibrosis.

PULMONARY VALVE DISEASE

Pulmonary stenosis is almost always congenital. Pulmonary regurgitation may be due to Marfan's syndrome or other diseases of connective tissue, and it may follow pulmonary valvotomy and repair of tetralogy of Fallot. Functional pulmonary regurgitation may be secondary to severe pulmonary arterial hypertension. Congenital absence of the pulmonary valve is an unusual association of tetralogy of Fallot, causing severe pulmonary regurgitation and marked dilatation of the right ventricular outflow and central pulmonary arteries.

MITRAL VALVE DISEASE

Mitral atresia is part of the hypoplastic left heart syndrome. Congenital mitral stenosis may occur in isolation, but is usually associated with aortic atresia or coarctation of the aorta. In 'parachute' mitral valve there is stenosis due to the chordae tendinae of both mitral leaflets attaching to a single papillary muscle.

Mitral regurgitation occurs in atrioventricular septal defects, corrected transposition, endocardial fibroelastosis, hypertrophic cardiomyopathy and in any condition in which there is severe left ventricular dilatation. Mitral valve prolapse rarely causes any signs or symptoms in childhood. It may be associated with Marfan's syndrome and ASD. Echocardiography is diagnostic.

AORTIC VALVE DISEASE

Aortic stenosis in children and infants is almost always congenital. Aortic regurgitation in childhood may be due to congenital anomalies of the aortic root (e.g. aortic sinus aneurysm, aortic sinus-to-left ventricle fistula), disease of the aortic wall (e.g. Marfan's syndrome) or lesions of the aortic cusps (e.g. rheumatic or infective endocarditis, mucopolysaccharidoses). It may also occur secondary to subaortic VSD. Most cases are not symptomatic, but severe aortic regurgitation may cause heart failure, when the chest radiograph may show an enlarged heart with a left ventricular shape and signs of pulmonary venous hypertension. The cause can often be determined by two-dimensional echocardiography, and the size and function of the left ventricle can be assessed. The severity of regurgitation can usually be estimated by Doppler scanning.

REFERENCES

Been M, Kean D, Smith M A, Douglas R H B, Best J J K, Muir A L 1985 Nuclear magnetic resonance in hypertrophic cardiomyopathy. British Heart Journal 54: 48–52
Edwards J E 1948 Anomalies of the derivatives of the aortic arch system. Medical Clinics of North America 32: 925
Martin R P, Rakowski H, French J, Popp R L 1978 Localisation of pericardial effusion with wide-angled phased array echocardiography. American Journal of Cardiology 42: 904–912
Olson M C, Posniak H V, McDonald V et al 1989 Computed tomography and magnetic resonance imaging of the pericardium. Radiographics 9: 633–649
Philp T, Summerling M D, Fleming J, Grainger R G 1972 Aberrant left pulmonary artery. Clinical Radiology 23: 153
Shapiro L M, McKenna W J 1983 Distribution of left ventricular hypertrophy in hypertrophic cardiomyopathy: a two-dimensional echocardiographic study. Journal of the American College of Cardiologists 2: 437–444
Stark D D, Higgins C B, Lanzer P et al 1984 Magnetic resonance imaging of the pericardium: normal and pathological findings. Radiology 150: 469–474

3

The gastrointestinal tract

V. Donoghue, H. Carty

NEONATAL GASTROINTESTINAL TRACT *V. Donoghue*

INTRODUCTION

Radiological investigation remains one of the most important sources of information for the clinician in his evaluation of neonatal gastrointestinal disorders, but the need for such examinations should be carefully considered.

Cassettes equipped with rare-earth screens and compatible fast films should be used so as to minimize radiation dose and movement artefacts. Films should be carefully collimated.

The initial radiographic evaluation should include a chest radiograph and supine abdomen without gonadal protection. These should be reviewed and supplemented, if necessary, by a decubitus view of the abdomen, which is preferable in the sick neonate and can be satisfactorily performed in an incubator.

3.1 CONTRAST MEDIA

Iso-osmolar water-soluble contrast media are the contrast media of choice in the initial evaluation of the neonatal gastrointestinal tract. These media are isotonic with blood containing 170 mg of iodine per millilitre. If they enter the peritoneal cavity or the bronchial tree, they are quickly absorbed and are much less hazardous than barium sulphate suspensions or the older hyperosmolar water-soluble contrast media, which adversely affected fluid and electrolyte balance. Retention of barium, particularly in the colon in the neonate, is highly undesirable. With the iso-osmolar water-soluble contrast media no significant fluid shift or hypovolaemia is associated with gastrointestinal administration. There is minimal absorption from the gut with prolonged visualization of the intestinal tract, and good contrast maintained for several days. These contrast media can be diluted in the ratio 2 : 1 with isotonic saline or water, without significant loss of radiographic contrast. All contrast media administered to neonates should be warmed, ideally to blood temperature.

The therapeutic effect of gastrografin is still required for the treatment of meconium ileus, some infants with milk curd syndrome, meconium plugs or the small left colon syndrome. Although this medium is frequently diluted 1 : 1, it remains hyperosmolar and fluid and electrolyte balance must be carefully monitored in infants so treated before and after radiography, and an intravenous infusion should be established before the examination.

REFERENCES

Belt T, Cohen M D 1984 Metrizamide evaluation of the oesophagus in infants. American Journal of Roentgenology 143: 367–369
Cohen M D 1987 Choosing contrast media for the evaluation of the gastrointestinal tract of neonates and infants. Radiology 162: 447–456
Dutton R V, Singleton E B 1987 Use of low osmolar contrast for gastrointestinal studies in low-birth-weight infants. American Journal of Diseases in Childhood 141: 635–638
Fleay R F, Fox R A, Sprague P L, Adams J P 1984 Dose reduction in paediatric radiology using rare earth filtration. Pediatric Radiology 14: 332–334
Harris P D, Neuhauser E B D, Gerth R 1964 The osmotic effect of water-soluble contrast media on circulating plasma volume. American Journal of Roentgenology 91: 693–698
Lutzker L G, Factor S M 1976 Effects of some water-soluble contrast media on the colonic mucosa. Radiology 118: 545–548
McAlister W H, Siegel M J 1984 Fatal aspirations in infancy during gastrointestinal series. Pediatric Radiology 14: 81–83
Robinson A, Dellagrammaticas H D 1983 Radiation doses to neonates requiring intensive care. British Journal of Radiology 56: 397–400

3.2   THE OESOPHAGUS

OESOPHAGEAL ATRESIA AND TRACHEO-OESOPHAGEAL FISTULA

Oesophageal atresia was first described in 1670 by Durston, A Narrative of a Monstrous Birth at Plymouth'. The first successful end-to-end anastomosis was achieved in Ann Arbor, Michigan, by Cameron Haight. The approximate incidence is 1 in 4000 births, and today most infants with oesophageal atresia can be successfully surgically treated. Associated anomalies, however, remain important causes of morbidity and mortality. The respiratory system is an outgrowth of the foregut at approximately the fourth week of fetal life. The aetiology of oesophageal atresia and tracheo-oesophageal fistula is not completely understood but faulty separation of the primitive trachea and oesophagus is the most widely accepted theory.

Classification (Fig. 3.2.1)

A. Oesophageal atresia without fistula (5–10%)
B. Oesophageal atresia with upper fistula only (1%)
C. Oesophageal atresia with low fistula (80–90%)
D. Oesophageal atresia with both low and high fistulas (2–3%)
E. H-fistula with no atresia (5–8%).

A very rare form of oesophageal atresia has been reported where there is membranous atresia of the oesophagus associated with an intramural fistula. Distal oesophageal stenosis also has been reported in some patients with oesophageal atresia with tracheo-oesophageal fistula. Atresia with overlapping proximal and distal fistulas have also been reported. The incidence of oesophageal atresia in twins is increased.

Clinically affected infants usually present early with excessive oral secretions and choking. Feeding difficulties with choking occur in infants with H-type fistulas, but the diagnosis may be delayed even for years with presentation as repeated chest infections.

In the majority of patients, the site of the atresia is between the proximal and middle thirds of the oesophagus. The proximal oesophagus forms a blind pouch which is distended with air, indicating the diagnosis. Confirmation can be accomplished by passing a radiopaque feeding tube through the nose to the level of the atresia. This usually curls when it approaches the blind end (Fig. 3.2.2). Chest films should include the upper abdomen to assess the presence of air in the stomach, which indicates the presence of a distal fistula, frequently accompanied by marked generalized gaseous distension of the gut. If a lateral film is obtained, there is usually considerable anterior displacement of the upper trachea, but this view is not routinely indicated. When there is a proximal fistula, it is located in the anterior wall of the oesophagus and in such cases the proximal pouch is not distended.

The length of the gap between the oesophageal segments varies. In oesophageal atresia with a distal fistula, the gap is usually short and primary repair is possible. When there is atresia and no distal fistula, there is usually a long gap (in the order of five vertebral bodies) between the proximal and distal oesophageal segments and primary repair with end-to-end anastomosis is not possible. Contrast studies are not indicated at the time of primary diagnosis of oesophageal atresia. The H-type fistula can be at any level, although the majority seem to occur between C7 and T2.

Radiological examination of infants with possible H-type fistula should be performed under fluoroscopic control in a prone position. The infant is placed prone on a pad on the step of an erect fluoroscopic table and firmly held if horizontal fluoroscopy is otherwise impossible. A feeding tube with end holes is introduced through the nose. The examination is begun with the tip of the tube in the distal oesophagus. Low osmolar contrast medium is injected through the tube, with enough pressure to distend the oesophagus as the tube is slowly withdrawn. The examination is recorded on video and spot films obtained, if possible. If contrast appears in the trachea or lungs, it is very important to be certain if the contrast went through a fistula or was aspirated. If the examiner is uncertain, the examination must be repeated after the trachea is cleared of contrast. The H-type fistula characteristically runs an upwardly oblique course, but rarely other paths are demonstrated (Fig. 3.2.3). Even though H-type fistulas may be demonstrated by fluoroscopy, bronchoscopy is a more sensitive method of showing them and if suspected on clinical grounds, the child should be referred for bronchoscopy. This is particularly so in older children when this form of examination is inappropriate, and when a conventional barium swallow is normal.

A right-sided aortic arch occurs in approximately 5% of patients with oesophageal atresia and, if detected preoperatively, influences the choice of side for thoracotomy. The normal thoracotomy approach to repair of atresia is via the right side. If a right-sided arch is present, a left thoracotomy is performed. The position

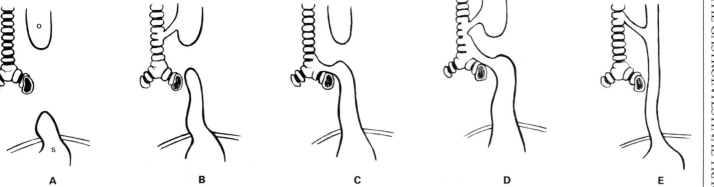

Fig. 3.2.1 Oesophageal atresia and tracheo-oesophageal fistula. **A** Atresia without fistula. **B** Atresia with upper fistula. **C** Atresia with low fistula. **D** Atresia with both low and high fistulas. **E** H-fistula with no atresia. o = oesophagus, s = stomach.

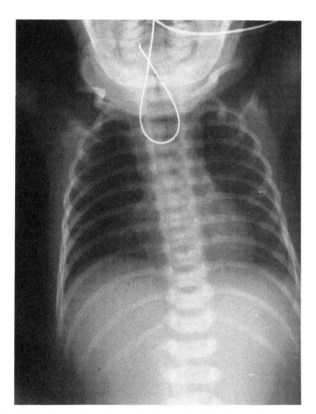

Fig. 3.2.2 Oesophageal atresia without fistula. Note radiopaque tube curls when it approaches the blind end. No air is present in the stomach and therefore there is no fistula.

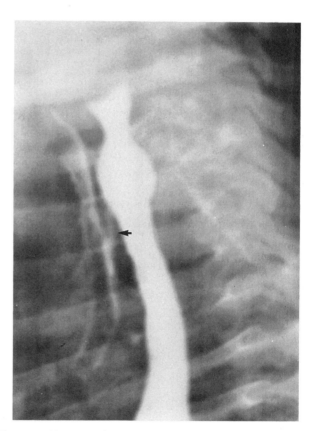

Fig. 3.2.3 H-type tracheo-oesophageal fistula. Barium enters the trachea through a fistula (arrow). Note the absence of barium in the proximal trachea.

of the arch can usually be determined by ultrasound. It may also be better shown by a high KV filtered film with an air-gap technique. CT has been used to demonstrate the fistulas but is not used routinely (Fig. 3.2.4).

Evaluation of the length of a distal pouch and thereby the intervening gap is necessary following primary closure of the fistula alone with the establishment of a gastrostomy. This can be performed by a 'refluxogram', with contrast medium introduced into the stomach via the gastrostomy and reflux promoted by gaseous distension of the stomach, gravity and suckling. The proximal pouch length is defined with an opaque nasogastric tube. Alternatively, stiff feeding tubes or bougies can be introduced orally into the proximal pouch and into the distal pouch via the gastrostomy (Fig. 3.2.5A).

Various techniques for promoting elongation of the oesophageal segments have been tried. The upper and lower oesophageal pouch can be elongated by bouginage (Fig. 3.2.5B), which may allow successful primary oesophageal reconstruction. Complications include mediastinitis, oesophageal perforation and necrosis of the pouch with subsequent scarring. If primary anastomosis is impossible, oesophageal replacement with a gastric interposition, gastric tube or colon transplant is performed. The gastric tube is made from the greater curvature of the stomach and is usually placed in the anterior mediastinum. In colonic replacement, a portion of the colon is interposed between the proximal oesophagus and stomach.

A common complication following repair is a leak at the site of the anastomosis. A chest drain is usually inserted at the time of operation. A water-soluble contrast swallow examination using low osmolar contrast medium is commonly performed about 5–7 days postoperatively to exclude anastomotic leak (Fig. 3.2.5C). Later complications of the often repetitive surgery are pleural thickening, rib deformities and scoliosis.

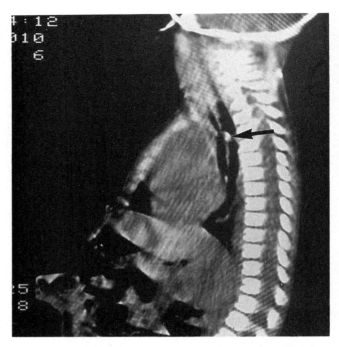

Fig. 3.2.4 Sagittal CT demonstrating tracheo-oesophageal fistula (black arrow).

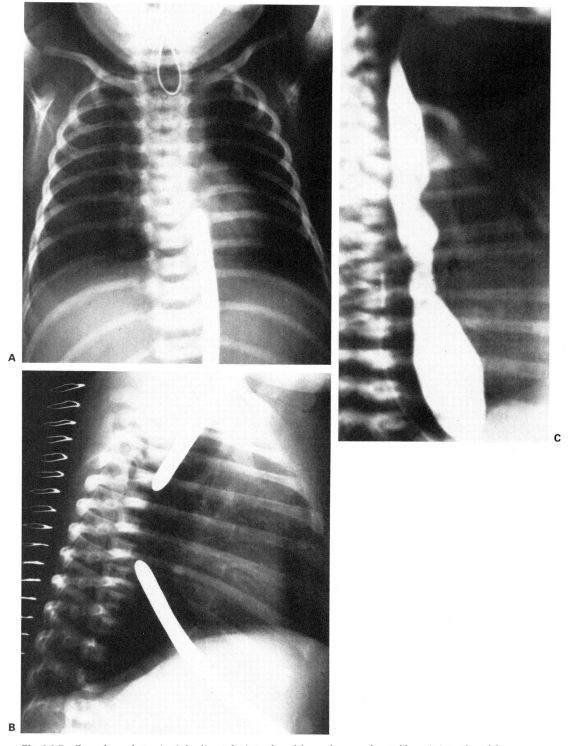

Fig. 3.2.5 Oesophageal atresia. **A** feeding tube introduced from above and metal bougie introduced from below to determine length of atretic segment. **B** Same infant some weeks later, showing a smaller gap. Radiopaque marker is included to allow for magnification. **C** Water-soluble contrast study after operation showing satisfactory anastomosis.

Shortening of the distal oesophagus is common in patients with oesophageal atresia after surgical repair. Associated hiatus hernia and gastro-oesophageal reflux are frequent. Oesophageal peristalsis in the distal oesophagus is almost always abnormal after repair of the atresia, and is best appreciated during supine studies. Gastro-oesophageal reflux is common. A stricture at the anastomotic site may be apparent as early as 1 week. Delayed stricturing may also occur in those patients with gastro-oesophageal reflux and who have not had antireflux procedures. Traditionally, dilatation has been performed with bougies at oesophagoscopy under general anaesthesia. An alternative is dilatation with inflatable balloon catheters (Fig. 3.2.6). Recurrent fistulas (Fig. 3.2.7) are a rare complication. The children present with choking during feeding and repeated chest infections. A missed proximal fistula presents in the same way. Any child with recurrent pneumonia or difficulty during feeding following repair of atresia should be suspected of having one of these conditions or a stricture or gastro-oesophageal reflux.

Tracheomalacia is another problem in these infants, thought by some to be due to chronic intrauterine compression of the trachea by a distended upper oesophageal pouch. Fluoroscopy allows dynamic evaluation of the degree of tracheal collapse during respiration and the efficiency of therapeutic procedures such as aortopexy.

Associations VATER, VACTER, VACTERL

Children with oesophageal atresia and tracheo-oesophageal fistula may have no other associated lesions, but a very significant number have multiple anomalies which are described as the VACTER association. The incidence of this anomaly is 1.6 in 10,000 live births. A common denominator of the VACTER association is suggested to be a defective mesodermal development during embryogenesis occurring before the seventh week of pregnancy. These associated defects may be lethal and may be a source of great morbidity. Particularly important are cardiac and renal defects. Echocardiography, ideally preoperatively, is important and routine, early, renal ultrasound is desirable. The increased incidence of other gastrointestinal atresias is another source of significant morbidity (Fig. 3.2.8).

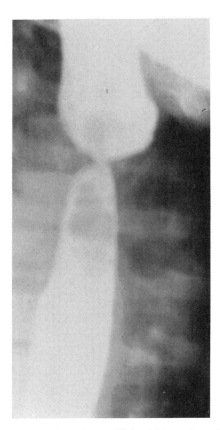

Fig. 3.2.6 Postoperative stricture. Tight stricture at anastomotic site.

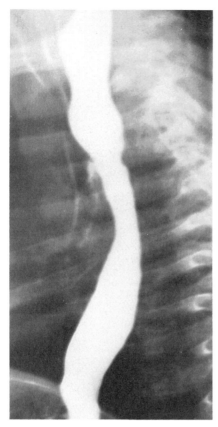

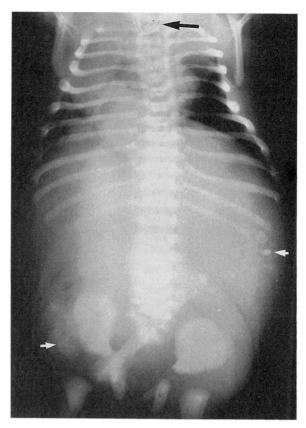

Fig. 3.2.7 Recurrent fistula. Contrast examination of oesophagus shows filling of trachea through recurrent fistula at anastomotic site.

Fig. 3.2.8 VACTER association with oesophageal atresia (black arrow), dextrocardia, lower lumbar and sacral vertebral anomalies. The infant also had an ectopic anus. There is calcification of meconium in the peritoneal cavity, the result of associated perforation (white arrows). There is a left pneumothorax.

Table 3.2.1   VACTER associations

	Common	Uncommon
Cardiovascular	Patent ductus arteriosus Ventricular septal defect	Right aortic arch Atrial septal defect Fallot's tetralogy Dextrocardia Double aortic arch Total anomalous pulmonary venous drainage Coarctation of the aorta Transposition of the great vessels
Skeletal	Vertebral Rib Radial	Sternal Congenital dislocation of the hip Club feed Polydactyly
Pulmonary		Lobar hypoplasia Lobar agenesis Unilateral pulmonary hypoplasia Unilateral pulmonary agenesis Pulmonary sequestration Tracheal agenesis Tracheal stenosis Oesophageal lung
Gastrointestinal	Anorectal atresia Duodenal atresia	Duodenal stenosis Malrotation of bowel Hypertrophic pyloric stenosis Oesophageal duplication cyst Congenital oesophageal stenosis Anal stenosis
Genitourinary	Unilateral renal genesis Renal dysplasia	Horseshoe kidney
Miscellaneous	Down's syndrome	Pierre Robin syndrome Goldenhar anomaly

Table 3.2.1 lists the major components of this constellation of anomalies.

Antenatal diagnosis

The diagnosis of oesophageal atresia may be suspected at antenatal ultrasound by the presence of polyhydramnios, reduced intraluminal liquid in the fetal gut and anomalies in other systems.

REFERENCES

Barnes J C, Smith W L 1978 The VATER association. Radiology 126: 445–449

Benson J E, Olsen M M, Fletcher B D 1985 A spectrum of bronchopulmonary anomalies associated with tracheoesophageal malformations. Pediatric Radiology 15: 377–380

Chetcuti P, Dickens D, Phelan P 1989 Spinal defects in patients born with oesophageal atresia and tracheoesophageal fistula. Archives of Diseases in Childhood 64: 1427–1430

Ein S H, Stringer D A, Stephens C A, Shandling B, Simpson J, Filler R M 1983 Recurrent tracheoesophageal fistulas. Seventeen-year review. Journal of Pediatric Surgery 18: 436–441

Goldthorn J F, Ball W S Jr, Wilkinson LG, Seigel R S, Kosloske A M 1984. Esophageal strictures in children: treatment by serial balloon catheter dilatation. Radiology 153: 655–658

Johnson A M, Rodgers B M, Alford B, Minor G R, Shaw A 1984 Esophageal atresia with double fistula: the missed anomaly. Annals of Thoracic Surgery 38: 195–200

Kirk J M E, Dicks-Mireaux C 1989 Difficulties in diagnosis of congenital H-type tracheo-oesophageal fistulae. Clinical Radiology 40: 150–153

Puri P, Blake N, O'Donnell B, Guiney E J 1981 Delayed primary anastomosis following spontaneous growth of esophageal segments in esophageal atresia. Journal of Pediatric Surgery 16: 180–183

Thomason M A, Gay B B 1987 Esophageal stenosis with esophageal atresia. Pediatric Radiology 17: 197–201

Uehling D T, Gilbert E, Chesney R 1983 Urologic implications of the VATER association. Journal of Urology 129: 352–354

LARYNGOTRACHEO-OESOPHAGEAL CLEFT

This is a rare anomaly with a cleft of variable size through the larynx, cricoid cartilages and part of the trachea. The most severe form is a common tube for the trachea and oesophagus (oesophagotrachea). Presentation is early with choking on feeding, excessive mucus and cyanosis, aspiration and respiratory distress. Anomalies such as oesophageal atresia and tracheo-oesophageal fistula may be associated. The diagnosis is made by laryngoscopy. Although contrast medium studies are not indicated for the condition, the diagnosis of cleft larynx should be considered if contrast medium easily fills the upper trachea on a swallow.

REFERENCES

Burroughs N, Leape L L 1974 Laryngotracheoesophageal cleft: report of a case successfully treated and review of the literature. Pediatrics 53: 516–522
Morgan C L, Grossman H, Leonidas J 1979 Roentgenographic findings in a spectrum of uncommon tracheoesophageal anomalies. Clinical Radiology 30: 353–358

GASTRO-OESOPHAGEAL REFLUX AND HIATUS HERNIA

Normally the lower oesophageal sphincter lies below the level of the diaphragm. It is shorter in infants than in adults. In addition, it is functionally immature. The pressure in newborns increases and is normal within 6–7 weeks, irrespective of the maturity of the child at birth. Until such time, gastro-oesophageal reflux in the neonate is a common problem but is usually 'benign'. Most cases of neonatal reflux cease spontaneously. A few infants, however, have persistent significant reflux with oesophagitis and hiatus hernia (Fig. 3.2.9). Bronchopulmonary dysplasia is a predisposing factor for severe gastro-oesophageal reflux in the premature infant. Brain damaged infants and infants with apnoea are predisposed to severe gastro-oesophageal reflux. Oesophageal dysmotility, swallowing dysfunction, antral dysmotility, nasopharyngeal reflux and aspiration into the airway may also be present in neurologically damaged infants, but dysmotility accompanies reflux even in normal children.

Gastro-oesophageal reflux may also be manifest by deteriorating pulmonary function, failure to thrive and occasional haematemesis and anaemia in the neonate.

In the neonatal period, the exclusion of gastric outlet obstruction, and, in particular, malrotation of the small bowel is an essential part of the fluoroscopic evaluation of gastro-oesophageal reflux and hiatal hernia.

While barium studies are needed to demonstrate the dynamics of swallowing and hiatus hernia, they do not always demonstrate reflux, particularly in infants with apnoeic attacks thought to be due to reflux. These children should also have an isotope 'milk scan' which is more sensitive in excluding reflux.

REFERENCES

Hrabovsky E E, Mullett M D 1986 Gastroesophageal reflux and the premature infant. Journal of Pediatric Surgery 21: 583–587
Haney P J 1983 Infant apnoea: findings on the barium esophagogram. Radiology 148: 425–427

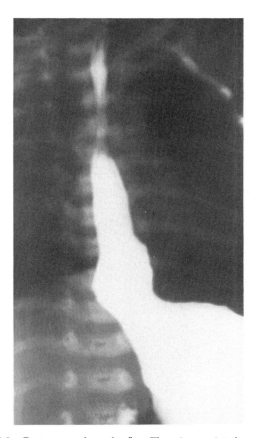

Fig. 3.2.9 Gastro-oesophageal reflux. There is associated oesophageal irregularity suggesting oesophagitis, and a small hiatus hernia.

PHARYNGEAL AND OESOPHAGEAL DIVERTICULA

Traumatic oesophageal and posterior pharyngeal diverticula usually result from mucosal perforation of the oesophagus as a complication of intubation (Fig. 3.2.10).

REFERENCE

Astley R, Roberts K D 1970 Intubation perforation of the esophagus in the newborn baby. British Journal of Radiology 43: 219–222

OESOPHAGEAL DUPLICATIONS

The oesophagus is the second most common site of gastrointestinal duplication. Non-communicating cysts usually present as posterior mediastinal masses. They may cause airway obstruction and feeding problems and extrinsic oesophageal compression. Histologically they may be lined with either oesophageal, gastric, intestinal or respiratory epithelium. When gastric mucosa lines the cyst, ulceration may occur leading to haemorrhage with sudden increase in size of the cyst. Those cysts containing gastric mucosa may be identifiable with isotope studies using ^{99m}Tc-Pertechnetate which is taken up by gastric mucosa.

REFERENCE

Ildstad S T, Tollerud D J, Weiss R G, Ryan D P, McGowan M A, Martin L W 1988 Duplications of the alimentary tract. Clinical characteristics, preferred treatment and associated malformations. Annals of Surgery 208: 184–189

OESOPHAGEAL WEB

Congenital webs are rare and may be associated with tracheo-oesophageal fistula and are considered to be a variant of oesophageal atresia. Cartilaginous remnants may be histologically seen within them. Webs may arise in prolonged gastro-oesophageal reflux.

REFERENCES

Azimi F, O'Hara A E 1973 Congenital intraluminal mucosal web of the esophagus with tracheoesophageal fistula. American Journal of Diseases of Children 125: 92–95

Jona J Z, Belin R P 1977 Intramural tracheoesophageal fistula (TEF) associated with esophageal web. Journal of Pediatric Surgery 12: 227–232

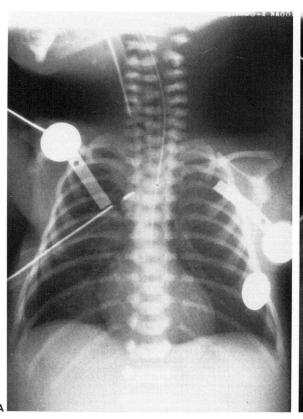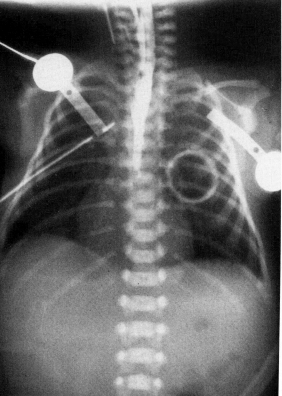

Fig. 3.2.10 **A** Plain film showing arrest of a nasogastric tube in the midthorax. This is too low for an oesophageal atresia and fistula. **B** Contrast instilled via a nasogastric tube is clearly outside the lumen of the oesophagus and lies in the mediastinum. Diagnosis – perforation of the pharynx by the nasogastric tube.

3.3 THE STOMACH

MICROGASTRIA

Congenital microgastria is a very rare abnormality in which fetal rotation of the stomach fails and the greater and lesser curves are not distinguishable. The stomach is midline in position (Fig. 3.3.1). Gastro-oesophageal reflux is common and the oesophagus is dilated and takes over the storage function of the stomach. The abnormality may be associated with the situs inversus asplenia-polysplenia syndromes, skeletal malformations and malrotation of the intestine. It has also been seen in association with oesophageal, duodenal and anal atresia and with Hirschsprung's disease.

REFERENCES

Gorman B, Shaw D G, 1984 Congenital microgastria. British Journal of Radiology 57: 260–262
Hockberger O, Swoboda W 1974 Congenital microgastria. A follow-up observation over six years. Pediatric Radiology 2: 207–208
Shackelford G D, McAlister W, Brodeur A E, Ragsdale E F 1973 Congenital microgastria. American Journal of Roentgenology 188: 72–76

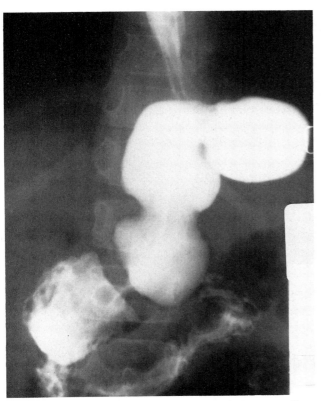

Fig. 3.3.1 Congenital microgastria. Barium meal shows small tubular stomach.

GASTRIC ATRESIA AND MEMBRANES

Almost all cases of gastric atresia occur at the pylorus or the antrum. They are thought to be due to localized vascular occlusion in fetal life and not to failure of recanalization of the intestinal tract. There are three types:

1. Complete atresia with no connection between the stomach and duodenum
2. Complete atresia with a fibrous band connecting stomach and duodenum
3. Gastric membrane or diaphragm (antral membrane).

In the diaphragmatic type, sometimes familial, obstruction is often incomplete as there is an opening in the centre of the diaphragm. Radiographs may show air in the dilated stomach with little or no distal gas.

Gastric atresia may be associated with multiple other atresias, particularly of the colon, and contrast medium enemas should be a routine part of preoperative investigation.

Neonatal presentation of severe epidermolysis bullosa is associated with atresia.

REFERENCES

Bell M F, Ternberg J L, McAlister W, Keating J P, Tedesco F J 1977 Antral diaphragm – a cause of gastric outlet obstruction in infants and children. Journal of Pediatrics 90: 196–202
Melham R E, Salem G, Mishalany H, Slim M, Der Kaloustian V M 1975 Pyloro-duodenal atresia – a report of three families with similarly affected children. Pediatric Radiology 3: 1–5
Orense M, Garcia Hernandez J, Celorio C, Canga C 1987 Pyloric atresia associated with epidermolysis bullosa. Pediatric Radiology 17: 435

GASTRIC HYPOTONIA

The radiographic appearances with distended stomach and little distal gas in the bowel may mimic those of gastric atresia and stenosis. Sepsis and central nervous system disease and generalized disorders of gastrointestinal motility should be considered as possible diagnoses.

GASTRIC PERFORATION

Although reported in association with indomethacin therapy, the aetiology of this condition is unsure. Presentation is of an acutely collapsed neonate with gross pneumoperitoneum and the perforation is found at surgery or, frequently, at post-mortem.

REFERENCES

Garland J S, Nelson D B, Rice T, Neu J 1985 Increased risk of gastrointestinal perforations in neonates mechanically ventilated with either face mask or nasal prongs. Pediatrics 76: 406–410
Rosser S B, Clark C H, Elechi E N 1982 Spontaneous neonatal gastric perforation. Journal of Pediatric Surgery 17: 390–394

GASTRIC DUPLICATIONS

These are uncommon and usually do not communicate with the stomach, and, if located at the gastric antrum, may produce gastric outlet obstruction.

REFERENCES

Alschibata T, Putnam T C, Yablin B A 1974 Duplication of the stomach simulating hypertrophic pyloric stenosis. American Journal of Diseases of Children 127: 120–122
Ildstad S T, Tollerud D J, Weiss R G, Ryan D P, McGowan M A, Martin L W 1988 Duplications of the alimentary tract: clinical characteristics, preferred treatment and associated malformations. Annals of Surgery 208: 184–189

PYLOROSPASM

In this condition, peristalsis is present in the stomach but the distal antrum and pylorus fail to relax to allow emptying of the stomach. Ultrasound of the pylorus shows normal dimensions. This is not common in the neonatal period but may be seen in infants with adrenogenital syndrome and adrenal insufficiency. Vomiting may be projectile in nature and associated with poor feeding.

REFERENCES

Byrne W J, Kangarloo H, Ament M E, Clifford W L, Berquist W, Foglia R, Fonkalsrud E W 1981 'Antral dysmotility'. An unrecognized cause of chronic vomiting during infancy. Annals of Surgery 193: 521–524
Weens H S, Golden A 1955 Adrenal cortical insufficiency in infants simulating high intestinal obstruction. American Journal of Roentgenology 74: 213–219

INTERPRETATION OF THE NEONATAL ABDOMINAL RADIOGRAPH

In the normal newborn, gas is present in the stomach by 30 minutes after birth, in the proximal small bowel by 1 hour, the distal small intestine by 3 hours, in the caecum by 4 hours, the descending colon by 6 hours and in the rectosigmoid colon by 24 hours. The diagnosis of obstruction is based on the interruption of the progression of air. Delayed passage of gas through the neonatal gut may occur following a traumatic delivery, septicaemia, hypoglycaemia or brain damage. If there is an intestinal obstruction, the onset of symptoms will depend on the location of the obstruction. High obstruction, such as duodenal or jejunal atresia, will present in the first 12 hours of life, while lower lesions such as ileal atresias will present at 24–36 hours.

An AP supine radiograph is the most important examination of neonatal gastrointestinal radiology. It is often performed in the neonatal intensive care unit with portable radiographic equipment. A supine lateral shoot through examination is often part of the initial plain film examination. This is valuable for detecting fluid levels and pneumoperitoneum. Absence of gas in the bowel may be noted in mechanically ventilated neonates severely affected by any cause of respiratory distress, particularly if neuromuscular paralytic drugs have been administered and in cases of continuous nasogastric suction.

3.4   THE DUODENUM

The differentiation of small from large bowel on plain radiographs can be impossible due to the absence of distinguishing features such as haustral folds. The sigmoid colon in a neonate can be an inferior relation of the liver, and the sigmoid, unlike in later life, can lie predominantly in the right side of the abdomen (Fig. 3.4.1). Although the rectum can be identified, particularly on a lateral view, the presence of gas within the rectum may be the result of digital rectal examination and should not be taken to indicate continuity of the gut. In the presence of clinical signs of high intestinal obstruction such as bilious vomiting and plain abdominal radiographs which are not characteristic of complete duodenal obstruction, contrast medium studies are indicated to provide information about the location and type of obstruction, of which malrotation and duodenal stenosis are the most likely causes. Corroborative signs of high obstruction are to-and-fro movement of contrast medium in the duodenum with duodeno-gastric reflux. The causes of duodenal obstruction in the newborn are listed in Table 3.4.1.

Table 3.4.1   Causes of duodenal obstruction in the newborn

Intrinsic	Extrinsic
Duodenal atresia	Ladd's bands
Duodenal stenosis	Midgut volvulus with malrotation
Duodenal web or diaphragm	Annular pancreas
	Duplication
	Haematoma
	Preduodenal portal vein

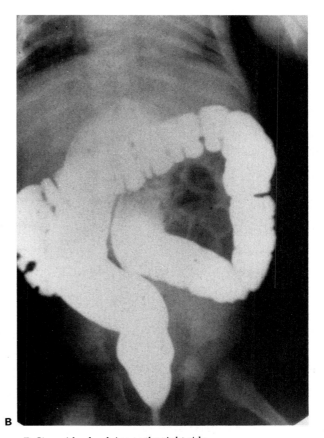

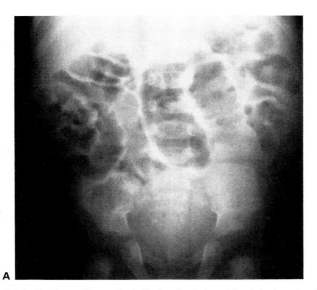

Fig. 3.4.1   Supine radiograph. **A** Redundant sigmoid colon at contrast enema. **B** Sigmoid colon lying to the right side.

DUODENAL ATRESIA AND STENOSIS

The aetiology of these conditions is thought to be failure of recanalization of the duodenum, between approximately the ninth and eleventh week of gestation. They do not appear to be related to intrauterine vascular accidents as in jejunal and ileal atresia and stenosis. Infants with atresia present in the first few hours of life with vomiting. The clinical findings in those with stenosis depend on the degree of the stenosis. The vomiting is usually bile stained, as the obstruction is usually at or below the ampulla of Vater.

The abdominal radiograph is usually diagnostic in duodenal atresia. Gas is present only in the stomach and the dilated first part of the duodenum, the characteristic 'double bubble' sign (Figs 3.4.2, 3.4.3). Occasionally, the hepaticopancreatic duct bifurcates in a Y-fashion at its insertion into the duodenum, with one branch inserting above the site of the atresia and one below, allowing a small amount of air to bypass the duodenal obstruction. There is no place for oral contrast agents if complete duodenal obstruction has been diagnosed by plain film radiography. An upper gastrointestinal series adds no further information.

Associated abnormalities are present in about 50% of the patients. Approximately 30% have Down's syndrome. Other anomalies include malrotation of the small bowel, oesophageal atresia (Fig. 3.4.2), congenital heart disease, imperforate anus, small bowel atresia, biliary atresia, annular pancreas, and renal anomalies. Some familial cases have been reported. Polyhydramnios is present in approximately 40% of patients and the diagnosis is frequently made antenatally by ultrasonography.

REFERENCES

Astley R 1969 High congenital duodenal stenosis. British Journal of Radiology 42: 385–386

Crowe J E, Sumner T E 1978 Combined esophageal and duodenal atresia with tracheoesophageal fistula: characteristic radiographic changes. American Journal of Roentgenology 130: 167–168

Nixon H H, Tawes R 1971 Etiology and treatment of small intestinal atresia; analysis of a series of 127 jejunoileal atresias and comparison with 62 duodenal atresias. Surgery 69: 41–51

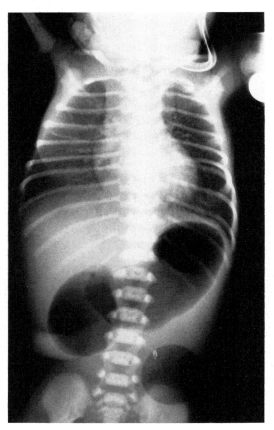

Fig. 3.4.2 Duodenal atresia. Supine radiograph showing the characteristic 'double bubble' sign. Note associated oesophageal atresia and incubator hole in lower left adbomen.

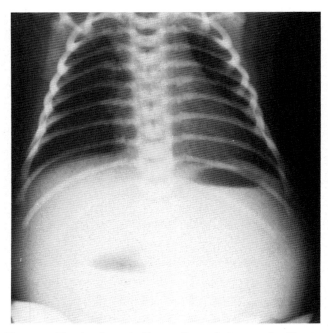

Fig. 3.4.3 Duodenal atresia. Erect radiograph showing fluid level in the stomach and first part of duodenum. Note oesophageal atresia.

ANNULAR PANCREAS

Annular pancreas is believed to result from failure of rotation of normal pancreatic tissue around the duodenum. It usually presents with symptoms of duodenal stenosis in the neonatal period, though it may be asymptomatic until late adulthood. Radiographically the findings are those of duodenal atresia or stenosis. It is found in association with duodenal atresia, duodenal stenosis, intrinsic duodenal diaphragm, malrotation and congenital absence of the gall bladder.

REFERENCES

Free E A, Gerald B 1968 Duodenal obstruction in the newborn due to annular pancreas. American Journal of Roentgenology 103: 321–325
Merrill J R, Raffensperger J G 1976 Paediatric annular pancreas: twenty years experience. Journal of Pediatric Surgery II: 921–925
Heij H A, Niessrn G T 1987 Annular pancreas associated with congenital absence of the gallbladder. Journal of Pediatric Surgery 22: 1033

DUODENAL DIAPHRAGM OR WEB

The aetiology is not certain but is probably due to failure of complete duodenal recanalization, usually at the level of the ampulla of Vater. There may or may not be an opening within the diaphragm. Clinical symptoms and age of presentation depend on the presence and size of the opening. If there is complete obstruction, a 'double bubble' configuration can be seen. Diagnosis is usually made with contrast studies (Fig. 3.4.4). The diaphragm is often difficult to demonstrate, but in some cases it becomes so stretched that an 'intraluminal' or 'wind-sock' diverticulum is formed in later life. It can occur in conjunction with duodenal bands, duodenal atresia, malrotation, situs inversus, Down's syndrome and diaphragms in other portions of the gastrointestinal tract. The surgical procedure is excision of the diaphragm with protection of the adjacent bile ducts.

REFERENCES

Hicks M C, Kalmin E H 1963 Congenital diaphragm of the descending duodenum. Radiographic demonstration of such lesion. Radiology 80: 946–948
Pratt A D 1971 Current concepts of the obstructing duodenal diaphragm. Radiology 100: 637–643

PREDUODENAL PORTAL VEIN

This is a rare abnormality where the portal vein lies anterior to the duodenum and can produce indentation and compression. It is an abnormality of development of the anastomotic channels between the right and left vitelline veins which drain venous blood from the primitive foregut, resulting in the development of the portal vein from the caudal ventral anastomosis which is anterior to the duodenum. Over 85% of patients with preduodenal portal vein have associated malformations which may be multiple. These include malrotation with bands, situs inversus, intrinsic duodenal obstruction, biliary atresia and annular pancreas. Radiographically the findings depend on the degree of obstruction. Plain films often show some degree of obstruction, and in some cases even a 'double bubble'. Diagnosis depends on demonstration of an indentation on the duodenum between the first and second portions. Surgically it is important that the vein is not transected, especially if it is contained in a peritoneal band.

REFERENCES

McCarten K M, Teele R L 1978 Preduodenal portal vein, venography, ultrasonography and review of literature. Annales de Radiologie 21: 155–160
Ziv Y, Lumbrozo R, Dintsman M 1986 Preduodenal portal vein with situs inversus and duodenal atresia. Australian Paediatric Journal 22: 69–70

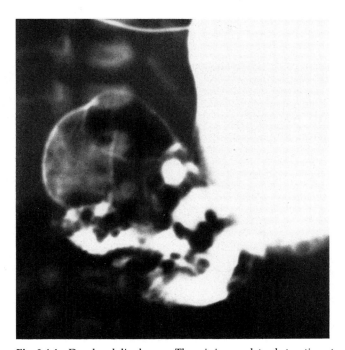

Fig. 3.4.4 Duodenal diaphragm. There is incomplete obstruction at the level of the ampulla of Vater. There is dilatation of the more proximal duodenum. An incomplete diaphragm was found at operation.

3.5   THE SMALL BOWEL

The small intestine of the neonate is quite different in appearance from that of the older child. It is difficult to identify the valvulae conniventes and it is difficult to distinguish jejunum from ileum. Peristalsis is usually quite marked and the transit time to large bowel is often shorter than in the older child or adult.

JEJUNO-ILEAL ATRESIA AND STENOSIS

It is now accepted that fetal intestinal ischaemia causes atresias in the small bowel distal to the duodenum, though there are some reports that the septal or diaphragmatic type may be due to failure of complete recanalization. Atresias have been reported in association with ergotamine ingestion during pregnancy, supporting the theory of a vascular injury, and may arise at varying times in pregnancy. Other anomalies of the gastrointestinal tract are seldom encountered with these atresias. The type of atresia varies from a membranous atresia to atretic blind ends with a fibrous connection or without any connection. A rare form of small bowel atresia is the 'apple-peel' small bowel. This consists of proximal small bowel atresia

which is long, with absence of the dorsal mesentery. The distal small intestine is spiralled around its vascular supply and resembles an apple peel. The result is a very short intestine and a high mortality. In some instances the condition is recessively inherited.

Multiple gastrointestinal atresias with intraluminal calcification are even rarer, and may be familial and with autosomal recessive inheritance.

Abdominal radiographs usually demonstrate small bowel obstruction. If high, only one or two loops are visualized (Fig. 3.5.1). If low, many loops are present (Fig. 3.5.2). Multiple air-fluid levels are usually present in the erect or decubitus projection. In some instances, gas mixed with meconium can produce a 'soap-bubble' appearance, although this is usually more common with meconium ileus. Occasionally, and mainly in ileal atresia, a loop of small intestine proximal to the atresia becomes grossly distended and filled with fluid and faeces producing a mass (Fig. 3.5.3). The bowel proximal to the loop is only mildly dilated. The fluid-filled loop may also contain meconium and give a bubbly appearance which can be confused with meconium ileus in cystic fibrosis.

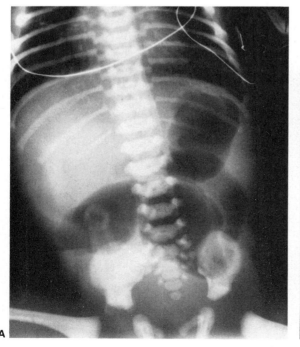
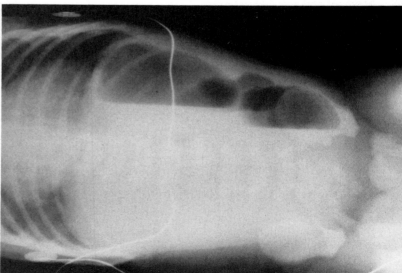

A

Fig. 3.5.1 Jejunal atresia. **A** Supine radiograph showing two dilated loops of bowel. **B** Air-fluid levels on decubitus radiograph confirming the high intestinal obstruction.

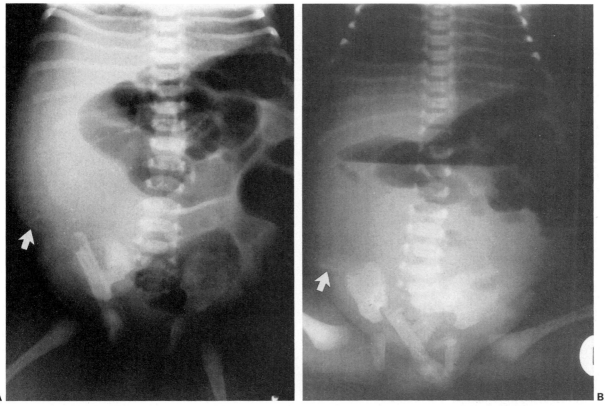

Fig. 3.5.2 Ileal atresia. **A** Supine radiograph showing many dilated loops of bowel. **B** Erect film showing multiple fluid levels in keeping with atresia. Note calcification of meconium in peritoneal cavity from previous perforation, most likely the result of a vascular accident (arrow).

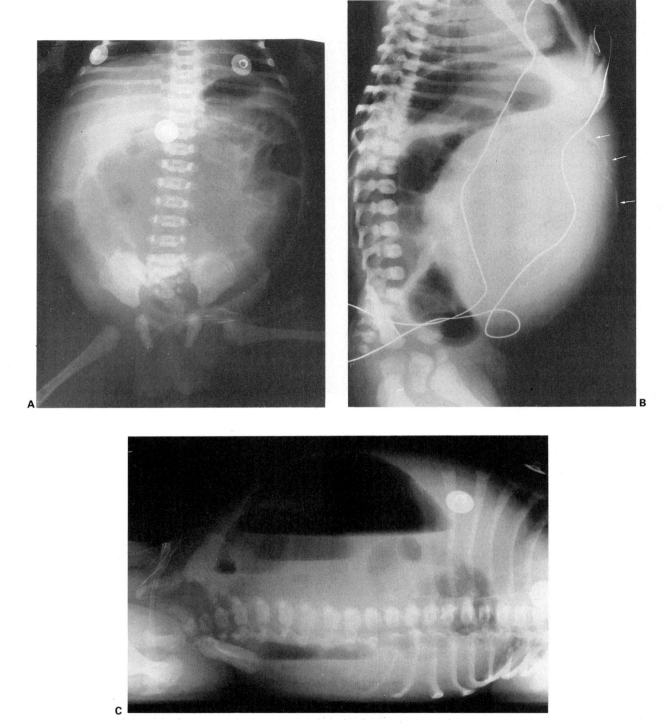

Fig. 3.5.3 Ileal atresia with pseudocyst formation. **A, B** Grossly distended loop of small bowel filled with fluid causing mass effect. Note calcification of meconium from meconium peritonitis (small white arrows). **C** Lateral decubitus film showing large air-fluid level in pseudocyst.

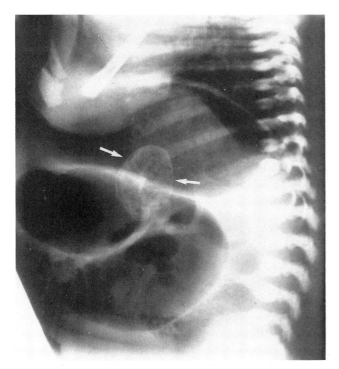

Fig. 3.5.4 Ileal with atresia intraluminal calcification of meconium within small intestine (arrows).

Even though there is an atresia, children may pass meconium if the vascular insult that caused the lesion occurred late. Passage of meconium is often taken clinically to equate with patency of the gastrointestinal tract, hence the delay in diagnosis.

Calcification of meconium peritonitis due to in utero bowel perforation is present in approximately 12% of atresias (Fig. 3.5.3B). This can be diagnosed antenatally using sonography. Rarely, extensive intraluminal calcification may occur (Fig. 3.5.4).

If the obstruction is thought to be high, contrast studies are not required. When doubt exists, a contrast enema is indicated. In infants with ileal atresia a microcolon will be present (Fig. 3.5.5). The rectum is typically distensible, unlike children with Hirschsprung's disease. Contrast will not enter dilated bowel and stops at the atresia. The ileocaecal valve is rarely competent in the neonate and in normal infants contrast medium, once it enters the small bowel, will flow freely.

Surgical treatment consists of an end-to-end anastomosis of small bowel with resection of non-viable bowel.

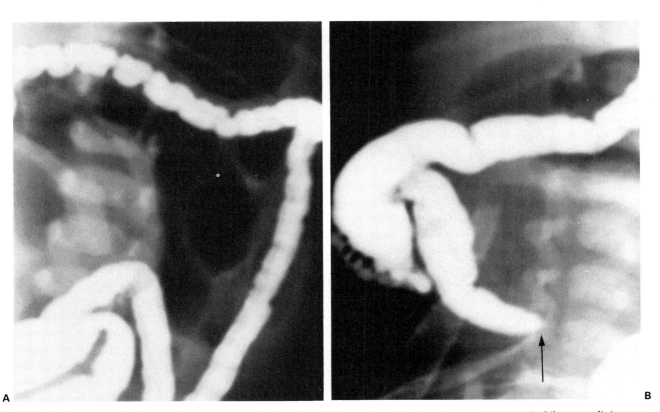

Fig. 3.5.5 Ileal atresia. **A** Small unused colon, the so-called functional 'microcolon'. **B** Reflux of contrast into terminal ileum, outlining area of atresia (arrow).

REFERENCES

Aharon M, Kleinhaus U, Lichtig C 1978 Neonatal intramural intestinal calcifications associated with bowel atresia. American Journal of Roentgenology 130: 999–1000

Carty H, Brereton R J 1983 The distended neonate. Clinical Radiology 34: 367–380

Coradello H, Ponhold W, Lubec G, Pollak A 1982 Disappearance of bowel gas in newborn infants on mechanical ventilation. Pediatric Radiology 12: 11–14

Daneman A, Martin D J 1979 A syndrome of multiple gastrointestinal atresias with intraluminal calcification. A report of a case and a review of the literature. Pediatric Radiology 8: 227–231

Foster M A, Nyberg D A, Mahoney B S, Mack L A, Marks W M, Raabe R D 1987 Meconium peritonitis: prenatal sonographic findings and their clinical significance. Radiology 165: 661–665

Graham J M Jr, Marin-Padilla M, Hoefnagel D 1983 Jejunal atresia associated with cafergot ingestion during pregnancy. Clinics in Pediatrics (Philadelphia) 2: 226–228

Seashore J H, Collins F S, Markowitz R I, Seashore M R 1987 Familial apple peel jejunal atresia: surgical, genetic and radiographic aspects. Pediatrics 80: 540–544

Yousefzadeh D K, Jackson J H Jr, Smith W L, Lu Ch H 1984 Intraluminal meconium calcification without distal obstruction. Pediatric Radiology 14: 23–27

MECONIUM ILEUS

This condition is usually associated with cystic fibrosis of the pancreas (mucoviscidosis) in the neonate and is the earliest manifestation of the disease. It can however occur with abnormalities of the pancreatic ducts. Clinically, infants have quite marked abdominal distension, often visible peristalsis, do not pass meconium and have bilious vomiting within the first 24 hours of life. In meconium ileus, obstruction is due to impaction of thick, tenacious meconium in the distal small bowel. Complications include ileal atresia or stenosis, perforation and meconium peritonitis and volvulus.

Plain radiographs in the uncomplicated case demonstrate numerous dilated air-filled loops of bowel (Fig. 3.5.6). Although historically it has been suggested that there is usually a paucity of fluid levels in this condition, in practice multiple air-fluid levels are a common feature. Admixture of gas with meconium, particularly in the right side of the abdomen, may give rise to a 'soap-bubble' appearance which, in practice, is relatively rare and not pathognomonic (Fig. 3.5.6). Peritoneal calcification secondary to meconium spillage may occur with meconium ileus, but can occur with any type of obstruction and in utero perforation.

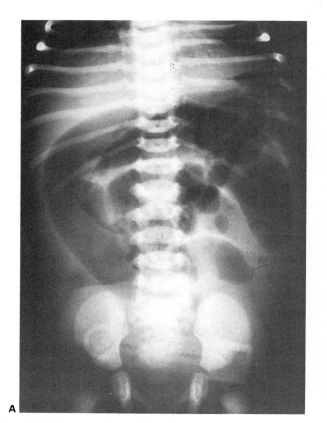

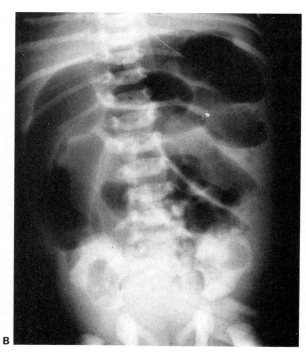

Fig. 3.5.6 Meconium ileus. **A** Supine radiograph showing numerous dilated air-filled loops of bowel. **B** Erect radiograph showing a paucity of fluid levels, in keeping with meconium ileus. Note 'soap-bubble' appearance in the left side of the abdomen.

A further pattern is that of gross abdominal distension with a central opacity and a few surrounding gas shadows (Fig. 3.5.7A). The central opacity represents a collection of meconium within which faint calcification may be seen. The meconium may be in grossly distended bowel or may be situated in the localized peritoneal collection, and associated volvulus and bowel infarction is common with a very poor prognosis. Ultrasonography may be useful in detecting such complications antenatally or delineating such collections in the presence of a relatively gasless abdomen (Fig. 3.5.7B, C). Intestinal perforation is commonly seen in meconium ileus (Fig. 3.5.7D).

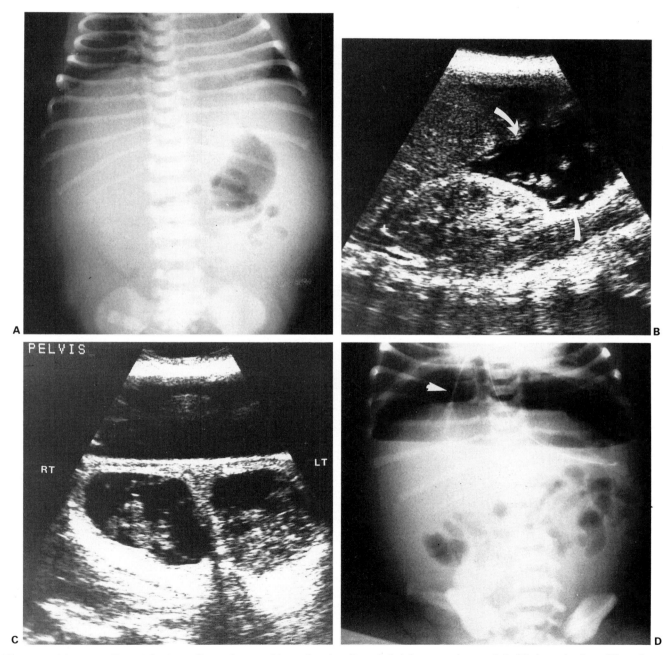

Fig. 3.5.7 Meconium ileus. **A** Supine radiograph at age 1 hour showing distended abdomen and normal air-filled proximal small bowel loops. **B** Abdominal ultrasonography at the same time showing free peritoneal fluid anterior to the right kidney and inferior to the liver and containing echogenic material (arrows). **C** Transverse image of scrotum showing fluid containing debris, having entered through a patent processus vaginalis. Appearances are in keeping with meconium perforation. **D** Erect abdominal film some hours later showing a pneumoperitoneum and therefore perforation. The infant had cystic fibrosis. Note the ligamentum falciparum outlined by air.

For further radiological management diagnostic enemas are frequently required, before which the child must be adequately resuscitated with intravenous infusions established and maintenance of adequate fluid and electrolyte balance ensured. A low osmolar contrast medium is used, and in both meconium ileus and ileal atresia will show a functional microcolon. When the medium refluxes into the terminal ileum, differentiation will be possible (Fig. 3.5.8). In meconium ileus, pellets of meconium will be outlined. These pellets, when passed, have a characteristic grey-buff colour. Having established the probable diagnosis of meconium ileus, the contrast medium is changed to gastrografin at a 1:1 dilution with sterile water. The detergent effect, in association with the considerable osmotic effect of this medium, even in diluted form, helps the passage of the sticky meconium pellets and so relieves obstruction. The aim is to introduce the gastrografin into the dilated small bowel beyond the obstructing intraluminal pellets of meconium. An initial attempt may not achieve this aim, and if the child is in a stable condition the examination may be repeated some hours later. Success will be shown by improving clinical signs with less distension and passage of meconium. If signs of obstruction are not relieved, or signs of peritonitis develop, further attempts at therapeutic enema should be abandoned. In such cases there may well be associated atresias in addition to the meconium obstruction.

REFERENCES

Abramson S J, Baker D H, Amodio J B, Berdon W E 1987 Gastrointestinal manifestations of cystic fibrosis. Seminars in Roentgenology 22: 97–113

Noblett H R 1969 Treatment of uncomplicated meconium ileus by gastrografin enema. Journal of Pediatric Surgery 4: 190–197

Willi U, Reddish J M, Teele R L 1980 Cystic fibrosis: its characteristic appearance on abdominal sonography. American Journal of Roentgenology 134: 1005–1010

ANOMALIES OF INTESTINAL ROTATION AND FIXATION

Malrotation encompasses a wide variety of anomalies of intestinal rotation and fixation – non-rotation, malrotation, reversed rotation and in association with, for instance, diaphragmatic hernia and omphalocele.

The midgut develops as an extension of the yolk sac. At 6 weeks of age, the gastrointestinal tract is a tubular structure, divided into foregut, supplied by the coeliac artery, the midgut supplied by the superior mesenteric artery and the hindgut supplied mainly by the inferior mesenteric artery. During growth of the bowel the duodenum and caecum rotate 270 degrees anticlockwise to assume the adult configuration. The gastrointestinal tract rotates along the axis of the superior mesenteric artery. Before 6 weeks' gestation, the duodenum initially rotates 90 degrees anticlockwise to lie to the right of the superior mesenteric artery (Fig. 3.5.9A). The caecum also rotates 90 degrees in the same direction to lie to the left of the superior mesenteric artery. During the sixth week, the liver is growing rapidly and fills the greater part of the abdominal cavity. Accommodation for the bowel is sought elsewhere and is found within the umbilical cord. During this period, the duodenum rotates another 90 degrees to lie posterior to the superior mesenteric artery (Fig. 3.5.9B), while the rest of the midgut is in the umbilical cord. By the tenth to the twelfth week of gestation, the intestine slides back into the peritoneal cavity where the final 90-degree rotation of the duodenum and 180-degree rotation of the caecum occurs (Fig. 3.5.9C). The right colon is the last portion of the gastrointestinal tract to complete rotation so the caecum descends into the right lower quadrant (Fig. 3.5.9D). Normally the small bowel mesentery is broad based, with its attachment extending from the ligament of Trietz to the ileocaecal valve. This wide base prevents the small intestine from twisting around the superior mesenteric artery.

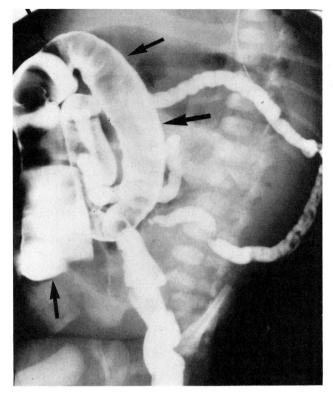

Fig. 3.5.8 Meconium ileus. Contrast enema outlining a functional microcolon. Contrast outlines a very dilated terminal ileum filled with meconium (arrows). Note small pellets of meconium frequently found in the microcolon.

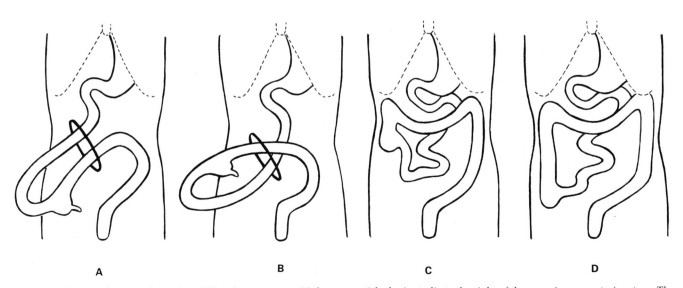

A   B   C   D

Fig. 3.5.9 Stages of intestinal rotation. **A** Duodenum rotates 90 degrees anticlockwise to lie to the right of the superior mesenteric artery. The distal large bowel also rotates 90 degrees anticlockwise. **B** Duodenum rotates another 90 degrees anticlockwise. The duodenojejunal flexure lies in the midline posterior to the superior mesenteric artery. **C** Duodenum has rotated its last 90 degrees anticlockwise with the duodenojejunal flexure lying to the left of the midline. The caecum continues rotating. **D** Normally rotated bowel.

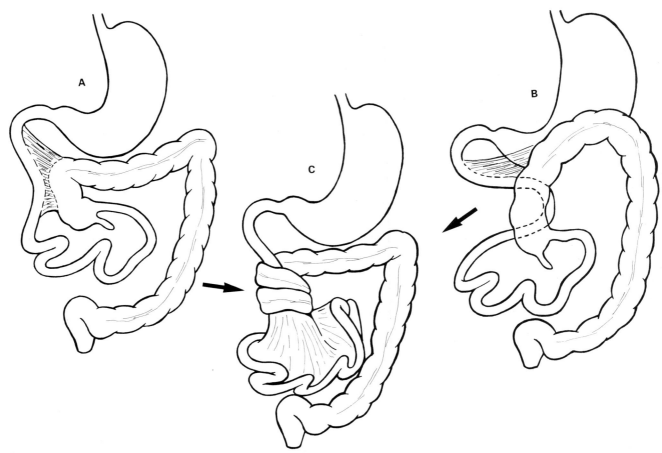

Fig. 3.5.10 Midgut volvulus (**C**) may develop from non-rotation (**A**) or incomplete rotation (**B**).

Omphalocele (exomphalos) occurs when the intestine does not return from the umbilicus and there is almost complete failure of rotation of the mid-gut. In non-rotation, the small bowel lies entirely to the right of the spine and the colon on the left (Fig. 3.5.10). The patients are often asymptomatic, although the root of the mesentery is short and may predispose to volvulus. Reversed rotation is where the duodenum passes anterior to the superior mesenteric artery, and the hepatic flexure and left transverse colon pass behind the superior mesenteric artery. The caecum is usually malrotated and medially placed. Obstructing bands and midgut volvulus can also occur with this form of rotational abnormality. In malrotation, positioning of the gastrointestinal tract is somewhere between the normal and complete non-rotation. Generally the caecum and the terminal ileum are displaced upwards and medially (Figs 3.5.10, 3.5.11).

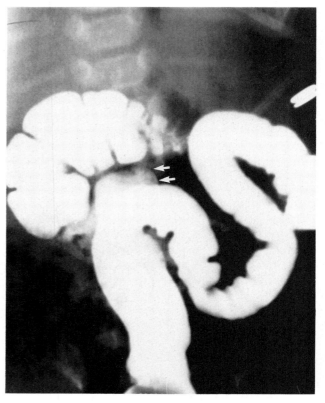

Fig. 3.5.11 Malrotation. The caecum is displaced upwards and medially on contrast enema examination (arrows).

In some cases, the caecum is mobile. In others, the ligament of Trietz or the caecum are poorly fixed and the small bowel is predominantly right sided. Duodenal bands are commonly present and the associated short mesentery predisposes to midgut volvulus. When this occurs, the entire gut twists around the superior mesenteric artery and impairs the vascular supply. This may be intermittent, causing bouts of abdominal distension and pain, or permanent and lead to bowel necrosis and perforation.

Clinical presentation is usually with bilious vomiting, but abdominal distension and tenderness are indications of bowel ischaemia. Radiographically, in infants with intestinal malrotation, obstructing volvulus and duodenal bands, a high partial or complete obstruction is noted (Fig. 3.5.12A). If the volvulus is complicated by ischaemia, the distal abdomen may be distended by fluid-filled compromised bowel (Fig. 3.5.12B). Intramural gas is rarely seen but, if present, indicates bowel necrosis. If the

diagnosis is not obvious on plain films, any infant with bilious vomiting should have a prompt contrast examination. A contrast meal using low osmolar water-soluble contrast is performed initially to demonstrate the level and nature of the obstruction. In malrotation this is usually in the second or third portion of the duodenum. The obstruction may be total with no contrast passing into the distal duodenum, making it impossible to distinguish malrotation from duodenal atresia. Urgent surgery is indicated, as with obstruction, as at this level volvulus may result in small bowel necrosis. In approximately 10% of patients with malrotation an intrinsic duodenal obstruction such as a web is found. Precise identification of the ligament of Trietz at the duodeno-jejunal flexure is easiest with the passage of the first bolus of contrast through the duodenum. In the normal supine infant, it is located to the left of the spine, almost at the level of the first part of the duodenum. When a volvulus is present, a 'cork-

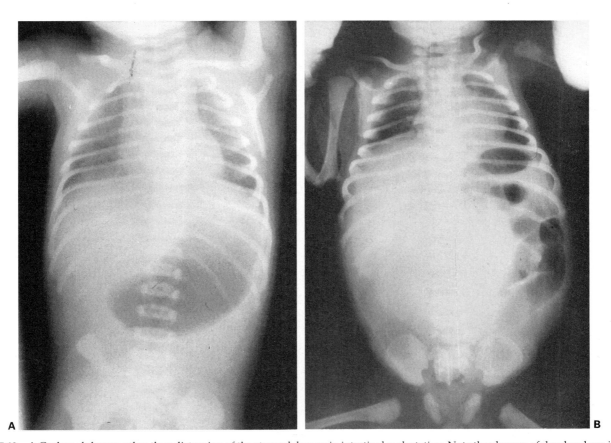

Fig. 3.5.12 **A** Gasless abdomen other than distension of the stomach by gas in intestinal malrotation. Note the absence of duodenal gas in contradistinction with the usual findings in intrinsic duodenal obstructions. **B** Infant with localized perforation, malrotation and volvulus, and bowel ischaemia secondary to malrotation. Note the normal bowel loops displaced to the left abdomen surrounding a gasless mass. Localized pneumoperitoneum seen in the lower right quadrant.

'screwing' appearance of the small intestine is seen as it twists around the superior mesenteric artery (Fig. 3.5.13). This is seen in the midline or to the right of the midline. Thickened mucosal folds indicating oedema and bowel ischaemia may also be seen. Ultrasound can be helpful in equivocal cases. In the normal infant the superior mesenteric vein lies to the right of the superior mesenteric artery (Fig. 3.5.14). In malrotation it is either anterior or to its left.

An abnormally low position of the duodenojejunal flexure projected below the gastric antrum or at a similar level to the third part of the duodenum, where it passes under the superior mesenteric artery in the midline, may be an incidental finding. Chronic distension of the colon or partial small bowel obstruction, do not necessarily imply significant underlying abnormality of mesenteric fixation. A redundant first and second part of the duodenal loop may also give a false impression of a malrotation. A normal duodenojejunal flexure is mobile in neonates and can be displaced manually to the right of the vertebral column. Although barium enemas have been advocated for ascertaining the position of the caecum, which is commonly high in malrotation, this is such a variable and frequent finding it is not a reliable diagnostic feature of upper intestinal malrotation. In suspected malrotation of the small bowel, there is no doubt that an upper gastrointestinal examination is more accurate than examination of the colon.

The accepted surgical procedure is Ladd's operation. This includes untwisting of the volvulus and placing the small bowel in the right abdomen and the colon on the left, the non-rotated position. The mesentery of the small intestine is spread from right to left with a broad attachment to prevent recurrent volvulus. The condition may be associated with other abnormalities such as Hirschsprung's disease, intussusception (Waugh's syndrome) and atrial isomerism with asplenia.

REFERENCES

Berdon W E, Baker D H, Bull S, Santuilli T V 1970 Midgut malrotation and volvulus. Which films were not helpful? Radiology 96: 375–383

Gaines P A, Saunders A J S, Drake D 1987 Midgut malrotation diagnosed by ultrasound. Clinical Radiology 38: 51–53

Hayden C K Jr, Boulden T F, Swischuk L E, Lobe T E 1984 Sonographic demonstration of duodenal obstruction with midgut volvulus. American Journal of Roentgenology 143: 9–10

Katz M E, Siegel M J, Shackelford G D, McAlister W H 1987 The position and mobility of the duodenum in children. American Journal of Roentgenology 148: 947–951

Potts S R, Thomas P S, Garstin W I H, McGoldrick J 1985 The duodenal triangle: a plain film sign of midgut malrotation and volvulus in the neonate. Clinical Radiology 36: 47–49

Taylor G A, Littlewood Teele R 1985 Chronic intestinal obstruction mimicking malrotation in children. Pediatric Radiology 15: 392–394

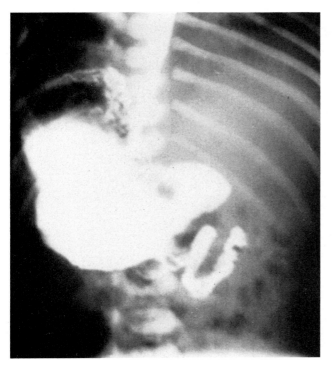

Fig. 3.5.13 Malrotation. Upper gastrointestinal contrast examination outlining cork-screwing of the proximal small bowel as it twists around the superior mesenteric artery.

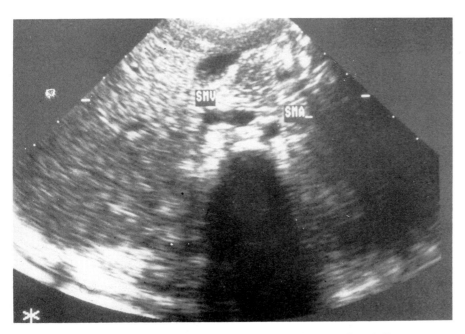

Fig. 3.5.14 Normal relationship of the SMA and SMV. In malrotation the vein lies anterior to or to the left of the artery.

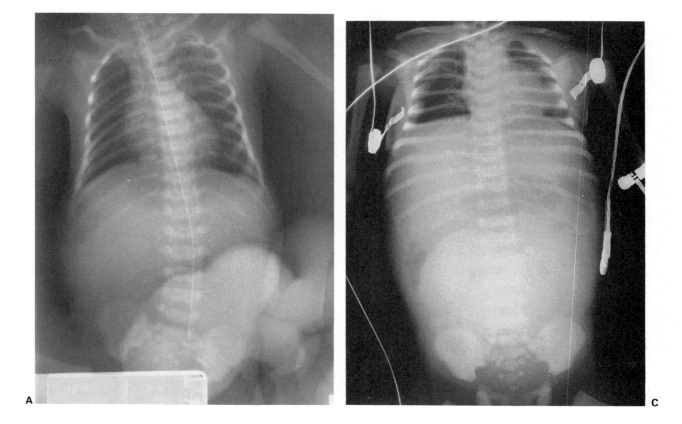

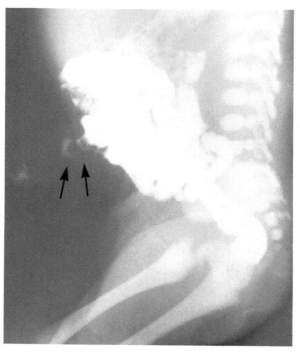

Fig. 3.5.15 **A** Large exomphalos. **B** Neonate with small omphalocele (exomphalos) contrast follow-through examination showing the extent of bowel herniation. **C** Plain abdomen (same child as in **A).** Post repair film. Note elevated diaphragms and paucity of abdominal gas. The repositioning of the contents of the exomphalos leads to these features.

EXOMPHALOS

In omphalocele (exomphalos) there is herniation of viscera into the base of the umbilical cord. Routine preoperative radiographs are usually unnecessary but the contents, particularly the liver, can be easily determined on ultrasonography if there is doubt. Contrast follow-through examinations can occasionally be of value to demonstrate the extent of bowel herniation (Fig. 3.5.15). Of more importance in these infants is the detection of associated anomalies which occur in 60% of infants. These most commonly include gastrointestinal, cardiac and chromosomal abnormalities.

GASTROSCHISIS

This condition in which there is a central abdominal wall defect above the umbilicus has similar radiological connotations and complications as exomphalos. Upper anterior abdominal wall defects are sometimes associated with defects involving the diaphragm, sternum, heart and pericardium.

Following repair of either exomphalos or gastroschisis, numerous complications may develop. Postoperative radiographs often show a distended abdomen with featureless distended bowel loops which may persist unaltered for many days (Fig. 3.5.15C). The difficulty is in distinguishing these from the similar appearance that may occur in necrotizing enterocolitis.

These infants are also often very slow to recommence absorption of food from the intestine. Contrast studies done to exclude strictures, and partial blind loops, show a slow passage of contrast through adynamic featureless bowel.

Long-term complications include those associated with short bowel, as extensive resection of necrotic bowel is often necessary during primary repair.

REFERENCES

Blane C E, Wesley J R, Dipietro M A, White S J, Coran A G 1984 Gastrointestinal complications of gastroschisis. American Journal of Roentgenology 144: 589–591

Gilbert W M, Nicolaides K H 1987 Fetal omphalocele: associated malformations and chromosomal defects. Obstetrics and Gynecology 70: 633–635

INTUSSUSCEPTION

Intussusception may occur in the neonatal period (Fig. 3.5.16). The symptoms are often restricted to vomiting, abdominal distension and blood-stained stools. These symptoms closely mimic necrotizing enterocolitis and the two conditions may coexist. It has been shown also in association with jejunal atresia.

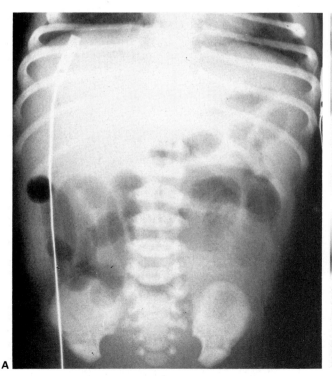
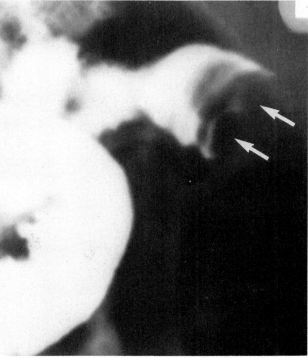

Fig. 3.5.16 A Neonate who presented with abdominal distension and bleeding per rectum and who had intussusception. Supine radiograph showing dilated loops of small bowel suggesting obstruction. **B** Contrast enema examination outlined an intussusception (arrows) which was successfully reduced hydrostatically.

Plain film findings are variable but generally will show a low small bowel obstruction. It has presented with a pneumoperitoneum and as fetal-neonatal abdominal ascites. Intussusception at this age is more likely to be due to a lead point such as Meckel's diverticulum, polyp, tumour, etc. If intussusception is suspected, reduction should be attempted, with caution. Obstruction may have been present for a long time, a lead point may be present and the reduction rates are lower than in older infants.

REFERENCES

Cipel L, Fonkalsrud E W, Gyepes M T 1977 Ileo-ileal intussusception in the newborn. Report of a radiologically diagnosed case. Radiology 6: 39–42
Gluk B, Alpan G, Vinograd I, Udassin R, Mogle P, Eyal F 1985 Meconium plugs and intussusception in a premature infant. American Journal of Perinatology 2: 67–69
Patriquin H B, Afshani E, Effman E et al 1977 Neonatal intussusception: report of 12 cases. Radiology 125: 463–466
Smith V S, Giacoia G P 1984 Intussusception associated with necrotising enterocolitis. Clinics in Pediatrics (Philadelphia) 23: 43–45

SEGMENTAL DILATATION OF SMALL BOWEL

Segmental dilatation of the small bowel is a rare congenital condition in which the calibre of the bowel lumen increases locally without obstruction to the lumen and without thickening of the muscle coat. The passage of intestinal contents throughout the dilated segment is not delayed unless there is a coexistent volvulus or exomphalos.

Segmental dilatation may coexist with other serious abdominal conditions in the neonatal period, such as exomphalos, malrotation of the midgut and Meckel's diverticulum. Local hamartomatous changes may be noted.

Plain radiographs of the abdomen may show an isolated loop of bowel containing an air-fluid level (Fig. 3.5.17). The characteristic finding on barium studies of the small bowel is a localized dilatation of the small bowel lumen (Fig. 3.5.18). In the absence of complications, the transit time of contrast medium through the small bowel is not delayed.

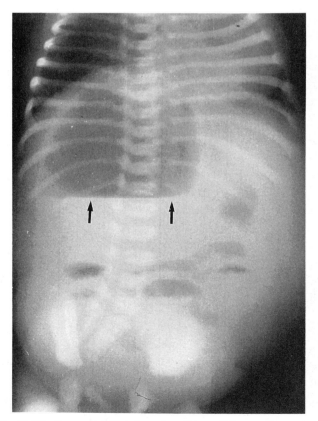

Fig. 3.5.17 Segmental dilatation of small bowel. Erect radiography showing dilated isolated loop of bowel containing air-fluid level (arrows). (Reprinted with permission from Br. J. Radiol.)

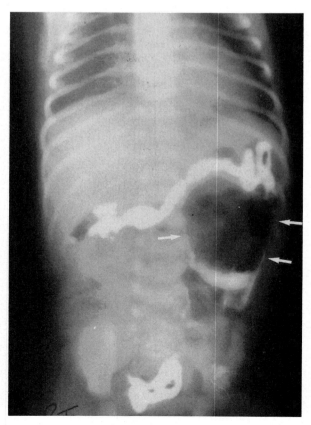

Fig. 3.5.18 Segmental dilatation of small bowel. Contrast examination showing barium has entered the localized area of dilatation (arrows).

REFERENCES

Bell M J, Ternberg J L, Bower R J 1982 Ileal dysgenesis in infants and children. Journal of Pediatric Surgery 17: 395–399
Brown A, Carty H 1984 Segmental dilatation of the ileum. British Journal of Radiology 57: 371–374
Ratcliffe J, Tait T, Lisle D, Leditschke J F, Bell J 1989 Segmental dilatation of the small bowel: report of three cases and literature review. Radiology 171: 827–830

SHORT BOWEL SYNDROME

The small intestine may be congenitally short or as a result of surgical resection for conditions such as volvulus with small bowel ischaemia, congenital atresias or exomphalos. As a rule, there is some generalized dilatation of the small bowel loops (Fig. 3.5.19) and sometimes an increase in prominence of the mucosal folds. Motor activity of the bowel may be disordered. During screening, transit time should be recorded. Coexistent strictures should be sought.

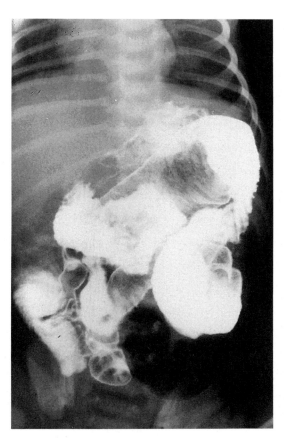

Fig. 3.5.19 Short bowel syndrome. Water-soluble upper gastrointestinal contrast examination outlining a short small bowel with dilatation of some of the loops.

Ultimate survival with normal growth, without parenteral nutrition, is now possible with as little as 11 cm of jejunoileum with an intact ileocaecal valve and as little as 25 cm of jenunoileum without an ileocaecal valve.

REFERENCES

Dorney S F, Ament M E, Berquist W E, Vargas J H, Hassall E 1985 Improved survival in very short small bowel of infancy with use of longterm parenteral nutrition. Journal of Pediatrics 107: 521–525
Tiu C M, Chou Y H, Pan H B, Chang T 1984 Congenital short bowel. Pediatric Radiology 14: 343–345
Touloukian R J, Smith G J 1983 Normal intestinal length in preterm infants. Journal of Pediatric Surgery 18: 720–723
Sansaricq C, Chen W J, Manka M, Dvis D, Snyderman S 1984 Familial congenital short small bowel with associated defects. A longterm survival. Clinics in Pediatrics (Philadelphia) 23: 453–455

DUPLICATION CYSTS

Duplication cysts occur most commonly in the small bowel near the ileocaecal valve, and are spherical or tubular structures lined with intestinal epithelium and with smooth muscle in their walls. Duplications of the small bowel have a mesenteric location. There are numerous suggested aetiologies: abnormalities of recanalization, vascular accidents and incomplete closure of neuroenteric openings. The child presents with a variety of symptoms including a palpable mass, a distended abdomen or signs of obstruction. Antenatal ultrasonographic detection is possible.

Plain abdominal films may show a soft tissue mass within the abdomen. Ultrasonography usually shows a well-defined cystic anechoic mass but may occasionally be echoic when it contains haemorrhage or inspissated material. It is usually unilocular. An echogenic inner rim is highly suggestive of a duplication. ^{99m}Technetium sodium pertechnetate is taken up by ectopic gastric mucosa which may be present in cystic duplications. As 15–20% of duplications contain gastric mucosa, this radionuclide may be of value in diagnosis but is only indicated when the diagnosis is uncertain. Barium studies may show displaced or obstructed loops of bowel but seldom produce filling of the cyst in the communicating variety.

REFERENCES

Ildstad S T, Tollerud D J, Weiss R G, Ryan D P, McGowan M A, Martin L W 1988 Duplications of the alimentary tract: clinical characteristics, preferred treatment, and associated malformations. Annals of Surgery 208: 184–189
Kangarloo H, Sample W F, Hansen G 1979 Ultrasonic evaluation of abdominal gastrointestinal tract duplication in children. Radiology 131: 191–194
Rose J S, Gribetz D, Krasna I H 1978 Ileal duplication cyst: the importance of sodium pertechnetate Tc^{99m} scanning. Pediatric Radiology 6: 244–246

MILK ALLERGY

This condition usually results from ingestion of cows' milk. Clinically the infant presents with diarrhoea and vomiting. Contrast studies demonstrate flocculation of barium, dilated small bowel loops and increased transit time similar to the appearances observed in coeliac disease.

REFERENCES

Liu H Y, Whitehouse W M, Giday Z 1975 Proximal small bowel transit pattern in patients with malabsorption induced by bovine milk protein ingestion. Radiology 115: 415–420
Walker-Smith J 1975 Cow's milk protein intolerance: transient food intolerance of infancy. Archives of Diseases in Childhood 50: 347–350

3.6 THE COLON

In the newborn the haustral pattern of the colon is less prominent than in the older child or adult, or absent. In addition, the sigmoid colon is often more redundant (Fig. 3.4.1) and often lies entirely to the right. The caecum may be higher and more medial than normal.

NECROTIZING ENTEROCOLITIS

The precise aetiology of necrotizing enterocolitis is unknown. It commonly affects premature infants but is seen in full-term infants. Although the aetiology is not known, the following are associated conditions that predispose to intestinal ischaemia: asphyxia, shock, hypoxia, respiratory distress, umbilical vessel catheterization, exchange transfusions, patent ductus arteriosus and other congenital heart lesions, dehydration, surgery, particularly cardiopulmonary bypass for cardiac lesions and intestinal obstruction.

Clinically the findings are usually bile-stained aspirates, abdominal distension and passage of blood per rectum, tachypnoea, tachycardia, apnoeic spells and hypotension. There is frequently neutropenia and thrombocytopenia. As soon as the disease is suspected treatment must be started. Oral feeding is discontinued, a nasogastric tube is used for decompression and intravenous antibiotics are commenced. An AP abdominal radiograph is first viewed and followed by a cross table lateral film if perforation is suspected.

Intramural gas is the radiological hallmark of necrotizing enterocolitis. It can take the form of a linear or bubbly collection of gas (Figs 3.6.1, 3.6.2). The bubbly appearance can, however, be difficult to differentiate from air mixed with meconium or faecal material. It can occur anywhere from oesophagus to rectum. The correlation between the presence and extent of intramural air and the severity of necrotizing enterocolitis is poor.

Non-specific radiographic findings include general small bowel dilatation and separation of the loops of bowel.

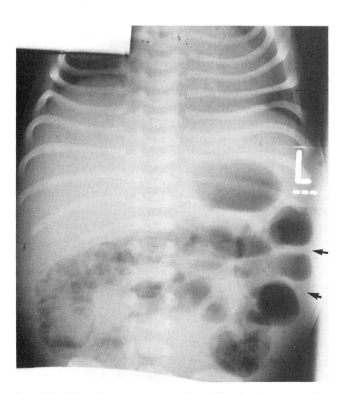

Fig. 3.6.1 Necrotizing enterocolitis. Erect film showing separation of bowel loops (arrows) and intramural gas.

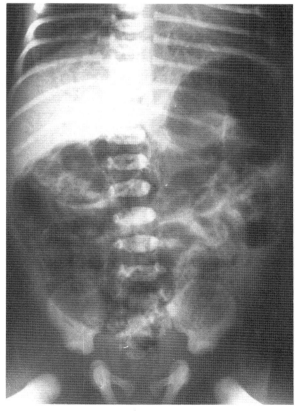

Fig. 3.6.2 Necrotizing enterocolitis with bowel loop distension, diffuse intramural air and portal venous gas.

The presence of portal venous gas (Fig. 3.6.2), originally described as a fatal sign, no longer indicates an irreversible disease process. It should be remembered that gas passing through an umbilical venous catheter may give rise to portal venous gas in the absence of necrotizing enterocolitis (Fig. 3.6.3). Ultrasound is highly sensitive in the detection of portal venous gas.

The role of radiology in necrotizing enterocolitis is to confirm the diagnosis and to monitor the course of the disease and detect complications.

Films are performed as clinically indicated. The supine radiograph may show evidence of free intraperitoneal air (Fig. 3.6.4). The appearances are those of hyperlucency of the entire abdomen, which is distended if the accumulation of free air is massive. In addition, both sides of the bowel wall may be visualized (Fig. 3.6.4) and the falciform ligament may be seen as an opaque line in the midabdomen or right upper quadrant. (Fig. 3.6.5). The cross table lateral view is often best to demonstrate bowel wall thickening, portal vein gas and free intraperitoneal air (Fig. 3.6.6).

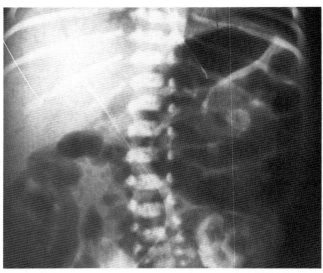

Fig. 3.6.3 Portal venous gas which has entered the liver through an umbilical venous catheter which is incorrectly placed.

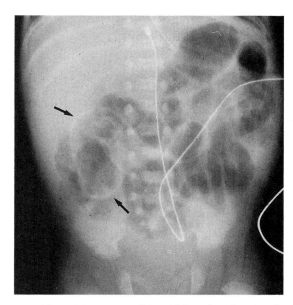

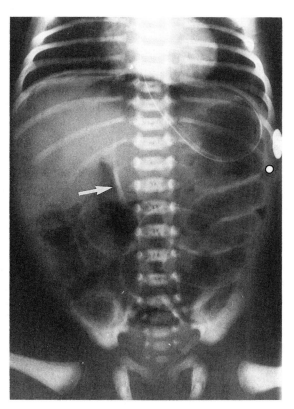

Fig. 3.6.4 Necrotizing enterocolitis with bowel perforation. Supine radiograph showing some increased lucency over the liver and discretely defined wall of small bowel (arrows).

Fig. 3.6.5 Necrotizing enterocolitis with bowel perforation. Supine radiograph showing falciform ligament (white arrow).

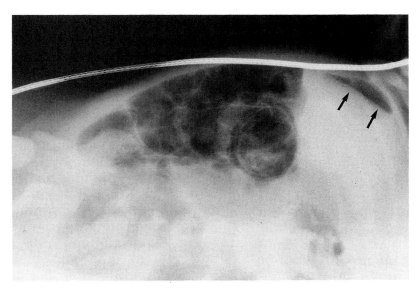

Fig. 3.6.6 Necrotizing enterocolitis. Lateral decubitus film. There is bowel wall thickening and intramural air. There is a small collection of air over the liver (arrows) indicating pneumoperitoneum.

In many infants with perforations no free air is detected but there is diminution of gas within the intestines and intestinal walls and an increase in density of the abdomen due to the presence of free intraperitoneal fluid, detectable by ultrasound. Air in Morison's pouch has recently been reported as an early sign of pneumoperitoneum and has the same significance as the more obvious signs of pneumoperitoneum. Persistent dilated loops of bowel have been found to correspond with necrotic segments found at operation, but are not an absolute indication for surgery. Ultrasonography is useful in the localization of abscess formation, resulting from a localized walled-off perforation, in the identification of gas in the portal venous system and in the assessment of bowel motility when differentiating bowel obstruction from ileus. In equivocal cases, water-soluble contrast medium examination has been advocated in the diagnosis of necrotizing enterocolitis, but it is not routine practice because of the risk of perforation and should be reserved for exceptional cases where the institution of therapy for nectrotizing enterocolitis would be otherwise detrimental. Idiopathic infantile arterial calcification is associated with necrotizing and presumed ischaemic enterocolitis (Fig. 3.6.7).

Strictures of the bowel, particularly the colon, are frequent following necrotizing enterocolitis and appear to be independent of the severity of the clinical disease (Fig. 3.6.8). These strictures, which may be variable in length, single or multiple, may resolve spontaneously. Clinically they may be associated with constipation, recurrent intermittent obstruction of the gut, or acute obstruction, sometimes with a history of continued low grade bleeding. When clinical symptoms suggest intestinal obstruction or plain radiographs reveal abnormally distended loops of bowel, a contrast enema should be carried out. This is particularly important if there has been a defunctioning enterostomy, before continuity of the bowel is re-established. As some strictures are very short, great care needs to be taken during fluoroscopy to show the continuity of the bowel lumen without overlapping loops obscuring pathology. At times, an upper intestinal study with follow-through films may be more revealing than an enema.

Balloon dilatation of colonic strictures is generally inappropriate following necrotizing enterocolitis. Rarer complications of enterocolitis include enterocyst formation, lymphoid hyperplasia, internal fistulas, adhesions and malabsorption. Associated septicaemias may result in osteomyelitis or septic arthritis in the newborn.

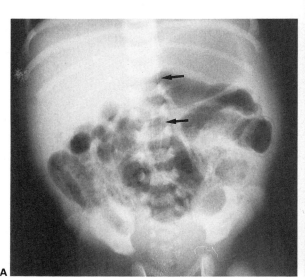
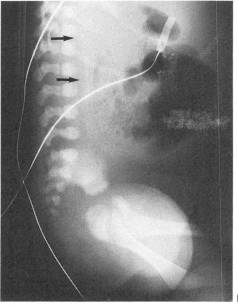

Fig. 3.6.7 **A & B** Necrotizing enterocolitis with intramural air and extensive calcification of the walls of the aorta (arrows).

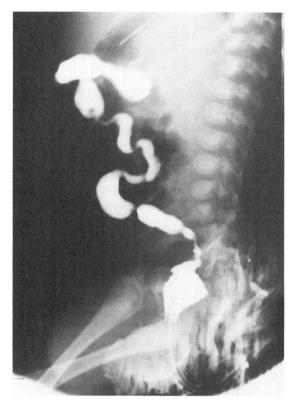

Fig. 3.6.8 Necrotizing enterocolitis. Colonic strictures which are multiple are present in this patient.

REFERENCES

Avni E F, Rypens F, Cohen E, Pardou A 1991 Pericholecystic hyperechogenicities in necrotizing enterocolitis: a specific sonographic sign? Pediatric Radiology 21: 179–181

Brill P W, Olson S R, Winchester P 1990 Neonatal necrotising enterocolitis: air in Morison pouch. Radiology 174: 469–471

Daneman A, Woodward S, De Silva M 1978 The radiology of neonatal necrotising enterocolitis (NEC). A review of 47 cases and the literature. Pediatric Radiology 7: 70–77

Donoghue V, Kelman C G 1982 Transient portal venous gas in necrotising enterocolitis. British Journal of Radiology 55: 681–683

Leonard T Jr, Johnson J F, Pettett P G 1982 Critical evaluation of the persistent loop sign in necrotizing enterocolitis. Radiology 142: 385–386

COLITIS IN THE NEONATAL PERIOD

In addition to necrotizing enterocolitis and the colitis associated with Hirschsprung's disease, a group of infants may present with a profuse bloody diarrhoea, most frequently viral in origin, but occasionally due to bacterial infection. The plain radiographs are typically non-specific, with perhaps mild dilatation of the bowel but without evidence of intramural or intrahepatic gas. Should a water-soluble contrast medium examination be performed, the findings may be unremarkable or there may be evidence of mucosal oedema and irregularity.

HIRSCHSPRUNG'S DISEASE

In Hirschsprung's disease, there is absence of normal myenteric ganglion cells in the involved segment of the colon. The length of aganglionosis is variable but always extends proximally from the anal canal. The condition most frequently presents in the full-term neonate, predominantly in males, with delayed passage of meconium, abdominal distension and bilious vomiting. Failure to pass meconium in the first 24 hours of life is a strong indication to exclude Hirschsprung's disease, as should diarrhoea, representing potentially lethal secondary enterocolitis, in a neonate.

The rectosigmoid area is involved in approximately 80% of cases. A long segment disease is less common. Total colonic aganglionosis may also involve a variable length of small bowel and accounts for approximately 5% of cases. Long segment Hirschsprung's disease has an increased familial incidence and a more equal sex distribution. A few cases of extensive intestinal aganglionosis have been reported; it appears that in total or near total intestinal aganglionosis, approximately 50% of siblings are affected. There have been a few reports of infants with coexistent Hirschsprung's disease and small bowel malrotation, and the association has been reported in many syndromes, including Down's syndrome, with congenital hypoventilation syndrome or Ondine's curse and congenital neuroblastoma.

It is important to diagnose the condition as early as possible, as complications include failure to thrive and Hirschsprung's enterocolitis which can lead to perforation, peritonitis and death.

Plain abdominal radiographs in the typical case of Hirschsprung's disease show some degree of low small bowel or colonic obstruction (Fig. 3.6.9), with more distension of large than small and few fluid levels. Indeed the presence of large bowel fluid levels should always suggest the diagnosis. When there is little or absent rectal gas, Hirschsprung's disease should be suspected though these findings may be seen in meconium plug syndrome and in premature infants. When Hirschsprung's disease is suspected clinically, histological verification is needed. Ideally, and if histopathological services are adequate and available, emergency rectal biopsy with subsequent intraoperative large bowel biopsies will allow accurate establishment of a defunctioning colostomy in the first instance. More typically, however, such ideal pathological services are not available and a barium enema will help in most patients to identify the level of

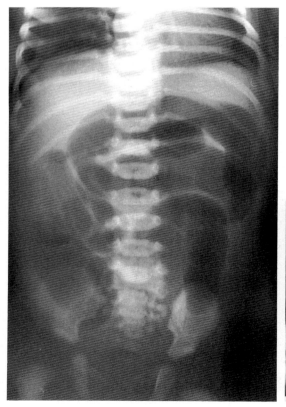

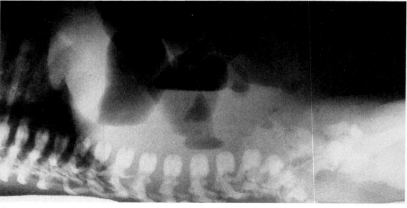

A   **B**

Fig. 3.6.9 Hirschsprung's disease. **A** Supine radiograph showing dilated loops of bowel with very little rectal gas. **B** Decubitus films: obstruction is confirmed by the fluid levels within the dilated loop.

aganglionosis and thus indicate a safe site for colostomy.

The choice of contrast medium is not critical, but in a critically sick infant, low osmolar contrast media are preferable. No bowel preparation before the examination should be performed and rectal examination is best avoided. A soft catheter is inserted just into the rectum and can be advanced to a higher level later if more practical. Initial high siting of the catheter may lead to the transition zone between normal and abnormally innervated bowel being missed. A balloon catheter should not be used. With the infant in the lateral position, the bowel is filled slowly. The diagnosis is suggested where there is a transition zone between relatively narrow and denervated and dilated, innervated bowel in the shape of an inverted cone (Fig. 3.6.10). When this is observed, the examination should be discontinued as filling of the more proximal dilated bowel beyond the transition zone may lead to impaction. A characteristic transition zone may not always be precisely demarcated. In such cases, abnormal contractions and irregular peristaltic activity of the aganglionic portion of the colon may be a useful indicator of disease. These can take the form of irregular thumb-printing or pointed serrations due to circular muscular contractions. The aganglionic bowel may be of normal calibre and appear narrowed only by comparison with the more proximally dilated bowel, but it often shows poor distensibility. Twelve-hour delayed postevacuation films are useful in cases of doubt, when contrast medium will be retained in the dilated bowel and may show better the transition zone.

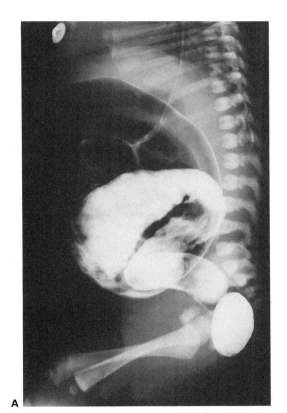

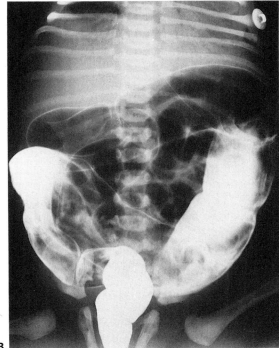

Fig. 3.6.10 Hirschsprung's disease. Lateral (**A**) and supine (**B**) films taken during contrast enema examination. The proximal sigmoid colon and descending colon are very dilated when compared to the distal sigmoid colon and rectum. The dilated segments are full of meconium. The transition zone is at proximal sigmoid colon level.

Enterocolitis is a recognized although uncommon complication of Hirschsprung's disease, presenting with profound, often bloody diarrhoea. The bowel wall and the mucosa become oedematous and inflamed and irregularity of the mucosa may be seen if an enema, which is generally contraindicated, is inadvertently performed (Fig. 3.6.11). Perforations are generally not a feature of this complication, which, if untreated, may be rapidly fatal. Progressive dilatation of the colon in such circumstances is a serious prognostic sign.

The rectosigmoid index relates the transverse diameter of the rectum to that of the sigmoid colon. Normally, this is a 1 : 1 relationship, or the rectal diameter is greater than the sigmoid diameter. If the rectal diameter is less than the sigmoid diameter, Hirschsprung's disease should be suspected. In practice, the sensitivity of this measurement is low. Manometric measurements of rectal pressures show that in Hirschsprung's disease there is absence of the normal relaxation of the internal sphincter, with a reduction in the intraluminal pressure in the anal canal when the rectum is distended with a balloon. This technique is of more relevance to older children.

Sometimes, rectal biopsies are performed for suspected Hirschsprung's disease and the diagnosis is not substantiated. A request for a contrast enema may then be made. Generally, this may be performed with safety after 24 hours following a suction biopsy. If a full thickness biopsy has been performed, if possible the examination should be delayed for 4 days and then be performed with a water-soluble contrast medium, but with care could be performed earlier if the clinical indication is strong enough.

Total colonic aganglionosis is difficult to diagnose radiologically. Plain films may demonstrate distal small bowel obstruction. A contrast enema may demonstrate a normal colon, a microcolon, or a short colon with less redundant flexures than normal. One indication of the diagnosis is irregularity of the colon wall and abnormal contractions seen throughout the colon, but these are easily overlooked when a normal colonic calibre lowers the threshold for observation. Another indication is impaction of meconium throughout the large bowel giving a double-contrast effect (Fig. 3.6.12).

Total intestinal aganglionosis is extremely rare and invariably fatal, and approximately half of the siblings with this condition are affected. When Hirschsprung's disease is combined with intestinal malrotation, potential complications include delayed diagnosis of the Hirschsprung's disease resulting in serious entero-colitis, or the delayed diagnosis of malrotation with resulting midgut volvulus and bowel ischaemia, or incorrect siting of the colostomy.

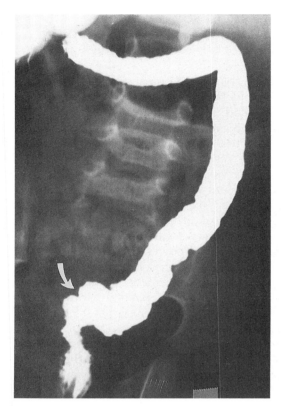

Fig. 3.6.11 Hirschsprung's disease involving rectum and distal sigmoid colon. Note irregularity of colonic mucosa above the transition zone (arrow), due to the onset of enterocolitis.

REFERENCES

Berdon W E, Baker D H 1965 The roentgenographic diagnosis of Hirschsprung's disease in infancy. American Journal of Roentgenology 93: 432–446

Berdon W E, Koontz P, Baker D H 1964 The diagnosis of colonic and terminal ileal aganglionosis. American Journal of Roentgenology 91: 680–689

Cremin B J, Golding R L 1976 Congenital aganglionosis of the entire colon in neonates. British Journal of Radiology 49: 27–33

De Campo J F, Mayne V, Boldt D W, De Campo M 1984 Radiological findings in total aganglionosis coli. Pediatric Radiology 14: 205–209

Filston H C, Kirks D R 1982 The association of malrotation and Hirschsprung's disease. Pediatric Radiology 12: 6–10

Rosenfield N S, Ablow R C, Markowitz R I et al 1984 Hirschsprung disease: accuracy of the barium enema examination. Radiology 150: 393–400

Roshkon J E, Haller J O, Berdon W E, Sane S M 1988 Hirschsprung's disease, Ondine's curse, and neuroblastoma – manifestations of neurocristopathy. Pediatric Radiology 19: 45–49

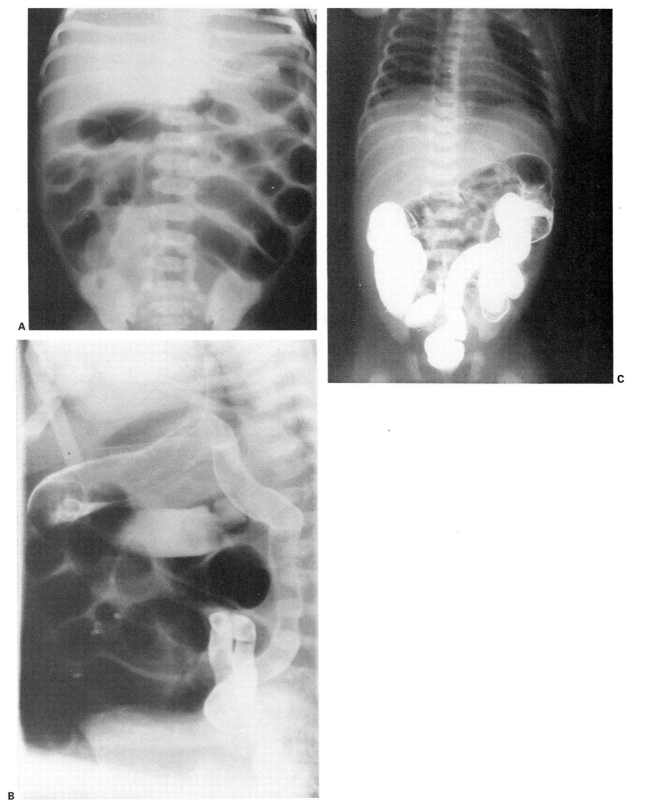

Fig. 3.6.12 **A**, **B** Plain film and enema in total colonic aganglionosis. **C** Another patient age 7 days with total aganglionosis showing a more normal calibre bowel.

NEURONAL DYSPLASIA

Increasingly, a condition of bowel dysmotility is being recognized in the neonatal period. Clinical presentation is with a distended abdomen and failure to pass meconium. The initial radiographs often suggest Hirschsprung's disease, and an apparent cone may be shown on contrast enema and indeed be apparent at laparotomy. Normal ganglia are shown on routine biopsy specimens, but with special histological staining techniques and tests three different forms of ganglion or muscular abnormality are found. The disease often extends into the small bowel and causes failure of food absorption. Peristaltic activity is present but incoordinated, and when observed on ultrasound is often vigorous. The children may require parenteral nutrition. The natural history is one of periods of improvement and relapse but slow improvement in symptoms occurs with maturity. The microcolon hypoperistalsis syndrome is thought to represent an extreme form of this lesion.

REFERENCES

Franken E A, Smith W L, Frey E E, Sato Y, Anuras S 1987 Intestinal motility disorders of infants and children: classification, clinical manifestation and roentgenology. Critical Reviews in Diagnostic Imaging 27: 203–236

Lake B D 1988 Observations on the pathology of pseudo-obstruction. In: Milla P J (ed) Disorders of gastrointestinal motility in childhood. John Wiley, Chichester, pp 81–90

Munakata K, Morita K, Okabe, Sueoka H 1985 Clinical and histologic studies of neuronal intestinal dysplasia. Journal of Pediatric Surgery 20: 231–235

Pollock I, Holmes S J K, Patton M A, Hamilton P A, Stacey T E 1991 Congenital intestinal pseudo-obstruction associated with a giant platelet disorder. Journal of Medical Genetics 28: 495–496

Puri P, Lake B D, Nixon H H, Mishalany H, Claireaux A E 1977 Neuronal colonic dysplasia: an unusual association of Hirschsprung's disease. Journal of Pediatric Surgery 12: 681–685

Scharli A F, Meier-Ruge W 1981 Localized and disseminated forms of neuronal intestinal dysplasia mimicking Hirschsprung's disease. Journal of Pediatric Surgery 16: 164–170

FUNCTIONAL OBSTRUCTIONS OF THE BOWEL

MECONIUM PLUG SYNDROME

Differentiation should be made between the meconium plug syndrome and meconium ileus. The latter term should be ideally reserved for the inspissated meconium characteristically collecting in the distal small bowel and proximal large bowel in children with cystic fibrosis of the pancreas (mucoviscidosis). The meconium plug syndrome is better reserved for the retention of meconium within a relatively normal calibre and normally innervated colon. Such plugs may occur commonly distally in the rectosigmoid region, but their distribution can be throughout the colon. Clinical presentation is of delayed passage of meconium and proximal intestinal dilatation with bile-stained vomiting at times. The meconium plug syndrome is not associated with a specific single disease entity or with any specific ganglionic pathology. It is a non-specific failure of bowel activity in response to a variety of conditions such as prematurity, septicaemia, diabetic mothers, hypothyroidism, hypoglycaemia, sedation, birth trauma and intracerebral haemorrhage. Physiological passage of meconium may be delayed in premature infants without any significant obstruction.

THE SMALL LEFT COLON SYNDROME

Original reports of this condition suggested an unduly high preponderance of diabetic mothers, but this localized relative narrowing of the descending colon with a fairly characteristic change in the diameter of the bowel in the region of the splenic flexure is not now believed to be particularly associated with maternal diabetes. The condition is believed to be due to a functional immaturity of muscular activity in the descending colon and rectum, which is typically transitory and self-limiting with maturation of neuromuscular function. Some cases, however, are, in reality, Hirschsprung's disease and because of this all such cases should have rectal biopsies (Fig. 3.6.13).

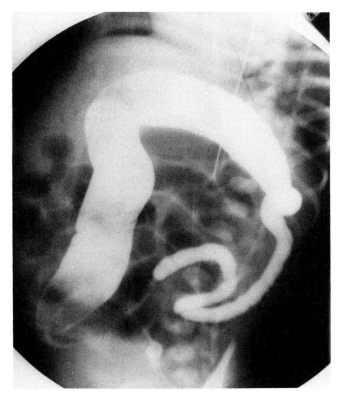

Fig. 3.6.13 Small left colon syndrome, typical appearance.

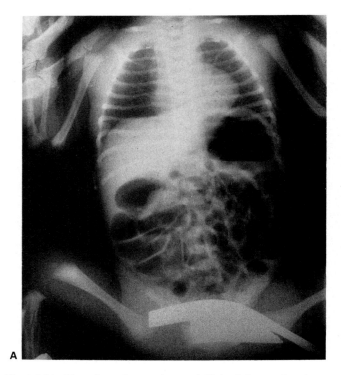

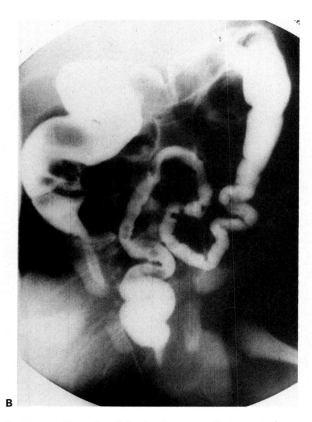

Fig. 3.6.14 Meconium plug syndrome. **A** Plain abdomen showing generalized bowel distension. **B** Contrast enema outlining cast of meconium in the transverse colon (same child as in **A**). **C** Another infant. (i) Plug impacted in rectosigmoid and descending colon. (ii) Left post evacuation. **D** Typical appearance of an evacuated plug.

Plain abdominal radiographs in both conditions are not specific, showing a variety of patterns varying from multiple gaseous distension to multiple air-fluid levels, but at times to relatively gasless abdomens, particularly in premature and critically sick infants (Fig. 3.6.14). A contrast medium enema can be both diagnostic and therapeutic. Water-soluble, low osmolar contrast medium may be used initially to show the intraluminal meconium, and frequently leads to evacuation of the plug during the examination. If desired, diluted gastrografin could be secondarily introduced, particularly for its detergent characteristics. Success rates in such functional obstructions are generally high, whereas in the meconium ileus associated with cystic fibrosis of the pancreas such therapeutic success by enemas is much lower. In the literature there has been considerable confusion between the two conditions and therefore also between the efficacy of therapeutic enemas. The calibre of the colon, particularly the rectosigmoid, in cases of functional obstruction is usually normal,

although some areas of the bowel may show significant narrowing (Fig. 3.6.14B). However, in the small left colon syndrome there is uniform narrowing of the rectosigmoid and typically of the descending colon to the region of the splenic flexure, where a typical transition zone to normal calibre colon can be seen (Fig. 3.6.13).

REFERENCES

Amodio J, Berdon W, Abramson S, Stolar C 1986 Microcolon of prematurity: a form of functional obstruction. American Journal of Roentgenology 146: 239–244

Berdon W E, Slovis T L, Campbell J B, Baker D H, Haller J O 1977 Neonatal small left colon syndrome; its relationship to aganglionosis and meconium plug syndrome. Radiology 125: 457–462

Le Quesne G E, Reilly B J 1975 Functional immaturity of the large bowel in the newborn infant. Radiologic Clinics of North America 13: 331–342

Pockaczesky R, Leonidas J C 1974 The meconium plug syndrome; roentgen evaluation and differentiation from Hirschsprung's disease and other pathologic states. American Journal of Roentgenology 120: 342–352

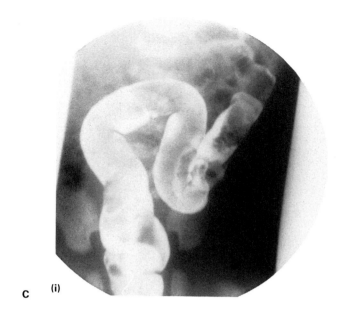

C (i)

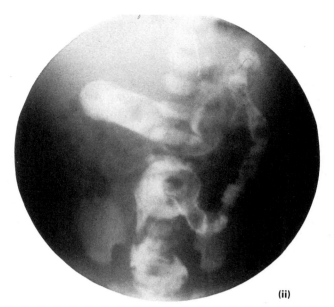

(ii)

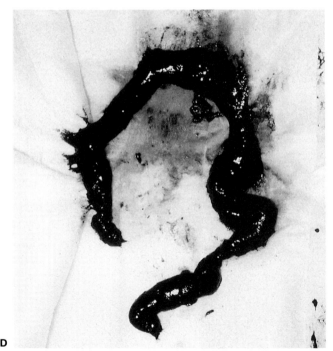

D

INSPISSATED MILK CURD SYNDROME

Intestinal obstruction secondary to milk curd is a condition resulting from feeding incorrectly reconstituted concentrated powder milks. It differs from other causes of neonatal intestinal obstruction in that there is normal passage of meconium before the obstruction develops. Bowel perforation and septic peritonitis have been reported.

Plain abdominal radiographs show distended loops in which the milk curds may be outlined by air (Fig. 3.6.15). Although surgical removal may be necessary, most infants can be managed conservatively. Introduction of dilute gastrografin per rectum into the region of the inspissated curds will help their evacuation, as will adequate rehydration and oral gastrografin. The intraluminal masses of milk curds may be associated with local mucosal necrosis and perforation needing surgical treatment (Fig. 3.6.16).

REFERENCES

Cook R C M, Rickham P P 1969 Neonatal intestinal obstruction due to milk curds. Journal of Pediatric Surgery 4: 599–605

Cremin B J, Smythe P M, Cywes S 1970 The radiological appearance of the 'inspissated milk syndrome'. A cause of intestinal obstruction in infants. British Journal of Radiology 43: 856–858

Koletzko B, Tangermann R, Von-Kries R, Stannigel H, Wilberg B, Radde I, Schmidt E 1988 Intestinal milk-bolus obstruction in formula fed premature infants given high doses of calcium. Journal of Pediatric Gastroenterology and Nutrition 7: 548–553

Konvolinka C W, Frederick J 1989 Milk curd syndrome in neonates. Journal of Pediatric Surgery 24: 497–498

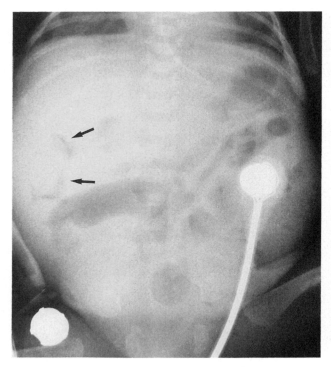

Fig. 3.6.15 Inspissated milk curd syndrome. Note very distended abdomen and intraluminal mass (inspissated curds) outlined by a rim of gas (arrows).

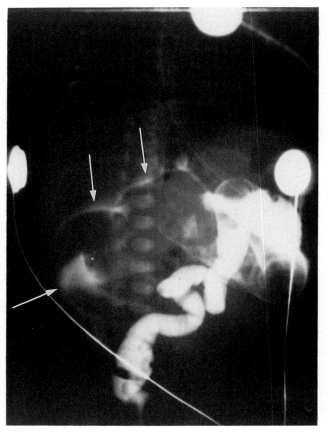

Fig. 3.6.16 Inspissated milk curd syndrome. Water-soluble contrast enema examination. Milk mass in distal transverse colon lumen causing obstruction at splenic flexure level. There is perforation with spill of contrast into the peritoneal cavity (arrows).

Table 3.6.1	Classification of anorectal anomalies
1. Ectopic anus	The terminal bowel opens at an abnormally high location such as the perineum, scrotum, vulva, vestibule, urethra, vagina or cloaca
2. Imperforate anus	The terminal bowel does not open at all. There are two types:
	a. Membranous imperforate anus
	b. Anorectal atresia (the anus and at least part of the rectum are absent)
3. Rectal atresia	The anus is present and open but a segment of the rectum is atretic
4. Anal stenosis and rectal stenosis	

From Gans SL 1970 Classification of anorectal anomalies: a critical analysis. Journal of Pediatric Surgery 5: 511–513.

MEGACYSTIS-MICROCOLON-HYPOPERISTALSIS SYNDROME

Megacystis-microcolon-intestinal-hypoperistalsis syndrome is a rare cause of intestinal obstruction in the newborn. The condition predominates in females and is generally fatal. There is abdominal distension caused by a distended, non-obstructed bladder. The bowel is shortened with a dilated proximal small bowel, narrowed distal small bowel, malrotated microcolon, absent or ineffective peristalsis and either a normal or increased number of ganglion cells. No mechanical bladder neck or urethral obstruction is present, and vesicoureteric reflux does not usually occur. The kidneys may by hydronephrotic. The exact aetiology is unknown.

REFERENCES

Berdon W E, Baker D H, Blanc W A, Gay B, Santulli T V, Donovan C 1976 Megacystis-microcolon-intestinal hypoperistalsis syndrome; a new cause of intestinal obstruction in the newborn. American Journal of Roentgenology 126: 957–964

Vintzileos A M, Gisenfield L I, Herson V C, Ingardia C J, Feinstein S J, Lodeiro J G 1986 Megacystis-microcolon-intestinal hypoperistalsis syndrome. Prenatal sonographic findings and review of the literature. American Journal of Perinatology 3: 297–302

ANORECTAL ANOMALIES

An anorectal anomaly occurs in approximately 1:5000 births and is slightly more common in boys than in girls. Various classifications and reviews of these lesions are reported, but that of Gans is the simplest. This classification was a compromise arrived at by an international symposium of paediatric surgeons in Melbourne in 1970 (Table 3.6.1). In this classification, ectopic anus refers to the most common abnormality and occurs in situations where there is failure of normal descent of the terminal bowel resulting in a lack of communication with the anus. The bowel as a result opens via a fistula at an abnormal location such as the perineum, scrotum, vulva, vestibule, urethra, vagina or cloaca. With imperforate anus, the terminal bowel ends blindly and no fistula exists. There are two types – membranous imperforate anus where only the anus or part of it is absent, and anorectal atresia where the anus and at least part of the rectum is absent. In rectal atresia, the anus is present and open but a variable segment of rectum above it is atretic. No fistula is present. Anal and rectal stenosis refer to cases of incomplete anal or rectal atresia. Deficiency of part of the sacrum is common in association with anorectal anomalies. Severe deficiencies are associated with failure of normal development of gluteal and perineal musculature and often contribute to incontinence following pull-through surgery.

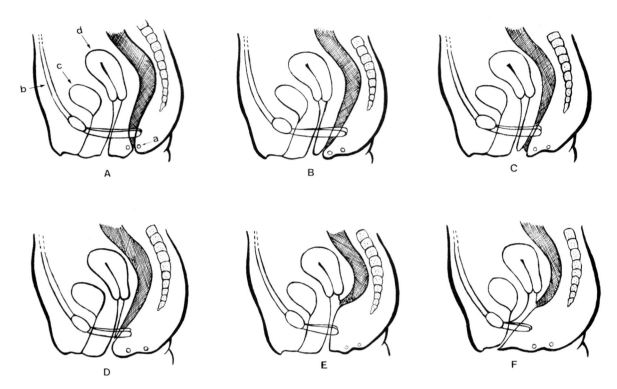

Fig. 3.6.17 Ectopic anus in female infant. **A** Normal female infant. **B** Anoperineal fistula. **C** Rectovestibular fistula. **D** Low rectovaginal fistula. **E** High rectovaginal fistula. **F** Rectocloacal fistula. a= external and sphincter, b= puborectalis sling, c = bladder, d = uterus.

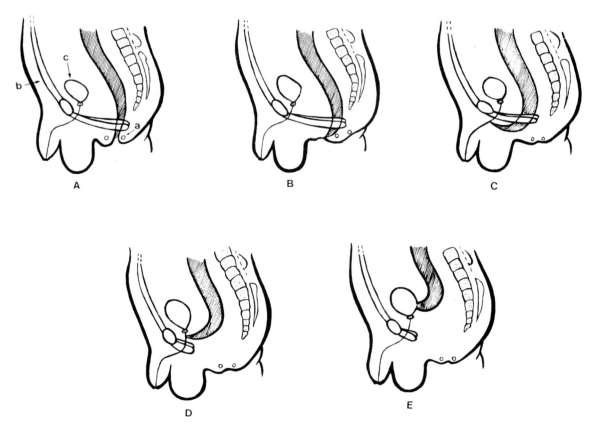

Fig. 3.6.18 Ectopic anus in male infant. **A** Normal male infant. **B** Anoperineal fistula. **C** Low rectourethral fistula. **D** High rectourethral fistula. **E** Rectovesical fistula. a = external sphincter, b = puborectalis sling, c = bladder.

In ectopic anus, the anal dimple and external sphincter of striated muscle will usually be found in the normal position, but development of the distal colon is arrested at a higher level with an ectopic opening through a fistula into the vagina or cloaca in females (Fig. 3.6.17) and bladder or urethra in males (Fig. 3.6.18) or onto the perineum. Anomalies which occur above the puborectalis are designated high or 'supralevator'. In these infants the sling is hypoplastic or absent and is usually functionally inadequate. Surgery is by a combined abdominoperineal approach to fashion a rectum and anus with subsequent hindgut pull-through. Lesions below the puborectalis muscle are low or 'translevator'. The sling is usually well developed and functional. These infants require a perineal surgical approach. A third group was introduced as an 'intermediate' in which the lesions were within the puborectalis sling. This group can be treated either by abdominal or perineal surgery. In simple anal membrane, incision of the membrane is all that is usually required. In anorectal atresia, colostomy with a later pull-through may be required, depending on the length of the atretic segment. In the presence of rectal atresia, calcified intraluminal meconium within the colon suggests the presence of a fistula to the urinary tract (Fig. 3.6.19).

In ectopic anus, in particular, other abnormalities of the gastrointestinal tract such as Hirschsprung's disease may occur, as may anomalies of the genito-urinary tract and the spine, in addition to sacral deficiency (Fig. 3.6.20). Anorectal anomalies may present as part of the VACTER association. Renal tract anomalies are very common. Investigation of the urinary tract initially by sonography is essential in all of these infants, as anomalies occur in 20% of infants with low ectopic anus and 40% of infants with high lesions.

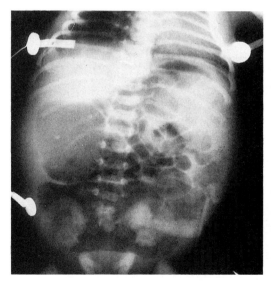

Fig. 3.6.19 Neonate with anorectal atresia. There is calcified meconium in the colon in the right upper quadrant. The child had a large rectourethral fistula and the calcification is due to the mixture of urine and meconium.

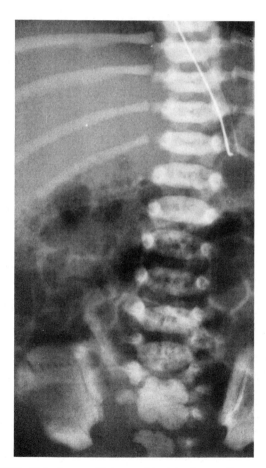

Fig. 3.6.20 Ectopic anus. Note sacral vertebral anomalies.

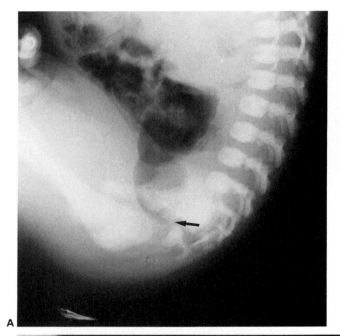

A

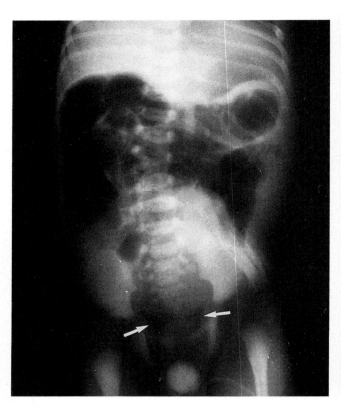

Fig. 3.6.21 Ectopic anus in a male infant. Note air in the bladder (white arrows).

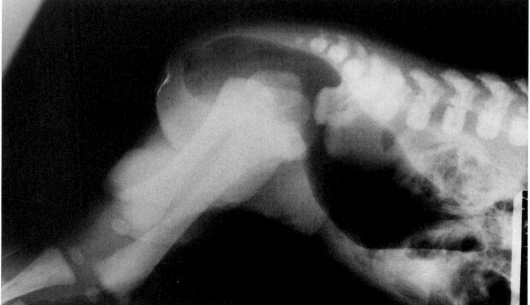

B

Fig. 3.6.22 **A** Ectopic anus. Lateral radiograph demonstrating an air-filled distal rectal pouch ending blindly above the ischium, indicating a high lesion (arrow). **B** Low lesion. Note the air in the distal pouch almost touches the barium on the anus.

Plain abdominal films usually show a low small bowel or colonic obstruction early in the neonatal period. In males, gas may be seen in the bladder (Fig. 3.6.21) and rarely in the vagina in female infants, confirming an associated fistula. A prone shoot-through radiograph is useful in determining the level of the atresia and allows assessment of the sacrum. The infant should be old enough for gas to have reached the rectum, over 12 hours. The infant is placed in the prone position with the buttocks on a pillow for 20 minutes before the study. Barium is painted onto the anal dimple and a lateral radiograph centred on the greater trochanter is obtained (Fig. 3.6.22). This projection is preferable to the 'invertogram' with hanging head and inverted body. The pubococcygeal line or a line drawn from mid pubic bone to sacro-coccygeal junction has been used, to classify lesions as high or low. This line is now believed to be too high, and the 'M' line running horizontally through the junction of the lower third and upper two-thirds of the ischia is suggested as a more accurate level of the puborectalis muscle (Fig. 3.6.23). There are potential errors in the radiographic assessment of the height of the lesion. A low lesion may appear high because of meconium in the distal rectum.

If plain radiography and clinical examination indicate a high lesion, most surgeons prefer immediate colostomy with a later elective investigation of the anatomy before abdominoperineal pull-through.

Sonography has been used to delineate the distance from the distal pouch to the perineum. Donaldson et al suggest that any child with a distance of less than 10 mm can be safely treated with a simple perineal anoplasty, but a distance of greater than 15 mm should definitely be diverted with a colostomy at birth. A distance of 10–15 mm should probably be diverted with a colostomy. The extent of bowel deficiency may be overestimated in the presence of much distal meconium.

Direct puncture of the anus and injection of contrast material is occasionally useful to outline the distal colonic pouch.

Following the establishment of a colostomy, most children with a high lesion will require cystography as part of the routine assessment of the urinary tract (Fig. 3.6.24). This will delineate most fistulas in the males and can be supplemented by local injections into fistulas if deemed appropriate. The defunctioned distal colostomy can also be delineated by water-soluble contrast material indicating bowel length and associated fistula.

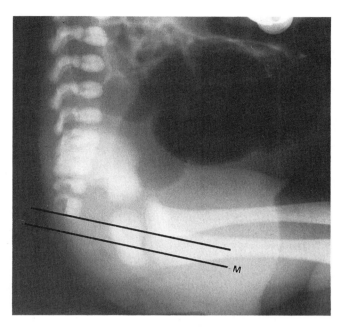

Fig. 3.6.23 Ectopic anus. 'M' line drawn through the junction of the upper two-thirds and lower one-third of the ischium. This corresponds to the level of the puborectalis muscle and determines the level of lesion.

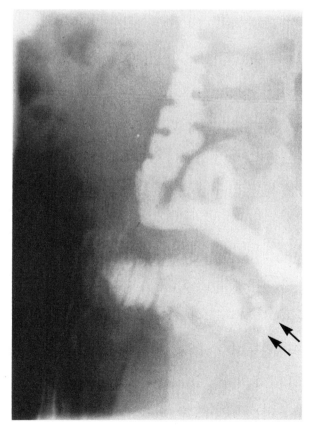

Fig. 3.6.24 Large rectovesical fistula in an infant with ectopic anus. It was impossible to perform a micturating cystogram because of the flow of contrast through the fistula.

Accurate diagnosis is essential in anorectal anomalies to determine the type of surgery. Damage to the pelvic floor with subsequent incontinence and impotence, persistence of undetected fistulas and damage to the urinary tract are potential complications of inappropriate surgery. In later life, in the investigation of incontinence following pull-through, the location of the rectum and anal canal relative to the levator ani muscles and their development can be demonstrated by direct coronal CT (Fig. 3.6.25), ultrasound or MRI.

REFERENCES

Berdon W E, Baker D H, Santuilli T V, Amoury R 1968 The radiologic evaluation of imperforate anus; an approach correlated with current surgical concepts. Radiology 90: 446–471

Cremin B J 1971 The radiological assessment of anorectal anomalies. Clinical Radiology 22: 239–250

Donaldson J S, Black T, Reynolds M, Sherman J O, Shkolnik A 1989 Ultrasound of the distal pouch in infants with imperforate anus. Journal of Pediatric Surgery 24: 465–468

Gans S L 1970 Classification of anorectal anomalies: a critical analysis. Journal of Pediatric Surgery 5: 511–513

Pouillade J M, Meyer P, Minh V T, Dodat H, Valla J S 1987 Enterolithiasis in two neonates with oesophageal and anorectal atresia. Pediatric Radiology 17: 419–421

Sato Y, Pringle K C, Bergman R A, et al 1988 Congenital anorectal anomalies: MR imaging. Radiology 168: 157–162

Taccone A, Martucciello G, Fondelli P, Dodero P, Ghiorzi M 1989 CT of anorectal malformation – a postoperative evaluation. Pediatric Radiology 19: 375–378

COLONIC ATRESIA

Three types of colonic atresia are recognized.

Type 1 – membranous occlusion
Type 2 – atresia connected by a thin atretic band
Type 3 – complete atresia with no connecting band.

In types 2 and 3, there is an associated mesenteric defect. Clinically, infants have symptoms of large bowel obstruction with vomiting, distension and failure to pass meconium. Radiographically, the colon proximal to the point of atresia is often massively dilated. Contrast enema examination usually reveals a distal microcolon (Fig. 3.6.26). In the membranous form, the membrane can bulge outwards and give a so-called 'wind-sock' sign. Colonic stenosis is rarer than atresia.

REFERENCES

Blank E, Afshani E, Girdany B R, Pappas A 1974 'Windsock sign' of congenital membranous atresia of the colon. American Journal of Roentgenology 120: 330–332

Bley W R, Franken E A Jr 1973 Roentgenology of colon atresia. Pediatric Radiology 1: 105–108

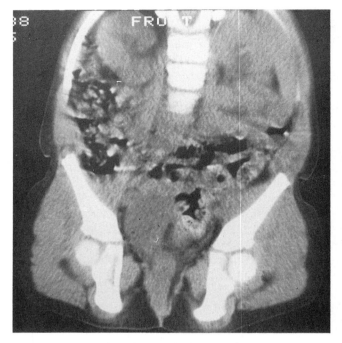

Fig. 3.6.25 Coronal CT showing the location of the rectum and anal canal after a pull-through operation.

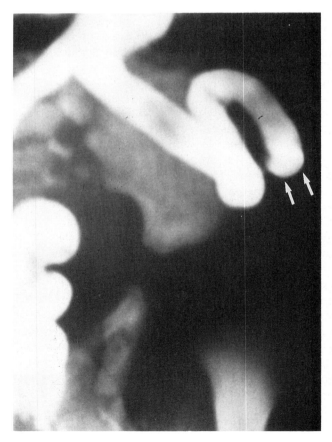

Fig. 3.6.26 Colonic atresia. The contrast enema outlines a microcolon ending abruptly (arrows), the site of atresia.

NON-NEONATAL GASTROINTESTINAL TRACT   *H. Carty*

3.7   SALIVARY GLANDS AND TONGUE

SALIVARY GLANDS

There are three main groups of glands producing saliva, the parotid, submandibular and sublingual glands. In young children the most frequent disorder that is likely to present for investigation is intermittent swelling of a parotid or submandibular gland, due to intermittent blockage of the duct. Sonography of the parotid gland is now the first line of investigation. It is possible to detect large cystic spaces in sialectasis, small areas of calcification in angiomatous malformations, and disordered sonographic patterns in tumours. Acinar enlargement has been found in children seropositive for the HIV virus. Definitive anatomical demonstration of sialectasis is still by sialography, which in complicated cases may be combined with CT (computed tomography). Tumours are best further investigated with CT and MRI (magnetic resonance imaging).

Plain radiographs before contrast sialography will demonstrate a calcified stone. An intraoral view is indicated in suspected submandibular pathology (Fig. 3.7.1). Sialography is carried out using water soluble low osmolar contrast (Fig. 3.7.2). A general

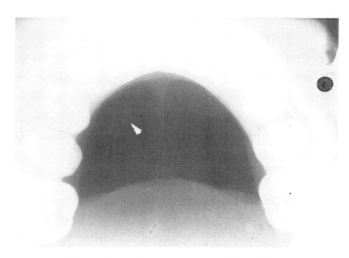

Fig. 3.7.1   Intraoral view showing stone in orifice of left submandibular gland (arrow).

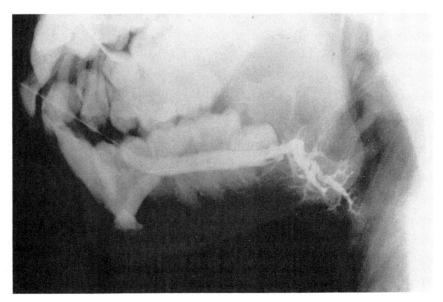

Fig. 3.7.2   Same patient as in Figure 3.7.1. There is gross dilatation of the main submandibular and branch ducts proximal to the obstructing stone.

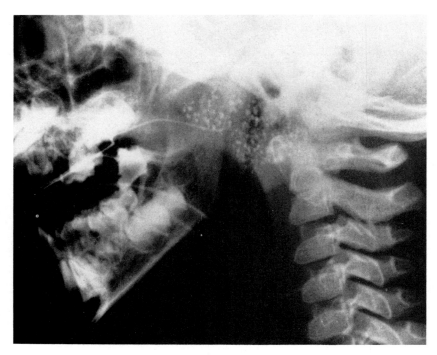

Fig. 3.7.3 Sialectasis of the parotid gland. There is dilatation of the acini which are filled with contrast. The duct is normal.

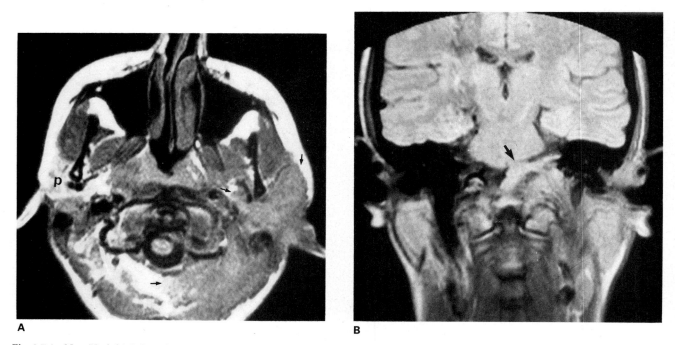

A   B

Fig. 3.7.4 Non-Hodgkin's lymphoma in a teenager, T1-weighted axial MRI. **A** shows the infiltrative tumour affecting both superficial and deep lobes of the parotid as well as the muscle planes in the back of the neck (arrows), compared with the normal fat planes and parotid (p) on the other side. **B** T2-weighted coronal sections show little difference in signal intensity between the normal and abnormal parotids but show extension of the tumour up through the foramen magnum into the posterior cranial fossa (arrow). The patient had a unilateral jugular foramen syndrome. (Courtesy of Dr Phelps.)

anaesthetic is rarely required, but if indicated the child must not receive atropine with the premedication. Contrast is injected until the child indicates a feeling of fullness in the gland. The orifice of the parotid duct lies in the cheek at the level of the second upper molar tooth. The submandibular orifice is in the raised mucosa sublingually, lateral to the frenulum.

In sialectasis, there is pooling of contrast in dilated acini within the gland (Fig. 3.7.3). The ducts may be normal or slightly irregular. Filling defects within the ducts are due to non-opaque stones or mucous plugs. Sialectasis has been reported in cystic fibrosis.

The commonest cause of salivary gland swelling in childhood is mumps, but these children do not present for radiological investigation. Suppurative infections are usually due to *Staphylococcus aureus*.

Chronic recurrent swelling of unknown aetiology also occurs. Some of these children may ultimately present with autoimmune disease. Recurrent viral infection can produce the same symptoms. Sialography, done to exclude sialectasis, is normal.

Neoplasia

Salivary tumours are rare in children. When they occur they are similar to those seen in adult practice, and include mixed tumours, teratomas, lymphomas (Fig. 3.7.4), carcinomas, neurofibromas and haemangiomas (Fig. 3.7.5). These latter are the most frequent. The vascular nature is well shown by ultrasonography, CT and MRI (Fig. 3.7.6), but angiography may be required to show the full extent preoperatively.

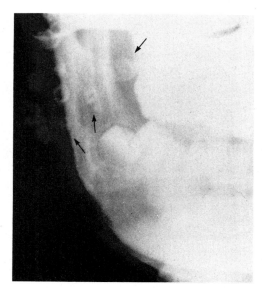

Fig. 3.7.5 Haemangioma of right parotid gland. Multiple calcified phleboliths are present.

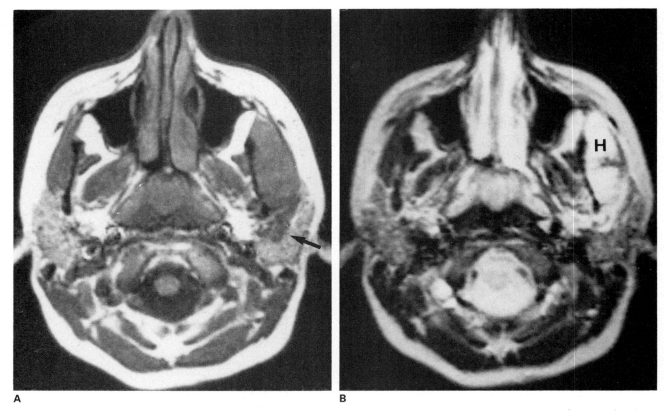

Fig. 3.7.6 A Haemangioma of parotid gland. T1-weighted MRI shows a low signal lesion in the parotid (arrow) with a bulky masseter muscle. **B** T2-weighted MRI shows a high signal from the haemangioma both within the parotid gland and extending throughout the masseter muscle. (Images courtesy of Dr Phelps.)

Ranula

Mucocoeles occur in the floor of the mouth and may, rarely, extend deeply to present as a mass in the neck. When simple, they are confined to the sublingual space, but the more complex ones may involve the submandibular space and extend to the parapharyngeal space. They rarely present for radiological investigation. On ultrasound, a ranula is of low echodensity, and cannot be distinguished from other cystic masses. At CT (Fig. 3.7.7) they are of low attenuation and have sharply marginated walls. The diagnosis is made on the aspirated fluid which is thick, clear and viscous, unlike the thinner aspirate from other cysts.

Sublingual dermoid and epidermoid lipomas

Another cause of midline swellings in the mouth is a sublingual dermoid cyst. The diagnosis of dermoid or lipoma may be suggested when a fat density of the contents is demonstrated at CT. Epidermoids are of homogeneous fluid density.

Plexiform neurofibroma

Plexiform neurofibromata may occur anywhere. When they occur in the mouth there is often bony as well as soft tissue involvement.

Tumours of the soft palate

Tumours of the soft palate in children are extremely rare and are mainly rhabdosarcomas and lymphomas (Fig. 3.7.8).

Salivary glands

REFERENCES

Bruns W T, Tang T T 1973 Submandibular sialolithiasis in a cystic fibrosis patient. American Journal of Diseases of Children 126: 685–686

Goddart D, Francois A, Ninane J, Vermylen Ch, Cornu G, Clapuyt Ph, Claus D 1990 Parotid gland abnormality found in children seropositive for the human immunodeficiency virus (HIV). Pediatric Radiology 20: 355–357

Gritzmann N 1989 Sonography of the salivary glands. American Journal of Roentgenology 153: 161–166

Herbert G, Ouimet-Oliva D, Ladouceur J 1975 Vascular tumours of the salivary glands in children. American Journal of Roentgenology 123: 815–819

Leake D, Leake R 1970 Neonatal suppurative parotitis. Pediatrics 46: 203–207

Rose P E, Howard E R 1982 Congenital teratoma of the submandibular gland. Journal of Pediatric Surgery 17: 414–416

Rubaltelli L, Sponga T, Candiani F, Pittarello F, Andretta M 1987 Infantile recurrent sialectatic parotitis: the role of sonography and sialography in the diagnosis and follow up. British Journal of Radiology 60: 1211–1214

Wilson W, Eavey R, Lang D 1980 Recurrent parotitis during childhood. Clinical Pediatrics 19: 235–236

Ranula

REFERENCES

Charnoff S, Carter B 1986 Plunging ranula: CT diagnosis. Radiology 158: 467–468
Coit W, Harnsberger H, Osborn A, Smoker W, Stevens M, Lufkin R 1987 Ranulas and their mimics: CT evaluation. Radiology 163: 211–216

THE TONGUE

Most abnormalities of the tongue are obvious clinically. The commonest disorder is a large tongue which may be isolated or seen as part of the Beckwith–Wiedemann syndrome or as a part of congenital hemihypertrophy. Radiological investigation of the associated abnormalities is required. The full syndrome is characterized by macroglossia, visceromegaly, hemihypertrophy, increased bone age, naevus flammeus, diaphragmatic hernia, omphalocele, umbilical hernia, adrenal and pancreatic hyperplasia, hyperglycaemia, polycythaemia and an increased incidence of both Wilms' tumour, neuroblastoma, hepatoblastoma and pancreatic neoplasm. Most children do not exhibit the full syndrome.

Neoplasm of the tongue occurs rarely. Rhabdosarcoma is the commonest malignant tumour. Lymphangiomas and haemangiomas are the most frequent benign lesions.

Involvement of the tongue by vascular malformation is difficult to treat clinically. These may be treated by direct injection of a thrombotic agent if they are venous, or be embolized if there is a large arterial supply. Careful patient selection is essential. Facilities for respiratory support must be available should they be required during the immediate post-treatment period when swelling can obstruct the airway. Considerable swelling of the tongue and the floor of the mouth can occur secondary to trauma and can also compromise the airway.

REFERENCES

Eaton A P, Maurer A 1971 The Beckwith–Wiedemann syndrome. American Journal of Disease of Children 122: 520–525
Gruner M, Guillaume A, Montagne J P, Faure C 1981 Nephroblastoma and Beckwith–Wiedemann syndrome. Annales de Radiologie 24: 39–42
Sotelo-Avila C, Gonzalez Grussi F, Fowler J 1980 Complete and incomplete forms of Beckwith–Wiedemann syndrome: their oncogenic potential. Journal of Pediatrics 96: 47–50
Tank E S, Kay R 1980 Neoplasms associated with hemihypertrophy, Beckwith–Wiedemann syndrome and aniridia. Journal of Urology 124: 266–268

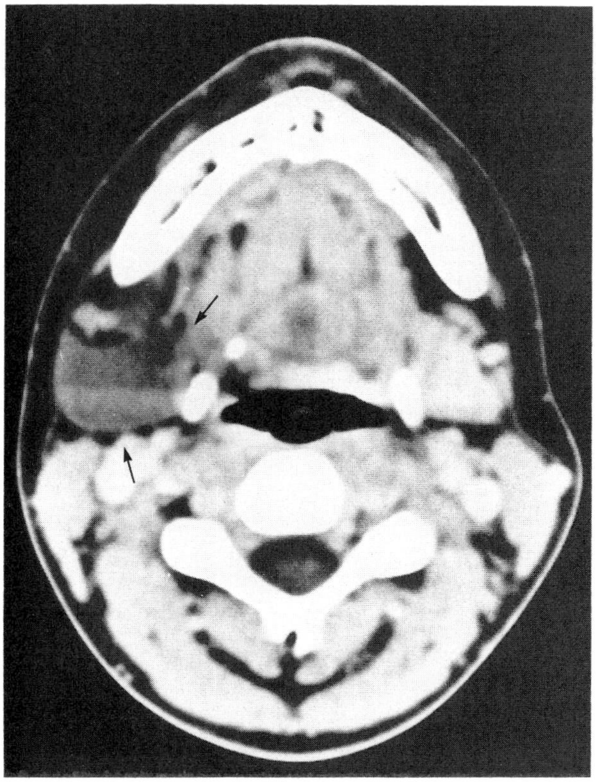

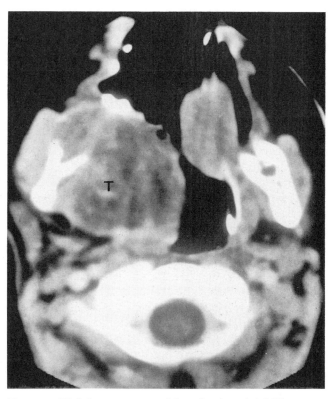

Fig. 3.7.7 Ranula. There is a low attenuation mass which does not enhance lying behind the angle of the right mandible, anterior to the great vessels. Aspirated material was clear, thick and viscous, which suggested the correct diagnosis. The patient presented with a recurrent painless swelling in the neck which fluctuated in size.

Fig. 3.7.8 Rhabdomyosarcoma of the soft palate. Axial CT scan showing a soft tissue mass (T) as non-homogeneous, but mostly of low attenuation. This could be due either to necrosis, which occurs in these tumours, or to myxomatous degeneration of the stroma. (Courtesy of Dr Phelps.)

3.8   THE PHARYNX

The pharynx is traditionally divided into three segments: the nasopharynx, which lies above the soft palate, the oropharynx, between the tonsils and larynx, and the hypo- or laryngopharynx, the region surrounding the larynx. The pharynx in the infant does not attain the more adult appearance until about the age of 6 years. Below this age, the retropharyngeal tissues, which in the adult are only 3 mm thick, are considerably thickened in a child–up to the width of two vertebral bodies if the neck is flexed. The width is influenced by the position of the patient, being greatest with flexion and with the mouth closed. This apparent thickening must not be mistaken for an abscess or tumour. Repeat films with neck extension will resolve most cases, as will fluoroscopy, when the mass will disappear with neck straightening. A child in pain with abscess or tumour will resist attempts at neck straightening. With abscess or tumour, the normal cervical lordosis is lost as muscle spasm and pain increase (Fig. 3.8.1). This is not lost in the normal child with pseudo-tumour appearances. In the normal child, during quite respiration with the head extended, the retropharyngeal tissues should not measure more than three-quarters of the width of the cervical vertebra. Careful correlation with the clinical history also reduces the misdiagnosis rate.

BRANCHIAL ARCH LESIONS

During embryological development a membrane separates the branchial clefts which arise from the ectoderm, from the pharyngeal pouches which arise from the endoderm. There are six arches in all, but the first and second are the most important pathologically, the fifth and sixth are rudimentary (Fig. 3.8.2). Developmental anomalies of the first arch cause cleft defects in the palate and lips, and mandibular hypoplasia. Developmental anomalies of the second arch result mainly from overgrowth of this arch in a caudal distribution and are more common than anomalies of the other five arches. The clinical presentation of anomalies of the branchial clefts depends on which portions remain patent. If a branchial cleft remains patent then there is a sinus draining to the skin surface (Fig. 3.8.3). The sinus is situated laterally on the neck at the anterior border of the sternomastoid muscle. Conversely a thyroglossal fistula is midline. The child presents with a recurrent mucosal discharge. Secondary infection can occur, but is more frequently found in blind cysts. A sinogram is indicated to outline the full extent before surgery. The orifice may need dilating before a fine catheter can be inserted.

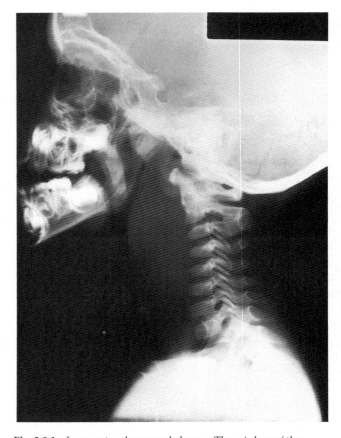

Fig. 3.8.1 Large retropharyngeal abscess. There is loss of the normal cervical lordosis. The abscess is displacing the normal pharyngeal air anteriorly.

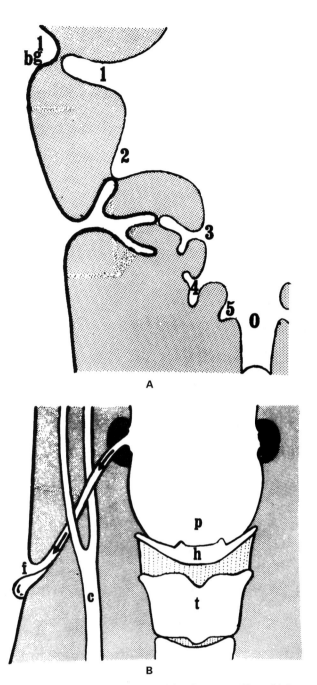

A

B

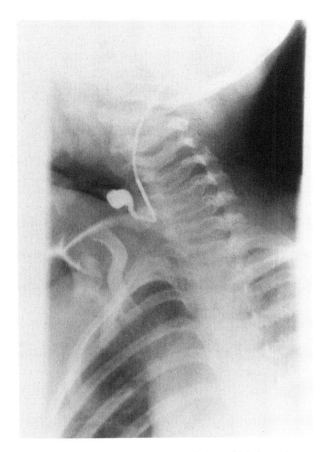

Fig. 3.8.3 Branchial sinus. Sinogram of a branchial sinus. A sialographic cannula has been inserted into the orifice and fills a fluid sac. The child presented with recurrent discharge.

Fig. 3.8.2 A Schematic drawing of development of branchial arches and grooves. This becomes the external acoustic meatus by term. The other grooves which lie opposite the second, third and four arches form the cervical sinus which is obliterated by term as the neck develops. bg = branchial grooves, o = oesophagus. **B** Schematic drawing of the position of a branchial sinus fistula. p = pharynx, h = hyoid bone, t = trachea, c = common carotid artery, f = fistula.

A branchial cyst, which arises when the central portion of the cleft remains patent, usually presents in an older child or adult when infection occurs in a blind cyst. A branchial cyst lies at the level of the hyoid bone, anterior to the carotid artery (Figs. 3.8.4, 3.8.5). The patient presents with soft tissue swelling of variable size. Calcification has been recorded. On plain radiographs there may be some displacement of pharyngeal soft tissues. Ultrasound will show the cystic nature of the mass, and its separate location from the thyroid gland. The diagnosis is based on the clinical presentation and the characteristic location of the mass.

If patency of a branchial cleft and its corresponding pharyngeal pouch coexist, a pharyngeal fistula will result. The discharging fistula becomes apparent soon after birth. A fistulogram will show the communication with the pharynx, at tonsilar level, as most arise from second arch level.

REFERENCES

Cavo J W, Pratt L L, Alonso W A 1976 First branchial cleft syndromes and associated congenital hearing loss. Laryngoscope 86: 739–745

Moore K 1982 The branchial apparatus and the head and neck. In: The developing human. Clinically oriented embryology. W B Saunders, Philadelphia, ch 10, pp 179–215

Shprintzen R J, Croft C, Berkman M D, Rakoff S J 1979 Pharyngeal hypoplasia in Treacher Collins syndrome. Archives of Orolaryngology 105: 127–131

Stovin J J, Lyon J A, Clemmens R L 1960 Mandibulofacial dysostosis. Radiology 74: 225–231

Telander R L, Deane S A 1977 Thyroglossal and branchial cleft cysts and sinuses. Surgical Clinics of North America 57: 779–791

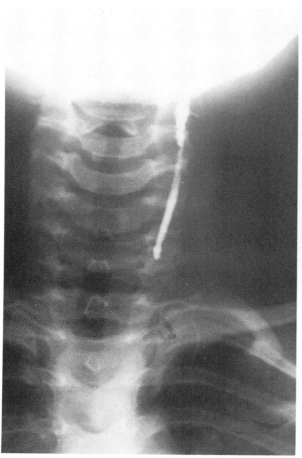

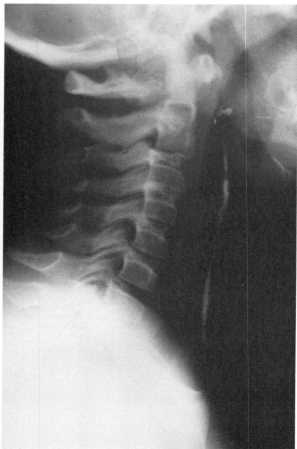

Fig. 3.8.4   AP (**A**) and lateral (**B**) view of sinogram of branchial sinus. The position of the track is anterior to the sternomastoid muscle.

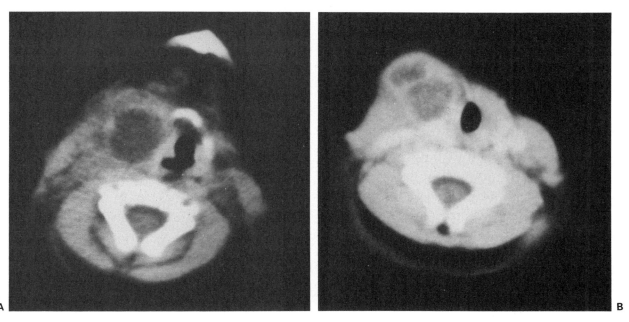

Fig. 3.8.5 Branchial cyst: **A** without contrast, **B** with contrast. Child age 6 months with recent onset of left neck mass. The mass was transonic on ultrasound and thought to be a cystic hygroma. CT done to show its extent and relationship to the great vessels. The mass has enhancement of the borders with contrast due to infection. There is some compression of the trachea. The cyst lies anterior to the carotid artery and anterior to the sternomastoid muscle.

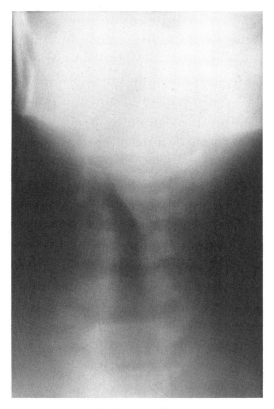

Fig. 3.8.6 Laryngocele. Twelve-year-old trumpet player who presented with soft neck mass. Tomography shows displacement of the airway by the unilateral mass.

LARYNGOCELES

These are rare in children and mostly occur in older children who play wind instruments, but they may be congenital (Fig. 3.8.6). The aetiology is unknown. On plain films one may see air within the lesion. Some are fluid filled and present for investigation as a high neck mass.

MICROGNATHIA

Generalized mandibular hypoplasia is seen as part of the many first arch syndromes – the commonest being Pierre Robin, Goldenhar's Syndrome, Treacher Collins syndrome and Weyer's mandibulofacial dysostosis. There are about 100 syndromes in total. It is also seen in association with some chromosomal lesions, especially trisomy 17/18 and 13/15. It is a feature of the cri du chat syndromes.

Isolated hypoplasia also occurs and can involve the whole or part of the mandible. It can be part of a more extensive anomaly – hemifacial microsomia, where there is associated temporomandibular joint dysfunction, facial hypoplasia and ipsilateral hearing defects.

The micrognathia leads to feeding and respiratory problems in infancy. As the child grows, there is spontaneous improvement. Radiological investigation is mainly directed at the demonstration of the mandibular anatomy and associated facial bone distortion prior to reconstructive surgery. This is best done by a combination of direct coronal CT scanning and axial CT with 3D reconstruction.

PHARYNGEAL POUCH

Congenital pharyngeal pouches are rare. They are discovered on investigation of swallowing disorders. Most arise from the second arch and therefore fill from the level of the tonsilar fossa. Secondary infection of the pouch may occur, as may overspill and pulmonary aspiration. Plain radiographs show a soft tissue mass in the neck which contains air. The barium swallow, in suspected cases, should be done with video recording, as indeed should all contrast swallows in children with swallowing disorders.

POST-TRAUMATIC PSEUDODIVERTICULUM OF THE PHARYNX

These lesions are far more frequent in children than true congenital lesions. They occur following perforation of the posterior wall of the pharynx. The incident is often not recognized at the time. Foreign body perforation and inadvertent perforation during passage of a nasogastric or endotracheal tube are two well-recognized causes (Fig. 3.8.7). The child presents with dysphagia. A retropharyngeal mass is seen on the plain radiograph, the mass filling with barium on contrast studies. Infection is a common complication. This may lead to mediastinitis and considerable fibrosis.

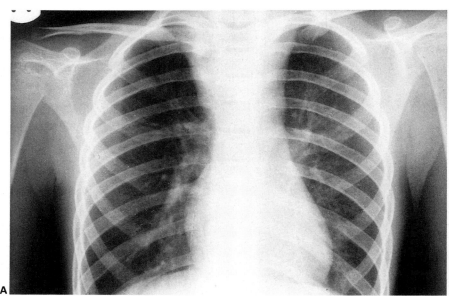

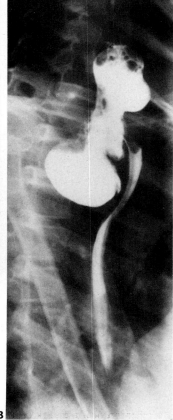

Fig. 3.8.7 A Widened mediastinum secondary to a mediastinal abscess from traumatic perforation of the pharynx. Three-month history of increasing dysphagia. **B** Contrast swallow (same child). A large pseudodiverticulum of the pharynx extends into the proximal thorax, and displaces the oesophagus anteriorly. At surgery a plastic toy coin was found in the pseudodiverticulum/abscess cavity. The child required a colonic interposition.

Pharyngeal perforation

Acute pharyngeal perforation may be due to direct trauma from a penetrating injury, e.g. by a lollipop stick when the child falls while sucking it, a swallowed sharp foreign body, e.g. a pin, or fishbone, or iatrogenic trauma during intubation. It can also result from a finger inserted into a child's mouth in an attempt to remove a foreign body. Pharyngeal perforation can result from child abuse, when a sharp object, such as a spoon, is forced into the mouth, when the frenulum may also be torn. Immediate manifestations of pharyngeal perforation are pain, subcutaneous emphysema and acute dysphagia. Later manifestations are a retropharyngeal abscess, mediastinitis and dysphagia. Traumatic carotid artery occlusion and hemiplegia have been described as a late sequel.

A water-soluble contrast swallow should be performed on all childern with suspected pharyngeal perforation to determine the site. Even though there may be a clear history of a foreign body, it is rare to see these on the plain radiograph unless they are of dense metallic or bony consistency. Aluminium ring-pulls off soft drink cans are of too low a metallic density to be reliably seen on plain radiographs.

REFERENCES

Ablin D, Reinhart M 1990 Esophageal perforation with mediastinal abscess in child abuse. Pediatric Radiology 20: 524–525
Hirsch M, Abramowitz H B, Shapira S, Barki Y 1978 Hypopharyngeal injury as a result of attempted endotracheal intubation. Radiology 128: 37–39
McDowell H P, Fielding D W 1984 Traumatic perforation of the hypopharynx. An unusual form of abuse. Archives of Disease in Childhood 59: 888–889
Pitner S E 1966 Carotid thrombosis due to intraoral trauma: an unusual complication of a common childhood accident. New England Journal of Medicine 274: 764–767

RETROPHARYNGEAL ABSCESS

The retropharyngeal lymph nodes receive drainage from the nose, pharynx and middle ear, three areas of frequent infection in childhood. A retropharyngeal abscess occurs from suppuration within the retropharyngeal lymph nodes, secondarily infected as a result of drainage of one of these areas. It can also occur secondary to a penetrating injury. Clinically, the child will present with some or all of these symptoms: fever, dysphagia, drooling, noisy breathing, torticollis and a stiff neck. A lateral radiograph of the neck shows widening of the retropharyngeal tissues, and loss of the normal cervical lordosis, with the neck held in slight flexion. Gas in the soft tissues indicates communication with the pharynx (Fig. 3.8.8). The abscess may be accompanied by subluxation of the vertebral bodies due to accompanying oedema of the anterior cervical ligaments. If present, the anaesthetist must be alerted so that he does not overextend the neck during intubation.

Retropharyngeal abscesses can extend into the mediastinum and have been recorded as communicating with the pleural cavity. Retropharyngeal abscess due to a secondary infection of the draining lymph nodes is confined to children, as these lymph nodes atrophy at approximately age 4.

REFERENCES

Ramilo J, Harris V J, White H 1978 Empyema as a complication of retropharyngeal and neck abscesses in children. Radiology 126: 743–746

RETROPHARYNGEAL MASSES

While a retropharyngeal abscess is an acutely presenting lesion, other masses may present with gradual onset of dysphagia or be noted on radiographs. These include cystic hygromas, haemangiomas, neurofibromas, either plexiform or dumb-bell type tumours, cervical neuroblastomas and lymphadenopathy, histiocytosis, tuberculosis and the rare sinus histiocytosis. Pouches, both congenital and post-traumatic, may also lead to widening of the retropharyngeal space.

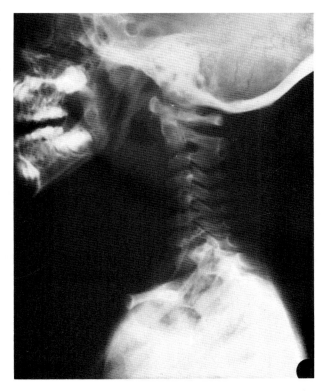

Fig. 3.8.8 Four-year-old boy with a retropharyngeal abscess. There is gas in the soft tissues at the level of C2 which indicates communication with the pharynx.

REFERENCES

McCook T, Felman A 1979 Retropharyngeal masses in infants and young children. American Journal of Diseases of Children 133: 41–43

Swischuck L E, Smith P C, Fagan C J 1974 Abnormalities of the pharynx and larynx in childhood. Seminars in Roentgenology 9: 283–300

PHARYNGEAL WEB

The discovery of asymptomatic mucosal webs in children is exceedingly rare, unlike adults, where they occur in about 5% of patients, with an increasing incidence in the elderly. These cricopharyngeal webs have an identical appearance in children and adults. They are seen as smooth anterior indentations of the barium column and are due to mucosal folds (Fig. 3.8.9). A few cases have been reported in children in association with dysphagia or iron deficiency anaemia (the Paterson–Kelly or Plummer–Vinson syndrome). They have also been reported in pemphigus, epidermolysis bullosa and dyskeratosis congenita.

REFERENCES

Borgstrom P S, Birch-Iensen M, Ekberg O 1988 Radiology of the pharynx and oesophagus in young adults. British Journal of Radiology 61: 909–913

Crawfurd M, Jacobs A, Murphy B 1965 Paterson–Kelly syndrome in adolescence: a report of 5 cases. British Medical Journal 1: 693–695

Nosher J L, Campbell W L, Seaman W B 1975 The clinical significance of cervical esophageal and hypopharyngeal webs. Radiology 117: 45–47

Puntis J W, Chapman S, Proops D W, Sartori P 1989 Dysphagia due to oesophageal web. Archives of Disease in Childhood 64: 141–143

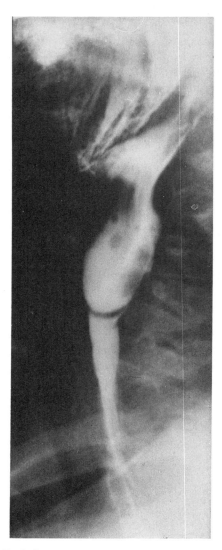

Fig. 3.8.9 Typical appearance of a cricopharyngeal web. Incidental finding in a mentally subnormal child undergoing contrast studies for the investigation of suspected gastro-oesophageal reflux.

TUMOURS OF THE PHARYNX

Primary tumours of the pharynx are very rare in children. Pedunculated tumours of the oropharynx and nasopharynx may prolapse into the hypopharynx and cause obstruction to breathing and swallowing. Polyps, dermoids, angiofibroma, hamartoma and lymphangiomas, persistent cevical thymus, lingual thyroid and neurofibromas have all been described arising in this region. All appear as a mass projecting into the pharynx on the lateral radiograph. There are no distinguishing features on the plain film, but contrast-enhanced CT will show which ones are vascular.

Involvement of the lymph node chains in the neck by lymphoma is very common. The glands are easily palpable. Burkitt's lymphoma can cause very extensive enlargement of the neck glands and lead to both dysphagia and dyspnoea.

Other masses in the neck that are not of gastrointestinal origin are carotid body tumours, arteriovenous malformations and jugular vein aneurysms. All are easily identifiable as vascular by both conventional and Doppler ultrasound and contrast-enhanced CT.

VELOPHARYNGEAL INCOMPETENCE

Fluoroscopy of the soft palate following coating with barium via nasal intubation provides useful information in the assessment of speech disorders. The examination must be recorded on video tape. When there is incompetence, the soft palate fails to reach the posterior wall of the pharynx (Fig 3.8.10), allowing nasal escape of air, or failure of lateral wall motion of the pharynx. During the examination, the patient pronounces a series of letters and sentences designed to show all palatal and pharyngeal movements associated with speech. The palate is outlined by barium, administered by nasal sniffing or by tube. Incompetence

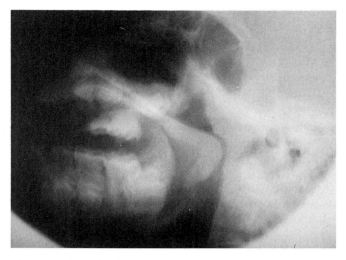

Fig. 3.8.10 Lateral radiograph of cricopharyngeal region shows failure of apposition of soft palate and posterior wall of the pharynx, as the patient says 'K' allowing escape of air.

occurs as a primary problem with congenital cleft disorders. While these are normally obvious at birth, a mild form in which there is a muscular defect at the midline of the soft palate, or the palate is hypoplastic, may go undetected until the onset of speech. Incompetence can also occur secondary to removal of large adenoids and with bulbar palsy.

REFERENCES

Barr L L, Hayden C K Jr, Hill L C, Swischuck L E 1989 Radiographic evaluation of velopharyngeal incompetence. American Journal of Roentgenology 153: 811–814
Stringer D A, Witzel M A 1986 Velopharyngeal insufficiency on video fluoroscopy: comparison of projection. American Journal of Roentgenology 146: 15–19

3.9 THE OESOPHAGUS

SWALLOWING DISORDERS – PHARYNGEAL LEVEL

Swallowing disorders in children require careful fluoroscopic studies with a good bolus of contrast and should always be recorded on video to allow repeated review. The sequence of movements during sucking and swallowing is fast and requires careful study to identify the problem. The sequence of events during swallowing has been described by Ardran and Kemp. There are six distinct events:

1. The tongue propels the bolus from front to back towards the pharynx.
2. The soft palate is elevated as the tongue reaches that area.
3. Pharyngeal constriction begins when the tongue is opposed to the soft palate. Apposition of the soft palate and pharynx prevents nasopharyngeal regurgitation (Fig. 3.9.1).
4. The larynx elevates to the level of the thyroid.
5. The larynx closes as the peristaltic wave reaches it preventing aspiration (Fig. 3.9.2).

6. The cricopharyngeus relaxes to allow the bolus to enter the oesophagus.

Incoordination of swallowing is a feature seen in infants with cerebral palsy, meningomyelocoeles, familial dysautonomia, oropharyngeal infection, intracranial tumours, collagen diseases, trauma and cranial nerve palsies. It may be transitory following trauma which may be directly penetrating, or secondary to ingestion of too hot a liquid or a toxic substance such as lye. Swallowing disorders due to collagen diseases occur more commonly in the mid and lower oesophagus. Swallowing problems can also be a manifestation of emotional disturbance, when contrast studies are done to exclude an underlying organic pathology.

Oral and pharyngeal infection will also lead to difficulty in swallowing. This is a particular problem in children who are immunosuppressed and infected with monilia and may be further complicated by mid and lower oesophageal dysphagia.

A prominent bulge on the posterior oesophagus

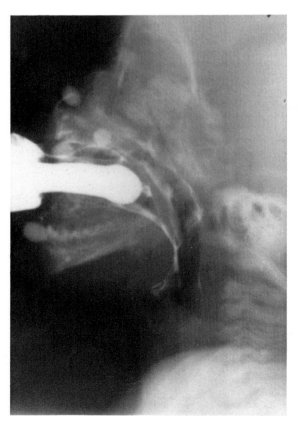

Fig.3.9.1 Nasopharyngeal reflux of barium due to incoordinated movements of pharynx and palate. The infant had bulbar palsy due to birth trauma.

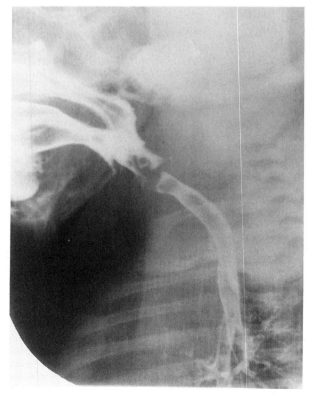

Fig. 3.9.2 Gross incoordination with gross nasopharyngeal reflux and failure of closure of the epiglottis allowing free aspiration of barium into the trachea. Infant with feeding difficulties and cerebral palsy.

is caused by contraction of the cricopharyngeal muscle and is an occasional finding in contrast studies in children. This is a normal finding and does not indicate an obstructive posterior pharyngeal bar (Fig. 3.9.3), and is referred to as achalasia of the cricopharyngeus. True achalasia of the cricopharyngeus does occasionally occur secondary to trauma, polio or cranial nerve damage. Failure of relaxation of the cricopharyngeus prevents the bolus of food entering the oesophagus and will cause aspiration of food into the trachea if glottic closure is imperfect.

Children who chronically aspirate food into the trachea and lungs do not gag and cough in the same way as a normal child would. They present with frequent chest infections and failure to thrive. Aspiration pneumonia is a serious complication of children with swallowing disorders and gastro-oesophageal reflux. The aspirated contents will be a mixture of saliva, gastric juices and the feed content. There are rare reports of fatalities resulting from aspiration of barium during investigation of children with recurrent vomiting.

Children who experience swallowing difficulties towards the end of feeding are described as suffering from 'fatigue aspiration'. It is seen in the collagen diseases, cerebral damage and myopathies, and will be missed at fluoroscopy unless the child is given a full feed.

Difficulty in swallowing can be an habitual problem in some young infants. There is no underlying organic pathology. The child will drink liquids normally, but gag and regurgitate solid food or lumps. The problem is one of feeding and is due to a faulty technique during the introduction of lumpy food during weaning. At fluoroscopy the child will drink fluids normally, but on being coaxed to take a solid lump (which has to be dipped in barium), it will gag as soon as the lump passes from the tongue to the back of the pharynx.

Micrognathia will also lead to difficulties with feeding and swallowing in early neonatal life. As the child matures, there is improvement.

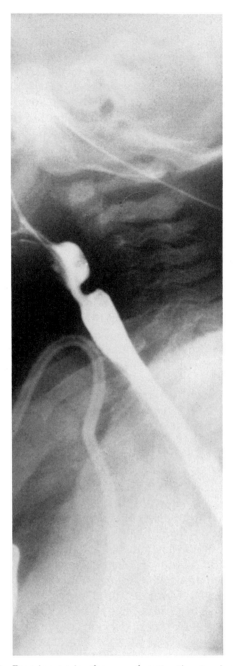

Fig. 3.9.3 Prominent cricopharyngeal contraction causing the posterior indentation of the oesophagus. 'Achalasia of the cricopharyngeus.'

REFERENCES

Ardran G M, Kemp F H 1956 Closure and opening of the larynx during swallowing. British Journal of Radiology 29: 205–208

Ardran G M, Kemp F H 1970 Some important factors in the assessment of oropharyngeal function. Developmental Medicine and Child Neurology 12: 158–166

Bishop H C 1974 Cricopharyngeal achalasia in childhood. Journal of Pediatric Surgery 9: 775–778

Borgstrom P, Birch-Ienson M, Ekberg O 1988 Radiology of the pharynx and oesophagus in young adults. British Journal of Radiology 61: 909–913

Cumming W, Reilly B 1972 Fatigue aspiration. A cause of recurrent pneumonia in infants. Radiology 105: 387–390

Curtis D J, Cruess D F 1984 Videofluoscopic identification of two types of swallowing. Radiology 152: 305–308

Dodds W, Logemann J, Stewart E 1990 Radiologic assessment of abnormal oral and pharyngeal phases of swallowing. American Journal of Rentgenology 154: 965–974

Dodds W, Stewart E, Logemann J 1990 Physiology and radiology of the normal oral and pharyngeal phases of swallowing. American Journal of Roentgenology 154: 953–963

Logemann J A 1988 Swallowing physiology and pathophysiology, in otolaryngology. Otolaryngologic Clinics of North America 21: 613–623

Lund W S 1990 Some thoughts on swallowing – normal, abnormal and bizzare. Journal of the Royal Society of Medicine 83: 138–142

Seaman W B 1976 Pharyngeal and upper esophageal dysphagia. Journal of the American Medical Association 235: 2643–2646

Steiner R M, Glassman L, Scwartz M W et al 1974 The radiological findings in dermatomyositis in childhood. Radiology 111: 385–393

ACHALASIA

Achalasia is a rare cause of dysphagia in children (only 3–4% of reported cases), and does not often present below the age of 6. Due to its rarity, there is often quite a delay in diagnosis. Familial cases have been recorded. The symptoms are similar to those in adults: dysphagia, vomiting of undigested food, halitosis and failure to thrive. In younger children, failure to thrive and repeated chest infection due to pulmonary aspiration are the presenting problems.

The primary pathology is failure of relaxation of the gastro-oesophageal sphincter, although the cause of this is not known. Absence of normal ganglion cells in Auerbach's plexus in the oesophagus sometimes extending to the gastro-oesophageal junction is the cause of the disordered motility.

On plain chest radiographs, there may be a dilated oesophagus with a fluid level and food debris, often easier to see on the lateral film, and an absence of the gastric air bubble. In children, dilatation is rarely as great as in adults, so the plain film is more frequently normal. At barium swallow, there is failure of relaxation of the gastro-oesophageal sphincter, absence of normal peristalsis, occasionally irregular contractions and a beaking of the distal oesophagus (Fig. 3.9.4). Emptying into the stomach is by gravity. If barium studies are equivocal, oesophageal manometry should be undertaken. In achalasia, there is aperistalsis or low amplitude contractions in the oesophagus with failure of relaxation of the lower sphincter and a raised resting pressure of the sphincter to 20 mmHg. Treatment is usually surgical, by Heller's operation, with division of the oesophageal muscle to the mucosal level. Even though there is an excellent functional result, the dilatation may persist on the chest radiograph. A complication of myotomy is reflux oesophagitis which may require fundal plication for its control. More recently, repeated pneumatic dilatation has been advocated, with surgical myotomy reserved for those who do not respond to balloon dilatation.

A rare association of ACTH insensitivity and alacrima has been reported in association with achalasia. This condition has an autosomal recessive inheritance.

Oesophagitis occurs secondary to the food retention, but is rarely demonstrated by barium studies, as the mucosal detail is obscured by food debris.

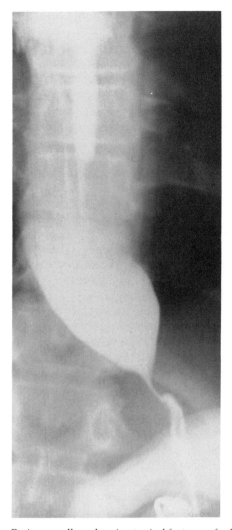

Fig. 3.9.4 Barium swallow showing typical features of achalasia. The oesophagus is dilated. The barium mixes with retained fluid. There is no gastric fundal air bubble. The pointed distal end of the oesophagus at the gastro-oesophageal junction is due to failure of relaxation of the sphincter.

REFERENCES

Ambrosino M, Genieser N, Bangaru B, Sklar C, Becker M 1986 The syndrome of achalasia of the esophagus, ACTH insensitivity and alacrima. Pediatric Radiology 16: 328–329

Berquist W E, Byrne W J, Ament M E, Fonkalsrud E W, Euler A R 1983 Achalasia: diagnosis, management, and clinical course in 16 children. Pediatrics 71: 798–805

Dellipiani A W, Hewetson K A 1986 Pneumatic dilatation in the management of achalasia – experience of 45 cases. Quarterly Journal of Medicine 58: 253–258

Donahue P E, Samelson S, Schlesinger P K, Bombeck C T, Nyhus L M 1986 Achalasia of the oesophagus – treatment controversies and the method of choice. Annals of Surgery 203: 508–511

Ehrich E, Aranoff G, Johnson W G 1987 Familial achalasia associated with adrenocortical insufficiency, alacrima, and neurological abnormalities. American Journal of Medical Genetics 26: 637–644

Hunter-Vaughan W, Williams J 1973 Familial achalasia with pulmonary complications in children. Radiology 107: 407–409

Mayberry J F, Mayell M J 1988 Epidemiological study of achalasia in children. Gut 29: 90–93

Patrick A, Campbell I W, Frazer M S, Smith D W, Walbaum P R 1984 Achalasia of the oesophagus presenting as foreign body obstruction. Archives of Disease in Childhood 59: 576–578

Starinsky R, Berlovitz I, Mares A, Versano D, Pajewsky M, Modai D 1984 Infantile achalasia. Pediatric Radiology 14: 113–115

CARDIOSPASM

Cardiospasm, a temporary entity, is present when there is failure of relaxation of the gastro-oesophageal sphincter, and, in this sense is similar to achalasia. The appearance of the distal oesophagus is similar to that in achalasia at barium examination. There is, however, no dilatation of the oesophagus with cardiospasm, and normal coordinated peristalsis is seen, unlike the aperistaltic or bizarre peristalsis in the oesophagus in achalasia. There is no retention of food or fluid. Treatment is by antispasmodics.

REFERENCE

Girdany B R 1963 The esophagus in infancy: congenital and acquired diseases. Radiologic Clinic of North America 1: 557–566

CHALASIA

There is failure of the normal closure of the distal oesophageal sphincter during the resting phase of oesophageal activity, with gastro-oesophageal reflux. The clinical presentation and treatment is similar to that of the infant with reflux, and for practical radiological purposes they are not separable.

IDIOPATHIC INTESTINAL PSEUDO-OBSTRUCTION

There have been occasional reports of oesophageal motility dysfunction in association with the idiopathic intestinal pseudo-obstruction syndrome. The patients present with dysphagia. At barium examination, there is absence of normal peristalsis with intermittent irregular contractions.

REFERENCE

Schuffler M, Pope C 1976 Esophageal motor dysfunction in idiopathic intestinal pseudo-obstruction. Gastroenterology 70: 677–682

LATE PROBLEMS OF THE OESOPHAGUS POST REPAIR OF A TRACHEO-OESOPHAGEAL FISTULA

Following successful primary anastomosis of the oesophagus for the repair of oesophageal atresia, stenosis may occur at the anastomosis (Fig. 3.9.5). Food impaction or impaction of other swallowed foreign bodies at the anastomosis is common. A filling defect is seen at the site of obstruction during barium swallow. There is no reliable correlation between the incidence of impaction and the calibre of the oesophageal anastomosis.

Motility disorders of the oesophagus are found in almost all children following repair of an atresia, though relatively few have symptoms related to this.

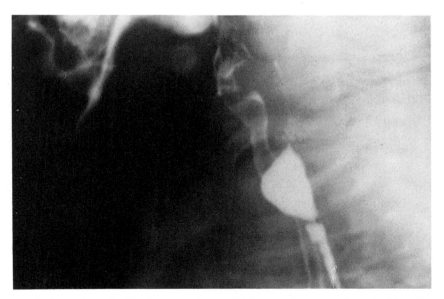

Fig. 3.9.5 Post repair of tracheo-oesophageal fistula: there is a severe stenosis at the site of the primary anastomosis. This child also had a recurrent fistula and pharyngeal incoordination with free passage of contrast into the trachea.

There is failure of the normal propulsive peristaltic wave, initiated during pharyngeal deglutition, just above the anastomosis. Forward movement through the anastomosis is mainly by gravity. Movement of the bolus distally is by peristalsis, but this is uncoordinated and leads to slow clearance of the bolus into the stomach (Fig. 3.9.6), incoordinated relaxation of the gastro-oesophageal function and 'yo yo' movement of food through the distal oesophagus. The basic defect is thought to be disruption of the normal innervation of the oesophagus due to the atresia. The coordination improves with age, but never returns to normal. The children adapt to the incoordination and relatively few have symptoms of dysphagia or pain related to it. The disordered motility has been confirmed by manometry.

An additional problem in these children is a higher incidence of gastro-oesophageal reflux than in the normal population, due in part to the same mechanism. There is also an increased incidence of hiatus hernia. Symptomatic reflux oesophagitis is a common problem and may cause failure to thrive in addition to pain and dysphagia. Both the reflux and disordered motility lead to increased risk of aspiration of gastric contents into the lungs leading to recurrent chest infection and bronchiectasis (Fig. 3.9.7). The diagnosis of reflux and oesophagitis is initially made by fluoroscopy, supplemented by scintigraphy, endoscopy and pH monitoring. It is important to identify the level to which reflux occurs during fluoroscopy and whether it is transanastomotic or not. The incidence of aspiration increases with the severity of the reflux. Careful attention is necessary to identify lower oesophageal strictures due to reflux and to identify their length. Mild stricture formation is easy to overlook in the presence of disordered motility and narrowing at the anastomosis. Detection of reflux by isotope scintigraphy is a very sensitive method of demonstrating reflux in these children. Demonstration

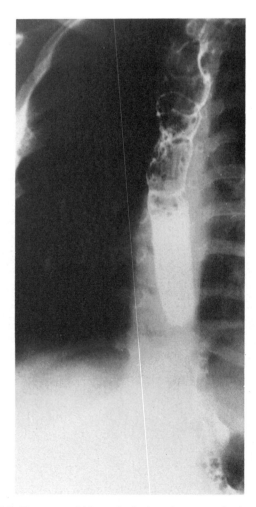

Fig. 3.9.6 Four-year-old boy who had a primary repair of a tracheo-oesophageal fistula as a neonate. Contrast swallow shows failure of clearing of barium due to disordered motility. There is no stricture at the anastomosis. No reflux is demonstrated during the barium study.

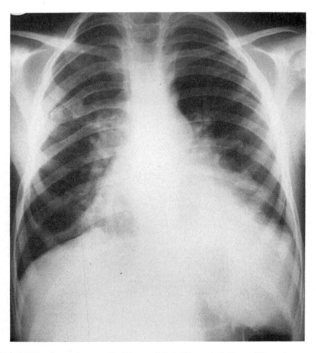

Fig. 3.9.7 Same boy as in Figure 3.9.6. There is bilateral basal collapse and bronchiectasis due to recurrent aspiration pneumonia from gastro-oesophageal reflux.

of radiopharmaceutical in the lungs provides conclusive proof of aspiration (Fig. 3.9.8).

Children with atresia without a fistula may have a colonic interposition as the primary surgical technique. Strictures at the upper anastomosis are common. The anastomosis is often tortuous and careful positioning during fluoroscopy is essential to demonstrate it, as is full distension with good bolus distension of the upper oesophagus. In general, children have most difficulty swallowing solid food, so during fluoroscopy it is important to observe the swallowing mechanism with food as well as liquids. The examination should be recorded on video. Passage of food through the intrathoracic colon is by gravity. Occasionally, there is stricture formation at the diaphragmatic area of the colonic interposition (Fig. 3.9.9). Dynamic assessment of hold up at this level should be made. The colonic gastric anastomosis is on the anterior stomach wall. This is only well demonstrated in a steep oblique or lateral position. Reflux of barium into the blind oesophageal stump is common and is usually asymptomatic, but occasionally oesophagitis is a complication.

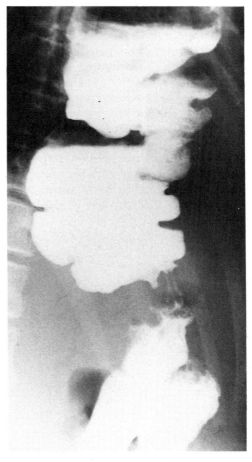

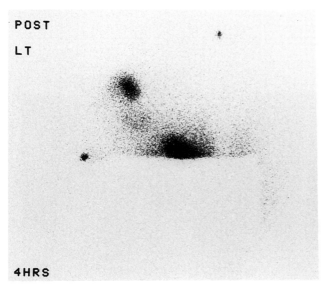

Fig. 3.9.8 Four-hour image of chest following radionuclide 'milk scan'. Extensive radiopharmaceutical is present in the left chest.

Fig. 3.9.9 Colonic interposition in a child who had oesophageal atresia. There is narrowing at the gastrocolic anastomosis.

The interposed colon lies retrosternally and usually in the left chest cavity. It can cause bizarre appearances due to the mixture of air, fluid and solid contents and must not be mistaken for pulmonary abscesses (Fig. 3.9.10). Adequate clinical details on the request form should prevent tragedies, with attempted aspiration of non-existent abscesses.

Recurrent fistula following repair usually occurs early. When suspected, it is usually most easily diagnosed by endoscopy and bronchoscopy, but may occasionally be seen at fluoroscopy. Strictures at both the proximal oesophago-colonic anastomosis, or at the site of anastomosis during primary repair, or associated reflux strictures may be treated successfully by balloon dilatation (Fig. 3.9.11) with an inflated balloon diameter of 10–15 mm. A suitable catheter is chosen, depending on the size of the patient and the degree of the stricture which is estimated from a previous contrast swallow examination. The balloon is sited so that it traverses the stricture. A soft-tipped flexible guide-wire inside the catheter facilitates the positioning because the guide-wire can pass the stricture easily. The balloon is slowly distended with contrast medium to a maximum pressure determined either by complete inflation or 'a feeling' of the pressure applied to the syringe. This pressure is maintained for approximately 30 seconds. The process is repeated several times until all the shouldering of the stricture has disappeared. The tube is withdrawn to above the site of the stricture, the guide-wire removed and the result assessed by contrast passing down the lumen of the tube. A formal programme of repeated ballooning is often required to relieve symptoms.

REFERENCES

Hoffer F, Winter H, Fellows K, Folkman J 1987 The treatment of post-operative and peptic esophageal strictures after esophageal atresia repair. A program including dilation with balloon catheters. Pediatric Radiology 17: 454–458

Jolley S G, Johnson D G, Roberts C C, Herbst J J, Matlock M E, McCombs A, Christian P 1980 Patterns of gastrooesophageal reflux in children following repair of oesophageal atresia and distal tracheooesophageal fistula. Journal of Pediatric Surgery 15: 857–862

McAlister W, Siegel M 1984 Fatal aspirations in infancy during gastrointestinal series. Pediatric Radiology 14: 81–83

Parker A F, Christie D L, Cahill J L 1979 Incidence and significance of gastroesophageal reflux following repair of esophageal atresia and tracheoesophageal fistula and the need for anti reflux procedures. Journal of Pediatric Surgery 14: 5–8

Shermeta D W, Whittington P F, Seto D S, Haller J A 1977 Lower oesophageal sphincter dysfunction in oesophageal atresia: nocturnal regurgitation and aspiration pneumonia. Journal of Pediatric Surgery 12: 871–876

Wolfson B, Allen J, Panitch H, Karmazin N 1989 Lipid aspiration pneumonia due to gastroesophageal reflux. A complication of nasogastric lipid feedings. Pediatric Radiology 19: 545–547

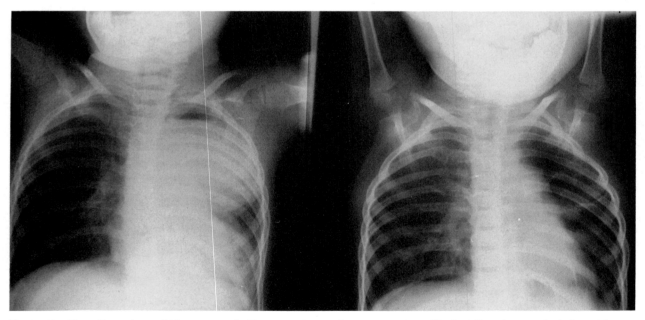

Fig. 3.9.10 Chest films taken at 24-hour intervals. The patient has a colonic interposition. The first film taken on admission with a respiratory tract infection followed a recent meal. The repeat film shows the air-filled colon. The pseudo-abscess appearance on the admission film is due to food and fluid in the colon.

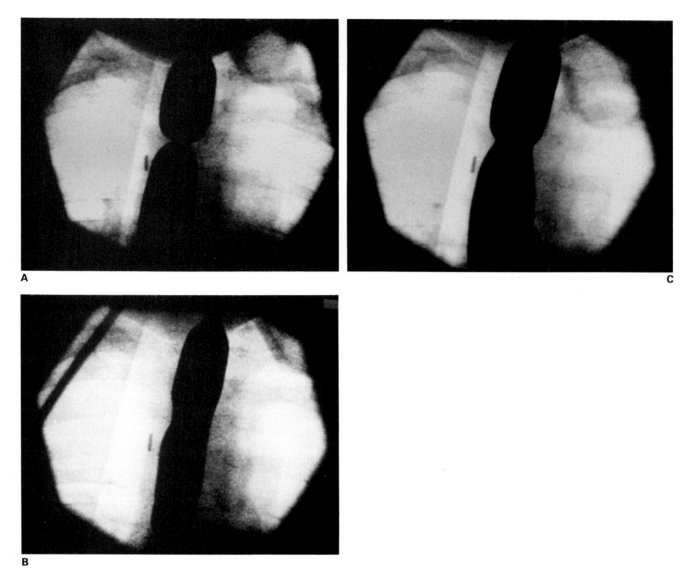

Fig. 3.9.11 Anastomotic stricture post repair of a tracheo-oesophageal fistula. Surgical clip on the azygos vein. **A** Initial size of stricture with balloon dilated. **B** Following 5 minutes of intermittent dilatation. **C** End result of dilatation.

RILEY–DAY SYNDROME (FAMILIAL DYSAUTONOMIA)

Recurrent respiratory infection and chronic relapsing pneumonia are found. Much of the chest disease is thought to be due to aspiration during swallowing or secondary to the dysfunction of the distal oesophagus where there is defective peristalsis and failure of emptying in the supine position. Other features of the syndrome include defective lacrimation, increased indifference to pain, excessive perspiration, drooling, emotional and motor instability, hypertension, absence of fungiform papillae on the tongue and skin blotching. Distension of the small bowel or colon are also described and this may be permanent.

REFERENCE

Grunebaum M 1974 Radiological manifestations in familial dysautonomia. American Journal of Diseases of Children 128: 176–178

CONGENITAL MYOTONIC DYSTROPHY

Steinert's myotonic dystrophy is an autosomal dominant hereditary condition which usually appears with clinical symptoms of muscle weakness and atrophy in adult life. Other features include cataracts, cardiac abnormalities, baldness and testicular atrophy. In the child, sucking and swallowing abnormalities and psychomotor retardation may occur. At barium study, there is hypotonia of the pharynx with poor clearance of barium, distension and hypotonicity of the oesophagus and impaired propulsive peristalsis. Other inherited myopathies have similar radiological appearances.

REFERENCE

Mabille J, Giroud M, Athias P 1982 Esophageal involvement in a case of congenital myotonic dystrophy. Pediatric Radiology 12: 89–91

GASTRO-OESOPHAGEAL JUNCTION ANATOMY

The anatomy of the infant's junction and sphincter differs in several respects from that of an adult. The most important of these is a shorter intra-abdominal course in childhood compared with adults. The sphincter surrounds the gastro-oesophageal vestibule and is held in place by a strong phrenicoesophageal membrane. Just above the vestibule and sphincter lies the ampulla of the distal oesophagus, which is often mistaken for a hernia by the inexperienced radiologist (Fig. 3.9.12). This can be avoided by identifying at fluoroscopy the non-distensible portion of the distal oesophagus. This lies at the distal oesophageal sphincter and should be just below the diaphragm. If it is above the diaphragm there is a sliding hiatus hernia which in infants is usually reducible (Fig. 3.9.13). The action of the diaphragm and the angle formed by the junction of the cardia and oesophagus all help to maintain competence of the gastro-oesophageal junction and prevent reflux.

In the normal infant, the muscle tone does not become mature for 7–8 weeks after birth. Thus, some reflux is common in all infants, and although almost physiological it can lead to oesophagitis and stricture formation even at this age. Fortunately, this is rare.

Persistent reflux with oesophagitis leads to scarring and fibrosis of the oesophagus with consequent shortening. The old concept of a congenitally short oesophagus has now been replaced by this more likely explanation. Similarly, the older description of an intrathoracic stomach is merely another description of an incarcerated sliding hiatus hernia.

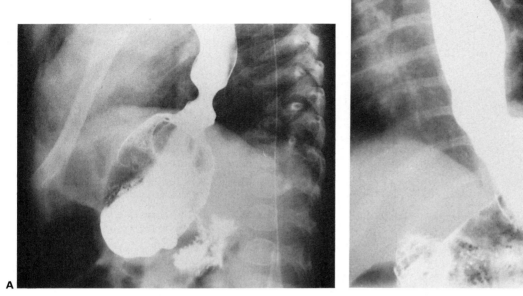

Fig. 3.9.12　**A** Distal oesophageal ampulla simulating a hiatus hernia. The gastro-oesophageal junction is at the diaphragm. **B** At the end of the examination there is gross gastro-oesophageal reflux. Compare with Figure 3.9.13.

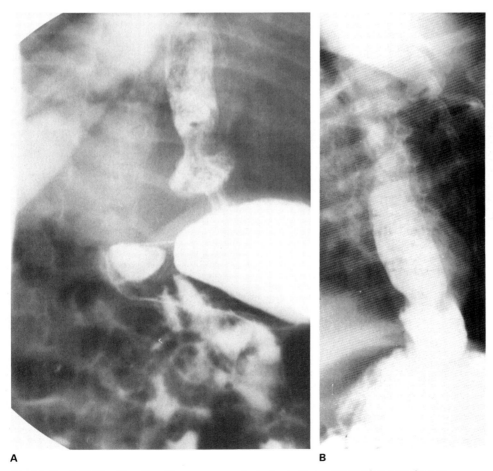

Fig. 3.9.13　**A** Child with reflux. The appearance is similar to Figure 3.9.12A but note the non-distensible portion is above the diaphragm. **B** This child has a small sliding hiatus hernia.

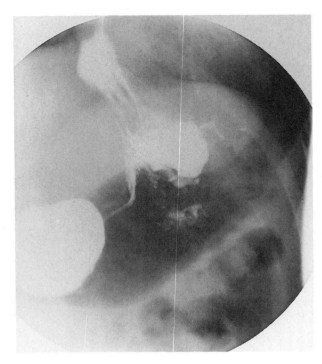

Fig. 3.9.14 Fixed sliding hiatus hernia.

HIATUS HERNIA

When the gastro-oesophageal junction lies above the diaphragm there is by definition a hiatus hernia. Initially, this is not fixed and is observed to slide up and down at fluoroscopy, giving rise to the name 'sliding hiatus hernia'. With continued reflux, oesophagitis and fibrosis of the distal oesophagus, the junction remains permanently above the diaphragam, giving rise to an irreducible hernia (Fig. 3.9.14). This is associated with incompetence of the lower oesophageal sphincter, giving rise to further reflux. During rest, the distal sphincter should remain closed and only open to admit a swallowed bolus of air, saliva, liquid or food. When it is incompetent, gastric contents gush into the oesophagus. This can occur even at rest. In less severe cases the reflux occurs only towards the end of oesophageal peristalsis during swallowing.

A rolling type of hiatal hernia occurs when a portion of the stomach herniates through the hiatus alongside the oesophagus (Figs. 3.9.15, 3.9.16). The gastro-oesophageal junction may be below the diaphragm or above. A rolling hernia may be large and cause symptoms through pressure and mass effect, but does not necessarily have associated reflux.

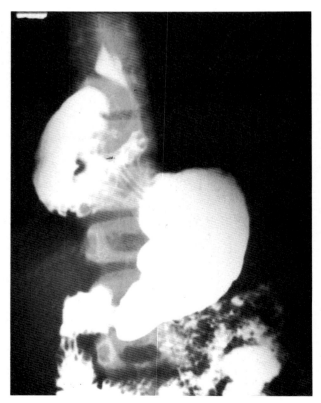

Fig. 3.9.15 Mixed para-oesophageal and sliding hiatus hernia. A large portion of the fundus of the stomach has herniated into the right chest through the foramen of Morgagni.

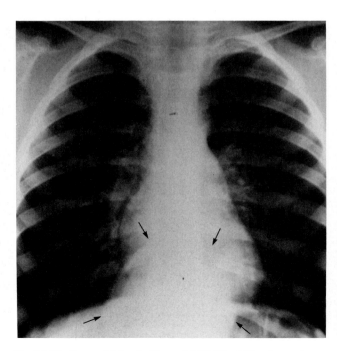

Fig. 3.9.16 Same child as in Figure 3.9.15. Chest film shows the hernia as a lower mediastinal central mass.

In general, medical treatment with thickened feeds, upright posture, metachlorpropromide, H^2 antagonists and antacids are tried before surgical measures are contemplated. Gross reflux and the presence of a large hiatus hernia usually require surgical correction. Paraoesophageal hernias require surgical repair.

There is a reported higher incidence of gastrooesophageal reflux and hiatus hernia in the UK and Europe than in the rest of the world. A familial incidence is reported.

PEPTIC OESOPHAGITIS

This is the result of gastro-oesophageal reflux. The radiological signs at fluoroscopy are irregularity of the mucosa with initially fine ulceration which eventually proceeds to a very irregular ragged mucosal appearance and thickening of the oesophageal wall (Figs. 3.9.17–3.9.19). By the time oesophagitis is easily seen on barium studies, it has been present for some time. The degree of involvement is best assessed at endoscopy. Occasionally, due to stricture, the endoscope cannot be passed. Under these circumstances, barium studies offer the only method of assessment of the distal oesophagus.

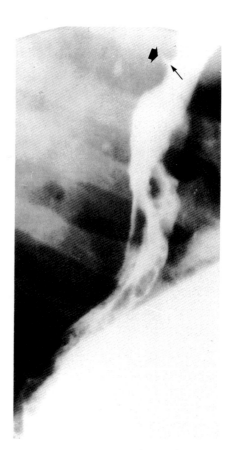

Fig. 3.9.18 Reflux oesophagitis with a large solitary mucosal ulcer (arrow).

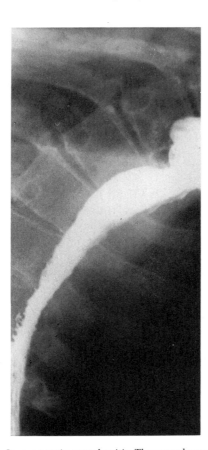

Fig. 3.9.17 Severe peptic oesophagitis. The oesophagus is dilated and baggy secondary to reflux. The mucosal wall is irregular due to extensive ulceration. This girl had severe spina bifida and gross kyphoscoliosis.

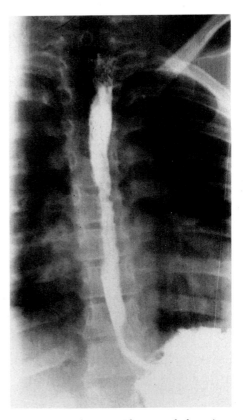

Fig. 3.9.19 Reflux oesophagitis with mucosal ulceration extending to the level of the carina. The narrow calibre is due to spasm.

GASTRO-OESOPHAGEAL REFLUX AND HIATUS HERNIA

Some degree of gastro-oesophageal reflux is a normal occurrence in all infants, manifest clinically by regurgitation during winding and during play. This, though socially a nuisance, is not significant and usually disappears with time and simple treatment by the use of thickened feeds and maintaining an upright posture following feeding. Clinical symptoms that suggest pathologically significant reflux include failure to thrive, recurrent chest infections due to aspiration, and persistent vomiting. The absence of vomiting does not preclude the presence of significant reflux. The decision to refer a child for radiological investigation of suspected reflux rests with the clinician, and the threshold for referral will vary considerably.

Investigation

There are many investigations for a suspected case of reflux, which in itself indicates that each has advantages and disadvantages. A logical investigation sequence would be to start with barium studies which provide a reliable method of excluding underlying anatomical abnormality in the oesophagus and stomach, or stomach outlet, and for demonstrating the presence of a hiatus hernia. Reflux associated with hiatal hernia is thought by some to be more significant than its presence without a hernia. During fluoroscopy the radiologist must identify the gastro-oesophageal junction, which is the non-distensible portion of the oesophagus, and the relationship of this to the diaphragm. Is it at, above, or below the diaphragm? If this lies above the diaphragm, then, by definition, there is a hiatus hernia which is usually of the sliding reducible type. Reflux through this is noted and the level to which the reflux rises recorded, as this, together with the frequency of the episodes, is an indication of the severity of reflux. Oesophagitis with mucosal ulceration is rarely seen in infants at barium examination, though often present at endoscopy.

Stricture formation should be noted and the full length of the stricture demonstrated by bolus swallowing in a 10–15° Trendelenburg position to maximize the chances of reflux distension of the distal oesophagus (Fig. 3.9.20).

Careful note is made of the gastric outlet and duodenum in all suspected refluxing children to exclude antral webs, pyloric or duodenal stenosis and malrotation, as causes of the reflux. In children with severe reflux, the gastro-oesophageal junction is often seen to be wide and lax, and the oesophagus rather baggy (Figs 3.9.12B, 3.9.13). Even if reflux is not demonstrated, these are signs strongly suggestive of reflux.

Reflux occurs more frequently with a full stomach, and it is good practice in an older infant to feed the child a normal meal and re-screen when the child has a full stomach, if reflux was not demonstrated initially.

Although reflux can be demonstrated by ultrasound it is a time-consuming examination, does not demonstrate the anatomy and is not recommended routine practice. There are simpler methods. Scintigraphy for gastro-oesophageal reflux is a very sensitive method of demonstration of the problem, but it does not demonstrate anatomical detail, merely the presence or absence of reflux, with some assessment of severity and frequency of the episodes (Fig. 3.9.21), and is usually the second line investigation. Two added advantages of this method are some assessment of gastric emptying and the late demonstration of radiopharmaceutical in the lungs, proving that reflux with aspiration is the cause of the recurrent chest infections. The test is more physiological than barium studies, and is probably the reason for the greater sensitivity. Nocturnal studies are important.

Continuous pH monitoring is particularly sensitive for detecting acid reflux but it is invasive as it involves placing the probe by a nasogastric route.

Technique of studies

The barium study is carried out with the infant in the lateral position and sucking on a bottle of dilute barium, and introduced by a catheter dummy. Pharyngeal coordination and motility, peristaltic activity of the oesophagus, and the position of the gastro-oesophageal junction are all actively scrutinized. Further screening is in the supine or oblique position. Compression of the abdomen and water siphoning, both of which were employed to induce reflux, have been abandoned. Intermittent screening is carried out until gastric emptying is observed and the position of the duodenojejunal flexure documented.

Scintigraphy is performed following a 4-hour fast.

The ultrasound examination is done supine or supine oblique away from the examiner. The reflux is shown as echolucent fluid refluxing from the stomach into the oesophagus and appearing as echogenic streaks.

REFERENCES

Arasu T S, Wyllie R, Fitzgerald J F, Franken E A, Siddiqui A R, Lehman G A, Eigen H, Grosfeld J L 1980 Gastroesophageal reflux in infants and children – comparative accuracy of diagnostic methods. Journal of Pediatrics 96: 798–803

Boix-Ochoa J M, Lafuente J M, Gil-Vernet J M 1980 Twenty-four hour esophageal pH monitoring in gastro-esophageal reflux. Journal of Pediatric Surgery 15: 74–78

Chen Y M, Gelfand D W, Ott D J, Munitz H A 1987 Natural progression of the lower oesophageal mucosal ring. Gastrointestinal Radiology 12: 93–98

Cleveland R H, Kushner D C, Schwartz A N 1983 Gastro esophageal reflux in children: results of a standardized fluoroscopic approach. American Journal of Roentgenology 141: 53–56

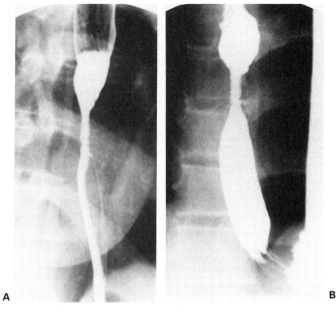

A

B

Fig. 3.9.20 Barium swallow. **A** Erect film showing a stricture of the oesophagus at approximately the level of the carina. There is poor distension of the distal oesophagus. **B** Swallow in the supine position showing distension of the normal distal oesophagus more clearly. The stricture was secondary to ingestion of caustic.

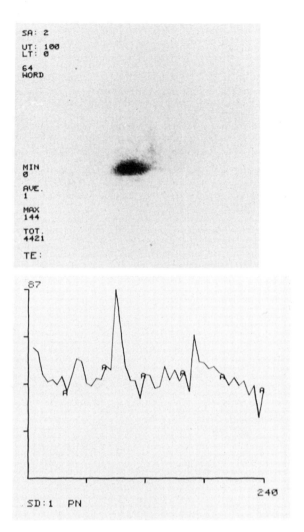

Fig. 3.9.21 'Milk scan.' Two episodes of reflux are seen as peaks on the time–activity curves. On the analogue image there is faint demonstration of contrast in the distal oesophagus.

Cohen M D, Beck J M 1980 Hiatus hernia: a complication of postero-lateral diaphragmatic herniation (Bochdalek Hernia) in infants. Clinical Radiology 31: 215–219

Friedland G W, Dodds W J, Sunshine P et al. 1974 The apparent disparity in incidence of hiatal herniae in infants and children in Britain and the United States. American Journal of Roentgenology 120: 305–314

Hampton F J, Macfadyen U M, Simpson H 1990 Reproducibility of 24 hour oesophageal pH studies in infants. Achives of Disease in Childhood 65: 1249–1255

Meyers W F, Roberts C C, Johnson D G, Herbst J J 1985 Value of tests for evaluation of gastro-esophageal reflux in children. Journal of Pediatric Surgery 20: 515–520

Newman B, Davis P 1989 Sonographic and magnetic resonance imaging of an anterior diaphragmatic hernia. Pediatric Radiology 20: 110–112

Seibert J J, Byrne W J, Euler A R, Latture T, Leach M, Campbell M 1983 Gastro-esophageal reflux – the acid test: scintigraphy or the pH probe? American Journal of Roentgenology 140: 1087–1090

Shub M D, Ulshen M W, Hargrove C B, Siegal G P, Groben P A, Askin F B 1985 Esophagitis: a frequent consequence of gastro-esophageal reflux in infancy. Journal of Pediatrics 107: 881–884

Stevenson G W 1989 Radiology of gastro-esophageal reflux. Clinical Radiology 40: 119–122

Ultrasound studies in gastro-oesophageal reflux

REFERENCES

Naik D R, Moore D J 1984 Ultrasound diagnosis of gastro-oesophageal reflux. Archives of Disease in Childhood 59: 366–367

Wright L L, Baker K R, Meny R G 1988 Ultrasound demonstration of gastroesophageal reflux. Journal of Ultrasound in Medicine 7: 471–475

REFERENCES

Fawcett H, Hayden C, Adams J, Swischuk L 1988 How useful is gastroesophageal reflux scintigraphy in suspected childhood aspiration? Pediatric Radiology 18: 311–313

Ham H, Piepsz A, Georges B, Delaet M, Rodesch P, Guillaume M, Cadranel S 1985 Evaluation of esophageal transit in children and in infants by means of Krypton -81m. Pediatric Radiology 15: 161–164

Martins J C, Isaacs P E, Sladen G E, Maisey M N, Edwards S 1984 Gastro-oesophageal reflux scintigraphy compared with pH probe monitoring. Nuclear Medicine Communications 5: 201–204

Paton J, Cosgriff P, Nanayakkhara C 1985 The analytical sensitivity of Tc ^{99m} radionuclide 'milk' scanning in the detection of gastro-oesophageal reflux. Pediatric Radiology 15: 381–383

Paton J, Nanayakkhara C, Simpson H 1988 Vomiting and gastro-esophageal reflux. Archives of Disease in Childhood 63: 837–838

CONDITIONS ASSOCIATED WITH GASTRO-OESOPHAGEAL REFLUX

Gastro-oesophageal reflux is mainly a disease in children under 2 years. Children with neuromuscular disease, hypotonia and cerebral palsy all have a higher incidence of reflux than the child with normal neuromuscular tone. These children are often mentally subnormal and do not complain as normal children would do. There is an increased incidence of peptic oesophagitis and stricture in these children. Fundal plication with control of the reflux can transform their lives, make them socially manageable and happier. They are often difficult to examine radiologically due to postural problems, and patience and ingenuity is required during fluoroscopy.

Sandifer's syndrome

The association of gross gastro-oesophageal reflux with involuntary torsion spasms of the head and neck and maintenance of abnormal posturing, e.g. torticollis or opisthotonos, is known as Sandifer's syndrome. These manoeuvres are related to attempts by the child to avoid episodes of reflux and are not due to neurological problems. The posturing disappears with treatment and relief of the reflux.

Apnoea attacks, cyanotic seizures, near-miss cot death and sudden infant death

In all of the above, gastro-oesophageal reflux with inhalation of gastric contents has been suggested as a possible mechanism. The relationship is not proven, but it may be a cause in some children, and most children presenting thus are investigated for reflux.

Recurrent chest infection, bronchiectasis and pulmonary fibrosis

There is no doubt that reflux with recurrent pulmonary aspiration can lead to permanent lung damage with bronchiectasis and, more rarely, pulmonary fibrosis. It can also cause severe bronchospasm and asthma. However, the mere demonstration of reflux in these children does not necessarily incriminate reflux as the cause of the pulmonary problem and the coexistence of the two conditions must not be overinterpreted. Other causes for pulmonary disease should be excluded. Demonstration of aspirated gastrointestinal contents by gastro-oesophageal scintigraphy is the best evidence that the pulmonary problems are due to reflux. While scintigraphy is highly sensitive in demonstrating reflux, it is not highly sensitive in reliably demonstrating aspiration. When documented it is worthwhile, but a negative test does not exclude aspiration.

Rare association

Rumination, the regurgitation of partially digested food, is described in association with reflux. Protein losing enteropathy and finger clubbing have been described in three children who had severe reflux oesophagitis, hiatus hernia and iron deficiency anaemia. This is an isolated report.

Anaemia

Children with reflux oesophagitis and a hiatus hernia may present with iron deficiency anaemia due to chronic slow blood loss. The symptoms of reflux may be minimal, absent, or not appreciated. A scintigram for identification of a Meckel's diverticulum should be done, in the presence of faecal occult blood. In scintigraphy for Meckel's, reflux of the radionuclide into the oesophagus following its secretion into the gastric lumen is frequently seen (Fig. 3.9.22). The significance of this must not be overlooked.

Barrett's oesophagus

The normal mucosal lining of the oesophagus is squamous epithelium. Rarely the oesophageal mucosa has columnar epithelium lining it for a variable length. In children this is rarely seen with a hiatus hernia. Stricture formation from reflux may occur at the junction of the squamous and columnar epithelium, away from the hernia, and can cause confusion.

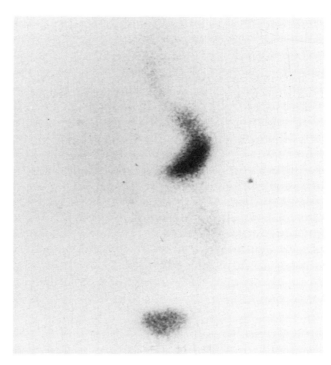

Fig. 3.9.22 Anterior view of a technetium pertechnetate scan in a boy who presented with anaemia. The scan was done to look for a Meckel's diverticulum. There is radionuclide in the oesophagus, due to reflux from the stomach following secretion of the pertechnetate.

Postural abnormalities and reflux

REFERENCES

Hadari A, Azizi E, Lernau O, Nissan S 1984 Sandifer's syndrome: a rare complication of hiatal hernia. A case report. Zeitschrift fur Kinderchirurgie 39: 202–203
Murphy N, Gellis S 1977 Torticollis with hiatus hernia in infancy. American Journal of Diseases of Children 131: 564–565

Barrett's oesophagus

REFERENCES

Barrett N R 1950 Chronic peptic ulcer of the oesophagus and 'oesophagitis'. British Journal of Surgery 38: 175–182
Karvelis K C, Drane W E, Johnson D A, Silverman E D 1987 Barrett oesophagus: decreased oesophageal clearance shown by radionuclide oesophageal scintigraphy. Radiology 162: 97–99
Yulish B S, Rothstein F C, Halpin T C 1987 Radiographic findings in children and young adults with Barrett's oesophagus. American Journal of Roentgenology 148: 353–357

REFERENCES

Byrne W J, Campbell M, Ashcraft E, Seibert J J, Euler A R 1983 A diagnostic approach to vomiting in severely retarded patients. American Journal of Diseases of Children 137: 259–262
Darling D, McCauley R, Leonidas J, Schwartz A 1978 Gastroesophageal reflux in infants and children, correlation of radiological severity and pulmonary pathology. Radiology 127: 735–740
Herbst J, Friedland G W, Zboralski F F 1971 Hiatal hernia and 'rumination' in infants and children. Journal of Pediatrics 78: 261–265
Herbst J, Johnson D, Oliveros M 1976 Gastroesophageal reflux with protein-losing enteropathy and finger clubbing. American Journal of Diseases of Children 130: 1256–1258
Mays E E, Dubois J J, Hamilton G B 1976 Pulmonary fibrosis associated with tracheobronchial aspiration: a study of the frequency of hiatal hernia and gastroesophageal reflux in interstitial pulmonary fibrosis of obscure etiology. Chest 69: 512–515
McFadyen U M, Hendry G M, Simpson H 1983 Gastro-esophageal reflux in near miss sudden infant death syndrome or suspected recurrent aspiration. Archives of Disease in Childhood 58: 87–91
Sondheimer J M, Morris B A 1979 Gastroesophageal reflux among severely retarded children. Journal of Pediatrics 94: 710–714

POSTOPERATIVE APPEARANCES AFTER FUNDAL PLICATION AND REPAIR OF HIATUS HERNIA

There are numerous types of surgical antireflux procedures. Each will have its own postoperative appearance on barium studies, and close understanding between the surgeon and radiologist will prevent incorrect interpretation of results. The essence of most primary repair procedures is fixation of the hernia in the abdomen with some form of fundal plication as an antireflux procedure. The most frequently performed operation is the Nissen fundoplication. Good long-term results are obtained. The appearance on barium swallow gives a mass-like appearance surrounding the distal subdiaphragmatic oesophagus, due to the wrapping of the fundus around the distal oesophagus to prevent reflux. (Fig. 3.9.23, 3.9.24).

On plain abdominal radiograph, the fundal wrap is seen as a solid 'pseudotumour', projecting into the gas bubble medially (Fig. 3.9.25).

If the wrap around is too tight, there is dysphagia, but, more distressing, failure of the normal belching ability and inability to vomit, which can lead to gastric distension needing re-operation. The stomach is air filled.

A further complication following Nissen repair is the development of a paraoesophageal hernia.

REFERENCES

Agha F P, Trenkner S W, Orringer M B, Vinh P N 1985 The combined Collis gastroplasty–Nissen fundoplication: surgical procedure and radiographic evaluation. American Journal of Roentgenology 145: 729–734

Blane C, Turnage R, Oldham K, Coran A 1989 Long-term radiographic follow up of the Nissen fundoplication in children. Pediatric Radiology 19: 523–526

Dedinsky G K, Vane D W, Black T, Turner M K, West K W, Grosfeld J L 1987 Complications and re-operation after Nissen fundoplication in childhood. American Journal of Surgery 153: 177–183

Festen C 1981 Paraoesophageal hernia: a major complication of Nissen's fundoplication. Journal of Pediatric Surgery 16: 496–499

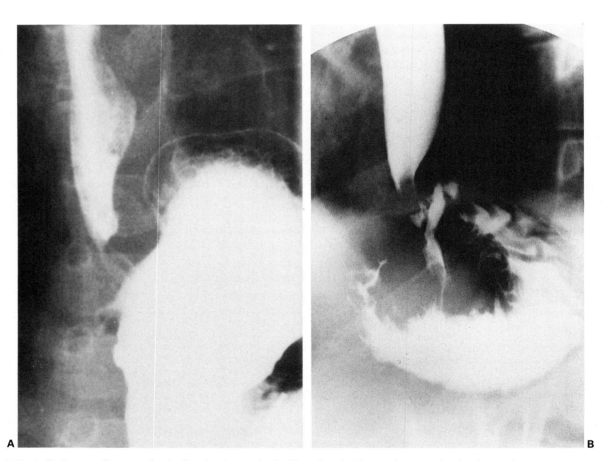

A   **B**

Fig. 3.9.23 **A** Barium swallow post fundoplication for repair of a hiatus hernia. The gap between the distal oesophagus and the fundus of the stomach is due to a portion of the stomach fundus being wrapped around the distal oesophagus. **B** Post Nissen repair. The fundal 'mass' is due to the plication.

TRANSVERSE FOLDS IN THE OESOPHAGUS – THE FELINE OESOPHAGUS

Fine transverse folds are occasionally demonstrated in a double contrast oesophagram in older children. These have been described in adults in association with gastro-oesophageal reflux. They are thought to be due to contraction of the muscularis mucosa and possibly represent an early stage of dysfunction. They are a transient phenomenon. They are described in the gastric antrum in adults but are not seen in children.

REFERENCES

Cho K, Gold B, Printz D 1987 Multiple transverse folds in the gastric antrum. Radiology 164: 339–341.
Williams S M, Harned R K, Kaplan P, Consigny P M 1983 Work in progress. Transverse striation of the oesophagus: associated with gastro-esophageal reflux. Radiology 146: 25–27

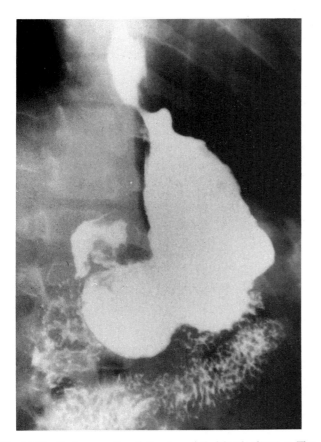

Fig. 3.9.24 Barium swallow following a failed fundoplication. The deformity at the gastro-oesophageal junction is due to a combination of a persistent hernia and fundal deformity due to the surgery.

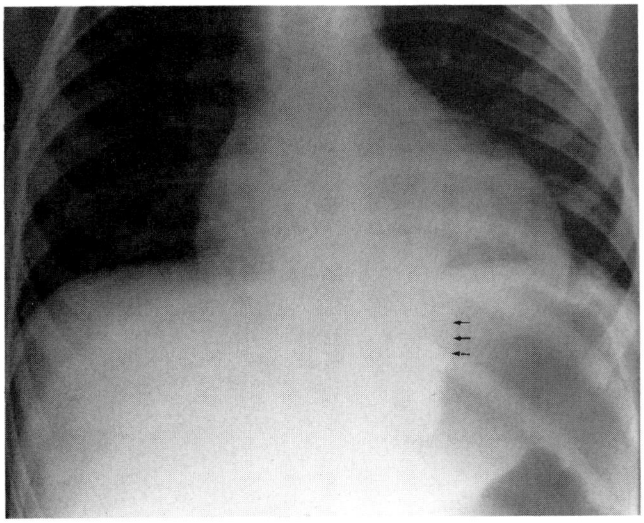

Fig. 3.9.25 Chest radiograph, post repair of a hiatus hernia by a Nissen fundoplication. The 'mass' projecting into the fundus of the stomach (arrows) is caused by the plication.

LATE-PRESENTING DIAPHRAGMATIC HERNIA

Congenital diaphragmatic hernias present most commonly in the newborn period and are discussed in detail in Chapter 1.

Later presentation is well recognized and the radiological features in the uncomplicated case are similar to those seen in the neonatal period. The child may present with clinical symptoms due to displacement of the abdominal contents into the chest through the congenital defect. This defect, particularly on the right where the liver has acted as a barrier between chest and abdominal contents, becomes unplugged during a bout of coughing with an associated chest infection (Fig. 3.9.26). There is often a dangerous delay in the clinical diagnosis, as the presence of the previously normal chest radiograph leads to confusion. The defect is often small and ischaemia of the herniated bowel may lead to perfora-tion with spillage of intestinal juices or faeces into the pleural cavity with resultant severe empyema and septicaemia. When unrecognized, this is a life-threatening condition.

Asymptomatic diaphragmatic hernias are an occasional incidental finding on radiographs of the chest or abdomen in children (Fig. 3.9.27). The most frequent of these are anterior with a mass, which will appear solid or air filled depending on its contents. These can be large yet cause few or no symptoms.

Volvulus of the intestine with ischaemic perforation is a well-known complication of diaphragmatic hernia and the child may present with a pneumonia and effusion, making it difficult to identify the underlying pathology. Ultrasound of the diaphragm is a useful tool in diagnosis. The defect is usually easily appreciated.

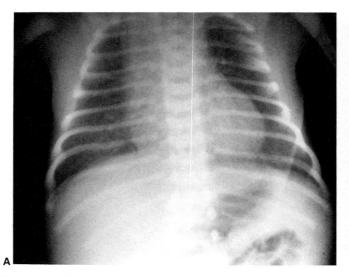
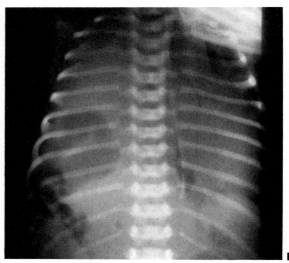

Fig. 3.9.26 **A** Two-month-old boy who presented with a chest infection. Radiograph on admission shows no evidence of a hernia. **B** Same child 48 hours later. There is now an opaque right hemithorax, displacement of heart and mediastinum to the left and bowel loops in the right chest. The child's condition had deteriorated. At operation a large defect was present in the right diaphragm through which the bowel had herniated. Part of the liver had also herniated through the defect. The child made an uneventful recovery.

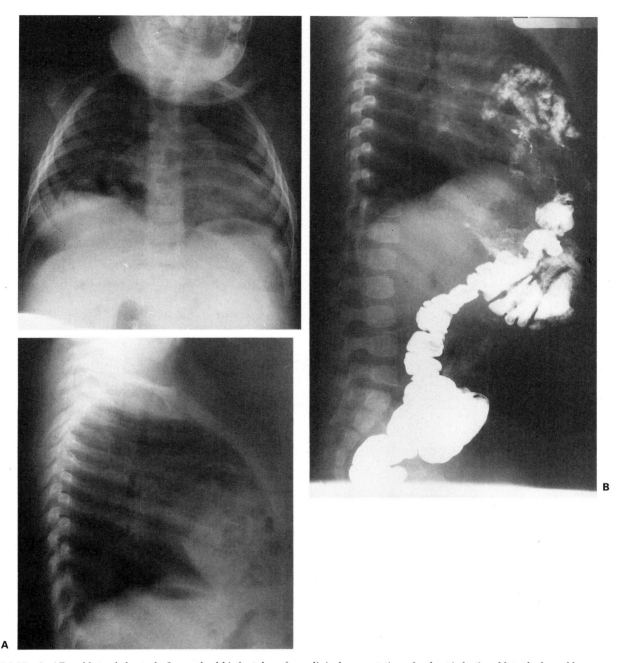

Fig. 3.9.27 A AP and lateral chest of a 3-month-old infant done for a clinical presentation of a chest infection. Note the bowel loops centrally and anteriorly. **B** Barium follow-through examination of the same child shows the hernia to contain mainly colon.

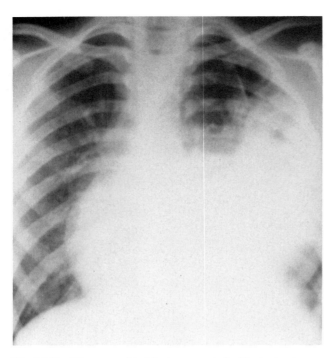

Fig. 3.9.28 Nine-year-old girl who presented with chest pain following a road traffic accident. The partially opaque left chest contains multiple fluid-filled loops of bowel. At surgery, much of the small intestine had herniated through a rupture in the diaphragm.

Traumatic rupture of the diaphragm as a consequence of falls, crushing or compression injuries is a rare, though well recognized, occurrence (Fig. 3.9.28). Traumatic rupture is most frequently seen following road traffic accidents, but may also result from a compression injury in child abuse. Most commonly, the diaphragmatic tear is on the left. It occurs in the central tendon and radiates to the periphery. Variable amounts of mesentery and intestine herniate through the rupture, with twisting of the neck of the hernia, ischaemia and perforation well known complications. If the tear is on the right, a portion of liver or the whole of the liver may herniate through the defect with twisting of the liver on its pedicle causing vascular compromise and ischaemic necrosis of the liver.

The kidney, or, more rarely, the spleen, may also herniate into the chest through a diaphragmatic defect, but more frequently there is an eventration of a portion of the diaphragm with a thin layer of muscle separating the kidney from the chest (Fig. 3.9.29). The condition is usually asymptomatic. There is a transdiaphragmatic paravertebral mass discovered as an incidental finding on a chest or abdomen film. The nature of the mass is identified by ultrasound and confirmed by intravenous urography. Delayed herniation of the kidney has been described following repair of a diaphragmatic hernia. Although usually an asymptomatic problem, occasional patients have been described who have hypertension, from stretching of the renal artery.

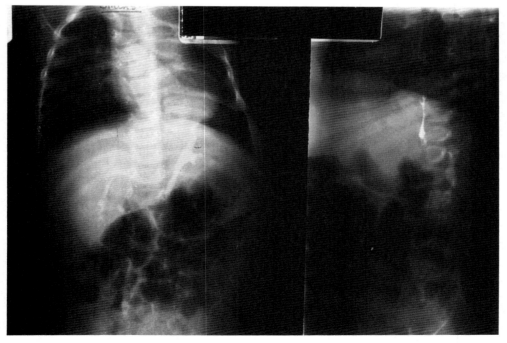

Fig. 3.9.29 Incidental finding of a paraspinal mass which subsequently proved to be a superior ectopic kidney in a child who had spinal radiographs for assessment of scoliosis. Rib and spinal anomalies are present.

REFERENCES

Berman L, Stringer D A, Ein S, Shandling B 1988 Childhood diaphragmatic hernias presenting after the neonatal period. Clinical Radiology 39: 237–244

Gaisie G, Young L, Oh K 1983 Late-onset Bockdalek's hernia with obstruction: radiographic spectrum of presentation. Clinical Radiology 34: 267–270

Liddell R M, Rosenbaum D M, Blumhagen J D 1989 Delayed radiologic appearances of bilateral thoracic ectopic kidneys. American Journal of Roentgenology 152: 120–122

Merten D F, Bowie J D Kirks D R, Grossman H 1982 Anteromedial diaphragmatic defects in infancy: current approaches to diagnostic imaging. Radiology 142: 361–365

Newman B, Davis P 1989 Sonographic and magnetic resonance imaging of an anterior diaphragmatic hernia. Pediatric Radiology 20: 110–112

CONGENITAL MALFORMATIONS

Oesophageal stenosis

Congenital oesophageal stenosis is a rare though well-described entity. Most cases of stenosis are secondary to trauma, systemic disease, infection or reflux. Primary stenosis is occasionally seen in the oesophagus distal to an atresia or tracheo-oesophageal fistula.

There are two forms of congenital stenosis. The more common is a 2–3 mm constriction in the mid oesophagus. Symptoms are due to food impaction at the site and the child does not usually present clinically until solid lumpy food is introduced. The less common form is a long narrowed segment which may occur at any point in the oesophagus. With this form, there is proximal dilatation, unlike the narrow band form where proximal dilatation is rare. Symptoms in children with the long form may occur at any age, and are often present at birth. The symptoms are those of constant drooling, difficulty in swallowing and aspiration.

Treatment of both types is by repeated dilatation, with surgery reserved for failure of this method.

Bars, cartilaginous rests and muscular hypertrophy

Intramural tracheobronchial cartilage containing rests are found as a cause of congenital oesophageal stenosis in some children (Fig. 3.9.30). Conversely, remnants of oesophageal muscle can cause tracheal or bronchial stenosis. These bars are all due to embryological maldevelopment and stem from incomplete separation of the tracheo-oesophageal septum. At barium study they usually appear as smooth areas of narrowing in the distal oesophagus with varying degrees of proximal dilatation. Obstruction can also occur due to congenital muscular hypertrophy or congenital epithelial hypertrophy and there has been a report of aberrant pancreatic tissue within the oesophagus causing stenosis. The barium studies cannot distinguish between the varying causes. Diagnosis is by biopsy.

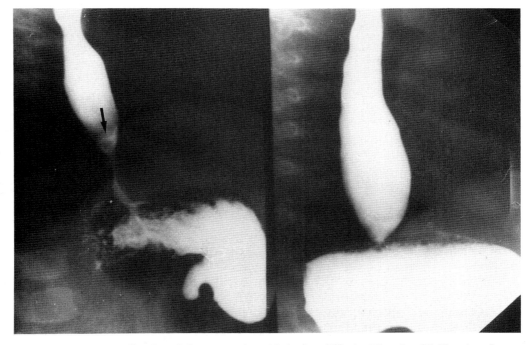

Fig. 3.9.30 Barium swallow in an infant presenting with feeding difficulty. There is mild dilatation of the oesophagus with a tight stenosis distally. The filling defect (arrow) was due to a cartilaginous rest which was causing the stenosis.

REFERENCES

Anderson L, Shackelford G, Mancilla-Jimenez R, McAlister W 1973 Cartilaginous esophageal ring: a cause of esophageal stenosis in infants and children. Radiology 108: 665–666

Blank E, Michael T 1963 Muscular hypertrophy of the esophagus: report of a case with involvement of the entire esophagus. Pediatrics 32: 595–597

Briceno L I, Grases P J, Gallego S 1981 Tracheobronchial and pancreatic remnants causing esophageal stenosis. Journal of Pediatric Surgery 16: 731–732

Dominguez R, Zarabi M, Oh K, Bender T, Girdany B 1985 Congenital oesophageal stenosis. Clinical Radiology 36: 263–266

Moore K L 1982 The respiratory system. In: The developing human. Saunders, Philadelphia, Ch II, pp 216–226

Todani T, Watanabe Y, Mizuguchi T, Uemura S, Matsuo S, Kimura T 1984 Congenital oesophageal stenosis due to fibromuscular thickening. Zeitschrift fur Kinderchirurgie 39: 11–14

Oesophageal webs

Congenital webs, though uncommon, are occasionally seen in association with tracheo-oesophageal fistula. They are thin diaphragms located at the level of the fistula. They are only appreciated at barium swallow or at endoscopy. Macroscopically the oesophagus appears normal. The web is seen on barium studies as a thin smooth transverse or oblique defect in the oesophagus. Webs also occur secondary to trauma either postoperatively or from corrosive ingestion or reflux and in association with epidermyolysis bullosa.

REFERENCES

Azimi F, O'Hara A E 1973 Congenital intraluminal mucosal web of the esophagus with tracheo-esophageal fistula. American Journal of Diseases of Children 125: 92–95

Fox P F 1978 Unusual esophageal atresia with tracheoesophageal fissure. Journal of Pediatric Surgery 13: 373

Hillemeier C, Touloukian R, McCallum R, Gryboski J 1981 Esophageal web: a previously unrecognised complication of epidermolysis bullosa. Pediatrics 67: 678–682

Vascular rings as a cause of dysphagia

A detailed description of the vascular rings and slings is found in Chapter 2 'The heart and great vessels'. Children with these rings may present with respiratory and gastrointestinal symptoms, with the respiratory symptoms usually overshadowing the symptoms of dysphagia. The respiratory symptoms depend on the degree of tracheal compression and the exact nature of the lesion, and include stridor, cough, costal recession, respiratory distress, especially when feeding, aspiration pneumonia and cyanosis. The barium swallow is carried out as a simple non-invasive method of confirming the suspected ring. There is a filling defect seen on the oesophagram due to the vascular anomaly (Fig. 3.9.31). The child should be examined in frontal, true lateral and both oblique projections. For adequate demonstration of the impression, there must be

adequate distension of the oesophagus. A contrast study done via a nasogastric tube in a paralysed ventilated child may give a false negative study. If the child is too ill to swallow a good bolus, contrast injected via a nasogastric tube situated just above the aortic arch usually provides the necessary distension.

Most children with significant rings present in the first few months of life. An aberrant right subclavian artery is the most frequent aortic arch anomaly with a reported incidence of 0.5% in the general population. It seldom, if ever, causes dysphagia and is commonly an incidental finding.

In the frontal projection, there is an oblique indentation of the oesophagus extending from left to right at just below the level of the aortic arch. On the lateral view, there is a posterior indentation on the oesophagus caused by the retro-oesophageal aberrant right subclavian artery (Fig. 3.9.32)

ACQUIRED DISEASES OF THE OESOPHAGUS

Foreign body ingestion

Infants and children of all ages swallow an infinite variety of foreign bodies, most inadvertently, but occasionally in the older child deliberately, either as an attention-seeking exercise, or as part of a suicidal attempt. Munchausen's syndrome, with repetitive swallowing of foreign bodies as a manifestation, has also been described in children.

Symptoms fall into two clear groups. Shortly after swallowing the foreign body the child complains of choking, a feeling of something stuck and dysphagia which may be partial or complete, depending on the degree of obstruction. Many children who have swallowed a foreign body complain of a continued feeling of something sticking, even when the foreign body has passed into the stomach, due probably to local spasm and trauma. Continued drooling and regurgitation imply impaction.

The second group of children have little or no symptoms related to the ingestion, but complain of progressive unexplained dysphagia, if the foreign body remains impacted. A more serious problem is the child who presents with respiratory difficulty, with or without dysphagia, due to mediastinitis and abscess formation from a silent perforation. This is similar to the retropharyngeal abscess with silent pharyngeal perforation. Radiological investigation depends on the nature of the foreign body. If it is likely to be radiopaque, then PA and lateral chest films are all that are required. Both views are required to fully appreciate the angle at which the foreign body lies to enable decisions about treatment, i.e. attempted removal by balloon catheter, endoscopic removal or forward propulsion of the foreign body into the stomach. Thin, low density foreign bodies may only be seen in one

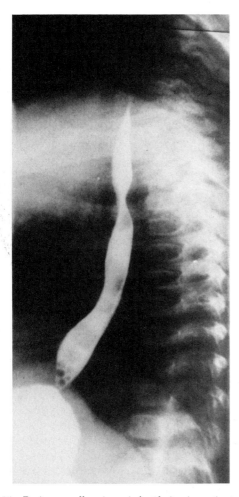

Fig. 3.9.31 Barium swallow in an infant being investigated for cyanotic attacks. Note the typical appearance of a constriction on both anterior and posterior surface of the oesophagus due to the vascular sling.

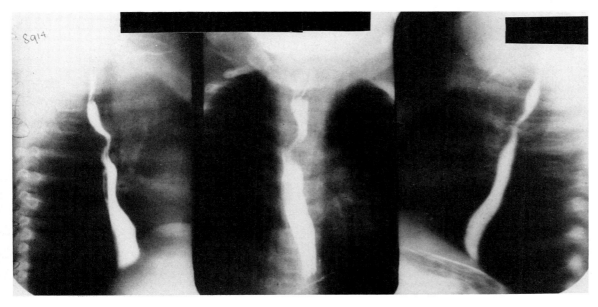

Fig. 3.9.32 Aberrant right subclavian artery causing an impression on the oesophagogram.

projection and need the increased radiographic density when the object is in the sagittal plane parallel to the X-ray beam before it can be identified. Commonly, this is described with the ring-pulls of soft drink cans, but may occur with any low density object. Though in theory pointed foreign bodies, e.g. open pins, nails, screws, etc., carry a hazard of perforation of the oesophageal wall, in practice this is rare and most can be safely recovered without open surgery.

If the swallowed foreign body is likely to be non-opaque, i.e. a food bolus, then a barium study is the primary investigation in order to confirm the diagnosis and locate the site of obstruction. Clinical indication of the site and feeling of sticking does not correlate well with the radiological location.

The site of impaction of all types of foreign bodies is usually at the level of the thoracic inlet (Fig. 3.9.33), the aortic arch or the gastro-oesophageal junction. Impaction elsewhere should raise a question of an underlying cause and follow-up studies, once the foreign body is removed and the acute oedema has settled, are prudent. Children with repaired oesophageal atresia or fundal plication are at increased risk of impaction. Most swallowed small foreign bodies are generally passed through the gastrointestinal tract without problem. Their passage usually occurs between 2 and 6 days, but may take up to 4 weeks. Delayed passage occurs when food is mistakenly withheld until the object is passed. Foreign bodies persisting in the duodenum after 6 days are unlikely to pass and if left may perforate into the right kidney.

There has been concern about the potential harm of swallowed button batteries, due to reports of oesophageal burns and subsequent stricture, or gastric perforation, if the seal between the two halves of the battery breaks and toxic chemicals are released. This has led to the development of magnet catheters for the removal of metallic foreign bodies, though it must be emphasized that most children will pass foreign bodies without complication, and once the object is in the stomach, the risk of leaving it to pass naturally is less than the risk of complications that may occur during attempted removal. These include perforation of the oesophagus and stomach by the instrumentation, aspiration of stomach contents during attempted removal, and aspiration of the foreign body itself.

Removal of foreign bodies

There are many reports of successful, non-operative, removal of foreign bodies, using a balloon catheter passed distal to the foreign body and then inflating the balloon to withdraw the foreign body as the catheter is removed. This is done under fluoroscopic control, in the Trendelenburg position and with full resuscitation facilities in case inhalation into the airways of the foreign body occurs during its passage through the pharynx. This technique is only suitable for a foreign body in situ for less than 24 hours, and should only be done by fully trained radiologists. Objects can be successfully pushed into the stomach by this technique as well without anaesthesia in a cooperative

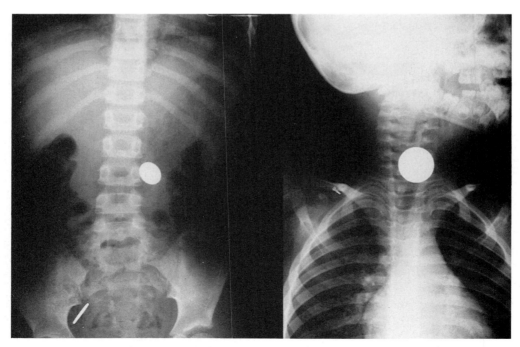

Fig. 3.9.33 Six-year-old boy who complained of choking and dysphagia. Symptoms were due to the coin impacted at the thoracic inlet. Previous coins had been swallowed without symptoms.

child. In general, it is not an appropriate method for removal of sharp, potentially penetrating, objects.

An alternative method of removal is direct grasping of the object and withdrawing it during endoscopy. The policy needs to be agreed locally and should not be a cause for conflict between hospital departments.

REFERENCES

Boothroyd A, Carty H, Robson J 1987 'Hunt the Thimble': a study of the radiology of ingested foreign bodies. Archives of Emergency Medicine 4: 33–38

Campbell J, Condon V 1989 Catheter removal of blunt esophageal foreign bodies in children: survey of the Society for Pediatric Radiology. Pediatric Radiology 19: 361–365

Campbell J, Quattromani F, Foley L 1983 Foley catheter removal of blunt esophageal foreign bodies. Experience with 100 consecutive children. Pediatric Radiology 13: 116–119

David T, Ferguson A 1986 Management of children who have swallowed button batteries. Archives of Disease in Childhood 61: 321–322

Eggli K, Potter B, Garcia V, Altman R, Breckbill D 1986 Delayed diagnosis of esophageal perforation by aluminum foreign bodies. Pediatric Radiology 16: 511–513

Paulson E, Jaffe R 1990 Metallic foreign bodies in the stomach: fluoroscopic removal with a magnetic orogastric tube. Radiology 174: 191–194

Towbin R B, Dunbar J S, Rice S 1990 Magnetic catheter for removal of magnetic foreign bodies. American Journal of Roentgenology 154: 149–50

Towbin R, Lederman H, Dunbar J, Ball W, Strife J 1989 Esophageal edema as a predicator of unsuccessful ballon extraction of esophageal foreign body. Pediatric Radiology 19: 359–360

Votteler T P, Nash J C, Rutledge J C 1983 The hazard of ingested alkaline disc batteries in children. Journal of the American Medical Association 249: 2504–2506

Scleroderma and dermatomyositis

About one-third of children with scleroderma have involvement of the oesophagus and suffer from pain and dysphagia. The lower two-thirds of the oesophagus are affected. Early signs are loss of normal motility with incoordination. This can progress to complete atony of the oesophagus, which becomes dilated, with emptying occurring by gravity. Sacculations can develop. As the gastro-oesophageal junction becomes more severely affected, reflux oesophagitis and stricture formation result. Barrett's oesophagus is a further complication.

In dermatomyositis, the pharynx and upper oesophagus are affected. Poor clearing of contrast from the pharynx is seen at barium examination, together with diminished peristalsis in the upper oesophagus and nasal regurgitation.

Aspiration of food into the lungs is a complication of both disorders, leading to aspiration pneumonia.

REFERENCES

Clements J L Jr, Abernathy J, Weens H S 1978 Atypical esophageal diverticula associated with progressive systemic sclerosis. Gastrointestinal Radiology 3: 383–386

Dabich L, Sullivan D B, Cassidy J T 1974 Scleroderma in the child. Journal of Pediatrics 85: 770–775

Grunebaum M, Salinger H 1971 Radiologic finding in polymyositis-dermatomyositis involving the pharynx and upper oesophagus. Clinical Radiology 22: 97–100

Recht M P, Levine M S, Katzka D A, Reynolds J C, Saul S H 1988 Barrett's esophagus in scleroderma: increased prevalence and radiographic findings. Gastrointestinal Radiology 13: 1–5

Steiner R M, Glassan L, Schwartz M W 1974 The radiological findings in dermatomyositis of childhood. Radiology 111: 385–393

Epidermolysis bullosa

This is a rare chronic skin disease affecting squamous epithelium and can affect the mouth, oropharynx and oesophagus, causing ulcers, fibrotic strictures and acquired oesophageal webs. Symptoms of oesophageal involvement include dysphagia and pain. At barium examination, there is loss of normal motility, varying degrees of stenosis and mucosal ulceration. Pyloric atresia has been reported in association with epidermolysis bullosa.

REFERENCE

Becker M H, Swinyard C A 1968 Epidermolysis bullosa dystrophica in children: radiologic manifestations. Radiology 90: 124–128

Behçet disease

Pyoderma, ulceration of the mucous membranes of the gastrointestinal tract and genitalia, uveitis and central nervous system involvement due to vasculitis are manifestations of this rare disease. Ulceration leads to a severe oesophagitis which can progress to stricture formation. Involvement of the ileum and colon closely resembles Crohn's disease.

REFERENCE

Baba S, Maruta M, Ando K, Teramoto T, Endo I 1976 Intestinal Behçet's disease: report of five cases. Diseases of the Colon and Rectum 19: 428–440

Granulomatous disease (neutrophil dysfunction)

Thickening of the gastric antrum is the most commonly described gastrointestinal manifestation of granulomatous disease. Similar thickening can occur in the distal oesophagus.

Mediastinitis with a dilated rigid oesophagus is also described.

REFERENCES

Markowitz J F, Aornow E, Rausen A R 1982 Progressive esophageal dysfunction in chronic granulomatous disease. Journal of Pediatric Gastroenterology and Nutrition 1: 145–149

Orduna M, Gonzalez De Orbe G, Gordillo M, Fernandez-Epifanio J, Serrano C, Collado J, Miralles M 1989 Chronic granulomatous disease of childhood. Report of two cases with unusual involvement of the gastric antrum and spleen. European Journal of Radiology 9: 67–70

DIVERTICULA

True congenital diverticula of the oesophagus are very rare. Diverticula may be present in association with duplications and are occasionally seen post repair of oesophageal atresia or following radiotherapy. Acquired pulsion or traction diverticula are also rare in children. These diverticula are due to herniations through congenitally potentially weak areas of the muscular wall of the oesophagus. The most frequent site is at the level of the carina. Granuloma formation in the carinal lymph nodes sets up an associated inflammatory reaction and subsequent fibrosis and causes traction on the anterior oesophageal wall. Histoplasmosis and tuberculosis are commonly associated diseases and rarely cause symptoms in children, but may be the site of impaction of a swallowed foreign body.

An epiphrenic diverticulum of the stomach is a very rare occurrence in children. When present they are frequently associated with obstruction at the gastro-oesophageal junction in adults, and have been reported in association with Ehlers–Danlos syndrome. A further rare type of diverticulum probably represents a *forme fruste* of an H-type fistula.

REFERENCES

Meadows J A Jr 1970 Esophageal diverticula in infants and children. Southern Medical Journal 63: 691–694
Nelson A R 1957 Congenital true esophageal diverticulum – report of a case unassociated with other esophagotracheal abnormality. Annals of Surgery 145: 258–264
Toyohara T, Kaneko T, Araki A, Takahashi K, Nakamura T 1989 Giant epiphrenic diverticulum in a boy with Ehlers–Danlos syndrome. Pediatric Radiology 19: 437

INTRAMURAL OESOPHAGEAL PSEUDODIVERTICULOSIS

In this condition there are outpouchings of the mucosa from the lumen into the oesophageal wall. These outpouchings have been shown to be dilated glands which have become obstructed due to desquamated squamous cells. Some underlying inflammatory process is the cause, often with associated monilial infection and caustic ingestion. Clinical symptoms are those of dysphagia of varying degrees. Contrast studies show numerous outpouchings of the mucosa, 2–3 mm deep, through an area of stricturing of the oesophagus. Dilatation of the stricture relieves symptoms.

REFERENCES

Braun P, Nussle D, Roy C, Cuendet A 1978 Intramural diverticulosis of the esophagus in an eight-year-old boy. Pediatric Radiology 6: 235–237
Cramer K R 1972 Intramural diverticulosis of the oesophagus. British Journal of Radiology 45: 857–859
Kim S, Choi C D, Groskin S A 1989 Esophageal intramural pseudodiverticulosis. Radiology 173: 418
Peters M, Crummy A, Wojtowycz M, Toussaint J 1982 Intramural esophageal pseudodiverticulosis. A report in a child with a sixteen-year follow-up. Pediatric Radiology 12: 262–263

OESOPHAGEAL VARICES

Varices in children are rarely discovered incidentally at barium examination. There is generally good clinical evidence of portal hypertension with splenomegaly and the barium studies are carried out to detect them, usually without smooth muscle paralysis. Varices appear as filling defects in the distal oesophagus, best seen on the partially filled oesophagus in the supine position (Fig. 3.9.34), and rarely ascend beyond the distal third. They may also be seen at the gastro-oesophageal junction, in the fundus of the stomach and in the first and second parts of the duodenum (Fig. 3.9.35). The oesophagus itself often looks atonic due to secondary degeneration of the muscularis mucosa. Although a site of bleeding, it is rare to see evidence of this on barium studies, and endoscopy is needed to isolate the site and, if appropriate, treat by sclerotherapy. There is an increased incidence of duodenal ulceration in these children. The differential diagnosis of varices on the oesophagram includes air bubbles, lymphoma deposits and granulation tissue resulting from oesophagitis. Neither lymphoma deposits nor granulation tissue will alter in response to posture or pressure changes associated with crying or the Valsalva manoeuvre. Congenital varices without portal hypertension have been described.

Oesophageal varices can be detected on CT studies and at ultrasound. Doppler imaging with colour flow mapping is a useful investigation in assessing the haemodynamics of the varices and the response to treatment.

REFERENCES

Balthazar E J, Naidich D P, Megibow A J, Lefleur R S 1987 CT evaluation of esophageal varices. American Journal of Roentgenology 148: 131–135

Harinck E, Fernandes J, Vervat D 1971 Congenital esophageal varices in identical twins without portal hypertension. Journal of Pediatric Surgery 6: 488–489

Rasinska G, Wermenski K, Rajszys P 1987 Percutaneous transsplenic embolization of esophageal varices in a 5 year old child. Acta Radiologica 28: 299–301

Sukigara M, Komazaki T, Yamazaki T, Anzai H, Koyama I, Omoto R 1987 Colour flow mapping of oesophagogastric varices and vessels in and around the liver with transoesophageal real time two dimensional Doppler ultrasound. Clinical Radiology 38: 487–494

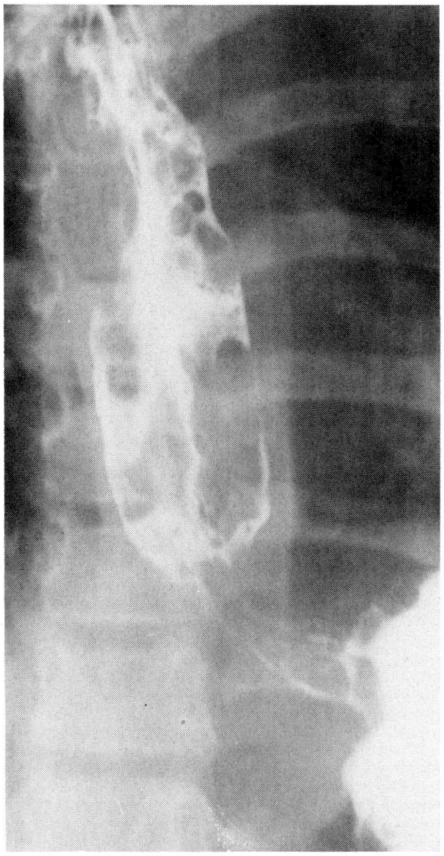

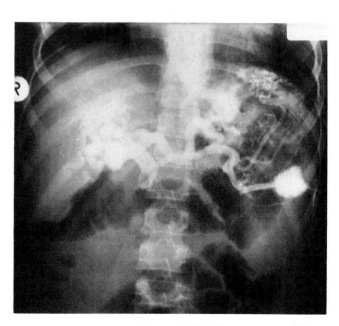

Fig. 3.9.34 Oesophageal varices. The numerous filling defects in the oesophagus and gastric fundus are due to varices. Note the dilated 'baggy' oesophagus.

Fig. 3.9.35 Same boy as in Figure 3.9.34. Splenoportogram. Major varices arise from the gastroduodenal vein at the gastric fundus and in the distal oesophagus. The portal vein is replaced by numerous large collateral veins.

INFECTIOUS DISEASES OF THE OESOPHAGUS

Moniliasis (candidiasis)

The most common infecting organism in children is *Candida albicans*, and, although a common systemic infection in neonates, is rare in the oesophagus. Children who are on immunosuppressive therapy are most at risk. Moniliasis is seen as a complication of steroid therapy. The earliest radiological finding is decreased motility of the oesophagus best demonstrated in the supine oblique position, when poor peristaltic activity and poor clearing of a swallowed bolus are observed. This is followed by demonstrable ulceration of the mucosa, initially seen as fine mucosal ulcers, but progressing to deep shaggy ulcers (Fig. 3.9.36), with a nodular mucosal appearance. The appearances may resemble intramural pseudodiverticulosis. There is rapid improvement with antifungal treatment. A serious complication is the development of a stricture (Fig 3.9.37), which may lead to stricturing of the whole of the oesophagus, needing colonic interposition. Other complications include perforation, mediastinitis and oesophagopleural fistulas.

Dysphagia is the presenting symptom. A small number of children may present with weight loss due to difficulty in swallowing, often with an insidious onset.

Late complications are food impaction at the site of stricture formation. In a small number of children, particularly in infants, stridor may be the presenting complaint.

Herpes simplex infection

Herpetic infection of the oesophagus, though much less frequent than candida infection, is the second common-

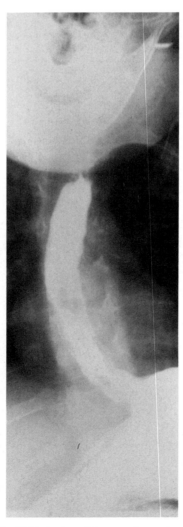

Fig. 3.9.36 Monilial infection of the oesophagus in a 4 year old on treatment for leukaemia. Mucosal ulceration is present throughout the oesophagus. Note the irregularity of the mucosal outline and filling defects in the oesophagogram.

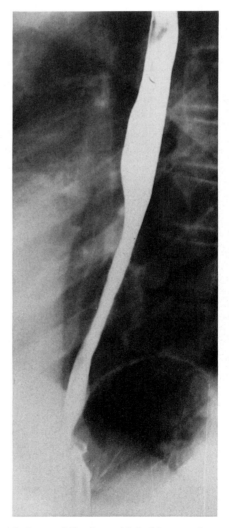

Fig. 3.9.37 Stricture of distal one-third of the oesophagus secondary to old monilial infection.

est oesophageal infection, and complicates systemic herpetic infection. The radiological findings are similar to those seen in candidiasis, i.e. motility disorders, spasm, mucosal ulceration, and stricture formation.

Other infections

Oesophageal involvement by tuberculosis, syphilis, histoplasmosis, meningococcal infection and cytomegalovirus have all been reported producing dysphagia. Decreased motility and varying degrees of ulceration are seen. Tuberculosis and histoplasmosis may cause fistulas to the pleural cavity or bronchi.

Other inflammatory diseases of the oesophagus

Inflammation associated with epidermolysis bullosa, Behçet's disease, scleroderma, chronic granulomatous disease and peptic oesophagitis are described elsewhere in this chapter. Inflammation, sometimes polypoidal, of the oesophagus is also reported in eosinophilic enteritis. Crohn's disease may occasionally affect the oesophagus, but there is usually evidence of this disease elsewhere.

Chagas' disease of the oesophagus

Systemic infection with *Trypanosoma cruzi* can cause an inflammatory disease of the oesophagus with destruction of the nerve cells leading to dysmotility, producing an appearance similar to achalasia. The two conditions cannot be differentiated. The diagnosis is made by isolating the organism. The disease is endemic in central Brazil, but occurs sporadically elsewhere in South America. As it can be transmitted from the mother during pregnancy, sporadic cases can occur anywhere in the world. The neonate may also suffer from hepatosplenomegaly jaundice, oedema, neurological symptoms and petechiae. Destruction of the neural plexus in the colon leads to a pseudo-obstruction with megacolon.

Oesophageal inflammation in AIDS

Infection with candida, mycobacterium, herpes, cytomegalovirus and tuberculosis have all been reported in adult patients with AIDS. In children, candida is the commonest oesophageal infection. The patients present with oral thrush, loss of appetite, dysphagia and refusal of food. The appearances on the oesophagogram are indistinguishable from those seen in children who have moniliasis of the oesophagus from other causes. Herpes infection, cryptococcus infection and cytomegalic oesophageal involvement show discrete ulcers on an otherwise normal mucosa but may be indistinguishable from candida on barium studies. There is usually other evidence of AIDS.

REFERENCES

Balthazar E J, Megibow A J, Hulnick D, Cho K C, Beranbaum E 1987 Cytomegalovirus esophagitis in AIDS: Radiographic features in 16 patients. American Journal of Roentgenology 149: 919–923

Bradford B, Abdenour G, Frank J, Scott G, Beerman R 1988 Usual and unusual radiologic manifestations of acquired immunodeficiency syndrome (AIDS) and human immunodeficiency virus (HIV) infection in children. Radiological Clinics of North America 26: 341–353

Forget P, Eggermont E, Marchal G, Geboes K, Jaeken J, Melchior S 1978 Eosinophilic infiltration of the oesophagus in an infant. Acta Paediatrica Belgica 31: 91–93

Goodman P, Pinero S, Rance R, Mansell P, Uribe-Botero G 1989 Mycobacterial esophagitis in AIDS. Gastrointestinal Radiology 14: 103–105

Guyer P B 1971 Candidiasis of the oesophagus. British Journal of Radiology 44: 131–136

Hamilton R, Mellow M, Braun N M, Polk G E 1977 Esophageal tuberculosis presenting with dysphagia. (Letter.) Journal of Pediatrics 91: 678–679

Haney P, Yale-Loehr A, Nussbaum A, Gellad F 1989 Imaging of infants and children with AIDS. American Journal of Roentgenology 152: 1033–1041

Kaufmann H J 1970 Candida esophagitis in children with malignant disorders. Annales de Radiologie 13: 157–162

Kirks D R, Merten D F 1980 Stridor in infants and children due to esophageal inflammatory disease. Gastrointestinal Radiology 5: 321–323

Lallemand D, Huault G, Laboureau J P 1974 Laryngeal and oesophageal lesions in patients with herpetic disease. Annales de Radiologie 17: 317–325

Levine M, Woldenberg R, Herlinger H, Laufer I 1987 Opportunistic esophagitis in AIDS: radiographic diagnosis. Radiology 165: 815–820

Matzinger M, Daneman A 1983 Esophageal involvement in eosinophilic gastroenteritis. Pediatric Radiology 13: 35–38

Simeone J F, Burrell M, Toffler R, Walker Smith G J 1977 Aperistalsis and esophagitis. Radiology 123: 9–14

Crohn's disease of the oesophagus

REFERENCES

Cynn W S, Chon H, Gureghian P A, Levin B L 1975 Crohn's disease of the esophagus. American Journal of Roentgenology 125: 359–364

Chagas' disease of the oesophagus

REFERENCES

Bittencourt A L 1976 Congenital Chagas disease. American Journal of Diseases of Children 130: 97–103

Winslow D J, Chaffee E F 1965. Preliminary investigations on Chagas' disease. Military Medicine 130: 826–834

OESOPHAGEAL TRAUMA

Chemical burns

The most severe oesophageal burns are caused by ingestion of alkaline chemicals, of which the most common is lye, which contains about 95% sodium and potassium hydroxide. The degree of damage to the oesophagus depends on the concentration of the alkali and its physical structure. Liquids burn the whole of the oesophagus, while ingested crystals will cause maximum damage in the mouth or pharynx. The depth of oesophageal burn varies from superficial ulceration to complete necrosis of the wall of the oesophagus with associated mediastinitis. Mediastinal abscess formation, tracheo-oesophageal and aortico-oesophageal fistulas are complications. Late effects include superior vena caval obstruction and periaortic fibrosis. It is unusual to find oesophageal burns without associated mouth burns. The admission chest radiograph is important in the early assessment. Mediastinal widening suggests perforation of the oesophagus, confirmed if there is an associated pneumomediastinum or a pleural effusion. Widening of the mediastinum or paraspinal pleural reflection can occur with an inflammatory reaction without perforation, and is a bad prognostic sign likely to indicate subsequent stricture formation.

Stricture formation occurs in up to one-third of patients, and occurs at the site of oesophageal spasm when the caustic is ingested. The length of the stricture is variable (Fig. 3.9.38), and may be multiple. Early contrast studies should be done with water-soluble contrast in case there is a perforation. Subsequent studies can be done with barium. The early changes following acute injury include diminished and irregular peristalsis, an air-filled atonic oesophagus, mucosal oedema and ulceration and occasionally aspiration. An air-filled atonic oesophagus is a bad prognostic sign as these patients will develop strictures.

The degree of damage may be underestimated by contrast studies and is better assessed by endoscopy but the risk of perforation at endoscopy is high.

Late contrast swallows following ingestion of alkali demonstrate areas of narrowing of the oesophagus, with smooth mucosa, pseudodiverticulae, diminished peristalsis and occasionally a hiatus hernia due to shortening of the oesophagus resulting from the stricture (Fig. 3.9.39).

When there is a severe stricture the contrast bolus may be insufficient to distend the normal part of the oesophagus and lead to a false assessment of the length of the stricture. Swallowing in the supine position helps to distend normal areas of the oesophagus and avoids an overestimation of stricture length. Balloon dilatations may be dangerous in alkali strictures.

Focal corrosive burns have been reported as a result of ingestion of Clinitest tablets, used by diabetics to test the urine, which are pure alkali. They are a pretty blue colour and are ingested by children in the belief that they are sweets. Ingestion of alkaline disc batteries has also led to oesophageal burns.

Tetracycline can produce a focal oesophagitis in children and is a complication of this treatment for acne. The radiological appearance is one of fine mucosal oesophageal ulceration.

REFERENCES

Amoury R A, Hrabovsky E E, Leonidas J C, Holder T M 1975 Tracheooesophageal fistula after lye ingestion. Journal of Pediatric Surgery 10: 273–277

Burrington J D 1975 Clinitest burns of the esophagus. Annals of Thoracic Surgery 20: 400–404

Franken E A 1973 Caustic damage of the gastrointestinal tract: roentgen features. American Journal of Roentgenology 118: 77–85

Maves M, Lloyd T, Carithers J 1986 Radiographic identification of ingested disc batteries. Pediatric Radiology 16: 154–156

Swischuk L 1989 Alimentary tract. In: Imaging of the newborn and young infant. Williams & Wilkins, Baltimore, ch 4, p 382

Other trauma

Oesophageal trauma can also result from blunt and penetrating injury, both rare in children. Iatrogenic trauma results from perforation during endoscopy or the passage of varying tubes and capsules, or during dilatation of strictures by bougies or balloons. The perforation is usually noticed at the time of injury and management instituted immediately. If not appreciated at the time, presenting symptoms include dysphagia, pain and subcutaneous emphysema. Radiographic findings will include mediastinal and subcutaneous emphysema, mediastinal widening and a hydropneumothorax. Contrast studies with water-soluble contrast are indicated to demonstrate the site and extent of the tear. Late symptoms due to a silent perforation will be those of dysphagia from stricturing or more rarely abscess formation and mediastinitis. Increased intraluminal pressure within the oesophagus may also lead to traumatic oesophageal injury similar to any other blunt injury such as blast injury. The rise in pressure within the oesophagus, particularly associated with violent retching against a close proximal end due to cricopharyngeal constriction, may lead to rupture of the wall or haematoma formation within the wall, as may rapid ingestion of effervescent drinks.

Intramural haematoma may also occur in children with blood dyscrasia and coagulation problems. The children present with chest or epigastric pain and dysphagia. An intramural mass will be demonstrated at barium swallow.

Spontaneous perforation of the oesophagus has

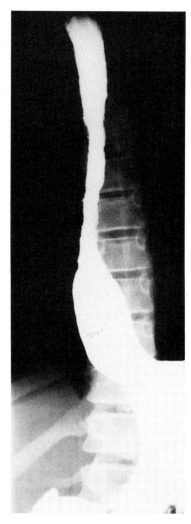

Fig. 3.9.38 There is a long stricture of the middle third of the oesophagus with mucosal ulceration, due to ingestion of alkali in the form of household caustic soda solution stored in a lemonade bottle.

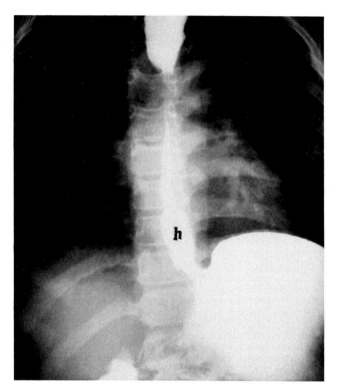

Fig. 3.9.39 Stricture of the middle third of the oesophagus post alkali ingestion. There is a little proximal dilatation. There is also a small irreducible hiatal hernia, secondary to shortening of the oesophagus from fibrosis. h = hernia.

been described more commonly in adults, but may occur in children, and is known as Boerhaave's syndrome. The tear is longitudinal and typically in the lateral wall of the lower third of the oesophagus.

Mallory–Weiss syndrome

In this syndrome there is a tear in the oesophageal mucosa and submucosa, but preservation of the muscular wall. The child presents with a history of violent retching followed by haematemesis. The history usually suggests the diagnosis. Bleeding may be profuse. At contrast examination, linear fissuring of barium is seen in the distal oesophagus.

Radiation injury

Fibrosis and stricturing of the oesophagus may result from mediastinal irradiation.

REFERENCES

Aaronson I A, Cywes S, Louw J H 1975 Spontaneous esophageal rupture in the newborn. Journal of Pediatric Surgery 10: 459–466

Baptist E C, Arenberg M E, Baskin W N 1981 Mallory–Weiss syndrome in a 16-week-old infant. Clinical Pediatrics 20: 59–60

Dubos J, Bouchez M, Kacet N, Liesse A, Lequien P, Remy J 1986 Spontaneous rupture of the esophagus in the newborn. Pediatric Radiology 16: 317–319

Freeman A H, Dickinson R J 1988 Spontaneous intramural esophageal haematoma. Clinical Radiology 39: 628–634

Goldstein H M, Rogers L F, Fletcher G H, Dodd G D 1975 Radiological manifestations of radiation-induced injury to the normal upper gastrointestinal tract. Radiology 117: 135–140

Harrell G, Friedland G, Daily W, Cohn R 1970 Neonatal Boerhaave's syndrome. Radiology 95: 665–668

Knauer C M 1976 Mallory–Weiss Syndrome. Characterisation of 75 Mallory–Weiss lacerations in 528 patients with upper gastrointestinal haemorrhage. Gastroenterology 71: 5–8

Lee S B, Kuhn J P 1976 Esophageal perforation in the neonate: a review of the literature. American Journal of Diseases of Children 130: 325–329

Perisic V, Ivanovski P, Mihailovic T 1988 Esophageal apoplexy. Pediatric Radiology 19: 51

OESOPHAGEAL TUMOURS

Both benign and malignant primary tumours are excessively rare in children and include hamartomas, carcinomas and leiomyomas, and laryngeal papillomatosis (Fig. 3.9.40).

Secondary involvement of the oesophagus by mediastinal or subcarinal nodes is more common, and may be due to malignancy or infection. Infective causes include tuberculosis and histoplasmosis. Inflammatory polyps have also been described.

Intrinsic tumours in children are mostly benign and appear as smooth indentations of the barium column usually with normal mucosa. The mucosa in carcinoma is usually ragged.

Extrinsic compression of the oesophagus by lymph node masses tends to be maximal in the upper mediastinum and carinal region, and usually extends over a longer length than an intrinsic intramural mass with more displacement of the oesophagus.

REFERENCES

Beckerman R C, Taussig L M, Froeder R C, Coulthard S W, Firor H, Tonkin I 1980 Fibromuscular hamartoma of the esophagus in an infant. American Journal of Diseases of Children 134: 153–155

Dieter R A Jr, Riker W L, Holinger P 1970 Pedunculated esophageal hamartoma in a child. Journal of Thoracic and Cardiovascular Surgery 59: 851–855

Jones T, Heller R, Kirchner S, Greene H 1979 Inflammatory esophagogastric polyp in children. American Journal of Roentgenology 133: 314–316

Kinnman J, Shin H I, Wetteland P 1968 Carcinoma of the oesophagus after lye corrosion: report of a case in a 15-year-old Korean male. Acta Chirurgica Scandinavica 134: 489–493

Schapiro R L, Sandrock A R 1973 Esophagogastric and vulvar leimyomatosis: a new radiologic syndrome. Journal of the Canadian Association of Radiology 24: 184–187

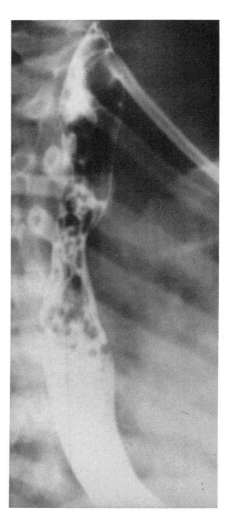

Fig. 3.9.40 Oesophageal papillomatosis. The multiple defects are due to tiny polyps. This child had involvement of the pharynx and upper airways as well.

DUPLICATION CYSTS

Duplication cysts usually present as posterior mediastinal masses and are discussed fully in Chapter 1 on the respiratory system. Dyspnoea is the most common presenting symptom, though many are discovered incidentally on routine chest radiographs, or during radiography for the assessment of scoliosis and vertebral anomalies. The oesophagus is the second most common site for duplications and most show no connection with the oesophagus. A small number extend below the diaphragm and may be associated with abdominal intestinal duplications. Complete duplication is very rare.

REFERENCES

Baker E 1989 Intrathoracic duplication cyst: a review of 17 patients. Journal of Medical Imaging 3: 127–134

Egelhoff J, Bisset G, Strife J 1986 Multiple enteric duplications in an infant. Pediatric Radiology 16: 160–161

Helund G, Bisset G 1989 Esophageal duplication cyst and aberrant right subclavian artery mimicking a symptomatic vascular ring. Pediatric Radiology 19: 543–544

Knight J, Garvin P J, Lewis E Jr 1983 Gastric duplication presenting as a double oesophagus. Journal of Pediatric Surgery 18: 300–301

BALLOON DILATATION OF OESOPHAGEAL STRICTURES

An alternative to surgical dilatation of strictures by bouginage is the dilatation by balloon catheters. Anastomotic strictures and peptic strictures are most suitable for this technique. Caustic strictures which tend to be more fibrotic are less successfully treated. The stricture length is identified by barium studies. Dilatation is done under heavy sedation or general anaesthesia. The balloon catheter is passed through the stricture over a guide-wire which may need endoscopic insertion. Dilatation is achieved using a series of graded balloon sizes inflated with contrast medium (Fig. 3.9.11), and should be repeated at regular 2–3-weekly intervals following the initial dilatation, the number of dilatations being dictated by the clinical response. Complications of dilatation by this method are few, but a serious complication is rupture of the oesophagus. The risk of this is minimized by gradual dilatation, using balloons of increasing diameter, and gentle hand inflation, so that inflation can be immediately stopped when undue resistance is felt.

Advantages of balloon dilatation over surgical bouginage include a reduced risk of perforation and concentric, even dilatation over the whole length of the stricture.

REFERENCES

Ball W S, Strife J L, Rosenkrantz J, Towbin R B, Noseworthy J 1984 Esophageal strictures in children: treatment by balloon dilatation. Radiology 150: 263–264

Dawson S L, Mueller P R, Ferrucci J T, Richter J M, Schapiro R H, Butch R J, Simeone J F 1984 Severe esophageal strictures: indications for balloon catheter dilatations. Radiology 153: 631–635

Goldthorn J F, Ball W S, Wilkinson L G, Siegel R S, Kosloske A M 1984 Esophageal strictures in children: treatment by serial balloon catheter dilatation. Radiology 153: 655–658

Hoffer F A, Winter H S, Fellows K E, Folkman J 1987 The treatment of postoperative and peptic esophageal strictures after esophageal atresia repair: a program including dilatation with balloon catheters. Pediatric Radiology 17: 454–458

Johnsen A, Ingemann Jenson L, Mauritzen K 1986 Balloon-dilatation of esophageal strictures in children. Pediatric Radiology 16: 388–391

Tam P, Sprigg A, Cudmore R, Carty H 1991 Endoscopy-guided balloon dilatation of esophageal strictures and anastomotic strictures after esophageal replacement in children. Journal of Pediatric Surgery 26: 1101–1103

3.10   THE STOMACH

The stomach in the infant and young child lies relatively horizontally compared with the more elongated J-shaped stomach demonstrated in anatomical illustrations. The size and shape is highly variable and depends on the amount of air and food contained within it. A full stomach in an infant's abdominal radiograph can produce an apparent upper abdominal mass with displacement of the other intestinal gas shadows. A similar confusing picture can be seen at ultrasound examination when there is a food-filled stomach with relatively little fluid and therefore little movement of contents on positional shift. Crying, with consequent swallowing of air, produces a larger air-filled stomach in the infant.

The stomach is divided anatomically into the fundus, the body and the antrum. The junction of the antrum and body is marked by the incisura on the lesser curve. The antrum and pylorus often have a more posterior orientation than in an adult. Steep, oblique and often lateral views are needed to demonstrate this properly in an infant both at barium study and ultrasound examination. The mucosal pattern is difficult to demonstrate by barium study in the infant due to the poor coating associated with excess mucus which is a normal finding in an infant's stomach. Double contrast barium studies are not indicated in young children and should be used only in the older child when looking for ulcers and erosions. Rugae are not commonly visible in the neonate. They develop as the child matures and are always more prominent on the greater than the lesser curve. These rugae are due to the normal folds of the gastric mucosa. Stomach emptying is very variable in infants and children and may take 15–20 minutes to commence. In the older child it is heavily affected by the child's psyche, the rate at which the barium is drunk and his like or dislike of the taste. Barium studies are unreliable in the assessment of gastric emptying, and overinterpretation of delayed emptying must be avoided.

In young infants there is often retropropulsion of food within the stomach during peristaltic activity. This must not be misinterpreted as a sign of outlet obstruction.

As the stomach lies in a relatively horizontal position in young children, during barium studies a common finding is to find a 'cup and spill' type stomach in which the fundus lies low. Barium enters this first and then cascades into the body and antrum from the overhanging fundus (Figs 3.10.1, 3.10.2). The gastric antrum and pylorus will remain in normal position, unlike an organoaxial volvulus when they will rotate upwards to lie in a high position.

CONGENITAL ANOMALIES

Microgastria, usually recognized during the neonatal period, is discussed elsewhere in this chapter.

Antral membrane

Gastric outlet obstruction can occur at the pylorus or in the gastric antrum due to the presence of an incomplete membrane. These, like those in the duodenum, represent incomplete forms of atresia. The membrane may be like a diaphragm with a central hole, or may be incomplete at either end. It consists of two mucosal layers enclosing a submucosal layer. Clinically the child presents with symptoms of partial gastric outlet obstruction, and is often thought to have infantile hypertrophic pyloric stenosis if presentation is at the appropriate age. The vomiting often begins when solid food is introduced to the infant's diet, but clinical symptoms may occur at any age. The two commonest presenting symptoms are cyclical postprandial vomiting, and episodes of transient vomiting.

The membrane is extremely difficult to demonstrate on barium studies and the diagnosis is usually suggested by finding delayed gastric emptying, poor filling of the duodenal cap, active peristalsis and failure to demonstrate the antral shouldering and elongated pyloric canal associated with hypertrophic pyloric stenosis. When the membrane is demonstrated, it is seen as a thin linear filling defect across the barium column. Persistent division of the gastric antrum into two chambers is another finding. A persistently dilated gas-filled stomach may be seen on the plain radiograph.

The precise causal relationship of an antral diaphragm and outlet symptoms must be determined by the severity of the clinical symptoms. Not all radiologically demonstrated diaphragms are clinically significant, and children may become asymptomatic without surgical excision.

REFERENCE

Jinkins J, Ball T, Clements J, Emler R, Weens H 1980 Antral mucosal diaphragms in infants and children. Pediatric Radiology 9: 69–72

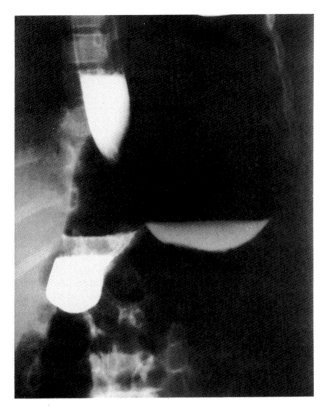

Fig. 3.10.1 Cup and spill type stomach. In this erect film the contrast first fills the fundus of the stomach and then cascades into the normal inferiorly positioned body and gastric antrum.

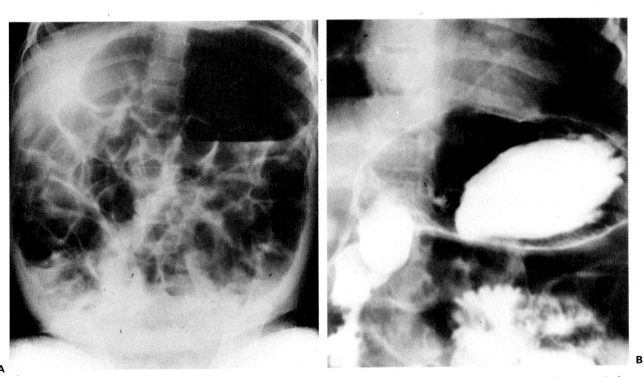

A   B

Fig. 3.10.2 Plain abdomen (**A**) and barium meal (**B**) of a child with a cup and spill stomach. The barium enters a dependent posteriorly placed gastric antrum and pylorus. Due to the rotation of the stomach and low-lying fundus, the normal position of the duodenojejunal flexure lying to the left of the midline and under the gastric antrum is not present. The flexure is low but is correctly positioned. This must not be misinterpreted as malrotation.

Volvulus

The normal stomach is maintained in position by four ligaments: the gastrohepatic, gastrophrenic, gastrosplenic and gastrocolic. The gastrophrenic ligament holds the stomach in position at the diaphragm. It is held in position inferiorly by the retroperitoneal position of the duodenum. Volvulus occurs when the fixation of the stomach is deficient either due to one of the ligaments being abnormal or the diaphragm being in an abnormal position as with eventration. Two types of gastric volvulus are described. In organo-axial volvulus, a complication of large hiatus hernia, there is transverse rotation around the axis of the stomach so that the greater curve lies uppermost (Fig. 3.10.3). Gastric outlet symptoms may occur. In mesentero-axial volvulus, the stomach rotates along an axis perpendicular to the transverse axis of the stomach which can lead to obstruction either at the oesophago-gastric junction or at the gastric outlet. The volvulus usually presents acutely with severe upper abdominal pain and vomiting if the obstruction is not at the gastro-oesophageal junction. If not relieved surgically, gastric necrosis and perforation may occur.

Symptomatic gastric volvulus in children is rare, although described with asplenia. Organo-axial volvulus must not be confused with the normal variant of a 'cup and spill' or 'waterfall' stomach.

REFERENCES

Aoyama K, Tateishi K 1986 Gastric volvulus in three children with asplenia syndrome. Journal of Pediatric Surgery 21: 307–310
Campell J B 1979 Neonatal gastric volvulus. American Journal of Roentgenology 132: 723–725
Ziprowski M N, Teele R L 1979 Gastric volvulus in childhood. American Journal of Roentgenology 132: 921–925

Gastric duplication

This is the least common of the varied enteric duplications forming less than 1% of the total. Three varieties are described. There is a cystic form which does not communicate with the gastric lumen. It presents as an extrinsic mass lesion indenting the stomach on the greater curve and is often mistaken for a pancreatic pseudocyst preoperatively (Fig. 3.10.4). The cyst is lined by a variety of gastric, intestinal and pancreatic epithelium. Secretions accumulate within the cyst to produce a symptomatic mass. Tubular duplication of the stomach is much rarer and may communicate with the main stomach cavity or with the small intestine. A further rare variety of duplication is a pedunculated cyst hanging from the stomach wall. Complications of all cysts include perforation due to ulceration within the gastric mucosal lining. The symptoms of vomiting often mimic those of hypertrophic pyloric stenosis. At ultrasound examination the cysts may be seen, but the

diagnosis can only be suggested as a differential diagnosis and is rarely reliably made preoperatively. Gastric duplication is one association of pulmonary sequestration. Carcinoma arising in a duplication cyst of the stomach has been described.

REFERENCES

Agha F P, Gabriele O F, Abdullah F H 1981 Complete gastric duplication. American Journal of Roentgenology 137: 406–407
Alschibaja T, Putnam T C, Yablin B A 1974 Duplication of the stomach simulating hypertrophic pyloric stenosis. American Journal of Diseases of Children 127: 120–122
Claudon M, Verain A, Bigard M, Boissel P, Poisson P, Floquet J, Regent D 1988 Cyst formation in gastric heterotopic pancreas:report of two cases. Radiology 169: 659–660
Egelhoff J, Bisset G, Strife J 1986 Multiple enteric duplications in an infant. Pediatric Radiology 16: 160–161
Hulnick D, Balthazar E 1987 Gastric duplication cyst: GI series and CT correlation. Gastrointestinal Radiology 12: 106–108
Mayo H W Jr, McKee E E, Anderson R M 1955 Carcinoma arising in reduplication of the stomach (gastrogenous cyst): a case report. Annals of Surgery 141: 550–554
Moccia W, Astacio J, Kaude J 1981 Ultrasonographic demonstration of gastric duplication in infancy. Pediatric Radiology 11: 52–54
Thornhill B A, Cho K C, Morehouse H T 1982 Gastric duplication associated with pulmonary sequestration: C T manifestations. American Journal of Roentgenology 138: 1168–1171

INFANTILE HYPERTROPHIC PYLORIC STENOSIS

Although hypertrophic pyloric stenosis is a very common disease in infants, occurring in 1 in 150 boys and 1 in 775 girls, the aetiology is unknown. The pathological process is that of spindle-shaped thickening and elongation of the circular muscle of the pylorus leading to elongation and constriction of the pyloric canal, causing symptoms of gastric outlet obstruction. The longitudinal muscle is unaffected. There is an abrupt demarcation between the hypertrophied muscle and the duodenal muscle, but proximally the transition from normal antral muscle to thickened muscle is gradual. While the typical presentation is of a male infant aged 3–5 weeks, the age ranges from about 10 days to 12 weeks. Infants born prematurely may present at a chronological age of up to 18–20 weeks, depending on the degree of prematurity. There is a significant familial history with up to 20% increased incidence in the children of affected parents. There is also an increased incidence in twins and triplets when one is affected, suggesting genetic predisposition. In addition there is said to be an increased incidence in children born with tracheo-oesophageal fistula. The presence of the outlet obstruction in these children may be overlooked as the vomiting is attributed to free gastro-oesophageal reflux.

While the aetiology is unknown, theories about its origin include functional or numerical abnormality in the neural cells of the myenteric plexus of the pylorus, but there is no histological evidence of this. Prolonged

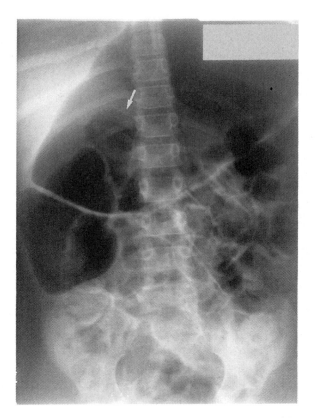

Fig. 3.10.3 Acute gastric volvulus organo-axial. The stomach is very distended. The greater curve lies uppermost and the gastric outlet and gas-filled duodenal cap lie in a high position (arrow points to duodenal cap).

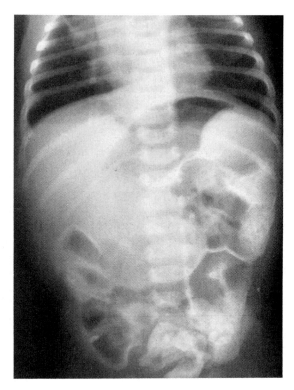

Fig. 3.10.4 Large gastric duplication cyst arising near the gastric antrum which is indenting the lower border of the stomach and displacing the transverse colon inferiorly.

pylorospasm and hyperacidity have also been suggested but are as yet unproven. Stress during the neonatal period has also been implicated. Pyloric stenosis has been reported resulting from the ingestion of erythromycin.

The diagnosis of pyloric stenosis is suspected clinically in an infant presenting with projectile vomiting, which usually begins as simple regurgitation and becomes more forceful and projectile as obstruction increases. Constipation is also a clinical feature, due to lack of passage of food into the intestine. Weight loss, dehydration and hypochloraemic alkalosis will develop as the vomiting persists if the child is untreated. The vomiting is usually non-bilious but in a small number of infants may contain bile. Jaundice is a feature in some infants. Haematemesis occurs rarely and may be caused by oesophagitis or superficial gastric ulceration in the region of the pyloric canal. In well developed cases the 'tumour olive' may be palpated clinically and this, in association with the history, is sufficient to proceed to surgery without further investigation, following metabolic stabilization. Traditionally, only doubtful cases were referred for radiological assessment prior to surgery, usually for barium studies. However, as ultrasonic diagnosis

is non-invasive, in many hospitals all patients are referred for ultrasonic confirmation of the diagnosis before surgery. Barium examination has largely been replaced by ultrasonic examination as the primary radiological procedure in specialized paediatric centres, with barium studies being reserved for those cases where the ultrasound studies are equivocal. This is a satisfactory arrangement in those institutions where there are sufficient numbers to allow adequate experience to develop. In smaller institutions with only two or three patients per year, barium studies may still be more reliable.

Ultrasound appearances

The examination is best done with the infant pacified by sucking a dummy. A 5 MHz or 7.5 MHz probe is needed. The examination is begun in the supine position, but the infant may need to be turned into either supine oblique position for a posteriorly facing pylorus to be brought into the pathway of the transducer. It the stomach is empty, due to nasogastric suction, it may be difficult to identify the length of the pyloric canal separately from the collapsed antrum. This problem can be eliminated by feeding the infant with an appropriate fluid of correct electrolyte balance such as Dioralyte. The features looked for at ultrasound examination are:

1. Elongation of the pyloric canal
2. Failure of opening of the canal during peristalsis.
3. Thickening of the muscle wall of the pylorus in both longitudinal and transverse sections

The normal pyloric muscle is less than 3 mm thick, the canal diameter 11 mm and the canal length 13 mm (Fig. 3.10.5). A canal length of 15 mm or more is elongated and indicates pyloric stenosis (Figs 3.10.6, 3.10.7). There is an area where normal and abnormal measurements overlap. In these circumstances, observation of the canal with assessment of its opening is important but this cannot be reliably done unless the infant is drinking. Failure of the canal to open is not a reliable sign of pyloric stenosis, if the stomach is empty, and peristaltic activity not stimulated. In an equivocal case, the patient should be re-examined after 24 hours. In many infants, the 'tumour' which was equivocal becomes easily visible within 24 hours. If doubt still persists, a barium study should be undertaken.

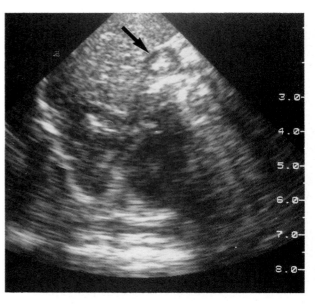

Fig. 3.10.5 Normal pylorus in cross-section (arrow). The muscle wall which is the dark ring is only 2 mm thick. The bright central echoes are from the air contained in the canal.

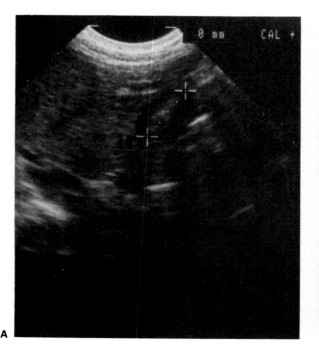

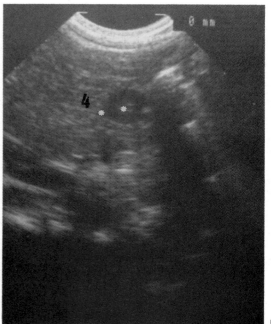

Fig. 3.10.6 **A, B** Pyloric stenosis. The canal length measures 14 mm (between crosses) and muscle width (asterisk) 4 mm. This is a small 'tumour'.

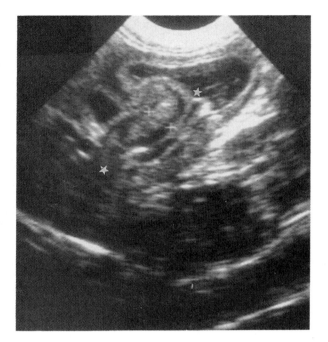

Fig. 3.10.7 Large pyloric tumour. Canal length 20 mm (between stars). Muscle thickness (between crosses) 6 mm.

Barium studies

In hypertrophic pyloric stenosis the stomach will distend and is slow to empty. By the time a barium study is done, the period of hyperactive peristalsis which occurs early in the disease has often ceased, and the stomach is then usually relatively atonic, with slow sinuous peristaltic activity progressing towards the pylorus, which has a beaked appearance if contrast does not pass into the canal (Fig. 3.10.8). This is followed by a slow reverse wave and the process repeated. Contrast medium may never enter the pyloric canal in a child with very hypertrophied muscle. Brief intermittent fluoroscopy with the infant lying on his/her right side should continue for 15 minutes before abandoning the examination. The beak sign is as reliable as the so-called 'string sign' with an elongated narrow canal curving upwards (Fig. 3.10.9).

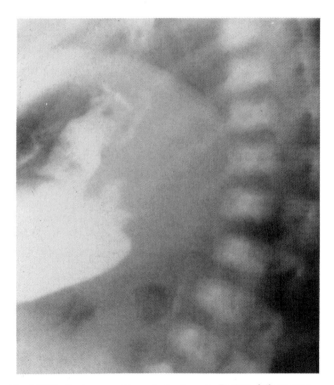

Fig. 3.10.8 Barium meal in pyloric stenosis. Barium fails to pass through the pyloric canal. The peristaltic wave forms a beak at the entrance to the obliterated canal lumen.

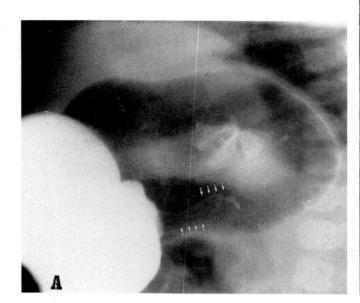
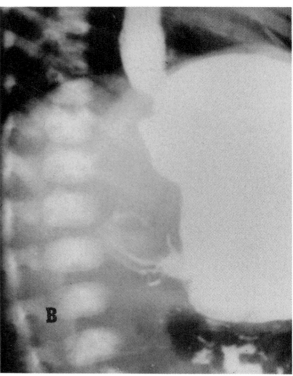

Fig. 3.10.9 **A** Pyloric stenosis. The stomach is distended. A little contrast has entered a thin canal forming the 'string sign' (arrows).
B A different infant with pyloric stenosis. There is a twin track appearance of the pyloric canal which is elongated, the 'string sign'. Some shouldering of the duodenum is also visible. Note gastro-oesophageal reflux due to the outlet obstruction.

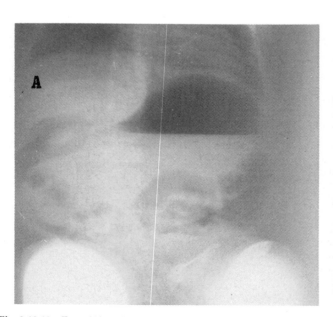
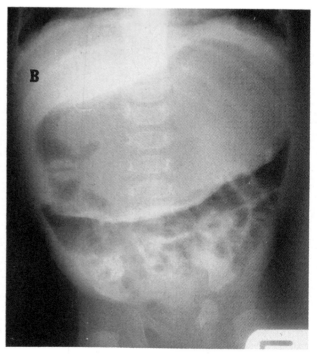

Fig. 3.10.10 Erect (**A**) and supine (**B**) plain radiographs of an infant with pyloric stenosis. There is an enlarged fluid-filled stomach which in the supine film is displacing the transverse colon inferiorly. Distal gas remains normal.

If barium passes through the canal, in addition to the elongated canal containing a thin channel of barium, indentation of the inferior border of the duodenum by the hypertrophic pyloric muscle will be seen. A twin track of barium is also frequently noted, with barium lying in channels between mucosal folds. This is only seen in hypertrophic pyloric stenosis and not with simple pylorospasm. As the distended barium-filled stomach overlies the pylorus and duodenal cap which are displaced posteriorly in pyloric stenosis, the infant needs to be in a steep oblique position to see the canal properly. Once contrast passes into the duodenum, it passes rapidly through the small bowel, and may well obscure a good view of the pylorus. Gastro-oesophageal reflux is a common accompaniment. Prolonged gastric emptying in infants is not unique to pyloric stenosis and occurs normally in some infants, with pylorospasm and in other causes of gastric outlet obstruction, e.g. antral membrane.

The plain abdominal supine radiograph, if done in an infant with a suspected diagnosis of pyloric stenosis, may demonstrate a dilated gas-filled stomach (Fig. 3.10.10), with an indentation due to peristalsis and relatively little distal bowel gas. The plain radiograph may be normal, especially following vomiting (Fig. 3.10.11).

The treatment is traditionally by pyloromyotomy. The postoperative barium appearance of the pylorus remains abnormal for some months. Shouldering and indentation of the duodenal cap persist and the canal remains rather flat and elongated, making interpretation difficult in the infant who continues to vomit. Early onset of gastric emptying is the best sign of successful surgery and suggests that the persistent vomiting is due to some other cause. Ultrasound will similarly show remaining hypertrophy for some time after pyloromyotomy, for about 12 weeks. Pyloromyotomy fails in a small number of infants needing further surgery. Balloon dilatation is under evaluation.

The diagnosis of pyloric stenosis is easy in a well-developed case, either clinically by ultrasound or by barium studies. There is a small group of infants who have a short segment pyloric stenosis with muscle hypertrophy, but as the canal is not very elongated at barium examination, the diagnosis is not obvious. These infants usually have equivocal measurements at ultrasound examination. The diagnosis in these infants should be made on a combination of clinical and radiological grounds.

There is a small group of children who present up to about 2 years of age with a history of repeated vomiting and failure to thrive. When they eventually have barium studies, some delay in gastric emptying with narrowing of the antrum but no shouldering of the duodenal cap is seen without muscle hypertrophy. These infants are diagnosed as 'burnt out' pyloric stenosis, presumably representing the mild end of a

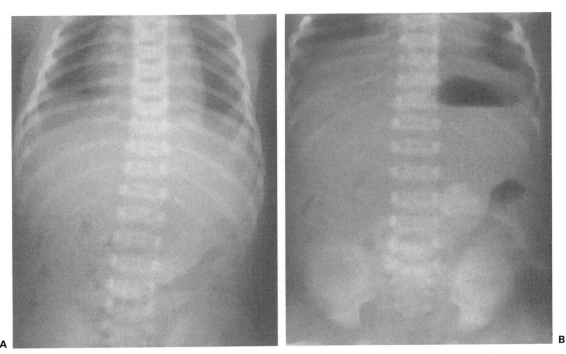

Fig. 3.10.11 A, B Same child as in Figure 3.10.6. Five-day history of vomiting. The erect and supine abdomen films are unremarkable.

spectrum of disease. Some children respond to antispasmodics but a few will need pyloromyotomy.

Few conditions mimic pyloric stenosis. Rarely, pyloric canal ulcers may cause similar symptoms, and these are diagnosed endoscopically. Antral membranes can cause similar symptoms, as can gastric duplications. Infants with a pyloric canal ulcer, or membrane, will have a normal ultrasound examination, while a duplication may be seen as a cyst at ultrasound. Symptoms may be mimicked by gastric tumours causing partial gastric outlet obstruction, but all are extremely rare in paediatric practice. In the young age group affected by hypertrophic pyloric stenosis, focal foveolar hyperplasia is most likely to be encountered, although adenomatous and hamartomatous polyps may occur. In endemic areas, tuberculosis of the antrum can cause clinical presentation of pyloric stenosis. Antral narrowing with symptoms similar to pyloric stenosis may be seen in chronic granulomatous disease, and antral stricture can occur secondary to foreign body and acid ingestion, but both occur in older children.

REFERENCES

Finsen V R 1979 Infantile hypertrophic pyloric stenosis – unusual familial incidence. Archives of Disease in Childhood 54: 720–721
Gillespie J C, Peterson G H, Lehocky R, Shearer L 1982 Occurrence of pyloric stenosis in triplets. American Journal of Diseases of Children 136: 746–747
Magilner A D 1986 Esophageal atresia and hypertrophic pyloric stenosis: sequential co-existence of disease. American Journal of Roentgenology 147: 329–330

Radiology

REFERENCES

Haran P, Darling D, Sciammas F 1966 The value of the double track sign as a differentiating factor between pylorospasm and hypertrophic pyloric stenosis in infants. Radiology 86: 723–725
Riggs W, Long L 1971 The value of the plain film Roentgenogram in pyloric stenosis. American Journal of Roentgenology 112: 77–82
Shopfner C E 1964 The pyloric tit in hypertrophic pyloric stenosis. American Journal of Roentgenology 91: 674–679
Swischuk L, Hayder C, Tyson K 1980 Atypical muscle hypertrophy in pyloric stenosis. American Journal of Roentgenology 134: 481–484

Ultrasound

REFERENCES

Blumhagen J D, Maclin L, Krauter D, Rosenbaum D M, Weinberger E 1988 Sonographic diagnosis of hypertrophic pyloric stenosis. American Journal of Roentgenology 150: 1367–1370
Carver R, Okorie M, Steiner G, Dickson J 1988 Infantile hypertrophic pyloric stenosis – diagnosis from the pyloric muscle index. Clinical Radiology 38: 625–627
O'Keefe F N, Stainsberry S, Swischuk L, Hayden C 1991 Antropyloric muscle thickness at ultrasound in infants: What is normal? Radiology 178: 827–831

Stunden R, LeQuesne G, Little K 1986 The improved ultrasound diagnosis of hypertrophic pyloric stenosis. Pediatric Radiology 16: 200–205

Complications

REFERENCES

Holgerson L O, Borns P F, Frouji M N 1974 Isolated gastric pneumatosis. Journal of Pediatric Surgery 9: 813–816
Spitz L, Batcup G 1979 Haematemesis in infantile hypertrophic pyloric stenosis: the source of the bleeding. British Journal of Surgery 66: 827–828
Swan·V M, Lussky R A 1966 Hypertrophic pyloric stenosis: a typical case complicated by massive hemorrhage. Archives of Surgery 93: 677–679
Watanabe A, Nagashima H M, Motoi M, Ogawa K 1979 Familial juvenile polyposis of the stomach. Gastroenterology 77: 148–151

Balloon dilatation

REFERENCES

Heymans H S, Bartelsman J W, Herweijer T J 1988 Endoscopic balloon dilatation as treatment of gastric outlet obstruction in infancy and childhood. Journal of Pediatric Surgery 23: 139–140
Tam P K, Carty H 1989 Non-surgical treatment for pyloric stenosis. (Letter) Lancet ii: 393

GASTRIC PNEUMATOSIS

Gastric pneumatosis is rare in children. Most commonly it is a manifestation of necrotizing enterocolitis, but is also recognized as a manifestation of gastric outlet obstruction. It has been reported in association with hypertrophic pyloric stenosis, duodenal stenosis and annular pancreas. When seen in association with gastric outlet obstruction, the pneumatosis is confined to the stomach wall but gas may be seen in the portal vein.

REFERENCES

Franquet T, Gonzalez A 1987 Gastric and duodenal pneumatosis in a child with annular pancreas. Pediatric Radiology 17: 262
Gupta A 1977 Interstitial gastric emphysema in a child with duodenal stenosis. British Journal of Radiology 50: 222–224
Leonidas J 1976 Gastric pneumatosis in infancy. Archives of Disease in Childhood 51: 395–398
Lester P, Budge A, Barnes J, Kirks D 1978 Gastric emphysema in infants with hypertrophic pyloric stenosis. American Journal of Roentgenology 131: 421–423

PYLOROSPASM

Pylorospasm is a common finding during barium examination in infants and young children. In the older infant and child, apprehension leads to pylorospasm, but in babies crying and general disturbance is a frequent association. In young infants, pylorospasm may be differentiated from hypertrophic pyloric stenosis by noting normal measurements of the pyloric muscle at ultrasound. In older children, patience, gaining the child's confidence, talking about favoured foods, and distracting the attention from his surroundings, will all eventually lead to relaxation and subsequent opening of the pylorus. Rarely, a pyloric canal ulcer will be seen, and the pylorospasm is due to associated inflammation.

REFERENCE

Lambrecht L, Robberecht E, Deschynkel K, Afschrift M 1988 Ultrasonic evaluation of gastric clearing in young infants. Pediatric Radiology 18: 314–318

FOCAL FOVEOLAR HYPERPLASIA

Focal foveolar hyperplasia is a polypoid gastric mass due to enlargement of the pits in the gastric mucosa into which the gastric glands empty, which become thickened and tortuous to give a polypoid mass, usually indenting the gastric antrum. At barium study, the mass produces narrowing of the antrum and pylorus, but there is no indentation of the duodenal cap (Fig. 3.10.12). At ultrasound examination, the mass is usually described as sonolucent but may also be echogenic and is seen separate from the gastric antrum and duodenum (Fig. 3.10.13)

REFERENCES

Katz M, Blocker S, McAlister W 1985 Focal foveolar hyperplasia presenting as an antral-pyloric mass in a young infant. Pediatric Radiology 15: 136–137
McAlister W, Katz M, Perlman J, Tack E 1988 Sonography of focal foveolar hyperplasia causing gastric obstruction in an infant. Pediatric Radiology 18: 79–81

COFFIN–SIRIS SYNDROME AND GASTROINTESTINAL SYMPTOMS

The Coffin–Siris syndrome consists of growth and mental retardation, coarse facial features, dysplastic fingernails, feeding and respiratory difficulties.

Duodenal and gastric perforation has been described secondary to peptic ulceration. Gastric outlet obstruction due to thickened antral mucosal folds has also been described. The antral mucosa is hyperechoic at ultrasound examination.

REFERENCE

Bodurtha J, Kessel A, Berman W, Hartenberg M 1987 Distinctive gastrointestinal anomaly associated with Coffin–Siris syndrome. Journal of Pediatrics 109: 1015–1019

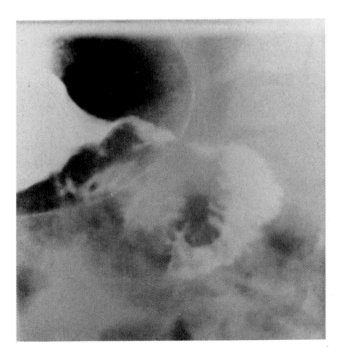

Fig. 3.10.12 Barium meal in a 3-month-old child with vomiting. There is narrowing and irregularity of the gastric antrum with indentation inferiorly due to the enlarged glandular pits.

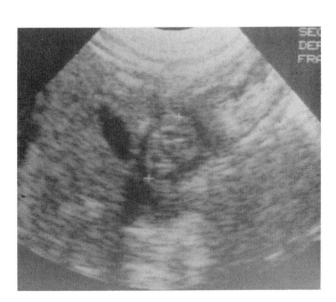

Fig. 3.10.13 Same child as in Figure 3.10.12. The ultrasound shows an enlarged mass of mixed echogenicity. At the examination gastric contents were observed to pass round this mass into the duodenum. Diagnosis: focal foveolar hyperplasia.

GASTRIC NEOPLASMS

All forms of gastric neoplasm, both benign and malignant, are extremely rare in children.

Gastric teratomas usually present in infancy as a mass lesion for investigation. About half contain calcification (Fig. 3.10.14). They are commoner in male infants and may cause respiratory embarrassment due to their size, and also cause haematemesis. Leiomyomas, leiomyoblastomas, leiomyosarcomas, lipoma, liposarcomas, neurofibromas, gastric carcinoma, hamartomas, haemangiomas and lymphangiomas have all been recorded. They present with varying symptoms which include nausea, indigestion, pain, haematemesis, anaemia from chronic blood loss and vomiting. The radiological features are similar to those seen in adults.

Children with ataxia telangiectasia who survive the respiratory and neurological problems of their disease have an increased incidence of lymphoma which is usually generalized but may affect the stomach or gastrointestinal tract throughout its length. There is also an increased incidence of carcinoma of the stomach in children who recover from treatment of other malignancies. They usually present with the second lesion in late teenage or young adulthood. Gastric polyps of differing histology have been reported in children with different syndromes, e.g. Coffin–Siris syndrome and Cowden's disease ('multiple hamartoma syndrome'). The coexistence of gastric and oesophageal leiomyoblastoma, pulmonary chondromas and functioning extraadrenal paragangliomas constitute Carney's triad, of which incomplete forms exist.

Inflammatory fibrous polyps are recorded. This group now includes those previously labelled as eosinophilic granulomas. Gastric inflammatory pseudotumour, also known as plasma cell granuloma, is due to a benign proliferation of myofibroblasts and inflammatory cells, and is being increasingly encountered in the abdomen and retroperitoneum. The cause is unknown. Presentation is with fever, pain, anaemia and sometimes failure to thrive. The irregular masses appear aggressive and simulate malignancy. Some patients have been reported to also have Castleman's syndrome, and also have lymphoid pseudotumours.

Pancreatic rests in the gastric mucosa may also mimic tumours.

Extrinsic indentation of the stomach by mass lesions of liver, spleen, pancreas and retroperitoneum is much more frequent in children than intrinsic neoplasm. Extrinsic masses cause smooth indentations of the mucosa and displacement of the stomach and do not cause mucosal destruction.

Gastric haematoma, a rare manifestation of haemophilia, may present as mass lesions.

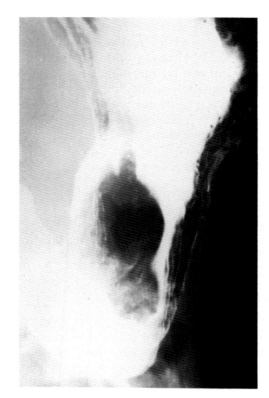

Fig. 3.10.14 Gastric teratoma. Note filling defect in the body of the stomach.

REFERENCES

Bodurtha J, Kessel A, Berman W, Hartenberg M 1987 Distinctive gastrointestinal anomaly associated with Coffin–Siris syndrome. Journal of Pediatrics 109: 1015–1019

Bowen B, Ros P, McCarthy M, Olmsted W, Hjermstad B 1987 Gastrointestinal teratomas: CT and US appearance with pathologic correlation. Radiology 162: 431–433

Buts J P, Gosseye S, Claus D, De Montpellier C, Nyakabasa M 1981 Solitary hyperplastic polyp of the stomach. American Journal of Diseases of Children 135: 846–847

Caberwal D, Kogan S J, Levitt S B 1977 Ectopic pancreas presenting as an umbilical-mass. Journal of Pediatric Surgery 12: 593–595

Cairo M S, Grosfeld J L, Weetman R M 1981 Gastric teratoma: unusual cause for bleeding of the upper gastro intestinal tract in the newborn. Pediatrics 67:721–724

Denzler T B, Harned R K, Pergam C J 1979 Gastric polyps in familial polyposis coli. Radiology 130: 63–66

Elliott S, Bruce J 1987 Submucosal gastric haematoma: a case report and review of the literature. British Journal of Radiology 60: 1132–1135

Esposito G, Cigliano B, Paludetto R 1983 Abdominothoracic gastric teratoma in a female newborn infant. Journal of Pediatric Surgery 18: 304–305

Gordon R A, D'Avignon M B, Storch A E, Eyster M E 1981 Intramural gastric haematoma in a haemophiliac with an inhibitor. Paediatrics 67: 417–419

Goto S, Ikeda K, Ishii E, Miyazaki S, Shimizu S, Iwashita A 1984 Carcinoma of the stomach in a 7 year old boy. Zeitschrift fuer Kinderchirurgie 39: 137–140

Haerer A F, Jackson J F, Evers C G 1969 Ataxia-telangiectasia with gastric adenocarcinoma. Journal of the American Medical Association 210: 1884–1887

Jakubowski A, Jakubowska K, Naumik A, Pietrou K 1970 Primary tumours of the stomach in children. Annales de Radiologie 13: 169–175

Kilman W J, Berk R N 1977 The spectrum of radiographic features of aberrant pancreatic rests involving the stomach. Radiology 123: 291–296

Mahour G H, Isaacs H Jr, Chang L 1980 Primary malignant tumours of the stomach in children. Journal of Pediatric Surgery 15: 603–608

Mazas-Artasona L, Romeo M, Felices R, Criado P, Espinosa H, Yanguela J, Peiron M 1988 Gastrooesophageal leiomyoblastomas and multiple pulmonary chondromas: an incomplete variant of Carney's triad. British Journal of Radiology 61: 1181–1184

Siegel M, Shackelford G 1978 Gastric teratomas in infants. Report of two cases. Pediatric Radiology 7: 197–200

Taylor A, Dodds W, Stewart E 1989 Alimentary tract lesions in Cowden's disease. British Journal of Radiology 62: 890–892

Watanabe A, Nagashia H, Motos M, Ogawa K 1979 Familial juvenile polyposis of the stomach. Gastroenterology 77: 148–151

Inflammatory polyps

REFERENCES

Eklof O, Lassrich A, Stanley P, Chrispin A 1973 Ectopic pancreas. Pediatric Radiology 1: 24–27

Jones T, Heller R, Kirchner S, Greene H 1979 Inflammatory esophagogastric polyp in children. American Journal of Roentgenology 133: 314–316

Livolsi V A, Perzin K H 1975 Inflammatory pseudotumors (inflammatory fibrous polyps) of the esophagus. A clinicopathologic study. American Journal of Digestive Diseases 20: 475–481

Maves C, Johnson J, Bove K, Malott R 1989 Gastric inflammatory pseudotumor in children. Radiology 173: 381–383

Salm R 1965 Gastric fibroma with eosinophilic infiltration. Gut 6: 85–91

Schroeder B, Wells R, Sty J 1987 Inflammatory fibroid polyp of the stomach in a child. Pediatric Radiology 17: 71–72

Shimer G R, Helwig E B 1984 Inflammatory fibroid polyps of the intestine. American Journal of Clinical Pathology 81: 708–714

GASTRIC INFLAMMATORY PSEUDOTUMOUR IN CHILDHOOD

An inflammatory pseudotumour is due to a proliferation of myofibroblasts and inflammatory cells, which form a mass which, though benign histologically, is frequently initially diagnosed as malignant. They are most commonly found in the lungs and retroperitoneum and are rare in children. Presenting complaints are non-specific and include fever, weight loss and a palpable mass. On barium studies, a mass lesion is seen within the stomach with irregular margins indistinguishable from a primary neoplasm. The diagnosis is only made histologically.

REFERENCE

Maves C, Johnson J, Bove K, Malott R 1989 Gastric inflammatory pseudotumor in children. Radiology 173: 381–383

GASTRIC ULCERS

It is unusual to demonstrate gastric ulcers in children. In young infants this is largely due to poor mucosal coating caused by excess mucus and fluid in the stomach. In older children it is probably due to a less meticulous double contrast technique than one applies to an adult barium examination, coupled with a low expectation of finding one, and a compromise method of performing the barium study when the examining radiologist is trying to combine examination of the stomach and the small bowel in response to the clinical information of non-specific abdominal pain.

The incidence of gastric ulcers in children is not known. Males have a higher incidence than females. Peptic ulcers are more frequent in children with blood group O and of Anglo Saxon or Scandinavian origin. Young infants may present with haematemesis, vomiting and anaemia due to chronic blood loss. Vomiting and haematemesis are more commonly due to gastro-oesophageal reflux. Perforation is a complication, and may be the presenting symptom, especially in infants. Ectopic pancreatic tissue in the stomach may also cause ulceration and bleeding. Food allergy may also induce ulceration.

The ulcer, when found, is usually in the lower part of the body of the stomach or in the antrum, or pyloric canal. The ulcer projects outside the lumen of the stomach (Fig. 3.10.15), with folds of gastric mucosa radiating into the crater. Rarely, there is such gross oedema that a neoplasm is simulated. Secondary signs of ulcer disease are pylorospasm, antral spasm and deformity. The irregularity and thickening of the gastric mucosa may be seen ultrasonically. Normal gastric mucosal thickness is less than 3.5 mm. In ulcer disease, the thickness is 4 mm or more. Muscle thick-

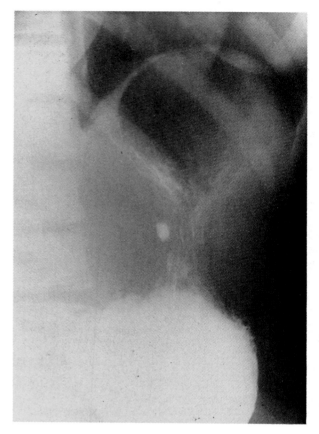

Fig. 3.10.15 There is a gastric ulcer on the lesser curve.

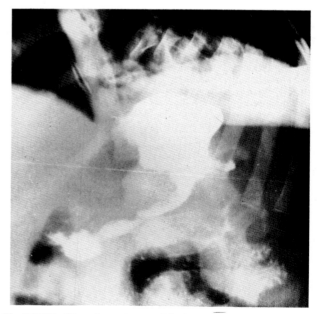

Fig. 3.10.16 There is a stricture of the lower part of the body of the stomach and the whole of the gastric antrum due to previous ingestion of iron tablets.

ness remains normal. In skilled hands, endoscopy is more reliable than barium studies in demonstrating gastric ulcers in children.

Gastric ulceration, scarring and fibrosis may also result from ingestion of toxic substances, caustic substances and some tablets – notably iron tablets (Fig. 3.10.16).

Stress ulcers are more common than peptic gastric ulceration in children. Stress ulcers occur in response to burns, fractures, trauma, sepsis, CNS disorders, steroidal treatment and shock. Erosive gastritis is caused by alcohol and drugs, particularly aspirin. The eponym Curling's ulcer is given to a stress ulcer associated with burns and Cushing's ulcer to those associated with CNS disease. Children with stress ulcers present with perforation or haematemesis and rectal bleeding, pain and vomiting being much less common than in peptic ulceration. Endoscopy is the best diagnostic procedure.

REFERENCES

Bell M J, Keating J P, Ternberg J L, Bower R 1981 Perforated stress ulcers in infants. Journal of Pediatric Surgery 16: 998–1002
Dunn S, Weber T R, Grosfeld J L, Fitzgerald J R 1983 Acute peptic ulcer in childhood. Archives of Surgery 118: 656–660
Eklof O, Lassrich A, Stanley P, Chrispin A 1973 Ectopic pancreas. Pediatric Radiology 1: 24–27
Hayden C K, Swischuk L E, Rytting J E 1987 Gastric ulcer disease in infants: ultrasound findings. Radiology 164: 131–134
Moody F G, Cheney L Y 1976 Stress ulcers: their pathogenesis, diagnosis and treatment. Surgical Clinics of North America 56: 1469–1478
Seagram C F G, Stephens C A, Cumming W A 1973 Peptic ulceration at the Hospital for Sick Children, Toronto, during the 20-year period 1949–1969. Journal of Pediatric Surgery 8: 407–413
Tomooka Y, Koga T, Shimoda Y, Kuroiwa T, Miyazaki S, Torisu M 1987 The ultrasonic demonstration of acute multiple gastric ulcers in a child. British Journal of Radiology 60: 290–292
Woodruff W, Merten D, Kirks D 1985 Pneumomediastinum: an unusual complication of acute gastrointestinal disease. Pediatric Radiology 15: 196–198

GASTRIC PERFORATION

Gastric perforation may occur spontaneously in the neonate and is well described (Fig. 3.10.17). In older children idiopathic perforation is very rare but has been described as a complication of gastric ulceration, chemical burns, acute dilatation secondary to trauma, mechanical ventilation or acute volvulus, or combined gastric outlet obstruction and gastro-oesophageal junction obstruction. The child presents with acute abdominal pain and abdominal distension with progression to peritonitis. In small tears, chest pain secondary to a pneumomediastinum occurs.

Traumatic rupture of the stomach due to external blunt trauma is much rarer than rupture of the duodenum or small bowel. Gastric perforation may also occur during instrumentation at endoscopy or rarely by a nasogastric tube.

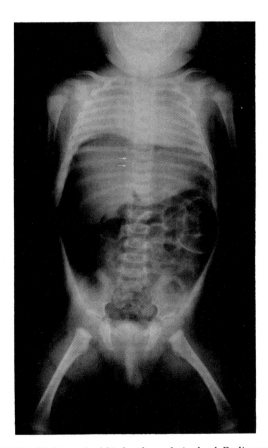

Fig. 3.10.17 Eight-week-old infant brought in dead. Radiograph pre post-mortem. There is a huge pneumoperitoneum with gas on both sides of the bowel lumen. This baby had had a spontaneous perforation of the stomach. The ligamentum falciparum is visible as a fine lucent line to the right of the midline.

DIVERTICULUM OF THE STOMACH

Gastric diverticula are very rare in children. They arise most commonly on the upper part of the lesser curve of the stomach, are outpouchings of the stomach wall lined by mucosa, and are usually an incidental finding on barium examination. The diverticulum fills with barium as the barium pours from the oesophagus into the body of the stomach. When full the barium spills from the diverticulum into the body of the stomach. They are of no clinical significance and are unrelated to symptoms of pain or vomiting. In adults, haemorrhage, volvulus and perforation have been recorded, but even in adults these are rare. There has been a report of a giant epiphrenic diverticulum in a boy with Ehlers–Danlos syndrome, and a further report of gastrointestinal diverticulosis in association with Marfan's syndrome.

REFERENCES

Fich A, Polliack G, Libson E 1989 Gastrointestinal diverticulosis in association with Marfan syndrome. Journal of Medical Imaging 3: 11–13

Toyohara T, Kaneko T, Araki H, Takahashi K, Nakamura T 1989 Giant epiphrenic diverticulum in a boy with Ehlers–Danlos syndrome. Pediatric Radiology 19: 437

GASTRIC VARICES

Varices occur within the submucosa of the fundus and upper part of the body of the stomach (Fig. 3.9.34). They are usually seen in association with oesophageal varices in patients with portal hypertension. When confined to the stomach, the aetiology is more commonly splenic vein occlusion with localized venous hypertension, rather than generalized portal venous hypertension. They may be seen on the plain radiograph as polypoid projections into the fundus of the stomach. At barium examination they appear as filling defects in the barium column.

REFERENCE

Cho K J, Martel W 1978 Recognition of splenic vein occlusion. American Journal of Roentgenology 131: 439–443

ACUTE GASTRIC DILATATION

Acute gastric dilatation represents an ileus in response to a variety of insults. Causes include trauma to the abdomen, remote trauma such as a head injury, and metabolic upsets such as diabetic ketoacidosis (Fig. 3.10.18). It also occurs postoperatively, particularly following scoliosis surgery, and can lead to respiratory distress. Prompt decompression by insertion of a nasogastric tube is indicated.

Gastric dilatation is also seen in neglected children who eat voraciously when exposed to food. A group of children with psychological disorders are recognized to have pathological aerophagia which may lead to abdominal distension. Following sedation, such gaseous distension frequently disappears.

Children with H-type tracheo-oesophageal fistulas show gaseous gut distension due to excess air passing through the fistula into the oesophagus and stomach (Fig. 3.10.19).

Portal venous gas has rarely been reported in association with acute gastric dilatation.

REFERENCES

Franken E A, Fox M, Smith J A, Smith W L 1978 Acute gastric dilatation in neglected children. American Journal of Roentgenology 130: 297–299

Gauderer M W L, Halpin T C, Izant R J 1981 Pathologic childhood aerophagia: a recognizable clinical entity. Journal of Pediatric Surgery 16: 301–305

Kasenally A T, Felice A G, Logie J R C 1976 Acute gastric dilatation after trauma. British Medical Journal 2: 21

Radin D, Rosen R, Halls J 1987 Acute gastric dilatation: a rare cause of portal venous gas. American Journal of Roentgenology 148: 279–280

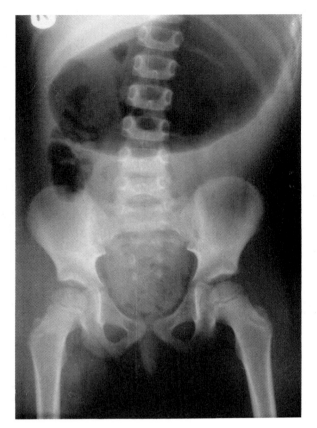

Fig. 3.10.18 Nine-year-old girl admitted with diabetic ketoacidosis. There is acute gaseous distension of the stomach with little distal intestinal gas.

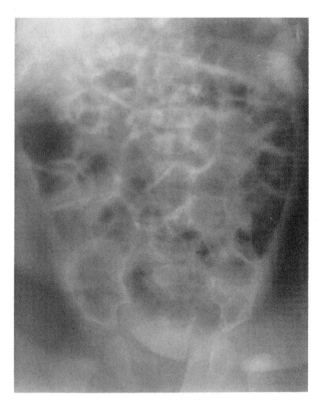

Fig. 3.10.19 Ten-week-old baby girl who presented with a distended abdomen, which on investigation proved to be due to a H-type tracheo-oesophageal fistula. She had no symptoms of choking or respiratory illness.

ADYNAMIC ILEUS OF STOMACH AND BOWEL: CHRONIC INTESTINAL PSEUDO-OBSTRUCTION

There is a small group of children who suffer from adynamic ileus of the bowel which may be either permanent, or intermittent with acute exacerbations. The underlying pathology is poorly understood. The children present with a variety of symptoms: failure to thrive, constipation and intermittent abdominal distension and a changing pattern of vomiting and constipation. In acute exacerbations there is often massive gastric dilatation (Fig. 3.10.20), with an outpouring of fluid into the gastric and small bowel lumen leading to abdominal distension and dehydration. Large nasogastric aspirates accompany this. Between exacerbations, some children can eat normally. Others have very poor absorption of food and require long-term intravenous feeding. Colonic emptying requires repeated enemas or suppositories. Mucosal and muscular biopsies of stomach and small bowel are normal on conventional histology and histochemical analysis. Abdominal radiographs in an acute phase show a distended fluid-filled bowel which resembles mechanical obstruction (Fig. 3.10.21). There is usually some air distally indicating incomplete obstruction, and bowel sounds are clinically absent. Massive stomach dilatation is sometimes seen without much evidence of distal dilatation.

REFERENCES

Byrne W J, Cipel L, Euler A, Halpin T, Ament M 1977 Chronic idiopathic intestinal pseudo-obstruction syndrome in children—clinical characteristics and prognosis. Journal of Pediatrics 90: 585–589

Lake B D 1988 Observation on the pathology of pseudo-obstruction. In: Disorders of gastrointestinal motility in childhood. John Wiley, Chichester, pp 81–90

Scharli A, Meier-Ruge W 1981 Localized and disseminated forms of neuronal intestinal dysplasia mimicking Hirschsprung's disease. Journal of Pediatric Surgery 16: 164–170

Schuffler M, Jonak Z 1982 Chronic idiopathic intestinal pseudo-obstruction caused by a degenerative disorder of the myenteric plexus: the use of Smith's method to define the neuropathology. Gastroenterology 82: 476–486

Shaw A, Schaffer H, Teja K, Kelly T, Grogan E, Bruni C 1979 A perspective for pediatric surgeons: chronic idiopathic intestinal pseudoobstruction. Journal of Pediatric Surgery 14: 719–727

Miyake T, Kawamori J, Yoshida T, Nakano H, Kohno S, Ohba S 1987 Small bowel pseudo-obstruction in Kawasaki disease. Pediatric Radiology 17: 383–386

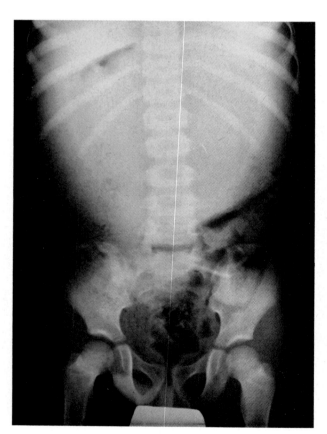

Fig. 3.10.20 Six-year-old boy with chronic intestinal pseudo-obstruction. A supine abdominal radiograph during an acute exacerbation shows a pseudoperforation appearance with the lucent appearance centrally due to air displaced anteriorly by a hugely distended fluid-filled stomach. He was dehydrated and in hypovolaemic shock.

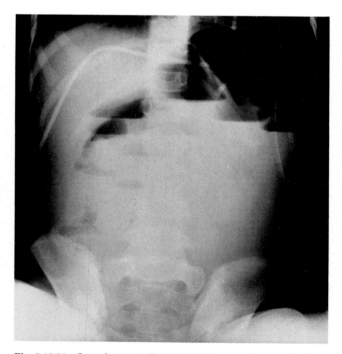

Fig. 3.10.21 Same boy as in Figure 3.10.20 on another admission. There is an ileus with multiple fluid-filled small bowel loops and marked abdominal distension. The pattern looks like mechanical obstruction. The diagnosis is not easy but the signs of obstruction were not present clinically. An awareness of the condition and the lack of correlation of clinical and radiological features lead to the correct diagnosis with avoidance of laparotomy.

CHRONIC GRANULOMATOUS DISEASE: GASTRIC INVOLVEMENT

Chronic granulomatous disease of childhood is a rare disease characterized by recurrent infections, with granuloma and abscess formation. Lungs, liver, spleen, lymph nodes and bones are most commonly affected. The basic defect is an inherited defective neutrophil function. The gastric antrum becomes narrowed, with thickening of the muscle due to granulomatous infiltration (Fig. 3.10.22). The child presents with symptoms of gastric outlet obstruction. Rarely, the body of the stomach and the fundus are involved. The thickening of the antral wall is seen at ultrasound examination. At barium studies, the antrum is noted to be narrow and stiff. When the body and fundus are involved, mucosal thickening is seen during barium examination.

REFERENCES

Hartenberg M, Kodroff M 1984 Chronic granulomatous disease of childhood. Probable diffuse gastric involvement. Pediatric Radiology 14: 57–58

Kopen P, McAlister w 1984 Upper gastro-intestinal and ultrasound examinations of gastric antral involvement in chronic granulomatous disease. Pediatric Radiology 14: 91–93

Orduna M, De Orbe G, Gordillo M, Fernandez-Epifanio J, Serrano C, Collado J, Miralles M 1989 Chronic granulomatous disease of childhood. Report on two cases with unusual involvement of the gastric antrum and spleen. European Journal of Radiology 9: 67–70

MENETRIER'S DISEASE

Hypertrophy of the gastric mucosa associated with prominence of the gastric folds is seen in children with Menetrier's disease. This hypertrophy is associated with excess mucus secretion and protein loss. At presentation the children usually look oedematous, with puffy eyes, and are frequently mistaken for nephrotics. Gastrointestinal symptoms, when present, are not prominent and consist of nausea, vomiting and loose bowel movements. There are two forms of the disease, an acute transient form, which is most common in children, and a chronic form, more common in adults. There is a reported increased risk of gastric carcinoma in adults with the disease, but not in children.

The radiological diagnosis is made by demonstration of the enlarged gastric mucosal folds during barium examination (Fig. 3.10.23). The enlarged folds are seen in the fundus and body of the stomach. The main differential diagnosis is lymphoma, but cytomegalovirus and campylobacter infection can produce a gastritis simulating Menetrier's disease radiologically.

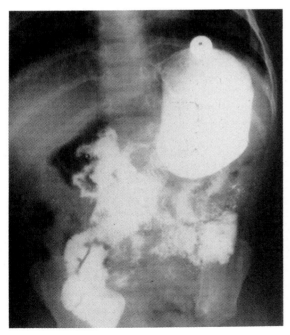

Fig. 3.10.22 Chronic granulomatous disease. Eight-month-old infant who presented with failure to thrive and recurrent infections. Current admission with vomiting. There is a stricture of the gastric antrum with an abrupt cut off at the body of the stomach. Film taken at 45 minutes. Note failure of gastric emptying.

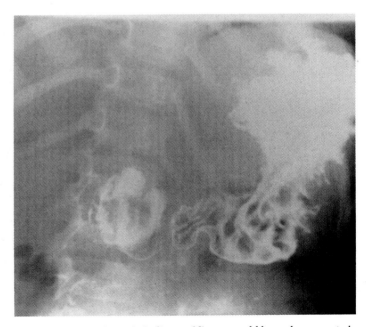

Fig. 3.10.23 Menetrier's disease. Nine-year-old boy who presented with oedema of face, hands and feet. He was initially diagnosed as having a nephrotic syndrome. Barium meal done for investigation of vomiting however shows marked thickening of the mucosa of the fundus and body of the stomach typical of Menetrier's disease. He recovered spontaneously.

REFERENCES

Baker A, Volberg F, Sumner T, Moran R 1986 Childhood Menetrier's disease: four new cases and discussion of the literature. Gastrointestinal Radiology 11: 131–134

Bar-Ziv J, Barki Y, Weizman Z, Urkin J 1988 Transient protein-losing gastropathy (Menetrier's disease) in childhood. Pediatric Radiology 18: 82–84

Burns B, Gay B B 1968 Menetrier's disease of the stomach in children. American Journal of Roentgenology 103: 300–306

Chaloupka J, Gay B, Caplan D 1990 Campylobacter gastritis simulating Menetrier's disease by upper gastro intestinal radiography. Pediatric Radiology 20: 200–201

Coad N A, Shah K J 1986 Menetrier's disease in childhood associated with cytomegalo virus infection: a case report and review of the literature. British Journal of Radiology 59: 615–620

Henderson S, Sprague P 1979 A case of hypertrophic protein losing gastropathy. Pediatric Radiology 8: 261–262

ZOLLINGER–ELLISON SYNDROME

This syndrome consists of a pancreatic islet cell tumour, severe peptic ulceration and gastric hypersecretion. The tumours produce high gastrin levels which cause the hypersecretion. Patients present with ulcer pain and watery diarrhoea due to the large volumes of gastric secretion. At barium examination, there is gross hypertrophy of the gastric rugal folds and often dilatation of the duodenum and small bowel. On follow-through examination, there may be a non-specific malabsorptive pattern and small bowel ulceration.

REFERENCE

Buchta R M, Kaplan J M 1971 Zollinger–Ellison syndrome in a nine-year-old child: A case report and review of this entity in childhood. Pediatrics 47: 594–598

EOSINOPHILIC GASTRITIS

Eosinophilic gastritis may accompany small bowel infiltration with eosinophils. There is a nodular appearance in the gastric antrum at barium examination.

REFERENCES

Jona J Z, Belin R P, Burke J A 1976 Eosinophilic infiltration of the gastrointestinal tract in children. American Journal of Diseases of Children 130: 1136–1139

Matzinger M, Daneman A 1983 Esophageal involvement in eosinophilic gastroenteritis. Pediatric Radiology 13: 35–38

Schulman A, Morton P, Dietrich B 1980 Eosinophilic gastroenteritis. Clinical Radiology 31: 101–104

Teele R T, Katz A J, Goldman H, Kettell R M 1979 Radiographic features of eosinophilic gastroenteritis (allergic gastroenteropathy) of childhood. American Journal of Roentgenology 132: 575–580

CAMPYLOBACTER GASTRITIS

Infection with campylobacter produces a chronic inflammatory process in which the mucosa of the gastric antrum is most severely affected. Radiologically enlarged gastric folds are seen, mostly in the antrum, but the body and fundus of the stomach may also be involved. Peptic ulceration may be demonstrated. The clinical presentation is non-specific and includes a history of nausea, fatigue, abdominal pain, weight loss and anorexia. The enlarged gastric folds may lead to a radiological diagnosis of Menetrier's disease. There is, however, no protein loss and serum proteins are normal.

REFERENCES

Chaloupka J, Gay B, Caplan D 1990 Campylobacter gastritis simulating Menetrier's disease by upper gastrointestinal radiography. Pediatric Radiology 20: 200–201

Morrison S, Dahms B, Hoffenberg E, Czinn S 1989 Enlarged gastric folds in association with campylobacter pylori gastritis. Radiology 171: 819–821

Yardley J 1989 Campylobacter pylori and large gastric folds. Radiology 171: 609–611

GASTRITIS: GRAFT VERSUS HOST DISEASE

Gastrointestinal manifestations of graft-versus-host disease, in patients who have had a bone marrow transplant, may be due to acute graft-versus-host disease or superimposed infection. Profuse watery diarrhoea is the main clinical presentation and the small bowel is most commonly involved. The characteristic small bowel pattern is one of mucosal thickening or effacement of the folds, and a featureless 'ribbon' bowel. Gastric involvement is manifested radiologically by dilatation, atony with delayed emptying, antral deformity and poor coating. Infecting organisms include rotavirus, Coxsackie and adenovirus.

REFERENCE

Jones B, Kramer S, Saral R, Beschorner W, Yolken R, Townsend T, Yeager A, Lake A, Tutschka P, Santos G 1988 Gastrointestinal inflammation after bone marrow transplantation: graft-versus-host disease or opportunistic infection. American Journal of Roentgenology 150: 277–281

AIDS: STOMACH INVOLVEMENT

Thickening of the pylorus and proximal duodenum are associated with cytomegalic virus infection in association with AIDS, leading to symptoms of gastric outlet obstruction.

Lymphadenopathy is the most frequent abdominal manifestation of AIDS and may involve any lymph node group. The enlargement may present clinically as an abdominal mass, or be detected during routine ultrasound examination. The enlargement may be a simple reactive enlargement, due to Kaposi's sarcoma, or due to infection, often with *Mycobacterium avium intracellulare*.

REFERENCES

Bradford B, Abdenour G, Frank J, Scott G, Beerman R 1988 Usual and unusual radiologic manifestations of Acquired Immunodeficiency Syndrome (AIDS) and Human Immunodeficiency Virus (HIV) infection in children. Radiologic Clinics of North America 26: 341–353
Haney P, Yale-Loehr A, Nussbaum A, Gellad F 1989 Imaging of infants and children with AIDS. American Journal of Roentgenology 152: 1033–1041

CHEMICAL GASTRITIS

Ingestion of large amounts of caustic substances, both acid and alkali, can lead to intense acute pylorospasm, with retention of the noxious substance in the stomach, causing mucosal ulceration, muscle necrosis and perforation with consequent peritonitis. Long-term effects include pyloric scarring and fibrosis with gastric outlet obstruction. The narrowed antrum is easily demonstrated at barium examination. Other causes of similar pyloric and antral fibrosis include drug overdose, especially aspirin and ferrous sulphate, taken in the form of iron tablets.

REFERENCES

Vuthibhagdee A, Harris N F 1972 Antral stricture as a delayed complication of iron intoxication. Radiology 103: 163–164
Franken E 1982 The stomach. In: Franken E A (ed) Gastrointestinal imaging in pediatrics, 2nd edn. Harper & Row, New York, Ch 5, pp 109–146

BEZOARS

When ingested materials collect in the stomach and proximal small bowel to form an intraluminal mass, the resulting mass is called a bezoar. There are two main types: trichobezoars or hair balls due to swallowed plucked hair, wool, fur etc., and phytobezoars due to aggregation of undigested food fibre. Trichobezoars are far commoner in children, and are usually found in emotionally disturbed children. Complications include gastric haemorrhage, gastric outlet obstruction and small bowel obstruction. Phytobezoars are described following ingestion of unripe persimmon and coconut. They also occur due to less exotic fibre accumulation in patients who have had a partial gastrectomy or gastrojejunostomy.

Lactobezoars, due to undigested milk curds, may form in children fed with an incorrectly reconstituted powdered milk, but more commonly lead to small bowel obstruction.

Aluminium hydroxide preparation used as antacids incorrectly reconstituted may form bezoars. Bezoars have also been reported following ingestion of a wide variety of bizarre substances, e.g. shellac, tar, bismuth, dirt and wax crayons.

Stomach bezoars appear as an intraluminal mass on the plain radiograph (Fig. 3.10.24). Air may be mixed within the mass giving it a mottled appearance. Following barium ingestion, the mass is outlined with small amounts of barium adhering to its surface (Fig. 3.10.25). Variable degrees of gastric outlet obstruction may be present. Occasionally, portions may project into the duodenum and jejunum. Surgical removal is usually necessary.

Clinically weight loss, anaemia, vomiting, bad breath and anorexia are present.

Lactobezoars are usually dissolved by fluid ingestion and rehydration.

Small bowel bezoars can also occur. They may be due to prolongation of a stomach bezoar into the small bowel. Trichobezoars are particularly likely to do this. They are also a well-known complication of surgery for peptic ulceration, either bypass surgery or vagotomy and pyloroplasty. Small bowel bezoars occurring in isolation are usually phytobezoars and due to undigested fibre from fruit seeds such as persimmon and sunflower seeds.

Small bowel obstruction is often visible on the plain radiographs. As in the stomach, the bezoar may appear as a mottled mass within the bowel lumen.

REFERENCES

McCracken S, Jongeward R, Silver T, Jafri S 1986 Gastric trichobezoar: sonographic findings. Radiology 161: 123–124

McGehee F, Buchanan G 1980 Trichophagia and trichobezoar: etiologic role of iron deficiency. Journal of Pediatric 97: 946–948

Newman B, Girdany B 1990 Gastric trichobezoars – sonographic and computed tomographic appearance. Pediatric Radiology 20: 526–527

Schreiner R, Brady M, Franken E 1979 Increased incidence of lactobezoars in low birth weight infants. American Journal of Diseases of Children 133: 936–940

Verstandig A, Klin B, Bloom R, Hadas I, Libson E 1989 Small bowel phytobezoars: detection with radiography. Radiology 172: 705–707

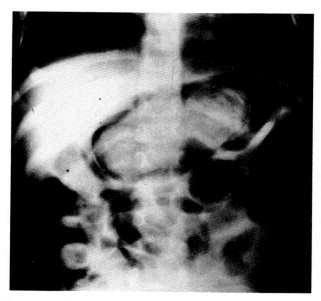

Fig. 3.10.24 There is a large intraluminal foreign body in the stomach due to a large trichobezoar.

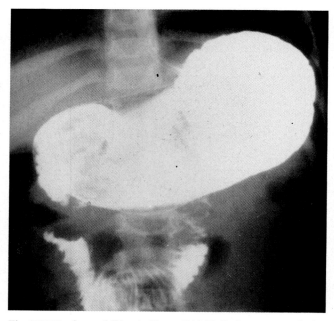

Fig. 3.10.25 Same child as in Figure 3.10.24. Barium surrounds the bezoar.

FOREIGN BODIES IN THE STOMACH AND INTESTINE

Children between the ages of 6 months and 5 years habitually put things into their mouths during play and accidentally ingest foreign bodies. In older children, ingestion is usually accidental or associated with psychiatric disease. The list of ingested foreign bodies is infinite and defies imagination. Similarly, though complications are very rare, migration of almost every swallowed foreign body across the bowel wall into the peritoneum has been described.

Most foreign bodies cause symptoms when impacted in the oesophagus or due to the corrosive effect of an ingested chemical substance, e.g. caustic or acid. Once non-corrosive foreign bodies reach the stomach, they are usually passed within 4–7 days, provided the child is fed normally. Occasionally, a foreign body may take longer to pass. Rarely, they impact in the duodenum, a Meckel's diverticulum (Fig. 3.10.26), or the appendix, but still more rarely cause symptoms. Long or sharp foreign bodies, i.e. plastic tooth picks, hair grips, or open safety pins, can impact in the duodenum, perforate it, or arrest at the ligament of Treitz. In practice, this is very rare and continued conservative management in the expectation of the object passing is preferable to surgical intervention. Non-opaque foreign bodies will, of course, not be seen on plain abdominal radiographs, so unless there is a history at presentation that suggests inhalation of a foreign body radiographs are not indicated.

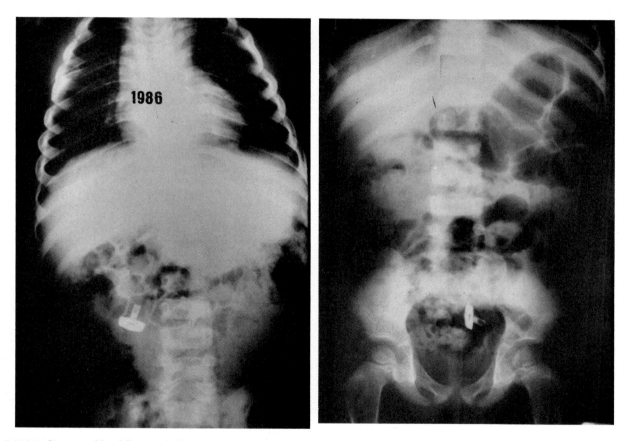

Fig. 3.10.26 Six-year-old mildly retarded boy under annual surveillance in the orthopaedic clinic for a platyspondyly and abnormal gait. The clockwork key was noted in 1986 (**A**), and it was presumed that he had recently swallowed it and it was an incidental finding. As it had not passed 1 year later (**B**) it was presumed to be impacted in a Meckel's diverticulum in view of the variable position. At operation a Meckel's containing a key was removed.

Aluminium foreign bodies and some glass have low radiodensity and may not be seen. Some tablets are mildly radiopaque while in the stomach, but once mixed with bowel content are no longer visible. Swallowed button batteries (Fig. 3.10.27) can be hazardous, as discussed earlier in this chapter.

Complications following foreign body ingestion are rare, occurring in less than 1% of patients. Antral narrowing and stricture have been described following caustic and acid ingestion and ingestion of iron tablets. Perforation has been recorded following ingestion of sharp objects and live button batteries. Lead paint ingestion can cause lead poisoning. Incidental discovery of foreign bodies in the colon is common in daily paediatric practice, and is of no concern. The foreign body most commonly seen is gravel or dirt scattered through the colon. Gravel located in the fundus of the stomach can mimic adrenal calcification. Lead paint chips are dense particles (Fig. 3.10.28). Dental amalgam appears as flakes of metallic density (Fig. 3.10.29). Lead shot often lodges in the appendix, but this is not an indication for appendicectomy in the absence of symptoms.

The policy of investigation of swallowed foreign bodies should be adjusted according to clinical presentation. If the history suggests aspiration or impaction in the oesophagus, a lateral radiograph to include the soft tissue of the neck, together with a frontal chest radiograph, should form the initial examination. The position should be confirmed immediately before attempts at removal. If the object is metallic and likely to be in the abdomen, a supine radiograph of the abdomen is all that is indicated and, unless the object is valuable (e.g. a diamond ring), or potentially harmful, no further radiographs are indicated.

Endoscopic, balloon catheter and magnetic removal have all been discussed earlier.

REFERENCES

Boothroyd A, Carty H, Robson W J 1987 'Hunt the Thimble' : a study of the radiology of ingested foreign bodies. Archives of Emergency Medicine 4: 33–38

David T, Ferguson A 1986 Management of children who have swallowed button batteries. Archives of Disease in Childhood 61: 321–322

Kulig K, Rumack C, Rumack B 1983 Disc battery ingestion. Journal of the American Medical Association 249: 2502–2504

Mandell G, Rosenberg H, Schauffer L 1977 Prolonged retention of foreign bodies in the stomach. Pediatrics 60: 460–462

Volle E, Beyer P, Kaufmann H 1989 Therapeutic approach to ingested Button-type batteries. Magnetic removal of ingested button-type batteries. Pediatric Radiology 19: 114–118

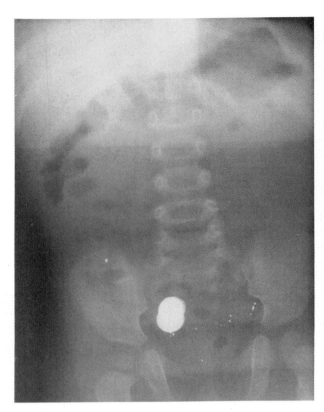

Fig. 3.10.27 Swallowed hearing aid battery. The child had diarrhoea and the radiograph was done to locate the battery. The intestinal juices have corroded the seal. Droplets of mercury have escaped into the intestinal lumen. The child was managed conservatively and recovered without harm.

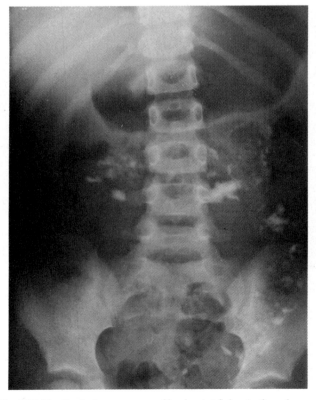

Fig. 3.10.28 Typical appearance of lead paint flakes in the colon.

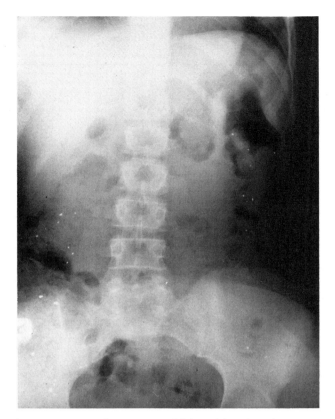

Fig. 3.10.29 Typical appearance of flakes of dental amalgam distributed throughout the colon.

CHEST PAIN OF GASTROINTESTINAL ORIGIN

Chest pain may result from a variety of gastrointestinal diseases, without obvious gastrointestinal symptoms, making diagnosis difficult. The pain is usually in the precordium or left chest, lasting in most cases between 1 and 60 minutes. Underlying causes include oesophagitis, diffuse oesophageal spasm and gastritis.

Pneumomediastinum is another rare complication of gastrointestinal disease and is associated with forceful retching and vomiting.

REFERENCES

Berezin S, Medow M, Glassman M, Newman L 1988 Chest pain of gastrointestinal origin. Archives of Disease in Childhood 63: 1457–1460

Woodruff W, Merten D, Kirks D 1985 Pneumomediastinum: an unusual complication of acute gastrointestinal disease. Pediatric Radiology 15: 196–198

AEROPHAGIA

Pathological swallowing of air leading to generalized abdominal distension, excessive flatus, and, on occasion, respiratory embarrassment has been described in a group of children suffering from psychological illness. The children are sent for investigation of abdominal distension. Gas is present throughout the bowel. Bowel sounds are normal or increased. Treatment is by counselling and relief of the underlying psychological problem.

3.11   THE DUODENUM

Anatomically the duodenum extends from the end of the pyloric canal to its junction with the jejunum. The first part is known as the duodenal cap or bulb and is mainly intraperitoneal. The remainder of the duodenum is retroperitoneal, the second part lying to the right of the head of the pancreas, the third part crossing the spine, and the fourth passing upwards to join with the jejunum at the ligament of Treitz. This normally lies to the left of the midline, under the gastric antrum at the level of the lesser curve of the stomach. The mucosa in the cap is smooth, but in the remainder is feathery. The loop of the duodenum forms a C shape, with the head of the pancreas contained within it. Normal extrinsic indentations of the duodenal mucosa seen at barium studies include the common bile duct which crosses the cap and the ampulla of Vater prominence on the medial wall, within the C loop. Both are usually only prominent in older children. A further normal variant is a circular fold in the duodenal cap which can be mistaken for a polyp (Fig. 3.11.1). Mistakes can be avoided by taking multiple spot films and using a muscle relaxant such as glucagon. Transit of contrast through the duodenum is rapid, once barium enters it. To-and-fro peristalsis may be seen in normal children, but it is not a prominent feature and, if vigorous, should suggest partial obstruction.

DUODENAL STENOSIS: ANNULAR PANCREAS: PRE-DUODENAL PORTAL VEIN – LATE PRESENTATION

Duodenal atresia presents in the neonatal period. Most patients with duodenal stenosis also present as neonates. A small number of children with congenital duodenal stenosis due to a diaphragm do not present until later childhood, particularly in Down's syndrome. In these children, the aperture is usually large. The diaphragm is usually at the level of the ampulla of Vater, but behaves as a wind-sock, with forward stretching as peristaltic waves pass distally. Symptoms are related to how much food passes through the central aperture, and are due to partial obstruction and include effortless vomiting, failure to thrive, abdominal pain, halitosis due to undigested food in the stomach, and occasionally awareness of a succussion splash.

On a plain radiograph one may see a double bubble with little distal bowel gas. The presence of gas visible in the duodenal cap in childhood should suggest the possibility of high partial intestinal obstruction.

Barium studies show dilatation of the first and second parts of the duodenum, which may be massive (Fig. 3.11.2). There is often gastric atony. There may be an associated malrotation of the small bowel.

Symptoms similar to duodenal stenosis due to a diaphragm occur with late presentation of annular pancreas (Fig. 3.11.3), or preduodenal portal vein. All three conditions may present at any age from birth to adulthood and the plain radiograph may be normal, or varying degrees of duodenal dilatation are seen. In patients with duodenal stenosis and diaphragm, the proximal duodenum can be hugely dilated. The dilatation may be so great that the duodenum extends far across the midline so that the point of obstruction appears to be in the distal duodenum or jejunum. Dilatation of the duodenum is less with annular pancreas and preduodenal portal vein. In annular pancreas concentric narrowing of the second part of the duodenum is seen (Fig. 3.11.3).

Postoperative studies following relief of the obstruction show a very slow return to a normal calibre duodenum with poor peristaltic activity in the proximal duodenum, a manifestation of the atony that ensues following prolonged distension of the proximal part.

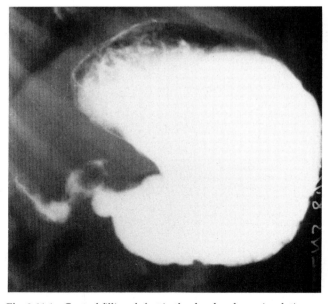

Fig. 3.11.1 Central filling defect in the duodenal cap simulating a polyp. Normal appearance on endoscopy.

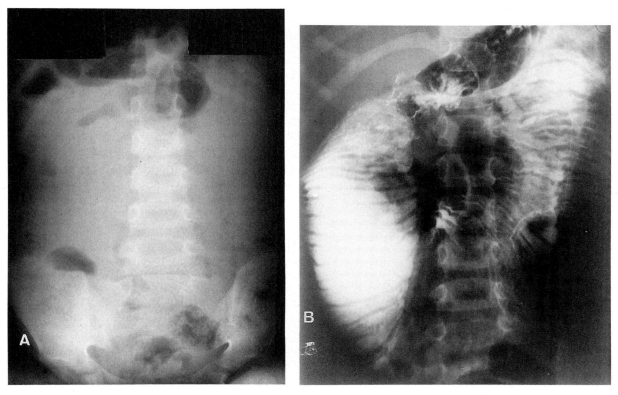

Fig. 3.11.2 Nine year-old girl who presented with failure to thrive. **A** Plain abdominal film. She had a succussion splash over the upper abdomen. **B** Barium studies. There is gross enlargement of the second and third parts of the duodenum due to a stenosis and wind-sock diaphragm. The distension on the plain abdominal film is due to a fluid-filled duodenum.

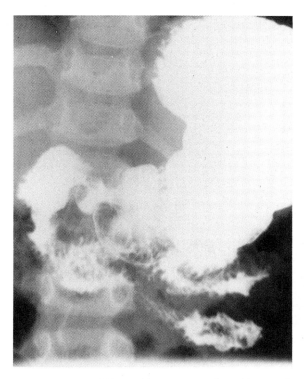

Fig. 3.11.3 Six-year-old boy with symptoms of vomiting attacks since birth. There is narrowing of the second part of the duodenum which was due to an annular pancreas. There was no associated malrotation in this boy.

MALROTATION AND NON-ROTATION – LATE PRESENTATION

Most children with symptomatic malrotation present in the neonatal period, or within the first few weeks of life, with bile-stained vomiting, and symptoms of volvulus. In a small number of patients, the presentation is less acute (F ig. 3.11.4). They present with intermittent vomiting, abdominal pain, failure to thrive and, rarely, a malabsorptive type illness (Fig. 3.12.9), thought to be due to chronic bowel wall congestion. Many of these children are labelled as psychosomatic and there is failure to investigate the cause of vomiting and pain. Some of the clinical presentations are very bizarre and unsocial, e.g. effortless vomiting during classroom work, and as the symptoms are intermittent it is not surprising that the children are labelled psychiatrically disturbed. The problem is further compounded by the difficulty in making the diagnosis at barium examination. The malrotation is seldom complete (Fig. 3.11.5). The fluoroscopic evidence may only be that of a low-lying duodenojejunal flexure, and a high-placed caecum. In some children the malrotation is intermittent and only demonstrable during an acute symptomatic episode.

Plain radiographs during a quiescent phase are normal. Barium studies may demonstrate a low-lying or midline duodenojejunal flexure with the initial position of jejunum to the right of the midline and a high caecum, but there is no dilatation of the duodenum. A high position of the caecum is a relatively common finding, and the diagnosis of malrotation should not be made on this finding alone. The two other signs, i.e. a low-lying duodenojejunal flexure and initial passage of jejunum to the right of the midline, are best appreciated on the first passage of the barium bolus, but become obscured rapidly. Unless actively looked for these signs are easily missed. During a symptomatic phase, dilatation of the duodenum with more obvious malrotation may be seen. Investigation policy should be to carry out a repeat examination during a symptomatic period, if investigation is negative during an asymptomatic period. The position of the superior mesenteric artery and vein can be assessed by ultrasound in an effort to help resolve difficult cases. In normal children the vein lies to the right of the artery (Fig. 3.11.6). In malrotation the vein lies anterior to the artery or to its left.

Non-rotation, that is the colon is in the left abdomen

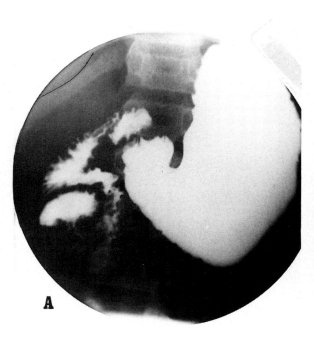

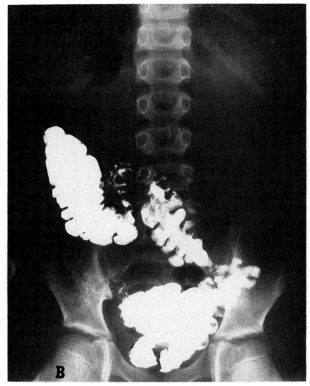

Fig. 3.11.4   Twelve-year-old boy with lifelong history of intermittent vomiting and abdominal pain. Diagnosis malrotation. **A** There is a spiral appearance of the duodenal loop with the duodenojejunal flexure lying to the right of the midline. **B** The caecum lies high in the subhepatic position, with the splenic flexure lying in the left iliac fossa.

and the whole of the small bowel in the right abdomen, is not usually associated with a midgut volvulus and may be asymptomatic. Reversed non-rotation is the mirror image of this. Reversed rotation occurs when the hepatic flexure and transverse colon lie behind the duodenum, and is very rare. Patients present with abdominal pain, and symptoms of intermittent obstruction.

REFERENCES

Houston C, Wittenborg M 1965 Roentgen evaluation of anomalies of rotation and fixation of the bowel in children. Radiology 84: 1–18

Katz M, Siegel M, Shackelford G, McAlister W 1987 The position and mobility of the duodenum in children. American Journal of Roentgenology 148: 947–951

Loyer E, Dunne Eggli K 1989 Sonographic evaluation of superior mesenteric vascular relationship in malrotation. Pediatric Radiology 19: 173–175

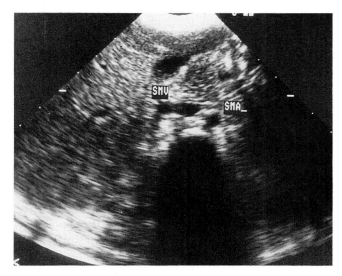

Fig. 3.11.6 Ultrasound in a patient with normal rotation.
SMA= superior mesenteric artery
SMV=superior mesenteric vein

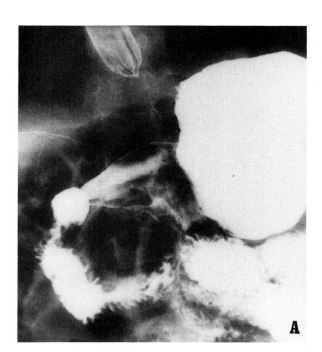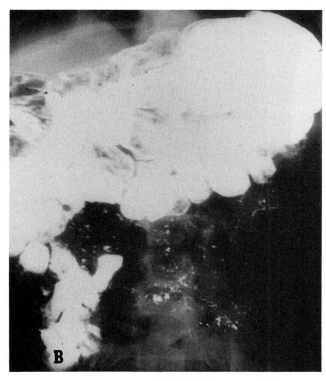

Fig. 3.11.5 **A** Upper gastrointestinal series in a child presenting with abdominal pain. The duodenojejunal flexure lies to the left of the midline but is low. **B** Film taken 12 hours later. The colon lies in transverse, malrotated position in the upper abdomen. Symptoms were relieved by fixation of the malrotation.

ABNORMALITIES OF SITUS

The position of liver, spleen, heart, etc. relative to the midline is known as situs and in normal patients the liver lies in the right upper quadrant, the spleen in the left upper quadrant, and the heart apex points to the left (Fig. 3.11.7). This normal position is known as situs solitus. Situs inversus is the mirror image of situs solitus. These individuals are also normal. Other forms of situs abnormalities – known as situs ambiguous – are associated with other congenital malformations, both of the heart, great vessels and the spleen. The cardiac implications of situs malposition are discussed in the cardiac chapter. The abnormal situs position may just be noticed on an abdominal radiograph and it is important to draw attention to the implications. Polysplenia and asplenia are associated with situs ambiguous.

PARADUODENAL HERNIA AND MESENTERIC HERNIA

Children with these internal hernias present with symptoms similar to those of late-presenting malrotation, e.g. intermittent abdominal pain, vomiting, which is often episodic, or occasionally acute intestinal obstruction.

In a paraduodenal hernia, rare in children, there is herniation of a segment of bowel into the retroperitoneum, either to the right or left of the second part (Fig. 3.11.8). A partial malrotation is present.

A more frequent internal hernia is herniation of bowel through a defect in the mesentery. The defect is most commonly in the ileal mesentery, and located between the ileocolic artery and its anastomosis with the last ileal artery. A sac of varying size may accompany the hernia.

These hernias are difficult to demonstrate by barium studies unless there is acute obstruction. Their presence may be suspected, by noting fixation of loops of bowel which cannot be displaced by palpation, or mild localized dilatation of a segment, or an unusual relationship of the loops of bowel related to the colon.

REFERENCES

Freund H, Berlatzky Y 1977 Small paraduodenal hernias. Archives of Surgery 112: 1180–1183

Harbin W, Andres J, Kim S, Borden S 1979 Internal hernia into Treves' field pouch: case report and review of the literature. Radiology 130: 71–72

Lough J, Estrada R, Wiglesworth F 1969 Internal hernia into Treves' field pouch: report of 2 cases and review of literature. Journal of Pediatric Surgery 4: 198–207

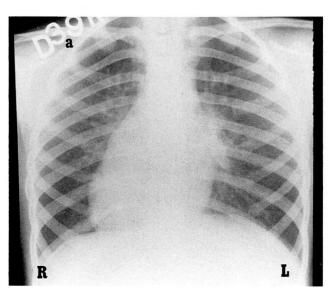

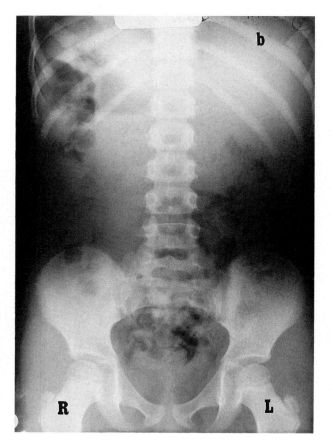

Fig. 3.11.7   **A**, **B** Incidental finding of total situs inversus in a girl of 10.

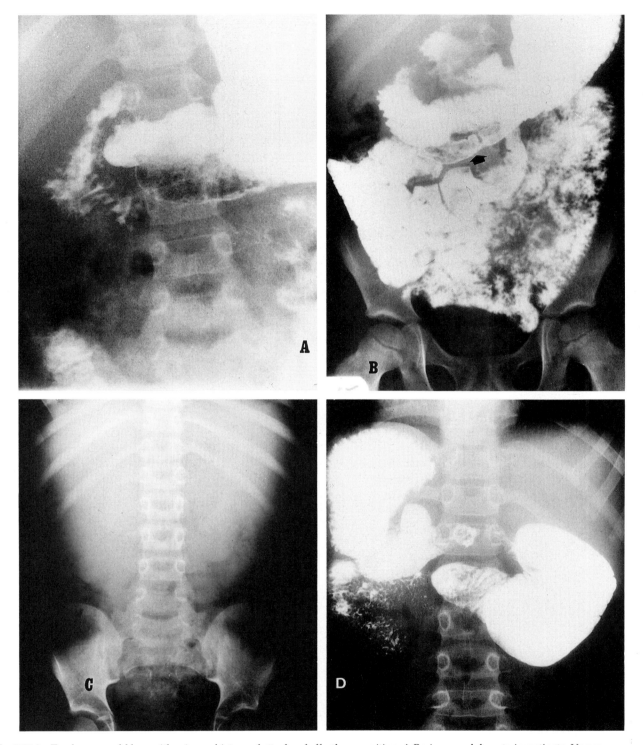

Fig. 3.11.8 Twelve-year-old boy with a 6-year history of attacks of effortless vomiting. **A** Barium meal done to investigate. Upper gastrointestinal tract normal. **B** Follow-through film at 1 hour. There is mild dilatation of the second and third parts of the duodenum. As this was only seen on this film it was assumed to be spurious. In retrospect there is an abnormal relationship of a loop of jejunum with the duodenum (arrow). **C** One year later. Plain abdominal film during an acute vomiting episode. There is an absence of upper gastrointestinal gas thought to be due to a mass. **D** Upper gastrointestinal study following the plain abdomen. There is incomplete obstruction of the third part of the duodenum. At operation a paraduodenal hernia was present which contained omentum and was causing the obstruction. (Films **C** and **D** courtesy of Dr R. Bissett, Booth Hall Children's Hospital, Manchester.)

SUPERIOR MESENTERIC ARTERY SYNDROME

Compression of the second part of the duodenum as it crosses the spine, by the superior mesenteric artery, leads to symptoms of high intestinal obstruction. It is usually only seen idiopathically in children with prolonged recumbency who are also thin and lose their retroperitoneal fat. It occurs acutely in children, placed in a body cast, following corrective surgery for scoliosis. The children present with retching and vomiting. Plain abdominal films show gastric distension with little distal gas. The gastric distension will not be seen if the child is on continuous nasogastric suction. Confirmation is by barium studies which show a distended stomach and first and second parts of the duodenum, with an abrupt cut off between the third and fourth parts. This examination may have to be done by portable radiography, without fluoroscopy, making it a very difficult diagnostic problem. Gastric perforation is a complication.

REFERENCES

Altman D, Puranik S 1973 Superior mesenteric artery syndrome in children. American Journal of Roentgenology 118: 104–108

Burrington J 1976 Superior mesenteric artery syndrome in children. American Journal of Diseases of Children 130: 1367–1370

Evarts C, Winter R, Hall J 1971 Vascular compression of the duodenum associated with the treatment of scoliosis. Review of the literature and report of eighteen cases. Journal of Bone and Joint Surgery 53A: 431–444

Ortiz C, Cleveland R, Blickman J, Jaramillo D, Kim S 1990. Familial superior mesenteric artery syndrome. Pediatric Radiology 20: 588–589

DUODENAL DUPLICATION

Duplications of the bowel are of two main varieties, tubular or, more commonly, cystic. Duodenal duplications represent about 6% of all duplications. They are most commonly cystic and are located on the mesenteric side of the first or second part of the duodenum on the anterior surface. Communication with the duodenal lumen is very rare. About 15% contain gastric mucosa.

The clinical presentation depends on the presence of a mass effect of the duplication. When large they may cause symptoms of obstruction. When they contain gastric mucosa, haemorrhage into the cyst with sudden enlargement is a complication. They are part of the differential diagnosis of cystic right upper quadrant masses discovered at ultrasound examination. At barium study they cause compression of the duodenum and may widen the duodenal loop (Fig. 3.11.9). Calcification within them has been demonstrated.

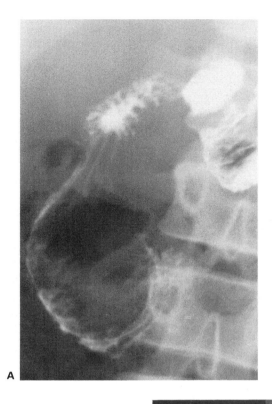

A

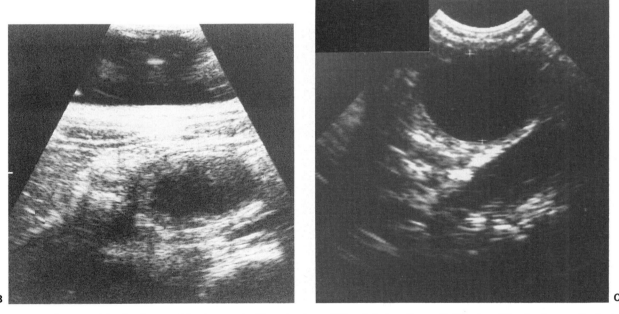

B   C

Fig. 3.11.9 Duplication of the duodenum: **A** barium study. There is a large filling defect on the medial border of the duodenum displacing and indenting the lumen. **B** Ultrasound. The mass is transonic and has a thick wall suggesting the diagnosis. This wall is unusually thick for a duplication cyst. More typical appearances are shown in **C** which is also a duplication cyst of the duodenum.

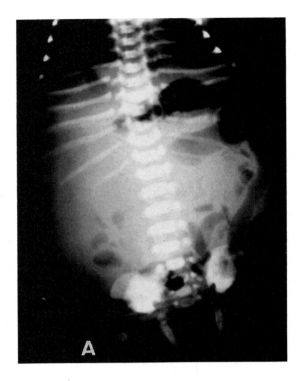

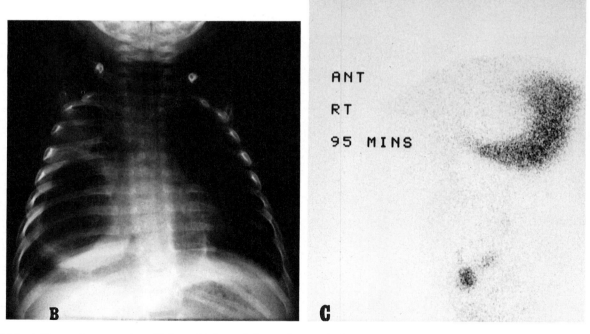

Fig. 3.11.10 **A** Neonatal presentation of infant with large abdominal mass which at operation was a duplication cyst of the jejunum. No connection seen at operation with the mediastinum. **B** Same infant presented at age 6 weeks with a chest infection. The cavitating mass was a further duplication cyst which had filled following the abdominal surgery. The chest radiograph as a neonate was normal. **C** Same child age 12. ^{99m}Tc-labelled pertechnetate scan done following complaints of recurrent abdominal pain. There are several areas of ectopic uptake of pertechnetate in the lower abdomen. At operation a long tubular duplication of the ileum was found, which had not been visible at the first operation.

Transsthoracic enteric duplications are tubular. The chest component is usually the clinically dominant portion, the infant presenting with a chest mass. The abdominal component is a tubular extension attached to the duodenum or proximal jejunum. Communication with the bowel lumen is rare. The duplication extends upwards from the bowel into the chest. It rarely communicates with the respiratory tract. Vertebral anomalies are often associated and communication through these with the neural tube may cause meningitis.

Duplications of the bowel, which may be multiple, are lined with alimentary epithelium, and their walls are composed of smooth muscle (Fig. 3.11.10).

REFERENCES

Alford B, Armstrong P, Franken E, Shaw A 1980 Calcification associated with duodenal duplications in children. Radiology 134: 647–648
Bowel R, Sieber W, Kiesewetter W 1978 Alimentary tract duplications in children. Annals of Surgery 188: 669–674
Egelhoff J, Bisset G, Strife J 1986 Multiple enteric duplications in an infant. Pediatric Radiology 16: 160–161
Hall C 1979 Transdiaphragmatic jejunal duplication: a report of five cases. Radiology 131: 663–667
Teele R, Henschke C, Tapper D 1980 The radiographic and ultrasonographic evaluation of enteric duplication cysts. Pediatric Radiology 10: 9–14

DUODENAL DIVERTICULUM

Congenital intraluminal duodenal diverticula are exceedingly rare in children. A diverticulum may be formed by an intraluminal wind-sock diaphragm.

Children present with symptoms of high intestinal obstruction, vomiting and abdominal pain. The dilated duodenum may be seen at ultrasound examination. The diverticulum will fill with contrast during barium studies, which distinguishes it from other intraluminal duodenal masses, such as intraluminal duplication cysts and choledoechoceles.

REFERENCES

Abdel-Hafiz A, Birkett D, Ahmed M 1988 Congenital duodenal diverticula: A report of three cases and a review of the literature. Surgery 104: 74–78
Heilbrun N, Boydon E 1964 Intraluminal duodenal diverticula. Radiology 82: 887–894
Newman A, Nathan M 1968 Intraluminal diverticulum of the duodenum in a child. American Journal of Roentgenology 103: 326–329

DUODENAL TUMOURS

Primary neoplasms of the duodenum in children are excessively rare. Haemangiomatous malformation and lymphangiohaemangiomas can affect any part of the gastrointestinal tract in children and the duodenum is not exempt.

REFERENCES

Bank E, Hernandez R, Byrne W 1987 Gastrointestinal hemangiomatosis in children: demonstration with CT. Radiology 165: 657–658
Hammoudi S, Corkery J 1985 Congenital haemangiopericytoma of the duodenum. Journal of Pediatric Surgery 20: 559–560
Mellish R W P 1971 Multiple hemangiomas of the gastrointestinal tract in children. American Journal of Surgery 121: 412–417
Shearburn E, Teja K, Botero L, Shaw A 1975 Pancreaticoduodenectomy in the treatment of congenital fibrosarcoma of the duodenum. Journal of Pediatric Surgery 10: 801–806

DUODENAL ULCERATION

Duodenal ulcers are rare in children but it is generally agreed that they occur more frequently than is traditionally taught, although the exact prevalence is not known. The aetiology of ulcers in children is the same as in adults, hyperacidity and stress, and there is often a strong family history. Symptoms in teenagers tend to be similar to those in adulthood – pain relieved by food and antacids – but in younger children the symptoms are very non-specific, e.g. vague abdominal pain and intermittent vomiting, or poor appetite. Haematemesis or melaena may be the presenting complaints, as indeed may perforation (Figs 3.11.11, 3.11.12). Children on steroids have an increased risk of duodenal ulceration. The radiological appearance of duodenal ulcers is the same in children as in adults. The crater is best seen on a double contrast examination with the duodenal bulb distended by air and paralysed. Associated deformity of the cap is present in longstanding cases (Fig. 3.11.13). Thickening of the antral and duodenal mucosal folds are indirect signs of ulceration. In acute exacerbations there may be considerable oedema. Postbulbar ulcers also occur in children as in adults (Fig. 3.11.14). Complete demonstration of the duodenal cap and loop is mandatory in any patient suspected of ulceration. One common pitfall is mistaking a normal circular fold in the duodenal bulb for ulceration (Fig. 3.11.1). Such children do not have spasm or thickening of the folds

and in a double contrast examination the fold will disappear.

Inflammation of the duodenal mucosa causes thickening and prominence of the folds without actual ulceration, and is named duodenitis. It is easier to diagnose endoscopically. Failure to demonstrate an ulcer at barium examination does not exclude duodenal ulceration and such children should have an endoscopy.

Aberrant pancreatic tissue within the duodenum may cause symptoms similar to peptic ulceration. The diagnosis is made when a nest of tissue with central umbilication is demonstrated in the second or third part of the duodenum. It too may be easier to diagnose by endoscopy.

Duodenal ulceration in children is commonly acute and resolves completely with appropriate medical management. Chronic deformity and intractable symptoms are rare in childhood and surgery is rarely required.

The decision to perform the initial investigation by endoscopy or barium studies is one that depends on local expertise. In skilled hands both methods of investigation are sensitive. Similarly, the choice of a modified single contrast or a formal double contrast study with smooth muscle paralysis will depend on the level of clinical suspicion of ulceration, and the age and tolerance of the child. A disadvantage of high density barium is that it is unsuitable for performing follow-through studies, should the upper gastro-

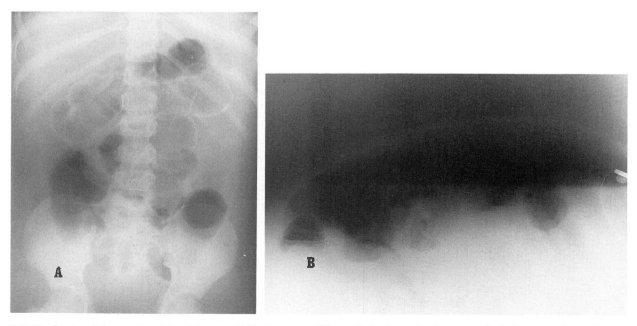

Fig. 3.11.11 Supine abdomen **A** and decubitus film **B.** Twelve-year-old boy who had sustained extensive body burns involving the abdominal wall. Abdominal distension was noted 1 week later, the boy being on a ventilator. The supine film shows gas on both sides of the bowel lumen. The decubitus film shows free fluid in the peritoneum. At operation there was a perforation of an acute gastric ulcer, but duodenal ulceration was also present.

intestinal investigation be negative. Erosions and shallow ulcers may well be missed by poor coating with low density barium and without paralysis.

REFERENCES

Agha F, Ghahremani G, Tsang T, Victor T 1988 Heterotopic gastric mucosa in the duodenum: radiographic findings. American Journal of Roentgenology 150: 291–294

Dunn S, Weber T, Grosfeld J, Fitzgerald J 1983 Acute peptic ulcer in childhood. Archives of Surgery 118: 656–660

Eklof O, Lassrich A, Stanley P, Chrispin A 1973 Ectopic pancreas. Paediatric Radiology 1: 24–27

Puri P, Boyd E, Blake N, Guiney E 1978 Duodenal ulcer in childhood: a continuing disease in adult life. Journal of Pediatric Surgery 13: 525–526

White A, Carachi R, Young D 1984 Duodenal ulceration presenting in childhood, long term follow-up. Journal of Pediatric Surgery 19: 6–8

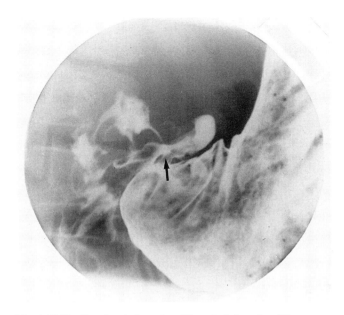

Fig. 3.11.13 Duodenal ulceration. There is deformity of the duodenal bulb with folds radiating into a central ulcer crater (arrow).

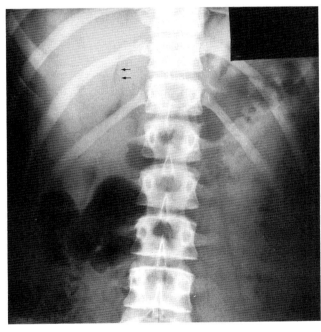

Fig. 3.11.12 Fifteen-year-old girl with 24-hour history of abdominal pain. There is gas in the lesser sac, seen as small streaks (arrows). A faint increased density is also visible over the liver due to free intraperitoneal air. At operation a perforated acute duodenal ulcer was found.

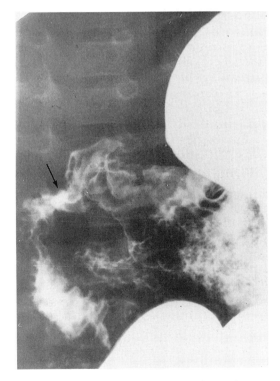

Fig. 3.11.14 Postbulbar ulcer (arrow) in an infant with recurrent vomiting and marked irritability.

DUODENAL HAEMATOMA

Blunt trauma to the upper abdomen which causes compression of the duodenum can result in a haematoma of the duodenum. The forces required are usually considerable, although sometimes apparently trivial injury causes bowel trauma. There is often associated injury of the liver and pancreas. The causes are most commonly road traffic accidents, non-accidental injury and 'fisticuffs' in older children. In non-accidental injury, the damage is sustained when the child is trampled on or punched. Duodenal haematomas may also occur spontaneously in children with Henoch–Schonlein purpura, haemophilia or children treated with anticoagulants. The most frequent presentation is vomiting due to partial obstruction of the duodenum. Pain may only be minimal. Occasionally, the child presents with a mass or perforation. The plain radiographic findings depend on the degree of injury. Perforation will cause free intraperitoneal air. Retroperitoneal perforation may be diagnosed by the presence of air outlining the psoas or kidney. The haematoma may be visible as a mass lesion in the upper abdomen. Retroperitoneal air and small amounts of free air may be more easily appreciated on CT. The haematoma may be seen at ultrasound examination and appear as a mass of mixed though generally low echodensity. Ultrasonic examination may also show injury to the liver, spleen, kidneys and pancreas if present. The haematoma presents as an intraluminal filling defect during barium examination (Fig. 3.11.15). The barium column curves round the mass, with splaying and stretching of the folds. Depending on the size of the haematoma, mass effect may be visible on the stomach and colon.

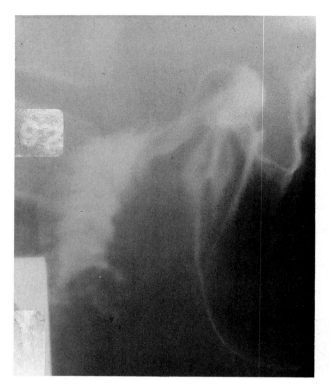

Fig. 3.11.15 Six-year-old girl who had fallen across the handlebar of her bicycle and presented with upper abdominal pain and vomiting. The filling defect in the lower second part of the duodenum is due to a haematoma.

REFERENCES

Bulas D, Taylor G, Eichelberger M 1989 The value of CT in detecting bowel perforation in children after blunt abdominal trauma. American Journal of Roentgenology 153: 561–564

Greenstein Orel S, Nussbaum A, Sheth S, Yale-Loehr A, Sanders R 1988 Duodenal hematoma in child abuse: sonographic detection. American Journal of Roentgenology 151: 147–149

Hayashi K, Futagawa S, Kozaki S, Hirao K, Hombo Z 1988 Ultrasound and CT diagnosis of intramural duodenal hematoma. Pediatric Radiology 18: 167–168

Kleinman P, Brill P, Winchester P 1986 Resolving duodeno-jejunal haematoma in abused children. Radiology 160: 747–750

Miller J, Kemberling C 1984 Ultrasound scanning of the gastrointestinal tract in children: subject review. Radiology 152: 671–677

Miyamoto Y, Fukida Y, Urushibara K, Hohjoh H, Ayugase M, Nagase M 1989 Ultrasonographic findings in the duodenum caused by Schonlein–Henoch purpura. Journal of Clinical Ultrasound 17: 299–303

Raby N, Meire H 1986 Duodenal haematoma mimicking traumatic pancreatic pseudocyst. British Journal of Radiology 59: 279–281

Sivit C, Taylor G, Eichelberger M 1989 Visceral injury in battered children: a changing perspective. Radiology 173: 659–661

Winthrop A, Wesson D, Filler R 1986 Traumatic duodenal haematoma in the paediatric patient. Journal of Pediatric Surgery 21: 757–760

3.12   THE SMALL BOWEL

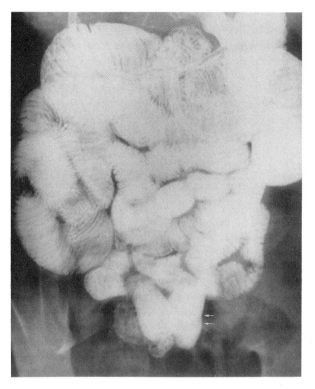

Fig. 3.12.1   Normal small bowel appearances during enteroclysis. Note the circular, smooth, delicate folds in the jejunum and the more featureless normal ileum (arrows).

The jejunum begins at the duodenojejunal flexure. In patients with normal situs it lies initially in the left upper quandrant crossing to mid abdomen. The transition between jejunum and ileum occurs imperceptibly. The iluem lies centrally in the lower abdomen and ceases where it enters the caecum at the ileocaecal valve. The normal mucosal pattern of the jejunum seen at barium examination is feathery and delicate (Fig. 3.12.1). That in the proximal iluem is coarser, but in the terminal ileum the mucosal folds are shallow and the mucosa is relatively featureless (Fig. 3.12.1). Mucosal folds in the jejunum and proximal ileum are circular but are longitudinal in the terminal ileum, especially in older children. A prominent almost cobblestone mucosal pattern may be seen at barium studies in some children and is due to lymphoid hyperplasia (Fig. 3.12.2). It can almost resemble Crohn's disease but is distinguished by the complete pliability of the bowel on palpation and absence of deep ulcers seen in profile views.

One cannot always distinguish jejunum from ileum on a plain abdominal radiograph with normal gas content (Fig. 3.12.3). In obstruction, and sometimes in

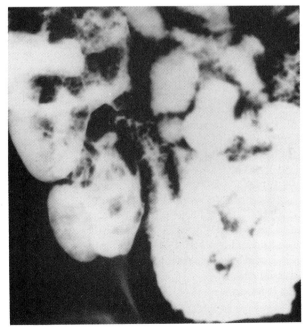

Fig. 3.12.2   Lymphoid hyperplasia of the terminal ileum. The nodular pattern is typical of this.

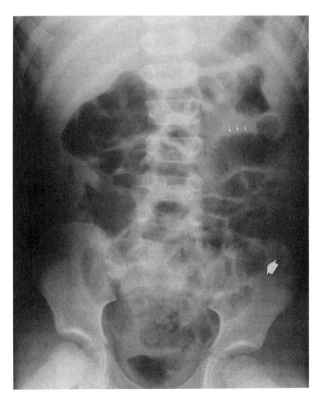

Fig. 3.12.3   Plain abdomen of a child with renal colic. Note the normal circular jejunal folds (arrows) and the more featureless ileum (arrowhead).

the normal abdomen, the finer jejunal folds formed by the valvulae conniventes can be seen outlined by air. Absorption of ingested food takes place through these mucosal folds. In a normal child gas is not seen in the body of the duodenum on a plain abdominal radiograph. Persistent gas in the duodenum is an indication of an abnormality.

The small bowel gas can be displaced by faecal loading of the colon, which can simulate displacement by a space-occupying lesion. In the young child the sigmoid colon normally lies within the abdominal cavity, the pelvis still being very shallow, and can displace normal small bowel gas around it.

The small bowel can be studied by barium follow-through examination or by small bowel intubation and enteroclysis. Each technique has its advocates. Intubation is unpleasant for children, and generally requires sedation. The tube must be placed in the duodenum beyond the ligament of Treitz to avoid gastro-oesophageal reflux with the hazard of aspiration in a sedated child. Local circumstances will dictate the choice of examination. In general, a follow-through is adequate as a simple examination in children who have small bowel studies to investigate non-specific abdominal pain. Enteroclysis should be reserved for children who will not drink an adequate volume of barium, in whom small bowel polyps are suspected and in whom resection of a previously identified isolated segment of Crohn's disease is being considered, provided the bowel is otherwise normal. For a successful barium follow-through, the child must drink a minimum of 250 ml volume of dilute barium quickly to ensure an adequate bolus for demonstration of the mucosa and assessment of peristalsis. Transit times vary enormously in normal children and range from half an hour to 6 hours from stomach to terminal ileum. Transit times are reduced in children with faecal loading of the colon. Some clumping and breaking up of the barium column is normal in children and must not be misread as indicating malabsorption. Transit of barium can be hastened by metachlorpropamide or more simply a drink.

Distinct feathery jejunal mucosa is generally not visible below 6 months. Measurements of mucosal height and thickness do not aid diagnosis in children. Assessment is subjective.

REFERENCES

Astley R, French J 1951 The small intestine pattern in normal children in coeliac disease. Its relationship to the nature of the opaque medium. British Journal of Radiology 24: 321–330

Lownerblud L 1951 Transit time through the small intestine: a roentgenologic study of normal variability. Acta Radiologica Supplementum (88) 1–85

Reiquam C, Allen R, Akers D 1965 Normal and abnormal small bowel lengths. American Journal of Diseases of Children 109: 447–451

Well J 1948 The mucosal pattern of the terminal ileum in children. Radiology 51: 305–309

INGUINAL HERNIA

During the third month of gestation the peritoneum extends from the abdomen into the scrotum as the processus vaginalis, which remains open in about 80% of infants at birth, but progressively closes so that by 2 years of age patency is only 20%. This patency may lead to the formation of an indirect inguinal hernia or hydrocoele of the cord, or scrotum. The patent processus only becomes detectable as a hernia when it contains abdominal viscera, usually small bowel. The diagnosis of an uncomplicated hernia is clinical and radiological investigation is not indicated. If the hernia incarcerates, it will lead to intestinal obstruction. This can occur at any age after birth and is the commonest cause of intestinal obstruction between 1 and 6 months of age in infants who have not had neonatal surgery. It is rare in females, less than 5% of all cases, and there is about an 80% right-sided dominance. The diagnosis is usually obvious clinically and the child proceeds straight to surgery. Occasionally, abdominal radiographs are requested to confirm the clinical suspicion of intestinal obstruction. An erect and supine, or a supine and decubitus view, are indicated, without gonadal protection. The plain films will show multiple fluid levels in distended bowel. Gas may be seen within the hernial sac, confirming the diagnosis (Fig. 3.12.4). However, in an incarcerated hernia, the bowel loops will be fluid filled and airless. The problem can be recognized by observing thickening of the inguinal scrotal folds on the affected side. In the normal infant, the inguino-scrotal folds form a symmetrical V. In an incarcerated hernia the affected side is thickened. This sign is also seen with hydrocoele of the cord, and communicating hydrocoele, and more rarely with undescended testis and lymphadenopathy. The combination of the clinical presentation, radiographs and ultrasound will usually suffice to distinguish the different causes.

Reduction en masse of a hernia can make clinical and radiological diagnosis of the cause of intestinal obstruction impossible (Fig 3.12.5). Contrast studies done preoperatively can be extremely helpful in ensuring the correct surgical approach, and are indicated provided the baby is clinically and haemodynamically stable. Water soluble contrast delivered by enema will demonstrate the site of obstruction in the inguinal canal.

Herniography

Injection of contrast medium into the peritoneum under aseptic conditions has been used in the past to

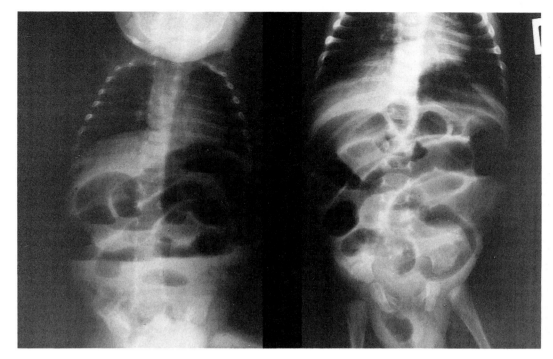

Fig. 3.12.4 Infant of 3 months who presented with a distended abdomen and bilious vomiting. There is small intestinal obstruction due to an inguinal hernia. Note the hernial gas projected over the scrotum. Note the normal left-sided scrotal shadows and their obliteration on the right.

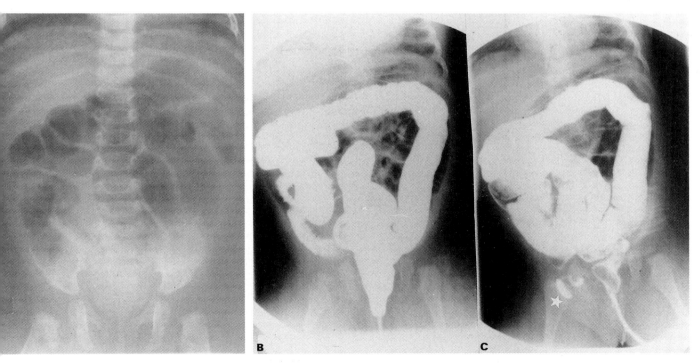

Fig. 3.12.5 **A** Four-month-old infant girl with abdominal distension and vomiting. There are distended loops of small bowel but there is still colonic gas. Child observed overnight. **B** Same child. Contrast enema 12 hours later shows an inguinal hernia which was reducible and appeared intermittently during the enema (star). Intermittent obstruction due to the hernia was the presumptive diagnosis. At operation this was confirmed. The neck of the sac was narrow and inflamed and oedematous bowel was found.

confirm a suspected hernia and to demonstrate a silent contralateral hernia in a patient with a clinically apparent lesion. The risk of development of a contralateral hernia is about 20%. The technique is no longer popular, and has never been extensively practised in Europe or the UK, and is not recommended.

Ultrasound

This can be valuable in demonstrating the contents of a groin, scrotal or mons mass. The defect in the canal is demonstrated, proving that the lesion is a hernia.

Umbilical hernia

Umbilical hernias are common in infants, particularly negroes, up to the age of 6 months. They are very rarely symptomatic. They regress spontaneously. On a supine radiograph they are seen as a round dense shadow in the central abdomen, which can be mistaken for a tumour (Fig 3.12.6). On the lateral view, bowel may be seen within them, but this is of no significance. Perforation has been described. They are a common finding in Beckwith's syndrome.

Other hernias, well known, though rare in adult practice, have been described in childhood, but they are even rarer. They include Spigelian hernia, herniation into the abdominal wall lateral to the rectus muscle, sciatic hernia into the sciatic notch and herniation into the foramen of Winslow.

REFERENCES

Currarino G 1974 Incarcerated inguinal hernia in infants: plain films and barium enema. Pediatric Radiology 2: 247–250
Franken E, Smith E 1969 Sciatic hernia: report of three cases including two with bilateral ureteral involvement. American Journal of Roentgenology 107: 791–795
Harbin W P, Andres J, Kim S H, Borden S 1979 Internal hernia into Treves' field pouch – case report and review of the literature. Radiology 130: 71–72
Hurlbut H, Moseley T 1967 Spigelian hernia in a child. Southern Medical Journal 60: 602–614
Murphy D 1964 Internal hernias in infancy and childhood. Surgery 55: 311–316
Oh K S, Dorst J P, White J J, Haller J A Jr, Heller R, James A, Johnson B, Strife J 1973 Positive-contrast peritoneography and herniography. Radiology 108: 647–654
Schwarz H 1977 Herniation through the foramen of Winslow: report of a case. Diseases of the Colon and Rectum 20: 521–523
Townsend E, Sahler C 1965 Perforation of an umbilical hernia. Journal of Pediatrics 66: 801–803
Walker J, Carty H 1989 A radiological feature to assist in the diagnosis of intestinal obstruction. British Journal of Radiology 62: 1105–1106

DUPLICATION

The term duplication of the bowel encompasses many previously used terms, described as separate entities. These include enteric and enterogenous cysts, diverticula, giant diverticula, atypical Meckel's diverticulum and duplex jejunum and ileum. Most duplications of the small bowel are cystic with a smaller number being tubular. They are lined with intestinal epithelium but the epithelium is not necessarily that of the adjacent normal bowel. They may contain gastric mucosa or pancreatic rests, either of which may haemorrhage causing sudden enlargement of the cysts. They may occur anywhere from mouth to anus but are commonest near the terminal ileum. They may be multiple and extend transdiaphragmatically. There is an equal sex incidence.

Clinical presentation includes a palpable abdominal mass, intermittent abdominal pain, vomiting, failure to thrive, anaemia, symptoms of intermittent intestinal obstruction or, rarely, but dramatically, sudden increase in size of the mass with exsanguination due to haemorrhage into it. Sixteen per cent of small bowel duplications contain gastric mucosa. Surgery is indicated even in the asymptomatic child if one is found incidentally. Cystic duplications do not communicate with the bowel lumen, tubular ones may.

A mass may be seen on the plain abdominal radiograph with loops of bowel displaced around it. Isolated case reports of calcification within the cyst are recorded. At ultrasound examination, the cyst has a well-defined wall. One can usually identify both the muscle wall and a separate mucosa giving a double outline. This, when present, helps to distinguish them from other cysts which have only a single wall (Fig. 3.12.7). It may contain a few septae. The content varies from being echolucent, to fluid containing echoes, due to haemorrhage and debris within it. If contrast examinations are done, barium-filled loops of bowel will be displaced around the cyst (Fig 3.12.8).

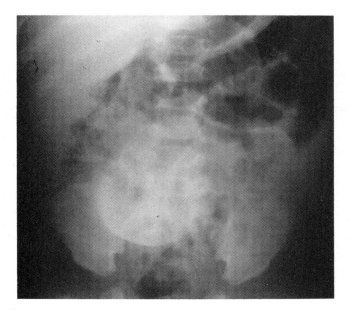

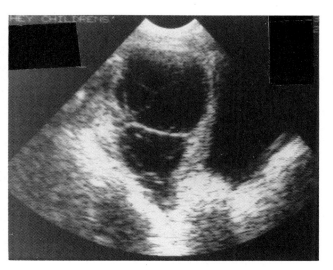

Fig. 3.12.6 The central dense shadow is due to a large umbilical hernia.

Fig. 3.12.7 Multiloculated duplication cyst of the ileum. This pattern is less common than the unilocular mass with a sharply defined wall. (See Figs 3.11.9C and 3.12.8).

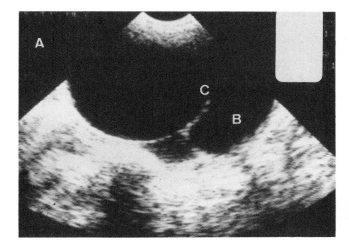

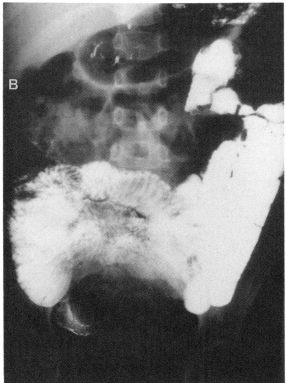

Fig. 3.12.8 **A** Typical duplication cyst (C) of the ileum sitting above the bladder (B). **B** Barium follow-through on the same child done before the ultrasound. Note the displacement of loops of ileum by the cyst.

Contrast is not routinely indicated if the plain film and ultrasound examination are diagnostic. Tubular duplications are a more difficult diagnostic problem. One may see a mass both on the plain film and at ultrasound, but both are often normal. At contrast studies, the bowel loops may be separated by the non-opacified duplicated segment. If there is communication, contrast is seen in both lumina, but may be missed as the duplicated length is thought to be a normal bowel loop. Barium may be retained in the duplication after it has passed through the normal bowel. The tubular duplication is often blind and bacterial overgrowth may be a problem. Many duplications contain gastric mucosa, which can be demonsrated by technetium pertechnetate scanning. This is particularly helpful in demonstrating the tubular lesions (Fig. 3.11.10C, 3.12.9).

Transdiaphragmatic extension of a duplication is well known and should be carefully looked for in all cases, particularly in duodenal and jejunal lesions. An extension of a soft tissue mass proximally may be seen on the plain radiograph. Asymptomatic duplications are discovered during antenatal ultrasound.

The differential diagnosis of a cystic abdominal mass in children should always include duplication, especially if there are intestinal symptoms. Choledochal cysts are usually unilocular, are situated in the right upper quadrant and are frequently associated with jaundice. Ovarian cysts may be impossible to distinguish as they are variable in site, particularly when they are pedunculated. Omental or mesenteric cysts are usually larger and septate, and do not fill with contrast. They may contain calcification but may be so large as to mimic gross ascites. Omental cysts lie anterior to the small bowel. Retroperitoneal lympangiomas are usually large, septate, and displace bowel anteriorly.

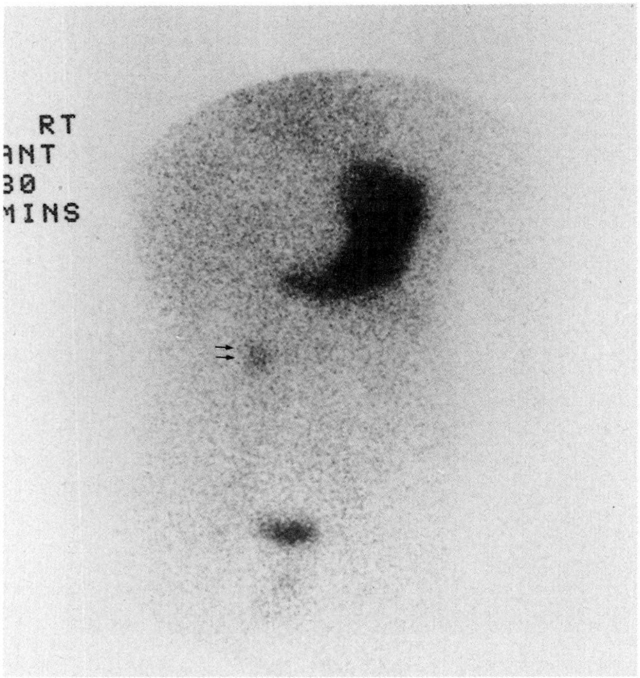

REFERENCES

Avni E, Godart S, Isreal C, Schmitz C 1983 Ovarian torsion cyst presenting as a wandering tumour in a newborn: antenatal diagnosis and post natal assessment. Pediatric Radiology 13: 169–171

Bastable J 1964 Intestinal duplication with calcification. British Journal of Radiology 37: 706–708

Egelhoff J, Bisset G, Strife J 1986 Multiple enteric duplications in an infant. Pediatric Radiology 16: 160–161

Hall C 1979 Transdiaphragmatic jejunal duplication: a report of 5 cases. Radiology 131: 663–667

Hitch D, Shardling B, Gilday D 1978 Tubular duplication of the bowel: use of technetium-99mTc pertechnetate in diagnosis. Archives of Disease in Childhood 53: 178–179

Miller J, Kemberling C 1984 Ultrasound scanning of the gastrointestinal tract in children: Subject review. Radiology 152: 671–677

Rose J, Gribetz D, Krasna I 1978 Ileal duplication cyst: the importance of sodium pertechnetate Tc99m scanning. Pediatric Radiology 6: 244–246

Teele R, Henschke C, Tapper D 1980 The radiographic and ultrasonographic evaluation of enteric duplication cysts. Pediatric Radiology 10: 9–14

Tschappeler H, Smith W 1977 Duplications of the intestinal tract: clinical and radiological features. Annales de Radiologie 20: 133–139

Fig. 3.12.9 Technetium pertechnetate scan in a child age 3 with a tubular ileal duplication. The child had intermittent abdominal pain for 9 months. The uptake seen in the right upper quadrant could lie in a high Meckel's diverticulum. At operation a 15-cm tubular ileal duplication was removed. It contained ulcerated gastric mucosa.

MECKEL'S DIVERTICULUM

A Meckel's diverticulum is a persistent remnant of the omphalomesenteric duct at its junction with the ileum. It is situated 30–45 cm proximal to the ileocaecal valve on the antimesenteric border. It is a common anomaly at autopsy occurring in 1–4% of patients, but has a much lower incidence of clinical presentation. The sexes are equally affected. The commonest clinical presentation is of melaena or recurrent anaemia, both caused by bleeding from ectopic gastric mucosa contained within the diverticulum. Rarely, blood loss can be catastrophic. Pain is not a prominent feature. Perforation may cause a clinical presentation of an acute abdomen. Local abscess formation may cause ilues and mimic appendicitis. Swelling of the anterior abdominal wall is a rare though classical clinical presentation. Volvulus may occur around a Meckel's diverticulum, following which the child will present with intestinal obstruction. It may also act as the lead point of an intussusception.

The plain radiographs are usually unhelpful in a patient suspected of having a Meckel's diverticulum. The ectopic gastric mucosa may be demonstrated by radionuclide scanning with technetium pertechnetate (Fig. 3.12.10). A negative scan does not exclude the presence of a Meckel's diverticulum but it is unlikely to contain gastric mucosa. Premedication with cimetidine, an H_2 antagonist, decreases gastric secretions, and is said to enhance the uptake of technetium pertechnetate by gastric mucosa, thus improving the diagnostic accuracy of 'Meckel's' scanning. Meckel's diverticula are best seen on anterior abdominal images, uptake in the gastric mucosa and in the ectopic tissue in the Meckel's occurring simultaneously. Images of the abdomen are taken at 5-minute intervals for 45 minutes after injection. An image with an empty bladder must be taken on completion, as a low lying Meckel's diverticulum may be obscured by a full bladder.

False-negative scans are found in children with a Meckel's diverticulum when they lack or contain insufficient gastric mucosa to take up the radionuclide. Similarly, impaired blood supply to the diverticulum due to twisting of the neck or dilution of the radioactivity in severe haemorrhage will produce a negative scan. Bleeding may also be identified by the use of radionuclide red cell labelling.

False-positive scans have been reported due to duplication cysts, abscess formation, regional enteritis and tumours. Occasionally, a foreign body (Fig. 3.10.26) or faecolith may be seen within the Meckel's diverticulum on a plain abdominal radiograph. Enteroclysis may sometimes demonstrate a Meckel's diverticulum but it is of more value in showing large lesions or 'giant' diverticula than the more usual small ones and is not generally advocated in children.

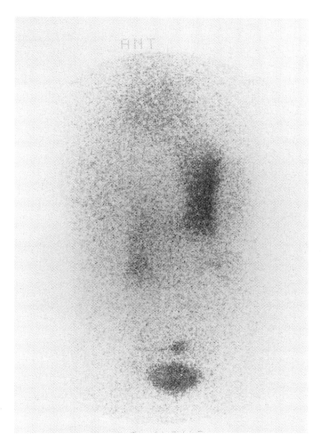

Fig. 3.12.10 Positive technetium pertechnetate scan in a 9-month-old infant who presented with anaemia. There is uptake in an area of ectopic gastric mucosa situated above the bladder. This is a typical site for a Meckel's diverticulum.

Occasionally, a Meckel's diverticulum is discovered incidentally when barium is noted trapped in the lesion when carrying out the examination for some other purpose.

Abdominal angiography, carried out during a phase of active bleeding, may also localize the bleeding point to a diverticulum, but is not helpful when there is no bleeding. It should only be carried out following negative scintigraphy.

Persistent omphalomesenteric duct

The omphalomesenteric duct connects the primitive midgut to the yolk sac during early embryonic life and is normally obliterated during the fifth to sixth week of fetal life. Persistence postnatally can lead to clinical presentation of a discharging sinus from the umbilicus or more rarely with persistence of the duct in toto – a fistula between the terminal ileum and umbilicus (Fig. 3.12.11). Sinography will demonstrate the depth of the sinus and the full fistula in the rare cases where this exists. Persistence of the ileal end of the duct leads to a Meckel's diverticulum. Another cause of umbilical discharge is a patent urachus.

REFERENCES

Baum S 1981 Pertechnetate imaging following cimetidine administration in Meckel's diverticulum of the ileum. American Journal of Gastroenterology 76: 464–465

Conway J 1980 Radionuclide diagnosis of Meckel's diverticulum. Gastrointestinal Radiology 5: 209–213

Daneman A, Reilly B, De Silva M, Olutola P 1982 Intussusception on small bowel examination in children. American Journal of Roentgenology 139: 299–304

Dixon P, Nolan D 1987 The diagnosis of Meckel's diverticulum: a continuing challenge. Clinical Radiology 38: 615–619

Hertzog M, Chacko A, Pitts C 1985 Leiomyoma of terminal ileum producing a false positive Meckel's scan. Journal of Nuclear Medicine 26: 1278–1282

Maglinte D, Elmore M, Isenberg M, Dolan P A 1980 Meckel's diverticulum: radiologic demonstration by enteroclysis. American Journal of Roentgenology 134: 925–932

Routh W, Lawdahl R, Lund E, Garcia J, Keller F 1990 Meckel's diverticula: angiographic diagnosis in patients with non acute hemorrhage and negative scintigraphy. Pediatric Radiology 20: 152–156

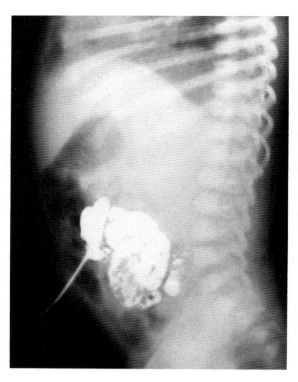

Fig. 3.12.11 Sinogram through a discharging umbilicus. A fistula through a persistent omphalomesenteric duct extends to the ileum.

ILEAL DYSGENESIS

The terms ileal dysgenesis, giant Meckel's diverticulum and segmental ileal dilatation have all been used to describe a developmental abnormality of the ileum at its junction with the vitelline duct. It is an anomaly due to persistence of a portion of the primitive gut rather than an abnormality of the vitelline gut. The dysgenetic bowel is situated on the antimesenteric border of the ileum. The size is very variable. Symptoms include anaemia, recurrent colicky abdominal pain, fatigue, failure to thrive, short stature, and occasionally diarrhoea due to bacterial overgrowth. Perforation and ulceration also occur. In the newborn period, children may present with symptoms of intestinal obstruction.

The plain radiograph is often normal, but subtle abnormalities with dilated air-filled bowel may be seen anywhere in the abdomen (Fig. 3.12.12). Barium studies again may be normal, but, on occasion, barium-filled saccular diverticula may be seen with a wide neck connecting it to the normal bowel lumen. The diagnosis is often missed at initial examination but seen retrospectively when the surgical findings are known. The abnormal saccular bowel is more easily seen by a study done following enteroclysis than by conventional follow-through.

REFERENCES

Bell M, Ternberg J, Bowen R 1982 Ileal dysgenesis in infants and children. Journal of Pediatric Surgery 17: 395–399
Leinster S, Hughes L 1981 Segmental mega ileum presenting as anaemia. British Journal of Surgery 68: 417–419
Miller D, Becker M, Eng K 1981 Giant Meckel's diverticulum. A cause of intestinal obstruction. Radiology 140: 93–94
Morewood D, Cunningham M 1985 Segmental dilatation of the ileum presenting with anaemia. Clinical Radiology 36: 267–268
Orenstein S, Magill H, Whitington P 1984 Ileal dysgenesis presenting with anemia and growth failure. Pediatric Radiology 14: 59–61
Ratcliffe J, Tait J, Lisle D, Leditschke J, Bell J 1989 Segmental dilatation of the small bowel. Report of 3 cases and a literature review. Radiology 171: 827–830

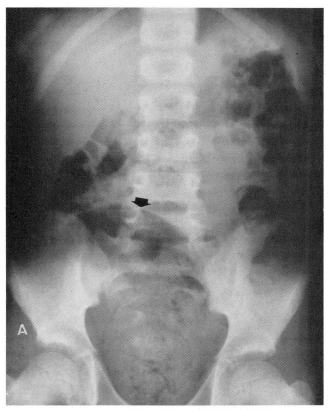

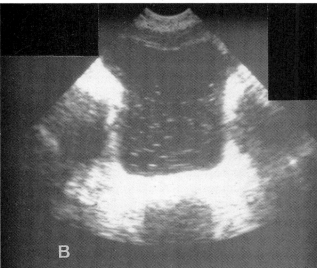

Fig. 3.12.12 **A** Ileal dysgenesis or Giant Meckel's diverticulum. Note the distended loop of ileum projected over the right sacroiliac joint and sacrum (arrow). **B** Ultrasound of the same child. The fluid-filled structure which contains echogenic material due to stagnant bowel content is the 'Giant Meckel's'. This was surgically confirmed.

DIVERTICULA

Diverticula of the small bowel, other than Meckel's diverticula, are almost unknown in children. True diverticula contain all bowel layers, mucosa, submucosa, serosa and muscle. False diverticula do not contain a normal muscle layer.

Jejunal diverticulosis, seen in adults, is an acquired disease and does not occur in children. There are rare reports of small bowel diverticula occurring in Noonan's, Ehlers–Danlos and Marfan's syndromes. Traction diverticula occasionally occur secondary to inflammatory disease. Many of the isolated diverticula discovered in children probably represent forms of duplication.

REFERENCES

Caplan L, Jacobson H 1964 Small intestinal diverticulosis. American Journal of Roentgenology 92: 1048–1062
Cumming W, Simpson J 1977 Intestinal diverticulosis in Noonan's Syndrome. British Journal of Radiology 50: 64–65
Fich A, Polliack G, Libson E 1989 Gastrointestinal diverticulosis in association with Marfan Syndrome. Journal of Medical Imaging 3: 11–13
Parulekar S 1972 Diverticulosis of the terminal ileum and its complications. Radiology 103: 283–287

SHORT BOWEL

Congenital short bowel with malrotation or non-rotation without atresia is very rare. Survival with a short bowel following surgical excision is becoming increasingly common with improvement in parenteral nutrition. Extensive small bowel resection is defined as removal of at least 30% of the small bowel but resection can involve more than this. The normal bowel length in infants is about 300 cm. It lengthens with age and by adulthood measures approximately 500 cm. Transit time of barium varies enormously in healthy children and ranges between 30 minutes and about 5 hours. Transit time is delayed by a large faecal residue in the colon. It is also significantly influenced by the quantities and type of barium administered, being slower with high density barium administered in small volumes and increased with a large bolus of a dilute rapid transit barium. Transit time can, however, be reliably documented by contrast studies, and this, together with observation of intestinal peristalsis, provides useful information in assessing clinical symptoms that may be related to a short bowel. Symptoms include diarrhoea, malabsorption, pain, recurrent obstruction, anaemia and failure to thrive. There is an increased incidence of gallstones in patients who have had a terminal ileal excision. Renal stones due to excessive resorption of oxalate also occur after ileal resection.

The intestinal transit time is related both to total length of bowel and the length of remaining ileum. The more extensive the ileal excision, the more rapid the transit. Secondary dilatation of the remaining bowel occurs. This is in part related to a general increase in mucosal area which develops as a means of improving nutritional absorption and in part due to the greater volume of intestinal content than normal contained within the shortened segment. Preanastomotic dilatation occurs early after surgery but should not persist. Motility disturbance with spasmodic peristalsis is quite common. Fragmentation of the barium column and transient intussusception have all been noted. There is frequently a change in the mucosal appearance, especially in the ileum, which develops folds more typical of jejunal mucosa. This occurs particularly after jejunal resection. Distension of the segment proximal to the anastomosis should suggest bacterial contamination, especially if contrast passes through the anastomosis easily. If contrast has difficulty in passing the anastomosis, proximal dilatation is more likely to be due to stenosis of the anastomosis. Fistula formation is a further complication and should be carefully looked for at fluoroscopy.

REFERENCES

Howarth E, Hodson C, Joyce C, Pringle E, Solimaro G, Young W 1967 Radiological measurement of small bowel calibre in normal subjects according to age. Clinical Radiology 18: 417–421
Kalifa G, Devred P H, Ricour C, Duhamel J, Fekete C, Sauvegrain J 1979 Radiological aspects of the small bowel after extensive resection in children. Pediatric Radiology 8: 70–75
Pellerin D, Bertin P, Nihoul-Fekete C, Ricour C 1975 Cholelithiasis and ileal pathology in children. Journal of Pediatric Surgery 10: 35–41
Tiu C, Chou Y, Pan H, Chang T 1984 Congenital short bowel. Pediatric Radiology 14: 343–345

MALABSORPTION

The symptoms of malabsorption are mainly failure to thrive, poor weight gain, and frequent stools which classically are described as pale, bulky, offensive and float in the lavatory pan, due to steatorrhoea. Abdominal distension also is present in severe cases. Many of the causes of malabsorption are shown in Table 3.15.6. The clinical symptoms and presentation and biochemical data will often lead to a swift diagnosis. Once a malabsorptive state is clinically suspected, a jejunal biopsy should be carried out jointly by the gastroenterologist and radiologist under fluoroscopic control. The biopsy should be taken when the capsule is in the proximal jejunum. The Crosby capsule is most in favour for small infants but as the child grows older the varying guided systems may be used. The tubing of the capsule may be stiffened by using an angiographic guide-wire which aids manipulation. Aspiration of duodenal contents for enzyme assay and culture may be carried out at the same examination if the capsule is passed with a nasogastric tube.

In most children presenting with clinical symtoms of malabsorption, plain abdominal radiographs are normal. Occasionally, in a fulminant presentation, there will be distended fluid-filled loops of bowel (Fig. 3.12.13). In protein-losing states ascites may be detectable on plain radiographs, but is much more easily detected by ultrasound. Ultrasonic examination is usually normal in malabsorption, but in severe cases, disturbed motility and fluid-filled bowel loops may be found.

Barium studies of the small bowel are rarely conducted nowadays as the primary method for diagnosing malabsorption. Histological studies from the biopsy will be positive earlier than barium studies and are more specific in indicating the precise cause of the malabsorption. However, the radiologist should be able to recognize a malabsorptive pattern on barium examination and be able to consider an appropriate differential diagnosis.

REFERENCES

Ament M E 1972 Malabsorption syndromes in infancy and childhood. Part I. Journal of Pediatrics 81: 685–697
Ament M E 1972 Malabsorption syndromes in infancy and childhood. Part II. Journal of Pediatrics 81: 867–884
Swischuk L, Welsh J 1986 Roentgenographic mucosal patterns in the 'malabsorption syndrome'. A scheme for diagnosis. American Journal of Digestive Diseases 13: 59–78
Tully T, Feinberg S 1974 A roentgenographic classification of diffuse disease of the small intestine presenting with malabsorption. American Journal of Roentgenology 121: 283–290

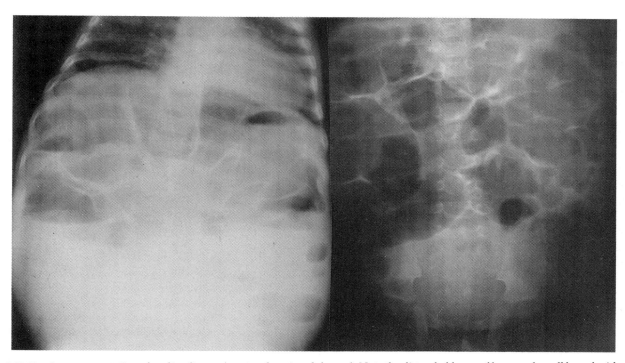

Fig. 3.12.13 Acute presentation of coeliac disease (erect and supine abdomen). Note the distended loops of large and small bowel with multiple fluid levels but no obstructive pattern.

COELIAC DISEASE

Thisis the most common cause of malabsorption and is due to intolerance to gluten protein, found mainly in grain crops. The age of onset of symptoms is variable but most present by 1 year. The severity of symptoms is also variable and ranges from mild to life threatening. The usual symptoms are of bulky, smelly, frequent stools and failure to gain weight. A rare presentation is that of a fulminant onset diarrhoea which can lead to life-threatening dehydration and electrolyte imbalance. With this presentation, a dilated fluid-filled bowel may be seen on plain abdominal radiographs (Fig. 3.12.13). In milder presentations, the plain radiographs are normal or may show mild bowel distension with liquid faeces in the colon. Muscle wasting of the limbs and buttocks with a protuberant abdomen is a classic picture. The degree of abnormality seen on barium studies parallels the clinical severity of the disease. The jejunal and ileal loops are mildly dilated, peristalsis is poor, and transient intussusceptions may be noted (Fig. 3.12.14). The normal feathery mucosal pattern in the jejunum is lost, to be replaced by a featureless bowel most commonly, so that it is difficult to distinguish jejunum and ileum. Occasionally, mildly thickened folds are visible (Fig. 3.12.14). The hallmark of malabsorption is fragmentation of the column of barium with flocculation. The fragmentation and flocculation are most prominent in the distal jejunum and ileum. There is failure to clear the barium normally from proximal bowel loops, leaving a stippled appearance due to small lumps of barium (Fig. 3.12.15B). The excess bowel secretions are responsible for all these changes. In spite of the clinical presentation of frequent stools, transit time is delayed to a variable degree on barium studies. Once treatment is instituted there is a rapid return to a normal appearances.

Children with coeliac disease have an increased incidence of lymphoma and carcinoma in later life.

Non-tropical sprue

Originally described as a gluten enteropathy which presents in adolesence or adulthood, and thought to represent a different condition to coeliac disease, it is now regarded as the same condition as coeliac disease, with a similar cause. Symptoms include steatorrhoea, weakness, weight loss and anorexia.

Tropical sprue

This is a form of malabsorption relatively common in the tropics with similar clinical, radiological and biopsy findings to gluten enteropathy (coeliac disease), but the patients do not respond to a gluten-free diet. Treatment is with tetracycline and folic acid.

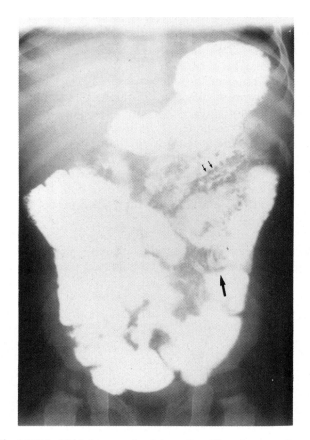

Fig. 3.12.14 Mild changes of malabsorption. There is coarsening of the jejunal folds and a transient intussusception (arrow).

REFERENCES

Anderson C, Astley R, French J, Gerrard J 1952 The small intesine in coeliac disease. British Journal of Radiology 25: 526–530

Collins S, Hamilton J, Lewis T, Laufer I 1978 Small-bowel malabsorption and gastrointestinal malignancy. Radiology 126: 603–609

Howarth E, Hodson C, Pringle E, Young W 1986 The value of radiological investigations of the alimentary tract in children with the coeliac syndrome. Clinical Radiology 19: 65–76

EOSINOPHILIC GASTROENTERITIS

Eosinophilic gastroenteritis is a disease mainly of adults but with sporadic reports of presentation in childhood. Pathologically there is infiltration of the gastrointestinal tract, mainly the stomach and small intestine, by eosinophils, with a peripheral eosinophilia. Involvement of oesophagus and colon is rare. Both the muscle layer and the serosa may be infiltrated. Clinical presentation depends on the site of involvement. Nausea, vomiting, periumbilical cramping pain, loose stools, watery diarrhoea, failure to thrive, weight loss, anaemia, and steatorrhoea are all described with small bowel involvement. The disease, in an individual patient, may present with acute exacerbations and quiescent periods. There is frequently an associated history of atopy in the family and the patient, but specific allergens in an individual patient are not normally identified.

Radiologically, stomach involvement is manifest by nodularity in the mucosa and rigidity of the gastric outlet when there is muscle wall involvement. In the small bowel, there is thickening of the walls of affected segments, with widening of the mucosal folds and sometimes a nodular mucosal pattern, especially in the duodenum. The combination of the radiological findings with the peripheral eosinophilia should lead to the correct diagnosis. Treatment is with steroids which effects both clinical and radiological improvement.

REFERENCES

Jona J, Belin R, Burke J 1976 Eosinophilic infiltration of the gastrointestinal tract in children. American Journal of Diseases of Children 130: 1136–1139

Matzinger M, Daneman A 1983 Esophageal involvement in eosinophilic gastroenteritis. Pediatric Radiology 13: 35–38

Schulman A, Morton P, Dietrich B 1980 Eosinophilic gastroenteritis. Clinical Radiology 31: 101–104

Teele R, Katz A, Goldman H, Kettell R 1979 Radiographic features of eosinophilic gastroenteritis (allergic gastroenteropathy) of childhood. American Journal of Roentgenology 132: 575–580

ALLERGIC ENTEROPATHY

Allergy to a variety of food proteins may produce malabsorption. Cows' milk allergy is probably the most frequently encountered. The child presents with some or all of the following symptoms – diarrhoea, failure to thrive, vomiting, macroscopic and occult blood loss, protein-losing enteropathy, eczema and respiratory symptoms with occasionally near fatal bronchospasm. Occasionally, it can present as acute intestinal obstruction. Unlike gluten enteropathy of coeliac disease, where barium examination is usually abnormal, barium studies in cows' milk allergic enteropathy are normal.

REFERENCES

Iyngkaran N, Robinson M, Prathap K, Sumithran E, Yadau M 1978 Cows' milk protein-sensitive enteropathy. Archives of Disease in Childhood 53: 20–26

Kuitunen P, Visakorpi J, Savilhati E, Pelkoneni P 1975 Malabsorption syndrome with cows' milk intolerance. Archives of Disease in Childhood 50: 351–356

Mcilhenny J, Sutphen J, Block C 1988 Food allergy presenting as obstruction in an infant. American Journal of Roentgenology 150: 373–375

DISACCHARIDASE DEFICIENCY

Normal carbohydrate absorption requires normal enzyme activity in the salivary glands, pancreas and intestinal mucosa. Dietary carbohydrate contains many disaccharides which have to be reduced to monosaccharides in the intestine for normal absorption. Lactase, maltase and sucrase are the intestinal disaccharides responsible for carbohydrate absorption. Congenital deficiency of any one of these may occur as an inborn error of metabolism, or deficiency may be acquired secondary to small bowel disease. In clinical practice, lactase deficiency, acquired or congenital, is common and renders the patient intolerant to milk or dairy products. Symptoms of diarrhoea, abdominal bloating and cramp are the most frequent. Diagnosis is by enzyme assay of the intestinal juices recovered by intubation or biopsy. The diagnosis can be made by barium examination of the small bowel. 50 g of lactose is added to the barium prior to oral administration (Fig. 3.12.15). In normal children, this has no effect on the small bowel pattern. In children deficient in lactase, the barium is diluted, the bowel distended and there is rapid transit with cramps.

REFERENCE

Tully T, Feinberg S 1974 A roentgenographic classification of diffuse diseases of the small intestine presenting with malabsorption. American Journal of Roentgenology 121: 283–290

HEREDITARY ANGIONEUROTIC OEDEMA

This is a rare familial disorder in which the child presents in mid to late childhood with episodes of oedema of the skin, mucous membranes and viscera, which causes cramping abdominal pain. The latter may occur as a presenting symptom. If barium studies are done during an acute attack, bowel oedema with mucosal thickening and separation of loops of bowel are seen. Onset of symptoms is usually in mid to late childhood. Laryngeal involvement can lead to death.

REFERENCE

Pearson K, Buchignani J, Shimkin P, Frank M M 1972 Hereditary angioneurotic edema of the gastrointestinal tract. American Journal of Roentgenology 116: 256–261

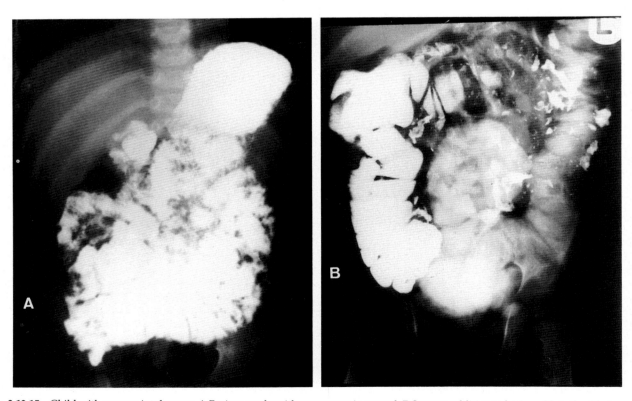

Fig. 3.12.15   Child with sucrose intolerance. **A** Barium study without sucrose is normal. **B** Sucrose addition to barium. Note the dilution of the barium, and retention of flocculated barium in the small bowel with failure of normal clearing. These are typical features of malabsorption.

ABETALIPOPROTEINAEMIA

This is an autosomal recessive disease in which the child develops steatorrhoea, retinitis pigmentosa, acanthocytosis and progressive neurological deterioration. The presenting features are usually steatorrhoea, abdominal distension and failure to thrive, in most cases leading to a clinical diagnosis of coeliac disease initially, but mucosal biopsy is diagnostic, the cytoplasm being filled with triglycerides. Thickening of the mucosa of the duodenum and jejunum with some dilution and clumping are found at barium examination.

REFERENCE

Weinstein M, Pearson K, Agus S 1973 Abetalipoproteinaemia. Radiology 108: 269–273

LYMPHANGIECTASIA OF BOWEL

Intestinal lymphangiectasia is a developmental abnormality of the intestinal lymphatics which results in excessive loss of protein into the bowel lumen in the small intestine. When severe the patient presents with symptoms of malabsorption, failure to thrive, and peripheral oedema secondary to the hypoproteinaemia. Chylous ascites occurs in some patients. Though a congenital defect, symptoms may start at any stage in childhood. The earlier symptoms start, the worse the prognosis.

Intestinal disease may be isolated or may occur as part of a more generalized disease with involvement of the lungs, the limbs or bones, or in Noonan's syndrome, or neurofibromatosis.

The definitive diagnosis is made by jejunal biopsy. Dilated lymphatic channels are visible within the mucosa, distorting the villi, macroscopically. Hypoproteinaemia, diminished immunoglobulin levels and lymphocytopenia are other laboratory findings.

At barium examination, diffuse thickening of the valvulae conniventes is seen in the majority of patients. The calibre of the bowel lumen is normal or minimally dilated. Dilution of barium, as seen in malabsorptive states, is not a feature, and if present is very mild (Fig. 3.12.14). There is often a disturbance of peristalsis with a to-and-fro pattern.

The differential diagnosis includes those other diseases that produce mucosal thickening and hypoproteinaemia without significant dilatation of the bowel lumen or dilution of the barium. The two main ones are nephrotic syndrome and cirrhosis of the liver.

There has been a report of a 15-year-old boy with constrictive pericarditis in association with intestinal lymphangiectasia and immunoglobulin deficiency whose symptoms disappeared and immunodeficiency resolved following pericardectomy. Chronic malrotation can lead to lymphatic obstruction.

Other causes of protein-losing enteropathy include allergic gastroenteropathy, regional enteritis, infectious mononucleosis, polyarteritis nodosa, systemic lupus erythematosus, progressive systemic sclerosis, neuroblastoma, giardiasis, graft-versus-host disease, eosinophilic gastroenteritis and immunodeficiency syndromes. The clinical and laboratory data usually serve to distinguish the lesions.

REFERENCES

Butler M, Carlton L, De Green H, Teplick S, Metz J 1974 Transient malabsorption in infectious mononucleosis. American Journal of Roentgenology 122: 241–244

Fisher C, Oh K, Bayless T, Siegelman S 1975 Current perspectives on giardiasis. American Journal of Roentgenology 125: 207–217

Gerdes J, Katz A J 1982 Neuroblastoma appearing as protein-losing enteropathy. American Journal of Diseases of Children 136: 1024–1025

Gorske K, Winchester P, Grossman H 1969 Unusual protein losing enteropathies in children. Radiology 92: 739–744

Herzog D, Logan R, Kooistra J 1976 The Noonan syndrome with intestinal lymphangiectasia. Journal of Pediatrics 88: 270–272

Nelson D, Blaese R, Strober W, Bruce R, Waldmann T 1975 Constrictive pericarditis, intestinal lymphangiectasia, and reversible immunologic deficiency. Journal of Pediatrics 86: 548–554

Schussheim A 1972 Protein-losing enteropathies in children. American Journal of Gastroenterology 58: 124–132

Shimkin P, Waldmann T, Krugman R 1970 Intestinal lymphangiectasia. American Journal of Roentgenology 110: 827–841

Tsukahara M, Matsuo K, Kojima H 1980 Protein losing enteropathy in a boy with systemic lupus erythematosus. Journal of Pediatrics 97: 778–780

HAEMANGIOMATOSIS OF THE BOWEL

Gastrointestinal haemangiomas may be multiple, small and scattered throughout the gastrointestinal tract, or may be solitary, large, cavernous haemangiomas. Either may present with intestinal bleeding which can be life threatening. The larger ones may act as a lead point of an intussusception or cause intestinal obstruction. Skin lesions may be associated. Haemangiomas are difficult to diagnose radiologically and may be invisible at laparatomy. Plain radiographs are usually normal, or show a degree of ileus if there has been a large bleed. Large lesions, usually hypoechoic, may be identified by ultrasound examination. Occasionally, phleboliths are seen on the plain radiograph. Thumb printing due to mucosal oedema, and intraluminal filling defects due to blood clots may be seen on barium studies but these are usually normal. Dynamic CT may show contrast medium enhancement of the bowel wall if prior administration of oral contrast medium is omitted. They are a cause of a false-positive scan during scintigraphy for Meckel's diverticulum. Labelled red blood cell scintigraphy will frequently show the presence of bleeding and localize it to a quadrant of the abdomen (Fig. 3.12.16), improving localization at surgery or suggesting the correct vessel for selective angiography.

Solitary lesions are best treated by surgical excision. Embolization of bleeding points is the preferred treatment for multiple lesions.

Apart from general disease such as hereditary telangiectasia, gastrointestinal haemangiomas in children are found in association with the blue rubberbled naevus syndrome, Klippel–Trenauney–Weber syndrome, Maffucci's syndrome and diffuse neonatal haemangiomatosis.

REFERENCES

Baker A, Kahn P, Binder S, Patterson J 1971 Gastrointestinal bleeding due to blue rubber bled naevus syndrome. Gastroenterology 61: 530–534

Bank E, Hernandez R, Byrne W 1987 Gastrointestinal haemangiomatosis in children: demonstration with CT. Radiology 165: 657–658

Dorfman G, Dronan J, Staudinger K 1987 Scintigraphic signs and pitfalls in lower gastrointestinal hemorrhage: the continued necessity of angiography. Radiographics 7: 543–562

Lewis R, Ketcham A 1973 Maffucci's syndrome: functional and neoplastic significance. Journal of Bone and Joint Surgery 55: 1465–1479

Smith R, Copely D, Bolen F 1987 Tc99m RBC scintigraphy: correlation of gastrointestinal bleeding rates with scintigraphic findings. American Journal of Roentgenology 148: 869–874

Stillman A, Hansen R, Hallinan V, Strobel C 1983 Diffuse neonatal haemangiomatosis with severe gastrointestinal involvement. Clinical Pediatrics 22: 589–591

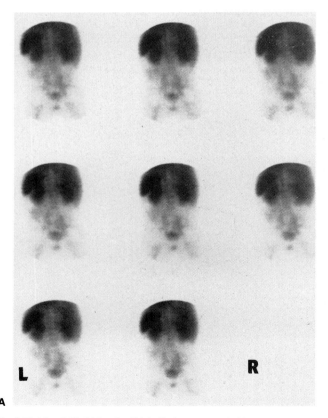

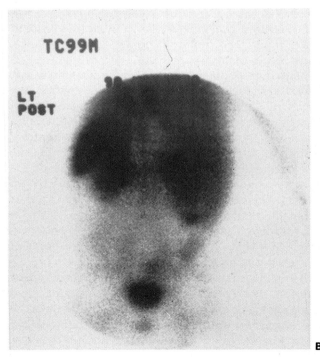

Fig. 3.12.16 **A** Red blood cell labelled scan in a child with recurrent gastrointestinal bleeding following bone marrow transplant. The images are taken at 5-minute intervals. Note the appearance of increased activity in the right iliac fossa during the sequential images. **B** A magnified view shows this to be in bowel. At surgery a 10-cm length of ileum was excised. At histology, there was a diffuse capillary angiomatous malformation of the mucosa.

WHIPPLE'S DISEASE

This is a bacterial disease largely found in adult practice but with occasional presentation in childhood. It is characterized by clinical features of intermittent arthritis, abdominal pain, weight loss and steatorrhoea. The diagnosis is made by biopsy with the finding of large macrophages filled with glycoprotein which are PAS positive. Radiologically, the findings are non-specific. There is mild to moderate thickening of the mucosal folds of the small bowel.

REFERENCES

Bayless T, Knox D 1979 Whipple's disease: a multisystem infection. New England Journal of Medicine 300: 920–921
Philips R, Carlson H 1975 The roentgenographic and clinical findings in Whipple's disease. American Journal of Roentgenology 123: 268–273

PROTEIN-LOSING ENTEROPATHY

Causes of protein-losing enteropathy include intestinal lymphangiectasia, occasionally in association with Noonan's syndrome, allergic gastroenteropathy, neuroblastoma, Whipple's disease, infectious mononucleosis, Crohn's disease, systemic lupus erythematosus, scleroderma, other collagen diseases, constrictive pericarditis, Menetrier's disease, ulcerative colitis and giardiasis.

The radiological findings attributable to the protein loss are similar, with thickened mucosal folds, and loss of normal motility. There may be additional features of the specific disease to aid diagnosis, but the general findings are non-specific.

REFERENCES

Burke J 1975 Giardiasis in childhood. American Journal of Diseases of Children 129: 1304–1310
Butler M, Carlton L, Degreen H, Teplick S, Metz J 1974 Transient malabsorption in infectious mononucleosis. American Journal of Roentgenology 122: 241–244
Gerdes J, Katz A 1982 Neuroblastoma appearing as a protein-losing enteropathy. American Journal of Diseases of Children 136: 1024–1025
Gorske K, Winchester P, Grossman H 1969 Unusual protein-losing enteropathies in childhood. Radiology 92: 739–744
Herzog D, Logan R, Kooistra J 1976 The Noonan syndrome with intestinal lymphangiectasis. Journal of Pediatrics 88: 270–272
Nelson D, Blaese R, Strober W, Bruce R, Waldmann T 1975 Constrictive pericarditis, intestinal lymphangiectasia, and reversible immunological deficiency. Journal of Pediatrics 86: 548–554
Tsukahara M, Matsuo K, Kojima H 1980 Protein losing enteropathy in a boy with systemic lupus erythematosus. Journal of Pediatrics 97: 778–780

KWASHIORKOR

Rarely do children with kwashiorkor undergo radiology, as the diagnosis is usually all too evident clinically. Small bowel studies have shown bowel dilatation, fragmentation and flocculation of the barium as seen in gluten enteropathy.

REFERENCE

Kowalski R 1967 Roentgenologic studies of the alimentary tract in kwashiorkor. American Journal of Roentgenology 100: 100–112

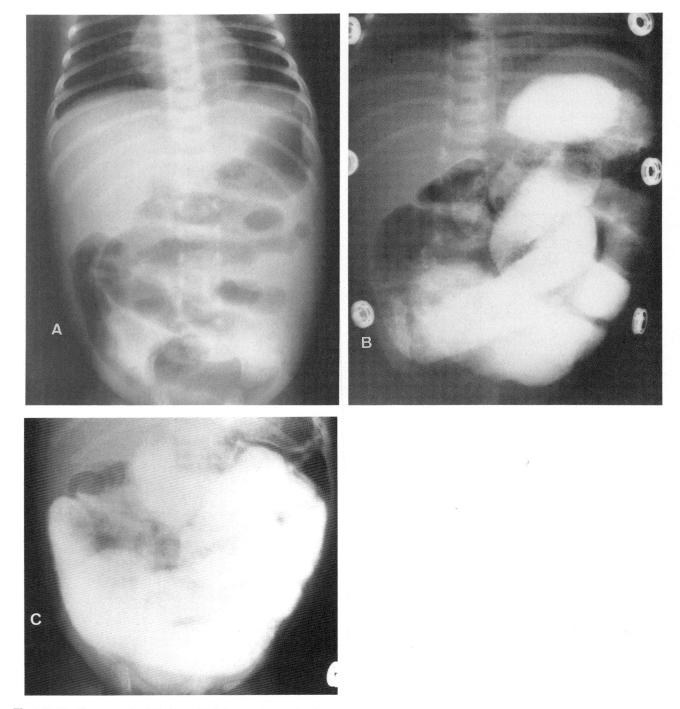

Fig. 3.12.17   Three-month-old infant with failure to thrive, diarrhoea and perineal ulceration. The eventual diagnosis was that of a complex immunodeficiency. **A** Plain abdomen with thickening of the bowel wall, separation of the loops and distension. At ultrasound there was ascites. **B**, **C** Two views from a barium follow-through showing dilated featureless bowel.

IMMUNODEFICIENCY SYNDROMES

In many patients with immunodeficiency, and, in particular, those with IGA deficiency, there are clinical symptoms of malabsorption and, occasionally, pseudo-obstruction (Fig. 3.12.17). Some of these children are infected with *Giardia lamblia* or strongyloides, which may be recovered from the stools. The radiological features are similar to those found in general malabsorptive states.

Giardiasis

While giardia affects immunocompromised children, it can also affect immunologically competent patients and presents with diarrhoea and symptoms of malabsorption (Fig. 3.12.18). Severe protein loss may occur with severe infestation. The radiological signs are non-specific and resemble those in other malabsorptive states.

REFERENCES

Burke J 1975 Giardiasis in childhood. American Journal of Diseases of Children 129: 1304–1310
Logalbo P, Sampson H, Buckley R 1982 Symptomatic giardiasis in 3 patients with X-linked agammaglobulinaemia. Journal of Pediatrics 101: 78–80

ENDOCRINE DISEASE

Bowel manifestations of endocrine disease in childhood are rare, with the exception of intestinal symptoms associated with neuroblastoma, from vasoactive polypeptides. Diarrhoea is a feature of hyperthyroidism and constipation of hypothyroidism. Diarrhoea and malabsorption are reported in a few cases of longstanding childhood-onset diabetes mellitus, probably attributable to a neuropathy. Acute gastric dilatation may be seen in diabetic ketoacidosis. Oesophageal stricture, possibly due to reflux oesophagitis during coma associated with ketoacidosis, has been occasionally reported. There are also rare reports of mild malabsorption states in association with hypoadrenalism, primary hypoparathyroidism, pseudohypoparathyroidism and the Zollinger–Ellison syndrome.

REFERENCES

Campbell J 1982 The small bowel, diffuse diseases. In: Franker E A (ed) Gastrointestinal imaging in pediatrics. Harper & Row, Philadelphia, pp 222–223

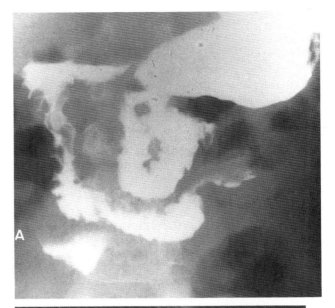

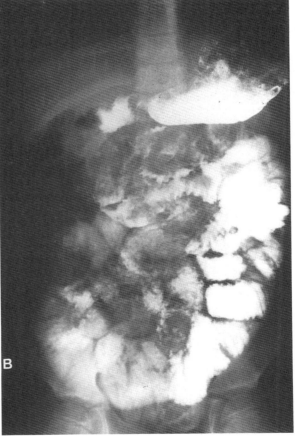

Fig. 3.12.18 Twelve-year-old boy with abdominal pain and diarrhoea due to proven giardiasis. All symptoms resolved following treatment. **A** Coarsening of the duodenal folds due to duodenitis. **B** Malabsorptive pattern with dilated loops of bowel, dilution of barium and coarsening of the mucosal folds. (Courtesy of Dr Chandran, Leighton Hospital, Crewe.)

BLIND LOOP SYNDROME

The small bowel has very little indigenous flora. If a segment is isolated from normal peristaltic activity, bacterial overgrowth may occur with resulting stasis and lead to malabsorptive symptoms which may be accompanied by vitamin B_{12} deficiency. Causes include inadvertent incorrect surgical anastomosis, fistula formation and, probably most commonly, partial isolation of a loop by adhesions (Fig. 3.12.19). Barium studies are the most reliable method of demonstrating the abnormal loop, but these must be done with great care under fluoroscopic control if the problem is to be identified. Management is surgical to relieve the abnormal intestinal circulation.

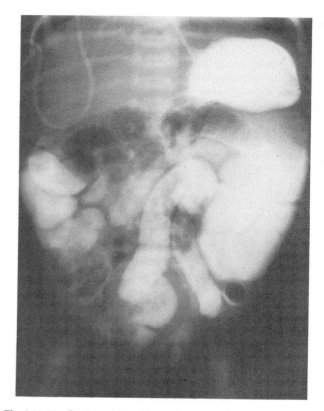

Fig. 3.12.19 Contrast follow-through on a child presenting with anaemia, diarrhoea and abdominal pain. Previous neonatal abdominal surgery for resection of ileal atresia. There is a large distended loop of bowel in the left abdomen, which at surgery was a loop of proximal ileum which was partially obstructed by adhesions. Following relief of the obstruction and antibiotics to cure the contamination in the trapped loop, the child made a full recovery.

SHWACHMAN'S SYNDROME

Pancreatic insufficiency associated with thymo-lymphopenia and metaphyseal chondrodysplasia is known as Shwachman-Diamond syndrome.

Children with this syndrome have short stature, failure to thrive, steatorrhoea and some, though not all, have chondrodysplasia of the metaphyses, mainly at the proximal femora and knees. The steatorrhoea varies in severity, as does the neutropenia.

REFERENCES

Shwachman H, Diamond L, Oski F 1964 The syndrome of pancreatic insufficiency and bone marrow dysfunction. Journal of Pediatrics 65: 645–663
Stanley P, Sutcliffe J 1973 Metaphyseal chondrodysplasia with dwarfism, pancreatic insufficiency and neutropenia. Pediatric Radiology 1: 119–126

COLLAGEN DISEASES

Small bowel involvement in the varied collagen diseases is usually only seen after many years of the clinical disease. Therefore, manifestations are rare in childhood. The bowel becomes infiltrated and loses its normal motility. The patient complains of pain, diarrhoea and weight loss. Small bowel barium examination will show thickening of the mucosal folds, separation of the loops, and pseudodiverticula on the antimesenteric border. Stress peptic ulcers with perforation are a well-known complication of steroid treatment of the disease.

REFERENCE

Magill H, Hixson S, Whitington G, Igarashi M, Hannissian A 1984 Duodenal perforation in childhood dermatomyositis. Pediatric Radiology 14: 28–30

GRAFT-VERSUS-HOST DISEASE

Gastrointestinal inflammation after allogenic bone marrow transplantation may be due to acute graft-versus-host disease or superinfection with viral or bacterial opportunistic infections. The infecting organisms include rotavirus, coxsackie and adenovirus. In graft-versus-host disease there is severe mucosal inflammation of the gastrointestinal tract with profuse watery diarrhoea. Involvement of the gastrointestinal tract is usually accompanied by skin and other systemic manifestations. Findings on barium studies include gastric atony, dilatation, retained secretions and delayed emptying, antral deformity, thickening of the mucosal folds in the duodenum, effacement of the folds, or replacement of the normal folds by a shaggy contour. Similar changes occur in the small bowel, with, in addition, separation of the loops and ribbon-like loops. Intestinal pneumatosis has also been reported. In the colon, there is enlargement of the haustral folds, or loss of the normal pattern, mucosal ulceration and spasm. The degree of involvement and the radiological findings are very variable. It is impossible to differentiate graft-versus-host disease from graft-versus-host disease with superinfection on radiological grounds.

REFERENCES

Jones B, Kramer S, Saràl R, Beschorner W, Yolken R, Townsend T, Yeager A, Lake A, Tutschka P, Santos G 1988 Gastrointestinal inflammation after bone marrow transplantation: graft-versus-host disease or opportunistic infection. American Journal of Roentgenology 150: 277–281
Yeager A, Kanof M, Kramer S, Jones B, Saral R, Lake A, Santos G 1987 Pneumatosis intestinalis in children after allogeneic bone marrow transplantation. Pediatric Radiology 17: 18–22

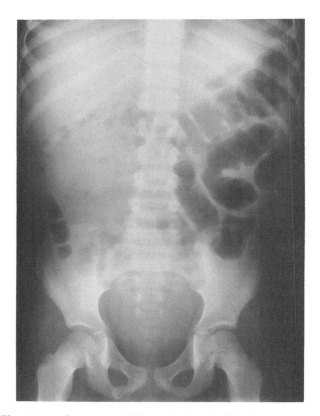

Fig. 3.12.20 Seven-year-old boy with Henoch–Schönlein purpura. The plain abdominal features are a localized ileus in the left abdomen with oedema of the bowel wall and some pneumatosis. The radiographic appearances are non-specific and could occur with the haemolytic uraemic syndrome or infarction.

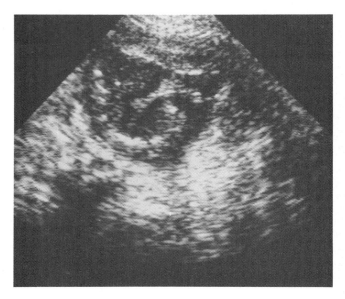

Fig. 3.12.21 Ultrasound of the affected region shows thickening of the bowel wall.

HAEMOLYTIC URAEMIC SYNDROME

The haemolytic uraemic syndrome, a condition of variable severity, encompasses haemolytic anaemia, thrombocytopenia and renal failure. A small number of patients present with gastrointestinal symptoms before the onset of the other manifestations. The abnormal symptoms include pain, vomiting, diarrhoea which may be bloody, and rectal bleeding. Both small and large bowel may be affected. Radiographic features on plain abdominal film include submucosal oedema with 'thumbprinting' (Figs. 3.12.20, 3.12.21), segmental ischaemic changes and ileus or obstruction if the oedema is very severe. On contrast studies of the small or large bowel submucosal oedema, spasm and mucosal ulceration may be seen (Fig. 3.12.22). Colonic strictures may form as a result of the ischaemia. The radiological features may be indistinguishable from those seen in Henoch–Schönlein purpura.

REFERENCES

Kawanami T, Bowen A, Girdany B 1984 Enterocolitis: prodrome of the haemolytic uraemic syndrome. Radiology 151: 91–92
Kirks D 1982 The radiology of enteritis due to hemolytic-uremic syndrome. Pediatric Radiology 12: 179–183

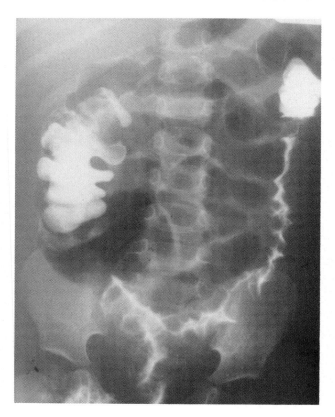

Fig. 3.12.22 Ischaemic colitis in a girl with haemolytic uraemic syndrome. The child presented with abdominal pain and blood per rectum. There is severe mucosal oedema, and a long colonic stricture due to the vascular insult. Note also dilated thickened small bowel.

HENOCH–SCHÖNLEIN PURPURA (ANAPHYLACTOID PURPURA)

Gastrointestinal manifestations of abdominal pain, vomiting and bloody diarrhoea may precede cutaneous lesions, leading to diagnostic confusion. Purpuric patches in the gut may lead to intussusception. In severe cases with small bowel involvement, barium studies will show changes very similar to those in Crohn's disease; areas of stenosis and dilatation, separation of bowel loops due to oedema, thickening of the mucosal folds and filling defects due to the submucosal haematomas. Transient intussusception may be observed during the examination. Many of the radiological features resolve with steroid treatment.

REFERENCE

Glasier C, Siegel M, McAlister W, Shackelford G 1981 Henoch–Schonlein syndrome in children: gastro intestinal manifestations. American Journal of Roentgenology 136: 1081–1085

DISTAL ILEAL OBSTRUCTION SYNDROME (MECONIUM ILEUS EQUIVALENT)

Children with cystic fibrosis require pancreatic enzyme supplements. Inadequate supplementation, or failure to take the enzymes, can lead to impaction of undigested food in the ileum, with obstruction. Complaints are of abdominal bloating, constipation and cramping pain. If the partial obstruction is not relieved, frank small bowel obstruction may follow. On the plain radiographs there is a mass of inspissated faecal material in the region of the terminal ileum and caecum (Figs. 3.12.23, 3.12.24), with variable distension of the proximal small bowel. The faecal mass is often palpable in the right iliac fossa.

The obstruction may be relieved by oral gastrografin, adjusting the enzyme intake and the administration of N-acetylcysteine. In severe cases repeated gastrografin enemas may also relieve the obstruction, but large volumes of fluid will be required, and the child will require constant coaxing to retain the fluid.

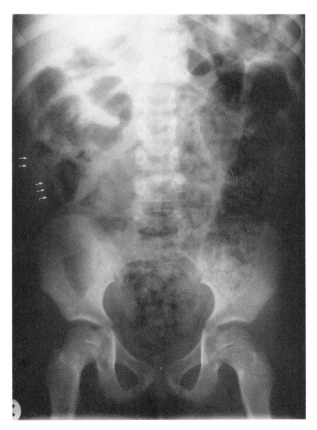

Fig. 3.12.23   Girl with cystic fibrosis. The whole of the colon is full of bubbly faecal content, typical of children with cystic fibrosis and inadequate pancreatic supplementation. She has a high caecum (arrows) due to neonatal resection. There is a little proximal small bowel dilatation.

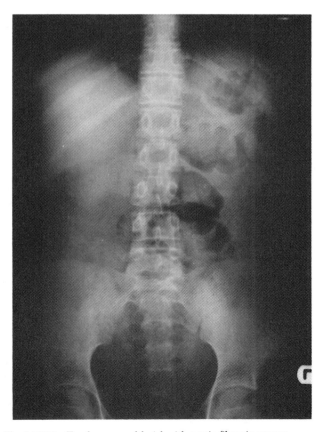

Fig. 3.12.24   Twelve-year-old girl with cystic fibrosis, severe recurrent abdominal pain and right iliac fossa mass. The right abdomen has bowel packed with thick faeces. There is little air mixed with the faeces making it difficult to see.

The aim is to get the contrast medium proximal to the impaction and into the ileum. Several enemas may be required, each one relieving part of the obstruction. Gastrografin diluted 1:1 with warm water is an appropriate contrast medium.

Children with cystic fibrosis may have other causes of abdominal pain, which should be excluded before attributing the cause of pain to the distal ileal obstruction syndrome. Such causes include duodenitis, appendicitis, ovarian cyst, gallstones, volvulus around adhesions, and strictures due to previous surgery and associated other pathology such as Crohn's disease (Fig. 3.12.25). Careful scrutiny of plain radiographs, and ultrasound examination of the abdomen is essential.

Most children who present with the distal ileal obstruction syndrome are known to have cystic fibrosis, but occasionally it may be the presenting symptom. Intussusception is a complication of cystic fibrosis, with the inspissated bowel content forming the lead point.

REFERENCE

Baxter P, Dickson J, Variend S, Taylor C 1988 Intestinal disease in cystic fibrosis. Archives of Disease in Childhood 63: 1496–1497

Dalzell A, Heaf D, Carty H 1990 Pathology mimicking distal intestinal obstruction syndrome in cystic fibrosis. Archives of Disease in Childhood 65: 540–541

Djurhuus M, Lykkegaard E, Pock-Steen O 1973 Gastrointestinal radiological findings in cystic fibrosis. Pediatrics Radiology 1: 113–118

O'Halloran S, Gilbert J, McKendrick O, Carty H, Heaf D 1986 Gastrografin in acute meconium ileus equivalent. Archives of Disease in Childhood 61: 1128–1130

Pilling DW, Steiner GM 1981. The radiology of meconium ileus equivalent. British Journal of Radiology 54: 562–565

Willi U, Reddish J, Teele R 1980 Cystic fibrosis: its characteristic appearance on abdominal sonography. American Journal of Roentgenology 134: 1005–1010

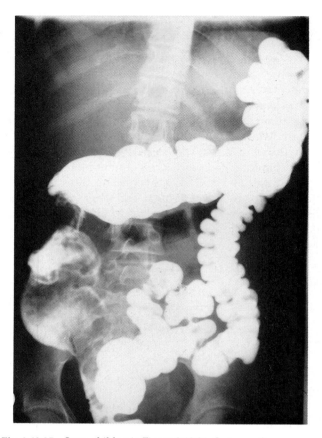

Fig. 3.12.25 Same child as in Figure 3.12.24. Gastrografin enema done to relieve the obstruction. This shows a stricture in the high ascending colon with proximal faecal impaction. At histology, this proved to be a Crohn's stricture.

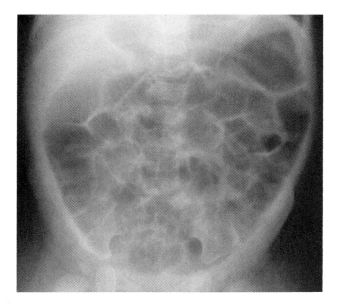

Fig. 3.12.26 Seven-month-infant with profuse watery diarrhoea. There is a gaseous distension of the whole of the large and small bowel. No evidence of bowel wall oedema. This is one pattern seen in gastroenteritis.

GASTROENTERITIS

Bacterial infection of the bowel, with vomiting and diarrhoea, is a common cause for hospital admission. Incorrectly treated gastroenteritis may be life threatening, with dehydration and even death. In clinically obvious cases, the child does not present for radiological investigation. Many children, however, have atypical clinical presentations and may present with abdominal distension without diarrhoea, or abdominal distension with confusing bowel sounds, or even bloody diarrhoea. The clinical problem is to exclude an underlying sepsis such as abscess or appendicitis, or an atypical mechanical obstruction. Plain radiographs show a very variable pattern, most frequently an ileus with gas distributed throughout the bowel (Fig. 3.12.26), with long air fluid levels in fluid-filled rather than air-filled distended bowel as is found in mechanical obstruction. In some, the features mimic mechanical obstruction (Fig. 3.12.27). In a small number of children there may be a gasless distended abdomen due to fluid-filled loops of bowel. In others, the abdomen may be almost gasless with short fluid levels in collapsed bowel (Fig. 3.12.28). The patterns are non-specific and can be very bizarre.

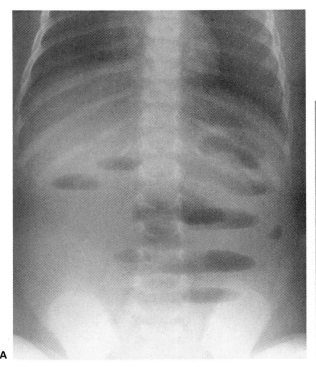

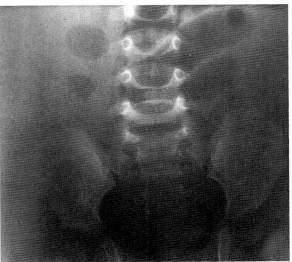

A   **B**

Fig. 3.12.27 Erect **A** and supine **B** abdomen in a very ill child with gastroenteritis. The supine film shows a few distended oedematous loops of small bowel in an almost gasless abdomen. Multiple long fluid levels are present in well-separated loops of bowel. There is distension of the flank stripes due to the fluid within the bowel.

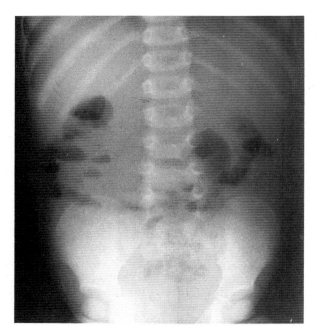

Fig. 3.12.28 Two-year-old boy with gastroenteritis. The abdomen contains very little gas. There are multiple short fluid levels in collapsed small bowel and transverse colon. This is a further pattern of gastroenteritis.

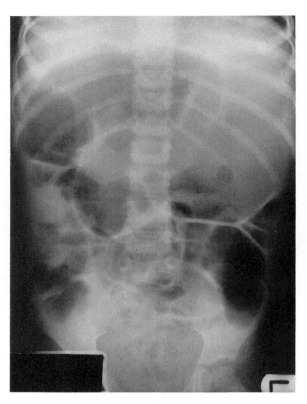

Fig. 3.12.29 Cryptosporidium gastroenteritis. There is marked gaseous distension of the transverse colon but no oedema of the bowel wall. This pattern is not specific to cryptosporidium infection but could occur with any gastroenteritic infection.

The radiological features may precede the onset of diarrhoea, or persist as clinical recovery takes place. In most cases there is no pattern specific to the infecting organism on stool culture. Cryptosporidium infection tends to produce severe distension of the large bowel (Fig. 3.12.29). In any child it is prudent to carry out an ultrasound examination to exclude an abscess or a missed appendicitis. Distended fluid-filled bowel loops are found in gastroenteritis. There may be a small amount of free fluid due to a transudate from the inflamed bowel.

Secondary malabsorption may follow severe gastroenteritis due to mucosal damage. Rarely, a necrotizing pattern is found on the plain abdominal radiograph secondary to severe gastroenteritis (Fig. 3.12.30).

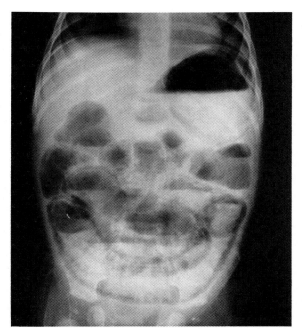

Fig. 3.12.30 Infant from the Middle East with gastroenteritis which was fatal. There is pneumatosis of both stomach and the entire small bowel.

SPECIFIC INFECTIONS

There are increasing reports of radiological abnormalities associated with specific organisms such as *Yersinia enterolytica*, campylobacter, cytomegalovirus, salmonella and *Salmonella typhi*.

Salmonella typhi

Thickening of the walls of the caecum and terminal ileum with mesenteric lymph gland enlargement is common in *Salmonella typhi*, but is seen also in campylobacter and yersinia infection. Life-threatening haemorrhage can occur due to necrosis and mucosal sloughing of affected bowel.

Yersinia enterocolitica

Infection with *Yersinia enterocolitica* can be radiologically and clinically indistinguishable from Crohn's disease with ulceration of the terminal ileum and colon. Affected children may have joint and ocular involvement.

Salmonellosis

Salmonella infection may cause lymph gland enlargement and hepatosplenomegaly which mimic lymphoma.

Cytomegalovirus infection

Infection with cytomegalovirus can lead to inflammatory lesions in any portion of the gastrointestinal tract where it may be associated with other infecting organisms such as candida. In all areas mucosal ulceration may be seen, with loss of normal mucosal folds, interruption of normal peristalsis and thickening of the mucosal folds in the small bowel. Ulceration may be deep and lead to profound haemorrhage. Cytomegalovirus infection is found in immunosuppressed debilitated patients and is common in AIDS. Pyloric outlet obstruction and thickening of the pyloric mucosa has also been noted.

Campylobacter

Infection with campylobacter may produce bloody diarrhoea with a proctocolitis indistinguishable from idiopathic ulcerative colitis, although the caecum and terminal ileum may also be affected.

Sonographically, thickening of the walls of the caecum and terminal ileum and lymph node enlargement are found in infection with campylobacter and *Salmonella typhi*.

REFERENCES

Blaser M, Reller L 1981 Campylobacter enteritis. New England Journal of Medicine 305: 1444–1452
Bradford B, Abdenour G, Frank J, Scott G, Beerman R 1988 Usual and unusual radiologic manifestations of acquired immunodeficiency syndrome (AIDS) and human immunodeficiency virus (HIV) infection in children. Radiologic Clinics of North America 26: 341–353
Brodey P, Fertig S, Aron J 1982 Campylobacter enterocolitis: radiographic features. American Journal of Roentgenology 139: 1199–1201
Haney P, Yale-Loehr A, Nussbaum A, Gellad F 1989 Imaging of infants and children with AIDS. American Journal of Roentgenology 152: 1033–1041
Kohl S, Jacobson J, Nahmias A 1976 Yersinia enterocolitica infections in children. Journal of Pediatrics 89: 77–79
Mahmoud H, Magill L, Pui C-H 1990 Salmonellosis mimicking abdominal lymphoma in a young boy. Pediatric Radiology 20: 193
Puylaert J, Kristjansdottir S, Golterman K, De Jong G, Kneckt N 1989 Typhoid fever: diagnosis by using sonography. American Journal of Roentgenology 153: 745–746
Rubin C, Fairhurst J 1988 Life-threatening haemorrhage from typhoid fever. British Journal of radiology 61: 415–416
Shrago G 1976 Yersinia enterocolitica ileocolitis findings observed on barium examination. British Journal of Radiology 49: 181–183
Teixidor H, Honig C, Norsoph E, Albert S, Mouradian J, Whalen J 1987 Cytomegalovirus infection of the alimentary canal: radiologic findings with pathologic correlation. Radiology 163: 317–323

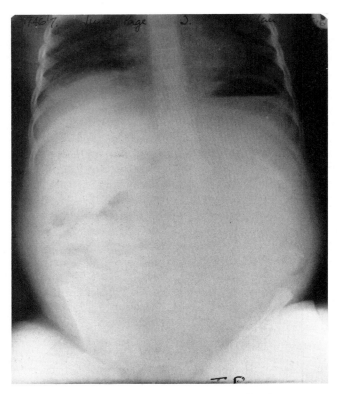

Fig. 3.12.31 Infant with tuberculous peritonitis. The plain abdominal film shows central displacement of the abdominal gas, distension of the flanks and a general lack of air. The appearances are due to ascites.

TUBERCULOSIS

Gastrointestinal tuberculosis may be endemic, but may appear sporadically, when it is frequently misdiagnosed as Crohn's disease. Symptoms depend on the region affected and extent of the intestine or mesentery involved. The symptoms include abdominal pain and weight loss, presentation with acute obstruction due to stricture, abdominal distension due to tuberculous ascites and a palpable abdominal mass. Diarrhoea is common initially. Ascitic fluid has a high protein content and should be cultured. Radiographic evidence of associated pulmonary tuberculosis is often absent.

The plain abdominal film may show evidence of ascites, distension of the properitoneal fat lines, and central location of bowel loops (Fig. 3.12.31). There may be calcified tuberculous nodes and calcification elsewhere in the mesentery, liver and spleen. (Figs 3.12.32, 3.12.33). Mass lesions due to enlarged nodes with displacement of bowel gas are common. Incomplete bowel obstruction is also frequent. On barium studies, areas of distension proximal to strictured bowel segments, displaced loops of bowel around nodal masses, and fixed bowel loops due to plastic peritonitis are found. Strictures are commonest in the ileocaecal region and can be identical to Crohn's disease. A malabsorptive small bowel pattern is also occasionally seen due to lymphatic obstruction. Occasionally filiform polyps are present.

The mass lesions, matted bowel loops and ascites may all be seen at ultrasound examination. CT will also show the lesions and give further information

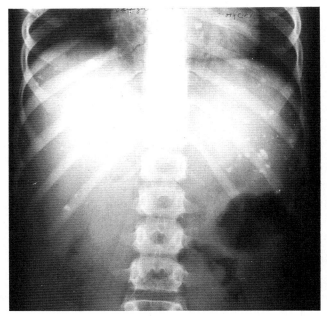

Fig. 3.12.32 Calcified tuberculous granulomas in the liver and spleen due to previous infection.

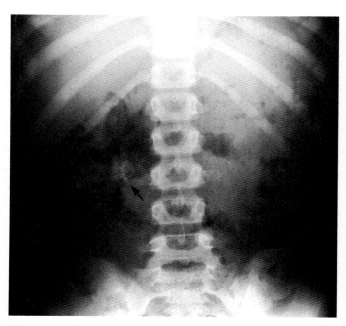

Fig. 3.12.33 Old calcified tuberculous glands in the right abdomen due to previous infection.

about peritoneal involvement and loculation of the ascites. The high protein content of the fluid gives a CT number higher than that of water.

The main differential diagnosis is Crohn's disease but in areas in which tuberculosis is endemic, this is the more likely diagnosis. Histoplasmosis may produce similar appearances.

REFERENCES

Balthazar E, Gordon R, Hulnick D 1990 Ileocecal tuberculosis: CT and radiologic evaluation. American Journal of Roentgenology 154: 499–503
Epstein B, Mann J 1982 CT of abdominal tuberculosis. American Journal of Roentgenology 139: 861–866
Peh W 1988 Filiform polyposis in tuberculosis of the colon. Clinical Radiology 39: 534–536
Werbeloff L, Novis B H, Bank S, Marks I N 1973 The radiology of tuberculosis of the gastrointestinal tract. British Journal of Radiology 46: 329–336

PARASITIC BOWEL INFECTION

Giardia lamblia is increasingly recognized as a cause of chronic diarrhoea, occurring most commonly in immunodeficiency states, but increasingly being reported in children who are immunologically normal who have drunk contaminated water. In severe infection, frank malabsorptive states can occur. On barium examination, there is thickening of the mucosal folds mainly in the duodenum and jejunum, with disturbed peristalsis (Fig. 3.12.19).

REFERENCES

Ament M 1975 Immunodeficiency syndromes and gastrointestinal disease. Pediatric Clinics of North America 22: 807–825
Burke J 1975 Giardiasis in childhood. American Journal of Diseases of Children. 129: 1304–1310
Fisher C, Oh K, Bayless T, Siegelman S 1975 Current perspectives in giardiasis. American Journal of Roentgenology 125: 207–217

Ascaris

Ascaris infestation may cause a variety of clinical complaints ranging from vague abdominal pain, general malaise due to interference with normal nutrition by the worms, to frank intestinal obstruction by an obstructing mass of intraluminal worms. Barium studies are characteristic. The cylindrical worm is seen displacing barium, often with a thin track of barium in the worm's intestine (Fig. 3.12.34). Perforation of the intestine has been recorded. In endemic areas the differential diagnosis is between ascaris infection and appendicitis in children presenting as an abdominal emergency. Pancreatic and biliary involvement by ascaris is well recognized.

REFERENCES

Bean W 1965 Recognition of ascariasis by routine chest or abdomen roentgenograms. American Journal of Roentgenology 94: 379–384
Katz M 1975 Parasitic infections. Journal of Pediatrics 87: 165–178

Trichuriasis

Whipworm infection is found mainly in warm climates and is usually acquired by eating contaminated food. Blood-stained diarrhoea is a finding in heavy infestation and diagnosis is by isolation of the worm from stools. If barium studies are done, the finding of granular mucosa with excessive colonic mucus is said to be characteristic.

REFERENCE

Reeder M M, Astacio J E, Theros E G 1968 An exercise in radiologic – pathologic correlation. Radiology 90: 382–387

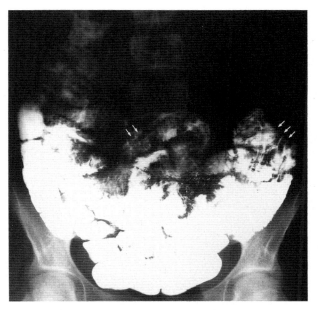

Fig. 3.12.34 Ascaris infection. Numerous worms are present in the ileum. Arrows point to the ascartis worms.

Hookworm

Hookworms cause clinical symptoms of anaemia and malnutrition due to their effect on the mucosal villi of the small bowel. Flattening of the mucosal folds with thickening may be discovered during barium examination for the investigation of anaemia.

REFERENCE

Katz M 1975 Parasitic infections. Journal of Paediatrics 87: 165–178

Strongyloidiasis

Strongyloides infection may occur in immunocompromised children or occur as a primary complaint. The clinical symptoms are epigastric pain resembling duodenal ulceration and malnutrition. Duodenal dilatation, stasis and partial obstruction are described, as is mucosal thickening in the duodenum and jejunum.

REFERENCE

Smith S, Schwartzman M, Mencia L, Blum E, Krogstad D, Nitzkin J, Healey G 1977 Fatal disseminated strongyloidiasis presenting as acute abdominal distress in an urban child. Journal of Pediatrics 91: 607–609

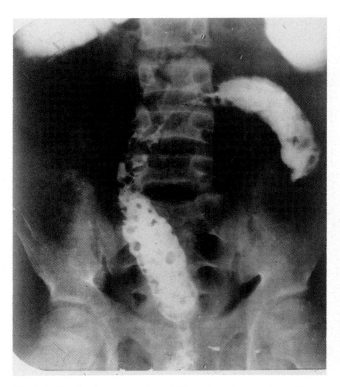

Fig. 3.12.35 Barium enema in a child with schistosomiasis. There are multiple inflammatory polyps due to the infection.

Schistosoma

All four species of schistosomal trematodes can cause intestinal lesions. The infection is acquired when cercariae in water penetrate the skin and enter the lymphatics and veins, where most are filtered out, but those that escape enter the portal venous system and lodge in the intestinal wall and mesenteric veins. Eggs then pass through the bowel and bladder wall and are excreted in faeces and urine, with associated bloody diarrhoea, iron deficiency anaemia and protein-losing enteropathy. Eggs that fail to pass through the bowel wall incite areas of fibrosis and stricture formation may be seen on barium studies. Schistosoma infection causes mucosal ulceration and inflammatory polyp formation in the small bowel and colon (Fig. 3.12.35). Coarsening and irregularity of the mucosa folds may also be found. The small bowel is mainly affected by *Schistosoma japonicum* and the large bowel by the other species.

REFERENCE

Chawla S 1979 Alimentary system. In: Cockshott C U, Middlemiss H (eds) Clinical Radiology in the Tropics. Churchill Livingstone, Edinburgh, pp 88–148

CROHN'S DISEASE

Crohn's disease, also known as regional enteritis, is a chronic disease of unknown origin characterized histologically by non-caseating granulomatous lesions, with fibrosis and stenosis in advanced cases. Any part of the gastrointestinal tract may be affected, though the terminal ileum is most commonly involved, affecting 50% of patients. Aphthous ulceration of mouth and perianal regions may be a presenting feature.

The disease most commonly presents in the age group 20–40 years, but may present at any age. Childhood presentation is common, and is probably increasing. Most children present above the age of 10 years, but it can present in younger children, usually as isolated cases without a family history, but there are well-documented families with cases crossing several generations.

Presenting symptoms include abdominal pain 75%, with diarrhoea 70%, bloody stools and perianal disease 40%. Pyrexia of unknown origin in association with the gastrointestinal symptoms is frequent. Presentation with a clinical picture of acute appendicitis is also common, the diagnosis being made at laparotomy, when a swollen terminal ileum is found with a normal appendix. These children tend to have a better prognosis and may not have further disease.

While abdominal pain and diarrhoea are the most frequent presenting complaints, non-gastrointestinal manifestations include joint pains, fever of unknown origin, anorexia without gastrointestinal symptoms, malaise, anaemia, failure to thrive, small stature, skin rash, uveitis, erythema nodosum and urinary tract symptoms, such as pneumaturia and passage of faeces per urethram or per vaginam due to fistula formation. A very rare presentation is with kwashiorkor type symptoms of a distended abdomen, peripheral oedema and an enlarged liver due to malnutrition. Children with Crohn's disease may present from any clinic in the hospital for investigation, including the psychiatric clinic, because of the sometimes bizarre symptoms.

Barium examination is the method of choice for demonstration of the extent of the disease. The choice of barium technique will depend on the clinical symptoms. If there is a history of vomiting it is important to examine the stomach and duodenum carefully, and a conventional barium meal is indicated, with a follow-through study of the small bowel after further barium. A combination of fluoroscopy and overcouch pictures is required. If symptoms are related only to the small bowel, then either the above technique or enteroclysis is suitable. Some reserve enteroclysis, usually done under sedation, for those children who will not drink adequate quantities of barium to ensure a good examination, where there is a strong clinical suspicion of Crohn's disease and previous studies have been negative, and when surgical removal of an involved segment is planned, provided there is no other affected segment.

Thickened bowel wall may be visible on CT and must not be confused with neoplastic thickening. In general, bowel wall thickness in inflammatory disease is less than 1 cm. CT is also very helpful in demonstrating complex abscess formation, identified on ultrasound, especially if multilocular and before drainage. The colon should be examined separately if it is thought to be involved. In cases in which there is

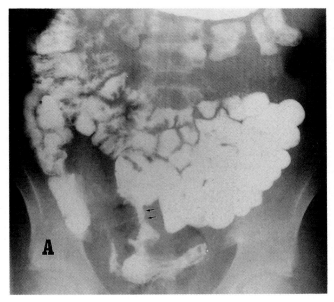
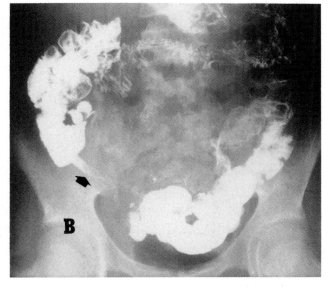

Fig. 3.12.36 **A** Crohn's disease of the distal ileum. There is a stricture (arrows) with a loop of bowel fixed in the pelvis, a narrow terminal ileum and separation of the loops due to thickening and oedema. **B** Same child. The arrow points to an ileocaecal fistula.

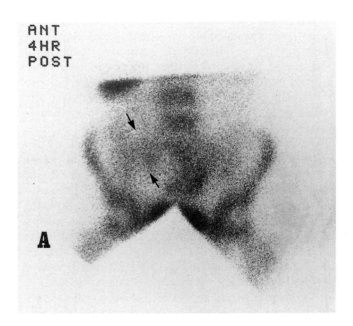

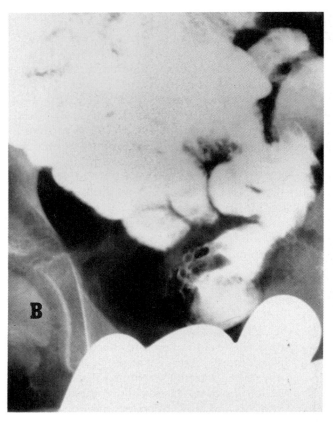

Fig. 3.12.37 **A** Twelve-year-old boy with persistent anaemia. ^{99m}Tc-labelled HMPAO scan of bowel done because of symptoms and negative barium studies in another establishment. Shows an area of increased radionuclide accumulation in the right iliac fossa (arrows). **B** Film of a loop of ileum in the pelvis showing a fixed loop with cobblestone mucosa.

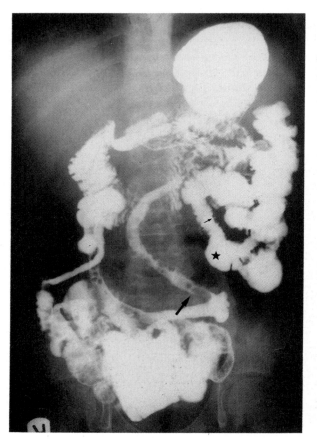

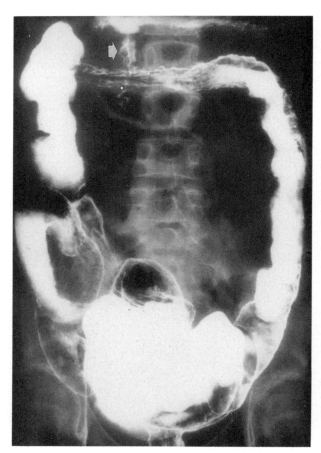

Fig. 3.12.38 This child shows most of the radiological features of extensive Crohn's disease. There are deep ulcers (small arrow), pseudodiverticulum formation (asterisk), and bowel strictures with cobblestone mucosa (large arrow).

Fig. 3.12.39 Crohn's disease of the colon with a gastrocolic fistula (arrowhead).

strong clinical suspicion of Crohn's disease, examination of the small bowel using white cell scanning with ^{99m}Tc-labelled HMPAO is a very satisfactory method for detecting inflammatory foci.

The radiological findings depend on the stage and extent of the disease. The typical appearance is of a narrow rigid segment of bowel with a thickened wall (Fig. 3.12.36), mucosal abnormalities, often described as cobblestone, and deep ulcers. A nodular appearance of the mucosa is also found, which is difficult to distinguish from lymphoid hyperplasia (Fig. 3.12.37). In general, when the bowel is affected by Crohn's disease, it loses its pliability, while bowel with lymphoid hyperplasia remains mobile. The disease may be confined to one segment, or there may be several affected areas with 'skip' lesions, normal bowel being present in between. Stricture formation may affect a whole segment or affect the mesenteric border with pseudodiverticulum formation (Fig. 3.12.38). Bowel loops become separated by thickening. Fistula formation and extramural abscess formation with compression of loops may also be found. Fistulae may be from one local intestinal loop to another but may be gastrocolic (Fig. 3.12.39), ileocolic, involve the bladder or vagina, or be directly to the skin with external sinus formation. Sinograms may demonstrate the lesions more fully. A rarer appearance is of diffuse infiltration of the bowel giving an appearance which suggests lymphomatous infiltration (Fig. 3.12.40). Crohn's disease of the upper gastrointestinal tract in children usually occurs in association with small bowel disease. Oral aphthous ulcers may be a presenting symptom. Oesophageal involvement is clinically manifest by dysphagia and aphthous ulceration may be seen on a double contrast oesophagogram. Very severe involvement may progress to stricture formation. Aphthous ulceration may also be visible in the stomach and duodenum. Other duodenal manifestations include cobblestone mucosa, nodular mucosa and stricture formation (Fig. 3.12.41). Fistula formation and perianal disease are features of Crohn's disease and are rare in ulcerative colitis. However, backwash ileitis and filiform polyps may also be found in both conditions. Percutaneous drainage of abscesses is often required and will usually save repeated laparotomies.

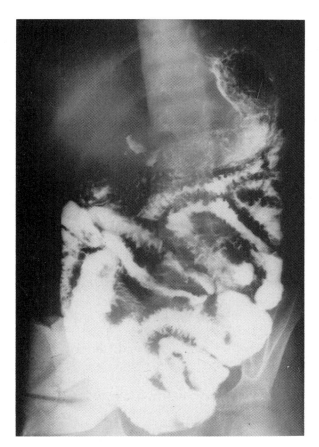

Fig. 3.12.40 Diffuse infiltration of the whole of the small bowel with Crohn's disease. There is separation of bowel loops, with areas of ulceration and extensive mucosal irregularity. This appearance can easily be confused with malignant infiltration.

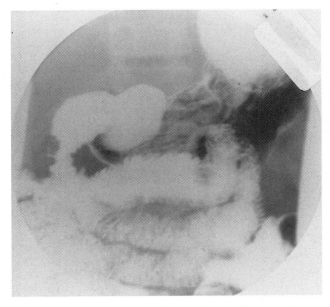

Fig. 3.12.41 Crohn's disease of the duodenum. There is stricture formation of the second part of the duodenum with one deep ulcer. This boy's only symptom was vomiting in the middle of a meal, following which he returned and finished his meal. He was thought to be psychiatrically disturbed.

When the colon is affected by Crohn's disease, the ulcers are deep and tend to be deeper than in ulcerative colitis (Fig. 3.12.42). There may be skip lesions. These features with sparing of the rectum help to distinguish it from ulcerative colitis, but the differentiation can be difficult and may be dependent on histology. Pseudopolyps may be present on the plain abdominal film (Fig. 3.12.43). In quiescent disease, stricture formation with pseudodiverticular formation may result (Fig. 3.12.44).

Complications of Crohn's disease include acute intestinal obstruction, blind loop states and malabsorption due to fistulas, and gallstones due to interruption of the enterohepatic circulation due to ileal disease or extreme resection. Toxic dilatation of the colon is less frequent than in ulcerative colitis. Abscess formation is relatively common, and may lead to hydronephrosis if the ureter is affected. Systemic complications include uveitis, sacroiliitis, and generalized arthritis, which may precede the onset of bowel symptoms. Later sequelae include growth retardation, delayed onset of maturity and, rarely, amyloid disease. Carcinoma of the small bowel has been described in adults. Psychiatric disturbance is common. The disease has been described in infants under 6 months, but this is very rare.

The differential diagnosis of Crohn's disease includes yersinia infection, ulcerative colitis and histoplasmosis. Lymphoma may produce a radiological appearance similar to Crohn's disease but there are usually other diagnostic features. Ischaemic bowel changes due to Henoch–Schönlein purpura may be similar.

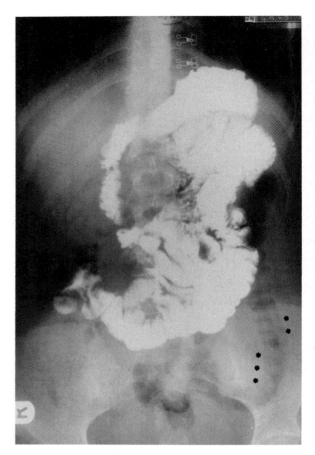

Fig. 3.12.43 Part of follow-through examination in Crohn's disease. Note the pseudopolypoid formation in the descending colon.

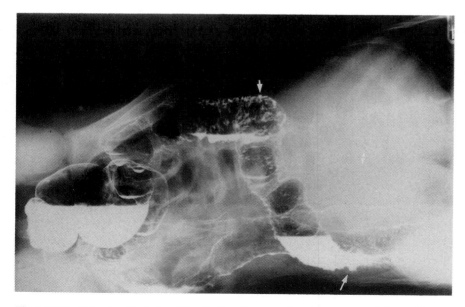

Fig. 3.12.42 Extensive Crohn's colitis affecting the ascending, transverse and descending colon. The rectum is normal. Note deep ulcer seen 'en face' (long arrow). Small arrow points to ulcerated mucosa.

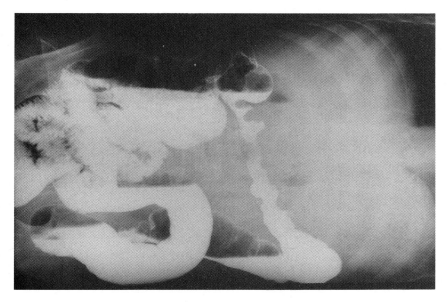

Fig. 3.12.44 Stricture formation of the transverse colon with mild pseudodiverticulum formation.

REFERENCES

Ajzen S A, Gibney R G, Cooperberg P L, Scudamore C H, Miller R R 1988 Enterovenous fistula: unusual complication of Crohn's disease. Radiology 166: 745–746

Ament M E 1975 Inflammatory disease of the colon: ulcerative colitis and Crohn's disease. Journal of Pediatrics 86: 322–334

Balachandran S, Hayden C, Swischuk L 1984 Filiform polyposis in a child with Crohn's disease. Pediatric Radiology 14: 171–173

Ferguson A 1984 Crohn's disease in children and adolescents. Journal of the Royal Society of Medicine (Supplement 3) 77: 30–34

Glick S, Teplick S, Goodman L, Clearfield H, Shanser J 1984 Development of lymphoma in patients with Crohn's disease. Radiology 153: 337–339

Guttman F 1974 Granulomatous enterocolitis in childhood and adolescence. Journal of Pediatric Surgery 9: 115–122

Kirks D, Currarino G 1978 Regional enteritis in children: small bowel disease with normal terminal ileum. Pediatric Radiology 7: 10–14

Levine M 1987 Crohn's disease of the upper gastrointestinal tract. Radiologic Clinics of North America 25: 79–91

Lindsley C B, Schaller J G 1974 Arthritis associated with inflammatory bowel disease in children. Journal of Pediatrics 84: 16–20

Lipson A, Bartram C, Williams C, Slavin G, Walker-Smith J, 1990 Barium studies and ileoscopy compared in children with suspected Crohn's disease. Clinical Radiology 41: 5–8

Puylaert J, Van Der Werf S, Ulrich C, Veidhuizen R 1988 Crohn's disease of the ileocaecal region: ultrasonic visualization of the appendix. Radiology 166: 741–743

Siegel M, Evans S, Balfe D 1988 Small bowel disease in children: diagnosis with CT. Radiology 169:127–130

Sty J, Chusid M, Babbitt D, Werlin S 1979 Involvement of the colon in chronic granulomatous disease of childhood. Radiology 132: 618

RADIATION ENTERITIS

Radiation-induced injury to the bowel is now less common as dosage schedules have become more refined and also with the advent of better and more sophisticated chemotherapy. Permanent damage is unlikely with doses below 5000 rads. Cramping abdominal pain and diarrhoea is mirrored by motility disturbance during barium examination. Mucosal ulceration may occur with doses of 40 Gy. Above 50 Gy, permanent narrowing and stricture formation may ensue and occasionally surgical resection is required for intermittent obstruction. During acute radiation damage, distended loops of thickened bowel with fluid levels are seen.

REFERENCE

Roswit B 1974 Complications of radiation therapy: the alimentary tract. Seminars in Roentgenology 9: 51–63

TRAUMA

As with duodenal haematomas, jejunal and ileal haematomas may also be caused by blunt abdominal trauma, either accidental or non-accidental. Spontaneous haematomas develop in a variety of diseases, including Henoch–Schönlein purpura, leukaemia, idiopathic thrombocytopenic purpura, haemophilia, with anticoagulant therapy, or other bleeding diatheses. Children present with abdominal pain and vomiting and may develop complete intestinal obstruction. Bleeding per rectum may occur due to the bleeding diathesis itself or when a haematoma ruptures into the bowel lumen. Gastrointestinal symptoms may be the presenting feature of Henoch–Schönlein purpura. Rarely, a small bowel intussusception occurs as a complication.

The plain abdominal radiographic appearances are variable and may be normal. Localized ileus in the affected area may be present and appear as a distended, isolated loop of bowel. Oedema of the mucosa will cause visibly thickened valvulae. Thumbprinting is occasionally present. The presence of a mass lesion with displacement of normal gas-filled loops around it and proximal obstruction is rarer than in duodenal trauma. Frank small bowel obstruc-tion occurs occasionally. The mass can sometimes be demonstrated at ultrasound examination.

Rupture of the bowel is a complication of duodenal or jejunoileal injury. Free intraperitoneal gas may be visible on an erect or decubitus radiograph, and on occasion outlines the falciform ligament (Fig. 3.12.45), but the leak of air is often slow and only small amounts may be present. CT examination of the abdomen is often appropriate for these children, as there are usually multiple injuries. Intraluminal contrast medium should be given before starting the examination. Signs of perforation include free air in the peritoneum, free fluid in the peritoneum without free air and thickening of bowel loops. Extraluminal contrast is also sometimes seen. In hypovolaemic shock, a hypoperfusion complex with dilatation of a fluid-filled intestine and abnormally intense contrast enhancement of bowel wall, mesentery and kidneys, with decreased calibre of aorta and inferior vena cava and free fluid may be seen, carrying a bad prognosis.

REFERENCES

Bulas D, Taylor G, Eichelberger M 1989 The value of CT in detecting bowel perforation in children after blunt abdominal trauma. American Journal of Roentgenology 153: 561–564

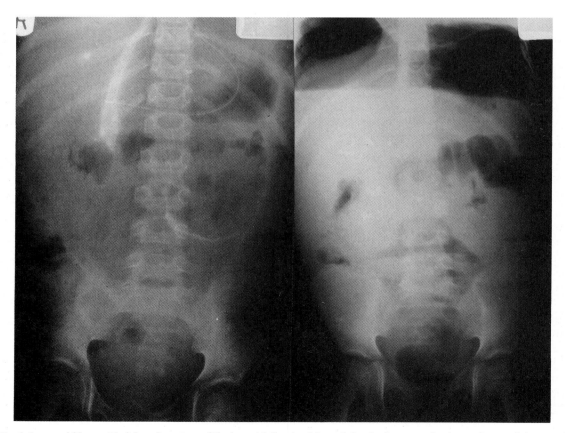

Fig. 3.12.45 **A** 6-year-old boy with delayed rupture of the bowel following blunt abdominal trauma. Supine and erect abdomen: there is a large pneumoperitoneum with air outlining a thick falciform ligament.

Burrell M, Toffler R, Lowman R 1973 Blunt trauma to the abdomen and gastrointestinal tract: plain film and contrast study. Radiologic Clinics of North America 11: 561–578

Filiatrault D, Longpre D, Patriquin H, Perreault G, Grignon A, Pronovost J, Boisvert J 1987 Investigation of childhood blunt abdominal trauma: a practical approach using ultrasound as the initial diagnostic modality. Pediatric Radiology 17: 373–379

Glasier C M, Siegel M J, McAllister W H, Shackelford G D 1981 Henoch-Schönlein syndrome in children: gastrointestinal manifestation. American Journal of Roentgenology 136: 1081–1085

Rodriguez-Erdmann F, Levitan R 1969 Gastrointestinal and roentgenological manifestations of Henoch-Schönlein purpura. Gastroenterology 54: 260–265

Scatarige J, Disantis D 1989 CT of the stomach and duodenum. Radiologic Clinics of North America 27: 687–706

Sivit C, Taylor G, Eichelberger M 1989 Visceral Injury in battered children: a changing perspective. Radiology 173: 659–661

Taylor G, Fallat M, Eichelberger M 1987 Hypovolemic shock in children: abdominal CT manifestations. Radiology 164: 479–481

Taylor G, Guion C, Potter B, Eichelberger M 1989 CT of blunt abdominal trauma in children. American Journal of Roentgenology 153: 555–559

ABDOMINAL PAIN

Abdominal pain is very common in childhood, and may be due to skeletal, gastrointestinal, urinary tract and ovarian pathology. It may also be due to referred pain from pneumonia or due to metabolic or haematological disease. Abdominal pain and fever occur as an 'abdominal crisis' in patients with sickle cell disease, when veno-occlusive disease is the cause. Infarction alone may cause pain but secondary infection is common and CT has a major role in the difficult distinction of the two.

The decision to investigate a child for abdominal pain is clinical. The investigations should be decided by consultation between radiologist and clinician. In general, an appropriate starting point is a supine abdominal radiograph, which should include the lung bases and an abdominal ultrasound examination with a full bladder. In examining the radiograph, the radiologist should look at the lung bases (Fig. 3.12.46), assess bowel gas for presence of constipation, evidence of malrotation, and hernias, look for gallstones, renal or ureteric stones, appendicolith, and observe the spine and pelvis for disc lesions, bone destruction and normality of the sacroiliac joints. With an ultrasound examination showing a normal liver, gallbladder, common bile duct, pancreas, kidneys and pelvis, no intussusception, mass lesion, abscess or abnormality of bowel wall or peristalsis, the radiograph will exclude most serious causes of abdominal pain and these are recommended as the first examinations. The plain abdominal radiograph should not include gonadal protection in girls.

It is useful to think of abdominal pain as acute or chronic and to relate this to the age of the child, as the causes will be different in differing ages. Some of the common causes are shown in Table 3.15.3.

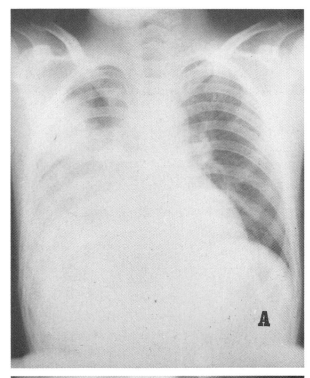

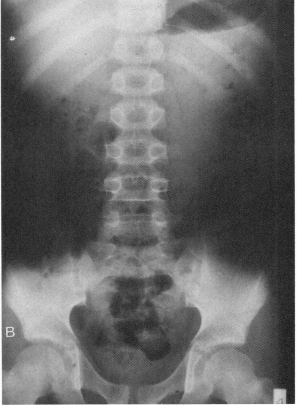

Fig. 3.12.46 Chest (**A**) and abdomen (**B**) of a 9-year-old girl presenting with right iliac fossa pain thought clinically to be due to appendicitis. She had referred pain from right lower lobe pneumonia.

Chronic abdominal pain in childhood is difficult to evaluate, as most of it is functional. Organic disease is evenly divided between the gastrointestinal and genitourinary tracts. The clinician treads a difficult path between labelling a child as having psychogenic illness who has real pathology, and overinvestigating hundreds of children. The combination of the plain abdominal radiograph and ultrasound examination will exclude most serious pathology.

REFERENCES

Bain H W 1974 Chronic vague abdominal pain in children. Pediatric Clinics of North America 21: 991–1000

Magid D, Fishman E, Charache S, Siegelman S 1987 Abdominal pain in sickle cell disease: the role of CT. Radiology 163: 325–328

Mendelson R, Lindsell D 1987 Ultrasound examination of the paediatric 'acute abdomen': preliminary findings. British Journal of Radiology 60: 414–416

Van Der Meer S, Forget P, Arends J, Kuijten R, Van Engelshoven J 1990 Diagnostic value of ultrasound in children with recurrent abdominal pain. Pediatric Radiology 20: 501–503

OBSTRUCTION

Acute small bowel obstruction in childhood is rare compared with adult practice, and has differing causes. Clinical symptoms are abdominal distension, vomiting and, depending on the length of symptoms, constipation and failure to pass flatus. High intestinal obstruction with repetitive profuse vomiting can lead to early electrolyte disturbance, less common with more distal lesions. Pain is variable, but is usually present, and is often spasmodic.

The radiological signs of distended loops of bowel proximal to the obstruction, with fluid levels, vary with the level of the obstruction (Fig. 3.12.47). The lower the obstruction, the greater are the number of fluid levels, described as having a 'ladder' pattern. The presence of gas distal to an obstruction depends on the timing of radiography relative to the onset of symptoms. Supine and erect or decubitus films are required for full assessment.

In viewing the radiograph, the level of the obstruction can be identified by assessing the number of dilated loops. Evidence of air trapped in the hernial orifices, the presence of free air, a mass lesion, or appendicolith should be sought. In high mechanical obstruction there will be few fluid levels. If there is doubt about the diagnosis or the level, a water-soluble contrast medium study can be invaluable. The contrast of choice is non-ionic, low osmolar contrast, which may be diluted equally with water. The choice of oral or rectal administration depends on the suspected level of obstruction. In general, rectal administration is preferable in suspected low lesions. A specific feature of obstruction due to a volvulus around an adhesion or a Meckel's diverticulum or twisted bowel due to incarceration in a hernial orifice is the 'beak sign', where the contrast comes to an abrupt V-shaped beak (Fig. 3.12.48).

The radiological features of air-fluid levels forming a 'ladder' pattern will be altered by continuous nasogastric suction which deflates the bowel proximal to the lesion. In these circumstances a water-soluble contrast medium study is invaluable. Air-fluid levels in the small bowel will also occasionally be absent, especially if the bowel is very full of fluid, and this is often seen in high intestinal obstruction or in closed loop obstructions. The condition is difficult to diagnose on the plain radiographs. Features to suggest it include a distended abdomen with the fluid-filled bowel loops just discernible by the contrast of the wall against the fluid. Ultrasonic examination will demonstrate the fluid-filled loops.

Common causes of obstruction in childhood are intussusception, incarceration in a hernia, adhesions due to previous surgery, and volvulus around a Meckel's diverticulum. Rare causes included obstruction due to parasites and swallowed foreign bodies. Many obstructions due to adhesions are incomplete and are managed conservatively by intravenous fluid replacement and nasogastric suction. Monitoring of recovery is both clinical and radiological. Gas returns to the distal bowel, and passage of flatus recommences as improvement occurs.

Unrelieved obstruction will lead to death, which may be due to electrolyte disturbance, perforation of the bowel wall due to impaired blood supply, and peritonitis.

REFERENCES

Clemett A R, Inkeles D A 1971 Differentiation of acute non-specific jejunitis from mechanical small bowel obstruction. Radiology 101: 87–91

Goh D W, Buick R G 1987 Intestinal obstruction due to ingested Vaseline. Archives of Disease in Childhood 62: 164–168

Levin B 1973 Mechanical small bowel obstruction. Seminars in Roentgenology 8: 281–297

Walker J, Carty H 1989 A radiological feature to assist in the diagnosis of intestinal obstruction. British Journal of Radiology 62: 1105–1106

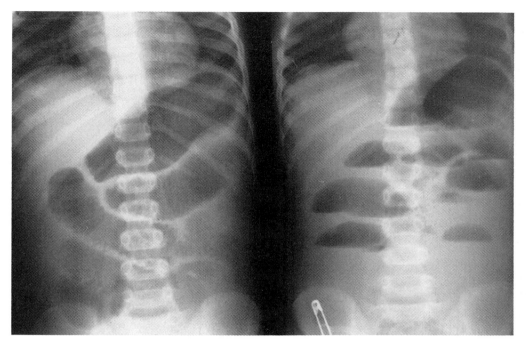

Fig. 3.12.47 Infant 6 days post laparatomy for appendicitis. There is a mechanical small bowel obstruction with distended loops of jejunum.

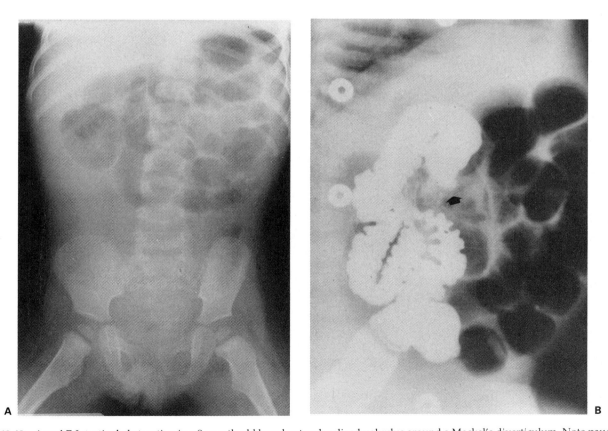

A   B

Fig. 3.12.48 **A** and **B** Intestinal obstruction in a 9-month-old boy due to a localized volvulus around a Meckel's diverticulum. Note paucity of gas in the right iliac fossa on the plain abdominal radiograph. A water-soluble enema shows the point of obstruction at the twisted bowel (arrow). (Figs. reproduced by courtesy of the Editors: British Journal of Radiology.)

ILEUS

Adynamic or paralytic ileus due to interruption of normal coordinated propulsive intestinal peristalsis, results in dilatation of loops of bowel, usually involving both large and small, with accumulation of both gas and fluid. Presentation is with a distended abdomen. Pain is not usually a presenting feature, but may occur as distension increases. Vomiting and nausea are early clinical features. Bowel sounds are absent on auscultation. There is usually relative constipation, but there may be passage of liquid stool, especially in ileus secondary to peritonitis and pelvic abscess. In the older child, distinguishing ileus from obstruction is relatively easy, but both clinical and radiological difficulty is compounded as prolonged mechanical obstruction can result in ileus.

Radiologically, the two conditions are differentiated by observing dilated bowel loops with fluid levels proximal to the obstruction in mechanical obstruction forming the 'ladder' pattern, and an absence of distal bowel gas, or normal calibre bowel gas distal to the obstruction. In ileus, there is distension of both small and large bowel (Fig. 3.12.49). The fluid levels are longer, and the degree of distension of an individual loop less than in mechanical obstruction. The plain abdominal radiographs should include a supine and erect or decubitus film. In cases of ileus, the plain radiographs may be supplemented by an abdominal ultrasound examination to exclude abscess collections in the subphrenic spaces or pelvis. If doubt persists, a water-soluble contrast medium examination of the small bowel will help to distinguish the conditions. This is important as it may be detrimental to submit a patient with ileus to surgery.

The major causes of ileus in children are abdominal or spinal surgery, trauma and peritonitis, but it is also a consequence of septicaemia and gastroenteritis. Rarer causes include the mucocutaneous lymph node syndrome, potassium depletion, some autonomic nervous system diseases, and the rare idiopathic pseudo-obstruction syndromes.

REFERENCES

Franken E A, Kleiman M B, Norins A L, Smith J A, Smith W L 1979 Intestinal pseudo obstruction in mucocutaneous lymph node syndrome. Radiology 130: 649–651
Schuffler M D, Lowe M C, Bill A H 1977 Studies of idiopathic intestinal pseudo obstruction in hereditary hollow visceral myopathy. Clinical and pathological studies. Gastroenterology 73: 327–338

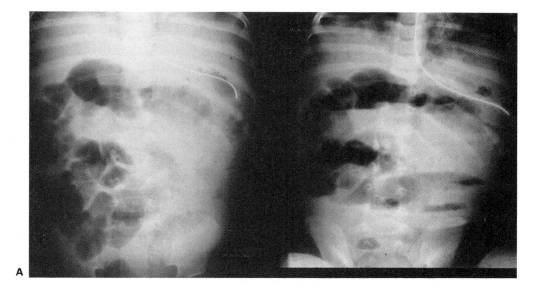

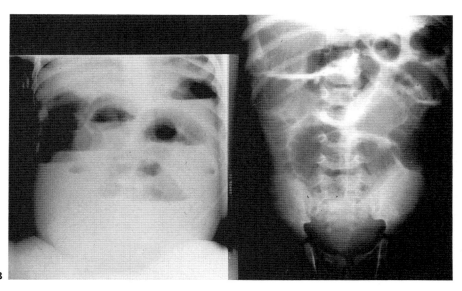

Fig. 3.12.49 **A** Two days post appendicectomy. There is postoperative ileus. Note the long fluid levels with air present throughout. **B** Six days later. There is now mechanical obstruction at the level of the ileum. Note the 'ladder' pattern, dilated bowel loops with valvulae coniventes and short fluid levels.

INTESTINAL PSEUDO-OBSTRUCTION

Functional obstruction in neonates is not uncommon, may be associated with a difficult delivery, jaundice and septicaemia, and is usually a transitory disease possibly associated with immaturity of the nerve plexus. Chronic intestinal pseudo-obstruction is recognized in a variety of clinical conditions including bacterial overgrowth, hypothyroidism, porphyria, scleroderma, amyloidosis and Chagas' disease, and Kawasaki's disease. It is characterized by recurrent attacks of small bowel obstruction, with abdominal distension, vomiting, pain and constipation or diarrhoea. The periodicity of the attacks and symptoms varies between patients. Occasionally symptoms commence in the neonatal period and persist, and normal bowel activity is never established. The outpouring of fluid into the bowel lumen may cause collapse with dehydration and electrolytic disturbance. Many patients require parenteral nutrition even between attacks as food absorption remains insufficient to sustain nutrition.

The radiographic appearances most commonly found are those of apparent mechanical obstruction of the small bowel, but there is usually some colonic air (Fig. 3.12.50). Bowel sounds are absent clinically. Acute gastric dilatation with litres of fluid in the stomach is a feature in some children (Fig. 3.10.20). The symptoms and radiological features often lead to exploratory laparotomy where no cause for the obstruction is found. Biopsy of mucosa and intestinal wall show normal neuronal innervation. The condition is usually sporadic, but there is one report of familial involvement.

Treatment is supportive. Ileostomy or colostomy do not relieve the symptoms.

Oesophageal motor dysfunction has been described in adults in association with the syndrome. It may also simulate Hirschsprung's disease.

Two patients have been seen who presented with episodic vomiting associated with pain, sweating and pallor, and had fluid-filled stomachs at clinical presentation during an acute episode. Barium studies between attacks showed a stomach which was normal in calibre when empty with very reduced peristalsis and delayed gastric emptying. The small bowel transit was normal.

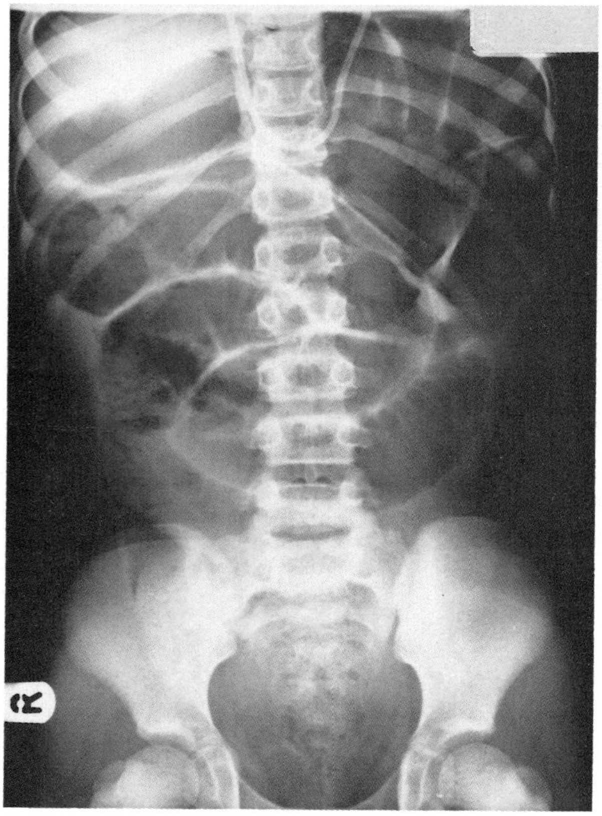

REFERENCES

Boruchow I B, Miller L D, Fitts W T 1966 Paralytic ileus in myxoedema. Archives of Surgery 92: 960–963

Brereton R J , Carty H M 1981 Functional intestinal obstruction in the neonate. Annals of the Academy of Medicine, Singapore 10: 494–501

Byrne W, Cipel L, Euler A, Halpin T, Ament M 1977 Chronic idiopathic intestinal pseudo-obstruction syndrome in children – clinical characteristics and prognosis. Journal of Paediatrics 90: 585–589

Franken E, Kleiman M, Norins A, Smith J, Smith W 1979 Intestinal pseudo obstruction in mucocutaneous lymph node syndrome. Radiology 130: 649–651

Kapila L, Haberkorn S, Nixon H 1975 Chronic adynamic bowel simulating Hirschsprung's disease. Journal of Pediatric Surgery 10: 885–892

Lake B D 1988 Observations on the pathology of pseudo-obstruction. In: Miller P J (ed) Disorders of gastrointestinal motility in childhood. John Wiley, Chichester, pp 81–90

Peachey R, Creamer B, Pierce J 1969 Sclerodermatous involvement of the stomach, and the small and large bowel. Gut 10: 285–292

Schuffler M, Jonak Z 1982 Chronic idiopathic intestinal pseudo-obstruction caused by a degenerative disorder of the myenteric plexus: the use of Smith's Method to define neuropathology. Gastroenterology 82: 476–486

Tschudy D P, Valsamis M, Magnussen C R 1975 Acute intermittent porphyria: clinical and selective research aspects. Annals of Internal Medicine 83: 851–864

Fig. 3.12.50 Chronic intestinal pseudo-obstruction. Seven-year-old boy. Note distended loops of jejunum but gas is present down to the rectum. The appearances suggest an incomplete mechanical obstruction of the bowel at jejunoileal level. A history of repeated attacks was present. (Same boy as in Fig. 3.10.20.)

CHILIADITI'S SYNDROME

Interposition of colon between liver and diaphragm and anterior abdominal wall is known as Chiliaditi's syndrome (Fig. 3.12.51). It is of no clinical significance, but it can create a mistaken appearance of a loculated pneumoperitoneum. The appearance is often transient and is more common in children prone to aerophagy, particularly those who are physically chairbound or mentally subnormal.

INTRA-ABDOMINAL ABSCESS

Inra-abdominal abscess formation may occur in a variety of sites. The most frequent of these are the pelvis, the subphrenic spaces, the subhepatic space and the right iliac fossa. Abscess formation may be the presenting feature of appendicitis. The commonest causes of abscess formation in children are peritonitis due to a ruptured appendix, perforation of a Meckel's diverticulum, peritonitis following abdominal trauma and postoperative peritoneal infection.

The symptoms depend on the degree of peritoneal inflammation and the location of the abscess. Most children will have fever and abdominal pain but this is often not well localized. Pelvic abscess may present with infective diarrhoea. Patients with subphrenic abscess may have chest or shoulder tip pain and symptoms more suggestive of chest infection than abdominal sepsis. Occasionally the presenting symptom will be of a urinary tract infection. The spread of infection within the peritoneum is influenced by the position of the peritoneal ligaments and mesentery.

Once an abscess is suspected clinically the child should have a supine abdominal and an erect chest radiograph, supplemented by erect or decubitus abdominal views, if indicated. All patients should have an ultrasound examination, done with a full bladder.

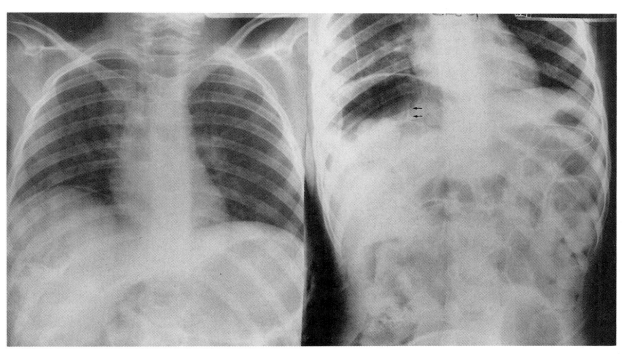

Fig. 3.12.51 Pseudoperforation appearance. Chest and abdominal radiograph of a mentally subnormal child who presented with a 24-hour history of abdominal pain. There is gaseous distension of the abdomen – a frequent finding in mentally subnormal children. The air under the right diaphragm is due to interposition of colon between it and the liver. Note a haustral marking within the subdiaphragmatic air (arrows), not reaching the wall. If there were free air the bowel wall would be visible.

Signs of abscess formation include a mass lesion with displacement of bowel loops, localized ileus formation (Fig. 3.12.52), abscess gas (Fig. 3.12.53), air-fluid levels in an extraluminal distribution and air-fluid levels in the subphrenic spaces.

On ultrasound examination, an abscess is seen as a low density mass lesion (Fig. 3.12.54). It may contain small bubbles of gas, and, depending on the degree of liquefaction, fluid contained in an irregular thick walled cavity may be seen, with debris within the liquid moving as the child's position is altered. Localized reduced bowel peristalsis is common. Mild hydronephrosis of the kidneys may be present in young children, due to ureteric compression at the peritoneal reflection.

If a CT examination is performed on a child with an abscess it should be done following adequate oral contrast medium with intravenous contrast medium administered either just before or during the examination, when enhancement of the abscess walls is seen. The CT density of the fluid varies with its protein content but is usually 1–15 Hounsfield units. The abscess may contain gas if in communication with the bowel lumen or be due to gas-forming organisms.

Percutaneous drainage of intra-abdominal abscess has in many instances replaced open surgical drainage, and may be done under ultrasound or CT control. Drainage of unilocular abscesses is more likely to be successful than drainage of multiloculated lesions, but it is worth attempting drainage of these, even if requiring more than one procedure.

A rarer manifestation of abdominal sepsis in children is swelling of the abdominal wall (Fig. 3.12.55).

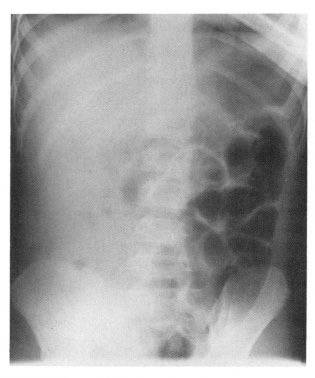

Fig. 3.12.52 Large right iliac fossa abscess due to a gangrenous appendix. Note paucity of gas in the right abdomen and displacement of distended bowel to the left.

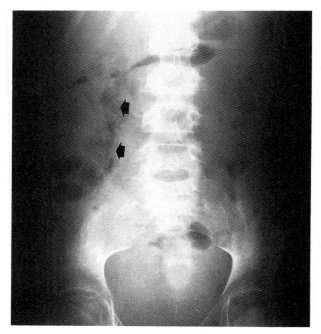

Fig. 3.12.53 Fifteen-year-old girl on treatment with steroids for dermatomyositis. She developed 'silent appendicitis' and presented with fever and shock. Note abscess gas in the right abdomen (arrows) due to a perforated appendix and abscess formation.

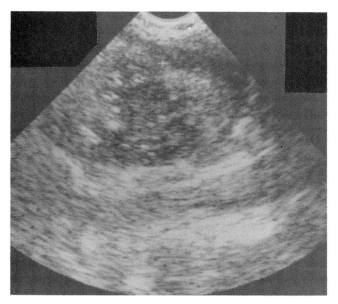

Fig. 3.12.54 Ultrasound examination of a right-sided abscess in the subhepatic region secondary to a perforated appendix. The child presented with a recurrence of fever 7 days post surgery. The abscess is unilocular, and contains small bright bubbles due to gas from an *E. coli* infection. This was successfully drained percutaneously.

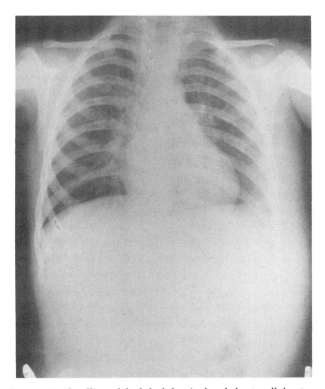

Fig. 3.12.55 Swelling of the left abdominal and chest wall due to intra-abdominal infection.

SUBPHRENIC ABSCESS

Subphrenic abscesses can accumulate if there is infection in the peritoneum, either due to postoperative problems, breakdown of an anastomosis or due to perforation of the bowel with release of intestinal contents and air into the peritoneum. The child presents with pyrexia, is generally unwell, and often complains of referred shoulder pain secondary to diaphragmatic irritation. A typical radiological sign is an air-fluid level under the diaphragm seen on an erect chest or abdominal radiograph (Fig. 3.12.56). There is splinting of the diaphragm with reduced respiratory movement, and frequently basal pulmonary consolidation with a small pleural effusion. The collection may be visible with ultrasound (Fig. 3.12.57), or CT before it is evident on a plain radiograph. Most collections at this site are suitable for percutaneous drainage.

Subhepatic collections are also common in paediatric practice, and are best seen by ultrasound or CT as they are rarely visible on plain radiographs.

Left subphrenic collections (Fig. 3.12.58) are more difficult to diagnose both at ultrasound examination and plain films, as the stomach, splenic flexure and abscess gas shadows can be confusing. Contrast medium studies may correctly establish the location of the gas shadows

REFERENCES

Meyers M, Oliphant M, Berne A, Feldberg M 1987 The peritoneal ligaments and mesenteries: pathways of intraabdominal spread of disease. Radiology 163: 593–604
Van Sonnenberg E, Wittich G, Edwards D, Casola G, Hilton S, Self T, Keightley A, Withers C 1987 Percutaneous diagnostic and therapeutic interventional radiologic procedures in children: experience in 100 patients. Radiology 162: 601–605

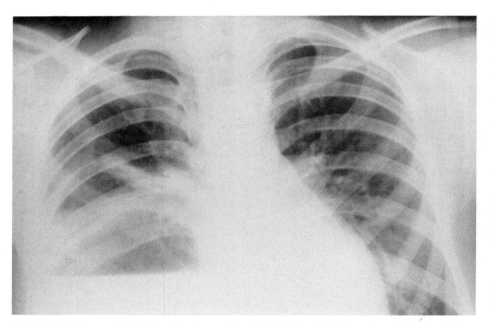

Fig. 3.12.56 Large right subphrenic abscess. Note air-fluid level, right basal consolidation and thickened abscess wall.

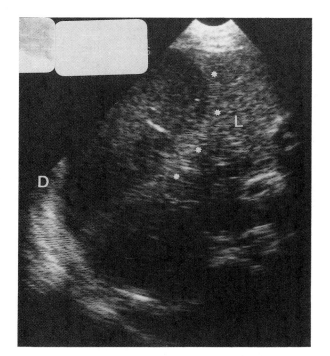

Fig. 3.12.57 Same child as in Figure 3.12.56. Ultrasound examination. There is a large abscess between the liver and the diaphragm. The bright echoes are due to bubbles of gas. L = liver, D = diaphragm. Asterisks outline the edges of the abscess.

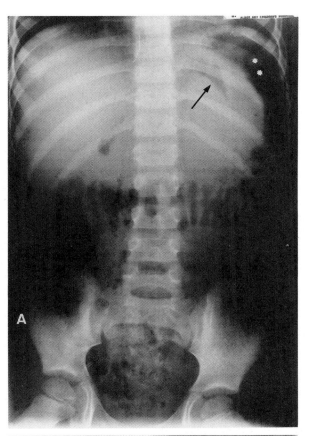

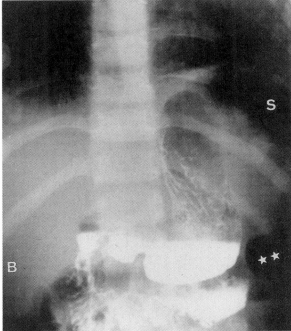

Fig. 3.12.58 **A** Left subphrenic collection. There is a collection of air (asterisks) in the left upper quadrant, which is displacing the splenic flexure distally. The stomach bubble (arrow) is seen separately. **B** Contrast study shows the separation of the stomach, bowel (stars) and subphrenic abscess (S).

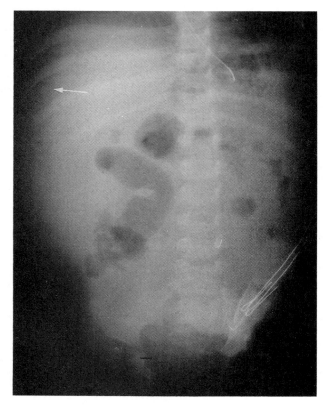

Fig. 3.12.59 Infant who presented with ascites due to portal vein thrombosis from prolonged dehydration. There are swabs on a colostomy dressing on the left (previous presentation with anorectal atresia). Note the liver edge (arrow) displaced medially by the ascites. The bowel loops are displaced centrally – a typical feature of ascites.

ASCITES

The term ascites refers to fluid in the peritoneal cavity, which may be a clear exudate or transudate, or be blood, urine, chyle, bile or lymph, often mixed.

Ascitic fluid may be a transudate or exudate. Exudate may be due to infections, tumours and peritonitis. Transudative ascites may result from portal hypertension, any cause of hypoalbuminaemia, lymphangiectasia and a variety of miscellaneous conditions which include hypothyroidism, biliary, urinary and chylous ascites, and pancreatitis.

Small amounts of ascitic fluid are not clinically detectable or visible on plain film, but are detectable by ultrasound examination, or by CT. Large volumes of ascites are recognizable on a plain abdominal film by observing the bowel loops lying central in the abdomen, a general grey appearance and lateral displacement of the properitoneal fat line and occasionally the liver edge displaced medially (Fig. 3.12.59). In general, 200–300 ml of fluid in the peritoneum needs to be present before it is reliably detectable on plain film.

At ultrasound examination, the location of fluid depends on the quantity. Small volumes under 20 ml are most easily seen in the pelvis, but with increasing volume fluid is found in the subphrenic space, the subhepatic space, the paracolic gutters and then between loops of intestine (Fig. 3.12.60). Non-infected ascites is trans-sonic. Echoes within the fluid suggest blood or infection depending on the clinical circumstances.

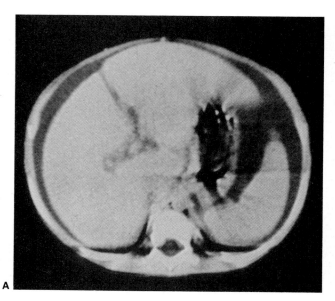

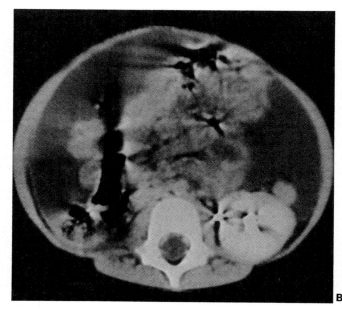

Fig. 3.12.60 Ascites due to hepatotoxicity from chemotherapy for Wilms' tumour. **A**, **B** Two frames from the CT examination. There is ascitic fluid distributed around the liver and spleen and in both paracolic gutters.

Ascitic fluid on CT is distributed similarly to that seen on ultrasound. Uncomplicated ascitic fluid measures less than 10 Hounsfield units.

REFERENCES

Grenier N, Filatrault D, Garel L, Dube J, Paille P 1986 CT features of peritoneal and mesenteric involvement in pediatric malignancies. Experience from thirteen cases. Annales de Radiologie 29: 275–285
Meyers M, Oliphant M, Berne A, Feldberg M 1987 The peritoneal ligaments and mesenteries: pathways of intraabdominal spread of disease. Radiology 163: 593–604

CHYLOUS ASCITES

Chylous ascites is relatively rare in children. It may be associated with chylothorax in the newborn period, or associated with trauma in older children. Other causes include parasitic infiltration, tuberculosis, neoplasm and lymphadenopathy. Chyle does not contain fat and therefore does not appear 'milky' if the patient is not consuming normal fat, sometimes leading to mistaken diagnoses.

REFERENCE

Niekel R, Zwemmer A, Schuur K 1987 Computer tomographic features of chylous ascites. Journal of Medical Imaging 1: 279–282

MESENTERIC VASCULAR INSUFFICIENCY

Acute mesenteric vascular insufficiency is rare in children, but can occur secondary to emboli in children with congenital heart disease. Other causes include vascular insufficiency due to collagen diseases, arteritis, polycythaemia and aortic catheterization. Acute occlusion can occur secondary to hypovolaemic shock, and with volvulus. Presentation is with acute abdominal pain, vomiting, abdominal distension and blood per rectum.

The radiographic appearances are very variable. The most frequent finding is of abdominal distension with air-fluid levels in the bowel simulating mechanical obstruction. This progresses to bowel wall oedema, 'thumbprinting' and ultimately intramural bowel wall gas and portal vein gas.

REFERENCE

Andersen J, Eklof O 1981 Segmental vascular occlusion of the colon. A tentative diagnosis in two pediatric cases. Pediatric Radiology 11: 5–7

INTESTINAL POLYPOSIS

Polyps in the small intestine in children are rare and occur most commonly in association with familial polyposis coli and the Peutz–Jegher syndrome. Rare causes include juvenile gastrointestinal polyposis associated with bloody diarrhoea, protein loss and electrolyte disturbance, with which macrocrania and intracranial cysts and a poor prognosis have been reported. Children with the blue rubber bleb naevus syndrome may have polypoidal haemangiomas in the stomach, small bowel and colon.

REFERENCES

Bhasin R, McAlindon J, Elliott H, Boskar D 1974 Recurrent juvenile duodenal polyposis. Journal of Pediatric Surgery 9: 553–554
McCauley R, Leonidas J, Bartoshesky L 1979 Blue rubber bleb nevus syndrome. Radiology 133: 375–377
Sachatello C, Hahn I, Carrington B 1974 Juvenile gastrointestinal polyposis in a female infant: report of a case and review of the literature of a recently recognised syndrome. Surgery 75: 107–113
Schwartz A, McCauley R 1976 Juvenile gastrointestinal polyposis. Radiology 121: 441–444

PEUTZ–JEGHER SYNDROME

Most of the polyps of Peutz–Jegher syndrome occur in the small intestine; colonic and stomach polyps are rare. The colonic polyps are adenomatous while the small bowel polyps are hamartomatous. In this condition multiple areas of dark mucocutaneous pigmentation are seen on the mucosa of the lips and over the digits. There is autosomal dominant inheritance, with an equal sex incidence.

The polyps vary in size and may be pedunculated or sessile, causing transient intussusceptions in the small bowel, with recurrent attacks of abdominal pain. Rectal bleeding may occur, particularly when colonic polyps are present. There is an increased risk of developing cancer but relative to the other polyposis syndromes it is low. Surgery is often required and may

result in the short bowel syndrome. The youngest recorded patient is 11 months.

There are no plain radiographic changes specific to polyps. The diagnosis is made on barium examination which is best done by enteroclysis in suspected cases when the polyps are seen as filling defects in the bowel lumen (Fig. 3.12.61). Transient intussusception during the examination is sometimes encountered.

REFERENCES

Morens D, Garvey S 1975 An unusual case of Peutz Jegher's syndrome in an infant. American Journal of Diseases of Children 129: 973–976

Tovar J, Elizaguirre I, Albert A, Jimenez J 1983 Peutz Jegher's syndrome in children: report of 2 cases and review of the literature. Journal of Pediatric Surgery 18: 1–6

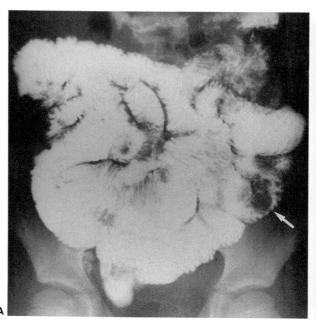
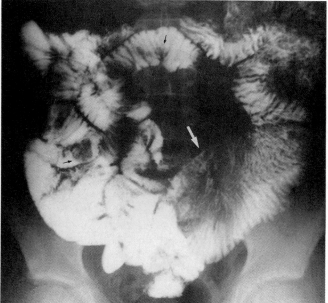

Fig. 3.12.61 Peutz–Jegher syndrome. **A, B** Two films from a follow-through examination in a 12-year-old boy with classical perioral pigmentation and recurrent abdominal pain. There are multiple small bowel polyps (arrows).

INTESTINAL LYMPHOMA

Lymphoma is the most frequent primary small bowel tumour in children, most often seen in early teenage. Secondary involvement of the bowel is rare but can occur in advanced Hodgkin's disease and occasionally in leukaemias (Fig. 3.12.62). Lymphoma of the bowel presents clinically with local symptoms and systemic disease is rare. Acute small bowel obstruction is the most frequent presenting symptom, the diagnosis often being made at laparatomy (Fig. 3.12.63). Subacute small bowel obstruction, abdominal mass, abdominal pain, intussusception, and, occasionally, malabsorption are other presenting features. Presentation is at any age in childhood.

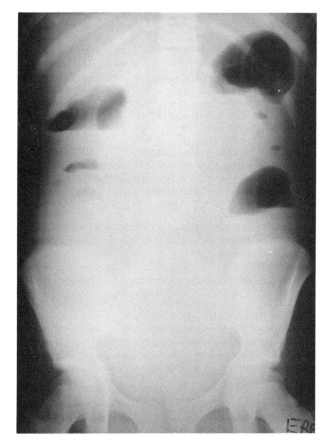

Fig. 3.12.63 Twelve-year-old boy with acute obstruction secondary to bowel lymphoma. Note the distended abdomen and some central displacement of the fluid-filled bowel loops secondary to ascites.

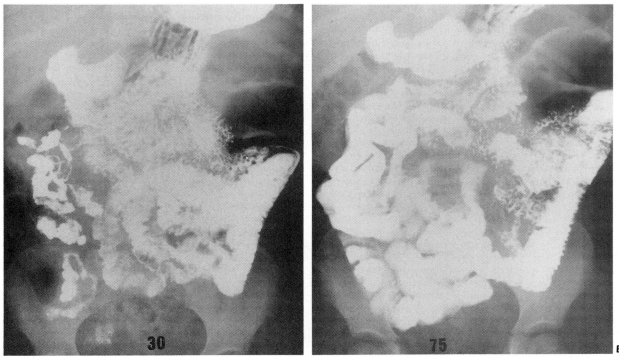

Fig. 3.12.62 Leukaemic infiltration of bowel. There is thickening and coarsening of the bowel mucosa. Separation of the loops and loss of normal peristalsis was noted on screening. (Films at 30 minutes (**A**) and 75 minutes (**B**).)

Signs of acute or subacute small bowel obstruction with or without a mass may be seen on the plain abdominal radiograph. At ultrasound examination a low echo density mass lesion with bowel loops enmeshed in it may be seen. A little free intraperitoneal fluid is often present. The liver and spleen are usually normal. Contrast studies of the small bowel show a variety of patterns:

1. diffuse infiltration of the bowel with separation of the loops, loss of pliability and mucosal thickening
2. a polypoid mass which may cause intussusception (Fig. 3.12.64)
3. single or multiple stenotic areas with shouldering of the walls resembling carcinomatous lesions
4. localized aneurysmal bowel dilatation with loss of mucosal pattern.

Primary mesenteric lymphoma or nodal masses within the mesentery will displace bowel loops. A rare presentation is lymphoma of the pancreas in which the infiltrated pancreas appears as a low echodensity mass on ultrasound examination and is usually a secondary manifestation.

Lymphoma can occur anywhere in the bowel, but has its highest incidence in the ileum. Colonic involvement is most frequent at the ileocaecal region, presenting as a mass lesion or intussusception.

The main differential diagnosis of bowel lymphoma is Crohn's disease. The two can be very difficult to distinguish radiologically, as can ileocaecal tuberculosis and appendix abscesses.

CT of the abdomen is required for full assessment of the disease. Peritoneal involvement is seen at CT by infiltration of the mesenteric fat, with increased attenuation, the presence of enlarged lymph nodes and loss of the normal pliability of the mesentery. Thickening of the bowel wall is also frequent (Fig. 3.12.65). Both lymphoma and inflammatory bowel disease can produce mass lesions, and cannot be reliably differentiated by CT. Percutaneous biopsy of a mass may obtain sufficient material for histology, and avoid surgery.

The prognosis for isolated small bowel lymphoma in children is good with many long-term survivors. Complications during treatment include fistula formation and malabsorption. Total parenteral nutrition during treatment may be needed.

REFERENCES

Angerpointner T A, Weitz H, Haas R J, Hecker W W 1981 Intestinal leiomyosarcoma in childhood – Case report and review of the literature. Journal of Pediatric Surgery 16: 491–495
Bartram C, Chrispin A 1973 Primary lymphosarcoma of the ileum and caecum. Pediatric Radiology 1: 28–33
Bessette J, Maglinte D, Kelvin F, Chernish S 1989 Primary malignant tumours of the small bowel: a comparison of the small bowel enema and conventional follow through examination. American Journal of Roentgenology 153: 741–745
Gourtsoyiannis N, Nolan D 1988 Lymphoma of the small intestine: radiological appearances. Clinical Radiology 39: 639–645
Grenier N, Filatrault D, Garel L, Dube J, Paille P 1986 CT features of peritoneal and mesenteric involvement in pediatric malignancies. Experience from thirteen cases. Annales de Radiologie 29: 275–285
Makepeace A, Fermont D, Bennett M 1987 Gastrointestinal non-Hodgkin's lymphoma. Clinical Radiology 38: 609–614
Miller J, Hindman B, Lam A 1980 Ultrasound in the evaluation of small bowel lymphoma in children. Radiology 135: 409–414
Siegel M, Evans S, Balfe D 1988 Small bowel disease in children: diagnosis with CT. Radiology 169: 127–130
Solomons N, Wagonfeld J, Thomsen S, Hill J L, Kirsner J 1976 Leiomyosarcoma of the duodenum in a 10 year old boy. Pediatrics 58: 268–273

CASTLEMAN'S DISEASE: ANGIOFOLLICULAR HYPERPLASIA

Castleman's disease, commoner in adults, is a condition of unknown cause with lymphoid tissue enlargement, presenting clinically as large nodal masses anywhere in the body, including the mesentery and retroperitoneum. With abdominal involvement there is often splenic enlargement. Clinical symptoms may also include fever, sweating and anaemia.

At ultrasound examination the nodal masses are of low echodensity. Lymphadenopathy and splenomegaly are seen at CT. Multiple sites may be involved.

REFERENCE

Libson E, Fields S, Strauss S, Bloom R, Okon E, Galun E, Polliack A 1988. Widespread Castleman disease: CT and US findings. Radiology 166: 753–755

OTHER MALIGNANT TUMOURS

Primary carcinoma of the small bowel in children is extremely rare. Secondary small bowel involvement by rhabdomyosarcoma, neuroblastoma, ovarian tumours and other lymphomas including Burkitt's also occurs. Carcinoid tumours most frequently occur in the appendix.

REFERENCES

Tankel J, Galasko C S B 1984 Adenocarcinoma of the small bowel in a 12-year-old girl. Journal of the Royal Society of Medicine 77: 693–694
Voegele L, Moncrief J 1975 Adenocarcinoma of the jejunum in an 18-year-old patient. Surgery 78: 251–253

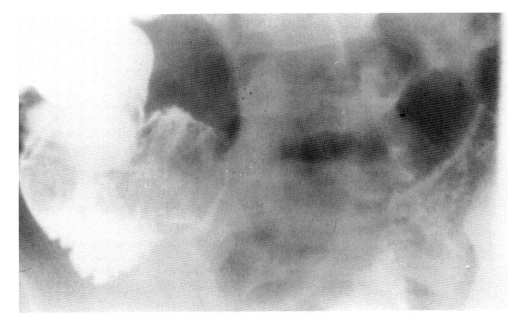

Fig. 3.12.64 Lymphoma of bowel. Note the intraluminal mass.

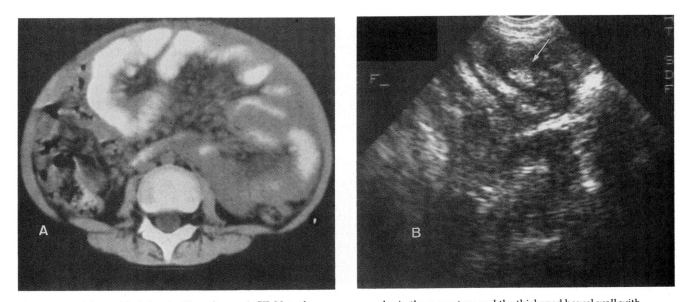

Fig. 3.12.65 A boy with abdominal lymphoma. **A** CT. Note the numerous nodes in the mesentery and the thickened bowel wall with separation of the loops. The bowel wall thickening may also be seen in Crohn's disease. **B** Ultrasound. Note thickened bowel (arrow).

PERITONEAL TUMOURS

Primary peritoneal tumours are very rare in children, with a few scattered reports of mesothelioma. Secondary involvement of the mesentery by direct infiltration from adjacent bowel, liver, pancreatic, pelvic or retroperitoneal tumours is not uncommon, particularly during recurrence or as a terminal event. Both primary and metastatic disease are characterized by deposits within the peritoneum and mesentery, and ascites. Both may be visible by ultrasound and CT, but CT gives a better appreciation of the extent of involvement. Pain, abdominal distension and symptoms of bowel obstruction are presentations.

REFERENCE

Kovalivker M, Motovic A 1985 Malignant peritoneal mesothelioma in children: description of two cases and review of the literature. Journal of Pediatric Surgery 20: 274–275

OMENTAL, MESENTERIC AND RETROPERITONEAL CYSTS

Cysts in these three areas are benign tumours of lymphatic origin, though sometimes of mixed lymphatic and haemangiomatous composition. They are variable in size but may be huge, and are being diagnosed with increasing frequency antenatally. The clinical presentation is related to the cyst size and location. Small, mesenteric cysts may cause the associated bowel segment to intussuscept. Larger ones cause abdominal pain or abdominal distension. The abdomen may have a 'doughy' feel on palpation.

Primary investigation is by ultrasound. The cysts are often multilocular with multiple septae. They are thin walled. The fluid is normally clear. Echoes within it often indicate haemorrhage, which is a complication and often leads to the clinical presentation as the cyst suddenly increases in size (Fig. 3.12.66). If they are complex, CT will enable full demonstration prior to surgery. An alternative method of treatment is percutaneous aspiration with sclerotherapy by intracavity tetracycline. Multiple aspirations may be necessary to achieve a cure. Failure of this technique is related to communication between adjoining cysts. The cyst content in uncomplicated cases is a clear, serous fluid, which foams due to a high protein content. The high protein content is also evident at MR imaging by a high signal on T1- and T2-weighted images.

The plain abdominal radiographic findings are related to the size of the cyst and its location. Displaced loops of bowel are seen with big lesions. In large cysts, the appearance may mimic ascites but, unlike ascites, the bowel loops are usually displaced laterally or upwards – not centrally. Calcification in the cyst wall is rarely seen.

The differential diagnosis of a cystic mass in the abdomen includes other cystic tumours, duplication cysts and ovarian cysts. In general, duplication cysts are unilocular and the muscular and mucosal wall should be identifiable. Complex large ovarian cysts may be difficult to differentiate, but may cause hydronephrosis, unusual with mesenteric cysts.

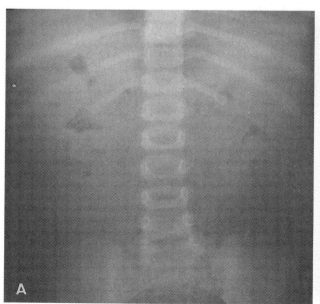
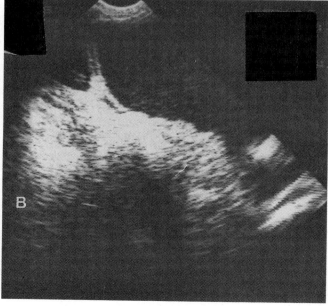

Fig. 3.12.66 A 3-year-old with recent onset of a distended abdomen but otherwise well. **A** Plain abdominal radiograph. The general greyness is due to a large mesenteric cyst displacing the bowel loops superiorly. **B** Ultrasound of the abdomen. There is a bilocular large mesenteric cyst. The echogenic content indicates previous haemorrhage into the cyst.

REFERENCES

Geer L, Mittelstaedt C, Stabb E, Gaisie G 1984 Mesenteric cysts: sonographic appearance with CT correlation. Pediatric Radiology 14: 102–104

Gyves-Ray K, Hernandez R, Hillemeier A 1990 Pseudoascites: unusual presentation of omental cyst. Pediatric Radiology 20: 560–561

Kelekis L, Kelekis D., Christopoulos S, Makridis K, Artopoulos J, Kelemouridis B 1980 Multiple mesenteric cysts in an infant. Computerized Tomography 4: 225–229

Leonidas J, Brill P W, Bhan I, Smith T 1978 Cystic retroperitoneal lymphangioma in infants and children. Radiology 127: 203–208

Prieto M, Casanova A, Delgado J, Zabalza R 1989 Cystic teratoma of the mesentery. Pediatric Radiology 19: 439

Ros P, Olmsted W, Moser R, Dachman A, Hjermsted B, Soblin L 1987 Mesenteric and omental cysts: histologic classification with imaging correlation. Radiology 164: 327–332

Shackelford G, McAlister W 1975 Cysts of the omentum. Pediatric Radiology 3: 152–155

ABDOMINAL WALL TUMOURS

The common abdominal wall tumours are lymphangiomas and haemangiomas, or mixed lesions, which may be isolated to the abdomen or more generalized extending to chest and limbs.

Rare tumours include desmoid tumours, abdominal wall dermoids, neurofibromas and fibromatosis. Infiltration with fibromatosis produces a generalized thickening of the muscles, which though not malignant, can be locally aggressive. A neurofibroma may be pedunculated. The rarer plexiform neurofibroma involves the muscle in an infiltrative pattern, and can arise in the retroperitoneum or pelvic floor causing obstruction of the ureters, bladder and blood vessels.

Desmoid tumours are proliferations of fibroblasts that arise from muscles or aponeuroses. They are locally invasive and represent a more discrete form of fibromatosis. There is an association with familial polyposis coli.

Lipomas may occur anywhere in the muscles and have increased echogenicity on ultrasound. If large enough, the fat content may be seen as a shadow of low density, on the plain radiograph. Ultrasound examination will show most lesions in the abdominal wall to be of lower echodensity than surrounding muscle. On CT they are seen as non-contrast enhancing lesions infiltrating the muscles but they may have the same CT number as normal muscles. The Hounsfield density of lipomas on CT is around minus 100. Lipomatosis of the pelvic organs is associated with multiple polypoidal lesions of the rectosigmoid colon.

REFERENCES

Baron R, Lee J 1981 Mesenteric desmoid tumours. Radiology 140: 777–779

Bowen A, Gaisie G, Bron K 1982 Retroperitoneal lipoma in children: choosing among diagnostic imaging modalities. Pediatric Radiology 12: 221–225

Jones I, Jagelman D, Fazio V, Lavery I, Weakley F, McGannon E 1986 Desmoid tumours in familiar polyposis coli. Annals of Surgery 204: 94–97

Mantello M, Haller J, Marquis J 1989 Sonography of abdominal desmoid tumors in adolescents. Journal of Ultrasound in Medicine 8: 467–470

Sulivan W, Wesenberg R, Lilly J 1980 Giant retroperitoneal lipoma in children. Paediatrics 66: 123–125

RETROPERITONEAL TERATOMA

Teratomas in the retroperitoneum may present at any age, but most commonly present in girls in the first year of life, and present either with a palpable mass, pain, weight loss or vomiting secondary to the mass. Most tumours are benign, and may contain fat, calcium, teeth or ossification. The fat content is more easily appreciated by ultrasound, CT or MRI. The lesions are typically solid with cystic spaces. Though easily seen on plain radiograph or ultrasound, the full extent should be assessed by CT before surgery.

REFERENCES

Bowen B, Ros P, McCarthy M, Olmsted W, Hjermstad B 1987 Gastrointestinal teratomas: CT and US appearance with pathologic correlation. Radiology 162: 431–433

Partlow W, Taybi H 1971 Teratomas in infants and children. American Journal of Roentgenology 112: 155–166

Schey W, Veseley J, Radkowski M 1986 Shard-like calcifications in retroperitoneal teratomas. Pediatric Radiology 16: 82–84

FETUS IN FETU

This is a very rare condition in which a mass composed of easily identifiable fetal parts, mainly limb bones and vertebras encased in a membrane, is found at surgery. Usually located within the retroperitoneum, this benign lesion is regarded as an inclusion of a monozygotic twin during fetal development. Clinical presentation is with an abdominal mass.

REFERENCES

Alpers C, Harrison M 1985 Fetus in fetu associated with an undescended testis. Paediatric Pathology 4: 37–46

Eng H L, Chuang J, Lee T Y, Chen W J 1989 Fetus in fetu: a case report and review of the literature. Journal of Paediatric Surgery 24: 296–299

George V, Khanna M, Dutta T 1983 Fetus in fetu. Journal of Pediatric Surgery 18: 288–289

Nocera R, Davis M, Hayden C, Schwartz M, Swischuk L 1982 Fetus-in-fetu. American Journal of Roentgenology 138: 762–764

INTRA-ABDOMINAL TESTIS

A further rare cause of an intra-abdominal mass is infarction of an intra-abdominal testis, which may present as a calcified opacity.

REFERENCES

Campbell J, Schneider C 1976 Intrauterine torsion of an intra-abdominal testis. Pediatrics 57: 262–264
Ein S H 1987 Torsion of an undescended intra abdominal benign testicular teratoma. Journal of Pediatric Surgery 22: 799–801
Smolko M, Kaplan G, Brock W 1983 Location and fate of the nonpalpable testis in children. Journal of Urology 129: 1204–1206

ABDOMINAL LYMPH NODES

Abdominal lymph nodes are situated close to the major organs around the coeliac axis, within the mesentery and along both iliac vessels. They are not seen on plain radiographs unless calcified. Calcified nodes result mainly from infection, most commonly tuberculosis. Occasionally they may resemble gallstones or renal stones if of an appropriate size and projection. Any clinical dilemma can easily be resolved by ultrasound and CT examination.

A thorough knowledge of normal CT anatomy and normal vessel variants is essential to avoid erroneous interpretation of nodal disease.

3.13   THE COLON

The structure of the colon is different from the small intestine, accounting for its distinct radiographic appearance. The sacculations which are normally present between the appendix base and rectum are due to the teniae coli, the longitudinal muscles which run in three bands along the length of the colon. The colonic wall is longer than the teniae, hence the sacculations. The haustral folds are incomplete, giving a characteristic appearance on the plain radiograph. In older children it is usually possible on a plain radiograph to identify the caecum, both flexures and the sigmoid colon and rectum (Fig. 3.13.1). Identification of the remainder of the colon depends on its content, and the degree of small bowel distension. Faeces in the right colon normally has a bubbly appearance. The faecal masses become more solid

from the hepatic flexure distally. The ileocaecal valve is located on the posteromedial wall of the caecum. It cannot be seen on plain radiographs but is frequently seen on barium studies. Its appearance is very variable and often prominent, and may resemble a tumour.

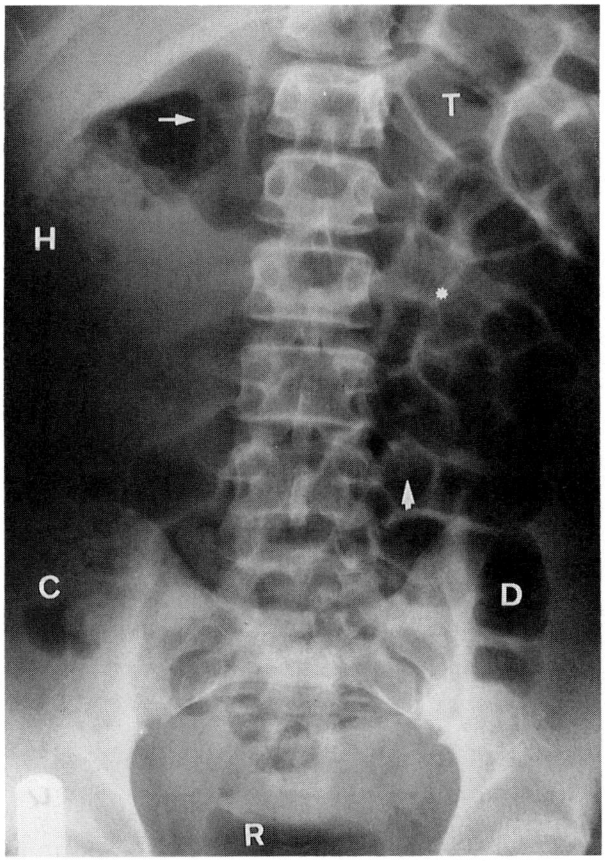

LYMPHOID HYPERPLASIA

Lymphoid hyperplasia is seen as multiple submucosal nodules, often umbilicated on double contrast examination of the colon (Fig. 3.13.2). They are most frequent at the flexures, transverse colon and rectum. They are a normal finding and not indicative of underlying pathology, but may give an appearance suggestive of small polyps. If there is doubt, the patient should undergo colonoscopy. In the past, lymphoid hyperplasia was cited as a cause of gastrointestinal bleeding, as it is frequent in patients who have a barium enema done during the course of its investiga-

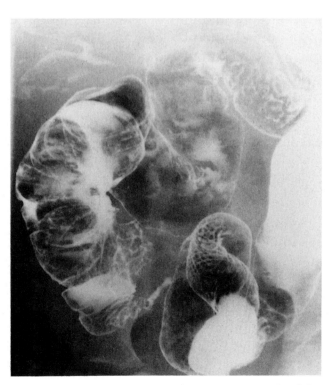

Fig. 3.13.1   Plain abdominal radiograph done following abdominal trauma. Note the characteristic appearance of bubbly faeces in the right abdomen, the haustral pattern in the transverse colon (arrow), the jejunum (asterisk) and ileum (arrowhead) and the descending colon and rectum. The relative lack of gas in the right upper quadrant was due to renal injury. C = caecum, H = hepatic flexure, T = transverse colon, D = descending colon.

Fig. 3.13.2   Lymphoid hyperplasia. Note the umbilicated nodular defects in the rectum. Film taken post reduction of intussusception, hence the caecal oedema.

tion. Current opinion is that they are not a cause of such symptoms and are of no clinical relevance.

REFERENCES

Byrne W, Jimenez F, Euler A 1982 Lymphoid polyps (focal lymphoid hyperplasia) of the colon in children. Pediatrics 69: 598–600

Capitanio M, Kirkpatrick J 1970 Lymphoid hyperplasia of the colon in children. Roentgen observations. Radiology 94: 323–327

Kenney P, Koehler R, Schackelford G 1982 The clinical significance of large lymphoid follicles of the colon. Radiology 142: 41–46

Laufer I, deSa D 1978 Lymphoid follicular pattern: a normal feature of the pediatric colon. American Journal of Roentgenology 130: 51–55

COLONIC DUPLICATION

Colonic duplication is much rarer than small bowel duplication. Duplications occur on the mesenteric border, and may communicate with the bowel lumen or be blind. Blind duplications presenting as mass lesions may be fluid filled or have mixed fluid and solid content. They cause symptoms by pressure, or mechanical interference with bowel function, and may cause intussusception. Though congenital, they may not present until later in childhood when they become symptomatic due to a sudden increase in size associated with bleeding into them. On plain radiographs, the only abnormality is a mass lesion displacing bowel around it. Ultrasound examination will show the mass to be fluid filled or of mixed echodensity.

Communicating duplications may be open at both ends or be blind proximally or distally. When in communication at both ends, they are often asymptomatic and are discovered incidentally (Figs 3.13.3, 3.13.4). When closed at one end, the duplication may become filled with gas and faeces, resulting in abdominal pain and distension. The gas- or faecal-filled mass may be visible on plain radiographs. Barium studies may show the communication, or simply extrinsic colonic pressure.

All duplications may contain ectopic gastric mucosa – hence their propensity to bleeding and sudden increase in size.

Many colonic duplications are associated with other anomalies of the body, mainly of the urinary tract, spine and abdominal wall.

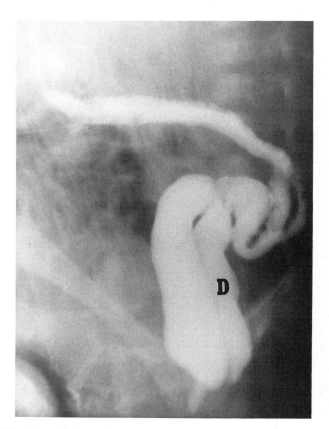

Fig. 3.13.3 Colonic duplication. Infant of 1 month. Barium enema done for investigation of bloody stools. There is a colonic duplication which is communicating with the normal channel at the rectosigmoid junction and filling retrogradely to the rectum. D = duplication.

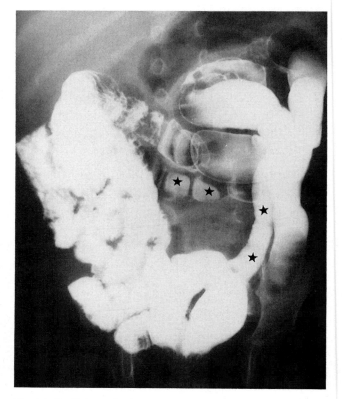

Fig. 3.13.4 Colonic duplication extending from the sigmoid colon to the hepatic flexure. This was in communication with the normal lumen at both ends. (Second channel marked by stars.)

REFERENCES

Baro P, Casas J, Sanchez D 1988 Colonic duplication in an adult. European Journal of Radiology 8: 199

Boothroyd A, Hall C 1990 Rectal duplications in children: a presentation of four cases. European Journal of Radiology 10: 38–41

Carr S, Shaffer H, De Lange E 1988 Duplication of the colon: varied presentation of a rare congenital anomaly. Journal of the Canadian Association of Radiology 39: 29–32

Singh S, Minor C 1980 Cystic duplication of the rectum: a case report. Journal of Pediatric Surgery 15: 205–206

Sonoda N, Matsuzaki S, Ono A, Taniuchi S, Iwase S, Kobayashi Y, Yamada T, Boku T 1985 Duplication of the caecum in a neonate simulating intussusception. Pediatric Radiology 15: 427–429

Yousefzadeh D, Bickers G, Jackson J, Benton C 1983 Tubular colonic duplication – review of 1876–1981 literature. Pediatric Radiology 13: 65–71

COLONIC DIVERTICULA

Colonic diverticula are acquired lesions and are very rare in paediatric practice, even in children with a prolonged history of constipation. There are occasional reports in children with poor collagen structure, e.g. Marfan's syndrome and Ehlers–Danlos syndrome.

MALROTATION

Symptoms due to malrotation with obstruction most commonly occur in the neonatal period due to duodenal obstruction and intermittent volvulus. However, an unexpected malrotation of the colon is an occasional finding during contrast enema examination for investigation of abdominal pain. In paediatric practice, this finding is always regarded as significant, and laparotomy with bowel fixation is undertaken prophylactically to avert a volvulus with bowel infarction. The position of the caecum is very variable and the discovery of a high or medial caecum must not be interpreted as indicative of malrotation.

SIGMOID VOLVULUS

Sigmoid volvulus is uncommon in children, and is most common in mentally subnormal, relatively immobile children. It is believed a congenitally short sigmoid mesentery allows the sigmoid to twist on itself, and if it rotates through 180°, the lumen obstructs. Acute symptoms are of pain, abdominal distension and absolute constipation. Perforation and faecal peritonitis occur rapidly if the obstruction is not relieved. Constipation and chronic abdominal pain are sometimes present with chronic presentation. The typical appearance is of two hugely dilated loops of colon arising from the pelvis, sometimes referred to as the 'coffee bean' sign (Fig. 3.13.5). A contrast enema shows the twisted obstructed sigmoid at the rectosigmoid junction.

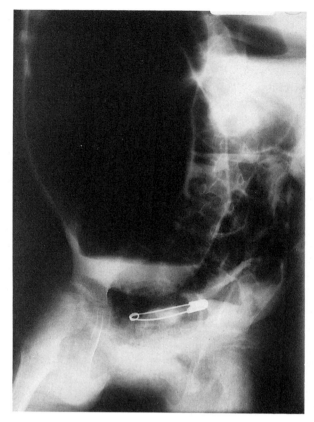

Fig. 3.13.5 Mentally subnormal girl with a 48-hour history of abdominal distension. The huge gas-filled bowel loop is the trapped sigmoid colon which has undergone volvulus. (Safety pin on a nappy.)

Volvulus of other parts of the colon have also been described, including splenic flexure, ascending and transverse colon.

REFERENCES

Andersen J F, Eklof O, Thomasson B 1981 Large bowel volvulus in children. Pediatric Radiology 11: 129–138

De-Castro R, Casolari E, Caal J, Rossi F, Federici S 1986 Sigmoid volvulus in children: a case report. Zeitschrift fuer Kinderchirurgie 41: 119–121

Janik J, Humphrey R, Nagaraj H 1983 Sigmoid volvulus in a neonate with imperforate anus. Journal of Pediatric Surgery 18: 638–638

Knight P, Morse T 1981 Splenic flexure volvulus. Journal of Pediatric Surgery 16: 744–746

Markowitz R, Shashikumar V, Capitano M 1977 Volvulus of the colon in a child with congenital asplenia (Ivemark's Syndrome). Radiology 122: 442

McCalla T, Arensman R, Falterman K 1985 Sigmoid volvulus in children. American Surgeon 51: 514–519

VOLVULUS OF THE CAECUM

Symptomatic caecal volvulus is rare in children, in spite of variable caecal position and the length of the caecal mesentery. Presentation may be acute with abdominal pain and intestinal obstruction, or chronic with symptoms of intermittent pain and colic. On plain radiographs, the grossly dilated caecum is seen to be in the centre of the abdomen or in the left upper quadrant, and usually has a fluid level. There is proximal small bowel obstruction. If there is doubt about the diagnosis, it can be confirmed by barium enema, but the plain radiographs are usually diagnostic.

REFERENCES

Berger R, Hillemeier A, Stahl R, Markowitz R 1982 Volvulus of the ascending colon: an unusual complication of non rotation of the midgut. Pediatric Radiology 12: 298–300
Kirks D, Swischuk L, Merten D, Filston H 1982 Cecal volvulus in children. American Journal of Roentgenology 136: 419–422

HIRSCHSPRUNG'S DISEASE

In Western society, most children with Hirschsprung's disease present in the neonatal period. Occasionally, a child will present beyond that period with a history of constipation and, during investigation of the constipation, radiological features of Hirschsprung's disease are found. The transitional zone between the ganglionated proximal bowel and the aganglionic distal bowel is usually at the rectosigmoid junction in these children (Fig. 3.13.6). In fact, the radiological signs are easier to appreciate at this age than in the neonatal period.

There is proximal distension of the faecal-filled colon which is of a fairly even calibre. This is in contradistinction to children with acquired megacolon in whom the maximum colonic distension and faecal loading are in the rectum and sigmoid colon, with a sharp decrease in colonic calibre proximal to this.

Proximal small bowel obstruction is not usually present, unless the child presents with Hirschsprung's enteritis, a very serious complication which may be associated with profound collapse.

Controversy has existed for many years about the presence of an ultra short segment Hirschsprung's disease, just proximal to the anus, said to lead to a clinical presentation of constipation. Barium enema cannot demonstrate this. Manometric rectal studies and defaecating proctography have been advocated for diagnosis in these cases.

Barium studies and rectal biopsy are the most appropriate method for investigating suspected late presenting Hirschsprung's disease. The patient should not be prepared with aperients or cleansing enemas.

The catheter tip should be placed just inside the anus and barium sulphate administered slowly by hand injection or carefully controlled flow from an enema reservoir. Balloon catheters must not be used. If a zone of transition is shown, contrast administration must immediately cease to avoid barium impaction proximally. In any child with a history of constipation, only enough contrast to show the zone of transition from undilated to dilated bowel, or the relationship of the faecal mass to the anus should be administered. If too much contrast is inadvertently administered, the ward staff should be informed and arrangements made for treatment with aperients and perhaps colonic lavage to avoid impaction.

Postoperative evaluation of the colon

The treatment of Hirschsprung's disease is colostomy on diagnosis, and subsequent surgery, usually by one of several surgical procedures:

1. Swenson pull-through in which the aganglionic segment is excised and there is an anastomosis between the normal colon and the anus.

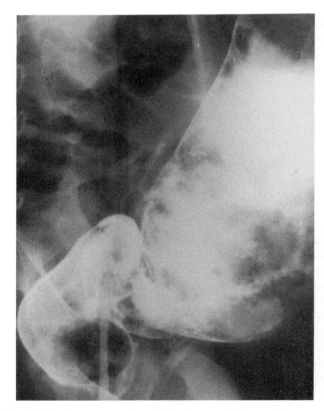

Fig. 3.13.6 Late presentation of Hirschsprung's disease. There is a transition zone at the rectosigmoid colon between distal aganglionic bowel and proximal ganglionic bowel. Boy age 4. Recent immigrant. Lifelong history of constipation.

2. Duhamel procedure, in which proximal ganglionic colon is anastomosed in an end-to-side anastomosis to a posterior preserved rectal wall (Fig. 3.13.7).

3. Soave procedure – the pull-through is tunnelled submucosally to the anus (Fig. 3.13.8).

There are others and all have their own postoperative appearances. In a Swenson pull-through, there is distortion of the perirectal space due to the surgery. In the Duhamel, retention of faeces anteriorly may compress the posterior rectum and cause an appearance of apparent twin channels. Postoperative leaks at the anastomotic sites and abscess formation may occur in the early postoperative phase. Continuing constipation, or faecal incontinence, is a late problem in many children, and such children may have a very sore perineum and great gentleness is required during contrast studies. Following the second stage surgery it is usual to leave the child with a colostomy to allow healing of the anastomoses. A distal bowel study is usually done before closure of the colostomy to ensure no leaks or stricture formation. Contrast studies are also often required later when fistula formation or abscess occurs.

All contrast studies done in the defunctioned bowel are best done with water-soluble contrast media to avoid formation of a barolith and minimize complications in the presence of a leak.

Associations of Hirschsprung's disease with malrotation and neuroblastoma have been described.

REFERENCES

Brereton R, Cudmore R, Carty H 1980 Hirschsprung's disease with intestinal malrotation: a dangerous combination. Zeitschrift fuer Kinderchirurgie 29: 2–4
Filston H, Kirks D 1982 The association of malrotation and Hirschsprung's disease. Pediatric Radiology 12: 6–10
Gaisie G, Oh K, Young L 1979 Coexistent neuroblastoma and Hirschsprung's disease – another manifestation of the neurocristopathy? Pediatric Radiology 8: 161–163
Mahboubi S, Schnaufer L 1979 The barium-enema examination and rectal manometry in Hirschsprung disease. Radiology 130: 643–647
Nagasaki A, Ikeda K, Hayashida Y 1984 Radiologic diagnosis of Hirschsprung's disease utilizing rectosphincteric reflex. Pediatric Radiology 14: 384–387

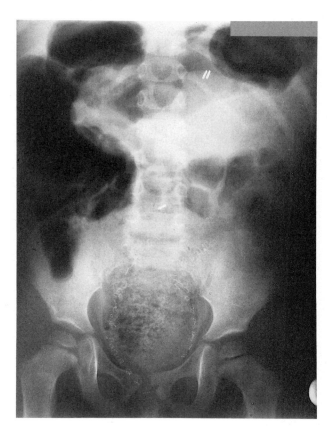

Fig. 3.13.7 Recurrent constipation post Duhamel procedure for Hirschsprung's disease. The staples outlining the resection are characteristic.

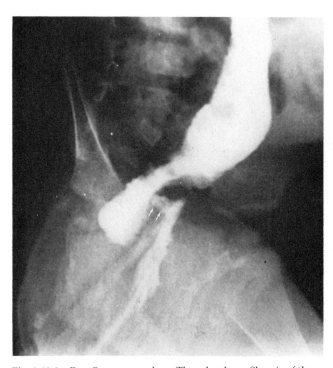

Fig. 3.13.8 Post Soave procedure. There has been fibrosis of the muscular channel and a fistula has formed to the presacral space which is in communication with the normal bowel. Contrast is in the defunctioned bowel which was being assessed prior to closure of colostomy.

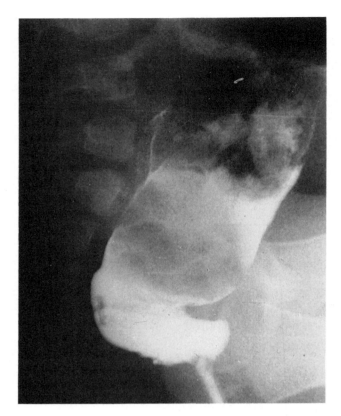

Fig. 3.13.9 Limited barium enema in a child being investigated for chronic constipation. Note the examination has been terminated once the relationship of the anus to the faecal mass has been shown.

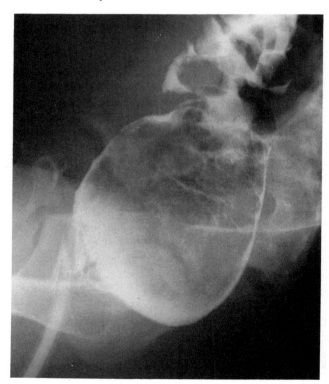

Fig. 3.13.10 Acquired megacolon. Note the ballooning of the rectum with a transition to more normal calibre sigmoid colon. Note also the ballooning of the rectum posteriorly so that the anus is apparently displaced anteriorly. This must be distinguished from a congenital anteriorly placed anus.

ACQUIRED MEGACOLON; ACQUIRED CONSTIPATION

Chronic constipation is a common symptom in children, and is generally a functional problem without underlying organic pathology. Children with this functional constipation usually are normal in the first year or so of life, unless they have anal fissures. The functional problem may be a manifestation of psychogenic illness or result from a previous fissure is ano. More rarely, it can be due to faulty diet. Constipation is common in the sedentary, mentally subnormal child, and is a constant feature of children with interruption of the normal neurogenic supply to bowel musculature, such as in spina bifida or sacral agenesis. It is also a feature of children with poor muscle tone, and certain endocrine disorders, in particular hypothyroidism. The clinical problem is to exclude organic pathology, in particular Hirschsprung's disease. Most children will be referred for a barium enema. Whilst constipation is the dominant presenting feature, overflow incontinence is common and may

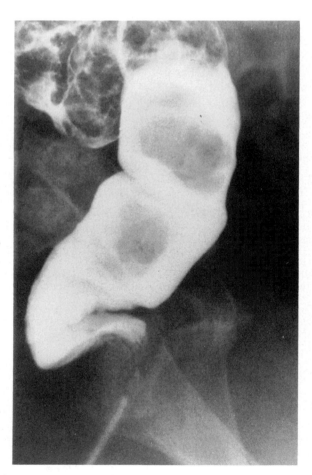

Fig. 3.13.11 Anterior displacement of the anus causing constipation. Defaecation is 'uphill'.

lead to a clinical referral for an enema to investigate diarrhoea! Good clinical liaison is necessary to ensure that the correct preparation for barium enemas is carried out. If there is doubt about the clinical history, a plain abdominal radiograph may save inappropriate management.

All investigations for constipation should be done without prior preparation. Only enough barium to show the relationship of the anal margin to the faecal mass should be injected (Fig. 3.13.9). In acquired constipation the rectum balloons mainly posteriorly so that it comes to lie distal to the anus (Fig. 3.13.10). There is no narrow segment of bowel, and usually a change in bowel calibre at the junction of sigmoid and descending colon, unlike Hirschsprung's disease. Another pattern is even distension of the rectum and the sigmoid colon without the ballooning (Fig. 3.13.9). Congenital anterior displacement of the anus also causes difficulty in defaecation with unremitting constipation (Fig. 3.13.11).

The degree of distension of rectum and sigmoid colon can be massive with dilatation extending to the diaphragm (Fig. 3.13.12), and may be sufficient to interfere with respiration. The bladder may also be displaced by the rectal mass (Fig. 3.13.13).

Treatment of this type of megacolon is entirely medical with initial clearing of the bowel and then appropriate dietary and bowel retraining.

Whilst Hirschsprung's disease is the main differential diagnosis, a small group of children will have chronic adynamic ileus of the colon, neuronal dysplasia or sacral anomaly. Radiographs must be assessed carefully for sacral anomaly or evidence of an intraspinal lesion, e.g. widening of the interpedicular distance. Very rarely severe constipation can lead to acute retention of urine but before attributing this to the constipation every effort must be made to exclude a neurogenic cause.

Rectal manometry is an adjunct to radiological investigation showing abnormal manometric relaxation in response to rectal distension.

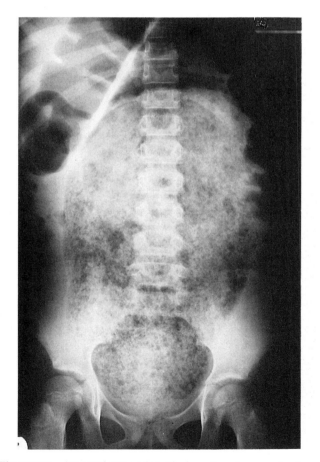

Fig. 3.13.12 Acquired megacolon. The huge faecal mass extends from the anus almost to the diaphragm. The calibre of the transverse colon is normal.

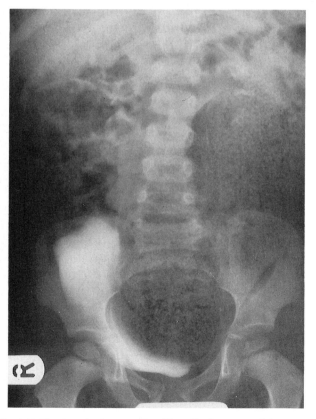

Fig. 3.13.13 Acquired megacolon. Note displacement of the bladder by the rectosigmoid mass of faeces.

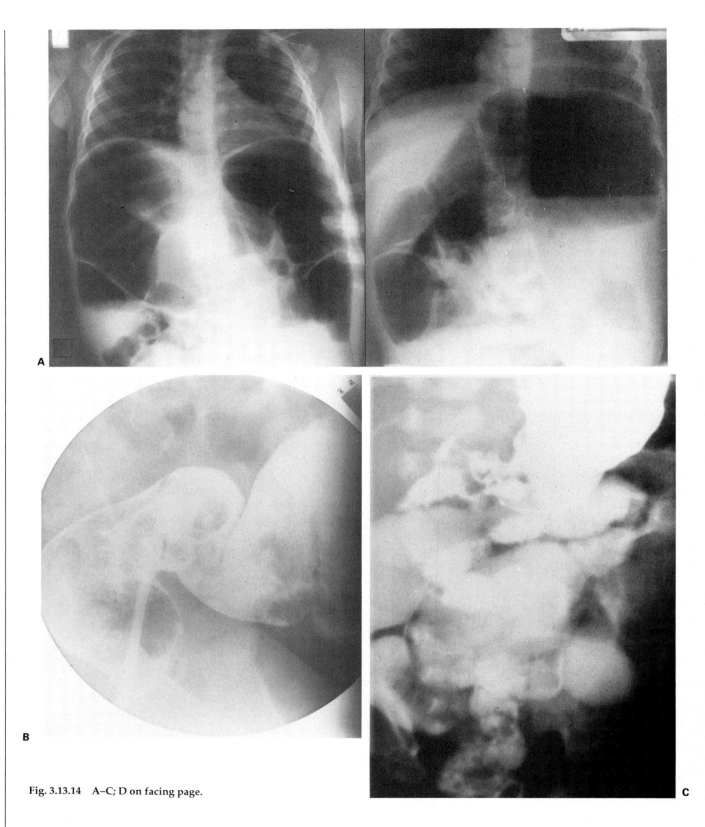

Fig. 3.13.14   A–C; D on facing page.

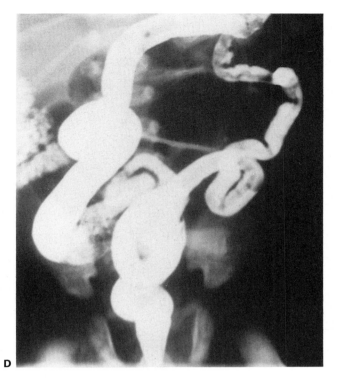

D

Fig. 3.13.14 **A** 3-year-old boy with neuronal dysplasia. **A** Erect and supine abdomen. He complained of recurrent attacks of abdominal distension and chronic constipation. Note the marked dilatation of the colon, without small bowel distension. The colonic appearance is similar to that seen in pseudo-obstruction. **B** Barium enema. There is an apparent transition zone at the rectosigmoid junction. An initial diagnosis of Hirschsprung's disease was made. All biopsies showed normal ganglia but more detailed examination showed histological features of neuronal dysplasia. **C** Neuronal dysplasia of small and **D**, large bowel in a neonate. Note general dilatation of the small bowel with normal calibre duodenum. The contrast enema shows a small colon with a distensible rectum. The infant presented with failure to pass meconium. Initial diagnosis was thought to be Hirschsprung's disease and a 'cone' was visible at operation in the terminal ileum. Histology and subsequent clinical behaviour proved neuronal dysplasia.

REFERENCES

Heij H, Moorman-Voestermans C, Vos A, Kneepkens C 1990 Triad of anorectal stenosis, sacral anomaly and presacral mass: a remediable cause of severe constipation. British Journal of Surgery 77: 102–104
Meunier P, Louis D, Jaunbert-De-Beaujeu M 1984 Physiologic investigation of primary chronic constipation in children: comparison with the barium enema study. Gastroenterology 87: 1351–1357

CHRONIC PSEUDO-OBSTRUCTION OF THE COLON

This is a rare condition presenting with constipation, abdominal distension and symptoms that suggest an acute colonic obstruction. On plain abdominal radiographs, distended large and small bowel is present with air-fluid levels throughout. A contrast enema will show no obstructing lesion. Routine rectal biopsy is normal. During enema, absent peristaltic activity gives the clue to the underlying problem.

REFERENCES

Franken E, Smith W, Frey E, Sato Y, Anuras S 1987 Intestinal motility disorders of infants and children. Classification, clinical manifestations and roentgenology. Clinical Reviews in Diagnostic Imaging 27: 203–236
Gilchrist A, Mills J, Russell C 1985 Acute large bowel pseudo obstruction. Clinical Radiology 36: 401–404
Kapila L, Haberkorn S, Nixon H 1975 Chronic adynamic bowel simulating Hirschsprung's disease. Journal of Pediatric Surgery 10: 885–892
MacMahon R M, Moore C C M, Cussen L J 1981 Hirschsprung-like syndromes in patients with normal ganglion cells on suction rectal biopsy. Journal of Pediatric Surgery 16: 835–839

NEURONAL COLONIC DYSPLASIA

In this condition, there is hypoplasia of the ganglion cells as opposed to complete absence. Clinically, the children present similarly to those with true Hirschsprung's disease, but usually later than the neonatal period. Radiologically, the features may be identical to Hirschsprung's disease, with a narrow non-distensible rectum and a transition zone to normal bowel demonstrated at contrast enema (Fig. 3.13.14).

Plexiform neurofibroma infiltrating the bowel can also mimic Hirschsprung's disease.

REFERENCES

Franken E A, Smith W L, Frey E E, Sato Y, Anuras S 1987 Intestinal motility disorders of infants and children: classification, clinical manifestations and roentgenology. Clinical Reviews in Diagnostic Imaging 27: 203–236
Lake B D 1988 Observations on the pathology of pseudo-obstruction. In: Milla P J (ed) Disorders of gastrointestinal motility in childhood. John Wiley, Chichester, pp 81–90
Munakata K, Morita K, Okabe I, Sueoka H 1985 Clinical and histologic studies of neuronal intestinal dysplasia. Journal of Pediatric Surgery 20: 231–235
Scharli A F, Meier-Ruge W 1981 Localised and disseminated forms of neuronal intestinal dysplasia mimicking Hirschsprung's disease. Journal of Pediatric Surgery 16: 164–170
Stone M M, Weinberg B, Beck A R, Grishman E, Gertner M 1986 Colonic obstruction in a child with von Recklinghausen's neurofibromatosis. Journal of Pediatric Surgery 21: 741–743

COLONIC STRICTURE

Stricture formation is a consequence of many anorectal operations, colonic resections, and may be a late complication of necrotizing enterocolitis, presenting with pain, failure to pass flatus, constipation and obstruction. When suspected, a constrast enema, before which knowledge of any surgical details is important, is indicated to identify the site of obstruction. Careful fluoroscopy with rotation into differing projections is essential to avoid overlapping of contrast-filled segments. Strictures can be short and easily missed. Balloon dilatation of postsurgical rectal strictures can be successful.

REFERENCE

Wilder W, Melhem R 1989 Balloon dilatation of post-surgical anorectal stricture in two infants. Pediatric Radiology 19: 527–529

FAECAL INCONTINENCE

Faecal incontinence is common with neurological impairment, and mental subnormality without underlying organic pathology. Overflow incontinence is a feature of gross constipation. Incontinence is also a frequent problem in inflammatory bowel disease. Incontinence may be a major problem following anorectal surgery, either for Hirschsprung's disease, anorectal malformations or colonic resection with ileorectal anastomosis, when failure of absorption of fluid is the problem. The discharge of ileal content can lead to severe excoriation of the perineum.

In both Hirschsprung's disease and anorectal pull through operations the problem is one of abnormal innervation, abnormal musculature and interruption of the normal anorectal sphincter. A contrast enema is indicated to assess the anorectal anastomosis, rectal peristalsis and continence during straining movements. More recent developments in investigation are the use of endorectal ultrasound to observe the sphincteric muscles, MRI examination and axial and direct coronal CT (Fig. 3.13.15), to assess the muscle and the location of the pull-through relative to the midline and puborectalis muscle sling. Defaecating proctography is occasionally helpful.

In all contrast studies, the following should be observed:

1. the anorectal angle and its position on straining
2. peristaltic activity and abnormal rectal wall movement.

During normal defaecation there is relaxation of the pelvic floor muscles, descent of the anorectal junction and widening of the canal. Failure of these movements is found in both constipation and following surgery.

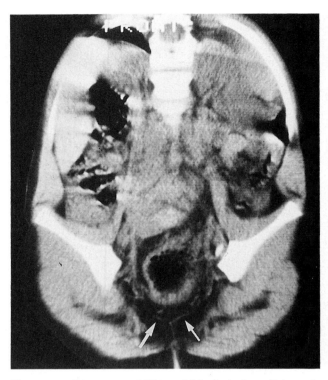

Fig. 3.13.15 Direct coronal CT in a child who had a pull-through for anorectal atresia. The arrows point to the levator ani muscles. Another cut showed the anal canal to lie centrally. These levator muscles are reasonably developed.

REFERENCES

1. Goei R 1990 Anorectal function in patients with defecation disorders and asymptomatic subjects: evaluation with defecography. Radiology 174: 121–123
2. Vade A, Reyes H, Wilbur A, Gyi B, Spigos D 1989 The anorectal sphincter after rectal pull-through surgery for anorectal anomalies: MRI evaluation. Pediatric Radiology 19: 179–183.

INTUSSUSCEPTION

Intussusception is invagination of a segment of bowel into the bowel distally. The two most common forms are ileo-ileocolic or ileocolic, accounting for over 90% of all cases. Ileo-ileal intussusception is rare as a primary presentation but is seen as a postoperative complication. Colo-colic intussusception is commoner in Africa but it is rare in Europe. Intussusception tends to occur seasonally and is most frequent during periods of viral respiratory illness and gastrointestinal infections. It is seen at all ages but is most frequent under the age of 2, with 75% of cases occurring under 2 years and 50% under 1 year. There is a male preponderance of 2 :1.

The invaginating bowel is known as the intussusceptum and the bowel surrounding it the intussuscipiens. Line diagrams of the different varieties are shown in Figure 3.13.16).

Colicky abdominal pain with drawing up of the legs to the abdomen is the commonest presentation (90%). Other common symptoms are vomiting (80%), blood per rectum with redcurrant jelly stools (60%) and an abdominal mass (60%). This mass is sometimes difficult to palpate in the tense abdomen. Diarrhoea is also a presenting feature. Abdominal distension may also be present even without frank bowel obstruction.

The natural history of the disease is progression to mechanical obstruction unless the intussusception is reduced. Bowel infarction may occur in the obstructed bowel due to vascular compromise. Children with obstruction or a compromised bowel may present in shock.

Aetiology

Most cases are idiopathic and are probably due to inflammation of Peyer's patches in association with a viral illness. Intussuscepting lead points include Meckel's diverticulum, duplication of the bowel, lymphoma, polyps (isolated or as part of syndromes such as Peutz–Jegher's), appendicitis, Henoch–Schönlein purpura and inspissated bowel content in patients with cystic fibrosis. It is rare to achieve successful hydrostatic reduction if there is a pathological lead point. Most children with a pathological lead point present above the age of 4 years. Isolated ileo-ileal intussusceptions are not usually reduced hydrostatically.

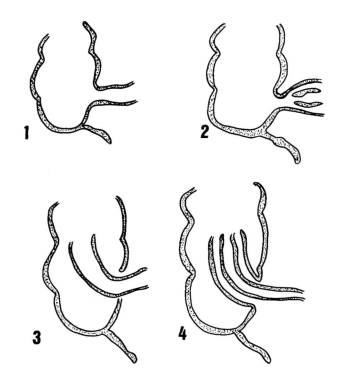

Fig. 3.13.16 Types of intussusception.
1 = Normal, 2 = ileo-ileal, 3 = ileo-colic, 4 = ileo-ileocolic.

Radiology

Emergency resuscitation must be instituted before any diagnostic or therapeutic procedures.

An initial supine abdominal radiograph should be supplemented by erect or decubitus views for assessment of obstruction. Perforation is rare at presentation. The typical appearance of intussusception on the plain radiograph is a soft tissue mass indenting the colon (Fig. 3.13.17), but this is present in only about 25% of patients. When present, it is seldom seen outside the region from the hepatic to splenic flexure (Fig. 3.13.18). Depending on the length of history and the degree of obstruction, a variable number of fluid levels in the small bowel may be associated. Two other frequent appearances are an absence of gas in the right upper quadrant with failure to identify the hepatic flexure gas pattern, and a non-specific right abdominal mass (Fig. 3.13.19). When there is significant obstruction the mass will not be appreciated, being obscured by bowel loops. A rarer appearance, particularly with an intussusception presenting in the rectosigmoid area, is an almost gasless abdomen. It is no longer accepted that the bowel distal to an intussusception is free of faeces. The plain film may be entirely normal in the presence of an intussusception.

Ultrasound

Ultrasound is a sensitive method of detecting intussusception and should be done where there is clinical suspicion and equivocal radiography, before proceeding to a diagnostic enema. The appearance is of a low density mass with a central target sign (Fig. 3.13.20). In ileo-colic intussusception a single bowel wall is seen around the central echo. In ileo-ileocolic intussusception it is possible to distinguish the two walls (Fig. 3.13.21), a bad prognostic sign for successful hyrostatic reduction as the ileo-ileal component is frequently not reduced hydrostatically. However, it is worth reducing the ileo-colic component as this makes surgery simpler.

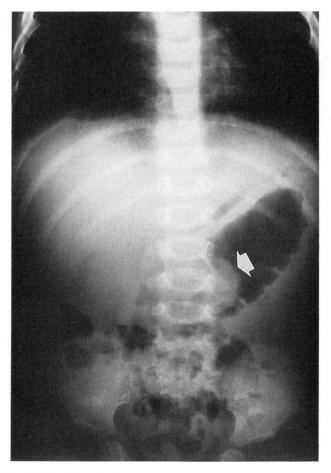

Fig. 3.13.17 Typical plain abdominal film of ileo-colic intussusception. The intussuscipiens (arrow) indents the colon.

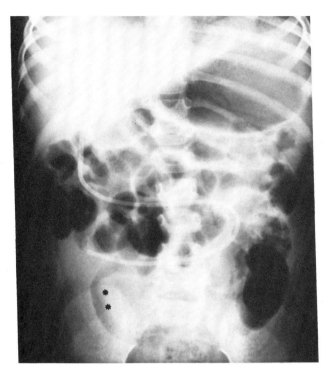

Fig. 3.13.18 Unusual though typical appearance of an intussuscepting mass in the lower abdomen. This was an ileo-ileal intussusception due to an inflammatory lesion around a Meckel's diverticulum (asterisks on intussuscipions).

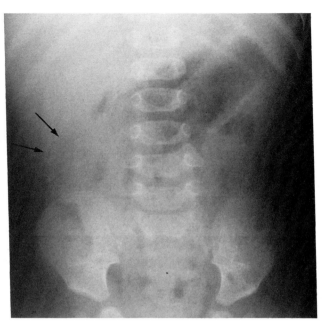

Fig. 3.13.19 Intussusception. Note right-sided mass (arrows) and absence of normal hepatic flexure outline.

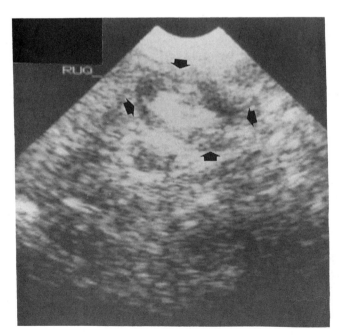

Fig. 3.13.20 Ileo-colic intussusception. The central bright echoes are due to air trapped in the intussuscipiens.

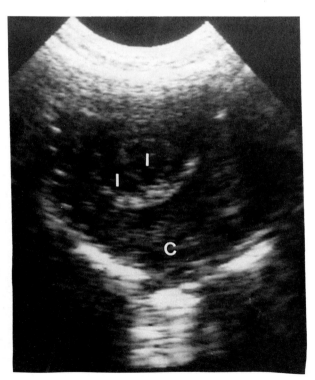

Fig. 3.13.21 Ileo-ileocolic intussusception. The central echoes have a double outline indicating an ileo-ileocolic intussusception. I = ileum, C = colon.

Reduction

Premedication with morphine sulphate will make the child less distressed and slightly improves the success rate of non-surgical reduction. Some centres use general anaesthesia but this is unnecessary.

Successful reduction of an intussusception may be achieved by hydrostatic means or by air insufflation. Neither should be attempted before discussion with the surgical team and until the child is haemodynamically stable. It has been traditional that closed reduction is not attempted in the presence of small bowel obstruction. This is no longer accepted. The only absolute contraindications to attempted closed reduction is persistence of shock following initial resuscitation, signs of peritonitis and demonstration of perforation. An intussusception presenting in the rectum is less likely to be reduced than one more proximally placed as it is difficult to achieve sufficient pressure for reduction (Fig. 3.13.22). However, it is worth attempting as it may succeed and any reduction diminishes the amount of bowel manipulation at

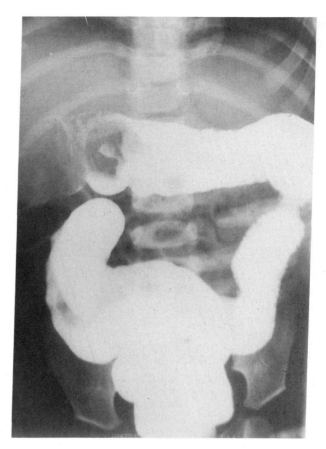

Fig. 3.13.23 Intussusception in the right upper quadrant. The coil spring appearance proximal to the head is due to barium trapped in the mucosal folds.

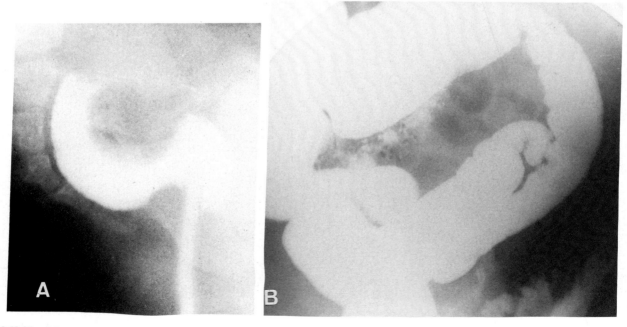

Fig. 3.13.22 **A** Intussusception presenting in the rectum. Despite this presentation, successful reduction was achieved. **B** Note barium in the small bowel indicating successful reduction.

subsequent surgery. A prolapsing intussusception cannot be reduced hydrostatically. Recurrent intussusception may be successfully reduced.

The choice of air or barium will depend on local practice and availability. Advantages of air are that it is quicker, cleaner, easier to see reflux through the ileocaecal valve, and has a substantially reduced radiation dose. There must be a reliable pressure valve in the system to maintain the pressure below 100 mmHg. Carbon dioxide, oxygen or room air may be used. For both hydrostatic and air reduction a catheter is placed in the rectum and the catheter taped to the bottom. For hydrostatic reduction, barium sulphate, diluted to approximately 1 : 3 with water, is gently and steadily introduced via the rectal catheter, with the enema bag being approximately 1 m above the table top. A typical appearance of an intussusception is shown in (Figure 3.13.23). Even, sustained pressure is more effective at achieving reduction than sudden bursts of pressure. Intermittent fluoroscopy will check on the progress of reduction. This frequently proceeds at an uneven pace and hold up is frequent in the region of the caecum and ascending colon. Pressure is sustained for 5 minutes then released and the colon refilled. Several attempts should be made before abandoning the examination. Successful reduction is confirmed when contrast flows through the ileocaecal valve into the terminal ileum. Care must be taken not to confuse the appendix with the terminal ileum. It is often easier to appreciate the small bowel contrast on a postevacuation film. If contrast flows round a loop of small bowel within the caecum, sufficient hydrostatic pressure cannot be sustained on the intussusception to achieve reduction and surgical intervention will be necessary (Fig. 3.13.24).

The ileocaecal valve may become very oedematous and it may be impossible to reflux contrast into the small bowel. The oedematous valve can look like a persistent unreduced intussusception, when in fact complete reduction has been achieved (Fig. 3.13.25). If this is the only residual defect, the child should not be referred for surgery. An expectant policy is advocated if there is no residual palpable mass. Severe caecal oedema is also sometimes found (Fig. 3.13.26). In both instances a normal ultrasound is also found but a good view may be obscured by air.

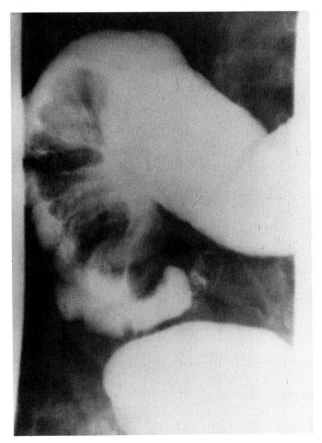

Fig. 3.13.24 A loop of ileum is present in the caecum, outlined by barium which is filling the appendix. This makes further reduction impossible.

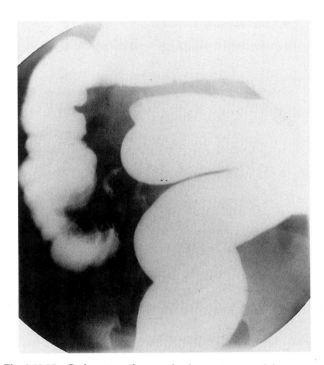

Fig. 3.13.25 Oedematous ileocaecal valve post successful reduction of intussusception.

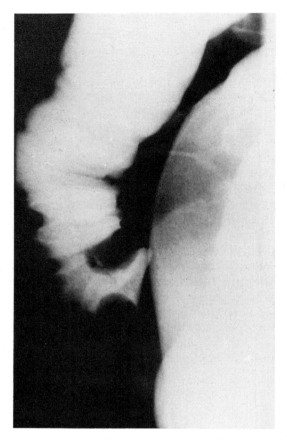

Fig. 3.13.26 Severe caecal oedema post successful reduction of intussusception.

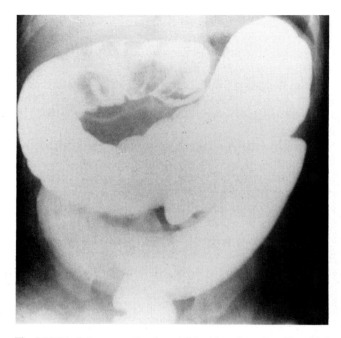

Fig. 3.13.27 Intussusception in a child with malrotation. Note high midline position of caecum. There is a loop of ileum contained within the caecum. The intussusception was irreducible.

Following reduction, the child is maintained on fluids for 12 hours and kept under close observation. It becomes rapidly clinically apparent if reduction has in reality been successful. A repeat ultrasound will confirm reduction. Children who have often been very fretful and distressed will suddenly calm down and often go to sleep on the table following successful reduction.

Even though glucagon and Buscopan act as bowel muscle relaxants, they have no effect on improving the success rate of hydrostatic reduction. The success rate of non-surgical reduction varies widely within reported series, and depends on the selection of cases and the experience of the radiologist. A realistic success rate for an experienced radiologist with an unselected group of patients is 70%.

Complications

Perforation during hydrostatic reduction is a rare complication. The examination must be immediately abandoned. Perforation may occur at the site of the intussusception where the bowel is compromised but is also well described in the normal bowel distal to the intussusception – the cause at this site is not known. If perforation occurs during air reduction, extensive air may enter the peritoneal cavity and lead to compromised diaphragmatic movement with respiratory embarrassment. Decompression of the peritoneum by inserting a trocar to allow escape of air may be necessary as emergency treatment. Barium peritonitis occurring as a result of perforation during hydrostatic reduction does not appear to lead to long-term complications provided careful peritoneal lavage and debridement is done at surgical exploration.

The association of intussusception and intestinal malrotation is known as Waugh's syndrome (Fig. 3.13.27).

REFERENCES

Armstrong E, Dunbar J, Graviss E, Martin L, Rosenkrantz J 1980 Intussusception complicated by distal perforation of the colon. Radiology 136: 77–81
Bisset G, Kirks D 1988 Intussusception in infants and children: diagnosis and therapy. Radiology 168: 141–145
Brereton R, Taylor B, Hall C 1986 Intussusception and intestinal malrotation of infants: Waugh's syndrome. British Journal of Surgery 73: 55–57
Campbell J 1989 Contrast media in intussusception. Pediatric Radiology 19: 293–296
De Campo J, Phelan E 1989 Gas reduction of intussusception. Pediatric Radiology 19: 297–298
Devred Ph, Faure F, Padovani J 1984 Pseudotumoral cecum after hydrostatic reduction of intussusception. Pediatric Radiology 14: 295–298
Eklof O, Hald J, Thomasson B 1983 Barium peritonitis. Experience of five pediatric cases. Pediatric Radiology 13: 5–9
Franken E, Smith W, Chernish S, Campbell J, Fletcher B, Goldman H 1983 The use of glucagon in hydrostatic reduction of intussusception. A double blind study of 30 patients. Radiology 146: 687–689
Hedlund G, Johnson J, Strife J 1990 Ileocolic intussusception: extensive reflux of air preceding pneumatic reduction. Radiology 174: 187–189
Jennings C, Kelleher J 1984 Intussusception: influence of age on reducibility. Pediatric Radiology 14: 292–295
Mahboubi S, Sherman N, Ziegler M 1984 Barium peritonitis following attempted reduction of intussusception. Clinical Pediatrics 23: 36–38
Paes R, Hyde I, Griffiths D 1988 The management of intussusception. British Journal of Radiology 61: 187–189
Patriquin H B, Afshani E, Effmann E, Griscom N, Johnson F, Kramer S, Rapp R, Reilly B 1977 Neonatal intussusception. Radiology 125: 463–466
Persoff M, Arterburn J 1972 Eosinophilic granuloma causing intussusception in a three year old child. American Journal of Surgery 124: 676–678
Stephenson C, Seibert J, Strain J, Glasier C, Leithiser R, Iqbal V 1989 Intussusception: clinical and radiographic factors influencing reducibility. Pediatric Radiology 20: 57–60
Stringer D, Ein S 1990 Pneumatic reduction: advantages, risks and indications. Pediatric Radiology 20: 475–477
Swischuk L, Hayden C, Boulden T 1985 Intussusception: indications for ultrasonography and explanation of the doughnut and pseudokidney signs. Pediatric Radiology 15: 388–391

ULCERATIVE COLITIS

Ulcerative colitis is an inflammatory disease of the colon of unknown aetiology. Most patients present in adult life. Childhood presentation is mainly over 10 years of age, but sporadic cases are reported younger than this, including the first year of life and neonates. There is a high familial incidence. There is an increased risk of development of carcinoma in patients with ulcerative colitis in whom the colon is not removed, starting at about 10 years from diagnosis and increasing with time. The clinical presentation is one of frequent loose stools, blood and mucus per rectum, colicky abdominal pain, weight loss and anaemia. Other symptoms include dehydration, poor growth, delayed physical and sexual maturation, and, more rarely, osteoporosis. Liver disease – fatty infiltration. sclerosing cholangitis and, ultimately, cirrhosis, may complicate the disease. Other extra-colonic manifestations include arthritis, skin rashes and uveitis and, rarely, cerebral thromboembolic disease. The arthritis affects the sacroiliac joints in most cases but may also affect the large and small joints in a pattern more suggestive of juvenile chronic arthritis. Occasionally the arthritic complaints antecede the bowel problems. Periosteal reaction has been rarely reported in ulcerative colitis.

The progress of the disease is very variable, some children pursuing a relentless course leading to early colectomy. Others may have periods of remission and exacerbation.

The initial ulceration is in the mucosa and submucosa, but it may spread to involve the muscle layer. Ulceration begins in the rectum and spreads proximally in a symmetrical fashion, unlike Crohn's disease, where involvement of one part of the bowel wall and not the whole circumference is common, together with disease affecting one segment and sparing another – 'skip lesions'. In the early stages of ulcerative colitis, the ulcers are small and even though contact bleeding is present on proctoscopy, no abnormality may be shown by barium studies. Barium studies should be done following bowel preparation unless the child is acutely ill and in shock, which suggests the complication of toxic megacolon. A double contrast technique is used. The earliest radiological sign is a fine granular appearance of the mucosa with fine ulceration of the wall when seen in profile (Fig. 3.13.28). This must not be confused with the filling of the normal crypts of Lieberkuhn, which are sometimes seen on postevacuation films in the normal colon. As the disease progresses the ulcers deepen and give a ragged edge to the colonic wall (Fig. 3.13.29). Tracking in the submucosal region gives 'collar stud abscess'. Later, there is progressive narrowing of the rectum, increase in the postrectal space, shortening of the colon, loss of haustra, and, ultimately, a short, stiff colon referred to as a 'lead pipe' colon (Fig.

3.13.30). In a healing stage, filiform mucosal polyps may be seen. Backwash ileitis is seen in some children due to incompetence of the ileocaecal valve.

The main differential diagnosis is Crohn's disease, and it is not always easy to separate the two conditions by barium enema alone. Other conditions that can simulate the radiographic changes of ulcerative colitis are amoebic and bacillary dysentery, yersinia and campylobacter colitis and pseudomembranous colitis.

Toxic megacolon is a complication generally seen in adult patients in which there is a diffuse dilatation of the colon and often pseudopolypoid appearance of the mucosa seen on the plain radiographs. In spite of the name, the degree of distension does not have to be very large. Signs of systemic toxicity occur in association with abdominal pain and distension. This is a serious complication and perforation and peritonitis are common if colectomy is not undertaken.

Management initially is by medical treatment but colectomy is required in many children with intractable symptoms. Two types of surgery are carried out – total colectomy with a permanent ileostomy and, increasingly, colectomy with endorectal pull-through to avoid permanent ileostomy. The

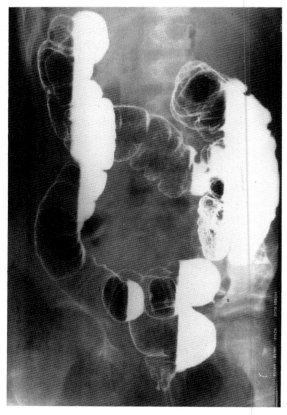

Fig. 3.13.28 Total colonic involvement with ulcerative colitis. There is a fine granular pattern visible in the rectum and descending colon but best seen in the transverse colon.

radiological appearances of a normal endorectal pull-through are a smooth mucosa with loss of the small bowel features, enlargement of the neorectum and enlargement of the presacral space. Recurrent disease in this region will show mucosal irregularity, narrowing and loss of distensibility.

REFERENCES

Arlart I P, Maier W, Leupold D, Wolf A 1982 Massive periosteal new bone formation in ulcerative colitis. Radiology 144: 507–508

Bank E, White S, Coran A 1986 The radiographic appearance of the endorectal pull-through. Pediatric Radiology 16: 216–221

Bar-Ziv J, Yagupsky P, Karplus M, Mares A, Maor E 1982 Congenital ulcerative colitis. Annales de Radiologie 25: 59–64

Chong S, Bartram C, Campbell C, Williams C, Blackshaw A, Walker Smith J 1982 Chronic inflammatory bowel disease in childhood. British Medical Journal 284: 101–103

Chong S, Walker-Smith J 1984 Ulcerative colitis in childhood. Journal the Royal Society of Medicine 77 (Supplement 3): 21–26

Ein S, Lynch M, Stephens C 1971 Ulcerative colitis in children under one year: a twenty year review. Journal of Pediatric Surgery 6: 264–271

Fernbach S, Lloyd-Still J 1984 The radiographic findings in severe rotavirus induced colitis. Journal of the Canadian Association of. Radiology 35: 192–194

Karjoo M, McCarty B 1976 Toxic megacolon of ulcerative colitis in infancy. Pediatrics 57: 962–965

Markowitz R, Ment L, Gryboski J 1989 Cerebral thromboembolic disease in paediatric and adult inflammatory bowel disease: case report and review of the literature. Journal of Pediatric Gastroenterology and Nutrition 8: 413–420

Stringer D 1987 Imaging inflammatory bowel disease in the pediatric patient. Radiologic Clinics of North America 25: 93–113

Winthrop J, Balfe D, Schackelford G, McAlister W, Rosenblum J, Siegel M 1985 Ulcerative and granulomatous colitis in children: comparison of double and single contrast studies. Radiology 154: 657–660

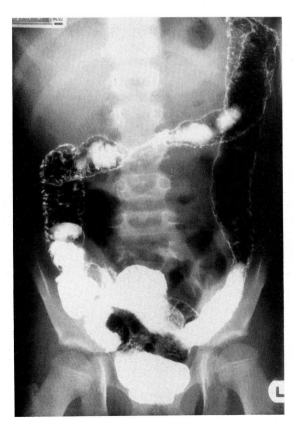

Fig. 3.13.29 Moderately severe ulcerative colitis. Note the ragged ulcerated edge of most of the colon with some collar stud abscesses in the transverse colon. Relative sparing of the rectum is due to local cortisone enemas.

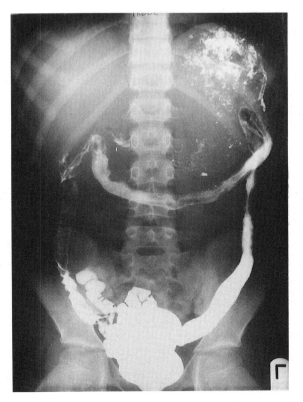

Fig. 3.13.30 Longstanding ulcerative colitis seen on follow-through examination. Note the featureless narrow colon which has not yet undergone shortening. (Barium in stomach is due to the earlier upper gastrointestinal study.)

THE PLAIN ABDOMINAL RADIOGRAPH IN INFLAMMATORY BOWEL DISEASE

Areas of bowel affected by inflammatory disease tend to be free of faeces. Careful review of the abdominal radiograph for segments of bowel free of faeces, particularly when associated with proximal bowel containing an abnormal faecal content, may suggest the presence of inflammatory bowel disease but will not distinguish between the differing types. Other features found include thickening of the bowel wall, mucosal oedema with a polypoid appearance ('thumbprinting'), abscess cavities, air in the bladder or kidneys due to fistula formation and, rarely in children, features of toxic megacolon, with dilatation of the transverse or whole colon, thickening of the bowel wall and mucosal oedema.

REFERENCE

Taylor G, Nancarrow P, Hernanz-Schulman M, Teele R 1986 Plain abdominal radiographs in children with inflammatory bowel disease. Pediatric Radiology 16: 206–209

PSEUDOMEMBRANOUS COLITIS

Pseudomembranous colitis is due to a colitis associated with a toxin produced by *Clostridium difficile* following antibiotic therapy. Shigella and staphylococcal infections have also caused a similar colitis. The condition is very rare in children, with fever, bloody diarrhoea and sometimes shock and collapse as presentations. On plain radiographs 'thumbprinting' of the large bowel, thickening of haustra and sometimes evidence of ascites, which is an exudative ascites secondary to the inflammation, may be seen. If a contrast enema is done, coarse ulceration with or without 'thumbprinting' is found (Fig. 3.13.31), but diagnosis is easier by colonoscopy where the yellowish mucosal plaques are seen.

REFERENCES

Kelber M, Ament M 1976 Shigella dysenteriae I: a forgotten cause of pseudomembranous colitis. Journal of Pediatrics 89: 595–596
Loughran C, Tappin J, Whitehouse G 1982 The plain abdominal radiograph in pseudomembranous colitis due to *Clostridium difficile*. Clinical Radiology 33: 227–281
Schussheim A, Goldstein E 1980 Antibiotic-associated pseudomembranous colitis in siblings. Paediatrics 66: 932–935
Stanley R J, Melson G L, Tedesco F J 1974 The spectrum of radiographic finding in antibiotic-related pseudomembranous colitis. Radiology 111: 519–524
Stringer D 1987 Imaging inflammatory bowel disease in the pediatric patient. Radiologic Clinics of North America 25: 93–113

TYPHLITIS (NEUTROPENIC COLITIS)

This is a form of colitis seen in immunocompromised patients due to bacterial overgrowth causing mucosal ulceration and ischaemia. Typhlitis strictly refers to caecal involvement, but there may be a pancolitis which can rapidly progress to perforation. The radiological manifestations are 'thumbprinting' of the bowel due to oedema, and in more severe cases submucosal and intramural gas, such as is seen in infants with necrotizing enterocolitis. Secondary small bowel dilatation may occur. Clinically the children present with pain and blood and mucus per rectum. Caecal involvement may cause clinical features similar to appendicitis. Thickening of the bowel wall is seen both on CT and ultrasound examination, neither of which is seen in appendicitis (Fig. 3.13.32). Severe gastrointestinal haemorrhage is a complication which can be life threatening. Its site may be localized by radioisotopic red cell scanning.

Whilst neutropenic colitis is most common in immunocompromised and severely neutropenic

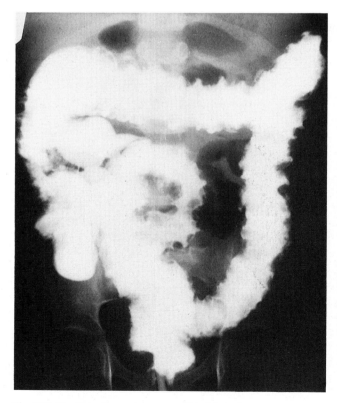

Fig. 3.13.31 Pseudomembranous colitis. Note the extensive coarse ulceration affecting the whole of the bowel.

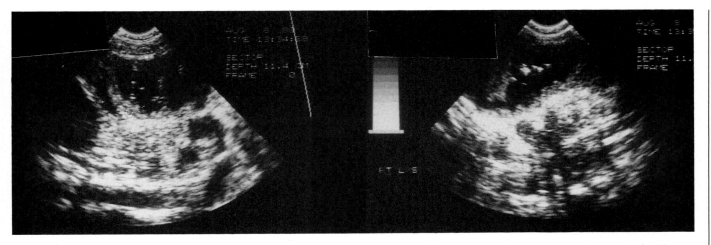

Fig. 3.13.32 Two frames from an ultrasound examination of the right abdomen in a child on treatment for leukaemia who presented with abdominal pain and blood per rectum. There is thickening of the bowel wall and mucosal irregularity typical of typhlitis.

patients due to leukaemia or its treatment, it has also been described following renal transplantation.

REFERENCES

Abramson S, Berdon W, Baker D 1983 Childhood typhlitis: its increasing association with acute myelogenous leukaemia. Report of 5 cases. Radiology 146: 61–64
Alexander J, Williamson S, Seibert J, Golladay E, Jimenez J 1988 The ultrasonographic diagnosis of typhlitis (neutropenic colitis). Pediatric Radiology 18: 200–204
Hunter T, Bjelland J 1984 Gastrointestinal complications of leukaemia and its treatment. American Journal of Roentgenology 142: 513–518
Meyerovitz M, Fellows K 1984 Typhlitis: a cause of gastrointestinal haemorrhage in children. American Journal of Roentgenology 143: 833–835
Yeager A, Kanof M, Kramer S, Jones B, Saral R, Lake A, Santos G 1987 Pneumatosis intestinalis in children after allogeneic bone marrow transplantation. Pediatric Radiology 17: 18–22

DETERGENT AND 'HOME' ENEMAS

Colitis is a complication of many unusual enema preparations used for a variety of reasons in many different cultures. The enema mixtures reported have contained a variety of detergents, caustic and herbal mixtures. The radiological manifestations in the acute phase include toxic dilatation of the colon, necrotizing colitis, ulceration and perforation. Long-term effects include strictures which may be multiple, and general shortening of the colon with loss of haustration akin to that seen in ulcerative colitis.

REFERENCES

Kirchner S, Buckspan G, O'Neill J, Page D, Burko H 1977 Detergent enema: a cause of caustic colitis. Pediatric Radiology 6: 141–146

Segal I, Solomon A, Mirwis J 1981 Radiological manifestations of ritual-enema-induced colitis. Clinical Radiology 32: 657–662

BEHÇET'S DISEASE

The clinical triad characterizing Behçet's disease consists of recurrent stomatitis, genital ulcerations and ocular symptoms. Some patients also develop gastrointestinal involvement with deep ulceration in the terminal ileum and colon, mimicking Crohn's disease. The disease is very rare in children.

REFERENCE

Stringer D, Cleghorn G, Durie P, Daneman A, Hamilton J 1986 Behçet's syndrome involving the gastrointestinal tract – a diagnostic dilemma in childhood. Pediatric Radiology 16: 131–134

AMOEBIASIS

Infection with *Entamoeba histolytica* is endemically acquired particularly in tropical areas, but patients present world-wide, due to ease of population movement. The acute clinical presentation is usually with amoebic dysentery in which diarrhoea, abdominal pain and tenderness occur. Severe involvement leads to mucosal ulceration with rectal bleeding. A fulminant form may have a clinical presentation of toxic megacolon. All clinical presentations and radiological features may mimic Crohn's disease or ulcerative colitis. The ascending colon is most frequently affected in amoebic colitis. Shallow aphthous type ulcers with associated colonic spasm are seen at contrast enema, as is irritability of a shrunken caecum with a normal terminal ileum.

Amoebomas appear as large fungating masses, resembling carcinoma. Complications of amoebic colitis include colonic strictures, fistula formation and a 'lead pipe' colon. Perforation may occur during the acute phase. Liver abscess is a serious complication.

REFERENCES

Gardiner R, Stevenson G 1982 The colitides. Radiologic Clinics of North America 20: 797–817
Martinez C R, Gilman R H, Rabbani G H, Koster F 1982 Amebic colitis: correlation of proctoscopy before treatment and barium enema after treatment. American Journal of Roentgenology 138: 1089–1093

CHAGAS' DISEASE OF THE COLON

Infection with trypanosoma can cause a megacolon. The colon can reach gigantic proportions in the older patient. Care must be taken not to fill the colon with barium should one inadvertently do an enema in such a patient, as is true for all patients with chronic constipation. There is an increased incidence of sigmoid volvulus.

REFERENCE

Ferreira-Santos R, Carril C F 1964 Acquired megacolon in Chagas' disease. Diseases of the Colon and Rectum 7: 353–364

COLITIS CYSTICA

In this condition there are intramural mucus containing cysts mainly in the rectal area, but they may be scattered throughout the colon. These cause irregular defects in the rectum on barium enema examination.

REFERENCE

Ledesma-Medina J, Reid B S, Girdany B R 1978 Colitis cystica profunda. American Journal of Roentgenology 131: 529–530

APPENDICITIS

The appendix extends medially from the base of the caecum. It usually projects in a mediocaudal position, but as it is very mobile and of variable length, its position is not constant and it can extend retrocaecally to lie behind the ascending colon, even reaching the liver. Symptoms of appendicitis occur when inflammation occurs, secondary to obstruction of the appendiceal lumen by faecoliths, lymphoid hyperplasia, foreign bodies or worms. Bacterial inflammation follows vascular engorgement of the appendiceal wall and mucosa. Perforation occurs when vascular compromise causes gangrene of the wall. This is followed variably by localized periappendiceal abscess formation, peritonitis, pelvic abscess, mechanical obstruction or ileus due to peritonitis. Localization of inflammation and abscess formation increase with age, but are poor in young infants, who often present with peritonitis and septicaemia.

The clinical presentation of appendicitis in the older child is similar to that in adults, abdominal pain, periumbilical pain localizing to the right iliac fossa, fever, vomiting and leucocytosis. Tenderness is present in the right iliac fossa, often with signs of localized peritonitis. In younger children and infants, the signs are very poorly localized – the child may simply present with fever and fretfulness. A pelvic abscess may produce signs suggestive of gastroenteritis. Peritonitis may cause a secondary urinary tract infection. The diagnosis is often delayed causing considerable morbidity and mortality. A lack of awareness that appendicitis can occur in an infant is the main cause of the delayed diagnosis.

The diagnosis, once suspected on clinical grounds, is often sufficiently positive that no radiological investigation is required. Plain abdominal radiographs are mostly negative in an uncomplicated case. In many of these children it is possible to demonstrate the inflamed appendix on abdominal ultrasound with compression scanning of the right iliac fossa, confirming the diagnosis (Fig. 3.13.33). A normal appendix diameter is 6 mm or less. The problem of intestinal gas interposed between the probe and the appendix can be overcome by scanning along the lateral wall of the abdomen with the probe projected under the caecal gas.

The discovery of a calcified faecolith in a suspected case of acute appendicitis confirms the diagnosis (Fig. 3.13.34). These are present in about 10% of acute presentations, and are projected in the region of the right iliac fossa or right pelvis. They may, however, be present anywhere along the line of a retrocaecal appendix and can mimic both a renal stone or gallstone, even having a laminated appearance (Fig. 3.13.35). Ultrasound will confirm the extrabiliary

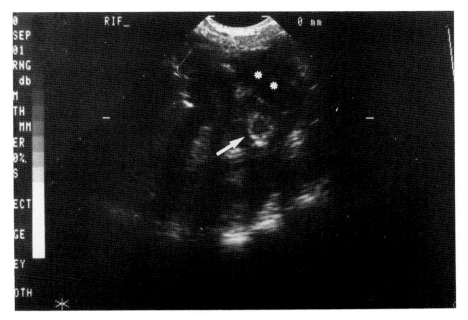

Fig. 3.13.33 Inflamed thickened appendix (arrow) is seen on a transverse section surrounded by oedematous bowel (asterisks) confirming the diagnosis of appendicitis.

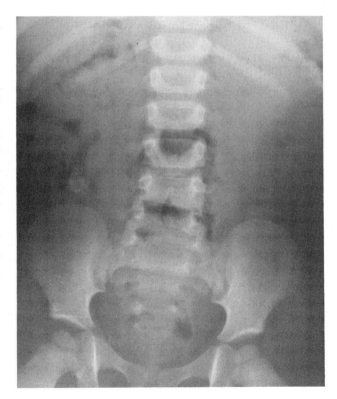

Fig. 3.13.34 Calcified faecolith in the right iliac fossa with air trapped in the appendix lumen proximally. The child presented with fever and abdominal pain.

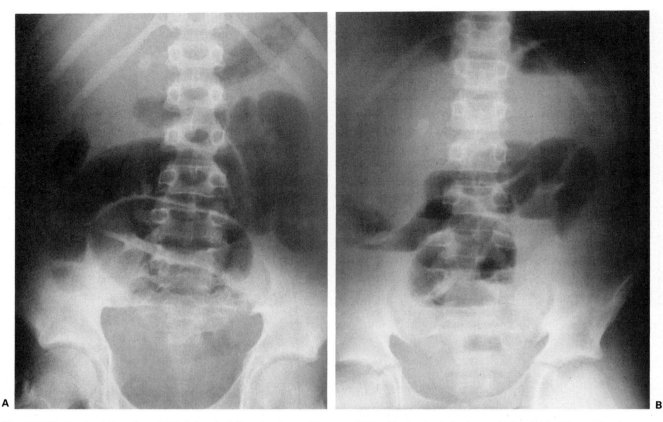

A   B

Fig. 3.13.35 Supine (**A**) and erect (**B**) abdominal films in a boy with appendicitis. The laminated calculus to the right of the midline was a faecolith which had migrated along the paracolic gutter from a ruptured appendix. The localized distal obstruction is due to peritonitis and an appendix abscess. Case surgically proven.

and extrarenal position. Faecoliths are quite commonly discovered as an incidental finding on plain abdominal radiographs in children, done for other reasons. Attention should be drawn to their presence, as elective appendicectomy is indicated. The faecolith is usually easy to see at ultrasound examination and casts a strong acoustic shadow.

Other plain film findings suggestive of appendicitis include a mass lesion with localized ileus in the right iliac fossa (Fig. 3.12.52), blurring of the properitoneal fat line, small bowel obstruction, or a mass with abscess bubbles and displaced caecal shadows in the right iliac fossa. Free peritoneal air is rare in a ruptured appendix. Plain film signs of a pelvic abscess are usually absent, though ileus may accompany peritonitis.

It has traditionally been taught that loss of the psoas outline is a reliable sign of peritonitis with appendicitis, but this is not so. Minor rotation and scoliosis can cause a similar appearance in normal children. Scoliosis concave to the right is a common finding in acute appendicitis, but is non-specific. Air visible in the appendicular lumen on plain radiography is an occasional normal finding.

In the past, non-filling of the appendix on barium enema has been regarded as diagnostic. This was not universally accepted, as non-filling can occur in asymptomatic children. With the advent of ultrasound, barium enema should no longer be performed. At ultrasound in a patient with acute appendicitis, the inflamed appendix is seen as a tubular structure with echo poor walls (Fig. 3.13.33). A faecolith may be seen within the lumen and casts an acoustic shadow (Fig. 3.13.36). Bowel movement around the inflamed appendix is often reduced or absent. Complications such as local, pelvic or subphrenic abscess formation are more easily identified than on plain abdominal radiographs. Their presence can significantly alter the clinical management to one of antibiotics and simple abscess drainage, leaving elective appendicectomy until the inflammation has settled.

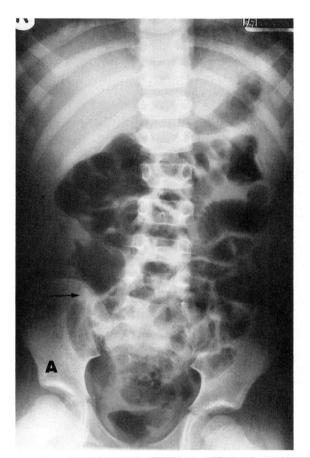

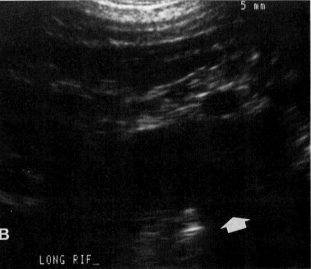

Fig. 3.13.36 Plain abdomen (**A**) and ultrasound (**B**) examination in a boy with appendicitis. On the plain abdomen there is a little medial displacement of the caecum, a small bubble of gas under the hepatic flexure and a mildly dilated small bowel often seen with early peritonitis. The faecolith is barely visible over the iliac blade (arrow). On ultrasound an acoustic shadow is cast by the faecolith and there is marked localized oedema.

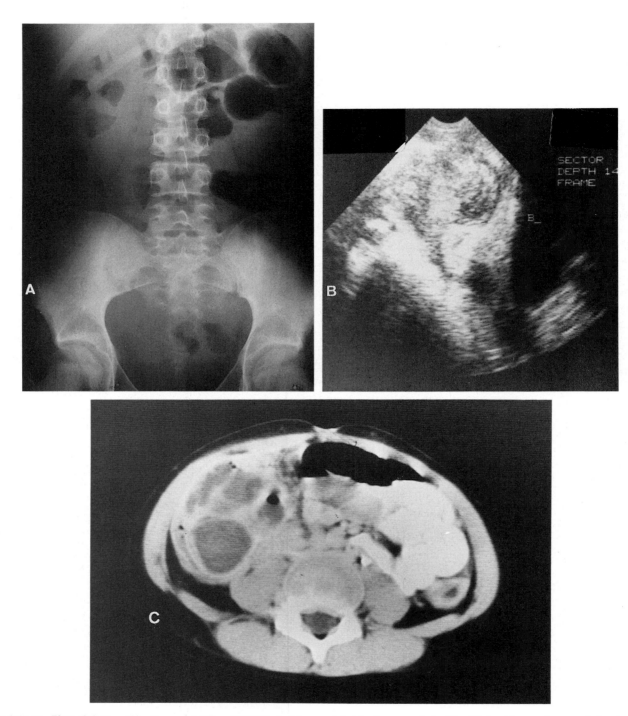

Fig. 3.13.37 Plain abdomen (**A**), ultrasound (**B**) and CT (**C**) of a 14-year-old girl who presented with a 10-day history of vague abdominal pain and malaise. The plain abdomen shows general lack of gas in the right abdomen but no diagnostic features. On ultrasound a complex mass was present behind the bladder (**B**) but extending proximally. No free fluid seen. The diagnosis of appendicitis, Crohn's disease and lymphoma were considered. CT shows a complex mass with enhancing walls and some gas which extended from the pelvis to kidney level. The diagnosis at surgery was appendicitis with extensive abscess formation.

CT is not indicated in the investigation of the uncomplicated case, but is very helpful when the presentation is that of a mass of unknown aetiology or in the identification of multiple abscesses (Fig. 3.13.37). The examination should be done with oral and intravenous contrast. The abscess walls will show contrast enhancement, but the appearances can be very bizarre and resemble a tumour. CT is more helpful in the assessment of postoperative complications than in the primary diagnosis.

In young infants who have a urinary tract infection secondary to the peritonitis or septicaemia, dilatation of the renal pelvis and ureters seen on urography or sonography, can occur down to the line of peritoneal reflection due to the peritonitis, leading to a continued mistaken diagnosis of a urinary tract infection (Fig. 3.13.38).

Postoperative complications are common in children who present with peritonitis and abscess formation. A subphrenic collection may be seen on the plain abdominal erect film as an air-fluid level under the diaphragm (Fig. 3.12.56). It can be difficult to distinguish a left subphrenic abscess from gastric or splenic flexure gas, and oral contrast may be necessary to distingish the varying gas shadows (Fig. 3.12.58). Many subphrenic collections have associated pleural effusions. Diaphragmatic movement is commonly restricted. All these findings may also be seen at ultrasound examination. The fluid collections can be accurately identified in relation to the position of the diaphragm. Percutaneous drainage of subphrenic collections or wound abscesses is probably preferable to further open surgery. The incidence of adhesions is significantly reduced and clinical recovery quicker than from laparatomy.

Crohn's disease, with terminal ileal involvement, and more rarely bowel lymphoma or appendiceal carcinoids, may also present as acute appendicitis, the diagnosis being made at surgery. There is probably no way of avoiding this type of mistaken diagnosis without overinvestigation of hundreds of children. Diarrhoea due to pelvic abscess formation can mimic gastroenteritis in young infants and toddlers, and delay diagnosis. Early ultrasound examination should avoid this. Abdominal pain that clinically mimics appendicitis can occur with right basal pneumonia. A further rare complication of appendiceal abscess is fistula formation.

Appendicitis and perforation have been described in the neonatal period but it is generally agreed that they most likely represent necrotizing enterocolitis.

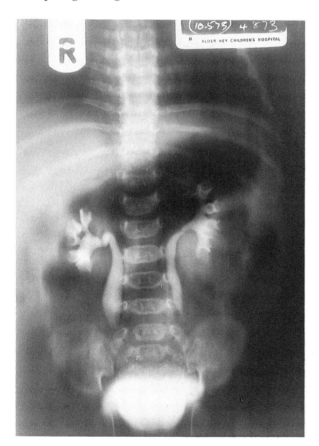

Fig. 3.13.38 Three month-old girl who presented with fever, diarrhoea and abdominal pain. An intravenous urogram done to investigate the urinary tract infection diagnosed by urine culture showed mild bilateral hydroureteronephrosis to the pelvis but normal distal ureters. Increasing abdominal distension led to laparotomy. A perforated gangrenous appendix and peritonitis were found.

REFERENCES

Baker D E, Silver T M, Coran A G, McMillin K I 1986 Post appendectomy fluid collections in children: incidence, nature and evolution evaluated using ultrasound. Radiology 161: 341–344
Bloom R, Gheorghiu D, Verstandig A, Pogrund H, Libson E 1990 The psoas sign in normal subjects without bowel preparation: the influence of scoliosis on visualisation. Clinical Radiology 41:204–205
Borushok K, Jeffrey R, Laing F, Townsend R 1990 Sonographic diagnosis of perforation in patients with acute appendicitis. American Journal of Roentgenology 154: 275–278
Hatch E, Naffis D, Chandler N 1981 Pitfalls in the use of barium enema in early appendicitis in children. Journal of Pediatric Surgery 16: 309–312
Jeffrey R, Laing F, Lewis F 1987 Acute appendicitis: high resolution real time ultrasound findings. Radiology 163: 11–14
Jeffrey R, Tolentino C, Federle M, Laing F 1987 Percutaneous drainage of periappendiceal abscesses: review of 20 patients. American Journal of Roentgenology 149: 59–62
Kao S, Smith W, Abu-Yousef M, Franken E, Sato Y, Kimura K, Soper R 1989 Acute appendicitis in children: sonographic findings. American Journal of Roentgenology 153: 375–379
Lister J, Tam P 1990 Meconium and bacterial peritonitis. In Lister J, Irving I M (eds) Neonatal surgery, 3rd edn Butterworth-Heinemann, London, Ch 35, pp 499–511
Maglinte D, Bush M, Aruta E, Bullington G 1981 Retained barium in the appendix: diagnostic and clinical significance. American Journal of Roentgenology 137: 529–533
Olutola P 1988 Plain film radiographic diagnosis of acute appendicitis: an evaluation of the signs. Journal of the Canadian Association of Radiology 39: 254–256

CARCINOID TUMOUR

Carcinoid tumour of the appendix or small bowel in childhood is rare, and symptomatic carcinoid is even rarer. Most carcinoids are discovered incidentally when the tumour mass leads to appendicitis or small bowel obstruction. Symptoms of carcinoid are due to raised serotonin levels causing flushing attacks and occur when liver metastases are present. Abdominal pain is due to intermittent obstruction. Radiographic changes on barium studies may resemble Crohn's disease. Localization of the tumor is possible with iodine-labelled MIBG scanning.

REFERENCES

Field J, Adamson L, Stoeckle H 1962 Review of carcinoids in children. Functioning carcinoid in a 15-year-old male. Pediatrics 29: 953–960

Hanson M, Feldman J, Blinder R, Moore J, Coleman R 1989 Carcinoid tumors: iodine-131 MIBG scintigraphy. Radiology 172: 699–703

Suster G, Weinberg A G, Graivier L 1977 Carcinoid tumor of the colon in a child. Journal of Pediatric Surgery 12: 739–742

DIRT EATING (GEOPHAGIA, PICA)

Frequently, multiple opaque fragments mixed with faeces are seen on plain abdominal radiographs due to dirt consumption. These fragments may be composed of a variety of substances, e.g. gravel, erasers, glass and metallic fragments. Such a finding is generally innocuous, but may be seen in psychologically disturbed children. Dental amalgam has a characteristic high radiographic density (Fig. 3.9.38). Lead paint fragments are also dense and may still be found where paint with a high lead content is present on dilapidated buildings (Fig. 3.9.39). Sufficient ingestion can cause lead poisoning and encephalopathy. Cartridge shot pellets from ingestion of game may localize in the appendix and have a characteristic round appearance. Some medicines – particularly enteric-coated capsules – can also be seen.

COLONIC POLYPS

Three kinds of polyps may occur in children – juvenile polyps, adenomas and hamartomas. Juvenile polyps are usually solitary, are composed mainly of connective tissue, do not contain epithelium, are not part of the syndromic polyposis conditions, and have no predisposition to malignancy. The polyps of familial polyposis coli are adenomas and are premalignant. Hamartomatous polyps are found in Peutz–Jegher syndrome, although most of the polyps in this condition are in the small bowel. Clinical presentation of colonic polyps in children is with painless rectal bleeding. If the polyps are large they may cause intussusception with abdominal pain and intermittent obstruction.

Juvenile polyps

Juvenile polyps are usually isolated. Over 60% are in the rectum and sigmoid colon. On double contrast barium examination they appear as smooth polyps on a stalk (Fig. 3.13.39). They sometimes spontaneously slough, after which the bleeding will stop. Most are discovered during investigation of rectal bleeding. Modern management is by colonoscopic removal.

Achieving adequate colonic cleansing in a young child is difficult in spite of aperients and washouts. The preparation can also be distressing. Retained faecal particles can simulate polypoid filling defects on contrast enema. A method of achieving a clean colon is described under Topic 3.15 in this chapter. Colonoscopy is a preferable method to double contrast barium enema for diagnosing the polypoid conditions in childhood. The polyp is directly visualized and biopsied or removed at a single examination. Colonic cleansing for colonoscopy has to be as thorough as for barium enema and the same regime can be employed. If the colonoscopy is technically unsatisfactory or impossible, arrangements should be made for the child to have a double contrast barium study while the colon is still clean, to avoid double preparation. Barium studies must not precede colonoscopy.

There are two variants of juvenile polyps. One is juvenile gastrointestinal polyposis, which presents with bloody diarrhoea, protein loss and electrolyte disturbances, and may be associated with macrocrania and intracranial cysts. It carries a poor prognosis. Polyps are present in both large and small bowel.

Juvenile polyposis of the colon is a distinct entity in which there are multiple polyps of the juvenile type scattered throughout the colon. The small bowel is not usually involved. Hundreds of sessile polyps are present throughout the colon. Pedunculated polyps may also be present. Chronic blood loss is a common

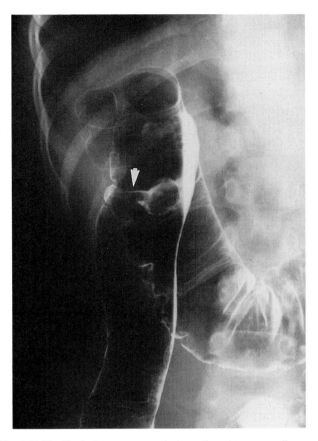

Fig. 3.13.39 Typical appearance of a juvenile polyp on a stalk (arrowhead).

clinical problem and may require colonic resection for its relief.

The blue rubber bleb naevus syndrome may have colonic involvement. The haemangiomas have a polypoid appearance indistinguishable from other polyps on barium enema, but at colonoscopy will appear blue.

There has been one report of generalized juvenile polyposis in association with pulmonary arteriovenous malformation and hypertrophic osteoarthropathy.

REFERENCES

Baert A L, Casteels-Van-Daele M, Broeckx J, Wijndaele L, Wilms G, Eggermont E 1983 Generalized juvenile polyposis with pulmonary arterio-venous malformation and hypertrophic osteoarthropathy. American Journal of Roentgenology 141: 661–662

Franken E A, Bixler D, Fitzgerald J F 1975 Juvenile polyposis of the colon. Annales de Radiologie 18: 499–504

Holgerson M O, Miller R E, Zintel H A 1971 Juvenile polyps of the colon. Surgery 69: 288–293

McCauley R, Leonidas J, Bartoshesky L 1979 Blue rubber bleb naevus syndrome. Radiology 133: 375–377

Sachatello C R, Hahn I S, Carrington C B 1974. Juvenile gastrointestinal polyposis in a female infant: report of a case and review of a recently recognised syndrome. Surgery 75: 107–113

Schwartz A, McCauley R 1976 Juvenile gastrointestinal polyposis. Radiology 121: 441–444

Familial polyposis coli

Familial polyposis coli is an autosomally dominant inherited condition, without sex predominance. It has an occurrence rate of 1:8000 births. There are hundreds or even thousands of polyps, distributed through the colon, more in the left than the right (Fig. 3.13.40). They are most commonly small sessile polyps initially and therefore appear thus in most children. As the patient grows older, larger pedunculated lesions may appear. These polyps are adenomatous and are premalignant; carcinoma will develop eventually in almost all cases if the colon is not removed. The time of appearance of the polyps varies, but the younger they appear, the earlier the onset of malignancy. Children may be asymptomatic, the disease being discovered during screening when a marker case is discovered in a family. Symptomatic children present with diarrhoea and blood per rectum. Double contrast barium enema is needed to demonstrate the polyps. The appearance in the early stages can be very confusing as the polyps may be very small and give the bowel an ulcerated appearance, or be difficult to distinguish from lymphoid hyperplasia. In the more developed case, the polyps are seen as mutiple, well-demarcated lesions on double contrast enema (Fig. 3.13.41). Carcinoma may be present in children, and is either of the annular constricting type or appears as a polypoid tumour. Colonoscopy is a better method than double contrast enema for screening a suspected family if facilities for paediatric colonoscopy are available. The polyps can be directly visualized and biopsied.

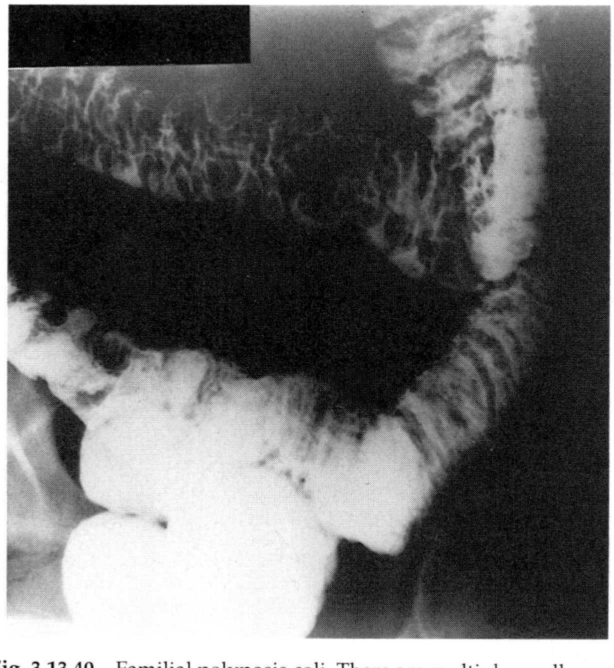

REFERENCES

Erbe R W 1976 Inherited gastrointestinal polyposis syndromes. New England Journal of Medicine 294: 1101–1104
Marshak R H, Lindner A E, Maklansky D 1977 Familial polyposis. American Journal of Gastroenterology 67: 177–189

Gardner's syndrome

Gardner's syndrome is an autosomally dominant inherited condition, consisting of multiple adenomatous polyps of the colon, osteomas in the bones, most frequently the facial bones, and multiple soft tissue tumours – fibromas, lipomas, epidermoid cysts and desmoid tumours. The desmoid tumours are especially frequent postoperatively. Not all patients have complete expression. The soft tissue and bony lesions may precede the colonic lesions. There is a high risk of malignancy in the colonic lesions, but there is also an increased risk of carcinoma of the pancreas and duodenum. Paediatric presentation is rare, but is

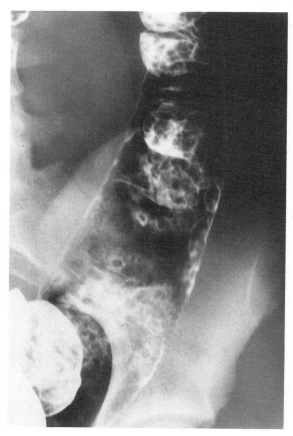

Fig. 3.13.40 Familial polyposis coli. There are multiple small polyps scattered throughout the mucosa.

Fig. 3.13.41 Familial polyposis coli. There are hundreds of tiny polyps present throughout the colon giving this granular appearance.

described in the early teenage years. Thyroid carcinoma has also been reported in association with Gardner's syndrome.

REFERENCE

Erbe R W 1976 Inherited gastrointestinal polyposis syndromes. New England Journal of Medicine 294: 1101–1104

CARCINOMA

Colorectal carcinoma is very rare in childhood, with only about 225 reported cases. The majority of cases arise in previously healthy individuals, but it can occur as a complication of ulcerative colitis, or the polyposis syndromes even in children, and has been reported from newborn to young adulthood. Tumours in the left colon tend to be annular, while right-sided tumours are more commonly ulcerative. Symptoms are similar to those in adult life-pain, rectal bleeding and bowel obstruction. Diagnosis in children tends to be delayed as it is rarely considered. The radiological appearances are similar to those in adults; strictures with shouldered edges in the constricting lesions, and ulcerating fungating tumours in the larger lesions. Invasion of adjacent organs is common. A typical 'target' sign may be seen at ultrasound examination, with echo poor walls surrounding an echoic centre. The lesions are often advanced or have metastasized by the time a diagnosis is made, and most are mucinous adenocarcinomas. There is an increased incidence in children or young adults who have had ureterosigmoidostomy, the tumours arising where the ureters are implanted into the colon.

REFERENCES

Cremin B, Brown R 1987 Carcinoma of the colon: diagnosis by ultrasound and enema. Pediatric Radiology 17: 319–320
Lamego C, Torloni H 1989 Colorectal adenocarcinoma in childhood and adolescence. Report of 11 cases and review of the literature. Pediatric Radiology 19: 504–508
Sooriyaarachchi G S, Johnson R O, Carbone P P 1977 Neoplasms of the large bowel following ureterosigmoidostomy. Archives of Surgery 112: 1174–1177

COLONIC LYMPHOMA

Colonic lymphoma is most commonly found in the ileocaecal region. Males are more frequently affected. Symptoms are vague and include abdominal pain, anaemia, occasionally a protein-losing enteropathy and malabsorption pattern. Often the diagnosis is made at laparatomy for acute obstruction. If a barium enema is done, the usual finding is a mass lesion with nodular defects indenting the bowel lumen. A variety of histological types of lymphoma have been reported.

Presentation can occur at any age, but in children is most frequent in the second decade.

REFERENCES

Bartram C, Chrispin A 1973 Primary lymphosarcoma of the ileum and caecum. Pediatric. Radiology 1: 28–33
Ein S H, Beck A R, Allen J E 1979 Colon sarcoma in the newborn. Journal of Pediatric Surgery 14: 455–457

COLONIC OBSTRUCTION

Large bowel obstruction is rarer in childhood than in adulthood, where carcinoma is a common cause. In children, acquired large bowel obstruction is most frequently due to adhesions or stricture formation at an anastomosis. It can occur secondary to sigmoid or caecal volvulus, pelvic tumours with displacement of the rectum and, rarely, due to constipation. It can of course occur in missed Hirschsprung's disease. Air-fluid levels with bowel distension throughout to the point of obstruction will be present on the plain radiographs, provided the radiological signs have not been altered by nasogastric suction. Removal of air and fluid by this method will deflate the bowel and alter the radiological appearance. If large bowel obstruction is suspected, a gentle single contrast barium enema to show the site and cause is indicated. If perforation is likely, water-soluble contrast should be used.

COLONIC TRAUMA

Colonic trauma due to blunt abdominal injury is much rarer than injury to the duodenum and small bowel; relative size and lack of fixation seems protective, so that if damage does occur it is often accompanied by other organ injury. Perforation of the colon due to blunt trauma is serious due to faecal contamination of the peritoneum, and the resulting pneumoperitoneum is large. Perforation from blunt trauma is usually at a relatively fixed position, e.g. the hepatic flexure. Plain radiographs show free air on the erect films. This may be suspected on supine film by noting a hazy collection of air centrally, 'the football sign', or outlining of the ligamentum falcifarum.

Direct colonic injury can also occur by penetrating objects inserted per rectum. Iatrogenic injury can take place during colonoscopy or barium enema. It can also occur due to insertion of solid objects during masturbation fetishes and, sadly, through anal penetration by the penis or fingers during sexual abuse. As well as intraperitoneal air, retroperitoneal air is common when perforation occurs by this method, often outlining the kidney and adrenal.

Haematomas of the colonic wall can cause vascular compromise and lead to stricture formation.

3.14 TRAUMA

The specific clinical features of trauma to the intra-abdominal organs are discussed in the relevant sections. It is, however, important to take a global view of the child admitted with abdominal trauma, a frequent occurrence in all accident and emergency departments.

Abdominal trauma is of two types, blunt and penetrating injury. A history of penetrating abdominal injury will usually be available and the wound clinically visible. Initial radiographs must include a supine and decubitus view to assess the presence of free air indicating perforation of a hollow viscus. Large amounts of free air suggest perforation of stomach or colon. If present, the child is referred for surgery. If there is no free air, then the principles of investigating blunt abdominal injury obtain.

In children with blunt abdominal trauma, the clinical condition of the child will dictate the nature and extent of radiological assessment. Where possible, conservative management has replaced immediate laparotomy in the stable child, and the current motto is 'Investigate aggressively but manage conservatively'. The underlying theme is that the surgeon does not mind waiting as long as he knows what is going on.

Following a decision to investigate, surgeon and radiologist decide between them the order of investigation, following review of emergency room radiographs. These should include a supine and decubitus view of the abdomen and a supine chest radiograph, unless the child is fit enough to sit up when an erect chest radiograph can replace the decubitus film. Attention to any accompanying head or skeletal injury is important as these can be more life threatening than the abdominal injury. Availability of ultrasound or CT dictate the next steps.

If CT is available, it is probably preferable to ultrasound as a complete picture of all abdominal contents is obtainable. If not, then ultrasound examination of liver, spleen, kidneys and pelvis will yield considerable information and show the presence of peritoneal fluid, liver and spleen haematomas, renal haematomas, contusions and perirenal fluid collections. Ultrasound may be difficult due to abdominal pain and tenderness, and intestinal gas may obscure a good view.

Radionuclide imaging has little part to play in the acute assessment but is ultimately invaluable in assessing renal function.

It cannot be overstressed that the presence of a functioning kidney on the contralateral side to the injury must be confirmed before any surgery is contemplated. This can be easily done during CT with contrast enhancement. If not available, then a single 'shot' intravenous urogram, if necessary on the operating table, must be done before nephrectomy.

After the plain radiographs, CT is the most valuable imaging method in trauma, in spite of the disadvantage of the radiation dose and the child having to be moved to the unit. All abdominal organs, peritoneal structures, retroperitoneal regions and bony structures can be seen at one examination. However, not all children need CT. In some, the injury is trivial and can be safely assessed by ultrasound. Others require immediate surgery. It is the seriously injured but moderately stable patient who benefits most from CT.

The CT should, if possible, be done following oral contrast to opacify the bowel lumen, making it easier to distinguish bowel from haematoma. If this cannot be done then CT, even without oral contrast, provides valuable information. All scans should be done with continuous or bolus intravenous contrast enhancement during the upper abdominal slices. A dose of 2 ml/kg of contrast is adequate. The child should be cooperative and, if necessary, sedated. Moving, restless scans are a waste of money and irradiation. During scanning, monitoring of vital signs should continue. Alternate slices of about 1 cm from diaphragm to pubis will provide adequate assessment, and reduce radiation. Contiguous slices can be done subsequently to clarify any region of ambiguity.

When reviewing plain abdominal radiographs in trauma, the following is a suggested method to identify most signs:

- Is there free air under the diaphragm or under the abdominal wall on the decubitus film?
- Is the gas distribution all within intestine?
- Are there any subhepatic collections or lesser sac collections?
- Is there any retroperitoneal air?
- Is there an air cystogram or pyelogram?
- Is there displacement of intestinal gas by a mass lesion to suggest haematoma?
- Is there acute gastric dilatation? If so, insertion of a nasogastric tube will deflate the stomach and make the patient more comfortable.
- Are the bones normal? In particular, look closely at the transverse processes and ribs for fractures.
- Is there any evidence of lung base consolidation which might indicate aspiration of abdominal food content?

Similar signs are looked for on CT but are easier to

appreciate. In addition, haematomas and lacerations of liver, spleen and kidneys can be seen. Free intraperitoneal fluid is also visible. Water has a Hounsfield number of 0–0 and fresh blood 30–40.

Once the extent of injury is established, and conservative management agreed, the child may be monitored by ultrasound, and repeat CT done to resolve any difficulties.

REFERENCES

Cook D, Walsh J, Vick C, Brewer W 1986 Upper abdominal trauma: pitfalls in CT diagnosis. Radiology 159: 65–69

Filiatrault D, Longpre D, Patriquin H, Perreault G, Grignon A, Pronovost J, Boisvert J 1987 Investigation of childhood blunt abdominal trauma: a practical approach using ultrasound as the initial diagnostic modality. Pediatric Radiology 17: 373–379

Kelly J, Raptopoulos V, Davidoff A, Waite R, Norton P 1989 The value of non-contrast-enhanced CT in blunt abdominal trauma. American Journal of Roentgenology 152: 41–46

Sivit C J, Taylor G A, Bulas D I, Bowman L M, Eichelberger M R 1991 Blunt trauma in children: significance of peritoneal fluid. Radiology 178: 185–188

Taylor G, Fallat M, Eichelberger M 1987 Hypovolemic shock in children: abdominal CT manifestations. Radiology 164: 479–481

Taylor G, Guion C, Potter B, Eichelberger M 1989 CT of blunt abdominal trauma in children. American Journal of Roentgenology 153: 555–559

3.15 GAMUTS, TECHNIQUES AND CONTRAST

ORDERED REVIEW OF ABDOMINAL RADIOGRAPH

A review of the abdominal radiograph should follow a systematic pattern. The following is suggested:

1. Check name, date and right and left markers.
2. Check bowel gas distribution for correct location of stomach, small bowel gas, position of caecum, position of colon.
3. Check both lung bases for consolidation and intact diaphragmatic outline.
4. Check position of liver and size of spleen.
5. Confirm normal position of kidneys and absence of mass lesions, both calcified and non-calcified.
6. Look carefully for stones in the kidneys, along the lines of the ureters and in the region of the appendix.
7. In females, look for evidence of ovarian cysts – fat content or tooth in dermoids or mass lesion noted by displacement of surrounding intestinal gas.
8. If distended loops of bowel are present, identify the level to which they extend and the presence of distal gas.
9. Look at faecal content for evidence of pancreatic insufficiency.
10. Check hernial orifices for evidence of hernial sac gas.
11. Look for displacement of properitoneal fat lines.
12. Check spine for presence of normal pedicles, congenital vertebral abnormalities and presence of normal disc spaces.
13. Check bony pelvis, spine and ribs for evidence of bone destruction.

GAMUTS

Table 3.15.1   Adynamic ileus

Inflammatory
  Sepsis
  Gastroenteritis
  Peritonitis
  Pancreatitis
  Pneumonia
Traumatic
  Accident
  Postoperative
Metabolic
  Hypokalaemia
  Hypoglycaemia
  Diabetic ketoacidosis
  Hypocalcaemia
Miscellaneous
  Scleroderma
  Henoch–Schönlein purpura
  Haemolytic uraemic syndrome
  Neurogenic ileus-autonomic dysfunction
  Intestinal pseudo-obstruction

Table 3.15.2   Ascites

Transudate
  Congestive cardiac failure
  Renal failure
  Liver failure
  Budd–Chiari syndrome
  Hypoalbuminaemia
  Peritonitis
Exudate
  Peritonitis (inflammatory including tuberculosis)
  Hollow viscous perforation
  Trauma
  Febrile relapsing
  Crohn's disease
  Malignant
  Pancreatitis
Chylous
  Lymphangiectasia
  Malignant
  Filariasis
Miscellaneous
  Biliary perforation
  Urinary tract perforation
  CSF ascites – from ventriculo-peritoneal shunt
  Ruptured ovarian cyst
  Peritoneal dialysis
  Myxoedema

Table 3.15.4   Intestinal obstruction

Postoperative adhesions
Incarcerated hernia
Congenital bands
Volvulus around a Meckel's diverticulum
Intussusception
Crohn's disease
Lymphoma
Duplication
Midgut volvulus with malrotation
Helminth infection
Cystic fibrosis
Bezoars

Table 3.15.3   Abdominal pain

Gastrointestinal origin
    Gastroenteritis
    Appendicitis
    Intussusception
    Bowel obstruction
    Crohn's disease
    Ulcerative colitis
    Tumour
    Ischaemia
    Helminth infection
    Malrotation
    Hernia
    Trauma
    Perforation
    Intestinal duplication
    Peptic ulceration
Hepatic and biliary
    Hepatitis
    Cholecystitis
    Cholelithiasis
    Liver congestion
Chest
    Basal pneumonia
    Ruptured diaphragm
Skeletal
    Discitis
    Spinal tumour
Renal
    Urinary tract infection
    Urinary tract obstruction
    Stones
Ovarian
    Ovarian cysts
Pancreas
    Pancreatitis
    Pancreatic pseudocyst
    Lymphoma
Retroperitoneal
    Tumour

Table 3.15.5   Intussusception

Idiopathic (Peyer's patch hypertrophy)
Meckel's diverticulum
Duplication cyst
Henoch–Schönlein purpura
Polyposis
Lymphoma
Cystic fibrosis

Table 3.15.6   Causes of malabsorption in children

Coeliac disease
Enteritis
Cystic fibrosis
Crohn's disease
Short bowel
Blind loop
Pancreatitis
Protein-losing enteropathy
Lymphangiectasia
Endocrine disease
Lymphoma
Kwashiorkor
Immunodeficiency
Lactase deficiency
Sucrase deficiency
Gastro/small bowel fistula

Table 3.15.7   Gastrointestinal bleeding: melaena or blood per rectum

Meckel's diverticulum
Anal fissure
Intussusception
Gastroenteritis
Angiomatous malformation
Crohn's disease
Ulcerative colitis
Colonic polyps
Henoch–Schönlein purpura
Uraemia
Disseminated intravascular coagulation
Duplication cysts
Hiatus hernia with reflux oesophagitis
Oesophageal varices
Gastric or duodenal ulceration
Bowel haematoma

CHOICE OF CONTRAST

The gastrointestinal tract in infants and children may be investigated satisfactorily by both barium sulphate and the water-soluble iodine-containing contrast. These latter fall into two categories:

1. Gastrografin – a hyperosmolar liquorice-flavoured medium which is rapidly diluted within the bowel lumen by the fluid drawn into the lumen from the extracellular compartment.

2. Low osmolar, isotonic compounds, used mainly for intravascular or intrathecal injection. These do not disturb the fluid balance and are therefore not diluted. They are the water-soluble contrast media of choice.

Gastrografin should be reserved for therapeutic indications in relieving meconium plugs in the newborn and in the treatment of distal ileal obstruction in cystic fibrosis patients. In the newborn, gastrografin enemas should not be attempted until the child has a satisfactory intravenous line in place, and careful monitoring of the infant's hydration is undertaken. Severe dehydration and hypovolaemic shock can occur. Dilution of gastrografin to 50% with water does not diminish the therapeutic effect but makes it safer.

Barium sulphate is the contrast of choice in most gastrointestinal tract contrast studies in children. Contraindications are few, but include known or suspected perforation, or fistulas, suspected aspiration, and potential for barium impaction such as could occur in adynamic ileus. Care must be taken not to fill the colon in children with constipation for fear of impaction. In general, barium should not be used in a defunctioned bowel as a barolith may form if the barium is not washed out.

Mucosal coating in the infant's and young child's stomach is poor due to the excess mucus and fluid normally present. High quality double contrast examinations of the upper gastrointestinal tract, such as are routinely indicated in adult examinations, are only indicated in children when investigating suspected gastric erosions or gastric and duodenal ulceration. In these circumstances, high density barium, gaseous distension and muscle paralysis with meta-chlorpropamide or glucagon are indicated. In most other situations, low density barium sulphate diluted to 30–50% with water is preferable and cheaper. The contrast may be flavoured with fruit juice of the child's choice to encourage acceptance.

SMALL BOWEL STUDIES

The small bowel may be examined by a follow-through examination after oral ingestion of a large volume of barium, 300–500 ml, dependent on the size of the child, to ensure good filling of the bowel loops, or it may be examined by enteroclysis, small bowel enema following jejunal intubation. Each technique has its advocates. Either technique correctly done can produce a satisfactory examination. However, enteroclysis with fluoroscopic monitoring of each bowel loop during filling is more sensitive in detecting small areas of Crohn's involvement and intestinal polyps. Intubation is unpleasant for the child, and should not be undertaken lightly. Indications for enteroclysis are a negative follow-through examination with a strong clinical suspicion of small bowel involvement with Crohn's disease, inadequate follow-through due to failure to drink adequate volumes of barium, and clinical suspicion of intestinal small bowel polyps or small bowel strictures and investigation of failure to thrive following neonatal surgery (Fig. 3.15.1).

The time taken for orally ingested barium to reach the ileum is very variable and ranges between 30 minutes and about 3 hours. Once the jejunum has been adequately examined, further passage can be expedited by giving the child a fizzy drink. When a follow-through examination is done, the examination must be monitored by a radiologist to determine the sequence of films and be supplemented by fluoroscopy and palpation as indicated.

CONTRAST ENEMA

A formal double contrast enema using high density barium, and air insufflation following adequate bowel preparation with dietary restriction and aperients, must be undertaken in children suspected of inflammatory bowel disease, unless symptoms are very acute, or bleeding from an intestinal polyp. An unprepared single contrast examination is all that is indicated in the investigation of constipation. The colon should not be filled and only enough barium to show the relationship of the faecal retention to the anus instilled.

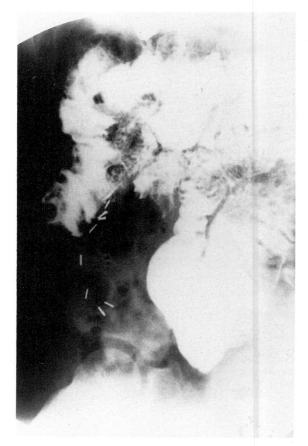

Fig. 3.15.1 Frame from intubated small bowel examination. Previous neonatal ileal resection for segmental dilatation. A follow-through examination done for investigation of short stature and failure to thrive was interpreted as normal. Persisting symptoms led to an intubated examination. A localized dilated loop was present with an abrupt change in calibre. On fluoroscopy, this loop had no peristaltic activity. This is an adynamic partially trapped loop and was thought to be acting as a 'blind loop' and causing symptoms.

Bowel preparation in children for double contrast should follow the same routine as in use for adults within the department, adjusting the dose of aperients to the weight of the child.

If the child is also having colonoscopy the same episode of bowel preparation can be used for both. Retained faecal content is a problem. In children in whom the clinical suspicion is one of a polyp, cleansing enemas will also be needed. One has to be cruel to be kind.

UPPER GASTROINTESTINAL TRACT STUDIES

The child is best examined following a 4-hour fast. This usually ensures hunger in infants and encourages drinking. A reluctant toddler is a challenge to all radiologists! The stomach and duodenum, and a search for reflux can be adequately examined following nasogastric intubation if required, but the swallowing mechanism and the presence of oesophageal lesions require adequate bolus swallowing. In all children, the examination should be initially directed to answer the clinical question posed and not done systematically as one would in a cooperative adult. The reluctant infant may take contrast from his own feeding cup or familiar teat when he won't use hospital issue.

In all children, if possible, an upper gastrointestinal series should be video recorded to allow repeated viewing. Careful observation of palatal movements is essential in any child with a history suggestive of aspiration or choking when feeding. The position of the gastro-oesophageal junction and its relationship to the diaphragm should be documented. The junction is identified by an area of non-distensibility which should remain below the diaphragm. It must not be confused with the phrenic ampulla, a temporary pouch at the lower oesophagus, and often mistakenly called a hernia. Counting the number of mucosal folds is not a reliable method of identifying stomach and oesophagus.

The pylorus in young children often points very posteriorly and steep, oblique projections may be needed to demonstrate it. The position of the duodenojejunal flexure must be identified, and documented in a true AP projection of the abdomen. Active assessment of peristaltic activity in the oesophagus and stomach is important.

ENEMA

The film sequence for double contrast studies should include a lateral film of the rectum to include the whole of the sacrum, so that the postrectal space may be assessed, oblique views of the rectosigmoid colon to award overlapping loops, and then overcouch prone, and both decubitus films, supplemented by erect spot films as indicated, so that the entire bowel is adequately seen.

IMMOBILIZATION

Wrapping a child securely in a blanket or using a commercially designed cradle are satisfactory for upper gastrointestinal examinations. The cradles are not generally as useful for children having enemas, as no amount of taping will keep a catheter in place in some infants, and it may need to be held in position by an attendant, taking care to keep the hands out of the fluoroscopic beam. Self-retaining balloon catheters should not be used.

SINOGRAMS

Sinography is often required when there are surgical complications following anastomoses. A plain abdominal radiograph should be done before the instillation of contrast. Soft disposable nasogastric tubes are the best catheters to use. Water-soluble contrast, fluoroscopic observation, skin markers to show the point of entry of a catheter and film at right angles to show the sinus tracks in perspective are indicated.

REFERENCES

Bell K E, McKinstry C S, Mills J O 1987 Iopamidol in the diagnosis of suspected upper gastro intestinal perforation. Clinical Radiology 38:165–168

Campbell J 1989 Contrast media in intussusception. Pediatric Radiology 19: 293–296

Cohen M 1987 Choosing contrast media for the evaluation of the gastrointestinal tract of neonates and infants. Radiology 162: 447–456

Maglinte D, Lappas J, Kelvin F, Rex D, Chernish S 1987 Small bowel radiography: how, when, and why? Radiology 163: 297–305

Margulis A, Thoeni R 1988 The present status of the radiologic examination of the colon. Radiology 167: 1–5

Ratcliffe J 1985 The use of low-osmolality water soluble contrast media in the paediatric gastrointestinal tracts: a report of 115 examinations. Radiology Now 8: 8–11

Ratcliffe J 1986 The use of low osmolality water soluble (LOWS) contrast media in the pediatric gastro-intestinal tract. A report of 115 examinations. Pediatric Radiology 16: 47–52

White M, Bartram C 1987 Technique and evaluation of the double contrast ileostomy enema. Clinical Radiology 38: 621–624

COMPLICATIONS DUE TO GASTROINTESTINAL CONTRAST AGENTS

Aspiration

Aspiration of small quantities of contrast into the trachea is common in children with pharyngeal incoordination and some infants with reflux or H-type fistula. Fatal aspiration has been described. Death is due to pulmonary oedema or pneumonia. If the clinical history is suggestive of aspiration, the initial swallow must be done with low osmolar, non-ionic contrast media, and care taken to allow the child to swallow only small amounts initially. Suction and suitable catheters should be available in the screening room when examining the child at risk, and gastrografin and the other high osmolar contrasts should be avoided in these children.

Barium impaction

Barium impaction is a potential complication in any child with a bowel motility disorder or a defunctioned bowel whose colon is filled with barium. Therefore, if barium is used in such situations, it is important to only use enough barium for diagnostic purposes in examining the constipated child to show the relationship of the constipation to the anus. There is seldom need to outline the whole colon. If this happens inadvertently, or is done deliberately for clinical reasons, then instructions must be given to the nursing staff about appropriate dietary and medical treatment to ensure adequate bowel clearing. Cleansing enemas may be required.

In a defunctioned bowel, as obtains following a colostomy, water-soluble contrast is the medium of choice for examining the defunctioned loop. There is a danger of barolith formation if the barium is not removed. Removal of a barolith, or its spontaneous passage, can lead to anal tears and rupture of anastomoses.

Barium peritonitis

Peritoneal contamination with barium is inevitable if perforation occurs during barium studies or is already present. Barium in the peritoneal cavity can cause granuloma formation and fibrous adhesions. Early mortality and morbidity, however, is due to the faecal contamination of the peritoneum that accompanies the barium extravasation, with the consequent peritonitis and septicaemia. Early reports suggested a high mortality, but modern management with antibiotics, peritoneal lavage and fluid replacement have made this a rare event in children. When barium is noted in the peritoneum during fluoroscopy, the examination should be immediately stopped and the child brought to surgery.

REFERENCES

Eklof O, Hald J, Thomasson B 1983 Barium peritonitis. Experience of five pediatric cases. Pediatric Radiology 13: 5–9
Fischer W, Nice C 1984 Barium impaction as a cause of small bowel obstruction in an infant with cystic fibrosis. Pediatric Radiology 14: 230–231
Friedman B, Hartenberg M, Mulroy J, Tong T, Mickell J 1986 Gastrografin aspiration in a three and three quarter year-old-girl. Pediatric Radiology. 16: 506–507
McAlister W, Siegel M 1984 Fatal aspirations in infancy during gastrointestinal series. Pediatric Radiology 14: 81–83
Walker C, Purnell G, Diner W 1989. Complications from extravasated retroperitoneal barium: case report and review of the literature. Radiology 173: 618–620

GASTROINTESTINAL ULTRASOUND

Ultrasound has been long established in the investigation of solid organ disease in the abdomen. It is increasingly the first line of investigation in the assessment of the child presenting with abdominal pain, either acute or chronic. A normal ultrasound examination, i.e. the demonstration of normal liver, gallbladder, kidneys, adrenals, pancreas and pelvic organs, and the absence of free intraperitoneal fluid, excludes many of the important causes of abdominal pain in children. It is also the first investigation in many instances in children presenting with abdominal trauma, where again a normal examination is reassuring. Ultrasound of the bowel itself is a more recent development. Bowel wall thickness (Fig. 3.12.21), appendicitis (Figs 3.13.33, 3.13.36, 3.13.37), localized bowel ileus, duplications (Fig. 3.11.9), hernial sac contents, pyloric stenosis (Fig. 3.10.7), intussusception (Figs 3.13.20, 3.13.21), and even mucosal irregularity such as occurs in typhlitis (Fig. 3.13.32), can be reliably assessed. Ultrasound machines are readily mobile and an ill child can easily be examined in the ward or intensive care unit.

Real time scanning using 5.0 mHz or 7.5 mHz probes is most appropriate in children under 10 years. Above this age, 3.5 mHz probes may be needed in addition. The abdomen should be examined with the bladder full. Gas may be displaced by using graded pressure scanning, or the bowel may be visualized under the gas by scanning with the probe placed laterally.

REFERENCES

Carroll B A 1989 Ultrasound of the gastrointestinal tract. Radiology 172: 605–608
Filiatrault D, Longpre D, Patriquin H, Perreault G, Grignon A, Pronovost J, Boisvert J 1987 Investigation of childhood blunt abdominal trauma: a practical approach using ultrasound as the initial diagnostic modality. Pediatric Radiology 17: 373–379
Mendelson R, Lindsell D 1987 Ultrasound examination of the paediatric 'acute abdomen': preliminary findings. British Journal of Radiology 60: 414–416
Miller J H, Kemberling C R 1984 Ultrasound scanning of the gastrointestinal tract in children: subject review. Radiology 152: 671–677
Ros P R, Olmsted W W, Moser R P Jr, Dachman A H, Hjermstad B H, Sobin L H 1987 Mesenteric and omental cysts: histological classification with imaging correlation. Radiology 164: 327–332
Stunden R, LeQuesne G, Little K 1986 The improved ultrasound diagnosis of hypertrophic pyloric stenosis. Pediatric Radiology 16: 200–205
Van Der Meer S, Forget P, Arends J, Kuijten R, Van Engelshoven J 1990 Diagnosis value of ultrasound in children with recurrent abdominal pain. Pediatric Radiology 20: 501–503

SCINTIGRAPHY FOR GASTROINTESTINAL BLEEDING

The location of a source of gastrointestinal bleeding in children is a difficult problem. Scintigraphy with ^{99m}Tc-labelled pertechnetate can be used to detect ectopic gastric mucosa in a Meckel's diverticulum or duplication cyst (Figs 3.11.10, 2.12.9, 3.12.10). ^{99m}Tc-labelled red blood cell scanning following in vivo labelling may locate a bleeding point. Thyroid blocking is not routinely used. Prior preparation with H$_2$ antagonists reduces gastric emptying, thus avoiding potential confusion with contrast entering the small bowel from normal passage of gastric contents.

The technique for scanning for ectopic gastric mucosa is as follows. An injection of pertechnetate is given following an overnight fast. Anterior and posterior views of the abdomen are taken at 10 minute intervals for an hour. Late views must be taken with an empty bladder in order that a Meckel's diverticulum behind the bladder is not missed. An uncooperative child will require sedation for a satisfactory scan. It is essential that the abdomen is clear of barium before carrying out abdominal scintigraphy, as barium blocks the transmission of gamma rays. A Meckel's diverticulum containing gastric mucosa becomes apparent as a hot spot in the abdomen appearing concurrently with the stomach uptake. A negative scan will occur with Meckel's diverticula that do not contain gastric mucosa, but they do not bleed. False-negative scans also occur, but failure to demonstrate a Meckel's diverticulum with scintigraphy makes it less likely to be the cause of bleeding. The diagnostic accuracy is about 90%.

Red blood cell scintigraphy is carried out following in vivo labelling of the patient's red blood cells. The technique involves an injection of methylene diphosphonate, followed in 30 minutes by an injection of ^{99m}Tc-labelled pertechnetate. Images of the whole abdomen are taken immediately after injection and at 10-minute intervals for 90 minute (Fig. 3.12.16). Further images, at hourly intervals up to 24 hours, should be taken if no bleeding is observed in the first 90 minutes. Further decisions about angiography for precise localization of the bleeding point are made depending on the clinical signs and symptoms. Bleeding rates of as little as 0.1 ml/min can be detected by this method.

REFERENCES

Dorfman G, Cronan J, Staudinger K 1987 Scintigraphic signs and pitfalls in lower gastrointestinal hemorrhage: the continued necessity of angiography. Radiographics 7: 543–562

Fries M, Mortensson W, Robertson B 1984 Technetium pertechnetate scintigraphy to detect ectopic gastric mucosa in Meckel's diverticulum. Acta Radiologica Diagnostica Stockholm 25: 417–422

Mitchell D, Stacy T, Grunow J, Leonard J 1988 Scintigraphic detection of an occult abdominal bleed in a child. Clinical Nuclear Medicine 13: 546–548

Smith R, Copely D, Bolen F 1987 Tc^{99m} RBC scintigraphy: correlation of gastrointestinal bleeding rates with scintigraphic findings. American Journal of Roentgenology 148: 869–874

Winzelberg G G, Froelich J W, McKusick K A, Strauss H W 1983 Scintigraphic detection of gastrointestinal bleeding: a review of current methods. American Journal of Gastroenterology 78: 324–327

Yeker D, Buyukunal G, Benli M, Buyukunal E, Urgancioglu I 1984. Radionuclide imaging of Meckel's diverticulum: cimetidine versus pentagastrin plus glucagon. European Journal of Nuclear Medicine 9: 316–319

Zwas S T, Czerniak A, Wolfstein I 1985 Unusual scintigraphic presentation of a shifting Meckel's diverticulum. Clinical Nuclear Medicine 10: 252–255

SCINTIGRAPHIC DETECTION OF GASTRO-OESOPHAGEAL REFLUX – 'MILK SCAN'

Gastro-oesophageal reflux may be detected by giving a drink of ^{99m}Tc-labelled sulphur colloid, administered in orange juice. The bottle is held in a lead shield, and the infant fed while in the nurse's arms. A further drink of juice is given to clear any activity from the mouth. The child is then laid in the right lateral position on the table with the gamma camera under the infant, and a series of 2-minute frames acquired. Time–activity curves are generated over the oesophagus. Reflux is seen as peaks in the graphs (Fig. 3.9.21). Following a full feed, the chest is subsequently scanned after a 2-hour period, the abdomen being masked off. The presence of radioactivity in the lungs indicates aspiration. The curves are very 'noisy' in a tachypnoeic infant, making it difficult to detect reflux. The technician should watch the examination on the acquisition screen and record visually observed episodes of reflux to overcome this problem. Long-term recording is sometimes useful and some late evening scans have shown higher rates of reflux.

REFERENCES

Fawcett H, Hayden C, Adams J, Swischuk L 1988 How useful is gastroesophageal reflux scintigraphy in suspected childhood aspiration? Pediatric Radiology 18: 311–313

Jona J, Sty J, Glicklich M 1981 Simplified radioisotope techniques for assessing gastroesophageal reflux in children. Journal of Pediatric Surgery 16: 114–117

Miller JH 1991 Upper gastrointestinal tract evaluation with radionuclides in infants. Radiology 178: 326–327

Paton J, Cosgriff P, Nanayakkara C 1985 The analytical sensitivity of Tc^{99m} radionuclide 'milk' scanning in the detection of gastro-oesophageal reflux. Pediatric Radiology 15: 381–383

ABDOMINAL CT

The main indications for abdominal CT in children are the investigation of tumours and other masses, lymph nodes, and the assessment of abdominal trauma. CT for the primary investigation of the bowel is rarely indicated but it can be valuable in the assessment of the extent of abscess formation.

There are inherent problems in examining the abdomen in children due to paucity of intra-abdominal fat, artefact from gaseous distension of stomach and colon (Fig. 3.12.60), and the conflicting requirements of sedation and the administration of oral contrast medium. There is no point in doing abdominal CT unless the child is cooperative, or sedated. An examination done on a wriggling child with motion artefact on the CT is a waste of equipment time and ionizing radiation. The child must be comfortable while being scanned; wrapping the child in a blanket and using sandbags to aid immobilization all help to reduce involuntary movement.

Sedation is usually required from about 4 months to 4 years. This is given 30 minutes before inserting a nasogastric tube, or it is put down the nasogastric tube. The child is then cuddled by the parent and contrast medium instilled through the tube. The volume of fluid is adjusted for age and weight, but in general is: 100 ml, up to age 6 months; 200 ml, 6 months to 1 year; 300 ml, 1–3 years; 700 ml, 3–10 years; 1000 ml for older children. A 2% solution of gastrografin or iopamidol is used. The contrast can be given in any medium the child wishes. Colonic opacification is usually achieved with this regimen by about 1 hour. All abdominal scans are done with intravenous contrast, administered as a continuous infusion during the first half of the examination; there will be sufficient contrast within the vascular tree during the second half. Prior scanning without contrast is decided upon an individual basis, but is done at least initially with mass lesions. It is not indicated in follow-up lymphoma surveys, or follow-up scans. Intravenous contrast is administered via long lines or drips if these are in situ. Care must be taken to use a scrupulously aseptic technique and flush the lines with heparin solutions if long lines are used. All intravenous contrast should be of the low osmolar, non-ionic variety. The dose of contrast is adjusted for age and scan area, but is of the order of 2 ml/kg, up to a maximum of 100 ml in a teenager. Scan times should be kept short, 2–4 seconds, dependent on the child's capacity to cooperate. Slice thickness is adjusted to the lesion under investigation, but should normally be the maximum width of the CT unit being used. Streak artefact from gas is reduced in the prone position and scanning in a decubitus position may reduce artefact over the left lobe of the liver from the gastric air, which can also be reduced by aspiration of the air. Barium in

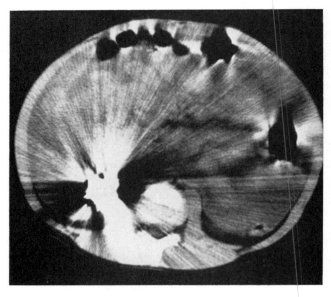

Fig. 3.15.2 Streak artefact from previous barium examination.

the scan plane generates streak artefact and renders the examination useless (Fig. 3.15.2).

REFERENCES

Kaufman R A 1989 Technical aspects of abdominal CT in infants and children. American Journal of Roentgenology 153: 549–554

Kelly J, Raptopoulos V, Davidoff A, Waite R, Norton P 1989 The value of non-contrast-enhanced CT in blunt abdominal trauma. American Journal of Roentgenology 152: 41–46

Scatarige J, DiSantis D 1989 CT of the stomach and duodenum. Radiologic Clinics of North America 27: 687–706

Siegel M, Evans S, Balfe D 1988 Small bowel disease in children: diagnosis with CT. Radiology 169: 127–130

Taylor G, Guion C, Potter B, Eichelberger M 1989 CT of blunt abdominal trauma in children. American Journal of Roentgenology 153: 555–559

RADIATION DOSE REDUCTION

Fluoroscopy or CT deliver the highest radiation doses to children during gastrointestinal investigation. There are simple measures which will produce significant dose reduction. The use of spotfilming devices, instead of image intensifier films, will reduce the dose for the procedure by a factor of 90%. The removal of the grid while screening will achieve a further dose reduction. The grid is only required in older children. The use of digital fluoroscopic systems with low dose scanning techniques can produce a dose reduction of about 80% compared with conventional fluoroscopy, but the films are 'grainy'. Conventional digital systems still achieve a significant dose reduction compared with non-digital systems. Carbon fibre table tops and cassette systems reduce dose levels. Cassette screen–film combinations should be chosen to give the minimum radiation dose possible. The use of video systems while screening allows repeated review of a procedure, rather than repeat fluoroscopy.

CT examination of the abdomen carries with it a significant radiation dose. If the examination is needed to resolve a clinical problem, then the dose involved is justified, but care must be taken to achieve a satisfactory examination from the beginning and not to have to repeat it because of poor preparation or lack of sedation. Protocols should be agreed that provide the appropriate information with minimum dose. The necessity for pre- and postintravenous contrast scanning should be carefully evaluated.

Where radionuclides are excreted by the kidneys, gonadal and bladder dose can be reduced by encouraging fluid intake, active bladder emptying and frequent nappy changes.

REFERENCES

Cohen G, Wagner L K, McDaniel D L, Robinson L H 1984 Dose efficiency of screen film systems used in pediatric radiography. Radiology 152: 187–193
Drury P, Robinson A 1980 Fluoroscopy without the grid : a method of reducing the radiation dose. British Journal of Radiology 53: 93–99
Kushner D, Herman T, Cleveland R, Kleinman R, Goosit M 1988 Reduction of radiation exposure during gastrointestinal biopsy procedures in children. Investigative Radiology 23: 211–215
Wesenberg R, Amundson G 1984 Fluoroscopy in children: low exposure technology. Radiology 153: 243–247

INTERVENTIONAL RADIOLOGY

Interventional radiological procedures in the child's abdomen are mainly of three kinds: percutaneous drainage of abscesses, percutaneous cyst aspiration for diagnostic purposes and, where appropriate, for sclerotherapy, and biopsy procedures – mainly of the liver and tumour masses. The techniques used in children are very similar to those in adults, although modified and adapted. In general, distances between lesions and vital organs are less, so greater care is required in precise positioning of needles and catheters to avoid puncturing the major vessels or bowel. When using spring-loaded 'triggered' biopsy needles, the distance travelled between the point of entry and end point of the needle must be known when planning the procedure. Biopsy specimen cores must be of a reasonable size for pathological analysis. Just because the child is small does not mean that the histopathologist needs a smaller bit for diagnosis! In general, these procedures should only be done by radiologists familiar with the techniques in children who have an understanding of the technical problems and are therefore more likely to avoid complications. Procedures must only be done following discussion with the referring clinician so that each has an understanding of the aims of the procedures and the likely complications. The radiologist should directly discuss the procedure with the child's parents and explain any likely problems, but keep them in perspective. Informed consent forms should be obtained and recorded.

Haematology

Fine needle aspiration procedures (needle gauge of 22 or less) do not require prior clotting screen unless the procedure is on a child at risk of bleeding. Patients requiring biopsy procedures using larger needles should have a recent clotting screen before the procedure and, where appropriate, the child should have prophylactic cover with plasma and platelets, which should be organized by the haematology department.

Specimen handling

Prior arrangement with the departments of microbiology, pathology, cytology and biochemistry should be made to arrange for the correct handling of the specimen.

Anaesthesia

The choice of local or general anaesthesia, or sedation regimens, will vary with the nature of the procedure, the cooperation of the child, his or his parents' wishes, and facilities available locally. If anaesthesia is required, as many procedures as possible should be coordinated under the one anaesthetic. With the advent of the spring-loaded biopsy devices, many biopsy procedures can now be done swiftly and almost painlessly under local anaesthesia and sedation.

Imaging control

Fluoroscopy, ultrasound and CT control are all appropriate for these procedures. Small lesions, where precision is required to ensure that the needle is in the lesion and major surrounding structures avoided, are best biopsied or drained under CT control, but procedures under CT are time consuming. Large lesions may be safely tackled under fluoroscopic or ultrasound control. MR controlled biopsy is technically more difficult.

Sclerosing agents

Intracavity administration of small amounts of intravenous tetracycline will cause some fibrosis and adherence of the walls of cysts and lymphangiomas.

Catheters

Drainage with catheter sheaths over needles, and catheters introduced by Seldinger's technique are satisfactory in children. Care must be taken to support the long needles, as muscle mass is so much less in children the needles tend to slip out of the lesion more easily than in adults. 5–6F catheters are adequate for drainage of non-viscous fluid collections but multiple holes are necessary for abscess drainage. Large double lumen sump drainage catheters are not appropriate for children. Simple aspiration of abscess collections is often as satisfactory as leaving a drainage catheter in situ, and removal of a pocket of pus by this technique will often achieve a dramatic improvement in the child's general well-being, with immediate fall in temperature. If necessary, the aspiration may be repeated. All abscess drainage procedures should be done under cover of intravenous antibiotics.

Biopsy size

The smaller the biopsy needle, the safer the procedure, but the larger the specimen, the easier it is for the pathologist to make a diagnosis. Most abdominal tumours can be safely biopsied using 14–18 gauge needles provided major vascular areas are avoided. The specimen must be taken from a solid point of the lesion and necrotic areas avoided for tissue diagnosis. 20 gauge needles are safer for pancreatic biopsy. Spring-loaded biopsy gun devices are particularly suitable for children's biopsy procedures. The procedure is so swift that tearing during the cutting is minimized, and respiratory motion is therefore less of a problem, and many biopsies are possible under local anaesthesia and sedation. Where the lesion is small, and great precision required in needle placement, or multiple passes are likely to be required for positioning as occurs with CT contrast, then it is better to plan the procedure under general anaesthesia.

REFERENCES

Amundson G, Towbin R, Mueller D, Seagram C 1990 Percutaneous transgastric drainage of the lesser sac in children. Pediatric Radiology 20: 590–593
Gaisie G, Jaques P, Mauro M 1987 Radiological management of fluid collections in children. Pediatric Radiology 17: 143–146
Hoffer F, Shamberger R, Teele R 1987 Ilio-psoas abscess: diagnosis and management. Pediatric Radiology 17: 23–27
Jaffe R B, Arata J A, Matlak M E 1989 Percutaneous drainage of traumatic pseudocysts in children. American Journal of Roentgenology 152: 591–595
Jeffrey R, Tolentino C, Federle M, Laing F 1987 Percutaneous drainage of periappendiceal abscesses: review of 20 patients. American Journal of Roentgenology 149: 59–62
Smith E H 1991 Complications of percutaneous abdominal fine needle biopsy. Radiology 178: 253–258
Towbin R R, Ball W S 1988 Pediatric interventional radiology. Radiologic Clinics of North America 26: 419–440

PERCUTANEOUS GASTROSTOMY

Percutaneous gastrostomy is an alternative technique to surgery for placing a feeding gastrostomy tube in position. The tube is inserted under local anaesthetic, following sedation. In one technique, gastric distension is achieved by injection of air via a nasogastric feeding tube. The nasogastric tube is replaced by a Dotter basket and sheath passed orally. Stomach puncture is performed through the abdominal wall, avoiding the left lobe of the liver. A wire is passed through the intragastric canula and gripped by the Dotter basket, and gently pulled into the mouth. Over this the gastrostomy tube is passed via the mouth over the guide-wire until the tip emerges from the stab wound. The intragastric portion of the tube is anchored in position by its crossbar or balloon depending in which system is used. The tube is fixed to the skin surface with sutures and fixing discs. The guide-wire is removed. If required, the feeding tube can be advanced coaxially into the jejunum.

REFERENCES

Towbin R, Ball W, Bissett G 1988 Percutaneous gastrostomy and percutaneous gastrojejunostomy in children: antegrade approach. Radiology 168: 473–476
Wills J, Oglesby J 1988 Percutaneous gastrostomy. Radiology 167: 41–43

COLONIC PREPARATION FOR BARIUM ENEMA

Preparation is contraindicated for the investigation of constipation. Good quality double contrast examination in children requires a clean colon. A suggested regimen is:

1. Low residue diet for 48 hours in all children
2. Aperient delivered in divided doses over the 48-hour period, the dose being adjusted for age:

0–2 years	one-quarter of adult dose
2–5 years	one-third of adult dose
5–10 years	one-half of adult dose
10–15 years	two-thirds of adult dose
15+	adult dose.

Instructions are given to double the fluid intake for the preparation period.

4

The liver, biliary tract and spleen

D. Pariente

INTRODUCTION

In the past few years, there has been a spectacular evolution in liver and biliary tract imaging with the advent of new imaging modalities, such as ultrasonography (US), computed tomography (CT) and magnetic resonance imaging (MRI). In spite of these relatively non-invasive techniques there is still a place for more invasive examinations, such as angiography and percutaneous transhepatic cholangiography (PTC).

As a result of these remarkable advances in technique, the paediatric radiologist plays a central role in the diagnosis, treatment and follow up of liver diseases in children.

4.1   IMAGING

ULTRASONOGRAPHY

Ultrasound is the ideal screening modality for liver diseases in children. There is no need for sedation and the examination is rapid, non-invasive and very informative.

Transducer frequency and resolution must be adapted not only to the size of the child but also the 'absorption' of the liver. The examination must be systematic and follow an ordered plan of the hepatic vessels in order to be reproducible and therefore capable of comparison on repeat examinations.

Pulsed Doppler has complemented US and yields important haemodynamic information. Quantitative values have been very disappointing to date and do not appear to be reliable. Colour Doppler is a significant advance in paediatric US, as it displays simultaneously morphological detail and flow imaging in a larger sector of the liver and therefore faster identification of anatomical structures.

COMPUTED TOMOGRAPHY

The technique for obtaining good quality CT scans of the liver in children is based on an aggressive attitude: the child must be correctly sedated or cooperative.

Bolus injection of IV contrast medium is mandatory. Opacification of the upper gastrointestinal tract is often required. The fastest scanning times are recommended to reduce motion artefacts and radiation dose.

MAGNETIC RESONANCE IMAGING

Experience with MRI of the liver in children is still limited to a few centres and to limited indications. Principles of sedation do not differ much from those used in CT scanning technique.

Advantages of MRI are multiplanar imaging capability, excellent tissue contrast differentiation, natural contrast of vessels and lack of ionizing radiation.

The main indication is the evaluation of liver tumours. The distribution of the lesion and its relationship to vascular structures are well shown. In generalized parenchymal liver disease, MRI has the potential to play a role, especially to evaluate the degree of iron overload.

The main disadvantages of MRI include the length of time of examination, the degradation of the image by movements such as respiration and peristalsis and the difficulty of monitoring sick infants and children.

RADIO-ISOTOPE IMAGING

The availability of radionuclide studies is very variable and therefore their use in paediatric liver disease is more sporadic than in adults. The expertise in both technique and interpretation is also variable.

There are two types of radiopharmaceuticals which are used to obtain static images of liver and spleen: colloid preparations which are taken up by macrophages, and radiopharmaceuticals which are actively transported by the hepatocytes into bile. They are given intravenously tagged to a gamma emitting isotope, usually ^{99m}Tc, but on occasion ^{123}I.

T_{99} sulphur colloid imaging

It reflects reticuloendothelial function and intrahepatic blood flow.

Filling defects on the scan may be due to a wide spectrum of lesions and it is less specific than US in the assessment of focal lesions.

Imaging of the biliary tree

^{99m}Tc-labelled iminodiacetic acid (IDA) derivates have replaced ^{131}I-labelled Rose Bengal in demonstrating biliary excretion and abnormalities in the biliary system. They also reflect hepatic function. ^{123}I-labelled Rose Bengal and ^{123}I-labelled bromosulphthalein have also been used, expecially for the diagnosis of biliary atresia.

ANGIOGRAPHY

Much of our current understanding of liver diseases is due to information gained from angiographic studies. Diagnostic angiographic studies are being replaced by US and CT, but there remain some indications such as preoperative work-up or as a prelude to embolization or other interventional procedures.

Digital subtraction angiography (DSA) has the advantage of showing better contrast in the late phases of superior mesenteric arteriograms with better visualization of the portal and hepatic venous system. It has to be emphasized that diagnostic angiography of the liver must include both opacification of the hepatic artery and portal vein. With the advent of DSA, the indications for *splenoportography* (SPG) have decreased, as visualization of the splenic vein may be obtained with good contrast on the venous phase of splenic arteriography. Splenoportography remains a safe and informative examination, if done carefully, taking account of the contraindications of ascites and coagulation disorders. It is generally performed under general anaesthesia, with a needle and an outer Teflon catheter (20–18 gauge needle). The splenic pressure can be recorded and corresponds to portal pressure.

Percutaneous transhepatic opacification of the portal or hepatic venous system can also be achieved, especially in Budd–Chiari disease.

CHOLANGIOGRAPHY

Oral cholecystography and IV cholangiography have been largely replaced by US. Only a few indications for IV cholangiography remain. The contrast may be improved and information gained increased by performing CT at the end of biliary contrast medium perfusion. Indications are the suspicion of biliary disease without cholestasis such as Caroli's disease and choledochal cyst.

On the contrary, percutaneous transhepatic cholangiography has gained wide acceptance in paediatrics and the technique does not differ from that in adults.

Percutaneous transhepatic cholecystography constitutes real progress and has allowed us to easily image non-dilated intrahepatic bile ducts. It is performed under ultrasound guidance.

When the gallbladder is small, opacification of the biliary tree may be obtained by simple puncture with a thin needle. When the gallbladder is large, a small catheter should be placed in its lumen to avoid displacement of the needle and bile leakage.

Endoscopic retrograde cholangio-pancreatography has been mainly used in older children. Recent advances in the equipment has allowed a few experts to use it in infantile cholestasis with success.

PERCUTANEOUS LIVER BIOPSY

This procedure often provides invaluable information on the nature and severity of liver diseases. It is always performed after less invasive imaging techniques which must exclude focal lesions such as haemangioma or hydatid cyst. Other contraindications include impaired coagulation and ascites.

Transjugular liver biopsy can be used in adult patients to avoid puncturing the liver capsule. However, sometimes the size of the specimen obtained is small and inadequate for diagnosis. Biopsies under ultrasound or CT guidance are more and more widely used, to avoid large vessels and to direct the needle to a focal lesion.

REFERENCES

Brunelle F, Chaumont P 1984 Percutaneous cholecystography in children. Annales de Radiologie 27: 111–116

Brunelle F, Riou J Y, Douillet P 1981 La cholangiographie transhépatique dans la dilatation des voies biliaires de l'enfant. Annales de Radiologie 2: 131–139

Carty H, Pilling D W, Majury C 1986[123] IBSP scanning in neonatal jaundice. Annales de Radiologie 29: 647–650

Doyon D, Roche A, Chaumont P 1978 Les examens vasculaires en pathologie digestive chez l'enfant. In: L'angiographie digestive chez l'adulte et l'enfant. Masson, Paris, p 121–169

Franken E A, Smith W L, Smith J A, Fitzgerald J F 1978 Percutaneous cholangiography in infants. American Journal of Roentgenology 130: 1057–1058

Guyes M T 1974 Angiography in infants and children. Grune and Stratton, New York

Kaufman R A 1989 Technical aspects of abdominal CT in infants and children. American Journal of Roentgenology 153: 549–554

Mowat A P (ed) 1987 Laboratory assessment of hepatobiliary disease. In: Liver disorders in childhood, 2nd edn. Butterworths-Heinemann, Oxford, p 366

Stanley P 1982 Pediatric angiography. Williams and Wilkins, Baltimore

Wilkinson M L, Mieli-Vergani G, Ball C, Portmann B, Mowat A P 1991 Endoscopic retrograde cholangio-pancreatography in infantile cholestasis. Archives of Disease in Childhood 66: 121–123

4.2 PORTAL HYPERTENSION

Portal hypertension in children may be due to a large variety of causes which can be classified as occurring at three anatomical levels of obstruction to portal blood flow: prehepatic (portal obstruction), intrahepatic and suprahepatic.

The main clinical signs of portal hypertension include splenomegaly, ascites and gastrointestinal bleeding which is the major clinical problem.

Ultrasonography (US) is the key to diagnosis, follow-up and postoperative assessment. Oesophagogastroduodenal endoscopy is the main method of assessing the risk of bleeding from varices. Angiography is performed only when a surgical portosystemic shunt is considered.

POSITIVE DIAGNOSIS OF PORTAL HYPERTENSION

It relies on the ultrasonic demonstration of a hepatofugal collateral circulation.

Gastro-oesophageal shunts are depicted in the lesser omentum which is studied on a longitudinal scan through the aorta. In normal non-obese children, its thickness at the level of the origin of the coeliac axis is a maximum size of one and half times the aortic diameter. In children with portal hypertension, the lesser omentum contains the dilated left gastric vein, its varicose collaterals and lymphatic stasis. Its thickness is greater than normal by up to three or four times (Fig. 4.2.1).

The visibility of a patent para-umbilical vein in the ligamentum teres is also specific for portal hypertension and indicative of an intra- or suprahepatic block (Fig. 4.2.2). Duplex sonography reinforces this diagnosis and shows the hepatofugal venous flow.

Spontaneous splenorenal shunts may also be demonstrated by Doppler US.

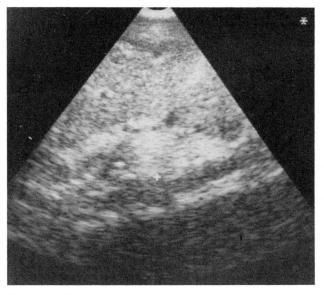

Fig. 4.2.1 There is a thickened lesser omentum, measured on a longitudinal scan, between the posterior aspect of the left lobe of the liver and the anterior aspect of the aorta (cross marks) at the level of the coeliac axis — diagnostic of portal hypertension.

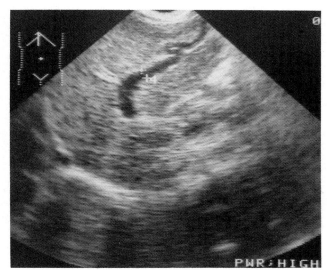

Fig. 4.2.2 There is a patent para-umbilical vein in the ligamentum teres, continuing the left portal vein — diagnostic of portal hypertension.

AETIOLOGICAL DIAGNOSIS

Prehepatic causes of portal hypertension

Portal obstruction is the single most frequent cause of portal hypertension in children.

Reported causes are:

- Traditionally neonatal venous catheterization has been said to be the main cause, but this no longer holds true and most cases are idiopathic.
- Some cases are due to malformations, associated with cardiovascular or urinary malformations.
- Omphalitis, hepatic abcesses and appendicitis have also been reported to be the cause of portal obstruction.

The liver is normal in size and function and ultrasonography is the best non-invasive method for diagnosis of portal obstruction: the normal bifurcation and the trunk of the portal vein are replaced by a hyperechogenic area where multiple tortuous vessels may be seen. These vessels correspond to hepatopetal collateral veins and are known as a portal cavernoma (Fig. 4.2.3). This sometimes contains a larger collateral vein which may simulate the normal portal vein.

Hepatopetal veins may be demonstrated in a thickened gallbladder wall. Angiographic study of the entire portal system is mandatory for precise mapping before surgery, as the extent of the cavernoma is highly variable. At the venous phase of superior mesenteric arteriography opacification of the superior mesenteric vein, extra- and intrahepatic portal cavernoma and, in most cases, the splenic vein (Figs 4.2.4, 4.2.5) are seen. If there is no reflux into the splenic vein, it should be visualized by selective splenic arteriography or in more detail by spleno-portography (Fig. 4.2.6).

In very rare instances, there may be an association of portal venous obstruction with intrahepatic bile duct dilatation. The presentation ranges from only mild laboratory changes to a clinical picture of obstructive jaundice. It is thought to be due to compression of the biliary tract by the portal cavernoma. Regression of bile duct dilatation after surgical portosystemic shunting has been reported (Fig. 4.2.7). The US diagnosis is difficult because of the numerous tubular channels present in the porta hepatis. It is easier since the advent of colour Doppler.

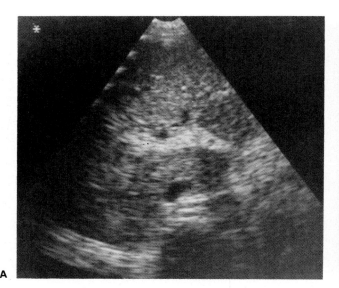
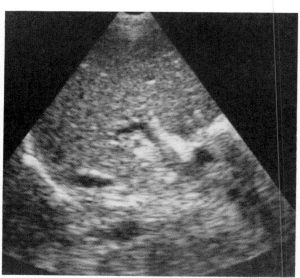

Fig. 4.2.3 Portal obstruction. Five-year-old boy presenting with gastrointestinal bleeding. **A** Transverse scan through the porta hepatis: the normal portal vein bifurcation is replaced by a hyperechogenic area with small tortuous vessels. **B** Longitudinal oblique scan through the portal vein trunk: a large hepatopetal collateral vein simulates a normal portal vein, but it is tortuous and surrounded by a hyperechogenic area.

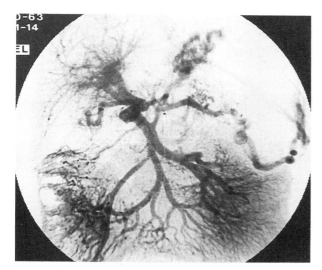

Fig. 4.2.4 Superior mesenteric arteriogram. Same case as Fig. 4.2.3. Preoperative work-up. At the venous phase, the intra- and extrahepatic portal obstruction is confirmed, but there is an intact superior mesenteric vein which will be used for mesocaval shunting.

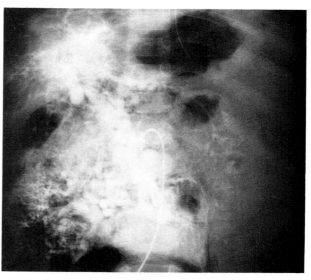

Fig. 4.2.5 Superior mesenteric arteriogram. In this case, the portal obstruction has extended to the superior mesenteric vein and no opacified vein suitable for use at surgery is demonstrated. Further work-up must be done to see the splenic vein, by digital splenic arteriography or splenoportography.

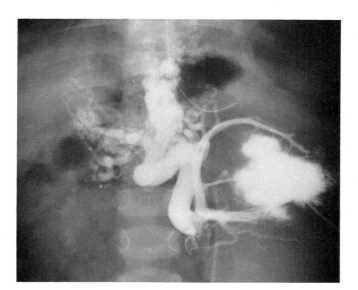

Fig. 4.2.6 Splenoportography. The splenic vein is large, but tortuous. There is portal vein obstruction with cavernomatous hepatopetal veins. Most of the contrast medium is diverted to a large coronary vein.

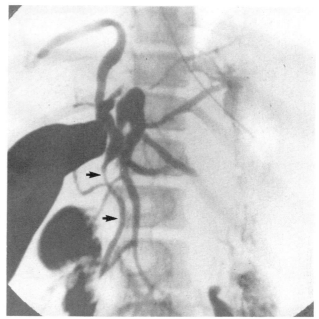

Fig. 4.2.7 Intrahepatic bile duct dilatation associated with portal vein obstruction. A 14-year-old girl, followed since 4 years of age for a well-tolerated portal obstruction, now has hepatomegaly with early biliary cirrhosis diagnosed on liver biopsy. A percutaneous transhepatic cholangiogram shows moderate intrahepatic bile duct dilatation with hypertrophy of the left lobe. The common bile duct (arrows) has a normal caliber but has a tortuous course. This was thought to be due to compression by the cavernoma. After surgical shunting biological findings returned to normal.

Intrahepatic causes of portal hypertension

Cirrhosis

The main causes of cirrhosis in childhood can be divided into three groups:

1. Biliary cirrhosis – the causes include biliary atresia, Byler's disease, paucity of intrahepatic bile ducts, cystic fibrosis, choledochal cyst, sclerosing cholangitis, alpha-1-antitrypsin deficiency,
2. Posthepatitic cirrhosis,
3. Metabolic cirrhosis — Wilson's disease, tyrosinaemia.

Ultrasound shows a normal portal venous system and normal hepatic veins. It may show dilatation of the bile ducts in some cases of biliary cirrhosis. Modifications of contours, surface and echostructure with macro- or micronodular appearance are highly suggestive of cirrhosis but the appearances are the same, irrespective of the cause (Fig. 4.2.8).

Congenital hepatic fibrosis

It is an autosomal recessive disease consisting in virtually all children of the association of hepatic and renal

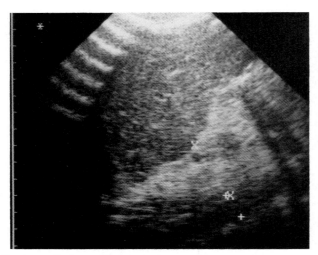

Fig. 4.2.8 Cirrhosis. There is thickening of the lesser omentum compared to aorta (cross marks). The inferior aspect of the liver appears macronodular.

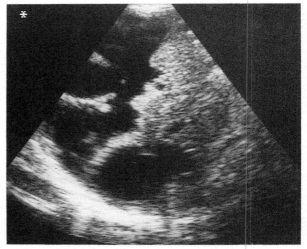

Fig. 4.2.9 Congenital hepatic fibrosis. There is a large cystic dilatation of the peripheral bile ducts in a 5-year-old boy with congenital hepatic fibrosis. Despite these impressive abnormalities of the bile ducts, liver function tests are normal.

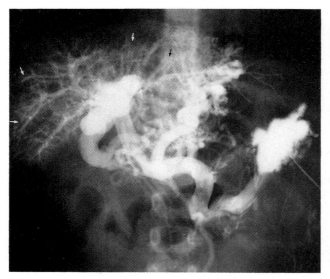

Fig. 4.2.10 Splenoportography in a patient with congenital hepatic fibrosis. Preoperative work-up before surgical shunting in a 12-year-old girl with congenital hepatic fibrosis and severe portal hypertension. Large hepatofugal veins are seen (arrows). There is also evidence of portal vein branch duplication, a characteristic but non-specific finding of congenital hepatic fibrosis.

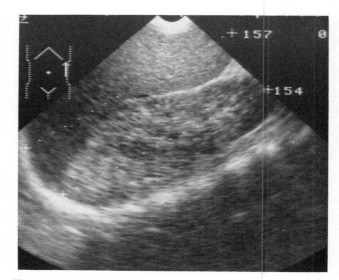

Fig. 4.2.11 Congenital hepatic fibrosis in an 8-year-old boy. There is striking enlargement of the spleen and kidneys. Normal renal echostructure has been replaced by global hyperechogenicity highly suggestive of the diagnosis of recessive type of renal polycystic disease.

lesions, ranging from purely histological abnormalities to severe clinical disease.

Hepatic lesions include portal fibrosis and biliary dysplasia with saccular dilatation of the peripheral bile ducts (Fig. 4.2.9). Two main complications are portal hypertension and rare but severe episodes of cholangitis. Bright echos in the portal spaces and cystic dilatations of the peripheral bile ducts may be seen on US.

On angiography duplication of the intrahepatic portal branches has been described in children with portal hypertension (Fig. 4.2.10). In a few cases hepatopetal collateral veins are seen along the normal portal vein, simulating a portal cavernoma. These two angiographic findings are characteristic. They are probably secondary to thrombosis or hypoplasia of the portal vein radicles which are described on liver biopsies.

Renal lesions correspond to polycystic renal disease of the infantile type. Nephromegaly with a hyperechogenic appearance of the entire parenchyma (Fig. 4.2.11) or limited to the medulla are the ultrasonic findings (Fig. 4.2.12). Small cysts may be visible. Persistent and streaky opacification of the dilated collecting tubules is seen on an intravenous pyelogram (IVP) (Fig. 4.2.13), but demonstration of this finding is not constant and the IVP is less sensitive than US for renal abnormalities.

REFERENCES

Bernard O, Alvarez F, Brunelle F, Hadchouel P, Alagille D 1985 Portal hypertension in children. Clinics in Gastroenterology 14: 33–35

Brunelle F, Alagille D, Pariente D, Chaumont P 1981 An ultrasound study of portal hypertension in children. Annales de Radiologie 24: 121–130

Choudhuri G, Tandon R K, Nundy S, Misra N K 1988 Common bile duct obstruction by portal cavernoma. Digestive Diseases and Sciences 33: 1626–1628

Day D L, Letourneau J G, Allan B T, Sharp H L, Ascher N, Dehner L P, Thompson W N 1987 Hepatic regenerating nodules in hereditary tyrosinemia. American Journal of Roentgenology 149: 391–393

Di Lelio A, Cestari C, Lomazzi A, Beretta L 1989 Cirrhosis: diagnosis with sonographic study of the liver surface. Radiology 172: 389–392

Freeman M P, Vick C W, Taylor K J W, Carithers R L, Brewer W H 1986 Regenerating nodules in cirrhosis: sonographic appearance with anatomic correlation. American Journal of Roentgenology 146: 533–536

Gibson R N, Gibson P R, Doulan J D, Clunie D A 1989 Identification of a patent paraumbilical vein by using doppler sonography: importance in the diagnosis of portal hypertension. American Journal of Roentgenology 153: 513–516

Patriquin H, Tessier G, Grignou A, Boisvert J 1985 Lesser omental thickness in normal children: baseline for detection of portal hypertension. American Journal of Roentgenology 145: 693–696

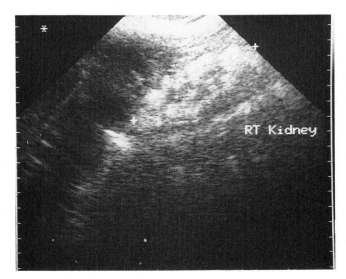

Fig. 4.2.12 Congenital hepatic fibrosis in a 5-year-old boy. Longitudinal scan through the right kidney showing another appearance which suggests kidney involvement and simulates nephrocalcinosis: there are hyperechogenic areas in the medulla.

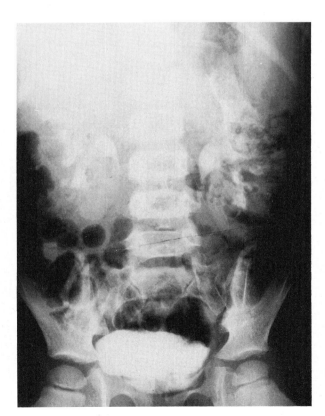

Fig. 4.2.13 Typical IVP appearance in congenital hepatic fibrosis and recessive type of renal polycystic disease: there is striking nephromegaly and linear precalceal opacification.

Suprahepatic causes of portal hypertension

The obstruction may be located in the centrilobular veins (veno-occlusive disease), hepatic veins or suprahepatic inferior vena cava (Budd–Chiari syndrome), or at the cardiac level.

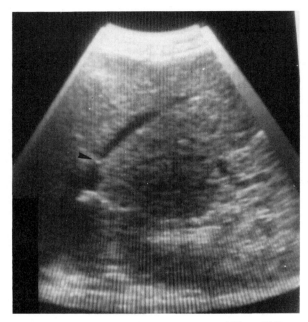

Fig. 4.2.14 Budd–Chiari syndrome in a 4-year-old boy. Oblique scan through the right hepatic vein shows dilatation above a stricture of the ostium (arrowhead).

BUDD–CHIARI SYNDROME

This is a rare occurrence in children and in most cases no causative factor is found. Budd–Chiari syndrome may be discovered in the presence of hepatomegaly, recurrent ascites, collateral venous circulation, or even fortuitously. Ultrasonic examination is the key of the diagnosis by showing abnormalities of the hepatic veins. They are not visible or replaced by an echogenic line, dilated above an abnormal ostium (Fig. 4.2.14), or tortuous, corresponding to intra- or extrahepatic collateral veins. Pulsed Doppler sonography may demonstrate an inverted flow in an hepatic vein, which is highly suggestive of the diagnosis (Fig. 4.2.15). US is not completely reliable in the assessment of inferior vena cava patency because it may be compressed by ascites and an enlarged caudate lobe (Fig. 4.2.16).

CT shows heterogeneous contrast enhancement of hepatic parenchyma with a patchy area of increased attenuation in the caudate lobe (Fig. 4.2.17). This pattern has also been reported in the other causes of hepatic venous congestion. At scintigraphy with sulphur colloid, the caudate lobe is preserved while the rest of the liver is abnormal.

Surgical treatment with portocaval shunt must be considered to relieve the venous congestion and avoid centrilobular fibrosis and cirrhosis.

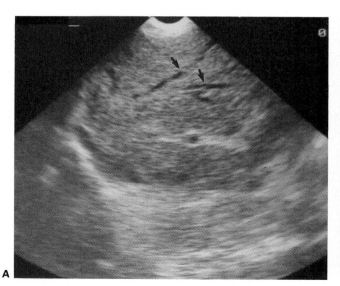

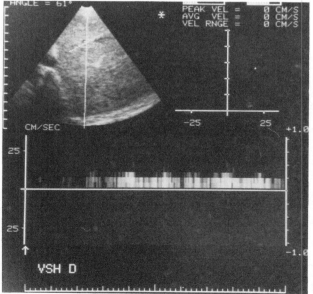

Fig. 4.2.15 An 8-year-old Tunisian girl, presenting with hepatomegaly and previous episodes of ascites. **A** The right hepatic vein appears tortuous with some collaterals and the ostium is not visible (arrows). **B** Duplex study demonstrates inverted flow in this right hepatic vein and therefore confirms the diagnosis of Budd–Chiari syndrome.

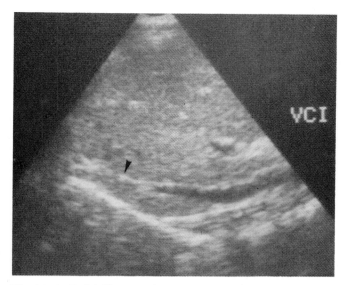

Fig. 4.2.16 Budd–Chiari syndrome. Fortuitous discovery in a 5-year-old boy presenting with mild hepatomegaly. The retrohepatic inferior vena cava appears as an echogenic line and was obstructed on cavography (arrowhead).

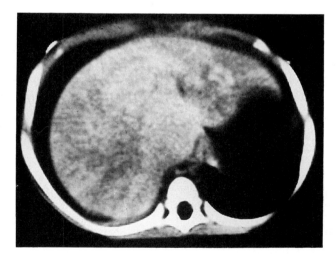

Fig. 4.2.17 A 3-year-old girl with Budd–Chiari syndrome. Ascites and heterogeneous contrast enhancement of the liver with hyperdensity of the caudate lobe are present on CT.

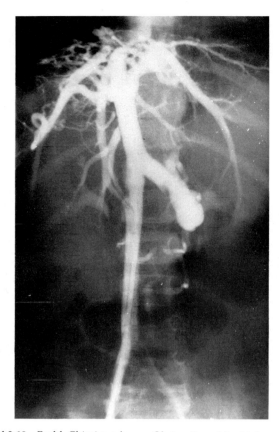

Fig. 4.2.18 Budd–Chiari syndrome. Obstruction of the high inferocardiac portion of the inferior vena cava and of main hepatic veins is demonstrated by cavography. There is abnormal contrast reflux in the left renal vein.

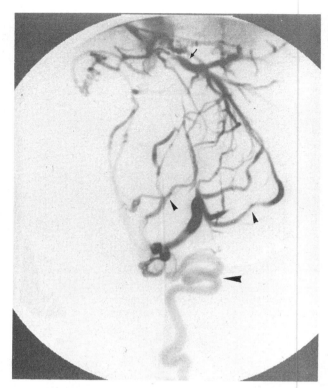

Fig. 4.2.19 Budd–Chiari syndrome. Retrograde phlebography. The catheter tip is introduced into the left hepatic vein (small arrow). A spider-web network of intrahepatic vein collaterals is opacified, typical of obstruction of the hepatic vein ostium (small arrowheads). Contrast drains by a tortuous extrahepatic parietal vein (large arrowhead).

Cavography is critical in surgical planning and the type of shunt will be mainly decided on inferior vena cava patency and pressure recording. In a few cases, a 'membranous obstruction' of the inferior vena cava has been reported, suggestive of a congenital malformation aetiology. Hepatic vein opacification should be attempted by retrograde phlebography via the inferior vena cava or superior vena cava (Figs 4.2.18, 4.2.19), and a transhepatic approach, guided by US, can be considered if ascites is not present (Fig. 4.2.20). A transluminal angioplasty may be performed for segmental obstruction or limited stenosis.

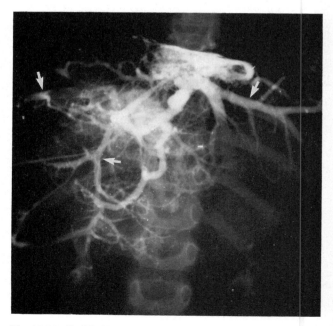

Fig. 4.2.20 Budd–Chiari syndrome. Transhepatic phlebography. A tortuous abnormal network of hepatic veins is opacified. Intact peripheral portions of right, middle and sagittal veins are seen (arrows), but the ostia are obstructed.

VENO-OCCLUSIVE DISEASE

It has been reported mainly in children of the Caribbean with ingestion of tea prepared from leaves containing pyrolizidine alkaloids. It occurs also as a consequence of radiation therapy, chemotherapy or bone marrow transplantation. Sporadic cases with no known aetiology are also reported in children. Diagnosis is made on histological findings.

Ultrasonography shows thin but patent and regular hepatic veins and CT may display heterogeneous contrast enhancement of the liver as in Budd–Chiari syndrome. Reversed portal flow has also been described with duplex examination.

Cardiac causes

They include constrictive pericarditis, congestive cardiac failure and also the exceptional cor triatriatum dextrum which may present as Budd–Chiari syndrome (Fig. 4.2.21).

REFERENCES

Lepage J R 1983 Cor triatriatrium dextrum and persistent muscle of Lower presenting as Budd Chiari syndrome. Angiology 34: 491–494

Lois J F, Hartzmann S, McGlade C T, Gomes A S 1989 Budd Chiari syndrome: treatment with percutaneous transhepatic recanalization and dilatation. Radiology 170: 791–793

Menu Y, Alison D, Lorphelin J M, Valla D, Belghiti J, Nahum H 1985 Budd Chiari syndrome: US evaluation. Radiology 157: 761–764

Pariente D, Gentil S, Brunelle F, Bernard O, Chaumont P 1987 Budd Chiari syndrome in children: radiologic investigation. Annales de Radiologie 30: 518–524

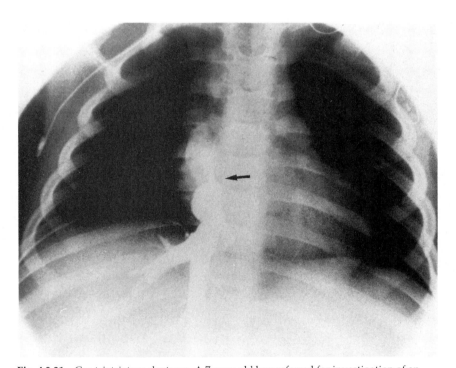

Fig. 4.2.21 Cor triatriatum dextrum. A 7-year-old boy referred for investigation of an episode of acute abdominal pain and hepatosplenomegaly. US shows large hepatic veins with patent ostia but liver biopsy is suggestive of Budd–Chiari syndrome. Contrast injection is performed in the inferior portion of the right atrium: there is a transverse membrane (arrow) dividing and obstructing the right atrium. There is also reflux of contrast medium into a large right hepatic vein. Pressure recording in the inferior vena cava and hepatic veins shows a striking increase = 20 mmHg. Resection of this membrane resulted in a cure.

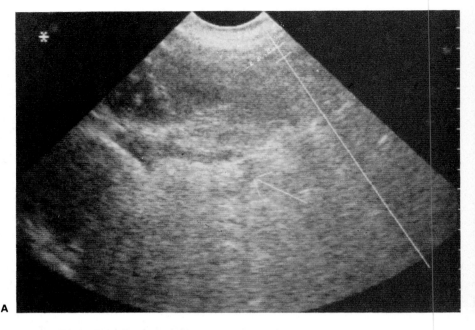

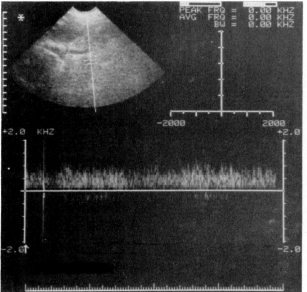

Fig. 4.2.22 Mesocaval shunt with interposed graft. **A** Visualization through the right kidney of the inferior vena cava and graft (arrow). **B** Doppler study shows satisfactory mesocaval flow through the graft.

DEMONSTRATION OF SURGICAL PORTOSYSTEMIC SHUNTS

The main indications for surgical portosystemic shunting include portal vein obstruction, Budd–Chiari syndrome and congenital hepatic fibrosis, with episodes of bleeding and severe varices on endoscopy.

The most common shunt performed is a mesocaval shunt with a jugular graft interposed between the superior mesenteric vein and the inferior vena cava. The other main types are a splenorenal shunt and, more recently, a direct portocaval shunt in the porta hepatis, done to protect the size of portal vein in intrahepatic blocks, with consideration of possible later liver transplantation.

The patency of the shunt can be established in the early postoperative period by ultrasonography. Demonstration of the regression of submucosal varices may be delayed on endoscopy for up to 6 months. Ultrasonic visualization of the shunt is obtained with a posterior approach through the kidney for the mesocaval shunt (Fig. 4.2.22) and through a trans-splenic or left transrenal approach for the splenorenal shunts (Fig. 4.2.23). Localization of the shunt can be helped by pulsed or colour Doppler which shows portosystemic flow. The presence of indirect signs of patency means that the shunt is haemodynamically functional:

— decrease in size and number of gastro-oesophageal collaterals and of the thickness of the lesser omentum;
— decrease of the portal flow with decrease of the size of the portal vein and, in some cases, hepatofugal flow with Doppler study;
— increase of the diameter of inferior vena cava; moreover the classical variations of the inferior vena cava diameter during the respiratory cycle are damped.

Angiography remains indicated when US and endoscopy fail to demonstrate patency of the shunt.

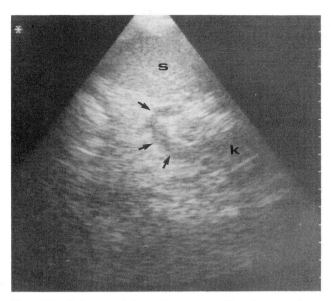

Fig. 4.2.23 Splenorenal shunt. Transverse axillary line scan shows the communication between the splenic and the left renal vein (arrows). (s = spleen; k = kidney.)

REFERENCE

Boucher D, Brunelle F, Bernard O, Forel F, Autrel D, Hadchouel P, Chaumont P 1985 Ultrasonic demonstration of portocaval anastomosis in portal hypertension in children. Pediatric Radiology 15: 307–310

4.3   LIVER TUMOURS

Liver tumours are rare in childhood, representing 1.5–3 % of all tumours, but current imaging techniques play a crucial role in diagnosis, therapeutic decision and follow-up. The clinical presentation is usually abdominal distension. Pain, fever, pallor, anaemia or jaundice occasionally occur. The main problem is the differentiation of malignant from benign tumours. Malignant types represent approximately 60% of liver tumours. Alpha-fetoprotein is elevated in about 90% of children with hepatoblastoma and 80% of hepato-carcinoma and therefore it is an essential test in diagnosis and follow-up of a liver tumour.

Because of its large availability and high sensitivity, US is the imaging modality of choice. When interpreted together with the clinical presentation it usually differentiates tumours from the other liver masses which mimic liver neoplasms, such as abscesses, hydatid cysts, haematoma, focal fatty infiltration (Fig. 4.3.1) and cirrhotic nodules. In most cases, a specific diagnosis can be suggested with US mainly based on a careful examination of intrahepatic vessels.

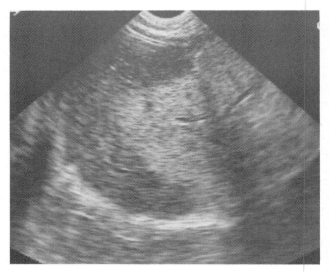

Fig. 4.3.1   Focal fatty infiltration in a 10-year-old boy. There is heterogeneous echogenicity of the liver parenchyma with an hyperechoic central area. There is no distortion of the hepatic vessels. The diagnosis was confirmed on guided liver biopsy.

REFERENCES

Boechat I, Kangarloo H, Gilsanz V 1988 Hepatic masses in children. Seminars in Roentgenology 23: 185–193

Boechat I, Kangarloo H, Ortega J, Hall T, Feig S, Stanley P, Gilsanz V 1988 Primary liver tumors in children: comparison of CT and MRI. Radiology 169: 727–732

Brunelle F, Chaumont P 1984 Hepatic tumors in children: ultrasonic differentiation of malignant from benign lesions. Radiology 150: 695–699

Leary D L, Weiskittel D A, Blaue C E, Goran A G 1989 Follow-up imaging in benign pediatric liver tumors. Pediatric Radiology 19: 234–236

Miller J H, Greenspan B S 1985 Integrated imaging in hepatic tumors in childhood. Radiology 154: 83–100

MALIGNANT TUMOURS

Hepatoblastoma

Hepatoblastoma is the most frequent malignant liver tumour and mainly occurs in children younger than 3 years.

The child usually presents with an abdominal mass. It has been described in association with hemihypertrophy (Beckwith–Wiedemann syndrome) and with a variety of paraneoplastic syndromes which include isosexual precocity, polycythaemia, hypoglycaemia, hypercalcaemia, thrombocytosis, osteomalacia, feminization, hyperlipidaemia. Elevation of alpha-fetoprotein serum level can be detected in nearly all patients.

Hepatoblastoma is most commonly located in the right lobe of the liver but in a few cases it may be multicentric. Several histological types have been recognized with differing prognosis, including epithelial (fetal or embryonal) mixed, mesenchymal-epithelial and anaplastic varieties. On US, its echogenicity is highly variable, mostly heterogeneous with frequent calcifications and areas of necrosis. Amputation or thrombosis of portal or hepatic vein branches are strongly suggestive of the diagnosis (Fig. 4.3.2). CT is required for more accurate demonstration of the extension of the tumour which usually appears hypodense with minimal or no enhancement compared with the rest of the liver (Fig. 4.3.3).

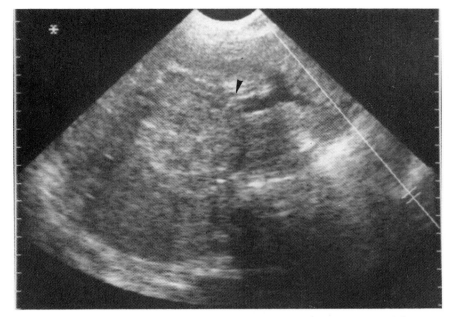

Fig. 4.3.2 Hepatoblastoma in a 12-year-old girl. There is a large heterogeneous right lobe mass with amputation of the right portal vein strongly suggestive of a malignant tumour (arrowhead).

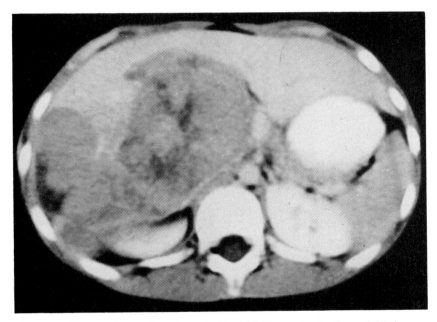

Fig. 4.3.3 CT scan of the patient shown in Fig. 4.3.2. The contrast-enhanced CT shows a lobulated hypodense mass involving the whole right lobe.

Following chemotherapy, angiography is indicated as a preoperative work-up to provide precise arterial and venous mapping (Fig. 4.3.4).

MRI when available may replace CT and even angiography. It shows the vascular relationship of the tumour and may be more accurate in demonstrating daughter nodules and small recurrences (Fig. 4.3.5).

REFERENCES

Brunelle F, Garel L, Harry G, Chaumont P 1979 L'angiographie portale des tumeurs hepatiques de l'enfant. Annales de Radiologie 22: 142–149

Dachman A, Pakter R L, Ros P R, Fishman E K, Goodman Z D, Kicktenstein J E 1987 Hepatoblastoma: radiologic–pathologic correlation in 50 cases. Radiology 164: 15–19

Tonkin I L D, Wrenn E I, Hollabaugh R S 1988 The continued value of angiography in planning surgical resection of benign and malignant hepatic tumors in children. Pediatric Radiology 18: 35–44

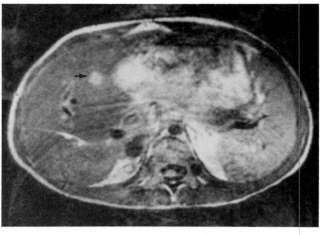

Fig. 4.3.5 Twelve-year-old girl with viral B hepatitis and hepatocarcinoma operated on 1 year before. Recent elevation of alpha-fetoprotein level has occurred. Negative US and CT examination. MRI (T_2-weighted image) demonstrates a small hyperintense nodule corresponsing to a small recurrence (arrow).

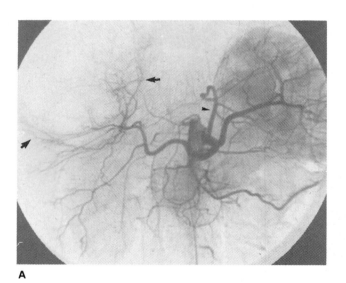

A

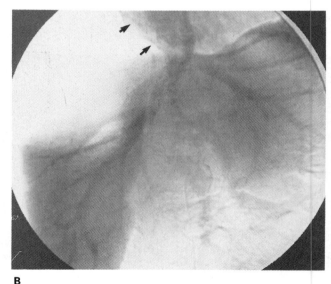

B

Fig. 4.3.4 Hepatoblastoma. Preoperative angiography. **A** Coeliac trunk injection shows multiple hepatic arteries with a left hepatic artery arising from the coronary artery (arrowhead). The tumour, located within the right lobe of the liver, presents with mild peripheral hypervascularity (arrows). **B** Late phase of superior mesenteric arteriogram: the defect seen on portography corresponds to the tumour. There is a filling defect in the inferior vena cava and inferior part of the right hepatic vein due to a thrombus confirmed at surgery (arrows).

Hepatocarcinoma

Hepatocellular carcinoma is rarer than hepatoblast-oma and usually arises in older children with chronic liver disease. The diseases include cirrhosis from any cause (biliary atresia, hepatitis, Byler's disease), adenomas particularly in glycogen storage disease, tyrosinaemia where there is a major risk after 3 years of age (Fig. 4.3.6) and the presence of hepatitis B surface antigen, even without cirrhosis; alpha-fetoprotein serum level is elevated in most patients.

Hepatocellular carcinoma is more often multicentric and invasive when compared with hepatoblastoma with evidence of tumoural thrombi in major portal or hepatic vein branches, so that prognosis is very poor (Fig. 4.3.7).

Preoperative investigation depends on the facilities available.

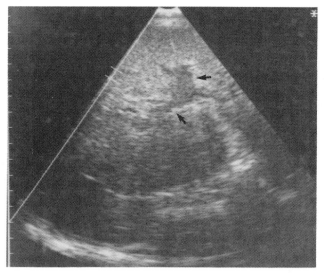

Fig. 4.3.7 Diffuse hepatocarcinoma with complete thrombosis of the portal vein (arrows). No signal is obtained on Doppler study.

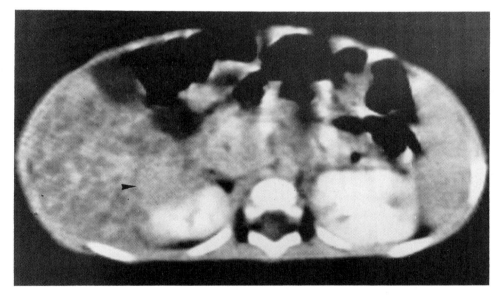

Fig. 4.3.6 One-year-old boy with tyrosinaemia. Contrast-enhanced CT shows heterogeneous density of the liver with a larger nodule in front of the right kidney (arrowhead), corresponding to a regenerating nodule. However there is a high risk of degeneration to hepatocarcinoma after 3 years of age.

The respective value of MRI, angiography and CT after intra-arterial lipiodol injection to define the extension and the resectability of this tumour (Fig. 4.3.8) is still a subject for debate.

A distinct variant of hepatocellular carcinoma with a more favourable outcome occurs in the non-cirrhotic liver of older children and young adults and has been called fibrolamellar carcinoma. There is no distinctive radiological finding to enable a conclusive preoperative diagnosis.

REFERENCES

Hayaski N, Yamamoto K, Tamaki N, Shibata T, Itoh K, Fujisawa I, Nakano Y, Yamaoka Y, Kobayashi N, Mori K, Titelbaum D S, Burke D R, Meranze S G, Saul S H 1988 Fibrolamellar hepatocellular carcinoma: pitfalls in non operative diagnosis. Radiology 167: 25–30
Ozawa K, Torizuka K 1987 Metastatic nodules of hepatocellular carcinoma: detection with angiography, CT and US. Radiology 165: 61–63

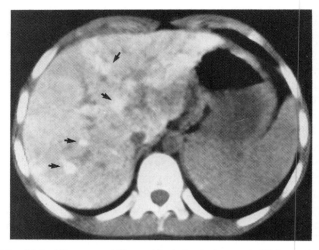

Fig. 4.3.8 Nine-year-old boy with cirrhosis due to viral B hepatitis. Alpha-fetoprotein levels are raised. US depicted one nodule, MRI two nodules and CT after intra-arterial lipiodol demonstrates multiple hyperdense nodules (arrows). Liver transplantation was performed and the child is doing well with a 2-year follow-up.

Sarcomas

Hepatic sarcomas are rare in children. Rhabdomyosarcoma may originate in the major bile ducts with a botryoid appearance with biliary tract dilatation and usually presents with jaundice (Fig. 4.3.9). When it arises from the distal intrahepatic duct, it is indistinguishable from other primary neoplasms of the liver.

Undifferentiated sarcoma may present with large cystic components suggestive of a benign lesion (Fig. 4.3.10). Percutaneous biopsy is indicated under US or CT guidance in the diagnosis of all the non-vascular non-secreting tumours for accurate histological diagnosis.

REFERENCE

Ros P R, Olmsted W W, Dachman A H, Goodman Z D, Ishak K G, Hartman D S 1986 Undifferentiated (embryonal) sarcoma of the liver: radiologic and pathologic correlations. Radiology 161: 141–145

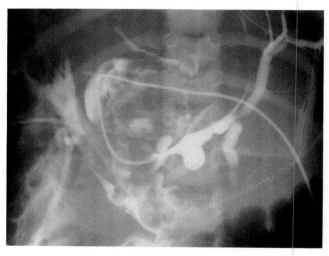

Fig. 4.3.9 Rhabdomyosarcoma of the biliary tree in a 6-year-old girl. There is a marked dilatation of the bile duct in the liver hilum with large filling defects, corresponding to the botryoid tumour. Percutaneous drainage was performed.

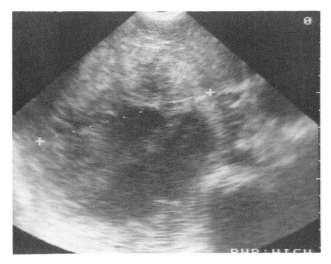

Fig. 4.3.10 Undifferentiated sarcoma of the right lobe of the liver in a 6-year-old boy. The lesion had large cystic components filled with gelatinous fluid at surgery.

Hepatic epithelioid haemangioendothelioma

This is a rare malignant type of vascular tumour mainly reported in adults with a female predilection. It can occur in older girls, and presents as a diffuse mass with invasion of hepatic veins and Budd–Chiari syndrome (Fig. 4.3.11).

REFERENCES

Furin S, Itai Y, Ohtomo K, Yamanchi T, Takenaka E, Lio M, Ibukuro K, Shichijo Y, Inone Y 1989 Hepatic epitheloïd hemangioendothelioma: report of 5 cases. Radiology 171: 63–68
Kirchner S G, Heller R M, Kasselberg A G, Greene H L 1981 Infantile hepatic hemangioendothelioma with subsequent malignant degeneration. Pediatric Radiology 11: 42–45

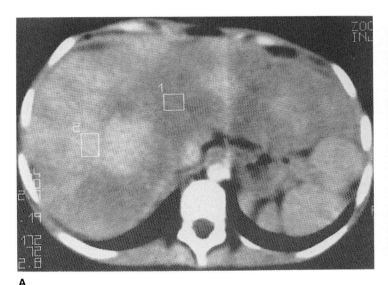

A

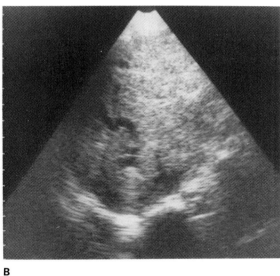

B

Fig. 4.3.11 Epithelioid haemangioendothelioma in a 12-year-old girl. **A** Contrast-enhanced CT shows diffuse multinodular involvement. **B** US demonstrates tortuous hepatic veins: Budd–Chiari syndrome secondary to tumoral involvement.

Metastases

Virtually any paediatric malignant neoplasm may produce them. Wilm's tumour, neuroblastoma and rhabdomyosarcoma are the most frequent sources of liver metastases. They usually present as hypoechoic nodules and the primary tumour is generally evident (Fig. 4.3.12) at presentation.

A special mention of *Pepper syndrome*, a form of liver metastases from neuroblastoma affecting small infants, must be made. Huge hepatomegaly is often the presenting sign. The primary tumour is seldom evident. It has a better prognosis than neuroblastoma presenting in older children and has a tendency to spontaneous regression. Liver involvement may present as diffuse homogeneous enlargement, or multiple solid nodules (Fig. 4.3.13) which in very rare instances may be cystic (Fig. 4.3.14). (See Neuroblastoma, Stage IV and IV S in Chapter 5.)

Leukaemia and lymphoma may also present as diffuse liver enlargement or as multiple hypoechoic nodules (Fig. 4.3.15).

REFERENCE

Yates C Y, Streight R A 1986 Focal fatty infiltration of the liver simulating metastatic disease. Radiology 159: 83–84

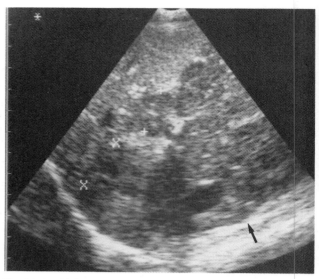

Fig. 4.3.12 Wilms' tumour of the right kidney with liver metastases in 4-year-old boy presenting with a right abdominal mass. US shows the right kidney tumour (arrow) and multiple hypoechoic nodules in the liver. Complete regression of the liver metastases occurred after chemotherapy.

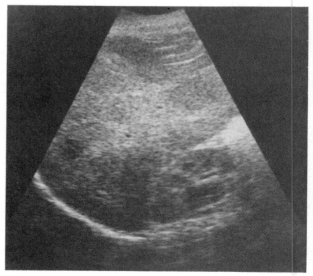

Fig. 4.3.13 Pepper syndrome. Four-month-old boy presenting with massive hepatomegaly. Multiple ill-defined hypoechoic nodules are visible. Increased catecholamine levels are present. The primary tumour was not found. The child recovered following treatment.

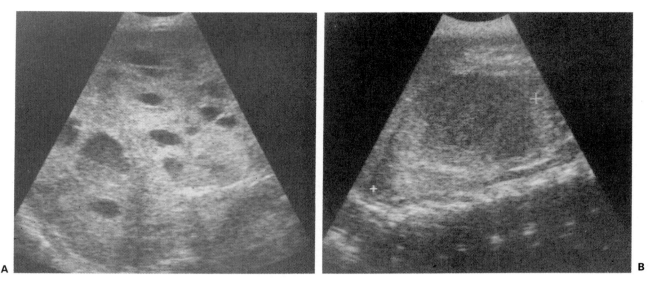

Fig. 4.3.14 Pepper syndrome. One-month-old baby girl with rapidly increasing hepatomegaly. **A** There are multiple cystic areas disseminated throughout the whole liver. **B** There is large left adrenal mass with a cystic component due to a primary neuroblastoma.

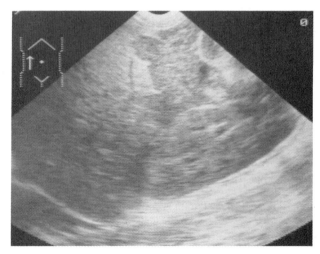

Fig. 4.3.15 Lymphoma with liver involvement in a 5-year-old boy with an abdominal mass. There is a large homogeneous and hypoechoic mass involving the liver. There is also nephromegaly with tumour in the upper pole of the right kidney.

BENIGN TUMOURS

Benign tumours comprise about a third of all primary liver tumours in childhood. They include haemangiomas, hamartomas, focal nodular hyperplasia and adenomas.

Haemangiomas

These mainly present in infancy, as a solitary form or as a diffuse one, also called haemangioendothelioma. Both types may be complicated by cardiac failure, hyperconsumptive coagulopathy (Kasabach–Merritt syndrome) and haemoperitoneum. The natural history is of spontaneous regression, provided the child can be kept alive while these complications occur.

In both types, hypervascularity with an enlarged hepatic artery and dilated hepatic veins (Fig. 4.3.16) are demonstrated by realtime and Doppler ultrasound.

A solitary haemangioma may be discovered antenatally or in the first days of life. It usually appears as a large heterogeneous mass and decreases in size spontaneously with the appearance of large areas of calcification (Fig. 4.3.17). A few years later, residual calcification may be found as a sequel.

The diffuse multinodular type of haemangioma is usually discovered later, in the first month of life. It is associated with cutaneous haemangiomas in 75% of cases. It may simulate a large liver tumour with multiple hypoechoic nodules on US (Fig. 4.3.18).

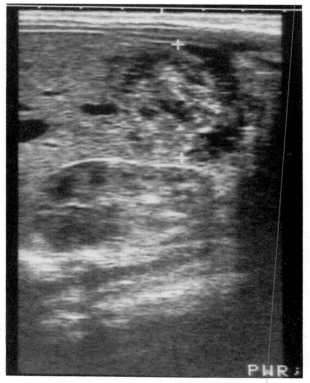

Fig. 4.3.17 Solitary haemangioma in a 1-month-old baby girl presenting with hepatomegaly. Alpha-fetoprotein level is normal. US shows a 3 cm heterogeneous mass with central calcifications, an enlarged hepatic artery and a dilated right hepatic vein. No treatment was required.

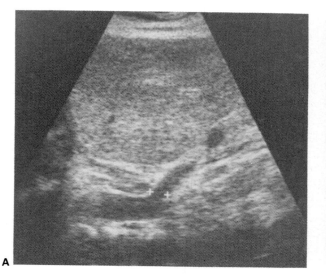
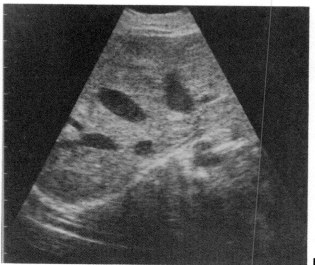

Fig. 4.3.16 Diffuse haemangioma in a 5-month-old girl presenting with cardiac failure. US shows diffuse involvement of the liver and findings of hypervascularity: **A** the hepatic artery is markedly enlarged (5 mm); **B** all the hepatic veins are strikingly dilated.

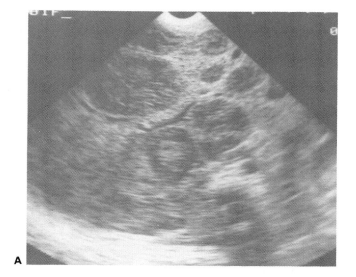

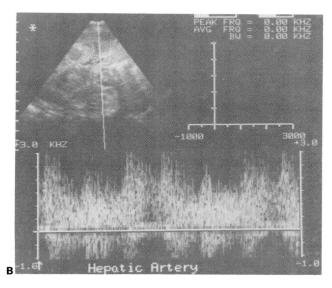

Fig. 4.3.18 Diffuse haemangioma in an 8-month-old girl with massive hepatomegaly. **A** Transverse scan through the portal bifurcation: multiple hypoechoic nodules simulating a tumour are present. **B** The hepatic artery is markedly enlarged with a turbulent signal indicative of high velocity flow.

Severe high output cardiac failure is frequent and may necessitate embolization. The natural history is for complete regression of the lesions, with calcification, but a few cases of late recurrence suggestive of malignant degeneration have been reported (Fig. 4.3.19). If the diagnosis remains uncertain with US, CT should be performed. Following bolus injection of contrast, typical marked peripheral enhancement of the lesions is found in both types (Figs. 4.3.20, 4.3.21).

Angiography is also performed as a prelude to therapeutic embolization when reduction of flow is required to control cardiac failure, thrombocytopenia or haemorrhage (Fig. 4.3.22). A very high intensity signal on the long T_2-weighted sequences is found on MRI but is not specific to haemangiomas (Fig. 4.3.19).

REFERENCE

Stanley P, Geer G D, Miller J H, Gilsanz V, Laning B H, Boechat I 1989 Infantile hepatic hemangiomas. Cancer 64: 936–949

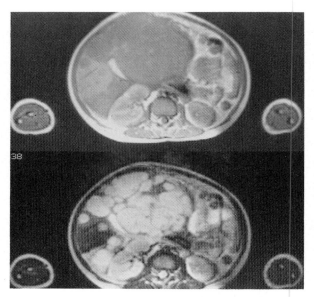

Fig. 4.3.19 Late recurrence of diffuse haemangioma in a 5-year-old girl with a history of diffuse liver haemangioma and multiple cutaneous haemangiomas in the neonatal period. There was regression of all lesions. This late recurrence presented with haemoperitoneum. Despite attempts at embolization and a left hepatectomy, the liver remained enormous with diffuse lesions, which were hyperintense on T_2-weighted MRI images. The child died soon after from massive bleeding.

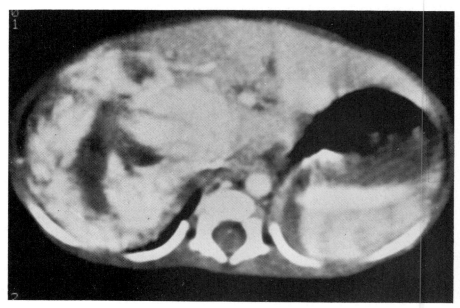

Fig. 4.3.20 Solitary haemangioma in a 2-week-old infant. This is the typical CT appearance of a solitary haemangioma with marked peripheral contrast enhancement.

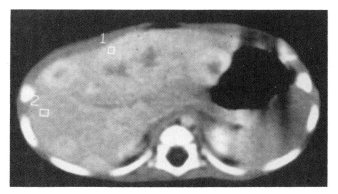

Fig. 4.3.21 Diffuse haemangioma. Six-month-old baby girl. The child has no clinical symptoms. Hepatomegaly was discovered on a routine developmental health check. CT confirms US findings: there is contrast enhancement of the multiple nodules. No treatment is indicated.

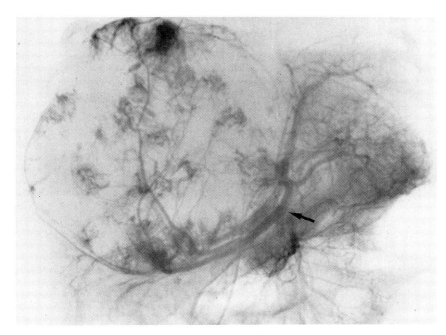

Fig. 4.3.22 Voluminous solitary haemangioma of the right lobe, in a child with cardiac failure. Angiography is performed as a prelude to embolization: the hepatic artery is markedly enlarged (arrow) and there is hypervascularity with typical puddling of contrast medium.

Mesenchymal hamartoma

This is a tumour composed of a mixture of hepatocytes, abnormal bile ducts and immature mesenchyme in variable portions.

It has been called a variety of names, including lymphangioma, cystic hamartoma and hepatic cyst, but the term of mesenchymal hamartoma is now generally accepted. It is thought to be a developmental anomaly rather than a true neoplasm.

It is usually discovered in the first 2 years of life and prenatal sonographic detection is possible. It may be very large. A uni- or multiloculated mass with cystic spaces and septa of variable size (Fig. 4.3.23) is seen on both US and CT.

This tumour has a good prognosis and is usually cured by excision.

REFERENCE

Ros P R, Goodman Z D, Ishak K G, Dachman A H, Olmsted W W, Hartman D S, Lichtenstein J E 1986 Mesenchymal hamartoma of the liver: radiologic–pathologic correlation. Radiology 158: 619–624

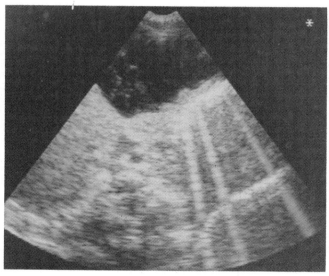

Fig. 4.3.23 Mesenchymal hamartoma in a 3-month-old baby girl with hepatomegaly. US shows a large cystic mass with multiple thin septations in the left hepatic lobe. Another smaller mass was also depicted in the right lobe. There are typical findings of mesenchymal hamartoma.

Focal nodular hyperplasia

It is characterized pathologically by a central dense fibrous scar from which radiate septa containing proliferating bile ducts and blood vessels. Between the septa there are normal hepatocytes.

It has been reported in all paediatric age groups with a female predominance.

It is usually asymptomatic and presents as a single large lobulated and well-defined mass. On ultrasound examination, it is homogeneous, generally isoechoic, and in some cases has a central fibrotic scar which is hyperechoic (Fig. 4.3.24). The mass is hypervascular with homogeneous enhancement on CT after bolus injection.

On angiography there is a fairly typical pattern with an enlarged hepatic artery and a peripheral network of hepatic veins. There is displacement but no amputation of portal branches. On MRI, the tumour appears isointense to the adjacent normal parenchyma with a central scar which is hyperintense on T_2-weighted sequences. This pattern is typical but not specific.

Percutaneous biopsy may be misleading if the sample only contains fibrotic septa or normal hepatocytes. However, the preoperative diagnosis is possible from the combination of all the clinical and radiological findings.

The pathogenesis is unknown. There may be a risk of increase in size at puberty or with contraceptive drugs.

Treatment of these benign but hypervascular masses is still debated.

REFERENCES

Stocker J T, Shak D G 1981 Focal nodular hyperplasia of the liver: a study of 21 pediatric cases. Cancer 48: 336–345
Toma P, Taccone A, Martinoli C 1990 MRI of hepatic focal nodular hyperplasia: a report of two new cases in the pediatric age group. Pediatric Radiology 20: 267–269

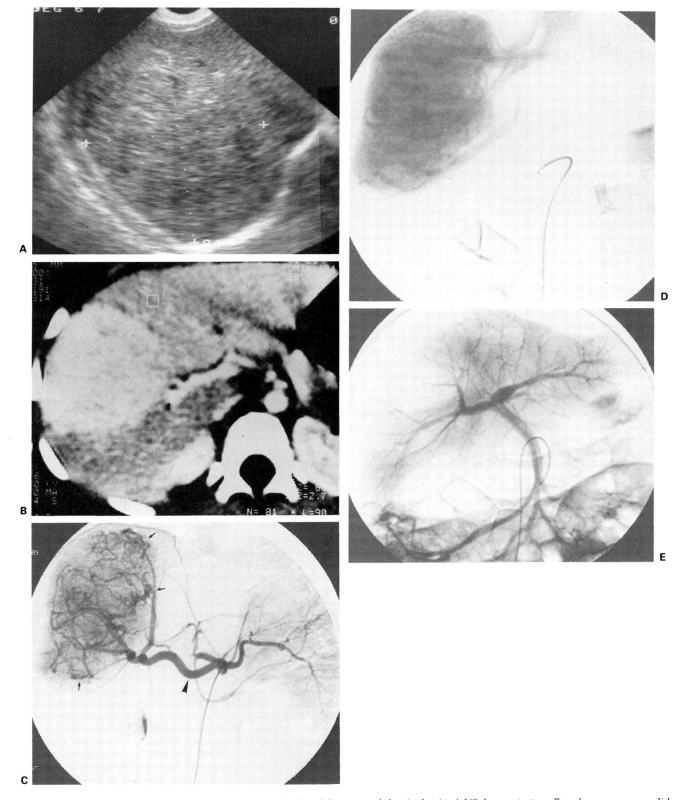

Fig. 4.3.24 Focal nodular hyperplasia. Two-year-old girl referred for vague abdominal pain. **A** US demonstrates a 7 cm homogeneous solid mass in the posterolateral segment of the right lobe. **B** CT with IV bolus injection shows marked homogeneous enhancement of the mass. **C** Preoperative arteriogram: the feeding artery is obviously enlarged (arrowhead). The mass is hypervascular with a fairly typical peripheral venous network (arrows). **D** Venous phase of selective injection shows rapid opacification of large hepatic veins (right and right inferior). **E** Venous phase of superior mesenteric arteriogram: segmental portal branches are displaced around the mass but are patent.

Adenomas

Histologically, adenomas consist of normal liver cells, but bile ducts and portal tracts within the tumour are absent. They usually present as hepatomegaly or mass, rarely with pain and haemorrage.

Adenomas are usually associated with glycogen storage disease (Fig. 4.3.25) or are secondary to anabolic steroids for treatment of Fanconi's anaemia. A few cases in otherwise healthy children have been reported. They may be multiple and degeneration into hepatocarcinoma is possible.

At ultrasound the echogenicity is variable, and areas of possible central haemorrage and calcifications may also be found.

CT shows most lesions as focal areas of decreased attenuation with heterogeneous contrast enhancement.

At angiography the vascularity of the lesion is highly variable.

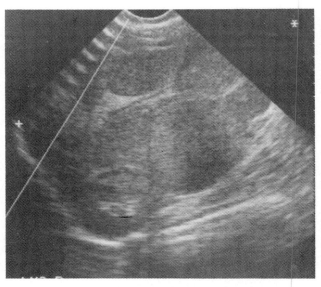

Fig. 4.3.25 Adenomas. Fifteen-year-old girl with type I glycogen storage disease. Multiple large adenomas involve the whole liver. On ultrasound examination they have a homogeneous isoechoic appearance compared with normal liver. These are indications for liver transplantation because of risk of malignant degeneration.

REFERENCES

Bourliere-Najean B, Panuel M, Guy S J M, Scheiner C, Devred M, Faure F, Padovani J 1989 Spontaneous liver adenoma in a child. Pediatric Radiology 20: 95

Brunelle F, Tammam S, Odievre M, Chaumont P 1984 Liver adenomas in glycogen storage disease in children. Pediatric Radiology 14: 94–101

Garel L, Kalifa G, Buriot D, Sauvegrain J 1981 Multiple adenomas of the liver and Fanconi's anaemia. Annales de Radiologie 24: 53–54

4.4   LIVER TRAUMA

Liver injury is a frequent event in blunt abdominal trauma in children, and represents 25–30% of visceral injuries. Hepatic injuries predominate in the right lobe (4/5) and in the posterior segments of the right lobe (2/3), probably because of compression against the surrounding ribs and spine.

Hepatic lesions include subcapsular haematoma, intrahepatic haematoma, laceration and contusion.

Recently non-operative management of hepatic as well as splenic injuries has become more commonplace. This is due to the accurracy of imaging modalities in evaluation of the lesions, coupled with careful serial clinical evaluation. Emergency exploratory laparotomy remains mandatory in a child with haemodynamic instability unresponsive to aggressive fluid replacement (Fig. 4.4.1). In this situation, the only investigation possible may be portable US in the intensive care unit (ICU) or operating room.

In haemodynamically stable children, US is still very useful to screen for haemoperitoneum and parenchymal lesions (Fig. 4.4.2). The sonographic appearance of liver contusions is variable and may be hypo- or hyperechoic. Ultrasound occasionally shows localized intrahepatic collections of fluid representing bile or blood, hypoechoic subcapsular lesions and blood in the gallbladder.

Constrast-enhancement CT represents the most accurate examination to precisely identify simultaneous liver, splenic and renal lesions (Fig. 4.4.3) and is strongly recommended when facilities are available.

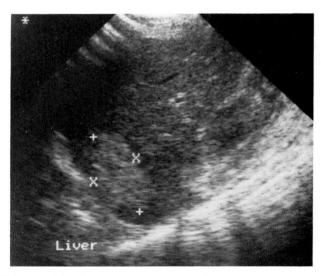

Fig. 4.4.2   Liver haematoma in an 8-year-old boy with mild abdominal trauma. US examination: a small echogenic haematoma is present in the periphery of the right lobe.

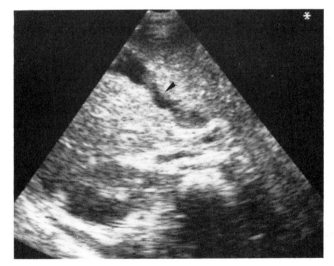

Fig. 4.4.1   Fracture of the liver in a 4-year-old boy with severe abdominal trauma. Surgery was undertaken as an emergency because of unstable haemodynamic status: a large fracture of the liver separating both lobes was found at surgery. The fracture was sutured. The child recovered completely. Postoperative US shows the lesion (arrowhead).

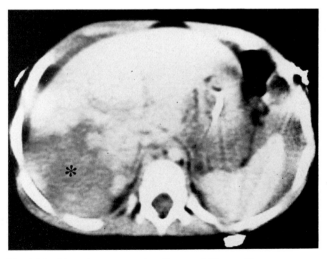

Fig. 4.4.3   Liver haematoma in a 2-year-old boy with severe abdominal trauma: contrast-enhanced CT shows a large hypodense haematoma extending to the hilum (*) and a haemoperitoneum. Conservative treatment.

On CT hepatic laceration and contusion appear as areas of decreased attenuation of variable shape. Subcapsular haematomas are low density fluid collections which are lenticular and may cause hepatic parenchymal compression (Fig. 4.4.4).

Infection is a complication of liver haematoma and may require percutaneous drainage of subsequent abscess formation. Biliary tract lesions are usually associated with deep complex lesions involving the hilum. However they may be isolated and are often of delayed identification. They include traumatic rupture of the gallbladder, rupture of the common bile duct at the pancreaticoduodenal junction or at the bifurcation of the hepatic duct. They may present with bile peritonitis or long-delayed biliary obstruction and jaundice.

Nowadays there is little indication for angiography in liver trauma. Its role is confined to the postoperative patient with continued bleeding directly into the peritoneal space or into the biliary system (haemobilia). Haemobilia should be clinically suspected when there is the association of abdominal pain, cholestasis and gastrointestinal haemorrhage. The vascular lesion may be demonstrated on Doppler ultrasound. Selective embolization in the case of a bleeding hepatic artery aneurysm or fistula formation with the portal system (Fig. 4.4.5) is often the treatment of choice.

Special mention has to be made of neonatal liver injury. Subcapsular haematoma is the most frequent injury, and it is usually secondary to obstetrical trauma. It is often associated with trauma to other organs (Fig. 4.4.6). It may be complicated by hypovolemic shock due to intraperitoneal rupture. It may reveal clotting disorders (Fig. 4.4.7). In most cases, treatment is conservative and consists of supportive measures.

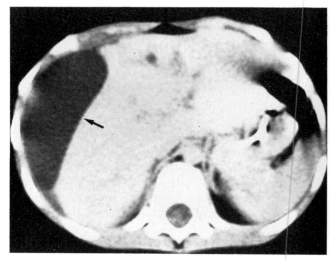

Fig. 4.4.4 Subcapsular haematoma in an 8-year-old girl with severe abdominal trauma. A large subcapsular haematoma is demonstrated on CT (arrow). Because of increasing size, it was drained percutaneously under US guidance without recurrence.

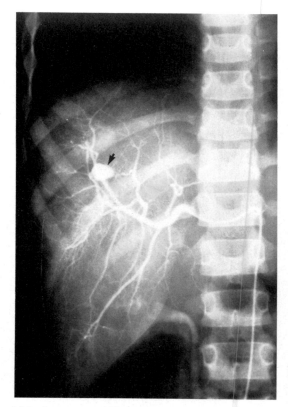

Fig. 4.4.5 Seven-year-old boy who presented with delayed haemobilia after abdominal trauma. Angiography shows an arterial aneurysm (arrow) which was successfully embolized (Dr Brunelle).

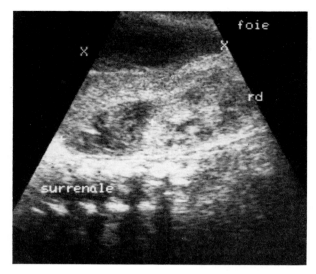

Fig. 4.4.6 Neonate who presented with severe anaemia at birth, following a traumatic delivery. Longitudinal scan through the right kidney shows a large subcapsular hepatic haematoma and right adrenal haemorrhage (crosses). (foie — liver, surrenale — above the kidney.)

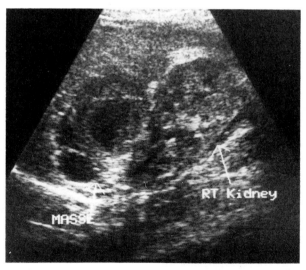

Fig. 4.4.7 Newborn baby boy presenting on day 1 with severe collapse, haemoperitoneum and anaemia. He was referred at day 8 with a diagnosis of liver tumour. Compared to the first CT scan, there was evident decrease in size of the mass. Diagnosis: liver haematoma in a haemophiliac newborn (probable obstetrical trauma).

REFERENCES

Brick S H, Taylor G A, Potter B M, Eichelberger M R 1987 Hepatic and splenic injury in children: role of CT in the decision for laparotomy. Radiology 165: 643–646

Brunelle F, Maurage C, Lacombe A, Chaumont P 1985 Emergency embolization in post traumatic hemobilia in a child. Journal of Pediatric Surgery 20: 172–174

Cohen J Y, Garel L, Sorin B, Roze J C, Mouzard A 1982 Subcapsular hematomas of the liver in the newborn. Annales de Radiologie 25: 34–40

Evans J P 1976 Traumatic rupture of the gallbladder in a 3-year-old boy. Journal of Pediatric Surgery 11: 1033–1034

Kaufman R A, Babcock D S 1984 An approach to imaging the upper abdomen in the injured child. Seminars in Roentgenology 19: 308–320

Kendall R S, Chapoy P R, Busutil R W, Koladny M, Ament M E 1980 Acquired bile duct stricture in childhood related to blunt trauma. American Journal of Diseases of Children 134: 851–854

Stalker H P, Kaufman R A, Towbin R 1986 Patterns of liver injury in childhood: CT analysis. American Journal of Roentgenology 147: 1199–1205

Veyrac C, Couture A, Baud C 1987 Less traumatismes des organes intraperitonéaux. In: Le traumatisme chez l'enfant. Cliniques de pédiatrie. Vigot, Paris, p 150–163

4.5 LIVER INFECTIONS

LIVER ABSCESS: PYOGENIC AND AMOEBIC

Liver abscess is an uncommon condition in childhood. Early diagnosis with US and aspiration, and treatment with appropriate antibiotic therapy and drainage in some cases have dramatically improved the prognosis.

Although mainly reported in immunocompromised children with chronic granulomatous disease, underlying malignancy and immunosuppression, pyogenic liver abscess can occur without any identifiable predisposing disease.

Liver abscess has been encountered in all age groups. In the neonatal period, it may be secondary to omphalitis, umbilical vein catheterization or abdominal surgery (Fig. 4.5.1). In older children, it may be secondary to other intra-abdominal sites of infection or to a systemic bacteraemia.

The clinical presentation is non-specific but hepatomegaly with tenderness, fever, leucocytosis, anaemia and a high sedimentation rate are present in most children. A raised hemidiaphragm with basal pneumonia, atelectasis or pleural effusion are frequently seen on chest films. US is the screening modality of choice, but it shows a broad spectrum of patterns ranging from a purely anechoic to a highly echogenic mass. The lesion may contain gas, have a thick wall or ill-defined borders. It may be isolated to one lobe or be multiple and involve both lobes (Fig. 4.5.2).

Scintigraphy has also been reported as a sensitive technique for abscess demonstration. Cold defects are seen with sulphur colloid scans. Scanning with white blood cells labelled with gallium-64 or indium-111 will show the area of increased uptake in the abscess. It is more time consuming than US, involves irradiation, and therefore should be reserved for difficult cases. The ultrasonic appearance is similar irrespective of the infecting organism which may be very variable and include staphylococcus, streptococcus, E. coli, klebsiella, pseudomonas, proteus, candida and amoebiasis. Amoebic abscess of the liver may occur in the absence of amoebic colitis. About half of the cases have a history of diarrhoea. It is most prevalent in children younger than 3 years with a peak incidence in the first year of life (Fig. 4.5.3). Delayed or absent seropositivity which are frequent in children may delay the diagnosis and increase the risk of extension or rupture to adjacent organs or spaces, pleura, lungs, pericardial sac, intra-abdominal, or abdominal wall. Hepatic candidiasis is a rare though serious complication seen in immunocompromised children. An unusual pattern of 'wheels within wheels' with diffuse microabscesses, involving the liver and also the spleen, may be seen on US.

The early identification of the infecting organism and prompt institution of treatment with appropriate antibiotics are mandatory. If blood cultures are negative, needle aspiration of the abscess under US guidance has to be performed as soon as possible.

Percutaneous drainage is recommended if there is failure to respond to antibiotic or metronidazole therapy and there are signs of impending rupture into adjacent structures, such as the pleural space and pericardium, with large abscesses. Failure to respond to percutaneous drainage is a clear indication for surgery but such cases should be very uncommon.

Resolution of the abscess cavity can be monitored by US and careful follow-up is especially recommended in neonates who are at risk of developing portal vein thrombosis and cavernoma (Fig. 4.5.1).

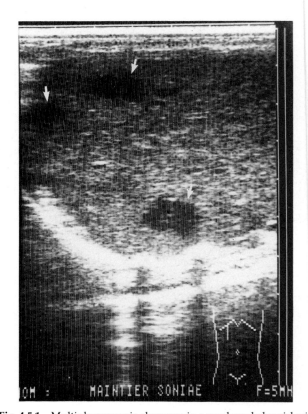

Fig. 4.5.1 Multiple pyogenic abscesses in a newborn baby girl with staphylococcus sepsis secondary to umbilical venous catheterization. There are multiple hypoechoic nodules consistent with abscesses (arrows). With antibiotic treatment, the abscesses resolved but portal cavernoma developed following portal vein thrombosis.

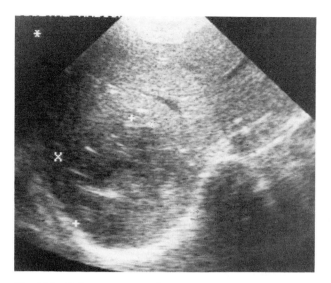

Fig. 4.5.2 Solitary pyogenic abscess in a 14-year-old girl presenting with painful hepatomegaly, fever and leucocytosis. US shows a large heterogeneous hypoechoic area which was aspirated and subsequently drained percutaneously (*Staphylococcus aureus*). No immune disorder was found.

REFERENCES

Bilfinger T V, Hayden K, Oldham K T, Lobe T E 1986 Pyogenic liver abscesses in non immunocompromised children. Southern Medical Journal 79: 37–40

Chusid M J 1978 Pyogenic hepatic abscess in infancy and childhood. Pediatrics 62: 554–559

Garel L A, Pariente D M, Nezelof C, Barral V J, Aboulker C, Sauvegrain J H 1984 Liver involvement in chronic granulomatous disease: the role of US in diagnosis and treatment. Radiology 153: 117–121

Merten D F, Kirks D R 1984 Amebic liver abscess in children: the role of diagnostic imaging. American Journal of Roentgenology 143: 1325–1329

Moore S, Millar A J W, Cywes S 1988 Liver abscess in childhood: a 13-year review. Pediatric Surgery International 3: 27–32

Moss T J, Pysher T J 1981 Hepatic abscess in neonates. American Journal of Diseases of Children 135: 726–728

Pastakia B, Shawker T H, Thaler M, O'Leary T, Pizzo P A 1988 Hepatosplenic candidiasis: wheels within wheels. Radiology 166: 417–421

Vachon L, Diament M J, Stanley P 1986 Percutaneous drainage of hepatic abscesses in children. Journal of Pediatric Surgery 21: 366–368

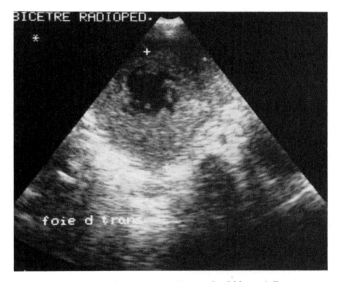

Fig. 4.5.3 Amoebic abscess in an 18-month-old boy. A 7 cm mass with central liquefaction. Percutaneous drainage was performed (foie d trans = right transverse liver).

HEPATIC TUBERCULOSIS

It is usually miliary, and is present in up to 80% of cases of pulmonary miliary disease. Macronodular tuberculous liver abscesses are extremely rare in children and are usually seen in debilitated patients.

The liver abscesses are generally found in association with caseating lymphadenopathy elsewhere in the abdomen, with splenic abscesses and ascites.

The CT findings in the active phase of the disease include high density ascites, low density nodal and hepatic masses with peripheral enhancement.

On healing the hepatic, nodal and splenic lesions show calcifications which may be seen on plain films.

REFERENCE

Moskovic E 1990 Macronodular hepatic tuberculosis in a child: computed tomographic appearances. British Journal of Radiology 63: 656–658

HYDATID DISEASE

The disease is common in sheep-grazing countries, such as Southern Europe and particularly the Mediterranean Basin. Man is infected by contact with the excreta of dogs. The ova are ingested, burrow through the intestinal mucosa and are carried in the portal vein to the liver where they develop into adult cysts. Cysts may also occur in the lungs, peritoneum, bones and brain.

Most cysts are clinically silent, but pain, abdominal distension and a palpable mass may be present.

The hydatid cysts are easily seen with US which is the method of choice in the diagnosis of the disease in the liver. There is a spectrum of findings depending on the stage of the lesion, which range from a simple anechoic cyst (Fig. 4.5.4) to a double-walled cyst with visibility of germinative membrane, cyst with septations and internal heterogeneous echoes (Fig. 4.5.5).

The diagnosis may be confirmed by serological tests such as the Casoni test in up to 80% of cases.

CT is useful to define the precise extension of the disease before surgery (Fig. 4.5.4), especially when there are multiple lesions.

Complications include intraperitoneal rupture of an intrahepatic cyst (Fig. 4.5.6), rupture into the biliary tract with, in a few cases, biliary obstruction and dissemination to other abdominal organs.

REFERENCES

Lewall D B, McCorkell S J 1985 Hepatic echinococcal cysts: sonographic appearance and classification. Radiology 155: 773–775

Lewall D B, McCorkell S J 1986 Rupture of echinococcal cysts: diagnosis, classification and clinical implications. American Journal of Roentgenology 146: 391–394

Marti-Bonmati L, Menor F, Ballesta A 1988 Hydatid cyst of the liver: rupture into the biliary tree. American Journal of Roentgenology 150: 1051–1053

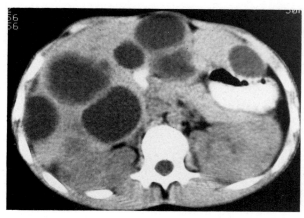

Fig. 4.5.4 Hydatid disease. Multiple hypodense hydatid cysts involve the whole liver: 16 cysts could be identified on CT.

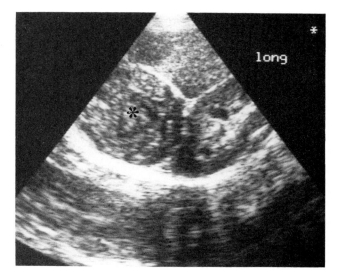

Fig. 4.5.5 Heterogeneous hydatid cyst presenting as a solid mass in a 4-year-old Algerian boy (*). Diagnosis was made at surgery.

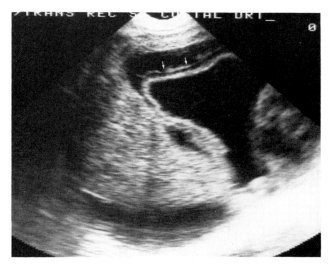

Fig. 4.5.6 Traumatic rupture of an unsuspected hydatid cyst. US shows fluid in the pouch of Douglas and a large cystic intrahepatic mass with a double wall corresponding to the germinative membrane (arrows).

ASCARIASIS

The normal habitat of the adult parasite *Ascaris lumbricoides* is the small intestine. The worms may migrate into the biliary system and cause one of the most severe complications of ascariasis which is much greater in children than in adults.

The clinical manifestations vary in severity depending upon the number of parasites in the biliary system: these include jaundice, fever, rupture of the hepatic or common bile duct with biliary peritonitis and abscess.

Two severe complications are infective phlebitis and embolization from IVC to the pulmonary artery.

Diagnosis is made by finding ova in the faeces, or the adult worm in the digestive tract. The worm may be seen in the gallbladder or dilated bile duct on US examination. The worm may also be seen on barium studies in the intestine, on endoscopy or on cholangiography in the biliary tree.

REFERENCE

Schulman A, Loxton A J, Heydenrych J T, Abdurahman K 1982 Sonographic diagnosis of biliary ascariasis. American Journal of Roentgenology 139: 435–489

FASCIOLIASIS

This is due to infection by a large leaf-shaped trematode common in Europe: *Fasciola hepatica*. Man acquires the infection by ingestion of aquatic plants, particularly watercress, or by drinking water containing the metacercariae (cystic form of the parasite). It migrates through the duodenum, enters the peritoneal cavity and reaches the capsule of the liver. The acute phase of the disease corresponds to migration through the liver: there is hepatomegaly, abdominal pain, fever and leucocytosis with marked eosinophilia.

US or CT may show superficial granulomas previously seen only on laparoscopy, or at surgery.

During the chronic phase, the parasite resides in the biliary tract. Patients may be asymptomatic or present with biliary obstruction or cholangitis. US may display the parasite in the gallbladder or in the common bile duct as an echogenic lesion without an acoustic shadow. It is sometimes mobile.

REFERENCE

Cauquil P, Pariente D, Loyer E, Lallemand D 1986 Unusual sonographic appearance of a case of hepatic fascioliasis. Journal of Radiology 67: 715–717

4.6 MISCELLANEOUS

PELIOSIS HEPATIS

This is a rare condition characterized by multiple cystic blood-filled spaces of varying size in the liver. It has been mainly reported in adults in association with various wasting diseases and after the administration of anabolic and corticosteroid therapy, azathioprine and contraceptives. Only a few cases have been described in children.

Depending on the size and the extent of the lesions, the clinical spectrum of peliosis hepatis ranges from subclinical disease incidentally diagnosed on liver biopsy to an acute diffuse form with hepatic failure and haemoperitoneum. The pathogenesis remains unclear and treatment is still debatable.

Angiography was the first reported imaging modality. It may demonstrate multiple collections of contrast material during the parenchymal and venous phases of hepatic arteriography or on wedge-hepatic venography.

The US appearances are rarely mentioned in the literature. Hypo- or hyperechoic areas are found, depending on the size and the age of the cavities (Fig. 4.6.1). The appearance is non-specific, but together with the clinical presentation it is suggestive of the diagnosis.

CT shows multiple low-attenuation areas without contrast enhancement.

REFERENCE

Cragg A, Castaneda-Zuniga W, Lund G, Salomonowitz E, Amplatz K 1984 Infantile peliosis hepatis. Pediatric Radiology 14: 340–342

CONGENITAL HEPATIC FISTULAS

These are rare disorders with variable severity and clinical presentation depending on the type of abnormal vascular communication.

US and Doppler studies can demonstrate these vascular malformations with accuracy.

Spontaneous portocaval fistula

This may be isolated and asymptomatic but is more often part of a malformation complex with facial dysmorphism and costal and spinal anomalies. This complex is close to Goldenhar's syndrome which has been reported associated with congenital absence of the portal vein.

In portocaval fistula, there is a large communication between the portal vein and the inferior vena cava (Fig. 4.6.2) and the intrahepatic portal branches are hypoplastic. Doppler studies document hepatofugal flow in the portal vein. No treatment is required.

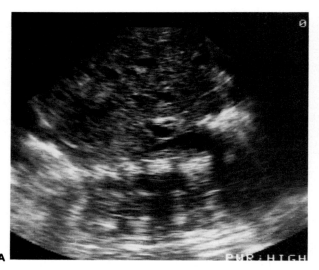 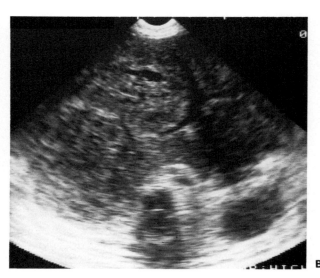

Fig. 4.6.1 Peliosis hepatis. Two-year-old girl referred for sudden onset of fever, hepatomegaly, anaemia, thombocytopenia, increased serum transaminase values and liver failure. US demonstrates multiple hypoechoic lesions in the whole liver with fluid in the pouch of Douglas. **A** Longitudinal scan. **B** Transverse scan. Surgical liver biopsy: peliosis hepatis. Slow recovery with supportive and antibiotic treatment. An associated *E. coli* urinary tract infection was found.

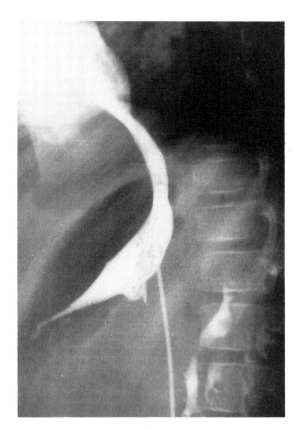

Fig. 4.6.2 Congenital portocaval fistula. Lateral view of cavogram. The catheter has been introduced into the communication between portal vein and IVC. In this 5-year-old girl this was associated with Budd–Chiari syndrome and gallstones.

Arterioportal fistula

This vascular malformation presents with portal hypertension, anaemia and gastrointestinal haemorrhage. There is intrahepatic communication between an enlarged hepatic artery and a dilated portal vein. Reversed flow in the portal vein is constant and may be seen with Doppler US. Treatment may be achieved with embolization but prognosis is poor.

Portal hepatic venous malformation

This has been previously reported in adult patients who mainly present with encephalopathy and hypoglycaemia. A few cases have been fortuitously discovered in children on US without any clinical finding.

US complemented by pulsed or colour Doppler demonstrates the abnormal communication between a portal vein branch and a hepatic vein usually located in the right lobe of the liver (Fig. 4.6.3).

REFERENCES

Charnsangavej C, Chin-Shiung Soo, Bernardino M E, Chuang V P, Wallace S 1983 Portal hepatic venous malformation: ultrasound, computed tomographic and angiographic findings. Cardiovascular and Interventional Radiology 6: 109–111

Helikson M A, Shapiro D L, Seashore J H 1977 Hepatoportal arteriovenous fistula and portal hypertension in an infant. Pediatrics 60: 921–924

Morse S S, Taylor K J W, Strauss E B et al 1986 Congenital absence of the portal vein in oculo auriculovertebral dysplasia (Goldenhar syndrome). Pediatric Radiology 16: 437–439

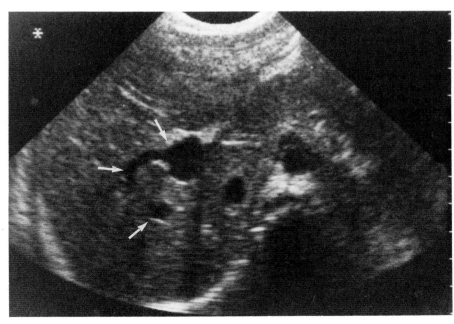

Fig. 4.6.3 Five-year-old boy with vague abdominal pain: fortuitous discovery on US of a fistula between an enlarged right portal vein (arrow) and the right hepatic vein, also arrowed.

LIVER CALCIFICATIONS

The cause of the calcification may be obvious (tumour, infection) but the calcifications are often discovered fortuitously on plain films or by US examination. The main causes of liver calcifications include:

Infections:
— tuberculosis
— brucellosis
— cytomegalovirus
— toxoplasmosis
— chronic granulomatous disease
— hydatid disease
Tumours:
— malignant: all tumour types,
— benign: haemangioma, adenoma, hamartoma
Trauma — haematoma

Vascular calcification:
— umbilical vein catheterization
— arterial or venous thromboembolism
— calculus in intrahepatic bile duct
— meconium peritonitis
— haemochromatosis.

REFERENCES

Felson B, Reeder M V 1987 Gamuts in radiology, 2nd edn, Audiovisual Radiology of Cincinnati Inc Ed., Cincinnati, Ohio
Mowat A P (ed) 1987 Liver disorders in childhood, 2nd edn. Butterworth-Heinemann, Oxford
Stringer D A 1989 Pediatric gastrointestinal imaging. B C Decker, Toronto, Philadelphia

FATTY INFILTRATION OF THE LIVER

Fatty infiltration of the liver has a variety of causes. These include metabolic disorders such as glycogen storage diseases, Reye's syndrome, diabetes, fructose intolerance and tyrosinaemia, acute starvation, severe malnutrition states, obesity, parenteral hyperalimentation, malabsorption syndrome, and steroid therapy.

This leads to increased liver radiolucency on plain abdominal radiographs.

At US the liver may be unusually bright, compared to the right kidney.

On unenhanced CT scan there is diffuse decrease in attenuation of the liver parenchyma and the intrahepatic vessels appear spontaneously hyperdense. Less commonly the fatty infiltration may be uneven, focal and mimic tumour. But there is no mass effect and no displacement of vessels (Fig. 4.6.1).

WILSON'S DISEASE

Wilson's disease or hepatolenticular degeneration is an inborn error of copper metabolism, characterized by defective biliary copper excretion and the accumulation of toxic amounts of copper in liver, brain, kidney and cornea. It is inherited as an autosomal recessive trait. Clinical features include cirrhosis of the liver, renal tubular injury, episodes of haemolytic anaemia and degeneration in the central nervous system.

The diagnosis is made on the presence of Kayser–Fleischer rings at the corneal limbus, or on serum caeruloplasmin, urinary copper and determination of the copper content of liver biopsy.

Cerebral CT findings consist of low density in the basal ganglia and variable cerebral white matter atrophy. MR findings consist of prolongation of T_1 and T_2 relaxation times in the basal ganglia and in the white matter. Bony manifestations of rickets have been reported.

HAEMOCHROMATOSIS

Haemochromatosis is characterized by cirrhosis or fibrosis of the liver with markedly increased iron stores, particularly in liver cells. Excessive iron storage occurs also in the heart, pancreas and endocrine organs. The congenital forms present in early infancy, those associated with chronic anaemia in late childhood.

On CT scans there is increased liver attenuation which correlates with liver iron concentrations.

On MRI the tissue iron greatly influences proton imaging because of its paramagnetic effect which results in decreased relaxation times of nearby hydrogen nuclei. There is decreased signal intensity of the liver compared to the intensity of the paraspinal muscles.

Following radiotherapy, an increase in the attenuation of the liver may be noted, although this may be preceded by a transitory decrease from fatty change. A similar increase in liver attenuation can result from chemotherapy, particularly that employing agents containing platinum. Uptake of radioisotopic colloid may be transiently decreased following radiotherapy and chemotherapy (Fig. 4.6.4).

REFERENCE

Hernandez R J, Sarnaik S A, Lande I, Aisen A M, Glaser G M, Chenevert T, Martel W 1988 MR evaluation of liver iron overload. Journal of Computer Assisted Tomography 12: 91–94

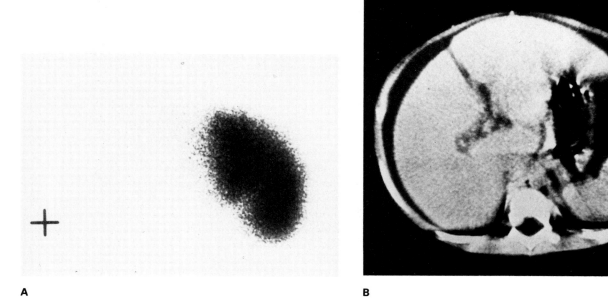

A
B

Fig. 4.6.4 **A** Sulphur colloid scan after radiotherapy to right renal bed and liver following Wilm's tumour. **B** Normal CT appearances of liver and spleen.

4.7   BILIARY TRACT

NEONATAL CHOLESTASIS

Neonatal cholestasis is a common clinical problem characterized by dark urine and discoloured stools and therefore it is easily distinguished from unconjugated hyperbilirubinaemia which may be physiological or due to haematological causes.

The main problem is to establish the cause of the cholestasis which includes lesions of the extrahepatic bile ducts (EHBD), the intrahepatic bile ducts (IHBD) or both. These are listed in the gamut.

EHBD =5%	Choledocholithiasis Choledochal cyst Perforation	'Surgical' causes
EHBD + IHBD = 40%	*Biliary atresia = 40%* Sclerosing cholangitis	
IHBD = 55%	Benign neonatal cholestasis Paucity of interlobular bile duct (hypoplasia) Byler's disease Alpha 1 antitrypsin deficiency Infections Cystic fibrosis Parenteral nutrition Niemann–Pick disease	'Medical' causes

Imaging has a major role to play in helping to distinguish the conditions.

The term 'neonatal hepatitis' has been replaced in the list by all the medical causes which may be nowadays identified.

Biliary atresia

This is the single most common cause of neonatal cholestasis, accounting for approximately half of the cases. The diagnosis should be established as soon as possible, as it has been proved that early treatment improves the prognosis.

Biliary atresia is a congenital anomaly, consisting of the interruption of the extrahepatic bile duct. The atresia may be complete or partial and it is currently thought to be an acquired progressive inflammatory disease of the biliary tract. Moreover the intrahepatic bile ducts have been shown to be always abnormal with a plexiform and moniliform appearance on preoperative or postoperative cholangiography (Fig. 4.7.1).

Multiple anatomical types of biliary atresia are described depending on the extent of the sclerotic process. The whole extrahepatic bile duct may be atretic (60%). This is the most frequent pattern. Other variations are shown in the line drawing. The gallbladder may be preserved, isolated or associated with a patent choledochus or a patent common bile duct (Fig. 4.7.1). A cyst may be found (= 10% of cases) on the remnant of the extrahepatic bile duct, composed almost exclusively of scar tissue, usually without an epithelial lining. Its size and location on the course of the extrahepatic bile duct is variable. It may or may not communicate with a patent gallbladder. These cystic forms have have been termed a 'correctable' form of biliary atresia and have a better prognosis.

Clinical presentation

In up to 80% of patients with biliary atresia the clinical presentation of persistent cholestatic jaundice with pale acholuric stools, and an enlarged and firm liver, strongly suggests the diagnosis.

In the other cases, these clinical findings are not as evident and further investigation is indicated to establish the diagnosis. These include ultrasonography, radionuclide studies, percutaneous cholangiography, percutaneous liver biopsy, PTC, and even exploratory laparatomy.

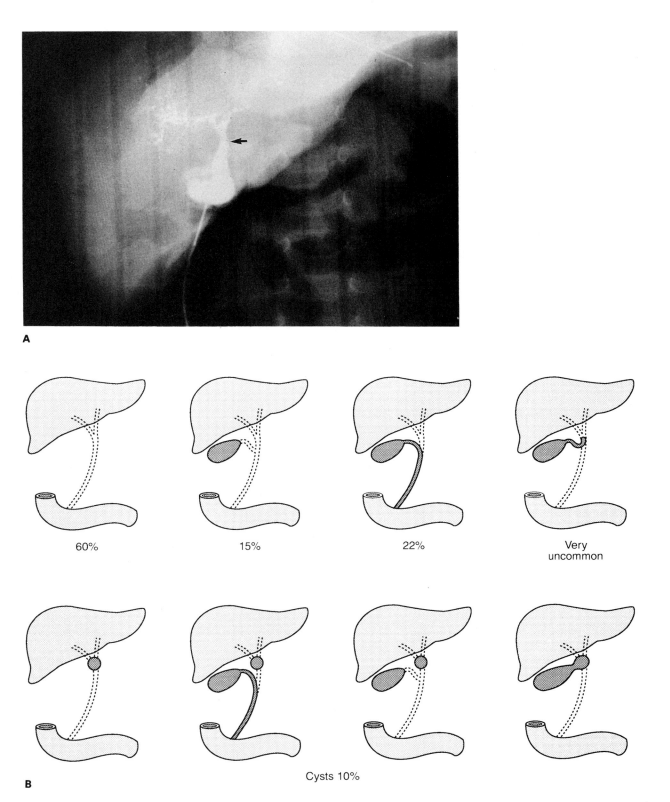

A

60%   15%   22%   Very
                                       uncommon

B   Cysts 10%

Fig. 4.7.1 **A** Biliary atresia. Peroperative cholangiography through the gallbladder. There is communication with a patent common hepatic duct (arrow) = uncommon form. **B** Typical appearance of extrahepatic bile ducts.

US findings

US in these infants must be done with high-resolution transducers. The normal common bile duct in newborns is rarely visible, unless it is dilated. It must not be confused with the hepatic artery of the newborn which is often prominent, measuring 2–3 mm. The hepatic artery is well identified by its horizontal course from the aorta (Fig. 4.7.2), by its indentation on the portal vein or with colour Doppler examination.

The presence or absence of the gallbladder is not a completely reliable diagnostic finding. A large gallbladder may be found in biliary atresia and emptying after a meal may even be demonstrated (Fig. 4.7.3). Failure to demonstrate the gallbladder is not specific to biliary atresia and may be found in other types of intrahepatic cholestasis, such as paucity of the intrahepatic bile ducts and benign neonatal cholestasis, but following a 4 hour fast, together with a clinical presentation, it is suggestive of biliary atresia. The findings of an anatomical anomaly as part of the non-cardiac polysplenia syndrome are diagnostic of biliary atresia. One or several anomalies of this malformation complex are present in 10–20% of cases. These include: polysplenia (Fig. 4.7.4), abdominal or thoracic situs inversus, preduodenal portal vein (Fig. 4.7.5), and azygous continuation of the inferior vena cava (Fig. 4.7.6).

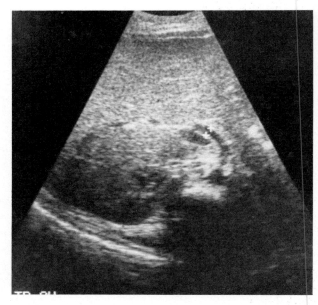

Fig. 4.7.2 Normal hepatic artery in a newborn: 2–3 mm in diameter; note the horizontal course and the origin from the aorta. The normal bile duct of a newborn with cholestatic jaundice is usually not seen unless it is dilated.

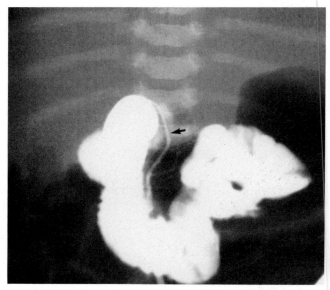

Fig. 4.7.3 Biliary atresia. A large gallbladder (3 cm in length) punctured under US guidance: there is a patent choledochus (arrow), but an atretic common hepatic duct.

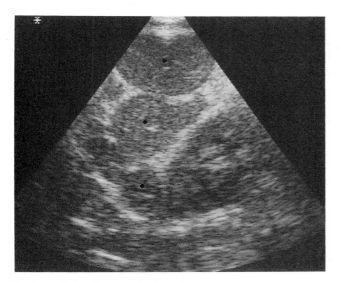

Fig. 4.7.4 Polysplenia. Multiple nodules of polysplenia in biliary atresia with malformation complex (*).

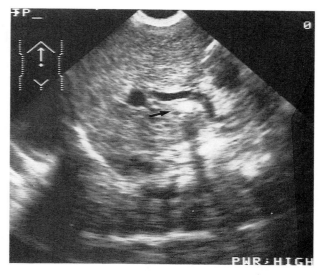

Fig. 4.7.5 Preduodenal portal vein. Abnormal course of the portal vein in front of the duodenal shadow (arrow) in biliary atresia with associated malformation complex.

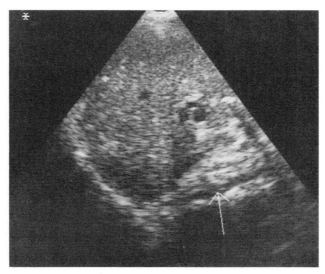

Fig. 4.7.6 Azygous continuation of IVC. This retrohepatic vessel corresponds to the azygos vein and does not join the inferior aspect of the right atrium.

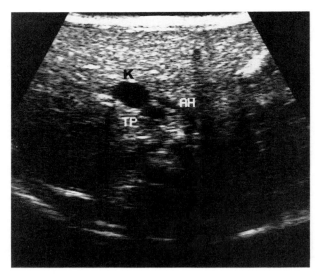

Fig. 4.7.7 Pedicular cyst of biliary atresia. There is a 1.5 cm cyst (K) located in the porta hepatis between the hepatic artery (AH) and the portal vein (TP).

Another diagnostic feature of biliary atresia which can be shown by ultrasonography is the presence of a biliary cyst in the porta hepatis (Figs 4.7.7, 4.7.8). Its differential diagnosis from a choledochal cyst is usually evident, as in a cholestatic infant choledochal cyst is always associated with intrahepatic bile duct dilatation and the communication may be demonstrated between the cyst and the bile duct. In summary, in neonatal cholestasis, US examination is useful to rule out other rarer causes of extrahepatic cholestasis with dilated bile ducts which represent only 5% of cases. Ultrasonography is diagnostic of biliary atresia only if it demonstrates elements of the polysplenia syndrome or a residual cyst in the porta hepatis. Failure to demonstrate a patent gallbladder in the presence of a typical clinical presentation is suggestive; but in the absence of these diagnostic elements, the diagnosis of biliary atresia cannot yet be confirmed and further investigations should be undertaken.

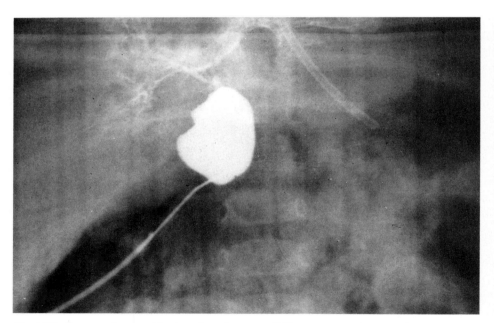

Fig. 4.7.8 Peroperative opacification of another case of biliary atresia with a cyst. This large cyst communicates with intrahepatic abnormal bile ducts. There is no communication with the duodenum.

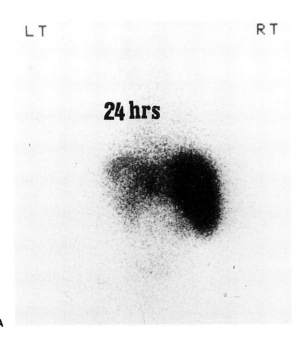

A

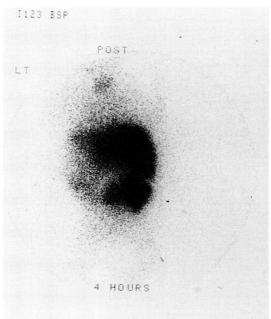

B

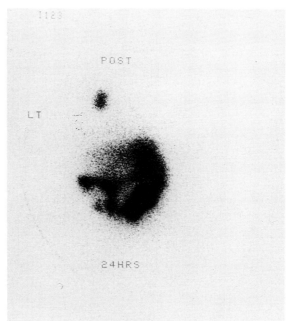

Isotopic studies

Isotopic studies are also of value.

The Rose Bengal faecal excretion test has been replaced by scanning procedures using IDA compounds. These labelled with ^{99m}Tc or ^{123}I can be demonstrated with a gamma camera to be concentrated in the liver and then excreted into the bile in the next 12 hours (Fig. 4.7.9). Excretion of the radiopharmaceutical from the liver into the bowel theoretically indicates a patent biliary tree, but a few false-positive studies have been reported. The absence of radionuclide in the intestine does not differentiate biliary atresia from severe intrahepatic cholestasis.

The next procedure is a *percutaneous liver biopsy*. Histological findings of biliary atresia are portal fibrosis, bile ductule proliferation and biliary thrombi. If a large gallbladder is present *percutaneous transhepatic cholecystography* can be performed to demonstrate the atretic common bile duct (Fig. 4.7.3).

Endoscopic retrograde cholangiopancreatography has been recently used by a few experts to make this diagnosis.

Fig. 4.7.9 **A** ^{123}I BSP scan. Biliary atresia. There is no excretion of radionuclide. **B** Neonatal hepatitis. Excretion is present at 4 and 24 hours but retention of radionuclide in the liver indicates liver damage.

Surgery

The current opinion is that surgery has to be undertaken before 60 days or ideally 40 days of life to provide the best chance, up to 80%, of clearing of jaundice and survival with a good quality of life, to at least 10 years of age, with the possibility then of liver transplantation.

Operative procedure depends on the anatomical type of biliary atresia. It consists of a porto-enterostomy (Kasaï procedure) with dissection of the bile duct fibrous remnant and small bowel anastomosis. The fundus of the gallbladder may be used for this anastomosis if the choledochus is patent (portocholecystotomy) (Fig. 4.7.10). A complication of the latter procedure is anastomotic leakage with bile peritonitis which requires surgery to repair it.

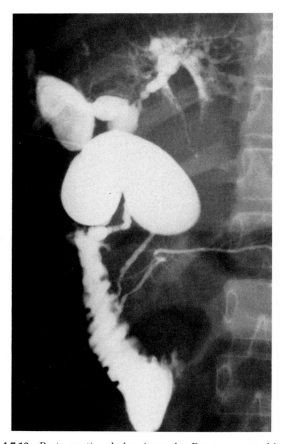

Fig. 4.7.10 Postoperative cholangiography. Fourteen-year-old girl with a history of biliary atresia and portocholecystostomy, presenting with episodes of cholangitis. PTC via the gallbladder shows a very small caliber of the choledochus with tiny intraluminal filling defects. Large intrahepatic cystic cavities are opacified corresponding to parenchymal necrotic areas filled with bile. She underwent liver transplantation a few months later.

Complications

Cholangitis, portal hypertension and biliary cirrhosis are the main complications following surgery.

Ultrasound plays an important role in the follow up of these patients. It may demonstrate intrahepatic cystic cavities, often filled with echogenic material, corresponding to bile-filled parenchymal necrotic areas (Fig. 4.7.10). If there is clinical evidence of cholangitis, these cavities may be punctured to obtain the infectious agent for culture and choice of antibiotic treatment.

The degree of portal hypertension and development of cirrhosis can be monitored by US. Pretransplantation work-up is also based on US. In longstanding biliary atresia without replacement treatment, vitamin-deficiency rickets with progression to fractures may develop. Hypertrophic osteoarthropathy has also been reported. It is characterized by periosteal reaction involving the shaft of the long bones, soft tissue swelling about the joints and digital clubbing. The pathogenesis is unknown.

REFERENCES

Abramson S J, Berdon W E, Altman R P, Amodio J B, Levy J 1987 Biliary atresia and non cardiac polysplenic syndrome: US and surgical considerations. Radiology 163: 377–380

Abramson S J, Treves S, Teele R S 1982 The infant with possible biliary atresia: evaluation by ultrasound and nuclear medicine. Pediatric Radiology 12: 1–5

Brun P, Gauthier F, Boucher D, Brunelle F 1985 Ultrasound findings in biliary atresia in children. Annales de Radiologie 28: 259–263

Carty H, Pilling D W, Majury C 1986 ^{123}I BSP scanning in neonatal jaundice. Annales de Radiologie 29: 647–650

Chaumont P, Martin N, Riou J Y, Brunelle F 1982 Percutaneous transhepatic cholangiography in extrahepatic biliary duct atresia in children. Annales de Radiologie 25: 94–100

Hussein M, Howard E, Mieli-Vergani G, Mowat A P 1991 Jaundice at 14 days of age: exclude biliary atresia. Archives of Disease in Childhood 66: 1177–1180

Kirks D R, Coleman R E, Filston H C, Rosenberg E R, Merten D F 1984 An imaging approach to persistent neonatal jaundice. American Journal of Roentgenology 142: 461–465

Laurent J, Gauthier F, Bernard O, Hadchouel M, Odievre M, Valayer J, Alagille D 1990 Long-term outcome after surgery for biliary atresia. Gastroenterology 99: 1793–1797

Mowat A P (ed) 1987 Liver disorders in childhood, 2nd edn. Butterworths-Heinemann, Oxford

Pariente D, Bernard O 1989 Diagnostic des cholestases du nouveau-né et de nourrisson. In: Radiopédiatrie: de la clinique à l'imagerie. Sauramps Med Ed, pp 61–74

Rothbert A D, Boal D K 1983 Hypertrophic osteoarthropathy in biliary atresia. Pediatric Radiology 13: 44–46

Serafini A N, Snoak W M, Hupf H B 1985 Iodine 123 Rose Bengal: an improved hepatobiliary imaging agent. Journal of Nuclear Medicine 16: 629–632

Torrisi J, Haller J, Velcek F 1990 Choledochal cyst and biliary atresia in the neonate. Imaging findings in 5 cases. American Journal of Radiology 155: 1273–1277

Williamson S L, Seibert J J, Butler H L, Golladay E S 1986 Apparent gut excretion of Tc-99m-DISIDA in a case of extrahepatic biliary atresia. Pediatric Radiology 16: 245–247

Other causes of neonatal cholestasis

Besides biliary atresia, *extrahepatic causes* of neonatal cholestasis are rare, representing 5% of the cases. They include:

— lithiasis of the common bile duct
— spontaneous perforation of the common bile duct
— choledochal cyst
— sclerosing cholangitis, which is usually a lesion of both intra- and extrahepatic bile duct and may present with a neonatal onset.

Intrahepatic causes of neonatal cholestasis are diverse and are listed in the gamut.

Imaging plays a minor role in the diagnosis of these entities which is mainly based on biological and histological findings.

Byler's disease is a familial progressive intrahepatic cholestasis of unknown cause, which often presents in infancy and progresses rapidly to hepatic failure. The gallbladder is often very large and percutaneous cholecystography shows a normal biliary tree.

Skeletal films may demonstrate metaphyseal lucent bands or lytic areas suggestive of congenital viral infections. Several elements of Alagille's syndrome (syndromic paucity of the interlobular bile duct) may also be found on radiological examinations. They include mainly the 'butterfly vertebrae' (Fig. 4.7.11) and pulmonary artery branch stenoses (Fig. 4.7.12). Other skeletal findings have also been reported: narrow lumbar spine, shortness of the ulna and radioulnar synostosis. The clinical features include a peculiar facies and posterior embryotoxon, found on slit lamp examination of the eyes.

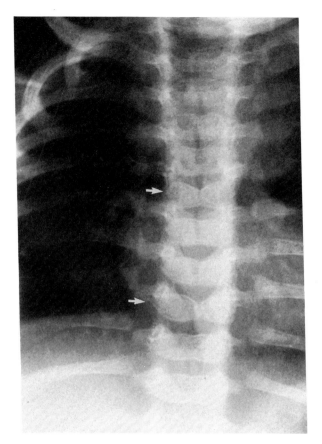

Fig. 4.7.11 'Butterfly' vertebrae (arrows) in a cholestatic newborn with cholestatic jaundice. The diagnosis is that of syndromic paucity of interlobular bile ducts (Alagille's syndrome).

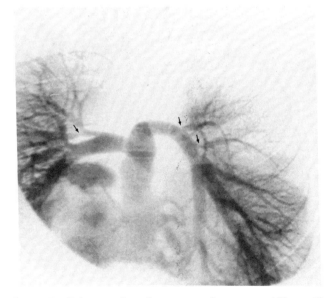

Fig. 4.7.12 Pulmonary branches stenoses. Seven-year-old boy with syndromic paucity of bile duct and cardiac murmur. Digital venous subtraction angiography shows multiple discrete stenoses with pulmonary hypoperfusion (arrows).

In syndromic and non-syndromic biliary hypoplasia, cholangiography (best performed via the gallbladder) demonstrates paucity and attenuation of intrahepatic bile ducts (Fig. 4.7.13).

REFERENCES

Alagille D, Estrada A, Hadchouel M, Gautier M, Odievre M, Dommergues J P 1987 Syndromic paucity of interlobular bile ducts (Alagille syndrome or arteriohepatic dysplasia): a review of 80 cases. Journal of Pediatrics 110: 195–200

Brunelle F, Estrada A, Dommergues J P, Bernard O, Chaumont P 1986 Skeletal anomalies in Alagilles's syndrome. Radiographic study in eighty cases. Annales de Radiologie 29: 687–690

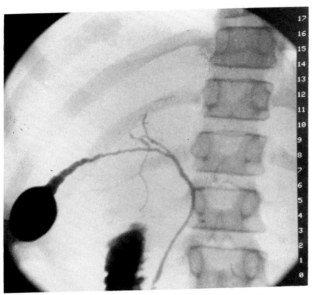

Fig. 4.7.13 The paucity of interlobular bile ducts is striking on percutaneous cholecystography performed in this 14-year-old boy with Alagille's syndrome.

COMMON BILE DUCT LITHIASIS IN INFANCY

This rare entity in infants first described as the 'bile plug syndrome' is more frequently diagnosed preoperatively since the advent of US.

The aetiology of the disease is still unclear. The calculi are pigment stones confirmed by morphology (blackish and crumbly at extraction) and by biochemical analysis. The following causative factors have been described: prematurity, infection, dehydration, parenteral nutrition, furosemide treatment and gastrointestinal dysfunction. This entity is probably due to a transient bile disturbance resulting from deficient glucurono-conjugation. Abnormal motility of the gallbladder and duodenum has also been advocated. The biliary tract is normal and there is no recurrence after treatment. The clinical presentation is non-specific with fluctuating jaundice and hepatomegaly.

Mild and even dilatation of the extrahepatic and intrahepatic bile ducts are present at US examination (Fig. 4.7.14). Sludge may be found in the gallbladder. In some cases, the calculcus may be depicted in the lower end of the common bile duct as an echogenic ball but does not always have acoustic shadowing. It may be obscured by the overlying bowel gas of the duodenum.

In a few cases, spontaneous resolution of the dilatation has been documented on US. This is probably secondary to passage of the calculus into the duodenum. However cholangitis and even liver abscesses may complicate this entity (Fig. 4.7.15) and the presence of fever is an indication for prompt treatment.

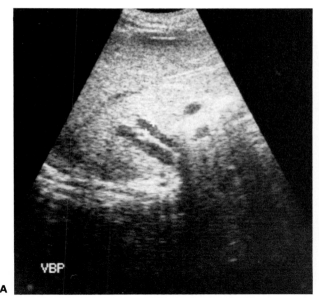

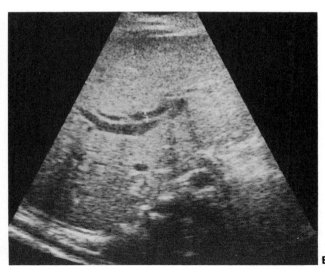

Fig. 4.7.14 Common bile duct lithiasis. One-month-old baby boy with fluctuating cholestasis. US shows mild and regular extra (**A**) and intra (**B**) hepatic bile duct dilatation. The distal choledochal lithiasis is not seen because of overlying duodenal gas.

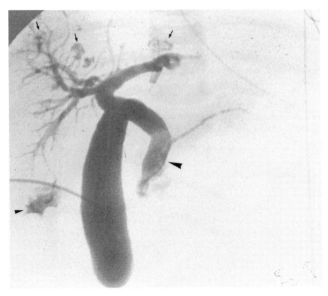

Fig. 4.7.15 Common bile duct lithiasis in a 3-week-old baby girl, with *E. coli* septicaemia and multiple hepatic abscesses. PTC obtained via gallbladder: there is obstruction of the common bile duct with a large intraluminal defect (large arrowhead). There is opacification of parenchymal cavities (arrows) and subcapsular leakage (small arrowhead). Clearing of the common bile duct and resolution of the abscesses were easily achieved by washing with saline.

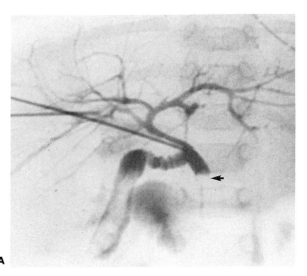
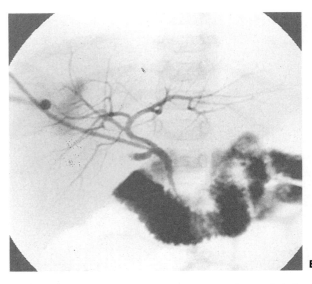

A   B

Fig. 4.7.16 **A** Common bile duct lithiasis (arrow) and sludge in the gallbladder in a 4-week-old baby boy, with mild intrahepatic bile duct dilatation. Placement of external drainage and washing with saline. **B** Two days later the stones have disappeared and the duct size has returned to normal.

Percutaneous cholangiography or cholecystography with flushing of the biliary tree in order to push the stone into the duodenum is the treatment of choice. The placement of an external drainage so that repeated washing may be done is recommended (Fig. 4.7.16). If this fails the infant will require surgery.

REFERENCES

Avni E F, Matos C, Van Gansbeke D, Muller F 1986 Atypical gallbladder content in neonates: ultrasonic demonstration. Annales de Radiologie 29: 267–273

Bernstein J, Braylan R, Brough J 1969 Bileplug syndrome: a correctable cause of obstructive jaundice in infants. Pediatrics 43: 273–276

Brunelle F 1987 Cholelithiasis in children. Seminars in Ultrasound, CT and MRI 8: 118–125

Brunelle F, Descos B, Bernard O, Valayer J, Chaumont P 1983 Common bile duct calculi in infants. Annales de Radiologie 26: 147

Cox K L, Chenng A T W, Lohse C L, Walsh E M, Iwahaski-Hosoda C K 1987 Biliary mobility: post-natal changes in guinea pigs. Pediatric Research 21: 170–175

Descos B, Bernard O, Brunelle F, Valayer J, Feldmann D, Hadchouel M, Alagille D 1984 Pigment gallstones of the common bile duct in infancy. Hepatology 4: 678–683

Holgersen L O, Stolar C, Berdon W E, Hilfer C, Levy J S 1990 Therapeutic and diagnostic implications of acquired choledochal obstruction in infancy: spontaneous resolution in three infants. Journal of Pediatric Surgery 25: 1027–1029

Keller M S, Markle B M, Laffey P A, Chawla J N, Jacir N, Frank J L 1985 Spontaneous resolution in cholelithiasis in infants. Radiology 157: 345–348

Lilly J R 1980 Common bile duct calculi in infants and children. Journal of Pediatric Surgery 15: 577–580

Man D W K, Spitz L 1985 Cholelithiasis in infancy. Journal of Pediatric Surgery 20: 65–68

Pariente D, Bernard O, Gauthier F, Brunelle F, Chaumont P 1989 Radiological treatment of common bile duct lithiasis in infancy. Pediatric Radiology 19: 104–107

SPONTANEOUS PERFORATION OF THE COMMON BILE DUCT

This is a rare disorder, with only about 80 reported cases. It has been reported from 1 week to 4 years of age, but is most frequent between 1 and 3 months. The pathogenesis is unknown. The perforation is located in almost all cases at the junction of the cystic and common bile duct. It has been suggested that there is an area of weakness in the bile duct wall at this point. Other recorded sites of perforation are the common hepatic duct, the common bile duct, the gallbladder and the cystic duct. The clinical presentation is variable, ranging from an acute surgical emergency to more commonly a chronic illness. Abdominal distension, ascites, hernia and fluctuating mild jaundice are the main findings.

At US examination ascites is found. In some cases a loculated fluid collection in and around the porta hepatis is also present. Bile duct dilatation is not constant. Hepatobiliary scintigraphy is diagnostic, showing free spillage of the radionuclide into the peritoneal cavity. Treatment is surgical and should not be delayed to avoid the complication of infection.

Most authors suggest that simple drainage of the biliary peritonitis with placement of a cholecystostomy tube are the surgical procedures of choice. Stenosis of the distal bile duct with the presence of stones has been demonstrated on preoperative cholangiography in some patients, giving rise to discussion as to whether the anomalies are cause or consequence of the perforation.

Spontaneous healing of the perforation with bile duct dilatation and accumulation of stones have also been described (Fig. 4.7.17).

REFERENCES

Bahia J O, Boal D K B, Karl S R, Gross G W 1986 Ultrasonographic detection of spontaneous perforation of the extrahepatic bile ducts in infancy. Pediatric Radiology 16: 157–159

Brunelle F, Descos B, Bernard O, Valayer J, Chaumont P 1983 Common bile duct calculi in infants. Annales de Radiologie 26: 147

Donahoe P K, Hendren W H 1976 Bile duct perforation in a newborn with stenosis of the ampulla of Vater. Journal of Pediatric Surgery 11: 823–825

Haller J O, Condon V R, Berdon W E, Sang O H K, Price A P, Bonen A D, Cohen H L 1989 Spontaneous perforation of the common bile duct in children. Radiology 172: 621–624

Hammoundi S M, Alanddin A 1988 Idiopathic perforation of the biliary tract in infancy and childhood. Journal of Pediatric Surgery 23: 185–187

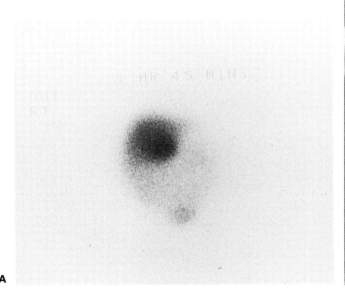

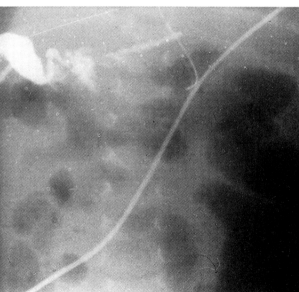

Fig. 4.7.17 A, B Infant with spontaneous perforation of the common bile duct, who presented with ascites which was bile stained. **A** Hida Scan showing circulation of Hida in the peritoneum. **B** Operative cholangiogram showing leak at the junction of the cystic common bile duct.

SCLEROSING CHOLANGITIS·

This is a rare cause of chronic progressive liver disease in children, characterized by an inflammatory obliterative fibrosis affecting the intra- and extrahepatic biliary tree. Fewer than 100 cases have been reported. The pathogenesis remains unknown. The disorder has an association with a variety of other diseases, including mainly chronic inflammatory bowel disease (= 50%), histiocytosis X (= 15%) (Fig. 4.7.18) and immuno-deficiency disorders (= 10%) (Fig. 4.7.19). Twenty-five per cent of cases are isolated and have no associated underlying condition. Neonatal onset has been noted in some of these idiopathic cases (Fig. 4.7.20). The clinical findings include hepatomegaly and jaundice. Liver function tests and histological changes are often non-specific. Cholangiography is essential to establish the diagnosis.

In some cases, dilatation of the bile ducts can be demonstrated by US and imaging obtained by percutaneous transhepatic cholangiography (PTC). If bile duct dilatation is not present at US examination, endoscopic retrograde cholecystopancreatography (ERCP) or percutaneous cholecystography especially in infants, should be attempted.

Typical cholangiographic anomalies include short annular strictures with intervening normal or dilated segments. The disease may be limited at the time of diagnosis to the intrahepatic bile duct.

The prognosis is poor with progressive evolution to biliary cirrhosis. Liver transplantation has been already performed in a few cases. There is no recurrence at 5 year follow-up.

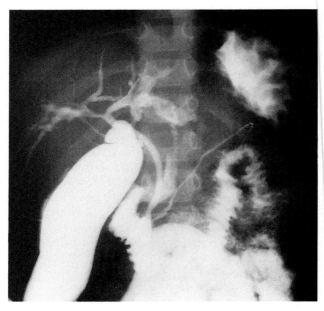

Fig. 4.7.18 Sclerosing cholangitis in a 3-year-old boy presenting with histiocystosis X (bilateral mastoiditis and diabetes insipidus). Percutaneous cholecystography shows multiple irregular dilatations of the intrahepatic bile ducts.

REFERENCES

Amédée-Manesme O, Bernard O, Brunelle F, Hadchouel M, Polonovki C, Bandon J J, Beguet P, Alagille D 1987 Sclerosing cholangitis with neonatal onset. Journal of Pediatrics 111: 225–229

Garel L, Brunelle F, Fisher A, Sirinelli D, Sauvegrain J 1985 Bile duct dilatation and immunodeficiency in children. Annales de Radiologie 28: 249–255

Leblanc A, Hadchouel M, Jehan P, Odièvre M, Alagille D 1981 Obstructive jaundice in children with histiocytosis X. Gastroenterology 80: 134–139

Pariente D, Bacadi D, Schmit P 1986 Biliary tract involvement in children with histiocytosis X. Annales de Radiologie 29: 641–645

Sisto A, Feldman P, Garel L, Seidman E, Brochu P, Morin C L, Weber A M, Roy C C 1987 Primary sclerosing cholangitis in children: study of five cases and review of the literature. Pediatrics 80: 918–923

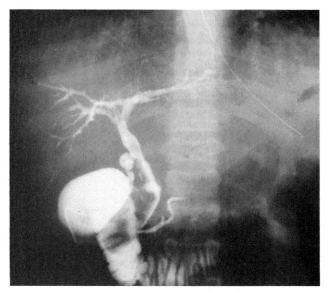

Fig. 4.7.19 Sclerosing cholangitis. Fourteen-year-old boy with severe congenital immunodeficiency and abnormal liver function. Percutaneous cholecystography: there is moderate bile duct dilatation with irregularities of peripheral bile duct and filling defect in the common bile duct corresponding to thick bile.

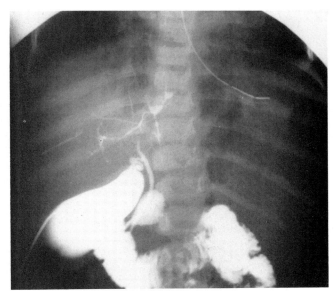

Fig. 4.7.20 Neonatal sclerosing cholangitis. Four-year-old boy with biliary cirrhosis and a history of neonatal cholestasis. Percutaneous cholecystography shows multiple stenoses of intrahepatic bile ducts interposed with dilated segments. There is also a pruned-tree appearance of the biliary tract.

CHOLEDOCHAL CYST

Although rare, this congenital entity represents the most frequent cause of extrahepatic cholestasis in childhood. It is mainly encountered in the first decade of life, with a female predominance, but antenatal and adult cases have been reported.

Various classifications have been proposed. The most commonly accepted is that proposed by Alonso-Lej's which is based on the type of cystic dilatation: fusiform type, pedunculated type (rare) and choledochocele (exceptional). The size of the cystic dilatation of the common bile duct is variable, as is the associated intrahepatic bile duct dilatation. The degree of dilatation is not related to the age of the child. The classical triad of features suggesting the diagnosis of choledochal cyst is abdominal pain, right upper quadrant mass and intermittent obstructive jaundice, which is rarely complete (10% of recent series). There is an increasing frequency of sonographic discovery in asymptomatic children whose US examination is done for some other purpose. Antenatal diagnosis has been reported as early as in the fifteenth week of gestation.

Single or recurrent episodes of pancreatitis is also a presenting finding (Fig. 4.7.21).

The diagnosis is made on US examination which demonstrates the cystic mass communicating with the bile duct. Pre- or peroperative cholangiography is performed to identify the precise anatomy of the lesion.

The precise aetiology is unknown but the most commonly accepted theory is the presence of an anomalous junction of the biliary and pancreatic channels with a long common duct, allowing reflux of pancreatic juice in the common bile duct (Fig. 4.7.22). Pancreatic enzymes have been found in the bile and raised levels have been demonstrated after IV cholecystokinin during percutaneous cholangiography.

Complications of choledochal cyst include: cholangitis, complete obstruction of the choledochus with lithiasis, biliary cirrhosis, traumatic and spontaneous rupture with biliary peritonitis and degeneration in late childhood.

Surgery consists of complete resection of the cyst and hepaticojejunostomy. In most cases the intrahepatic bile duct dilatation returns to normal after surgery and the prognosis is good. In a few cases there is persistent cystic dilatation of the intrahepatic bile ducts with episodes of cholangitis and formation of stones which raises the possibility of associated Caroli's disease.

Differential diagnosis

In the neonatal period, the main differential diagnosis is biliary atresia. The clinical presentation of biliary atresia is quite different with complete cholestasis, and US fails to show communication of the cyst with the bile ducts. Another rare diagnosis is duodenal duplication compressing the distal part of the choledochus (Fig. 4.7.23).

The antenatal *differential diagnosis of a subhepatic cystic mass* includes:

— choledochal cyst
— biliary atresia
— duodenal duplication
— ovarian cyst
— cystic pedunculated hamartoma of the liver
— omental cyst.

Caroli's disease is characterized by cystic, non-obstructive dilatation of the intrahepatic bile ducts. It is a complicated spectrum of diseases.

- Most cases in children are diffuse and associated with congenital hepatic fibrosis and recessive polycystic kidney disease.
- A few cases are associated with a choledochal cyst. The cystic dilatation of the intrahepatic bile ducts may be segmental and require surgery.
- Very rare cases have been described as the only hepatic lesion without portal fibrosis. Some authors believe that the term Caroli's disease should be restricted to those rare cases.

REFERENCES

Babbitt D D 1969 Congenital choledochal cyst. New etiological concept based on anomalous relationships of the common bile duct and pancreatic duct. Annales de Radiologie 12: 231–240

Bass E M, Cremin B J 1976 Choledochal cysts: a clinical and radiological evaluation of 21 cases. Pediatric Radiology 5: 81–85

Mowat A P (ed) 1987 Disorders of the gallbladder and biliary tract. In: Liver disorders in childhood, 2nd edn. Butterworth-Heinemann, Oxford, pp 337–355

Schroeder D, Smith L, Crichton Pain H 1989 Antenatal diagnosis of choledochal cyst at 15 weeks' gestation: etiologic implications and management. Journal of Pediatric Surgery 24: 936–938

Suarez F, Bernard O, Gauthier F, Valayer J, Brunelle F 1987 Biliopancreatic common channel in childhood. Pediatric Radiology 17: 206–211

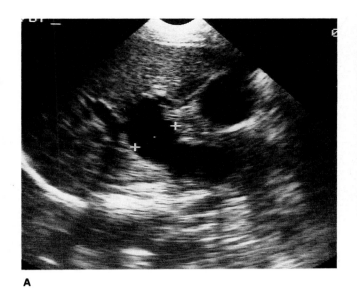
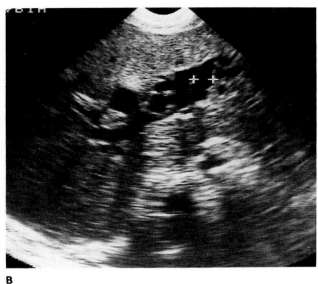

A

B

Fig. 4.7.21   A, B Choledochal cyst. Three-year-old girl presenting with an acute episode of abdominal pain and increased level of pancreatic enzymes. US demonstrates marked dilatation of the common bile duct (2 cm) (**A**) and intrahepatic bile ducts (**B**). No abnormality of the pancreas is found. PTC confirmed the diagnosis.

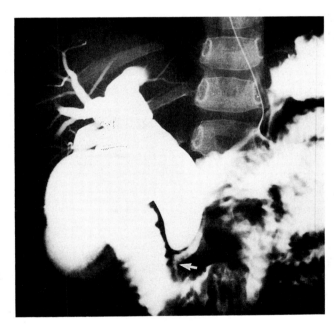

Fig. 4.7.22   Choledochal cyst in a 6-year-old boy with abdominal pain and mild jaundice. PTC shows a choledochal cyst with intrahepatic bile duct dilatation. An abnormal choledocho pancreatic common channel is evident (arrow).

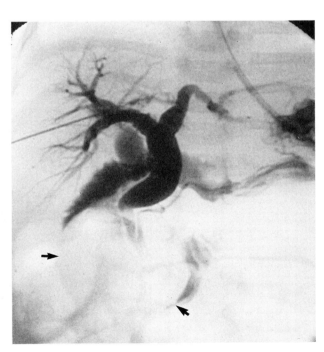

Fig. 4.7.23   Duodenal duplication. Two month-old baby girl with mild cholestasis. On US there is bile duct dilatation and a large cystic mass which appears distinct from the common bile duct. PTC shows the compression of the common bile duct by the duodenal duplication (arrows).

GALLBLADDER DISORDERS

Gallstones occur much more commonly in adult life than in childhood, but the frequency of the diagnosis in children has been increasing since the extensive use of US. Fetal and neonatal gallstones have also been documented with spontaneous resolution in most cases. This can occasionally occur in older children as well (Fig. 4.7.24). Symptoms of gallstones in children include right upper quadrant pain and episodes of obstructive jaundice. Passage of stones into the bile ducts is relatively rare compared with adult practice.

The diagnosis is made by US. Oral cholecystography is no longer indicated.

The main causes of gallstones in children are:

— haemolytic anaemia (spherocytosis, sickle-cell anaemia, thalassaemia)
— biliary cirrhosis (Byler's disease)
— cystic fibrosis
— Wilson's disease
— ileal disease (Crohn's disease) or resection
— parenteral nutrition
— furosemide, ceftriaxone (cephalosporin)
— biliary tract obstruction (choledochal cyst)
— obesity
— familial history
— metachromatic leukodystrophy.

Hydrops of the gallbladder

This is a rare disorder in which there is acute distension of the gallbladder without any mechanical obstruction of the cystic duct.

The age range is large with cases reported in the newborn period. There is a male predominance.

Clinical presentation includes upper abdominal pain, vomiting and rarely mild jaundice.

The diagnosis is based on US which shows a distended gallbladder with a thin wall and anechoic content. The pathogenesis is unknown. It may occur as an isolated finding with favourable outcome, or be associated with various diseases and sometimes is the initial presenting feature.
These include:

— scarlet fever and streptococcus infection
— Kawasaki disease
— leptospirosis
— salmonella and shigella infection
— extensive burning
— polyarteritis nodosa
— familial paroxysmal polyseritis
— prolonged parenteral hyperalimentation.

Spontaneous resolution is the usual outcome and it occurs in most cases in 1 or 2 weeks. Perforation is rare. Surgery is usually not necessary.

Thickening of the gallbladder wall is seen in the following conditions

— ascites
— hypoalbuminaemia
— cholecystitis: infectious and calculous
— portal hypertension
— viral hepatitis (Fig. 4.7.25)
— partial emptying of gallbladder.

REFERENCES

Benichou J J, Labrune B 1985 Les hydrocholécystes chez l'enfant. Archives Francaises de Pediatrie 42: 125–127

Heier L, Daneman A, Lowden J A, Cutz E, Craw S, Martin D J 1983 Biliary disease in metachromatic leukodystrophy. Pediatric Radiology 13: 313–318

Klingensmith W C, Cioffi-Ragan D T 1988 Fetal gallstones. Radiology 167: 143–144

Mowat A P (ed) 1987 Disorders of the gallbladder and biliary tract. In: Liver disorders in childhood, 2nd edn. Butterworth-Heinemann, Oxford, pp 337–355

Nzek D A, Adedoyin M A 1989 Sonographic pattern of gallbladder disease in children with sickle cell anaemia. Pediatric Radiology 19: 290–292

Patriquin H B, Di Pietro M, Barber F E, Teele R L 1983 Sonography of thickened gallbladder wall: causes in children. American Journal of Roentgenology 141: 57–61

Pracros J P, Descos B, Hermier M, Pouillaude J M, Tran-Minh V 1986 Ultrasonic study of pseudo-surgical viral hepatitis. Annales de Radiologie 29: 287–292

Robinson A E, Erwin J H, Wiseman H J, Kodroff M B 1977 Cholecystitis and hydrops of the gallbladder in the newborn. Radiology 122: 749–751

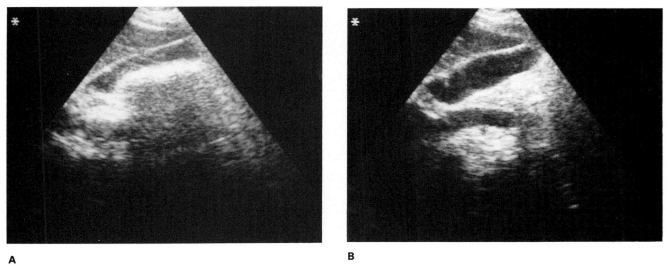

A   **B**

Fig. 4.7.24 Gallstones. **A** Nine-year-old girl with history of complicated appendicitis, referred for persistent abdominal pain and oliguria. Small stones are found in the kidney and in the gallbladder with acoustic shadowing. **B** One week later after surgical treatment of renal stones, there has been spontaneous resolution of gallstones.

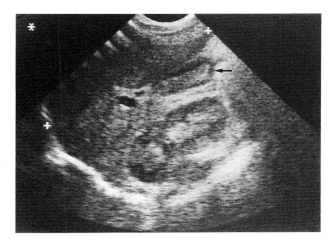

Fig. 4.7.25 Viral hepatitis. Seven-year-old girl with clinical presentation consistent with appendicitis. US showed fluid in the pouch of Douglas, thickening of the gallbladder wall and a small echogenic lumen (arrow). These findings are suggestive of acute hepatitis which was rapidly confirmed.

4.8   LIVER TRANSPLANTATION

Over the past few years, the remarkable results of liver transplantation have changed the management and prognosis of children with liver diseases.

The main indications include biliary atresia, Byler's disease, alpha-1-antitrypsin deficiency, chronic hepatitis, fulminant hepatitis, tyrosinaemia, glycogen storage disease type I with adenomas and metabolic disorders.

In most series, the rate of survival is approximately 80%, with a better prognosis when transplant is carried out electively than as an emergency.

Liver transplantation requires extensive use of imaging modalities and heavily involves the radiological team in the preoperative as well as in the postoperative work-up.

PREOPERATIVE RADIOLOGICAL WORK-UP

Preoperative work-up includes evaluation of cardiac and pulmonary status with chest film, echocardiography, scintigraphy and, in some cases, angiocardiography. Increased cardiac output, hypoxia due to pulmonary shunts and pulmonary arterial hypertension are well-known but unexplained complications of cirrhosis and portal hypertension. Their presence may hasten the need for transplantation or even preclude it (Fig. 4.8.1). Skeletal films are performed to assess bone maturation and mineralization. The nutritional status is often impaired in cholestatic diseases and should be corrected before transplantation to improve the prognosis.

Finally it is essential to evaluate the patency of the inferior vena cava and the diameter of the portal vein which represent critical anatomical information for surgical planning. This is adequately obtained with US and pulsed or colour Doppler in about 75% of patients in most series. However, angiography remains indicated in a few circumstances:

1. In cases of biliary atresia with an associated malformation complex, the so-called non-cardiac polysplenic syndrome which is present in 10–20% of cases. This includes one or several of the following anomalies:

— polysplenia
— thoracic or abdominal situs inversus with gastrointestinal malrotation (Fig. 4.8.2)
— preduodenal portal vein
— azygous continuation of the inferior vena cava. In this case hepatic veins directly enter the right atrium
— anomalous origin of the hepatic artery.

All these anomalies may be depicted on US, however vascular anatomy may be very complex. For most surgeons, precise arterial anatomy of the transplant candidate is not required since the arterial anastomosis will also depend on the anatomy of the graft.

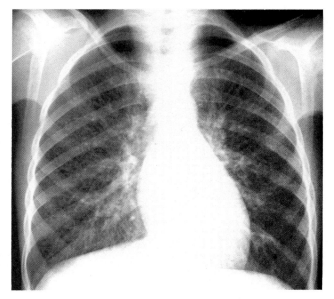

Fig. 4.8.1 Chest film of a 14-year-old girl with Budd–Chiari syndrome treated by mesocaval anastomosis. Secondary appearance of severe hypoxia. There is a spidery vascular network mimicking an interstitial pattern: multiple arteriovenous shunts are demonstrated on scintigraphy. Liver transplantation is planned.

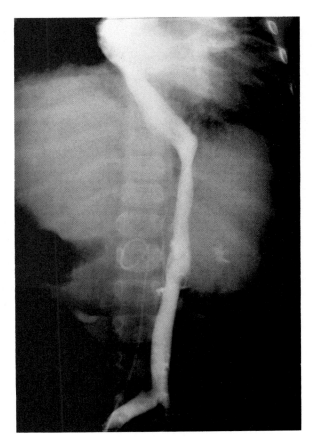

Fig. 4.8.2 Biliary atresia with malformation complex. Abdominal situs inversus and a left-sided inferior vena cava are present.

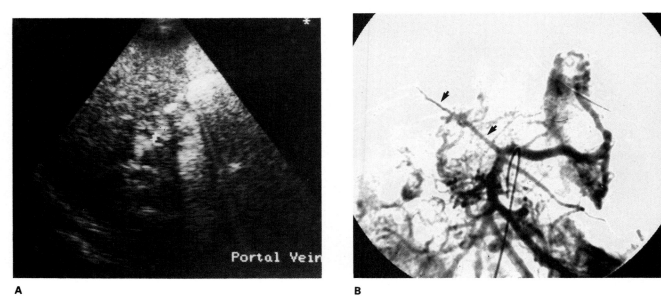

A　**B**

Fig. 4.8.3　Small portal vein. Sixteen-month-old boy with biliary atresia and failure of the Kasai procedure. **A** The portal vein appears very small on US and flow is very difficult to record on Doppler study. **B** Superior mesenteric arteriography (venous phase) confirms its small size (arrows) and patency of the superior mesenteric and splenic vein. Liver transplant was performed with a venous graft.

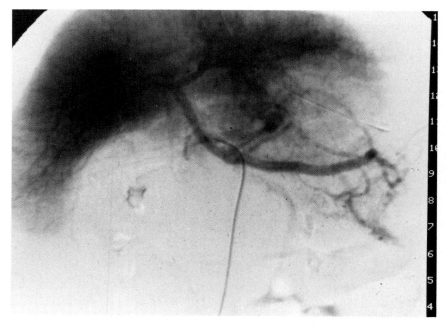

Fig. 4.8.4　Six-month-old girl with biliary atresia. Massive inverted portal flow is demonstrated on the late phase of the hepatic arteriogram.

2. Angiography is also indicated when the portal vein is not identified or its diameter is less than 4 mm. A decrease in the size of the portal vein is a frequent event in end-stage liver disease, as opposed to dilatation of the hepatic artery (Fig. 4.8.3). Inverted portal flow may be demonstrated in some cases on pulsed Doppler US. It is often so massive that it can be nicely demonstrated on the late phase of hepatic arteriography with slow injection of contrast medium (Fig. 4.8.4). If superior mesenteric and hepatic arteriograms fail to display the portal vein, it may be shown by fine needle transhepatic portography (Fig. 4.8.5). Portal vein thrombosis is rare and it no longer precludes transplantation, as surgeons are nowadays performing venous anastomoses with venous grafts placed on the superior mesenteric or splenic vein. Precise venous mapping is still required in these cases.

3. Cavography should be performed when the inferior vena cava is not identified (Fig. 4.8.2), or thrombosed. This does not preclude transplantation but the superior caval anastomosis of the graft will be achieved on the inferior part of the right atrium.

4. In cases of previous surgical portosystemic shunt, the anatomy of the portal vein will also require angiographic demonstration as transplantation will be more complicated.

MRI has been reported to be useful in this vascular work-up (Fig. 4.8.6). In our experience we have been disappointed in its ability to image complex anatomy in young children.

REFERENCES

Cardella J F, Amplatz K 1987 Pre operative angiographic evaluation of prospective liver recipients. Radiologic Clinics of North America 25: 299–308
Claus D, Clapuyt P H 1987 Liver transplantation in children: role of the radiologist in the pre operative assessment and the post operative follow-up. Transplantation Proceedings 19: 3344–3357
Day D L, Letourneau J G, Allan B T, Ascher N L, Hund G 1986 MR evaluation of the portal vein in pediatric liver transplant candidates. American Journal of Roentgenology 147: 1027–1030
Zajko A B, Campbell W L, Bron K M, Schade R R, Koneru B, Van Thiel D H 1988 Diagnostic and interventional radiology in liver transplantation. Gastroenterology Clinics of North America 17: 105–143

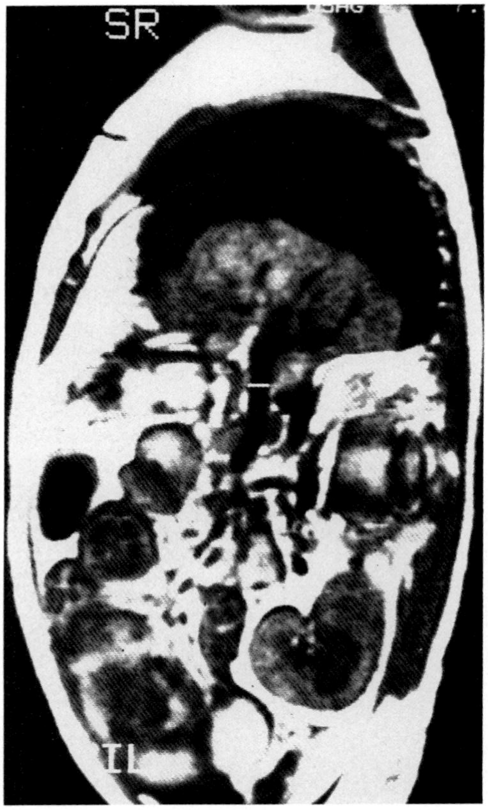

Fig. 4.8.6 MRI. Eight-year-old girl with decompensation of chronic hepatitis. Because of the massive ascites, the severe atrophy of the liver and its thoracic location, US failed to identify the portal vein. MRI non-invasively demonstrates a large patent portal vein (7 mm).

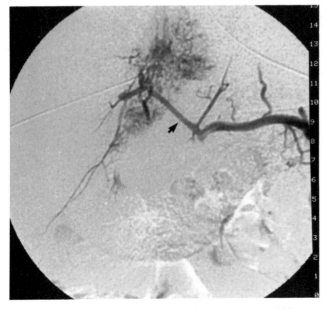

Fig. 4.8.5 Transhepatic portography. Nineteen-month-old boy with biliary atresia. US, splenoportography, superior mesenteric and hepatic arteriography have failed to demonstrate a portal vein. Fine needle transhepatic portography shows a 2 mm patent portal vein (arrow).

POST-OPERATIVE WORK-UP

After transplantation, US with pulsed or colour Doppler is the method of choice for detection of the main complications. It can be performed as a portable examination at the bedside in the early postoperative period in these critical patients. The clinical and biochemical findings are non-specific in the diagnosis of most of the complications.

Vascular complications

The patency of vascular anastomoses is accurately depicted by pulsed Doppler (Fig. 4.8.7).

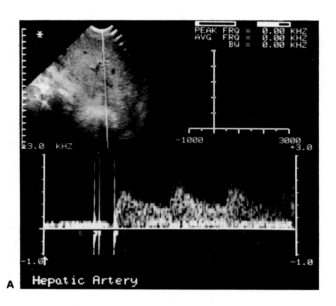

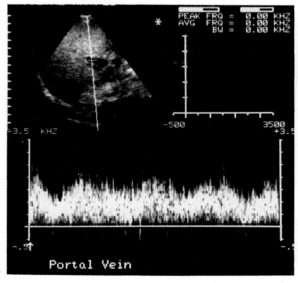

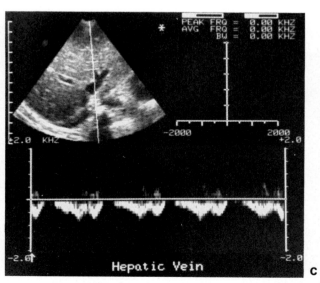

Fig. 4.8.7 The patency of the vascular anastomoses after liver transplant is assessed at the bedside by Doppler. **A** Normal intrahepatic signal of the hepatic artery. Because of respiratory motion there is successive recording of venous and arterial flow. **B** Normal portal vein flow above the anastomosis. **C** Normal triphasic hepatic vein flow.

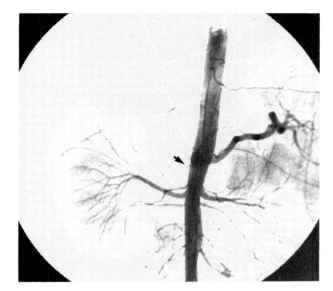

Fig. 4.8.8 Hepatic artery thrombosis. Global aortogram confirms Doppler study: there is complete obstruction of the hepatic artery (arrow).

Hepatic artery thrombosis

This is a frequent complication of paediatric liver transplantation, reported in approximately 10% of cases. It mainly occurs with infant donors or recipients.

It is usually a devastating condition, but its clinical presentation is highly variable and includes fulminant necrosis and septicaemia necessitating retransplantation on an emergency basis, or delayed biliary complications due to ischaemia of the biliary tract, or relapsing fever and bacteraemia.

The diagnosis is based on the absence of an intrahepatic arterial Doppler signal. Colour Doppler may facilitate this diagnosis. It has to be confirmed by angiography (Fig. 4.8.8), but the use of Doppler has avoided a lot of unnecessary angiograms.

Contrast-enhanced CT is the best method to evaluate the extension of parenchymal ischaemia which is variable, often predominant in the left lobe and is important in the prognosis (Fig. 4.8.9).

Bile duct necrosis may occur at any portion of the biliary tract or at the anastomosis, with the appearance of intra- or extrahepatic bilomas and of bile duct dilatation and stenosis. These complications are well depicted on US if one is aware of the frequent echogenic appearance of the dilated bile ducts filled with sludge and epithelial debris (Fig. 4.8.10).

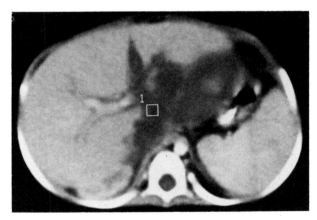

Fig. 4.8.9 Liver ischaemia after hepatic artery thrombosis. There is a large hypodensity in the left lobe without contrast enhancement corresponding to liver infarction, which is best evaluated by CT.

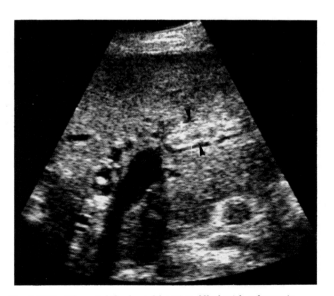

Fig. 4.8.10 There is bile duct dilatation filled with echogenic material which is identified with a high resolution transducer: this represents sludge and epithelial debris after hepatic artery thrombosis (arrowheads).

Cholangiography via an indwelling surgical drain or by a percutaneous approach has to be performed, to identify the precise extension of the lesions and to plan the treatment by percutaneous drainage, dilatation or surgery. Long-term drainage has proved useful in most cases as a treatment for the cholangitis and prior to retransplantation (Fig. 4.8.11). Arterial collateral circulation has been observed in all our children with hepatic artery thrombosis, 3 weeks to 1 month later on Doppler studies and on arteriography (Fig. 4.8.12). This collateral circulation carries a risk of massive haemorrhage during surgery and it does not seem to prevent delayed biliary complications, as these occur even with delayed hepatic artery thrombosis. Because dreadful complications seem to occur in all cases of hepatic artery thrombosis it is important to diagnose it as soon as possible and to perform surgical arterial recanalisation to save the graft.

The protocol of post-transplant work-up consists of a routine daily Doppler US examination during the first 2 weeks when the risk of hepatic artery thrombosis is at its greatest. Later on, US may be performed as clinically indicated.

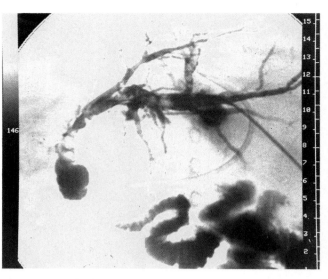

Fig. 4.8.11 PTC of the same patient with a reduced-sized graft (right hepatectomy) is performed via a left approach under US guidance. There is bile duct dilatation with intraluminal filling defects. An external drainage is placed to treat cholangitis before retransplantation.

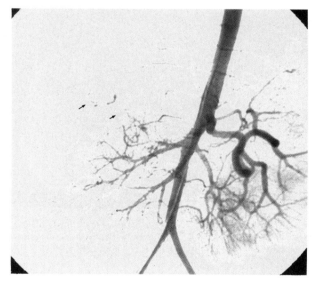

Fig. 4.8.12 Collateral arterial revascularization of liver (arrows), 2 months after hepatic artery thrombosis, is shown on this arteriogram.

Other vascular complications

Hepatic artery stenosis may be asymptomatic or may be complicated by biliary problems.

Portal vein thrombosis is fortunately a rarer complication than hepatic artery thrombosis and only a few cases have been reported. However it is a major complication as three out of our seven cases died (Fig. 4.8.13). Pulsed or colour Doppler are diagnostic and prompt surgical relief has been proposed. Portal vein stenosis is uncommon, and is secondary to a mechanical problem at the anastomotic site. It presents with the reappearance of the clinical and radiological signs of portal hypertension. However the portal anastomosis is often prominent on US, with an echogenic area of narrowing and sometimes with the impression of kink.

Inferior vena cava thrombosis in its retrohepatic portion may be encountered, especially with an adult reduced-size graft and an incongruous large inferior vena cava. In most cases, hepatic vein drainage is preserved and no complication occurs.

A few cases of secondary Budd–Chiari syndrome have been reported, which have been successfully treated by percutaneous angioplasty.

Arterial aneurysms are a very serious complication as they carry a risk of dissection with intractable haemorrhage. They may be secondary or associated with chronic infection ('mycotic aneurysms') or with severe rejection. They are very difficult to depict with US or CT and angiography is required if suspected.

REFERENCES

Flint E W, Sumkin J H, Zajko A B, Bowen A D 1988 Duplex sonography of hepatic artery thrombosis after liver transplantation. American Journal of Roentgenology 151: 481–483

Pariente D, Riou J Y, Schmit P, Verlhac S, Bernard O, Devictor D, Gauthier F, Houssin D 1990 Variability of clinical presentation of hepatic artery thrombosis in pediatric liver transplantation: role of imaging modalities. Pediatric Radiology 20: 253–257

Zajko A B, Calus D, Clapuyt P, Esquivel C O, Moulin D, Starzl T E, Deville de Goyet J, Otte J B 1989 Obstruction to hepatic venous drainage after LT: treatment with balloon angioplasty. Radiology 170: 763–765

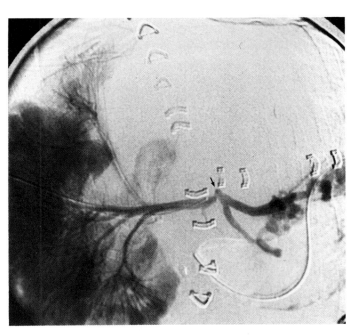

Fig. 4.8.13 Portal vein thrombosis is confirmed by superior mesenteric arteriography (arrow): there is diversion of contrast medium into a large coronary vein.

Biliary complications

These are frequent, and occur in about 15% of cases. Their severity is a function of the aetiology.

The main cause of biliary complication is hepatic artery thrombosis or stenosis and is due to necrosis of the biliary tract which is only vascularized by the hepatic artery in the transplanted liver: collaterals arising from the gastroduodenal artery are interrupted during surgery. Necrosis may occur at any portion of the biliary tract leading to bile leakage, stenosis and dilatation. On cholangiography dilated bile ducts have shaggy borders very suggestive of epithelial necrosis (Fig. 4.8.14). The prognosis is poor, even with multiple surgical procedures, percutaneous drainage and balloon dilatation, and in most cases retransplantation is required. Biliary anastomotic stenosis may occur in isolation. It has been observed with choledochocholedochostomy or choledochojejunostomy (Fig. 4.8.15). The diagnosis is made on US, as biochemical findings are often non-specific. Percutaneous dilatation may be successful and may avoid surgery. In some cases, this anastomotic stenosis may be due to a kink or plication during surgery and re-operation is necessary.

A few cases of obstructing bile sludge have been reported without a mechanical obstruction. These cases can be treated with cholangiography and lavage.

Formation of a mucocele of the cystic duct remnant is an uncommon event, which may compress the common bile duct and cause bile duct dilatation. The treatment is surgical. Cholangiography either by an indwelling surgical drain or by percutaneous approach has to be performed under antibiotic cover, as it carries a serious risk of cholangitis and septicaemia in these immunocompromised children. External drainage or immediate surgery is recommended if a significant obstruction is discovered.

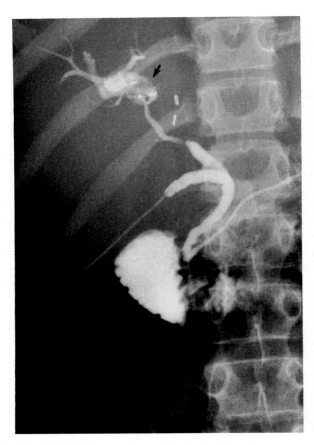

Fig. 4.8.14 Bile duct necrosis secondary to hepatic artery thrombosis. Opacification via an indwelling surgical drain shows the shaggy appearance of the bile duct junction (arrow).

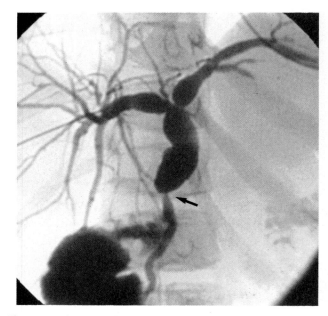

Fig. 4.8.15 Stricture of choledochocholedochostomy 1 month after liver transplantation (arrow). Successful treatment by percutaneous balloon dilatation.

Fluid collections

Right pleural effusions and ascites are common after liver transplantation. Trans-sonic collections around the ligamentum teres and the ligamentum venosus are nearly always present and represent transient lymphatic stasis (Fig. 4.8.16). Intraperitoneal fluid collections are easily demonstrated on US, but their nature is often difficult to predict without aspiration. They may represent abscess, haematoma, biloma or even loculated ascites in these multioperated patients (Fig. 4.8.17).

REFERENCES

Hoffer F A, Teele R L, Lillehei C W, Vacanti J P 1988 Infected bilomas and hepatic artery thrombosis in infant recipients of liver transplants. Radiology 169: 435–438

Letourneau J G, Hunter D W, Ascher N I, Roberts J P, Payne W D, Thompson W M, Najarian J S, Castaneda-Zuniga W K 1989 Biliary complications after liver transplantation in children. Radiology 170: 1095–1099

Pariente D, Bihet M H, Tammam S, Riou J Y, Bernard O, Devictor D, Gauthier F, Houssin D, Chaumont P 1991 Biliary complications after transplantation in children: role of imaging modalities. Pediatric Radiology 21: 175–178

Rejection

This is one of the most common complications of liver transplantation. It has to be recognized early to be effectively treated.

Unfortunately no imaging modality appears to be really reliable in making this diagnosis. Percutaneous liver biopsy has to be performed to demonstrate its presence. US is useful to guide the needle, especially in the reduced-sized livers with disturbed anatomy.

REFERENCE

Marden D M, De Marino G B, Sumkin J H, Sheahan D G 1989 Liver transplant rejection: value of the resistive index in Doppler US of hepatic arteries. Radiology 173: 127–129

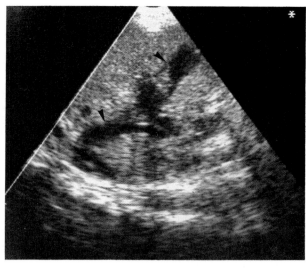

Fig. 4.8.16 Fluid collections around the ligamentum teres and the ligamentum venosus (arrowheads) representing lymphatic stasis.

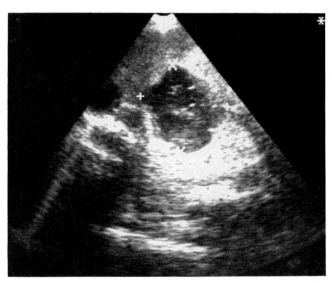

Fig. 4.8.17 Loculated ascites. This large subhepatic collection with echogenic material suspected to be an abscess, was non-infected loculated ascites.

4.9 SPLEEN

The spleen is part of the reticuloendothelial system and is therefore involved in many haematopoietic, lymphoid and multisystem disorders. It is also secondarily enlarged in liver disease due to its intimate relationship with the portal venous system.

The role of the spleen in regulating the immune system and the response to infection is well recognized, as is the importance of avoiding splenectomy when possible. Severe sepsis occurs in 1–2% of splenectomized patients and has a 50–70% mortality. Children are especially susceptible to this dreadful complication.

Splenic enlargement may be seen on plain abdominal radiographs. When enlarged, in mild cases, the splenic tip is seen below the rib ends. As enlargement progresses, the spleen enlarges distally and medially and displaces the abdominal gas distally, and the stomach bubble medially. The spleen may be imaged with US, CT and scintigraphy. The choice of modality depends on the clinical situation. Isotopic studies are performed with ^{99m}T-labelled sulphur colloid which is taken up by the reticuloendothelial system. More rarely imaging is done with labelled damaged red blood cells which are sequestered in the spleen when it is desirable to look at the functioning spleen alone without interfering activity from the liver. MRI may also prove useful in imaging of the spleen, but indications are not yet clear.

Needle puncture and aspiration for bacteriological or cytological diagnosis can be performed with a fine needle (20–22 gauge) without significant complications.

ANOMALIES

Asplenia

Asplenia has a marked male preponderance. It is usually associated with severe cardiovascular abnormalities and is called Ivemark's syndrome. There is also an associated high incidence of visceral heterotaxy and malrotation of the gastrointestinal tract which may be complicated by volvulus. The prognosis is poor, due to cardiac or infectious complications.

Exceptionally asplenia may occur as an isolated lesion and be discovered during investigation of a severe sepsis or meningitis.

The diagnosis is based on US, scintigraphy and the presence of Howell–Jolly bodies in the peripheral blood.

Polysplenia

This has a female preponderance and is less severe than asplenia. Its known associations include mild cardiovascular anomalies, bilobed lungs, dextrocardia and malrotation. In the non-cardiac polysplenia syndrome, there is an association with biliary atresia (Fig. 4.9.1).

Multiple nodules of spleen are demonstrated on US and CT.

Accessory spleens, fortuitously discovered in about 5% of children, are quite different and are easily recognized and differentiated from polysplenia. Accessory spleens are found as small splenic nodules of 1 cm diameter, localized near the hilum or the inferior pole of the spleen.

Wandering spleen

Owing to deficiency in ligamentous attachments and an abnormally long pedicle, the spleen may wander to an ectopic location.

The usual modes of clinical presentation are either as an abdominal mass, or as acute or chronic torsion. The diagnosis relies on US and on radionuclide scan. The discovery of a wandering spleen constitutes an emergency and requires urgent surgery to avoid complete infarction of the spleen (Fig. 4.9.2).

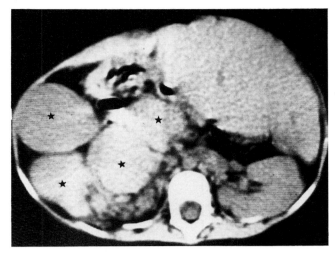

Fig. 4.9.1 Non-cardiac polysplenia (*) syndrome with biliary atresia and abdominal situs inversus.

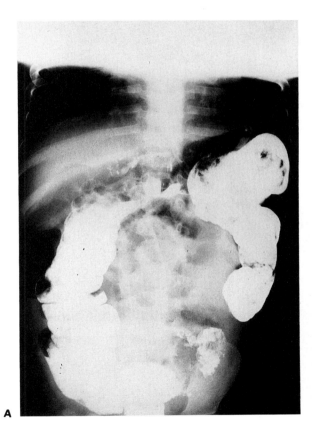

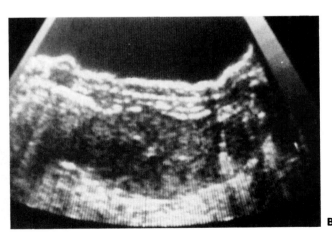

Fig. 4.9.2 Torsion of a wandering spleen. One-year-old boy presenting with acute abdominal pain and a paraumbilical mass. **A** Barium enema performed to rule out intussusception shows the left colonic angle occupying the whole left upper quadrant and the displacement of the descending colon by the mass. **B** US of the abdominal mass: homogeneous solid structure, corresponding to the spleen. Surgery with fixation achieved a cure.

INFECTION

Splenomegaly is present in multiple infectious processes such as typhoid, spirochete infection, mononucleosis and malaria and resolves with adequate treatment.

However direct splenic infection with abscess formation is more unusual. Infectious organisms are various, including amoebiasis, bacteria and candida. The commonest route is the haematogenous spread of bacteria from a focus elsewhere in the body, especially the liver (Fig. 4.9.3). Splenic abscess is seen rarely in immunocompetent children.

Splenic granulomas have also been reported in children with cat scratch disease (Fig. 4.9.4).

REFERENCES

Cox F, Perlman S, Sathyanarayana 1989 Splenic abscesses in cat scratch disease: sonographic diagnosis and follow-up. Journal of Clinical Ultrasound 17: 511–514

Quinn S F, Van Sonnenberg E, Casola G, Wittich G R, Neff C C 1986 Interventional radiology of the spleen. Radiology 161: 289–291

Shiels W E, Johnson J F, Stephenson S R, Huang Y C 1989 Chronic torsion of the wandering spleen. Pediatric Radiology 19: 465–467

Smith W L 1982 The spleen. In: Franken E A (ed) Gastrointestinal imaging in pediatrics, 2nd edn. Harper and Row, London, 469–472

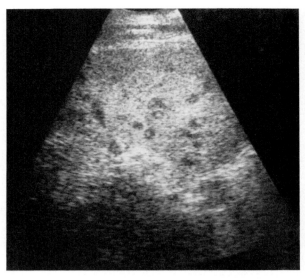

Fig. 4.9.3 Hepatosplenic candidiasis in a 14-year-old boy with leukaemia. Multiple round hypoechoic nodules are present involving the spleen and liver with central echogenic dots: 'wheels within wheels'.

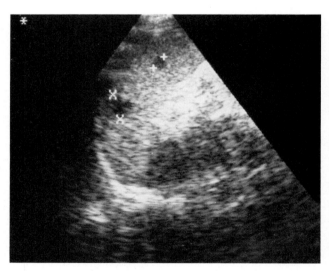

Fig. 4.9.4 Granulomas in cat scratch disease: hypoechoic nodules involving the spleen and also the liver.

TUMOURS

Primary tumours of the spleen are rare.

Benign tumours

Splenic cysts are the most common benign tumours.

Parasitic cysts, caused by hydatid disease, are present in the spleen in only 2–4% of cases (Fig. 4.9.5).

Non-parasitic cysts can be classified as 'true' cysts, containing an epithelial lining, and false or pseudo-cysts without an epithelial lining. 'False' cysts are presumed to be post-traumatic, post-infectious or post-ischaemic. 'True' cysts are epidermoid cysts and usually present as a mass. There is a strong female preponderance. They are usually solitary and may be huge. Clinical presentation is often an incidental finding of an enlarged spleen. The sonographic appearance is highly suggestive with irregular borders, wall trabeculation and calcification, and low-level internal echoes, corresponding to cholesterol crystals (Fig. 4.9.6).

Other benign tumours are rarer and include haemangioma, hamartoma and lymphangioma. The appearance of all these lesions is variable on imaging modalities, with large or small cystic cavities and possible calcifications.

REFERENCES

Dachman A H, Ros P R, Murari P J et al 1986 Non parasitic splenic cysts: a report of 52 cases with radiologic–pathologic correlation. American Journal of Roentgenology 147: 537–542

Pracros J P, Louis D, Tran-Minh V, Defrenne P 1983 Radiologic investigations in epidermoïd cysts of the spleen in children. Annales de Pediatrie 30: 159–165

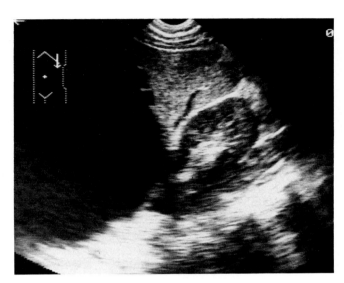

Fig. 4.9.6 Epidermoid cyst. There is a large splenic cyst with irregular borders and internal echoes, highly suggestive of the diagnosis.

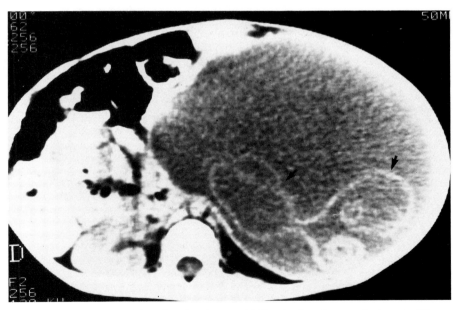

Fig. 4.9.5 Hydatid cyst of the spleen in a 9-year-old Algerian boy. Large splenic cyst with floating of the detached germinative membrane (arrows). Another cyst was present in the liver.

Malignant tumours

Primary malignant tumours are exceptional in childhood and are represented mainly by angiosarcomas. However the spleen is frequently involved in systemic malignancies such as lymphoma, leukaemia and histiocytosis X.

On US, the lymphomatous spleen may present with multiple hypoechoic nodules.

TRAUMA

Because of its fragility and its thoracoabdominal location, the spleen is frequently involved in trauma. Modern management is conservative with avoidance of excision when possible. Decisions are based on the haemodynamic condition of the child.

The main lesions found in trauma include haemoperitoneum, subcapsular haematoma, intraparenchymal haematoma or contusion and fracture (Figs 4.9.7, 4.9.8).

US is usually the first screening procedure because of its availability at the bedside. Examination may be difficult or impossible because of overlying painful rib fractures.

Nuclear medicine scans reliably demonstrate splenic trauma, but must be done as an emergency.

CT is probably the most accurate method of assessing the spleen. Rarely secondary splenic rupture with a normal early examination has been reported.

After trauma, particles of splenic tissue can implant within the chest and the abdomen and become functional as accessory spleens. This condition, referred to as splenosis, may be documented by US or CT.

REFERENCE

Pappas D, Mirvis S E, Crepps T J 1987 Splenic trauma: false negative CT diagnosis in cases of delayed rupture. American Journal of Roentgenology 149: 727–728

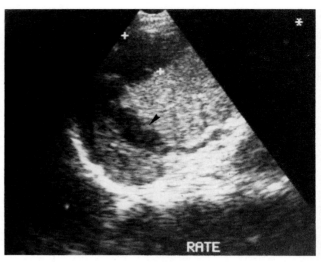

Fig. 4.9.7 Splenic trauma. Eleven-year-old boy with abdominal trauma. There is a fracture of the spleen (arrowhead) and a large perisplenic haematoma. Spontaneous resolution occurred without surgical treatment.

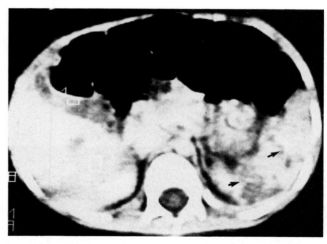

Fig. 4.9.8 Splenic trauma. Four-year-old boy. Multiple fractures of the spleen (arrows) and haemoperitoneum are present. Spontaneous complete healing.

MISCELLANEOUS

Splenic infarcts

They may occur as a complication of leukaemia, sickle cell anaemia, valvular heart disease and diffuse intravascular coagulation. There is a wide range of sonographic appearances reported, probably related to the age of infarct. They are hypoechoic in the earlier stages and hyperechoic in healed infarcts (Fig. 4.9.9). This evolution is suggestive of the diagnosis.

The lesion may be round or wedge shaped, simple or multiple.

REFERENCE

Maresca G, Mirk P, De Gaetano A, Barbaro B, Colagrande C 1986 Sonographic patterns in splenic infarcts. Journal of Clinical Ultrasound 14: 23–28

Gaucher's disease

Discrete focal lesions may be seen in the spleen of patients with Gaucher's disease. These lesions may be hypoechoic, corresponding to focal clusters of Gaucher cells, or hyperechoic and composed of Gaucher cells with fibrosis or infarction (Fig. 4.9.10).

REFERENCE

Hill S C, Reinig J W, Barranger J A, Fuik J, Shawker T H 1986 Gaucher disease: sonographic appearance of the spleen. Radiology 160: 631–634

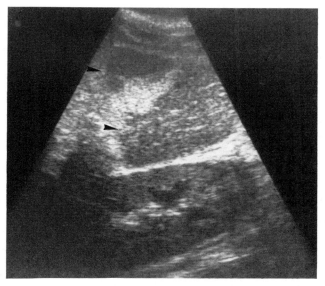

Fig. 4.9.9 Splenic infarct. Five-year-old boy with leukaemia who presented with left upper quadrant abdominal pain and splenomegaly: hypoechoic appearance of the lower pole of the spleen with sharp limits (arrowheads).

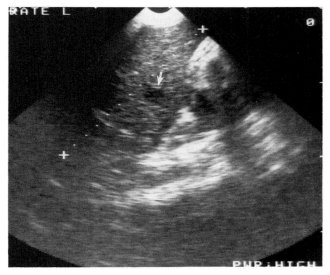

Fig. 4.9.10 Gaucher disease. Sixteen-year-old girl: mild splenomegaly with a few small hypoechoic nodules without significance (Gaucher cells) (arrow).

Splenic calcification

The main causes of splenic calcifications include:

— tuberculosis
— brucellosis
— hydatid cysts
— haemangiomas
— hamartomas
— sequelae of abscess and haematoma
— cat scratch granulomas
— infarction
— sickle cell anaemia
— haemosiderosis.

In longstanding portal hypertension the spleen may become fibrotic but remain large and have multiple linear echogenic structures (Fig. 4.9.11), which have no pathological significance.

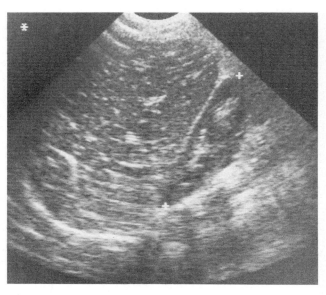

Fig. 4.9.11 Portal hypertension. Fourteen-year-old boy with biliary atresia and portal hypertension. Splenomegaly with multiple hyperechoic linear structures.

5

The urinary tract

E. F. Avni, C. Dicks-Mireaux, S. Neuenschwander, D. Van Gansbeke

INTRODUCTION

The practice of uroradiology in the paediatric population has changed a great deal recently. New imaging techniques have been developed, such as radioisotopes and ultrasound, which enable functional and anatomical information to be obtained in a relatively non-invasive fashion. The routine use of antenatal ultrasound has contributed to a greater understanding of urinary tract pathologies, and the presentation of children with urinary tract abnormalities is now very different. Newborns represent a larger group of patients requiring investigation and we have the opportunity to investigate and cure patients before complications occur.

The investigation of well-recognized diseases such as sepsis, malignant disease and lithiasis has also changed with the impact of new techniques.

5.1   IMAGING TECHNIQUES

Many techniques can be used to image the urinary tract. Ultrasound is widely used as the first imaging modality of any suspected anomaly. It is followed by many other techniques, both radiological and non-radiological. Each patient should have the investigations tailored to the clinical problem.

REFERENCES

Broyer M 1985 Développement pré- et périnatal des fonctions rénales. Journal d'Urologie (Paris) 91: 100–102.
Gonzales J 1985 Relation structure et fonction dans le développement de l'appareil urinaire du foetus. Journal d'Urologie (Paris) 91: 108–117.

ULTRASOUND

Ultrasound provides remarkably detailed information on the urinary tract of the fetus, newborn and child without the use of radiation or invasive venepuncture. It usually directs the further evaluation of most pathologies and has supplanted the intravenous urogram as the initial examination.

Indications

As mentioned above, most patients with suspected pathology relating to the urinary tract will have an ultrasound examination. However more specific indications are given in Table 5.1.1.

Table 5.1.1

Postnatal investigation of suspected antenatal abnormality
Congenital abnormalities, e.g. cloacal anomalies
Sepsis, including urinary tract infection, pyelonephritis
Neuropathic bladder – spina bifida
Hypertension
Haematuria, dysuria
Abdominal mass
Ascites
Renal transplant
Acute renal failure
Screening of patients at risk of developing renal tumours, e.g. spontaneous aniridia
Trauma
Malformation syndromes with urinary tract involvement, e.g. VATER
Nephrocalcinosis
Abdominal pain, e.g. pelviureteric junction obstruction

Technique

The patient should be examined without sedation. Bladder evaluation is an essential part of the assessment of the urinary tract and therefore whenever possible the child should drink prior to the examination and have a full bladder. In some cases, e.g. suspected neuropathic bladder, it may be useful to ask the patient to empty the bladder at the end of the examination and then to assess the postmicturition residue. In infants who are not toilet trained, the bladder should be examined at the beginning of the scan as many babies pass urine and empty their bladders during the examination. If the ureters are visualized this is most easily done on the transverse scan of the bladder. Dilated ureters are seen as cystic structures behind the bladder. Images of the kidneys are obtained in the prone, supine and oblique positions. An assessment of the renal length is possible and normal values are available. Doppler ultrasound and colour flow is used in the evaluation of the transplant kidney. The use of Doppler in the investigation of renal hypertension is more difficult due to respiratory movement.

Antenatal ultrasound: normal appearances (prenatal development of urinary tract)

The human urinary tract is derived from the ureteric bud and the metanephric blastema. During the fifth week of gestation, the ureteric bud arises from the mesonephric blastema, which is an area of undifferentiated mesenchyme in the nephrogenic ridge. The ureteric bud undergoes numerous divisions to form the calyces and tubules. By the end of the fifth month, the entire collecting system, consisting of ureter, renal pelvis, major and minor calyces and between approximately one and three million collecting tubules are formed. With the growth of the ureteric tree, there is proliferation of the metanephric blastema to form the nephrons. By 20 weeks of pregnancy approximately one-third of the nephrons are present and nephrogenesis is completed by 36 weeks.

The production of urine begins between the fifth and ninth week of gestation. The bladder is the first part of the fetal urinary tract to be visualized sonographically. It appears as a small cystic structure in the lower part of the fetal abdomen at around 13–14 weeks' gestation (Fig. 5.1.1). The presence of a filled bladder provides evidence of renal function. The fetal kidneys are visualized at around 16 weeks' gestation and appear as small echogenic masses in the lumbar areas. Mild dilatation of the renal pelvis assists in the identification of the kidneys (Fig. 5.1.2).

The renal length increases with gestational age (Fig. 5.1.3). The circumference of the kidney remains constant throughout gestation at one third to one-quarter of the abdominal circumference.

Corticomedullary differentiation appears gradually and is present after about 28 weeks' gestation (Fig. 5.1.4). Fetal lobulation of the kidneys is often seen and is a normal finding. The normal ureters are not seen antenatally. As the fetus micturates periodically in utero, the fetal bladder can be seen to fill and empty during the ultrasound examination.

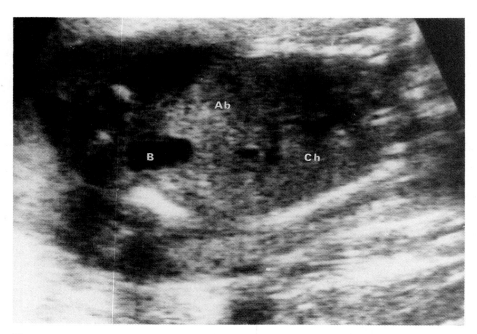

Fig. 5.1.1 Fetal bladder (16 weeks). Sagittal scan of fetal body. Ch = Chest, Ab = abdomen, B = bladder.

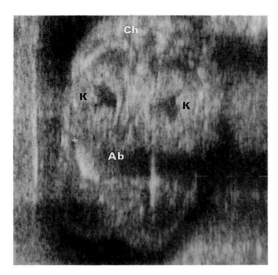

Fig. 5.1.2   Normal fetal kidneys (K) (± 16 weeks). Sagittal scan of fetal abdomen. Mild physiological dilatation is present. Ch = Chest, Ab = abdomen.

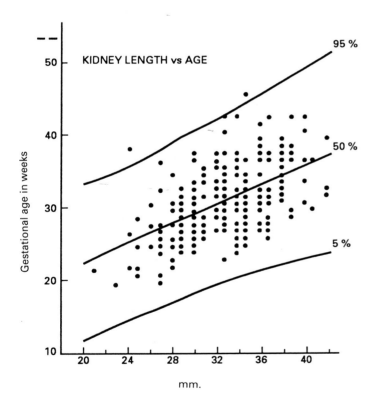

KIDNEY LENGTH vs AGE

95 %

50 %

5 %

Gestational age in weeks

mm.

Fig. 5.1.3   Renal length vs age: experimental values and polynomial regression, 5th and 95th percentites. (Reproduced with permission from Jeanty P, Dramaix-Wilmet M, Elkhazen M, Habinant C, Van Regemarter N 1982 Measurements of fetal kidney growth on ultrasound. Radiology 144: 159 –162.)

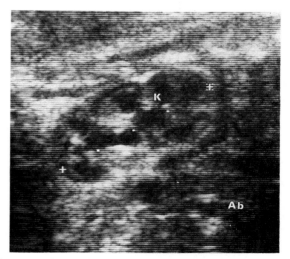

Fig. 5.1.4   Normal fetal kidney (K) (± 30 weeks) (magnified) (between crosses). Sagittal scan of fetal abdomen (Ab). A good corticomedullary differentiation is present.

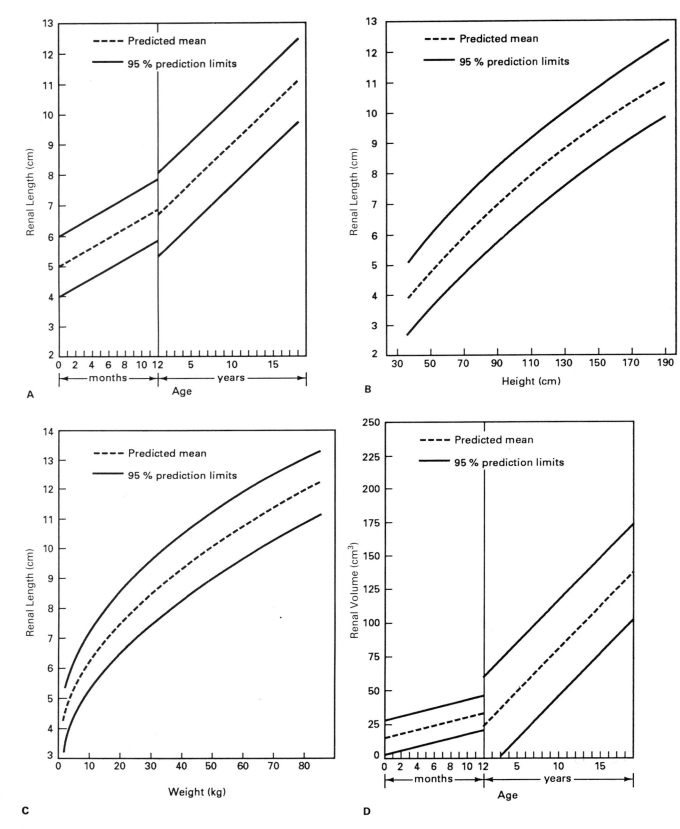

Fig. 5.1.5 Maximum renal length and volume vs age, height and weight. (Reproduced with permission from Han B K, Babcock D S 1985 Sonographic measurements and appearances of normal kidneys in children. American Journal of Roentgenology 145: 611–616.)

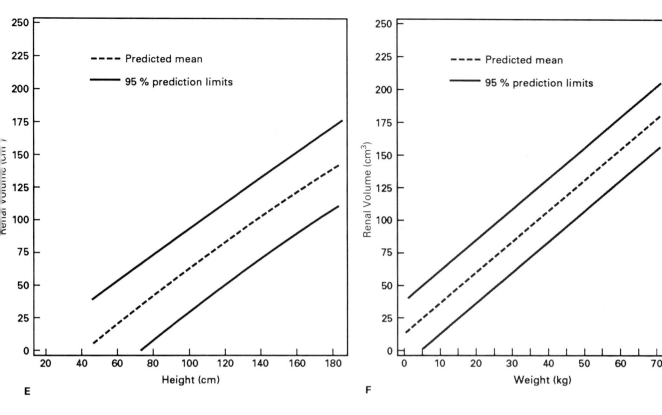

E

F

Postnatal ultrasound: normal appearances

After birth, kidney growth parallels the baby's growth in weight and height (Fig. 5.1.5).

Corticomedullary differentiation is evident in the newborn kidney. The cortex is relatively hyperechogenic and the medulla hypoechoic (Fig. 5.1.6). The cortical hyperechogenicity decreases gradually but corticomedullary differentiation may be seen in late childhood (Fig. 5.1.7). Lobulation of the renal outline is also seen in both fetus and neonate (Fig. 5.1.8). It usually disappears gradually in the neonatal period but may persist. The echogenicity of the renal hilum is low in the neonate and this increases with age due to

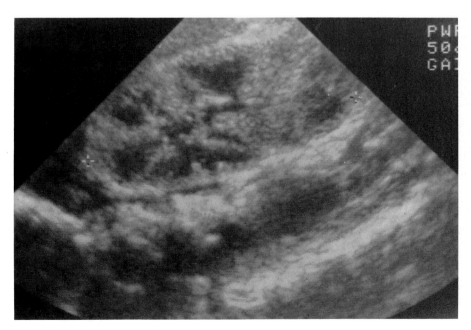

Fig. 5.1.6 Newborn kidney (between crosses). Sagittal scan.
Typical corticomedullary differentiation with relatively hyperechoic cortex.

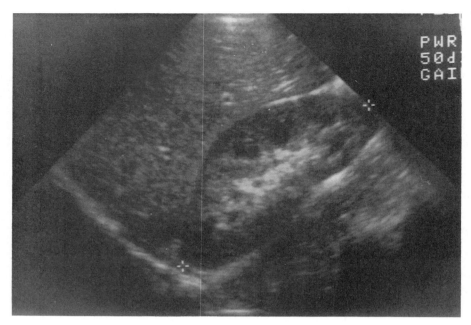

Fig. 5.1.7 Eight-year-old normal right kidney (between crosses). Sagittal scan. A corticomedullary differentiation is still present.

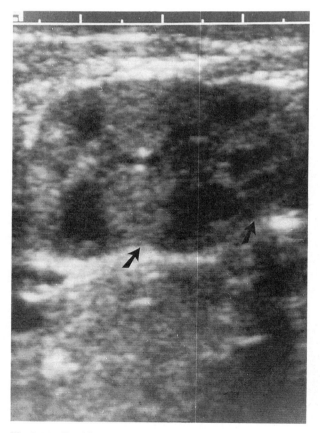

Fig. 5.1.8 Fetal lobulation of the kidney. Prone sagittal scan of a newborn kidney. Lobulation is seen on the anterior part (arrows).

fat deposition (Fig. 5.1.9). In a duplex system, two hilar complexes may be seen separated by a cortical band.

Slight distension of the renal pelvis may be seen in the normal child, and may be more obvious in the prone position. However, the pelvic diameter in the transverse plane should not exceed 5 mm (AP) (Fig. 5.1.9A). Dilatation extending into the calyces is abnormal. Hypertrophy of a column of Bertin (Fig. 5.1.10) is a common normal variant and usually detected in midsections of the kidney on transverse scans. It should not be mistaken for a renal mass.

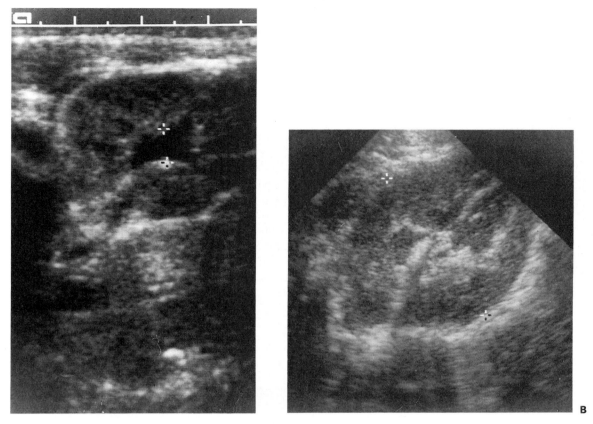

Fig. 5.1.9 Evolution of hilar fat deposition. Tranverse scans of the kidneys. **A** At birth (no fat is present). Mild dilatation of renal pelvis (4 mm). **B** At age 8. Hyperechoic hilum secondary to fat.

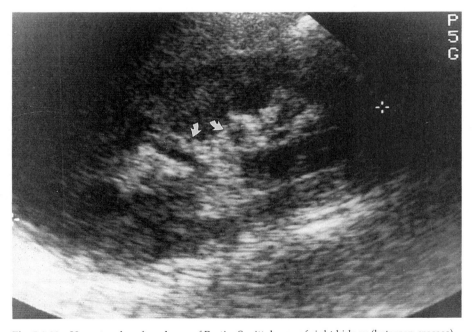

Fig. 5.1.10 Hypertrophy of a column of Bertin. Sagittal scan of right kidney (between crosses). A column of Bertin displaces hilar fat (arrows).

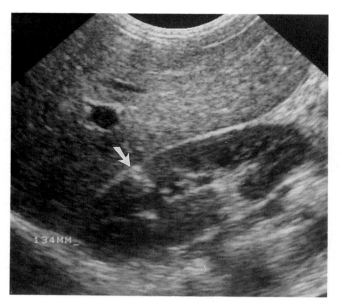

Fig. 5.1.11 Interrenicular junction. Sagittal scan of right kidney. Hyperechoic interrenicular junction is present at the upper pole (arrow).

The interrenicular plane between the upper and middle kidney can be seen as a triangular, or linear, hyperechoic area on the parasagittal scans, and should not be mistaken for a scar (Fig. 5.1.11).

Ureters of normal size are not routinely seen on ultrasound scans. Mild ureteral distension may occur in the normal child who has a very full bladder. It is possible to identify the normal vesicoureteric junction and the submucosal ureteral tunnel. Due to the jet phenomenon, entrance of urine into the bladder from the ureters may be seen as small echoes produced by turbulence (Fig. 5.1.12). This finding does not exclude the presence of vesicoureteric reflux. The typical appearance of the bladder is a round or oval fluid-filled structure (Fig. 5.1.12). Wall thickness, in a filled bladder, should not exceed 4 mm.

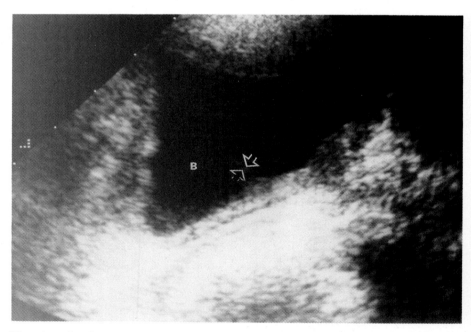

Fig. 5.1.12 Jet phenomenon. Sagittal scan of the bladder (B). The vesicoureteric junction can be localized due to urine entering into the bladder corresponding to the jet phenomenon (arrows).

Assessment of the normal renal vasculature at the renal hilum and at the level of the interlobar and arcuate vessels is possible with duplex Doppler and colour flow Doppler (Figs 5.1.13, 5.1.14). A systematic approach to the paediatric urinary tract, including the kidneys, bladder and ureters, is necessary in order to identify or exclude any pathology (Table 5.1.2).

Table 5.1.2 Renal ultrasound: interpretation

Size – renal length
Number of kidneys
Position
Dilatation of renal pelvis
Dilatation of calyces
Dilated ureters
Cortical thickness
Cortical echogenicity
Corticomedullary differentiation
   Present
   Absent
   Reversed
Cysts
Calcification
Renal masses
Bladder wall thickness
Postmicturition residue

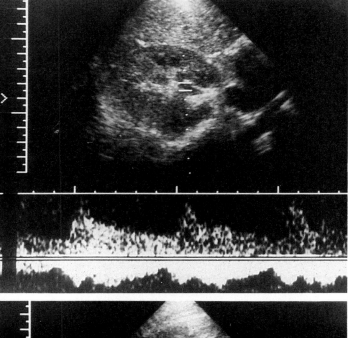

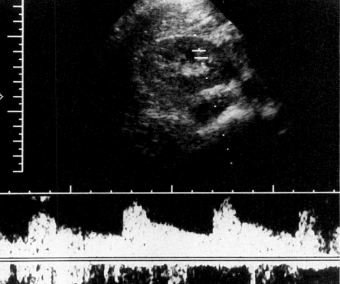

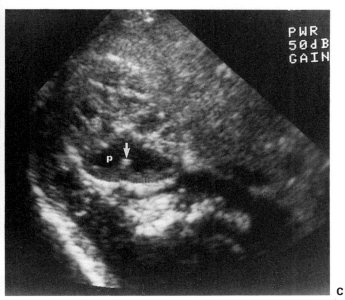

Fig. 5.1.13 Renal vascularization. Transverse scans. **A** Duplex Doppler at the renal hilum; both renal artery (systo-diastolic pattern) and vein (with normal respiratory variations) are evaluated. **B** Duplex Doppler of the interlobar artery. **C** Typical appearance of arcuate vessel (arrow) at the base of a large pyramid (p).

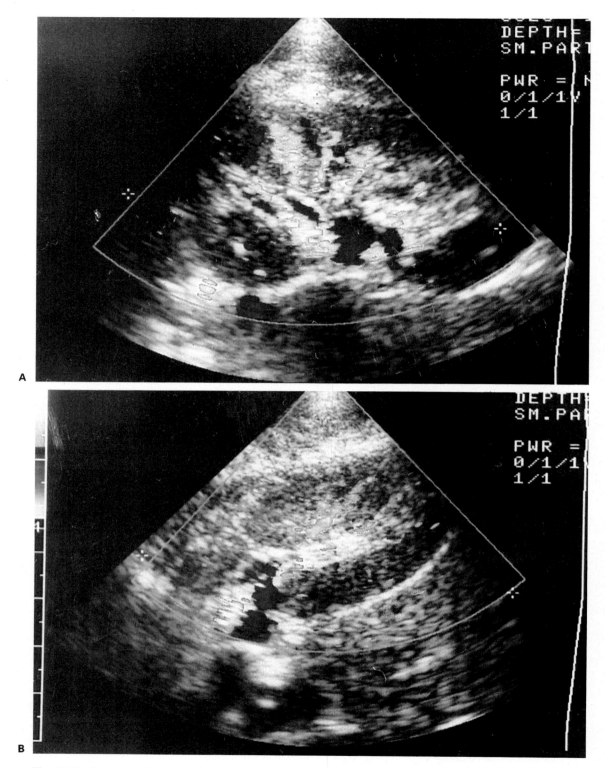

Fig. 5.1.14 Renal vascularization. Colour Doppler. Sagittal (**A**) transverse scans (**B**). Normal venous and arterial flow is displayed as far as the interlobar area.

REFERENCES

Avni E F, Brion L 1982 Ultrasound of the neonatal urinary tract. Urological Radiology 5: 177–181

Bowie J O, Rosenberg E R, Andreotti R F, Fields S I 1983 The changing sonographic appearance of fetal kidneys during pregnancy. Journal of Ultrasound in Medicine 2: 505–507

Carter A R, Horgan J G, Jennings T A, Rosenfield A T 1985 The junctional parenchymal defect: a sonographic variant of renal anatomy. Radiology 154: 499–502

Erwin B C, Caroll B A, Muller H 1985 A sonographic assessment of neonatal renal parameters. Journal of Ultrasound in Medicine 4: 217–220

Haller J O, Berdon W E, Friedman A P 1982 Increased renal cortical echogenecity: a normal finding in neonates and infants. Radiology 142: 173–178

Han B K, Babcock D S 1985 Sonographic measurements and appearances of normal kidneys in children. American Journal of Roentgenology 145: 611–616

Hardwick D, Hendry M A 1984 The ultrasonic appearances of septa of Bertin in children. Clinical Radiology 34: 107–112

Hoffer F A, Mari Hanabergh A, Teele R L 1985 The interrenicular junction. A mimic of renal scarring on normal pediatric sonograms. American Journal of Roentgenology 145: 1075–1078

Hricak H, Slovis T L, Callen C W, Callen P W, Romanski R W 1983 Neonatal kidneys: sonographic anatomic correlation. Radiology 147: 699–702

Jeanty P, Dramaix-Wilmet M, Elkhazen M, Hubinont C, Van Regemorter N 1982 Measurements of fetal kidney growth on ultrasound. Radiology 144: 159–162

Jecquier S, Rousseau O 1987 Sonographic measurements of the bladder wall in children. American Journal of Roentgenology 149: 563–566

Jones B E, Hoffer F A, Teele R L , Lebowitz R L 1990 Pitfalls in pediatric urinary sonography. Urology 35: 38–44

Lawson T L, Foley W D et al 1981 US evaluation of fetal kidneys. Radiology 138: 153–158

Marchal G J, Baert A L, Eeckels, Proesmans W 1983 Sonographic evaluation of the normal ureteral submucosal tunnel in infancy and childhood. Pediatric Radiology 13: 125–129

Marchal G J, Verbecken E, Oyen R, Moerman E, Baert A L, Lauwerijns J 1986 Ultrasound of the normal kidney. A sonographic, anatomic and histologic correlation. Ultrasound in Medicine and Biology 12: 999–1009

Sauvain J L, Pierrot V, Chambers R et al 1989 Echographie et Doppler pulsé des artères du parenchyme rénal au cours des syndromes obstructifs et des dilatations des cavités excrétrices rénales. Journal de Radiologie 70: 389–398

Schlesinger A E, Hedlund G L, Pierson W P, Null D M 1987 Normal standards for kidney length in premature infants: determination with US. Radiology 164: 127–129

Vade A, Lau P, Smick J, Harris V, Ryva J 1987 Sonographic renal parameters as related to age. Pediatric Radiology 17: 212–215

INTRAVENOUS UROGRAPHY

Although the role of the intravenous urogram (IVU) has diminished with the advent of new techniques, it continues to provide important anatomical information in certain specific cases, e.g. tuberculosis. The routine use of intravenous urography is no longer advocated and when it is performed the availability of other techniques may reduce the number of radiographs obtained during one examination.

Good quality images are difficult to obtain in neonates, because of immature renal function and abdominal gas obscuring the detail. Thick section tomography will improve detail. In this group, ultrasound rather than intravenous urography should be the imaging technique of choice. If an IVU is necessary it should if possible be postponed until the baby is 6–12 weeks of age.

Indications

- Anatomical detail, e.g. diverticula
- Diurnal enuresis and suspected ectopic ureter
- Papillary necrosis
- Urinary tuberculosis
- Postoperative evaluation.

Usually, when comprehensive ultrasonography, nuclear medicine and CT are available, the indications for intravenous urography are few. However in some institutions, the IVU is necessary in the further evaluation of the abnormal sonogram, haematuria and duplex systems.

Preparation

No sedation or preparation is required routinely. The use of purgatives is to be avoided in children. Dehydration, with the advent of non-ionic contrast media, is unnecessary and also discouraged.

Technique

A preliminary plain radiograph of the abdomen is performed in order to visualize nephrocalcinosis, calculi or associated skeletal malformations.

Non-ionic contrast media are used if possible as they are associated with less side-effects. Routinely, the dose used is 2–3 ml/kg.

The examination is tailored to the child's problem. In uncomplicated cases the first film obtained is a 5-minute view centred on the kidneys. In newborns and infants a bottle of liquid or a carbonated drink is given after the injection so that the stomach distends with gas and fluid; the tube is gently angled towards the feet and the kidneys are visualized through the distended stomach. A 12–15-minute film of the abdomen is then taken. Despite the routine use of higher concentrations of contrast media, gentle compression of the abdomen with a wide restraining band may be used prior to the 12-minute film to improve visualization of the pelvicalyceal system. This may also assist in the immobilization of the patient. A later 25-minute view of the abdomen is then taken, when compression has been removed (Fig. 5.1.15). On these views, the parenchyma should appear regular and cortical thickness even. The calyces are convex and clearly delineated. With non-ionic contrast media, precalyceal collecting tubules are sometimes physiologically opacified (Fig. 5.1.16). This should be distinguished from abnormal causes of this appearance (Table 5.1.3). On a normal IVU, the complete length of the ureter is not markedly opacified. In children, the bladder is partly intra-abdominal and lateral portions of the bladder ('ears') may lie in the inguinal areas. In cases of obstruction, particularly if function is poor, delayed films should be obtained.

Table 5.1.3   Visualization of precalyceal tubules on IVU
IVU with non-ionic contrast medium Medullary sponge kidney (Cacchi–Ricci) Autosomal recessive polycystic kidney disease Laurence–Moon–Biedl syndrome Ehlers–Danlos syndrome Beckwith–Wiedemann syndrome

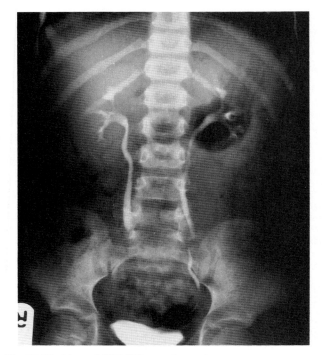

Fig. 5.1.15   Normal IVU. Fifteen-minute view.

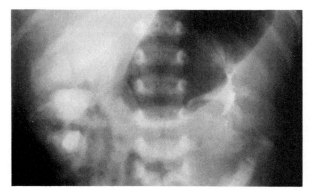

Fig. 5.1.16   IVU with low osmolarity contrast medium. Normal opacification of the precalyceal collecting ducts in the left kidney (case with right megaureter with uterocoele). The right kidney dilatation is due to distension from a ureterocoele.

Premedication and adverse reactions

Adverse reactions are infrequent in children. The examination should not however be performed in a dehydrated child. Non-ionic contrast agents are advocated in children, particularly if there is a history of allergy or previous reaction to contrast. In many institutions, with the falling number of routine IVUs, non-ionic contrast agents are used in all paediatric cases. If there is a clear history of asthma or a previous reaction to contrast, premedication with an antihistamine and oral prednisolone (0.5 mg/kg 6 hourly) should be given for 2 days prior to the examination, to reduce the incidence of adverse reactions. If a mild anaphylactoid reaction occurs (nasal stuffiness, itching, or urticaria) during the examination an antihistamine is effective when necessary, although most mild reactions are harmless. For severe anaphylactoid reactions, subcutaneous adrenaline is the drug of choice, with supplementary oxygen, intravenous fluids and other adrenergic drugs as necessary. A vasovagal attack with bradycardia and hypotension may be treated by laying the patient supine and elevating the lower limbs. It should be remembered that a busy radiology department is not an ideal situation for dealing with cardiorespiratory emergencies and the resuscitation team should be called whenever necessary.

Radiation dose

The gonadal radiation dose of an IVU is related to the number of films obtained and the age of the patient (Table 5.1.4).

Table 5.1.4 Gonadal radiation dose during IVU		
	Gonadal radiation dose (mR per film)	
	Male	Female
6 months		
AP	0.94–14	7.2–10
Pelvis	23–35	24–27
4 years		
AP	1.2–18	11–12
Pelvis	55–62	33–35
12 years		
AP	5.4–60	35
Pelvis	75–84	38–45
From National Council in Radiation Protection and Measurements No. 68 RP. *Pediatric Radiology* 81: 58–63.		

MICTURATING CYSTOURETHROGRAM (MCUG)

Micturating cystourethrography is an essential examination for the evaluation of the anatomy of the bladder and urethra. The presence of vesicoureteric reflux is demonstrated and in the young non-potty-trained infant, the MCUG is the only technique to demonstrate reflux.

If pressure recordings are taken during the examination, urodynamic information relating to bladder and sphincter function can be obtained (see 'urodynamics' below).

Indications/preparation

- Antenatal diagnosis of urinary tract abnormality
- Proven urinary tract infection, in boys and girls
- Enuresis, dribbling
- Trauma
- Duplex systems
- Posterior urethral valves
- Rectal agenesis: to identify a fistula
- Siblings of children with vesicoureteric reflux
- Cloacal anomalies
- Intersex problems.

Sedation is not normally used, and is strongly discouraged as it may affect the infant's ability to cooperate and pass urine.

Examination

If possible the child should void prior to the examination. The perineal and meatal area is washed with antiseptic solution. A 6 French gauge infant feeding tube which has been lubricated with local anaesthetic jelly is gently inserted in the meatus and advanced into the bladder. The procedure is performed with full sterile precautions.

Visualizing the urethra in girls may be difficult. Fusion of the labia minora is sometimes present. These can usually be gently separated, but if this is not possible, topical treatment with oestrogen cream prior to the examination is helpful. The catheter may be inserted into the vagina by mistake. The catheter should be left in place and then a second catheter is inserted into the urethra. The first catheter is then removed. In cases of intersex problems and cloacal anomalies, identification of the separate openings may be difficult. A catheter should be introduced into the most anterior orifice and contrast may be injected blindly in order to identify the urethra and vagina.

In boys, the use of local anaesthetic jelly is recommended to reduce urethral sensation. The foreskin should not be fully withdrawn in the neonate. The catheter should be gently inserted into the meatus. Resistance to the passage of catheter may be met at the level of the external sphincter or bladder neck. Gentle pressure usually overcomes this and the presence of urine in the catheter confirms that the bladder has been reached. A suprapubic approach with a catheter introduced via a suprapubic puncture is sometimes used in boys with a severe phimosis, urethral stricture or other catheter problems. The examination is performed under fluoroscopic control. Spot camera films are ideal, in order to reduce the radiation dose as much as possible. The average gonadal dose for a MCUG is 317 mR for girls and 68 mR for boys.

The bladder is filled with dilute contrast media, using either a continuous infusion from a bottle, or a hand injection with a syringe (Fig. 5.1.17). Mild vesico-ureteric reflux and intraluminal anomalies are not seen during filling. In the neonate and young infant, the bladder is filled until the patient is incontinent and passes urine around the catheter and the catheter is then removed. In the cooperative patient, the bladder is filled until the patient has a strong desire to void, the catheter is then removed and the child asked to void. Voiding films should be taken to demonstrate reflux but also the anatomy of the male urethra. Views in the oblique position are obtained to demonstrate reflux and in the lateral position to demonstrate the male urethra, vesicorectal fistulas and extrinsic displacement of the bladder. It is necessary to visualize the full extent of reflux and to demonstrate the presence of renal and intrarenal reflux and dilatation of calyces when present.

Normal urethral anatomy

The male urethra shows the following normal features which should not be misinterpreted as abnormalities (Fig. 5.1.18): verumontanum, sphincters. Normal sphincter contractions should not be misdiagnosed as stenoses (Figs 5.1.19, 5.1.20). A normal prostatic utricle is sometimes visualized.

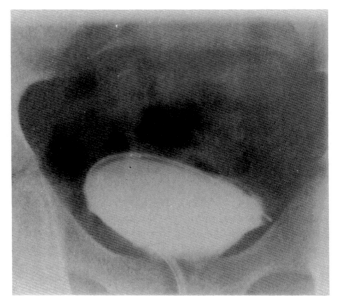

Fig. 5.1.17 MCUG. Partial filling of the bladder.

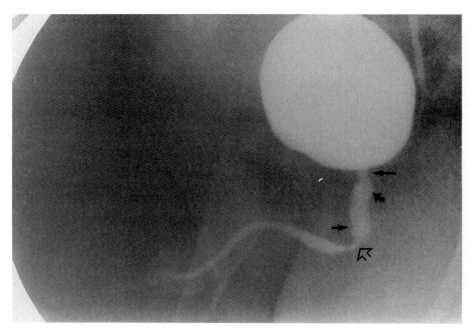

Fig. 5.1.18 MCUG . Normal male urethra. Normal indentations and narrowings related to bladder neck (long arrow), verumontanum (rounded arrow), external sphincter (short arrow) and urogenital membrane (open arrow).

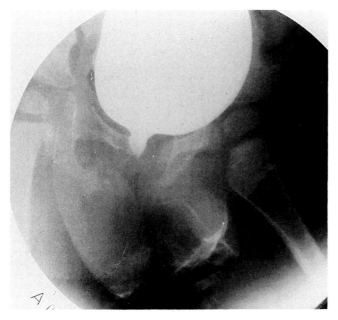

Fig. 5.1.19 MCUG. Male urethra. Normal contraction of the external sphincter. This must not be mistaken for valves.

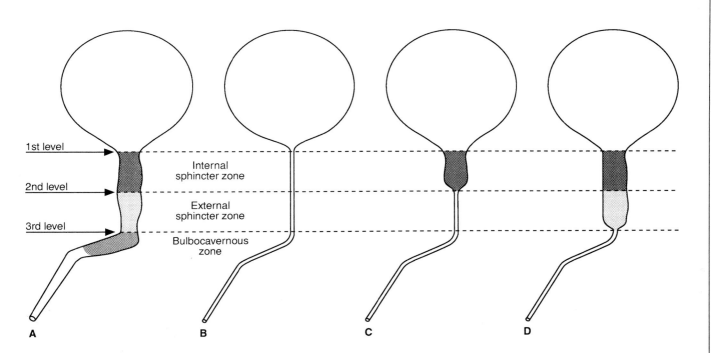

Fig. 5.1.20 Levels and zones of the urethral lumen by the sphincters. **A** Urethra distended during voiding and, **B**, undistended when not voiding. **C** Internal sphincter zone expanded to the second level when the external sphincter is voluntarily contracted during voiding. **D** The internal and external sphincter zones expanded but the lumen is constricted by the voluntary action of the bulbocavernosus muscle. (Reproduced with permission from Stephens F D 1963 Congenital malformation of the rectum, anus and genitourinary tracts. Churchill Livingstone, Edinburgh.)

The female urethra has a simpler anatomy (Fig. 5.1.21). Sphincteric contractions should not be misinterpreted as stenoses. In both sexes, in infancy the bladder may protrude into the inguinal canal to form bladder 'ears'. These protrusions must not be mistaken for diverticula (Fig. 5.1.22).

Complications

Most complications are secondary to poor sterile technique and catheterization. There is a small risk of urinary tract infection following catheterization, and some departments advocate the use of a short course of prophylactic antibiotics following the cystogram.

The catheter may enter and fill a giant utricle or an ureterocoele which may be misinterpreted as the bladder (Fig. 5.1.23). Forceful catheterization may lead to urethral damage and rupture, or bladder rupture. Contrast injected through a catheter in the vagina may lead to hysterosalpingography with peritoneal extravasation. Extravasation may also occur with incorrect placement of a suprapubic catheter.

In bladder outlet obstruction with marked reflux, overdistension of the collecting system, which is inevitable, may cause calyceal rupture and the formation of a urinoma.

Reflux of contrast into the vagina during voiding is a normal and fairly frequent finding.

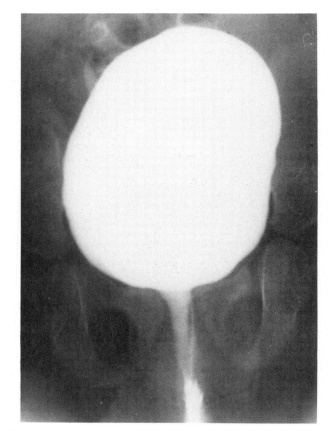

Fig. 5.1.21 MCUG. Normal female urethra.

REFERENCES

IVU and MCUG

Brinkman H 1985 Tolerance of non-ionic contrast media in children. In: Kaufman H (ed.) Contrast media in pediatric radiology workshop Berlin, August 22–24. Karger, Berlin, pp 56–62

Bush 1990 Treatment of systemic reactions to contrast media. Urology 35: 145–159

Fits F B, Herbert S G, Mellins H Z 1977 Criteria for examination of the urethra during excretory urography. Radiology 125: 47–52

Lebowitz R L 1985 Pediatric uroradiology. Pediatrics Clinics of North America 32: 1353–1362

Lebowitz R L 1986 The detection of vesicoureteral reflux in the child. Investigative Radiology 21: 519–531

Lebowitz R L, Ben Ami T 1987 Trends in pediatric uroradiology. Urologic Radiology 5: 135–147

Leibovic S J, Lebowitz R L 1981 Reducing patient dose in VCUG. Urologic Radiology 2: 103–108

Magill H L, Clarke E A, Fitch S J et al 1986 Excretory urography with iohexol: evaluation in children. Radiology 161: 625–630

Meradji M, Ben Gershom E 1984 Excretory urography with four different contrast media. Radiological and biochemical trials in 295 young infants. Annales de Radiologie (Paris) 27: 199–206

Ohlson L 1989 Normal collecting ducts: visualization at urography. Radiology 170: 33–37

Rawlinson B J, Hyde I, Williams J 1988 Quality of urograms in infants: a comparison of diatrizoale, metzizamide and Iohexol. British Journal of Radiology 61: 592–595

Wyly J B, Lebowitz R L 1984 Refluxing ureteral ectopic ureters. Recognition by the cycling VCUG. American Journal of Roentgenology 142: 1263–1267

Zerin M J, Lebowitz R L 1985 Catheter malposition during cystography: a cause of diagnostic errors. American Journal of Roentgenology 153: 363–367

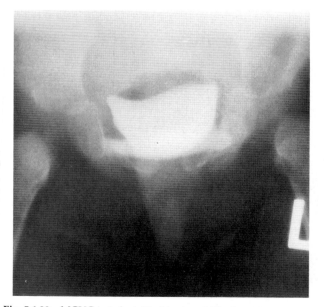

Fig. 5.1.22 MCUG in infant. Bladder 'ears'. The lateral outpouchings are due to herniation of a portion of the bladder into the inguinal canals.

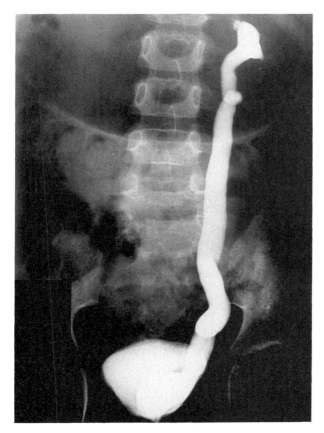

Fig. 5.1.23 MCUG. Complications. Inadvertent catheterization of an ureterocoele. There is also some contrast in the bladder.

ISOTOPES

Radioisotopes are widely used in the assessment of renal morphology and function. The advantages of radionuclide studies are a lower radiation dose when compared with conventional radiographic studies, increased sensitivity compared with radiographic examinations in cases of renal scarring, acute pyelonephritis and small kidneys, and their ability to collect information relating to renal physiology and function.

Preparation and technique

Most nuclear medicine examinations take place in general departments where no special paediatric facilities are available. In order to obtain good quality studies certain general principles should be considered. It is advisable to allow twice as much time for a paediatric study as for an equivalent adult examination. A selection of books, paper and coloured pencils will occupy the child prior to the examination and reduce the anxiety about the impending study. Some young children are unable to cooperate and will require sedation. The dose of radioisotope should be calculated on a body surface area/weight basis. A local anaesthetic cream, if available, should be applied to the proposed site of venepuncture in order to make the injection less painful. A butterfly needle and threeway tap is used so that the isotope syringe can be flushed without disturbing the needle. The child should be amused with books and music and immobilized with sand bags and velcro straps during the examination. The number of images should be reduced to a minimum and the most important images be obtained first. When possible, the camera should be placed with the collimator upwards, so that the child lies on top of the camera with nothing above. This is not possible in renal transplant studies.

Radioisotope studies of the renal tract can be divided into three groups: dynamic renal scintigraphy, static renal scans and radionuclide cystography.

Dynamic renal scintigraphy

These studies are carried out using either ^{99m}Tc-DTPA or ^{99m}Tc-MAG3. The major indications for these studies are:

- Assessment of differential renal function
- Investigation of renal tract dilatation and obstruction
- Evaluation of renal transplant
- Assessment of established systemic hypertension.

DTPA is not protein bound in blood and is filtered by the glomerulus without any tubular handling; MAG3 is 90% protein bound and actively secreted by the proximal tubules with no filtration. In most situations either DTPA or MAG3 can be used, however MAG3 should be used in children under 2 years of age as the high protein binding and increased renal extraction allows clearer visualization of the kidneys when compared with DTPA. The dynamic renal scan has virtually replaced intravenous urography in the investigation of hydronephrosis.. The advantage is the reduced radiation burden, the ability to quantify renal function and response to a diuretic stimulus, and also the lower morbidity and mortality from the radionuclide compared with contrast medium (Fig. 5.1.24).

Techniques of renography vary in detail. One technique is as follows. The isotope is injected intravenously, sixty 20-second frames are recorded and a blood sample is taken at 20 minutes, followed immediately by an injection of 1 mg/kg frusemide, into a different venepuncture site. Recording continues for a further 12 minutes and postmicturition images are taken. It is important to end the study with an image of an empty bladder, as a full bladder may impair drainage of the renal tract and give a false diagnosis of obstruction. Newer techniques, now widely practised in paediatic hospitals, have eliminated the need for a blood sample at 20 minutes. Instead, counts are taken over the heart to provide information for curve analysis. This is simpler to perform. Diuretic renography is difficult to assess in neonates because the immature kidney is unresponsive to frusemide, and little response is seen under 6 months of age so curves look flat. The renal function, be it ERPF or GFR is reliably calculated. In general most urologists will not operate on neonatal kidneys unless quantitative assessment shows diminished function.

In interpreting renograms for function it is important to view the images as well as the curves and to take note of both the three minute uptake and the final quantitative estimation of GFR or ERPF.

Static renal scans

Scanning with ^{99m}Tc-DMSA is sensitive for the detection of regional cortical impairment. The indications are:

- Diagnosis of a renal scar
- Follow-up reflux nephropathy
- Establishment of renal involvement in acute urinary tract infection
- Diagnosis of acute pyelonephritis
- Possible renal agenesis and small kidneys
- Renal fusion and ectopia
- Sustained systemic hypertension
- Diagnosis of hypertension
- Renal masses.

Images of the kidneys are taken 2 hours after intravenous injection of the isotope. In addition to the routine posterior views, anterior left and right oblique views are required (Fig. 5.1.25).

It is now well established that the DMSA scan is the most sensitive method for the detection of renal scars and has replaced intravenous urography in the investigation of urinary tract infection and reflux nephropathy. In acute renal involvement, there are areas of reduced uptake which may be single or multiple. In chronic reflux nephropathy, a small kidney with peripheral defects and a deformed outline is seen.

A DMSA scan with inhibition of the angiotensin converting enzyme (ACE) using captopril is useful in establishing a renovascular cause for hypertension.

Occasionally, reflux damage is manifest by a smooth, small kidney without focal scarring. A discrepancy in uptake between the kidneys of more than 10% is considered significant. DMSA scanning is an excellent method of monitoring progress (Fig. 5.1.26).

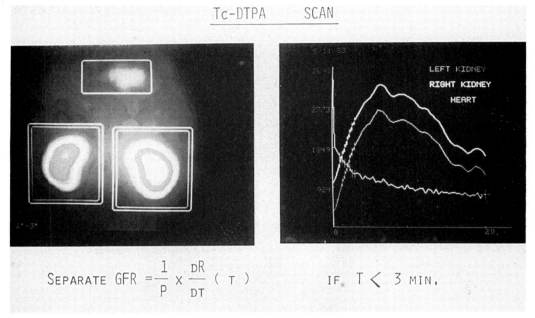

Tc-DTPA   SCAN

LEFT KIDNEY
RIGHT KIDNEY
HEART

$$\text{SEPARATE GFR} = \frac{1}{P} \times \frac{dR}{dT} \, (T) \qquad \text{IF} \; T < 3 \; \text{MIN.}$$

Fig. 5.1.24 ^{99m}Tc-DTPA isotope study. Glomerular filtration transit time, typical graph (right).

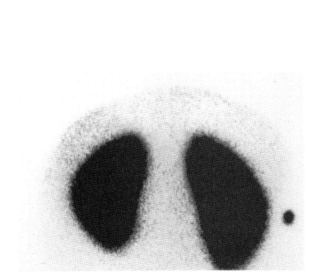

Fig. 5.1.25A   Normal DMSA isotope study. Posterior view shows bilateral normal functioning kidneys. Black dot is cobalt marker.

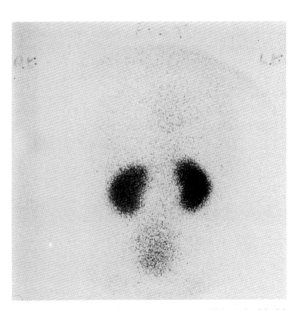

Fig. 5.1.25B   Normal DMSA scan at 6/52. DMSA in the bladder is due to renal immaturity and is normal at this age.

Radionuclide cystography

Vesicoureteric reflux may be detected with an indirect radionuclide cystogram (IRC) or with a direct radionuclide cystogram (DRC).

A DRC is similar to a MCUG and requires catheterization of the bladder. Saline and 500 µCi of ^{99m}Tc-pertechnetate are instilled into the empty bladder until the bladder is full and micturition occurs. The entire procedure is carried out, on top of, or in front of the gamma camera, with the renal areas and the bladder in the field of view at all times. This technique is very sensitive for the detection of reflux with a much lower radiation dose than a conventional MCUG.

Studies using ^{99m}Tc-DTPA or MAG3 suggest that an IRC cystogram is as sensitive as an MCUG in detecting vesicoureteric reflux. The study is carried out with ^{99m}Tc-MAG3 which is injected intravenously; 30 minutes later 70% of the activity is in the bladder and the child is asked to void, while placed in front of the gamma camera, with the renal areas and bladder in the field of view. The time activity curves are generated over these fields of interest (Fig. 5.1.27). ^{99m}Tc-MAG3 is used in preference to DTPA because of the higher kidney to background activity. The low radiation dose and avoidance of bladder catheterization make indirect radionuclide cystography a valuable technique for the detection of vesicoureteric reflux in the cooperative toilet-trained child.

REFERENCES

Boldrach N H, Ramos O L, Goldraich I H 1989 Urography versus DMSA scans in children with vesico-ureteral reflux. Pediatric Nephrology 3: 1–5

Conway J J, King L R, Belman B, Thorton T 1975 Direct and indirect radionuclide cystography. Journal of Urology 113: 689–693

Gordon I 1987 Indications for ^{99m}Technecium DMSA scans in children. Journal of Urology 137: 464–467

Piepsz A, Dobbeleir A, Erbsmann F 1977 Measurement of separate clearance by means of Tc DTPA complex and a scintillation camera. European Journal of Nuclear Medicine 2: 173–177

Piepsz A, Hall H, Ham H R, Permitter N, Collier F 1986 Radioisotopic evaluation of the renal parenchymal function in children with UPJ obstruction. A retrospective study. European Journal of Pediatrics 145: 207–210

Piepsz A, Ham H R, Roland J H et al 1986 Tc DMSA imaging and the obstructed kidney. Clinical Nuclear Medicine 11: 389–391

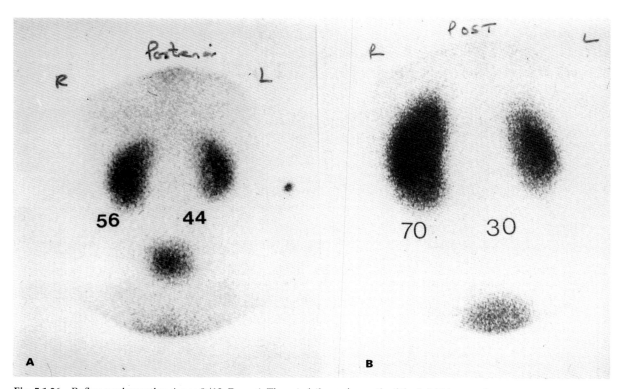

Fig. 5.1.26 Reflux nephropathy: **A** age 9/12, **B** age 4. There is failure of growth of the left kidney and compensatory hypertrophy of the right.

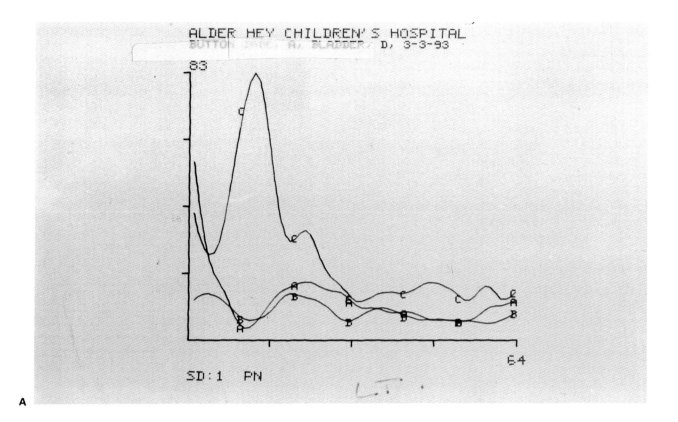

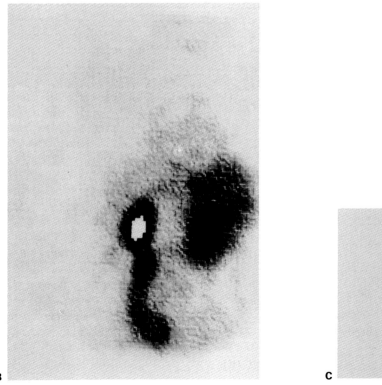

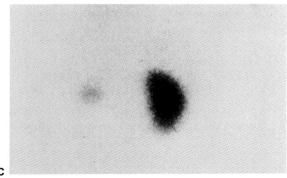

Fig. 5.1.27 Child with reflux damage on left. Indirect voiding cystogram: (**A**) Time activity curve over the left kidney. Note rise in counts in curve C due to reflux. (**B**) Image during voiding showing left reflux. Contrast in the right is due to prior renogram. (**C**) DMSA scan: there is virtually no left renal function.

COMPUTED TOMOGRAPHY (CT)

Faster scanning times and high resolution scanners have made CT scanning a useful technique for imaging paediatric renal disease.

Indications

- Renal masses:
  — staging and extent of tumours
  — renal abscesses
- Abdominal trauma
- Complications of renal transplantation
- Complicated renal cystic disease.

Preparation

Patients should be fasted for 3 hours prior to the examination.

Patients should not move during the examination and therefore sedation may be required. Many sedation regimens are in current practice, none of which are perfect.

Over the age of 3 years it may be possible to scan patients without sedation and each child should be assessed individually.

If oral contrast medium is required, this should be given 30–40 minutes prior to the scan to opacify the small intestine. In some cases, e.g. scans of the bladder, contrast is given 18–24 hours prior to the scan to opacify the rectum and distal colon.

Technique

This may vary according to the clinical indications. Contiguous slices, 10 mm thick, are obtained through the kidneys, including the liver and bladder if necessary. In cases of renal masses, images both before and after intravenous contrast medium are obtained; 3 ml/kg is given as a bolus and the scan is performed immediately after the injection with no interscan delay in order to obtain good constrast in the renal parenchyma and major vessels.

In cases of abdominal trauma, scans following intravenous contrast alone may be sufficient and again dynamic scans following a bolus injection are obtained.

At the end of the scan, it is often useful to obtain a plain abdominal radiograph to demonstrate the ureters.

Normal anatomy

Normal kidneys are easily identified with CT. The attenuation of renal parenchyma of normal kidneys on precontrast scans is slightly less than liver (Fig. 5.1.28), and enhances up to 80–120 HU with contrast (Fig.

5.1.29). Following contrast injection, the cortex enhances more than the medulla with corticomedullary differentiation that may last 1–3 minutes. Subsequently opacification of the pelvicalyceal system and ureters occurs. Layering of dense contrast may be seen in the bladder, obscuring intraluminal masses.

MAGNETIC RESONANCE IMAGING (MRI)

Advances in MRI have changed the approach to many paediatric conditions because excellent tissue-contrast differentiation, high resolution multiplanar capability and lack of ionizing radiation make it a very useful tool. Unfortunately at present MRI is not universally available, and because of lengthy scan times sedation is required in many cases.

Indications/preparation

Sedation in young children is required to obtain a good study, and in some cases general anaesthesia may be required. Indications are similar to CT. MRI has been demonstrated to be as good as CT in the evaluation of renal masses. It is also useful in the evaluation of complex congenital anomalies associated with cloacal anomalies and anorectal anomalies. The neuropathic bladder may be demonstrated and MRI of the spine is useful to look for underlying causes such as spinal dysraphism. In the majority of cases renal cystic disease is assessed with ultrasound; however MRI may be useful in difficult cases and in the demonstration of complications such as haemorrhage into the cysts. MRI may also have a role in renal transplant assessment, but at present is not routinely used in paediatrics. Multiplanar T_1-weighted images, particularly in the coronal plane, are the most useful in the assessment of the kidney and lower urinary tract. T_2-weighted images may be helpful if there is associated haemorrhage. Intravenous contrast, gadolinium-DTPA in combination with T_1-weighted sequences, may provide additional information in renal abscesses and tumours.

Normal appearances

The kidneys are clearly visualized on coronal T_1-weighted images, and because the renal medulla has a longer relaxation time than the renal cortex these two zones are differentiated in the normal kidney (Fig. 5.1.30). Signal intensity of the cortex is similar to the liver, and that of the medulla slightly less.

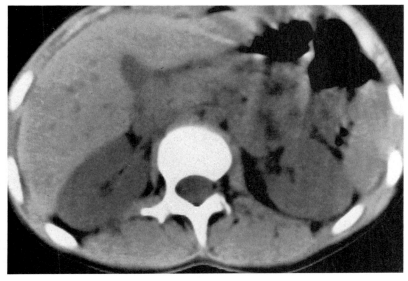

Fig. 5.1.28 CT. Normal non-enhanced appearance of the kidneys.

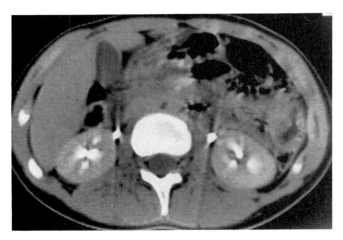

Fig. 5.1.29 CT of the kidneys. Appearance after contrast injection. Pyelocalyceal system and ureters are opacified.

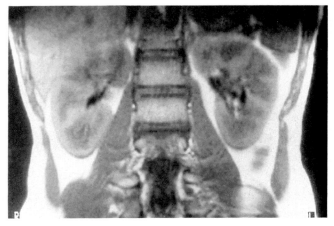

Fig. 5.1.30 MRI. T$_1$-weighted image. Frontal view of normal kidneys. Typical corticomedullary differentiation.

REFERENCES

CT and MRI

Boechat M I, Kangarloo H 1989 MR imaging of the abdomen in children. American Journal of Roentgenology 152: 1245–1250

Cohen M D 1988 Kidneys. In: Siegel M J (ed) Pediatrics body CT. Churchill Livingstone Edinburgh, pp 135–175

Dietrich R B, Kangarloo H 1986 Kidneys in infants and children. Evaluation with MRI. Radiology 159: 215–221

Dietrich R B, Kangarloo H 1987 Pelvic abnormalities in children. Assessment with MRI. Radiology 163: 367–370

Kaufman R A 1989 Technical aspects of abdominal CT in infants and children. American Journal of Roentgenology 153: 549–554

Kuhn J P, Berger P E 1981 Computed tomography of the kidney in infancy and childhood. Radiologic Clinics of North America 19: 445–458

Zeman R K, Cronan J J, Rosenfield A G et al 1986 CT of renal masses. Pitfalls and anatomic variants. Radiographics 6: 351–372

ANGIOGRAPHY

With the development of US, CT and MRI the need for conventional angiography has decreased dramatically. MRI is now able to provide angiographic images of the aorta and main renal arteries, and US with colour flow and Doppler yields considerable information about renal blood flow. However angiography remains important in the following situations:

- Renal hypertension
  — renal artery stenosis
  — fibromuscular hyperplasia
- Renal artery stenosis following renal transplant
- Renal arteriovenous malformations
- Connective tissue disorders, e.g. systemic lupus, polyarteritis nodosa.

In many instances arteriography is required not only for diagnosis but also for therapeutic reasons. Balloon dilatation of vascular stenosis, and embolization of arteriovenous malformations is possible in children.

URODYNAMICS

Urodynamic investigations are used to evaluate functional bladder problems. Several different techniques are available, ranging from an ultrasound assessment of postmicturition residual bladder volume, to formal videourodynamics with pressure studies.

Indications

- Assessment of neuropathic bladder, e.g. myelomeningocoele, spinal dysraphism
- Diurnal incontinence, urgency and frequency
- Assessment of bladder reconstruction, e.g. caecocystoplasty
- Voiding difficulties
- Prerenal transplant.

Ultrasound

An ultrasound examination is able to evaluate bladder capacity and in combination with a urinary flow rate, mean and maximum flow rates, flow pattern and postmicturition residual volume. Its advantages are that it does not need contrast administration or ionizing radiation and is much less frightening for a child than conventional videourodynamics. In the patient with a neuropathic bladder large postmicturition residues may be found, and may be the cause of incontinence. Abnormal flow rates are also seen in patients with urethral strictures. The urinary flow rate is influenced by the initial bladder volume and should be assessed with caution if less than 100 ml of urine is passed.

Similarly, some doubt has been expressed about the accuracy of ultrasound bladder volume measurements. However if these limitations are understood much useful information may still be gained from the examination.

Isotopes

Urodynamic assessment with pressure studies is possible if a small amount of isotope is introduced into the bladder, and images during filling and micturition obtained. The presence of reflux and bladder emptying can be demonstrated. The radiation dose to the patient is less than with a conventional video urodynamic study, but unfortunately insertion of a bladder catheter is required.

The indirect radionuclide cystogram (IRC), has also been shown to be capable of providing considerable information about bladder function. If the voided urine volume and activity are measured and correction factors applied for decay and attenuation, then quantification provides both full and residual bladder volumes and maximum urine flow rate.

Videourodynamics

Videourodynamics remains the standard investigation for evaluating the bladder. During the investigation pressure recordings of the pressure in the rectum and the pressure in the bladder are obtained. Continuous subtraction of these recordings provides a pressure reading known as detrusor pressure which reflects changes due to the tension in the bladder wall and is not affected by coughing or abdominal straining. The bladder is slowly filled with contrast medium via a urethral catheter, and a video mixing facility is used to display the pressure tracing and the image of the bladder on the television screen. In this way the visual record of the bladder behaviour can be interpreted in the light of pressure changes.

Abnormalities such as bladder neck weakness with incontinence, detrusor instability or the unstable bladder, reduced bladder compliance and dyssynergic bladder neck activity can be assessed. The full range of findings will not be discussed here and readers should refer to more specialized texts.

REFERENCES

Boothroyd A E, Dixon P J, Christmas T J, Chapple C R, Rickards D 1990 The ultrasound cystodynamogram – a new radiological technique. British Journal of Radiology 63: 331–332
Saxton H M 1990 Urodynamics: the appropriate modality for the investigation of frequency, urgency, incontinence and voiding difficulties. Radiology 175: 307–316
Van der Vis-Melsen M J, Baert R J, Rajnherc J R, Groen J M, Bemelmans L M, De Nej J J 1989 Scintigraphic assessment of lower urinary tract function in children with and without cutflow tract obstruction. British Journal of Urology 64: 263–269

5.2 ANOMALIES OF KIDNEY NUMBER, SIZE AND POSITION

ABNORMAL NUMBER OF KIDNEYS

Bilateral renal agenesis (1 : 4000 live births)

This condition is diagnosed in utero when no renal tissue is identified after 16–18 weeks' gestation. No urine is present in the fetal bladder. Oligohydramnios, pulmonary hypoplasia and characteristic facies with low-set ears (Potter's syndrome) are associated features. The adrenal glands appear larger than usual and may be mistaken for kidneys.

The differential diagnosis is renal hypoplasia but in most cases even small kidneys are visualized with a careful ultrasound examination.

Unilateral renal agenesis (1 : 450 live births)

In utero, no renal tissue is detected in one of the lumbar areas (Fig. 5.2.1). After birth, the diagnosis is confirmed by ultrasound examination. A ^{99m}Tc-DMSA scan should be performed in order to exclude a small functioning ectopic kidney which may not be visualized on ultrasound. Hypertrophy of the remaining kidney occurs. In left renal agenesis, the splenic flexure of the colon occupies the lumbar area and should not be mistaken for a kidney on ultrasound.

Renal agenesis is associated with many syndromes and with the Vater complex. Renal agenesis is also strongly associated with gynaecological anomalies in girls and to a lesser extent genital anomalies in boys. Cyst of the seminal vesicle ipsilateral to renal agenesis has been described. It is also established that there is a familial link between renal agenesis and dysgenesis. An ultrasonographic study of the first degree relatives of babies with agenesis or dysgenesis showed a 9% incidence of asymptomatic renal disease. It would therefore seem reasonable to screen siblings and parents of children with renal agenesis.

Renal agenesis has to be differentiated from a small involuted, multicystic, dysplastic kidney, and a kidney that is non-functioning as a result of a neonatal vascular accident.

Supernumerary kidney

This is a rare condition where a mass of renal tissue has no parenchymatous connection with the normal kidney. It lies caudal to the normal kidney and is usually small. The ureter either joins or enters separately into the bladder.

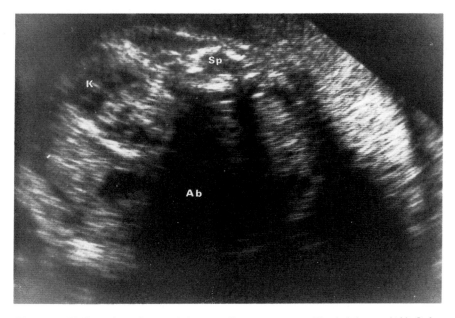

Fig. 5.2.1 Unilateral renal agenesis in utero. Transverse scan of fetal abdomen (Ab). Only one kidney (K) is seen. Sp = fetal spine.

ABNORMAL KIDNEY SIZE

As mentioned previously, the kidneys can be measured and compared with normal values established for age, height or weight. This leads to the detection of large or small kidneys. The spectrum of diagnosis is wide. US is the initial imaging modality in the assessment of the aetiology (refer to the various chapters for detailed descriptions).

Large kidneys See Tables 5.2.1, 5.2.2

Table 5.2.1 Unilateral nephromegaly
Obstruction
Duplex system
Inflammation/acute pyelonephritis
Trauma
Renal vein thrombosis
Tumours/tumour-like conditions
Wilms' tumour
Mesoblastic nephroma
Renal cell carcinoma
Abscess
Hydatid cyst
Renal cyst
Cystic duplication
Xanthogranulomatous pyelonephritis
Compensatory hypertrophy

Table 5.2.2 Bilateral nephromegaly
Nephrotic syndrome
Cystic diseases
Autosomal recessive polycystic kidney disease
Autosomal dominant polycystic kidney disease
Tuberous sclerosis
Acute pyelonephritis
Duplex systems (complicated or not)
Obstructed kidneys (pelviureteric junction, vesicoureteric junction)
Bilateral renal vein thrombosis (acute)
Bilateral Wilms'
Infiltration
Leukaemia
Lymphoma
Nephroblastomatosis
Amyloidosis
Glycogen storage disease

Small kidneys See Table 5.2.3

Table 5.2.3 Unilateral (U) or bilateral (B) small kidneys	
Congenital hypoplasia	U/B
Renal aplasia (Potter II$_B$)	U
Renal dysplasia	U/B
Sequelae of cortical necrosis	U/B
Sequelae of renal vein thrombosis	U/B
Sequelae of pyelonephritis	U/B
Postobstructive atrophy	U/B
Renal artery stenosis	U/B
Postoperative	U/B

Renal hypoplasia

Hypoplastic kidneys refer to congenitally small kidneys with less than the normal number of cells or nephrons. The condition may be unilateral or bilateral.

Unilateral conditions are usually asymptomatic. Ultrasound shows small kidneys with preserved corticomedullary differentiation. Renal function when assessed by isotopes, is good.

Bilateral renal hypoplasia is usually associated with chronic renal failure. In utero, polyhydramnios may be present. On US, in utero and after birth, both kidneys are small (Fig. 5.2.2) when compared with normal values. The cortex is hyperechoic or heterogeneous. The function on IVU or isotope studies may be poor. Histologically, there is a reduction in the total number of nephrons, large glomeruli and dilated tubules (so-called oligomegalonephric hypoplasia).

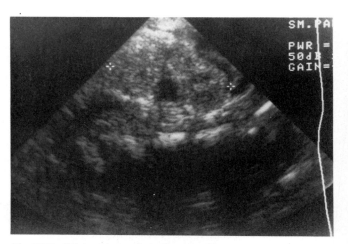

Fig. 5.2.2 Bilateral hypoplasia diagnosed in utero. US at birth. Sagittal scan of the kidney. Small kidney (2 cm between crosses) with poor cortico-medullary differentiation.

Renal dysplasia

Dysplasia is due to disordered differentiation of the metanephros, resulting in a poorly functioning kidney. Dysplastic renal tissue is found in multicystic dysplastic kidneys, renal cystic diseases, obstruction, vesicoureteric reflux and some congenital anomalies, e.g. Jeune's asphyxiating thoracic dystrophy, Zellweger's cerebrohepatorenal syndrome.

Insults to the developing kidney in utero or after birth may result in poor growth and renal dysplasia. Severe obstruction in utero may result in renal rupture and the formation of a urinoma. The result at birth is a dysplastic kidney (Fig. 5.2.3).

Renal dysplasia does not have a characteristic and diagnostic appearance on imaging, but there are features on US which are suggestive (Table 5.2.4, Fig. 5.2.4). Abnormal appearances on antenatal US may suggest the presence of dysplasia in the fetus. Renal function is best evaluated with isotope studies (DMSA). If function is very poor an MCUG demonstrating reflux and abnormal calyces may also suggest dysplasia (Fig. 5.2.5). The contralateral kidney may subsequently show compensatory hypertrophy resulting in an increase in size and diffuse (Fig. 5.2.6) or localized parenchymal hyperechogenicity thought to be the result of glomerular hyperfiltration. (See 5.16 'Renal transplant'.)

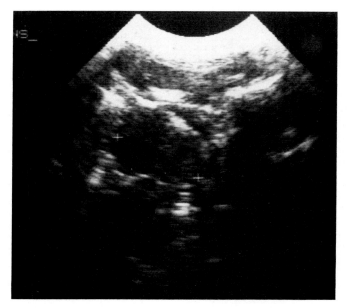

Fig. 5.2.3 Hypodysplastic kidney. US. 2 cm length kidney (between crosses). A resolving urinoma was seen in utero. This non-functioning kidney was removed.

Table 5.2.4 Dysplasia patterns (US)

Small or large kidneys
Thin cortex
Hyperechoic cortex – heterogeneous cortex
Cysts
    Diffuse
    Peripheral

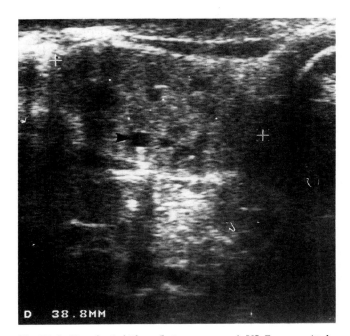

Fig. 5.2.4 Dysplastic kidney (between crosses). US. Prone sagittal scan. No corticomedullary differentiation. Hyperechoic cortex. Parenchymal cyst (arrowhead). Case with posterior urethral valves.

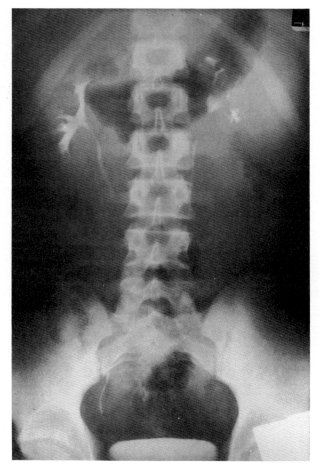

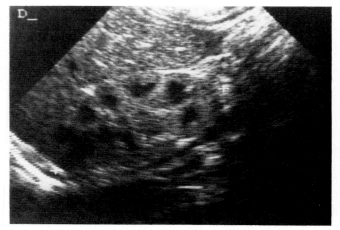

Fig. 5.2.5 Left renal hypoplasia. IVU in a 14 yr. old admitted with splenic trauma. At ultrasound a small left kidney was seen. This boy had never had urinary symptoms. The features of dysplasia are a small smooth kidney with abnormal calyces but no ureteric or pelvic dilatation. He did not have reflux on MCUG.

Fig. 5.2.6 Hyperfiltration. US. Sagittal scan at age of 6 months. Cortical hyperechogenicity with preserved corticomedullary differentiation.

ABNORMAL POSITION OF KIDNEYS

Abnormal orientation of individual kidneys

Abnormal orientation of kidneys is not uncommon and not usually of pathological significance.

Horseshoe kidneys and other types of renal fusion

Horseshoe kidney is the commonest form of renal fusion (1 : 312 live births) (Table 5.2.5). It may be associated with other congenital anormalies, e.g. Turner's syndrome. In most cases, the lower poles are fused and there is an isthmus, or 'bridge', which lies anterior to the spine. This may be difficult to visualize on US and is often better identified with DMSA isotope scanning (Fig. 5.2.7) or CT . On IVU, a horse-shoe kidney is suspected if there is convergence of the long axis of the kidneys or medially directed calyces (Fig. 5.2.8). Occasionally, patients with stones or obstruction are found to have horseshoe kidneys. One part of a horseshoe kidney may rarely present with a Wilm's tumour or a multicystic kidney.

Table 5.2.5 Classification of renal fusion

I *Monopolar fusion*
   A   Homopolar fusion
      1   'Horseshoe' kidney: it involves the inferior poles and is the most frequent variety of fusion
   B   Heteropolar fusion
      1   'L-shape' kidney: one kidney is in crossed ectopia lying transversally; it fuses its superior pole with the inferior pole of the contralateral kidney
      2   'Superimposed' kidney: one kidney is in crossed ectopia, lying vertically; it fuses its upper pole with the lower pole of the other kidney
      3   'Sigmoid' kidney: both kidneys are ectopic, lying transversly near the midline; one superior pole is fused with the inferior pole of the contralateral kidney

II *Bipolar fusion*   A   'Ring' kidney: both kidneys are ectopic; fusion occurs at the level of both poles

III *Medial fusion*
   A   'Cake' kidney (complete fusion): both kidneys are ectopic and totally fused medially
   B   'H-shaped' kidney (hilar fusion): the kidneys are mainly fused at the level of their hilar regions
   C   'Y-shaped kidney': hilar fusion with only one excretory system (our case)

Reproduced with permission from Ascoli R, Pavone C, Cavallo N 1988 Hilar fusion: a rare renal malformation. European Urology 14: 171–172.

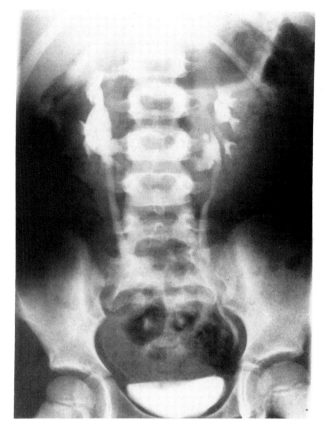

Fig. 5.2.7   Horseshoe kidneys. IVU. Typical orientation of renal axis.

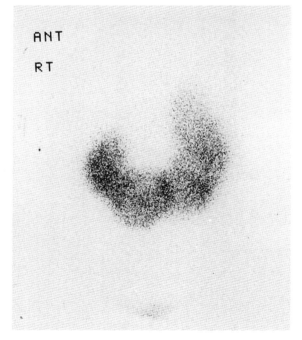

ANT

RT

Fig. 5.2.8   DMSA scan in horseshoe kidney. Note the axes of the kidneys and bridge of functioning renal tissue.

In crossed fused ectopia, the contralateral kidney usually lies lower than the normal kidney and their poles are more or less fused (Fig. 5.2.9). One ureter crosses the midline before entering the bladder at a normal level. The diagnosis is sugggested by US and confirmed by DMSA, isotope scanning and IVU. Vesicoureteric reflux is common.

Rarely, the fused kidneys form a single mass of renal tissue in an ectopic position, typically in the pelvis. This type of kidney has been called the 'discoid' or 'cake' kidney (Fig. 5.2.10).

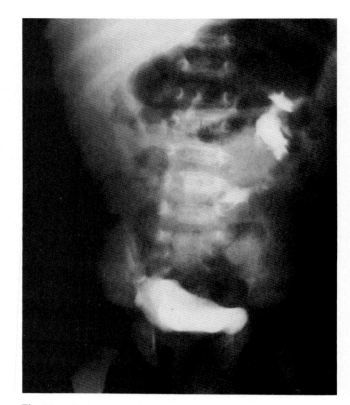

Fig. 5.2.9 Left crossed fused ectopia. IVU.

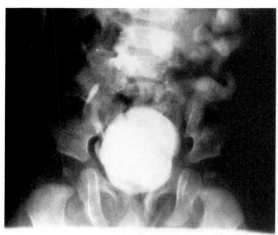

A

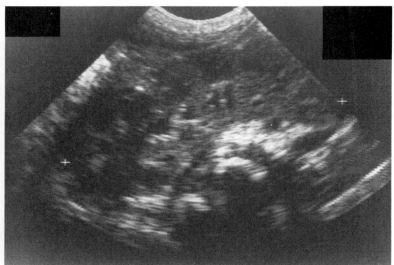

B

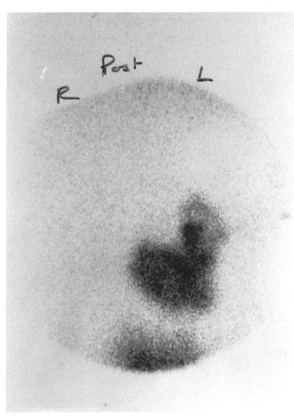

Fig. 5.2.10 Fused pelvic kidneys. **A** IVU. Dilated left part. Reflux was present in both parts. The ureteral orifices were both ectopic. **B** US. Transverse scan of the kidneys (between crosses) forming a banana-shape mass in front of the spine (sp). **C** Pancake kidney: DMSA scan. There is a mass of fused renal tissue in the pelvis.

C

Ectopic kidneys

A pelvic kidney is usually small. Calculi are important complications. Diagnosis is made by US, both postnatally and prenatally (Fig. 5.2.11), but can be missed because of bowel gas. In such cases isotope studies, DMSA and CT are useful (Fig. 5.2.12).

A thoracic kidney is a rare entity. It presents as a mass overlying the diaphragm on a plain chest radiograph (Fig. 5.2.13A). Diagnosis is suggested by US (Fig. 5.2.13B), and confirmed by isotope studies. (DMSA or IVU).

Late presentation of a thoracic kidney may occur following repair of congenital diaphragmatic hernia and may cause hypertension.

An ectopic kidney is otherwise asymptomatic.

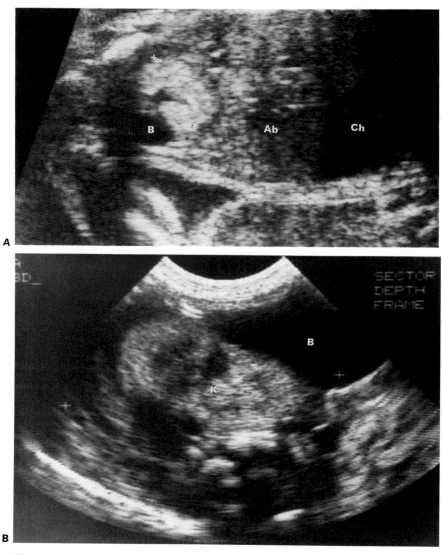

Fig. 5.2.11 US of pelvic kidney (in a case of a nephrotic-like syndrome). **A** In utero. Sagittal scan of fetal abdomen (Ab). The hyperechoic kidney (between crosses) is seen above the bladder (B). Ch = fetal chest. **B** At birth. Sagittal midpelvic scan. Abnormal hyperechoic kidney (K) can be seen above the bladder (B).

Fig. 5.2.12 Pelvic kidney. **A** CT. Contrast enhanced pelvic kidney in front of the sacrum (child with ventriculoperitoneal shunt). **B** DMSA scan in a child with a pelvic kidney. Note the need for separate images of the pelvic and normal kidneys as well as anterior and posterior views to evaluate scarring properly. The pelvic kidney is small and has a focal scar in its lower pole.

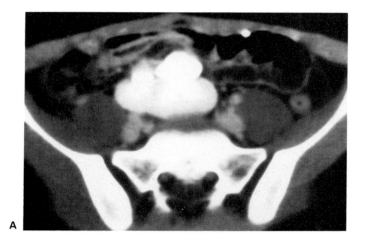

A

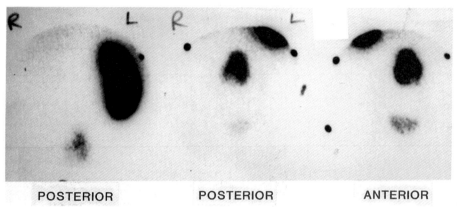

B   POSTERIOR   POSTERIOR   ANTERIOR

Fig. 5.2.13 Thoracic kidney. **A** Chest radiograph. Opacity superimposed on the left hemidiaphragm. **B** US. Transverse scan at the xyphoid level. Kidney (K) lies behind the left lobe of the liver (L) lateral to the spine (Sp).

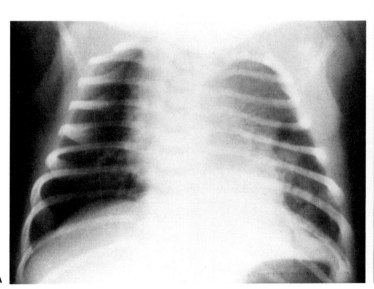

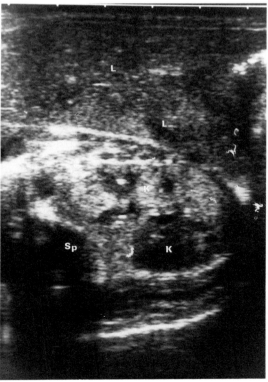

A   B

GENETICS OF CONGENITAL ABSENCE AND SEVERE RENAL DYSPLASIA

Congenital absence or significant dysgenesis of the kidneys have a familial basis. Parents and siblings of affected infants have a 15-fold higher chance of having a renal malformation.

Roodhooft and co-workers found occult urogenital anomalies in 9% of parents of bilaterally affected infants. Renal evaluation with US and isotope cystograms are recommended in parents and siblings of affected children.

REFERENCES

Aaronson I A, Cremin B J 1984 Anomalies of kidney number position and size. In: Aaronson I A, Cremin B (eds) Clinical pediatric uroradiology. Churchill Livingstone, Edinburgh, pp 52–75

Ascoli R, Pavone C, Cavallo N 1988 Hilar fusion: a renal malformation. European Urology 14: 171–172

Avni E F, Thoua Y, Van Gansbeke D et al 1987 Development of the hypodysplastic kidney: contribution of antenatal US diagnosis. Radiology 164: 123–125

Avni E F, Vansinoy M L, Hall M, Stallenberg B, Matos C 1989 Hypothesis: reduced renal mass with glomerular hyperfiltration, a cause of renal hyperechogenecity in children. Pediatric Radiology 19: 108–110

Bernstein J 1971 The morphogenesis of renal parenchymal maldevelopment (renal dysplasia). Pedatric Clinic of North America 18: 395–407

Brenbridge A N, Chevalier R L, Eldahr S, Kaiser D L 1987 Pathologic significance of nephromegaly in pediatric disease. American Journal of Disease in Childhood 141: 625–654

Chevalier R L, Campbell F, Brenbridge A N 1984 Nephrosonography and renal scintigraphy in evaluation of the newborn with nephromegaly. Urology 24: 96–103

Glassberg H I, Filmer R B 1985 Renal dysplasia, renal hypoplasia and cystic diseases of the kidneys. In: Kelalis King, Belman (eds) Clinical pediatric urology. Saunders, Philadelphia, pp 922–971

Goodman D, Norton K I, Can L, Yeh H C 1986 Crossed fused renal ectopia: US diagnosis. Urologic Radiology 8: 13–16

Lidell R M, Rosenbaum D, Blumhagen J D 1989 Delayed radiologic appearance of bilateral thoracic ectopic kidneys. American Journal of Roentgenology 152: 120–122

Nakada T, Furuta H, Kazama T, Katayama T 1988 Unilateral renal agenesis with or without ipsilateral adrenal agenesis. Journal of Urology 140: 933–937

Phokitis P 1964 The supernumerary kidney. Urologic Internationales 17: 265–293

Risdon R A, Young L W, Chrispin A R 1975 Renal hypoplasia: a radiological and pathological correlation. Pediatric Radiology 3: 213–225

Romero R, Cullen M, Grannum P et al 1985 Antenatal diagnosis of renal anomalies with US (III): bilateral renal agenesis. American Journal of Obstetrics and Gynecology 151: 38–43

Roodhooft A M, Birnholz J, Holmes L B 1984 Familial nature of congenital absence and severe dysgenesis of both kidneys. New England Journal of Medicine 310: 1341–1344

Sanders R C, Nussbaum A R, Sole Z K 1988 Renal dysplasia sonographic findings. Radiology 167: 623–626

5.3 CYSTIC DISEASE OF THE KIDNEY

Classification (Table 5.3.1).

Table 5.3.1 Classification of renal cystic diseases
1. Recessive polycystic disease (infantile, hepatorenal)
2. Dominant polycystic kidney disease (adult)
3. Dysplastic cystic disease
Multicystic dysplasia
Cystic dysplasia
4. Cortical cystic disease and cortical cysts
Glomerulocystic disease
Simple cyst
Multilocular cyst
5. Medullary cystic disease and medullary cysts
Medullary sponge kidney/Cacchi Ricci
Medullary cystic disease (nephronophthisis)
Microcystic disease
Pyelogenic cyst (calyceal diverticulum).
6. Renal cysts as part of hereditary or multidefects syndrome, e.g. Turner's syndrome
7. Renal failure

AUTOSOMAL RECESSIVE POLYCYSTIC KIDNEY DISEASE (ARPKD)

ARPKD is characterized by autosomal recessive inheritance and hepatorenal lesions. The incidence in the population is 1 in 40 000. Involvement is bilateral and the renal cystic lesions are not seen as classical cysts on imaging but correspond to dilated tubules that occupy the entire kidney with loss of the normal cortico-medullary differentiation. The collecting system is normal. Hepatic fibrosis with portal hypertension is associated with ARPKD and is a problem in patients presenting later in childhood.

Perinatal diagnosis

ARPKD can be diagnosed antenatally in the third trimester; the kidneys are large and hyperechoic. The kidneys may appear normal initially, the characteristic appearances only being seen in the third trimester. This is probably due to the evolution of urine production by the fetus and the volume of urine required to dilate the ectatic tubules. This results in an increased number of acoustic interfaces producing hyperechoic kidneys. In severe cases oligohydramnios with a small bladder is present.

At birth, the diagnosis is confirmed with US, demonstrating large, hyperechoic kidneys (greater than 8 cm renal length) with loss of corticomedullary differentiation. In some cases, US may show a hypo-echoic rim around the kidney representing a 'layer' of normal renal cortex (Fig. 5.3.1A). The larger this 'layer' the better the prognosis.

IVU displays a characteristic appearance of large kidneys with a radiating arrangement of opacified tubules seen on delayed films. The pelvicalyceal system is intact although distorted and splayed. The IVU is usually unnecessary to make the diagnosis. CT shows kidneys filling the abdominal cavity (Fig. 5.3.1B) in severe disease.

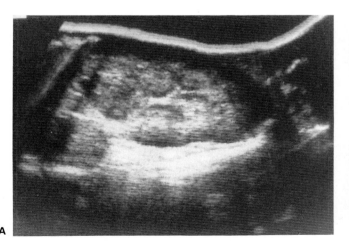

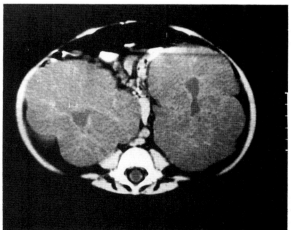

Fig. 5.3.1 Recessive PKD. **A** US at birth: sagittal section: large 8 cm kidney with a rim of hypoechoic cortex. **B** CT of ARPKD in a different child. The kidneys virtually fill the abdominal cavity.

597

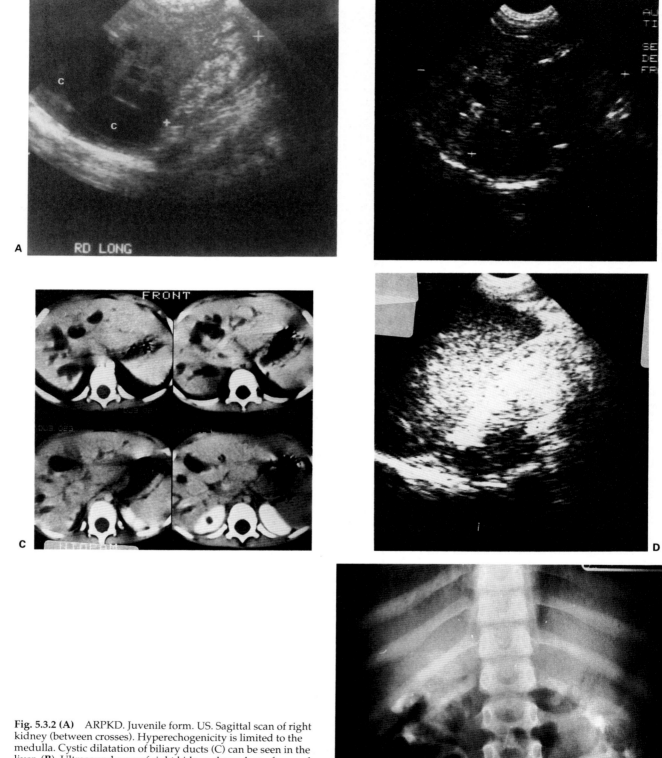

Fig. 5.3.2 (A) ARPKD. Juvenile form. US. Sagittal scan of right kidney (between crosses). Hyperechogenicity is limited to the medulla. Cystic dilatation of biliary ducts (C) can be seen in the liver. (**B**) Ultrasound scan of right kidney shows loss of normal architecture, with discrete cysts. Note cysts in liver. (**C**) CT scan same child. Note extensive liver cysts and one cyst in the right kidney on these cuts. (**D**) Older sister of this child who also has ARPKD who presented with a haematemesis due to varices and portal hypertension. The right kidney is diffusely echobright with almost complete loss of corticomedullary differentiation. (**E**) IVU (same child). Note persistent nephrogram, enlarged kidneys and persistent filling of the ectatic tubules, best seen in the left upper pole calyx.

Infants that survive the neonatal period usually present later with varying clinical presentations and milder involvement of the kidneys (juvenile form). A variety of ultrasound appearances are seen, ranging from cystic changes confined to the medulla to hyperechogenicity throughout the medulla (Fig. 5.3.2). This makes the diagnosis more difficult, as both the recessive intermediate, milder forms and the dominant type of polycystic kidney disease can have similar appearances.

Hepatic involvement and portal hypertension is diagnosed with US; splenomegaly, abnormal portal blood flow and cystic dilatation of the biliary ducts may be seen (Fig. 5.3.2).

AUTOSOMAL DOMINANT POLYCYSTIC KIDNEY DISEASE (ADPKD)

This type of renal cystic disease, with a dominant transmission, most frequently manifests after the third decade of life, but now is more frequently being diagnosed in infants and children. Any segment of the nephron can be dilated and progressive renal fibrosis, tubular atrophy and glomerular sclerosis occur. Associated abnormalities, such as hepatic and pancreatic cysts are common, with approximately one-third of all patients having one or more epithelial lined cysts of the liver. The incidence in the population is 1 in 1000.

ADPKD may be detected both antenatally and in the neonate. The cysts develop progressively and initially changes may be unilateral (Fig. 5.3.3), and consist of small intrarenal cysts with increased echogenicity or in other cases slightly larger renal cysts seen in the periphery of the kidney (Fig. 5.3.4). It may therefore be difficult to differentiate the early presentation of ADPKD from ARPKD. The IVU is sometimes helpful, demonstrating prompt excretion of contrast medium with nodular pooling of contrast medium in delayed films. Classical large, bilateral sonolucent cysts may be seen on US and the diagnosis is then easy, although these appearances are also found in tuberous sclerosis with renal involvement.

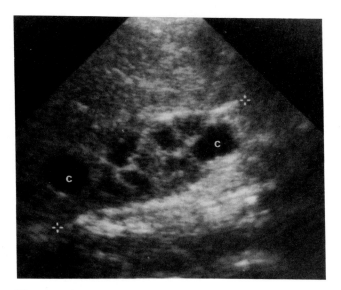

Fig. 5.3.3 Dominant PKD. US at 6 months. Sagittal scan of the right kidney (between crosses). Two cysts are present (C). The left kidney was normal. (US was normal in utero and at birth. The mother of this child was affected.)

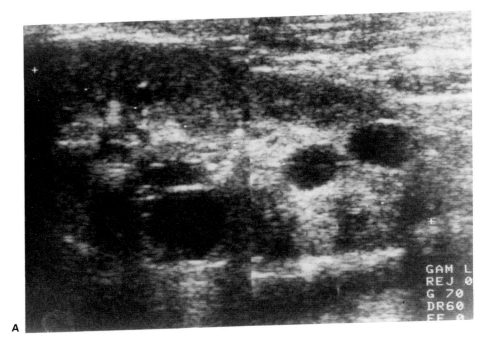

A

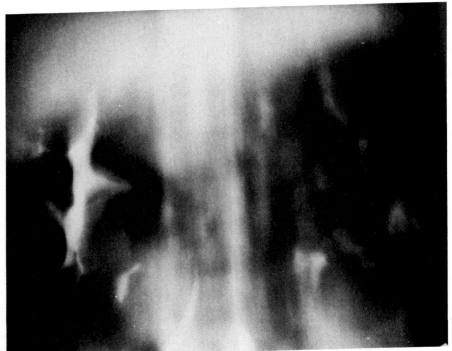

B

Fig. 5.3.4 Dominant PKD. US at the age of 2 years. Same case as Figure 5.3.3. Bilateral cysts are now present. **A** Sagittal scan of left kidney. **B** Typical IVU appearance of PKD in another child.

DYSPLASTIC CYSTIC DISEASE

Multicystic dysplastic kidney (MDK)

The multicystic dysplastic kidney is the most severe and commonest form of congenital cystic renal dysplasia. The pathogenesis is due to complete ureteric obstruction early in fetal life, usually before 8–10 weeks with an atretic ureter. Incomplete obstruction between the 10th and 36th week results in a hydronephrotic type described by Felson et al, and the pelvi-infundibular stenosis described by Lucaya et al may represent an intermediate form. These appearances probably represent a spectrum of changes due to obstruction in utero. The typical sonographic appearance in utero is that of a multicystic mass (Fig. 5.3.5),

with non-communicating cysts of variable size, without normal renal tissue and central arrangement (Fig. 5.3.6). The condition must be distinguished from a severe pelviureteric junction obstruction.

In utero, the diagnosis is only possible in the third trimester; earlier, the cystic part may not be detected. The condition is usually unilateral; bilateral disease or MDK with contralateral renal agenesis is lethal. Contralateral abnormalities, such as pelviureteric junction obstruction or reflux, occur in a third of cases.

After birth, the diagnosis is confirmed by US. A functional study preferably, with isotopes or an IVU, demonstrates no function in the affected kidney. An MCUG is performed to exclude contralateral reflux, which may be present.

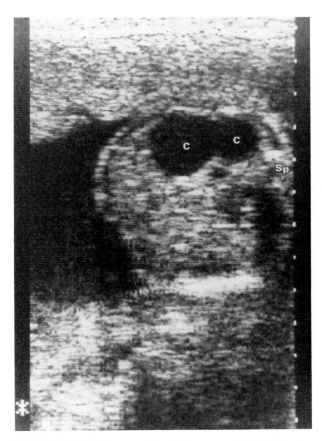

Fig. 5.3.5 MDKD in utero. Cysts (C) are seen in the left lumbar area. Sp = fetal spine.

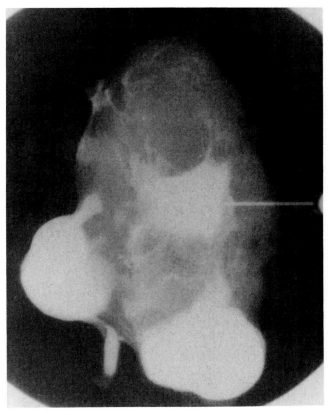

Fig. 5.3.6 Postnephrectomy opacification of an MDKD. Small connecting channels are seen between the cysts. (Courtesy of Dr F. Diard.)

If it is difficult to distinguish this condition from a severe pelviureteric junction obstruction, direct puncture of the cysts and opacification with radiopaque contrast medium may be necessary. MDKD may involve part of or the entire kidney. Typically the upper pole of a duplex system or one kidney in a horseshoe kidney may be affected. Associated abnormalities such as ureterocoeles or a Gartner duct remnant around the ureterovesical junction should be looked for (Fig. 5.3.7).

US may show involution of the MDK which can start in utero or after birth (Fig. 5.3.8). The time and duration of involution varies and probably represents resorption of fluid. Involution has usually started by 6 months. If involution occurs, US may eventually fail to demonstrate any mass (Figs 5.3.8, 5.3.9). Hypertrophy of the opposite kidney occurs and hyperfiltration may lead to hyperechogenicity of the renal cortex and increased corticomedullary differentiation.

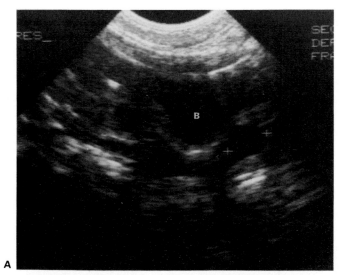

A

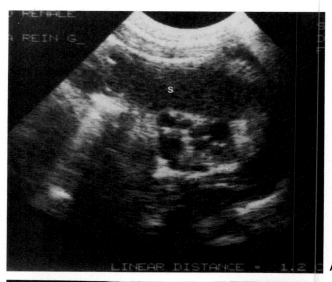

A

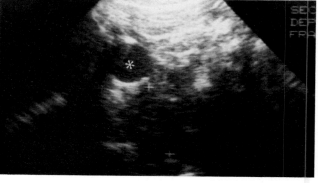

B

Fig. 5.3.7 Gardner duct remnant related to an MDKD presenting as a vaginal mass. **A** US. Sagittal scan of the bladder (B). A cyst (between crosses) is seen behind the bladder. **B** Opacification by puncture of the cyst reveals the connecting channel between the cyst and the MDKD.

Fig. 5.3.8 Involution of an MDKD. Same case as in Figure 5.3.5. **A** US at birth. Transverse scan of the left kidney (between crosses). Partial involution of the cystic part. S = spleen. **B** US at the age of 1 year. Aplastic kidney between crosses with no residual cysts.

Haemorrhagic foci related to perinatal asphyxia may occur in multicystic dysplastic kidneys, when US demonstrates increased echogenicity within the cysts and subsequent calcification. There is some concern that malignant change within a residual involuted multicystic kidney may occur with an increase in conservative and non-operative management although there is no definite evidence to support this.

Cystic dysplasia

Cystic dysplasia is related to other urinary tract abnormalities, usually obstruction. It is found in association with posterior urethral valves or marked pelviureteric junction obstruction. The kidneys are often small and US demonstrates increased echogenicity with small peripheral cysts (Fig. 5.3.10).

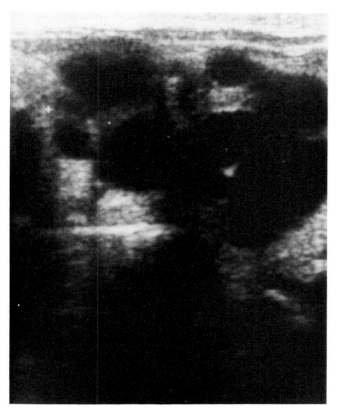

Fig. 5.3.9 MDKD in childhood. Four-year-old child. Typical sonographic appearance. Multicystic mass without any parenchyma.

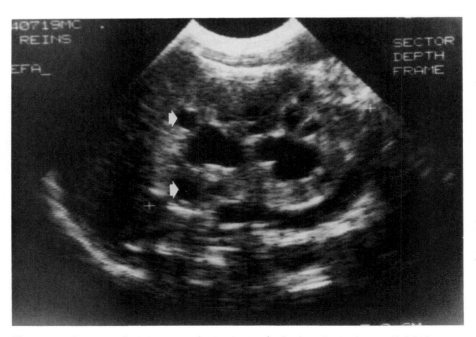

Fig. 5.3.10 Cystic dysplasia in a case of posterior urethral valves. Sagittal scan of left kidney (between crosses). Dilatation of the pelvicalyceal system. Hyperechoic parenchyma with macrocysts (arrows).

CORTICAL CYSTS

Glomerulocystic disease

Glomerulocystic renal disease is associated with numerous syndromes. The kidneys are enlarged and the glomerular spaces and tubules are dilated. Sonographically the appearances may be indistinguishable from ARPKD.

Isolated cortical cysts

Simple benign renal cysts are thought to be rare in childhood but with increasing use of US are being discovered more frequently. The aetiology is unclear and may be focal ischaemia, tubular obstruction or calyceal diverticula that have lost their communication in utero. The sonographic appearances are of a unilocular sonolucent mass without connection to the pelvicalyceal system (Fig. 5.3.11). Cases have been described in utero.

Large cysts may be confused with a duplex system, calyceal diverticulum or cystic Wilms' tumour. If septated, the cysts resemble a multilocular cyst.

US is diagnostic but, if there is any possibility of a solid tumour, CT is useful to demonstrate or exclude a solid component. Follow-up of uncomplicated cases is with US. Sclerotherapy under ultrasound control is a satisfactory method of treatment.

A number of syndromes are associated with cortical cysts. (See 'Renal cysts associated with syndromes' below.)

MEDULLARY CYSTS

Medullary cystic disease/nephronophthisis

This is an autosomal recessive disease with tubular nephropathy and progression to chronic renal failure. The US appearances are of a few medullary or corticomedullary cysts in normal or moderately small kidneys. There is loss of corticomedullary differentiation and increased parenchymal echogenicity (Fig. 5.3.12).

Medullary sponge kidney

This condition may be unilateral or bilateral and also consists of collecting tubule abnormalities but does not usually result in altered renal function. However, patients present with complications such as stone formation, bleeding or infection. Sonographically, the kidneys may be normal or demonstrate increased echogenicity of the renal pyramids (Fig. 5.3.13A). Intravenous urography demonstrates contrast medium concentrated in fan-shaped streaks beyond the calyces (Fig. 5.3.13B). The papillae may be enlarged. The differential diagnosis includes acute pyelonephritis and the normal tubular opacification on IVU with low osmolality contrast medium (Table 5.1.5).

Calyceal diverticulum (pyelogenic cyst)

A pyelogenic cyst is present in up to 3% of all IVUs with a typical appearance of a contrast-filled structure connected to a calyx. The appearance on US is characteristic but can resemble a simple cyst.

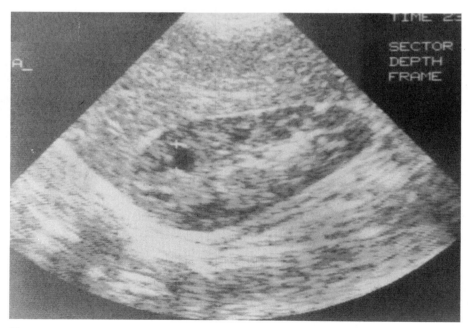

Fig. 5.3.11 Cortical cyst. US. Sagittal scan of right kidney An 8 mm cyst is visualized (between crosses). IVU was normal.

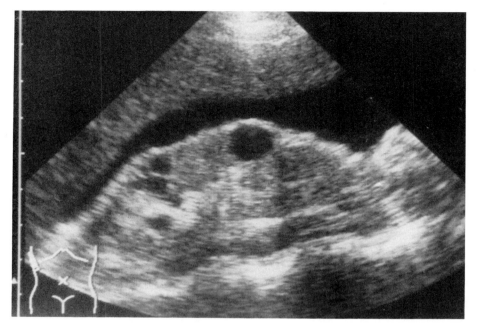

Fig. 5.3.12 Nephronophtisis. US appearance (8-year-old child). Sagittal scan of right kidney. Corticomedullary differentiation is absent. Diffuse macrocysts can be seen. Ascites is present.

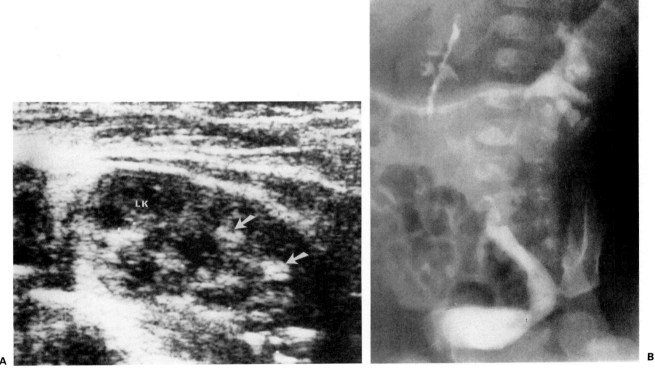

Fig. 5.3.13 Medullary sponge kidney/unilateral involvement. **A** US. Prone sagittal scan of left kidney (LK). Reversed corticomedullary differentiation with hyperechoic medulla (arrows). **B** IVU. Left precalyceal tubular opacification.

RENAL CYSTS ASSOCIATED WITH SYNDROMES

Syndromes associated with renal cystic disease and renal cysts are multiple (Table 5.3.2). Polycystic renal disease and central nervous abnormalities occur in Meckel's syndrome and may be detected by antenatal US (Fig. 5.3.14). Large cysts occur in tuberous sclerosis (Fig. 5.3.15) and von Hippel–Lindau disease; their sonographic appearance resembles ADPKD and may precede the neurological abnormalities. Small cortical cysts are found in Conradi's disease, Zellweger's syndrome, Turner's syndrome and other trisomies. Laurence–Moon–Biedl syndrome is frequently associated with medullary nephronophthisis.

Table 5.3.2	Syndromes of multiple defects with kidney involvement
Hereditary	**Non-hereditary**
Zellweger's	Dandy–Walker
Meckel's	Down's
Jeune's asphyxiating dystrophy	Ehlers–Danlos
Tuberous sclerosis	Congenital hemihypertrophy
Von Hippel–Lindau	Laurence–Moon–Biedl
	Trisomy 13–15, 18
	Turner's
	Vater association
	Beckwith–Wiedemann

Fig. 5.3.14 Meckel–Gruber's syndrome – 22 weeks pregnancy. Sagittal scan of fetal abdomen. Large hyperechoic kidney (between crosses) consistent with polycystic disease. A cervical meningocoele was also present. Sp = fetal spine, Ch = fetal chest.

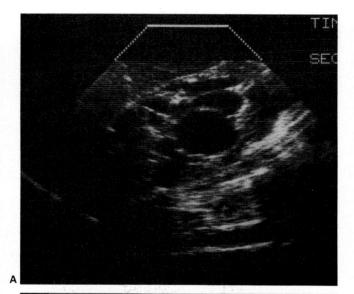

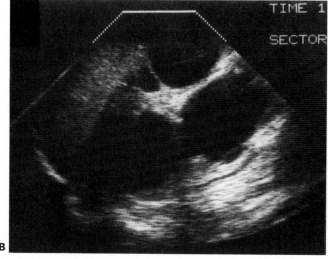

Fig. 5.3.15 Tuberous sclerosis. Bilateral cystic involvement. Sagittal scan of left (**A**) and right kidney (**B**).

MULTILOCULAR CYSTIC NEPHROMA

This is a cystic renal mass which presents as a palpable abdominal mass in a child younger than 4 years. It is also known as a 'cystic nephroblastoma', unilateral multilocular cyst or 'cystic partially differentiated nephroblastoma'. On US the mass presents as a well-defined, intrarenal septated cystic mass (Fig. 5.3.16). CT scanning confirms the multilocular, well-defined septated mass. Removal of the mass and careful histological examination of the specimen is required as the differential diagnosis includes a cystic Wilms' tumour.

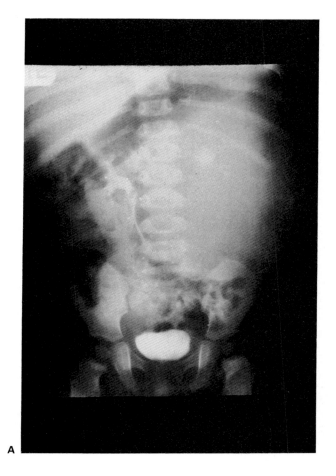

A

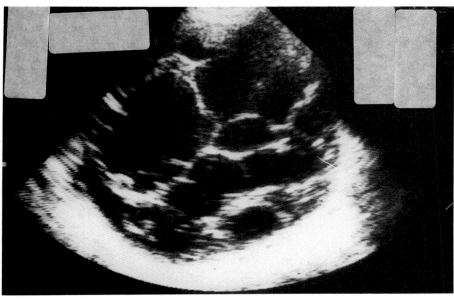

B

Fig. 5.3.16 Multilocular cystic nephroma. (**A**) IVU. (**B**) USS. The IVU shows an appearance indistinguishable from Wilm's tumour. The US shows well defined cysts which would not be seen in Wilm's tumour.

REFERENCES

Andriole J, Gouse J, Schultz C, Capur M 1986 Bilateral abdominal masses in an asymptomatic infant. Investigative Radiology 21: 355–359

Avni E F, Szliwoski H, Spehl M, Lelong B, Baudain P, Struyven J 1984 Renal involvement in tuberous sclerosis. Annales de Radiologie (Paris) 27: 207–214

Avni E F, Thoua Y, Lalmand B, Didier F, Droulle P, Schulman C C 1987 MDK: natural history from in utero diagnosis and postnatal FU. Journal of Urology 138: 1420–1424

Avni E F, Vansinoy M L, Hall M, Stallenberg B, Matos C 1989 Hypothesis: reduced renal mass with glomerular hyperfiltration, a cause of renal hyperechogenicity in children. Paediatric Radiology 19: 108–110

Bartholomeus T H, Slovis T L, Kroovand R L, Corbett D P 1980 The sonographic evaluation and management of simple renal cysts in children. Journal of Urology 123: 732–736

Beretsky I, Lankin D H, Rusoff J H, Phelan L 1984 US differentiation between the MDK and the UPJ obstruction in utero using high resolution RT scanners employing digital detection. Journal of Clinical Ultrasound 12: 429–433

Diard F, De Lambilly C, Nicolau A, Chafeil J F, Bondormy J M 1987 Le rein multikystique. Etude anatomo-radiologique de 19 pieces operatoires. Consequences pratiques et pathogeniques. Journal de Radiologie 68: 365–371

Diard F, Ledosseur P, Cardier L, Calabet A, Bondommy J M 1984 Multicystic dysplasia in the upper component of the complete duplex kidney. Pediatric Radiology 14: 310–313

Felson B, Crussen L J 1975 The hydronephrotic type of unilateral congenital MDK. Seminars in Roentgenology 10: 113–123

Fitsch S J, Stapelton R B 1986 US features of glomerulocystic disease in infancy. Similarity to infantile PKD. Pediatric Radiology 16: 400–402

Gagnadoux M F, Habib R, Levy M, Brunelle F, Broyer M 1988 Maladies kystiques renales de l'enfant. In: Broyer M (ed) Actualites nephrologiques. Flammarion, Paris, pp 39–58

Garel L A, Habib R, Pariente D, Broyer M, Sauvegrain J 1984 Juvenile nephronophthisis: sonographic appearance in children with severe uremia. Radiology 151: 93–95

Garret A, Carty H, Pilling D W 1987. Multilocular cystic nephroma. Report of three cases. Clinical Radiology 38: 55–57

Griscom N T, Vawter G F, Fellers F X 1975 Pelvi-infundibular atresia: the usual form of MDK: 44 unilateral and 2 bilateral cases. Seminars of Roentgenology 10: 125–130

Grossman H, Rosenberg E R, Bowie J D, Ram P, Merten D F 1983 Sonographic diagnosis of renal cystic diseases. American Journal of Roentgenology 140: 81–85

Glassberg K I, Stephens F D, Lebowitz R L et al 1987 Renal dysgenesis and cystic disease of the kidney: report of the committee on terminology, nomenclature and classification, section on urology, American Academy of Pediatrics. Journal of Urology 38: 1085–1092

Habif D V, Berdon W E, Ming Neng Y 1982 IPKD: in utero sonographic diagnosis. Radiology 42: 475–477

Kaariainen H, Jaaskelainen J, Kivissain L, Koskinies O, Norio R 1988 Dominant recessive PKD in children: classification by IVP, US and CT. Pediatric Radiology 18: 45–50

Kaplan B S, Kaplan P, Rossenberg H K, Lamothe E, Rosenblatt D S 1989 Polycystic kidney diseases in childhood. Journal of Pediatrics 115: 867–880

Kramer S A, Hoffman A D, Aydin G, Kelalis P P 1982 Simple renal cysts in children. Journal of Urology 128: 1259–1261

Lucaya J, Enriquez G, Delgado R, Castellate A 1984 Infundibulopelvic stenosis in children. American Journal of Roentgenology 142: 471–474

Luthy D A, Hirsch J H 1985 Infantile PKD observations from attempts at prenatal diagnosis. American Journal of Medical Genetics 20: 505–517

McAllister W H, Siegel M J, Schafelford G, Askin F, Kissanes J M 1979 Glomerulocystic kidney. American Journal of Roentgenology 133: 536–538

Paille P, Garel L, Grignon A, Allaire G, Sward P, Grenier N 1986 Dysplasie renale in utero. Six formes iconographiques individualisees a l'echographic avec correlation histologique: Annales de Radiologie (Paris) 29: 406–414

Patriquin H B, O'Regan S 1985 Medullary sponge kidney in childhood. American Journal of Roentgenology 145: 315–319

Pedicelli G, Jacquier S, Bowen A, Boisvert J 1986 MDK: spontaneous regression demonstrated with US. Radiology 160: 32–36

Porch P, Noe H N, Stapelton F B 1986 Unilateral presentation of adult type PKD in children. Journal of Urology 135: 744–746

Premkumar A, Berdon W E, Levy J, Amadio J, Abransom S J, Newhouse J H 1988 The emergence of hepatic fibrosis and portal hypertension in infants and children with RPKD. Initial and FU US and radiographic findings. Pediatric Radiology 18: 123–129

Pretorius D H, Lee M H, Manco Johnson M L, Weingast G R, Sedman A B 1987 Diagnosis of autosomal dominant PKD in utero and in the young infant. Journal of Ultrasound in Medicine 6: 249–255

Sanders R C, Hartman D S 1984 The sonographic distinction between neonatal MDK and hydronephrosis. Radiology 151: 621–625

Sanders R C, Nussbaum A R, Solez K 1988 Renal dysplasia: sonographic findings. Radiology 167: 623–626

Saxton M H, Golding S J, Chantler C, Haycock G D 1981 Diagnostic puncture in renal cystic dysplasia (MK). Evidence in the aetiology of the cysts. British Journal of Radiology 54: 555–561

Strand W R, Rushton H G, Markle B M, Sudesh K 1989 APKD in infants. Asymmetric disease mimicking an unilateral renal mass. Journal of Urology 141: 1151–1153

Wood B P, Goske M, Rabinowitz R 1984 MDK masquerading as UPJ obstruction. Journal of Urology 132: 972–974

Zenes K, Volpel M C, Weiss H 1984 Cystic kidneys. Genetics, pathologic anatomy, clinical picture of prenatal diagnosis. Human Genetics 68: 103–104

5.4 URINARY TRACT DILATATION

GENERAL CONSIDERATIONS

Dilatation of the urinary tract is common in newborn babies and children. Most cases are detected with US in the perinatal period, and the aetiology of the dilatation is usually congenital. Evaluation with US allows assessment of the level of the abnormality and of the renal parenchyma. However, US may be unable to differentiate some causes of dilatation, as in obstruction and vesicoureteric reflux, and it does not provide functional information and therefore further imaging is required.

An MCUG should be performed in all male infants and in young female patients, when urethral anomalies and reflux, particularly into duplex or complicated renal systems, need to be diagnosed.

IVUS are rarely performed in neonates because of the poor images obtained due to the transitional nephrology of the newborn (see '5.15 Oliguria in the newborn'). If an IVU is required the examination should be delayed at least up to the age of 1 month, and preferably 3 months. Delayed opacification of the pelvicalyceal systems, crescent-like opacification at the edge of dilated calyces on early films (Fig. 5.4.1) with subsequent opacification, a persistent dense nephrogram and finally opacification of the dilated calyces are the characteristic radiological appearances of obstruction.

Table 5.4.1 Prolonged nephrogram (IVU)

Acute renal failure
Extrarenal obstruction
Renal vein thrombosis
Intratubular blockade
  Tamm–Horsfall proteinuria
  Myoglobinuria
  Rhabdomyolysis (battered child)
  (Multiple myeloma)
Acute pyelonephritis

A persistent dense nephrogram is seen in various other conditions (Table 5.4.1) and the differential diagnosis should also be based on the clinical and sonographic appearances. Delayed films may be necessary to demonstrate the anatomy and point of obstruction. Prone films are better for demonstrating the ureter. The timing of films depends on the degree

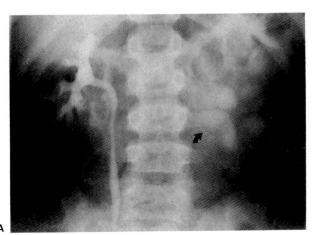

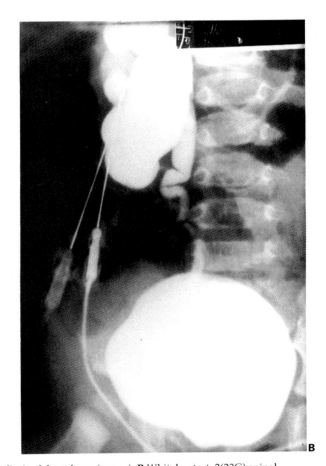

Fig. 5.4.1 A IVU. Obstruction pattern. Crescent-like opacification at the limit of the calyces (arrow). **B** Whitaker test: 2(23G) spinal needles are inserted into the kidney under US control and the kidney is perfused at a flow rate of 10 ml/min. In this patient there is a dilated renal collecting system and proximal ureter, but no pressure rise was demonstrated during perfusion. US and renography had suggested obstruction.

of dilatation, the greater this, the later should be the film. 24 hour films may be needed in severely dilated systems. However, IVUs are generally no longer indicated in the investigation of urinary tract dilatation as in most instances the combination of US and radionuclide renography will identify the site and cause of dilatation or obstruction.

Isotope studies with ^{99m}Tc-DTPA or MAG3 are essential in order to differentiate obstructive from non-obstructive cases.

If the diagnosis remains unclear, an antegrade pyelogram with direct opacification of the urinary tract after puncture with ultrasound guidance will help to further evaluate the pathology. Pressure measurement during the Whitaker test, will help to confirm or exclude obstruction in difficult cases (Fig. 5.4.16).

REFERENCES

Avni E F, Rodesch F, Schuman C C 1985. Fetal uropathies: diagnostic pitfalls and management. Journal of Urology 134: 921–925

Ball W S, Towbin R, Strife J L, Spencer R 1986. Intervention genito-urinary radiology in children. American Journal of Roentgenology 147: 791–796

Brown T, Mandell J, Lebowitz R L 1987. Neonatal hydronephrosis in the era of sonography. American Journal of Roentgenology 148: 959–963

Chopra A, Teele R L 1980. Hydronephrosis in children: narrowing the differential diagnosis with ultrasound. Journal of Clinical Ultrasound 8: 473–478

Cohen H L, Haller J O 1987. Diagnostic sonography of the fetal genito-urinary tract. Urologic Radiology 9: 88–98

Dunbar J S, Nogrady M B 1970. The calyceal crescent: a roentgenographic sign of obstructive hydronephrosis. American Journal of Roentgenology 110: 520–528

Friedland G W 1979. Pediatric urography. Urologic Clinics of North America 6: 375–393

Haller J O, Cohen H L 1987. Pediatric urosonography: an update. Urologic Radiology 9: 99–109

Hellin I, Person P 1986 Prenatal diagnosis of urinary tract abnormalities by US. Pediatrics 78: 879–883

Ransley P G 1976 Opacification of the renal parenchyma in obstruction and reflux. Pediatric Radiology 4: 226–232

Reuss A, Wladimiroff J W, Niermeiyer M F 1987 Antenatal diagnosis of renal tract anomalies by ultrasound. Pediatric Nephrology 1: 546–552

Riedy M J, Lebowitz R L 1986 Percutaneous studies of the upper urinary tract in children with special emphasis on infants. Radiology 160: 231–235

Rosenberg H K, Gefner W B, Lebowitz R L, Mahboubi S, Rosenberg H 1983 Prolonged dense nephrogram in children. Urology 31: 325–329

Rouse G A, Kaminsky C K, Saaly H P, Gerube G L, Fritzsche P J 1988 Current concepts in sonographic diagnosis of fetal renal disease. Radiographics 8: 119–132

Seeds J W, Mittelstaedt C A, Mandell J 1986. Pre- and post-natal ultrasonographic diagnosis of congenital obstructive uropathies. Urologic Clinics of North America 13: 131–154

Smith F G, Robillard J E 1989. Pathophysiology of fetal renal disease. Seminars in Perinatology 13: 305–319

Wantzell P G, Arnold A J, Carty H, Rickwod A M K 1988. Two needle modification of the Whitaker tests. British Journal of Urology 62: 388

PELVIURETERIC JUNCTION OBSTRUCTION

Pelviureteric junction obstruction is the commonest cause of upper urinary tract dilatation in children. On radioisotope functional studies some cases of pelvicalyceal dilatation do not demonstrate features of obstruction. When obstruction is present the causes vary. Operative findings suggest that local, intrinsic lesions, such as ureteric stenosis, or an adynamic segment are present in more than half the cases. Extrinsic lesions such as vascular impressions or angulation and kinking are present in the rest. However, the presence of pelviureteric dilatation and the role of these surgical abnormalities is unclear.

Perinatal diagnosis

In utero, the measurement of the fetal pelvicalyceal system should be performed on a transverse scan of the abdomen. Measurements of the transverse diameter of the pelvis are taken and dilatation less than 5 mm is considered normal and seen in many fetuses during the second and third trimester. Dilatation between 5 and 10 mm may also resolve spontaneously, but may be associated with vesicoureteric reflux, undetected megaureters and may increase. Therefore all these cases should have sonographic follow-up in utero and after birth; any sign of deterioration should lead to full uroradiological investigation. Dilatation greater than 10 mm is definitely abnormal and requires full investigation after birth (Fig. 5.4.2).

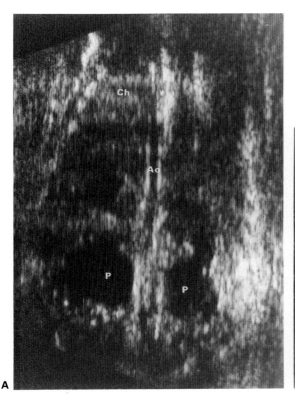
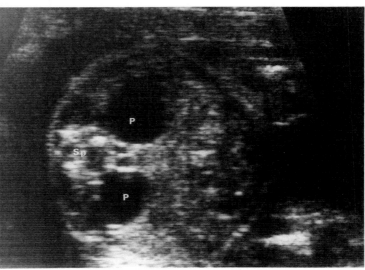

Fig. 5.4.2 Bilateral pelviureteric junction in utero. **A** Coronal view of fetal trunk. Bilaterally dilated pyelocalyceal system (P). Ch = fetal chest, Ao = Aorta. **B** Transerve scan of fetal abdomen. Dilated pyelocalyceal system (P) above 10 mm (12 and 20 mm). Sp = fetal spine.

After birth, US is performed to confirm the abnormality (Fig. 5.4.3). In mild cases, if neonatal dehydration is present, the dilatation will be underestimated. The examination should therefore be delayed until after the 5th day. Dilatation of the renal pelvis may be accompanied by varying degrees of calyceal dilatation; these cases, in contrast with those with dilatation of the pelvis alone, probably have worse function and a worse prognosis.

Renal parenchyma may also be demonstrated with US, and features suggestive of dysplasia demonstrated (Fig. 5.4.4). However, accurate assessments of function cannot be made from these appearances.

As mentioned, US cannot differentiate dilatation due to vesicoureteric reflux from obstruction and therefore a full radiological investigation must include an MCUG and radionuclide study. Most cases of pelviureteric junction obstruction do not have reflux, although they may coexist and reflux may be seen on MCUG. A radionuclide study with ^{99m}Tc-DTPA will demonstrate functional impairment, with measurements of the individual kidney's glomerular filtration rates. It is also able to determine whether obstruction and poor drainage are present, particularly if an intravenous diuretic, such as furosemide, is given and the images are reviewed as well as the curves (Fig. 5.4.5).

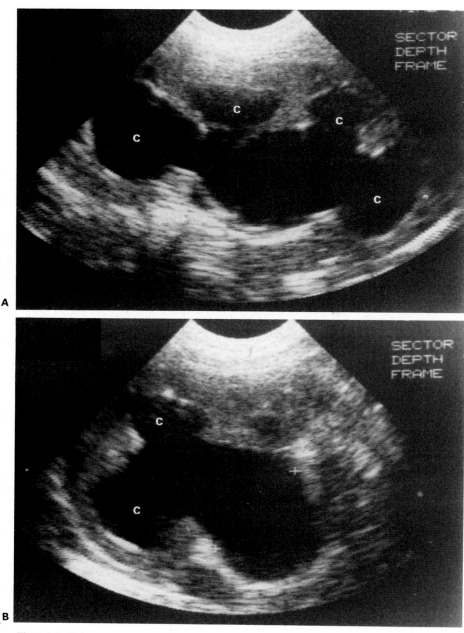

Fig. 5.4.3 Pelviureteric junction obstruction after birth. US. **A** Sagittal scan of the left kidney. Dilatation of renal pelvis and calyces. **B** Transverse scan (distance between crosses = 20 mm) of dilated kidneys. C = calyces.

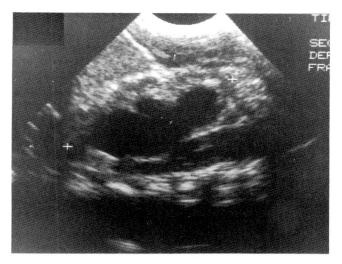

Fig. 5.4.4   Left ureteropelvic junction obstruction in a 2-month-old baby. US. Sagittal scan. Dilated pelvis. The kidney is small (30 mm). The parenchyma appears thin, irregular and heterogenous suggesting dysplasia.

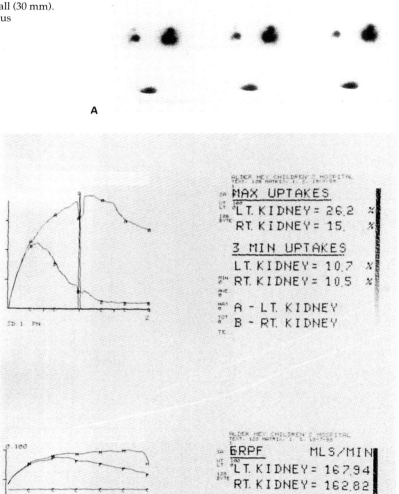

A

Fig. 5.4.5 A&B   Renograms in a boy with a left PUJ obstruction. The images (**A**) show a typical PUJ configuration on the left. The left curve (**B**) continues to rise even after a diuretic is given halfway through the examination. There is a little excretion in response to the diuretic. The appearances are typical of incomplete obstruction. Note that the three minute uptakes and the ERPFs are equal indicating no loss of function.

B

Intravenous urography may be used to demonstrate the anatomy of the pelviureteric junction and classical signs of obstruction are demonstrated (Fig. 5.4.6). Radiographs with the patient in the prone position may be useful.

Pressure measurements after puncture of the dilated renal pelvis under fluoroscopic control have been advocated by Whitaker in doubtful cases and is particularly useful beyond the neonatal period. However, little is known about the normal pressure measurements in neonates, and results in this group have been so variable that particular cases with obstruction and a poor outcome were not identified.

Following investigation, treatment may be surgical or conservative. If treatment is conservative, regular follow-up ultrasound and radionuclide studies (every 6 months for 2 years and then yearly for 5 years) are required to detect any deterioration in renal function.

Pelviureteric obstruction in older children

This group is becoming rarer as more cases are detected antenatally. They may present with a urinary tract infection, pain, a renal mass or haematuria. The diagnosis and investigations are the same as in the neonatal group.

Postoperative studies

Postoperatively an early nephrostogram through the surgical drain is usually required 7 days after surgery. This will detect any leak. Persistent postoperative pelvicalyceal dilatation is normal and secondary to oedema at the site of surgery. This gradually resolves in the next 6–12 months, and changes are monitored with follow-up US. Radionuclide studies confirm this improvement.

Increasing dilatation postoperatively is abnormal and may be due to secondary fibrosis and re-stenosis. Other early postoperative complications include urinomas following anastomotic leaks and haemorrhagic collections. US, intravenous urography and sinograms are useful in detecting and monitoring the complications. Postoperative renography at 6 months will confirm the residual renal function (Fig. 5.4.7A). Large collections may be drained percutaneously with ultrasound guidance (Fig. 5.4.7B).

Unusual causes of pelviureteric junction obstruction

Renal calculi, strictures, valves, abdominal vessels and intraluminal lesions such as polyps are potential causes of this (Fig. 5.4.8). Severe vesicoureteric reflux with kinking of the pelviureteric junction may result in

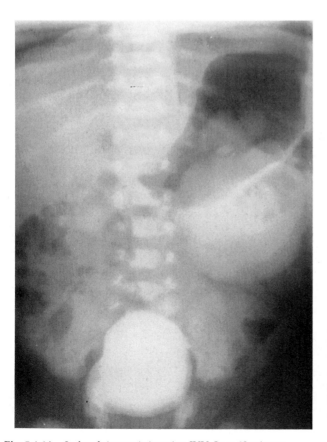

Fig. 5.4.6A Left pelviureteric junction IVU. Late 60 minute radiograph.

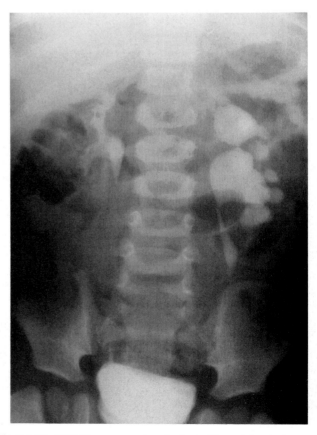

Fig. 5.4.6B IVU. One year post pyeloplasty. The pelviureteric junction is patent and functions satisfactorily.

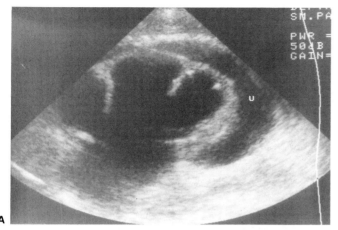

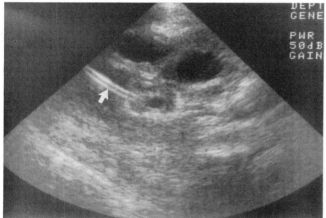

obstruction which resolves with treatment of the reflux. Pelviureteric junction obstruction and vesico-ureteric reflux may also coexist independently.

Differential diagnosis

Sonographically pelviureteric junction obstruction must be distinguished from vesicoureteric junction obstruction and multicystic dysplastic kidney disease (MDKD). In vesicoureteric obstruction a dilated ureter is seen behind the bladder, this is not present in pelviureteric junction obstruction. An IVU may be useful and will demonstrate the dilated ureter. In MDKD the sonolucent cystic structures do not communicate and are of varying sizes with the largest cyst often lying laterally, in pelviureteric junction obstruction, the largest 'cyst' in the pelvis lies medially and the pelvis and calyces are seen to communicate. Direct puncture of the 'cysts' and opacification with contrast medium may be useful.

Fig. 5.4.7 Pelviureteric junction obstruction. Postoperative urinoma. Sagittal scans of left kidney. **A** Dilated pyelocalyceal system with a perirenal collection (U). **B** Post percutaneous drainage. The collection has resolved. Arrow = nephrostomy tube.

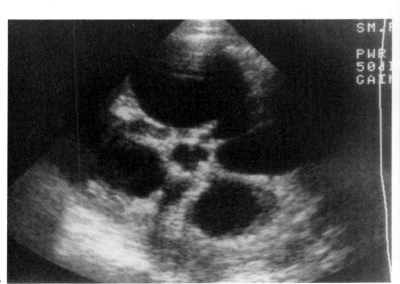

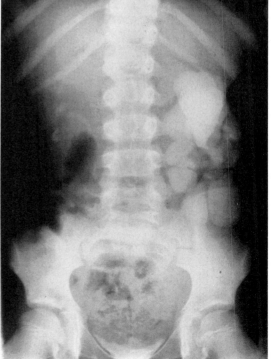

Fig. 5.4.8 Atypical pelviureteric junction obstruction. **A** US. Sagittal scan of left kidney. Appearance consistent with multicystic dysplastic kidney. **B** IVU. Left kidney is functioning. No renal pelvis is seen. At surgery, a vessel was crossing the renal hilum and compressing the pelvis.

Calyceal and pelvi-infundibular stenosis

A single, dilated upper calyx may be due to extrinsic, usually vascular, compression.

In pelvi-infundibular stenosis, obstruction occurs at a higher level with dilated calyces connected to a non-dilated renal pelvis. Both US and intravenous urography will demonstrate the abnormal appearances. This condition may represent an intermediate form between MDKD and hydronephrosis (Fig. 5.4.9).

Megacalicosis

Megacalicosis is an uncommon condition with dilatation of the minor calyces with a non-dilated pelvis and ureter. It is thought to be a congenital abnormality due to underdevelopment of the renal pyramids. Nuclear medicine studies do not demonstrate any evidence of obstruction, although stasis of isotope in the calyces may occur. Megacalicosis may be associated with polycalicosis, and multiple (up to 50) dilated calyces are seen on IVU (Fig. 5.4.10). Dilated calyces are also observed on ultrasound examination. Complications include infection and stones.

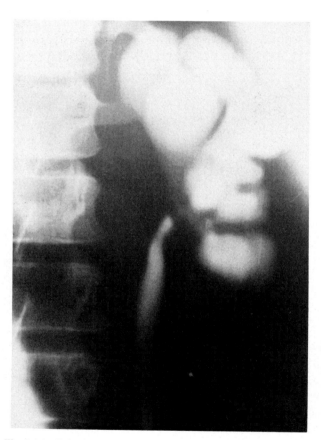

Fig. 5.4.9 Pelvi-infundibular stenosis. IVU. Tomogram. Dilated calyces. Renal pelvis is small. The pelviureteric junction is patent.

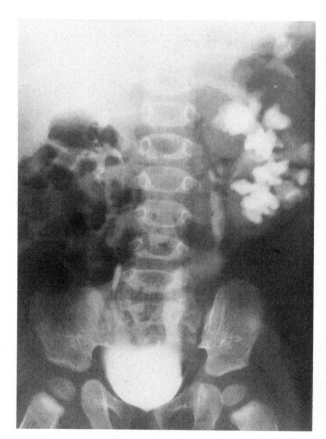

Fig. 5.4.10 IVU. Left megapolycalicosis.

REFERENCES

Arnold A J, Rickwood A M K 1990. Natural history of pelvi-ureteric obstruction detected by prenatal sonography. British Journal of Urology 65: 91–96

Bernstein G T, Mandell J, Lebowitz R L, Bauer S B, Colodny A H, Retik A B 1988. Ureteropelvic junction obstruction in the neonate. Journal of Urology 140: 1216–1221

Dinkel E, Dittrich M, Peters H et al 1985 Sonographic biometry in obstructive uropathy in children. Preoperative diagnosis and post-operative monitoring. Urologic Radiology 7: 1–7

Ebel K D, Bliesener J A, Gharib M 1988. Imaging of uretero-pelvic junction obstruction with stimulated diuresis. With consideration of the reliability of ultrasonography. Pediatric Radiology 18: 54–56

Galifer R B, Veyrac C, Faurous P 1988 Les anomalies congénitales de la jonction pyélourétérale chez l'enfant. Etude multicentrique de 985 observations chez 883 enfants. Annales de Pédiatrie (Paris) 35: 31–39

Grignon A, Fillion R, Filiatrault D et al 1986 Urinary tract dilatation in utero. Classification and clinical applications. Radiology 160: 645–647

Grignon A, Filiatrault D, Homsy Y et al 1986 Ureteropelvic junction stenosis: antenatal ultrasonographic diagnosis, post-natal investigation and follow-up. Radiology 160: 649–651

Hanna M K, Gluck R 1988 Uretero-pelvic junction obstruction during the first year of life. Urology 31: 41–45

Hoddik W K, Filly R A, Mahonny B S, Callen P W 1985 Minimal fetal renal pyelectasis. Journal of Ultrasound in Medicine 4: 85–89

Homsy Y L, Williot P, Danais S 1986 Transitional neonatal hydronephrosis: fact or fantasy? Journal of Urology 136: 339–341

Kleiner B, Callen P W, Willy R A 1987 Sonographic analysis of the fetus with ureteropelvic obstruction. American Journal of Roentgenology 148: 359–363

Laing F C, Burke V D, Wing V W, Jeffrey R B, Hashimoto B 1984 Post-partum evaluation of fetal hydronephrosis: optimal timing for follow-up sonography. Radiology 152: 423–424

Noe N H, Magill H L 1987 Progression of mild ureteropelvic junction obstruction in infancy. Urology 30: 348–351

O'Reilly P H 1987 Idiopathic hydronephrosis: diagnosis, management and outcome. British Journal of Urology 63: 569–574

Piepsz A, Hall M, Ham H R, Reilmutter N, Collier F 1986 Radioisotopic evaluation of the renal parenchymal function with UPJ obstruction: a retrospective study. European Journal of Pediatrics 145: 207–210

Piepsz A, Hall M, Ham H R, Verboren M, Collier F 1989. Prospective management of neonates with UPJ stenosis. Therapeutics strategy based on Tc DTPA studies. Scandinavian Journal of Urology and Nephrology 23: 31–36

Snyder H M, Lebowitz R L, Glodmy A et al 1980 Ureteropelvic junction obstruction in children. Urologic Clinic of North America 7: 273–295

Tsai T C, Lee H C, Huang F Y 1989 The size of the renal pelvis on ultrasonography in children. Journal of Clinical Ultrasound 647–651

Whitaker R H 1973 Methods of assessing obstruction in dilated ureters. British Journal of Urology 45: 15–22

URETERIC ABNORMALITIES AND DILATATION

Megaureters and abnormalities of the vesicoureteric junction

The initial diagnosis of a megaureter is usually made on US and may be confirmed with an IVU. Further imaging is required to assess the aetiology of the megaureter (Fig. 5.4.11) and to determine whether surgery is indicated. Imaging may therefore include US, micturating cystourethrography, IVU and nuclear medicine studies.

The most common type of megaureter is obstructive and is related to an aperistaltic segment at the vesicoureteric junction (primary megaureter). It has also been suggested that ureteral valves are the cause of vesicoureteric and pelviureteric junction obstruction. The second most common form of megaureter is due to gross vesicoureteric reflux.

Grossly dilated ureters are also seen in association with a ureterocoele, either as part of a duplex kidney or when related to a single system.

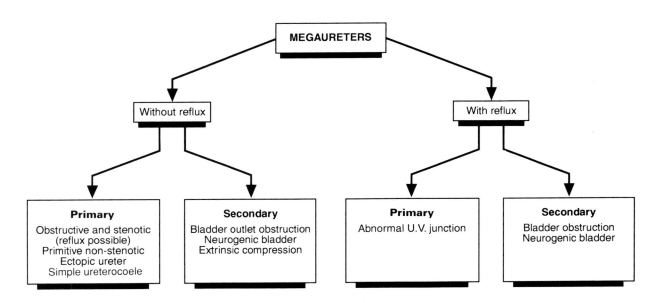

Fig. 5.4.11 Types of megaureters. (Adapted from F. Diard, Brussels, 1990, personal communication.)

Perinatal diagnosis

Normal fetal ureters are never seen on US, and if they are identified, imaging of the urological system is required after birth (Fig. 5.4.12). Antenatal imaging should include examination of both kidneys, the pelvicalyceal systems and the bladder. After birth, usually on the 5th postnatal day, ultrasound examination will demonstrate the dilated ureter as a tubular, anechoic structure which is visualized behind the bladder and also proximally at the level of the renal pelvis. The lumbar course of the ureter is harder to see. Dilatation of the pelvicalyceal system may be present, but this does not correlate with the degree of ureteric dilatation. Peristalsis may result in a varying calibre of ureter (Fig. 5.4.13).

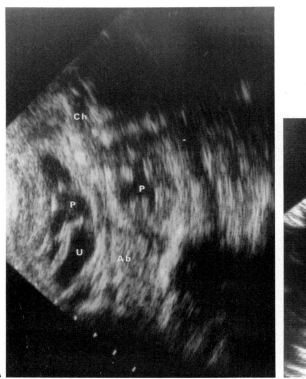

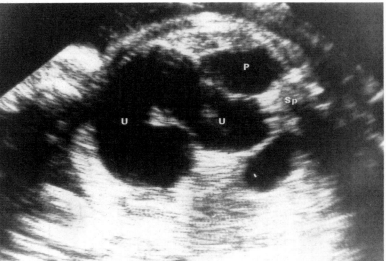

Fig. 5.4.12 **A** Coronal view of fetal trunk. Dilatation of right pelvicalyceal system (P) and ureter (U). The left renal pelvis is also visible (P). Ch = fetal chest, Ab = fetal abdomen. **B** Transverse scan of fetal abdomen. Markedly dilated ureter (U). Sp = fetal spine, P = dilated renal pelvis.

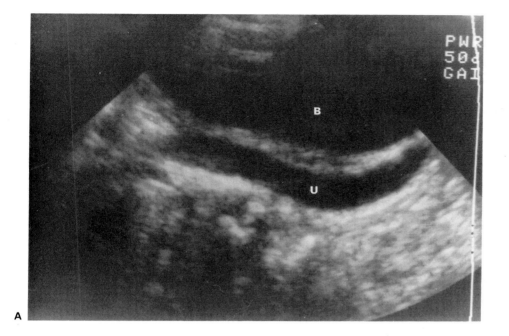

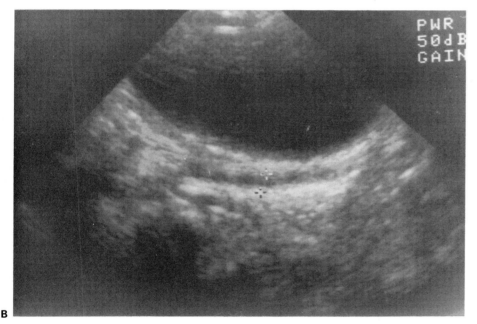

Fig. 5.4.13 Ureteral peristalsis after birth on ultrasound. **A** Sagittal scan of the bladder. A dilated ureter (U) is seen behind the bladder (B). **B** Same scan as in **A**. The ureter is almost invisible, following peristalsis.

Cystic dilatation of the intravesical portion of the ureter, often protruding into the bladder lumen, corresponds to a ureterocoele which may be related to a single system or upper pole of a duplex system.

Refluxing megaureters are diagnosed with an MCUG (Fig. 5.4.14).

Intravenous urography may be used to demonstrate the anatomy of the megaureter and may be useful in complicated cases with duplex kidneys. The megaureter will opacify, and may be seen only on delayed films. In primary megaureters, the lower end of the ureter has a typical convex distal tip (Fig. 5.4.15). Refluxing megaureters are large and atonic. A uretero-cele when present may or may not fill with contrast on an IVU, resulting in a characteristic 'cobra head appearance, or a filling defect within the bladder, which may then opacify and become indistinguishable in the bladder.

Progressive resolution of the dilatation occurs in the first 6 months in some megaureters, possibly through maturation of the vesicoureteric junction (Fig. 5.4.16). Progressive dilatation of a primary megaureter is uncommon. Some cases, depending on renography anatomical studies and clinical assessment, will require surgery.

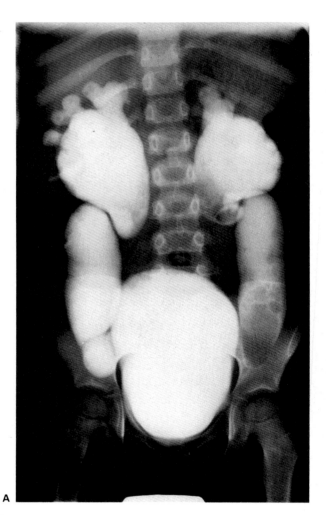

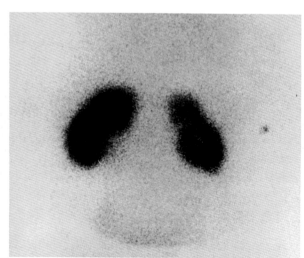

Fig. 5.4.14 **A** MCU. Refluxing megaureters. **B** DMSA scan with scarring of the upper pole of the kidney.

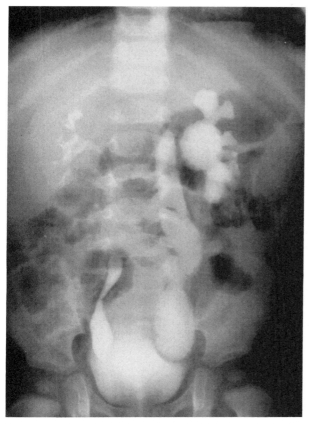

Fig. 5.4.15 IVU. Primary megaureter. Typical distal convex tip of left megaureter.

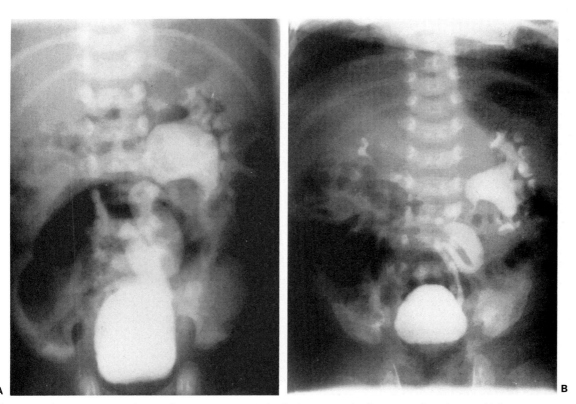

Fig. 5.4.16 Spontaneous resolution of a megaureter. **A** At birth. **B** At 1 month of age, partial resolution of left megaureter.

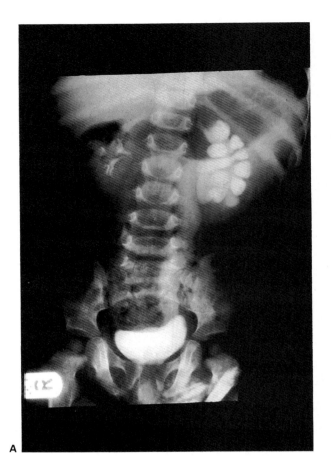

A

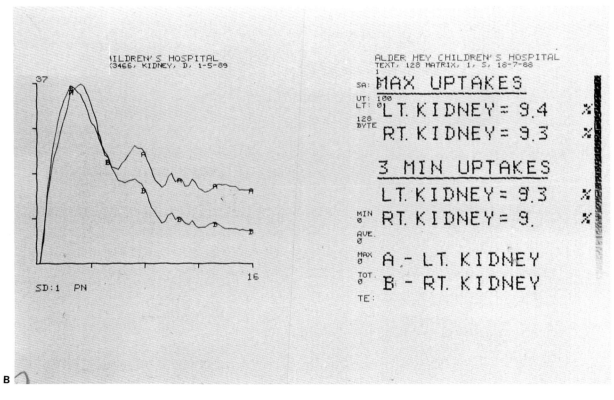

B

Fig. 5.4.17 Boy aged two presenting with UTI. **A** IVU: There is left hydroureteronephrosis with a megaureter. **B** Renogram: Diuretic given at the beginning of the examination. Both kidneys excrete but washout on the left is incomplete indicating partial obstruction.

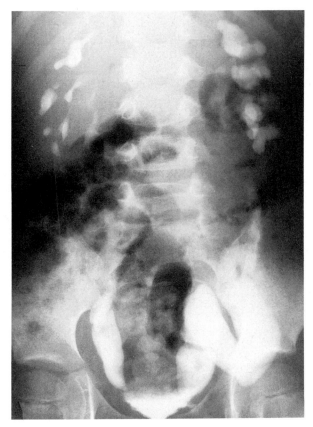

Fig. 5.4.18 IVU. Inguinal herniation of left megaureter.

Megaureters in older children

In older children, the diagnosis of a megaureter is usually made following a urinary tract infection (Fig. 5.4.17). Inguinal herniation of an extremely dilated ureter may present as a lump in the groin. US demonstrates a tubular structure connected to the urinary tract which is confirmed with an IVU (Fig. 5.4.18).

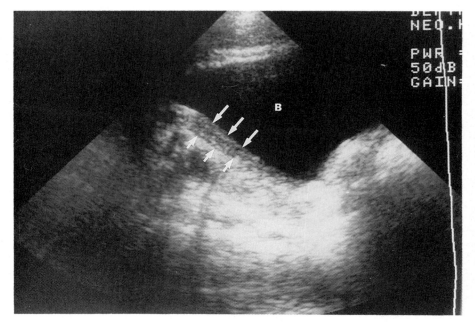

Fig. 5.4.19 US. Post reimplantation of ureter. Oblique scan of the bladder (B) shows posterior thickening (arrows) of the bladder wall.

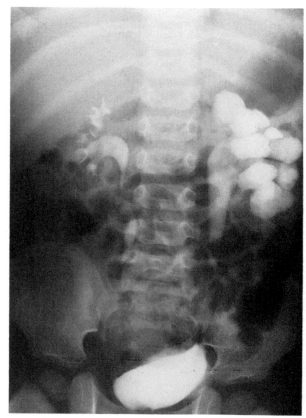

Fig. 5.4.20 IVU. Postoperative study. Tapering of the ureter with 'psoas hitch' procedure. Deviation and elongation of the bladder to the left.

Postoperative studies

Surgical treatment of a primary megaureter consists of ureteral tapering and reimplantation into the bladder. This results in thickening of the posterior bladder wall on US (Fig. 5.4.19). If the bladder is attached to the psoas muscle a typical bladder deformity is seen on an IVU (Fig. 5.4.20). Complications of surgery include increasing ureteric dilatation, urine leakage (Fig. 5.4.21) and secondary vesicoureteric reflux. Follow-up is with US and an MCUG if necessary.

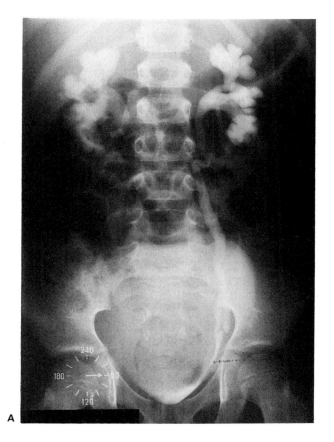

A

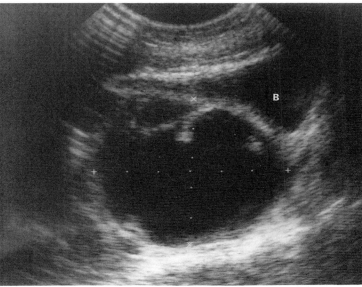

B

Fig. 5.4.21 Post reimplantation urinoma. **A** IVU. Post micturition. The small bladder is compressed by the urinoma which fills with contrast medium. Necrosis of the reimplanted ureter has occurred. **B** Sagittal ultrasound scan of the bladder (B). A 5 cm cystic mass (between crosses) is visible above the bladder.

Ureteric dilatation above the bladder

Dilatation of the upper two-thirds of the ureter may be seen in normal girls and in infants on an IVU, and is secondary to crossing of the iliac vessels.

Dilatation of the ureter above the bladder is otherwise uncommon. There may be dilatation of the proximal ureter and pelvicalyceal system of a retrocaval ureter. The dilated upper third of the ureter takes an abrupt medial turn seen on an IVU (Fig. 5.4.22). CT is also diagnostic, demonstrating the exact anatomical relationship between the inferior vena cava and the ureter.

Ultrasound is often unable to demonstrate the cause of mid or proximal ureteric dilatation because the ureter is not easily visualized between the pelviureteric junction and bladder.

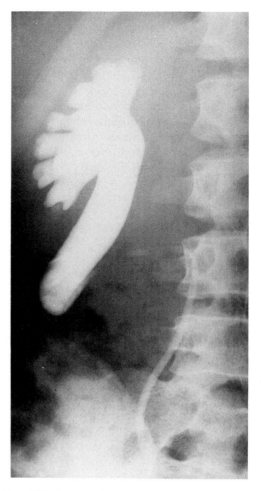

Fig. 5.4.22 IVU. Retrocaval ureter. Characteristic abrupt deviation of the proximal ureter.

'Congenital' strictures of the ureter are rare primary lesions and are considered to be secondary to an extrinsic vascular compression. The vessels involved are usually a persistent left umbilical artery or right ovarian vein (Table 5.4.2). Congenital ureteric diverticula are secondary to dilatation of a blind branch of the ureteric bud (Fig. 5.4.23), they may result in obstruction and infection. Cystic or tubular branching of the ureter is seen on IVU (Fig. 5.4.24). Primary or secondary retroperitoneal fibrosis is a rare cause of ureteric dilatation in children. Dilatation of the upper urinary tract is present and a soft tissue para-aortic mass encasing one or both ureters is demonstrated with CT. It may be secondary to trauma, vasculitis, chemotherapy and Henoch–Schönlein syndrome.

Table 5.4.2   Ureteric lesions (IVU)
Intramural
Inflammation
Ureteritis
Ureteritis cystica
Tuberculosis – schistosomiasis
Submucosal haemorrhage
Intraluminal
Valves
Blood clot
Calculus
Fungus disease
Polyp
(Air)
Extrinsic
Vascular notching
Normal vessels (iliac, hypogastric, ovarian)
Collateral artery (renal artery stenosis)
Collateral veins (renal vein or IVC obstruction)
Dilated vein without obstruction (arteriovenous malformation, varicocele)
Diverticulum (vesicoureteric junction)
Retroperitoneal fibrosis

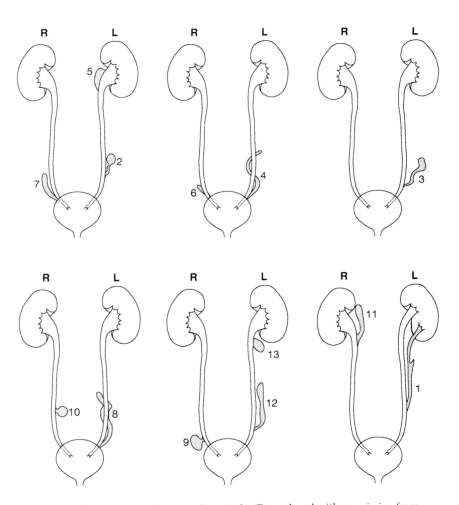

Fig. 5.4.23 Site and shape of ureteric diverticula. (Reproduced with permission from Sarajic M, Dursh Zivkovic B, Svaren E et al 1989 Congenital ureteric diverticula in children and adults. Classification, radiological and clinical features. British Journal of Radiology 62: 551–553.)

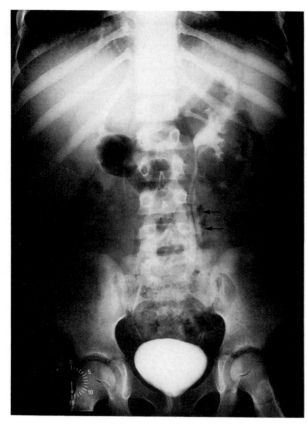

Fig. 5.4.24 IVU. Blind branching of the left ureter.

Unusual intraluminal lesions may also result in ureteric dilatation (Table 5.4.2). Lithiasis is the commonest cause and has a typical appearance on US and IVU; it should be differentiated from a blood clot, fungus ball or, rarely, a polyp.

REFERENCES

Pelvi-infundibular stenosis and hydrocalyces

Benz G, Willich E 1977 Upper calyx reno-vascular obstruction in children: Fraley's syndrome. Pediatric Radiology 5: 213–218

Lucaya J, Enriquez G, Delgado R, Catellote A 1984 Infundibulopelvic stenosis in children. American Journal of Roentgenology 142: 471–474

Megacalycosis

Holthussen W, Lundius B 1984 Megapolycalicosis with ureteric obstruction: a retrospective analysis of ten childhood cases. Annales de Radiologie (Paris) 27: 191–198

Kozakewich H P W, Lebowitz R L 1974 Congenital megacalyces. Pediatric Radiology 2: 251–258

Mandell G A, Snyder H M, Heyman S, Kalles M, Kaplan J M, Norman M E 1987 Association of congenital megacalycosis and ispilateral segmental megaureter. Pediatric Radiology 17: 28–33

Ureter dilatation, megaureter and abnormal UVJ

Belman A B, 1974 Megaureter: classification, etiology and management. Urologic Clinics of North America 1: 497–522

Docino S G, Lebowitz R L, Retik A B, Colodny A H, Bauer S B, Mandell J 1989 Congenital midureteral obstruction. Urologic Radiology 11: 156–160

Gearhart J P, Woolfenden K A 1982 The vesico-psoas hitch as an adjunct to megaureter repair in childhood. Journal of Urology 127: 505–507

Kaufman R A, Dunbar J S, Gole D E 1981 Normal dilatation of the proximal ureters in children. American Journal of Roentgenology 137: 945–949

Keating M A, Escala J, Mac Snyder H, Heynman S, Ducket J W 1989 Changing concepts in management of primary obstructive megaureter. Journal of Urology 142: 636–640

Kenavi M M, Williams D I 1976 Circumcaval ureter, a report of four cases in children with review of the literature and a new classification. British Journal of Urology 48: 183–192

King L R 1985 Ureter and uretero-vesical junction. In: Kelalis, King and Belman (eds) Clinical pediatric urology, 2nd edn. Saunders, Philadelphia, pp 486–512

Lautin E M, Haramati N, Frayer D et al 1988 CT diagnosis of circumcaval ureter. American Journal of Roentgenology 150: 591–594

Leiter E 1979 Persistant fetal ureter. Journal of Urology 122: 251–253

Maizels M, Stephens F D 1980. Valves of the ureter as a cause of primary obstruction of the ureter: anatomic embryologic and clinical aspects. Journal of Urology 123: 742–747

Mezza Coppa P M, Price A P, Kassner E G, Haller J O, Glassberg K I 1987 Cohen ureteral reimplantation: sonographic appearance. Radiology 165: 851–852

Peters C A, Mandell J, Lebowitz R L et al 1989 Congenital obstructed megaureters in early infancy diagnosis and treatment. Journal of Urology 142: 641–645

Pfister R C, Hendren W H 1978 Primary megaureters in children and adults. Clinical and pathophysiological features of 150 ureters. Urology 12: 160–176

Pollack H M, Popky G L, Blumbery M L 1975 Hernias of the ureter – an anatomic roengenographic study. Radiology 117: 275–281

Sarajic M, Dursh Zivkovic B, Svoren E et al 1989 Congenital ureteric diverticula in children and adults. Classification, radiological and clinical features. British Journal of Radiology 62: 551–553

Schneider K, Fendel H, Kohn M M 1985 Investigation of dilated ureters in children. Annales de Radiologie 29: 424–426

Sherman C, Winchester P, Brill P W, Minnsberg D 1988 Childhood retroperitoneal fibrosis. Pediatric Radiology 18: 245–247

Snyder M M, Johnston J H 1978 Orthoptic ureterocele in children. Journal of Urology 119: 543–546

Young D W, Lebowitz R L 1988 Congenital anomalies of the ureter. Seminars in Roentgenology 21: 172–187

LOWER URINARY TRACT OBSTRUCTION: POSTERIOR URETHRAL VALVES

Congenital urethral valves may result in the most severe obstructive uropathies of infancy. They may present later in childhood or even early adult life with renal failure, urinary infection or incontinence. The majority take the form of bicuspid or unicuspid mucosal folds at the level of the verumontanum.

Perinatal diagnosis

Urinary tract dilatation in utero may be due to bladder outlet obstruction. The main cause is posterior urethral valves. Antenatal US demonstrates a large thick-walled bladder which fails to empty in a male fetus. Mild or marked dilatation of the upper urinary tract is present (Fig. 5.4.25A). Usually there is thinning and increased echogenicity of the renal parenchyma and macrocysts may be seen (Fig. 5.4.25B). These features are suggestive of dysplasia and if present it is important to assess renal function.

In the second trimester the differential diagnosis includes urethral atresia which may be part of the prune belly syndrome. Urethral atresia may present earlier than posterior urethral valves in the pregnancy because of fetal growth retardation.

Ascites and renal dysplasia may be present and the outcome may be fatal. In later pregnancy the differential diagnosis includes the 'megacystis-megaureter syndrome', in which there is a large bladder with marked bilateral hydronephrosis secondary to reflux, but the chest development and amniotic fluid are normal.

Bladder outlet obstruction may also be secondary to urethral polyps or a diverticulum of the anterior urethra.

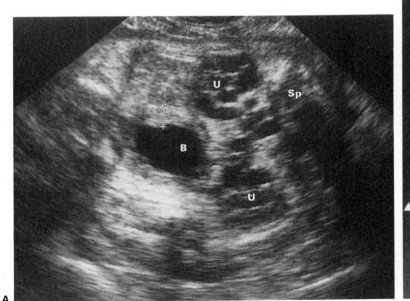

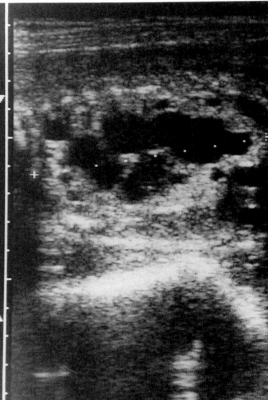

A   **B**

Fig. 5.4.25 Ultrasound. Posterior urethral valves in utero – 30 weeks. **A** Transverse scan of fetal abdomen with thickened filled fetal bladder (B), wall thickness 5 mm between crosses. U = bilateral dilated ureters, Sp = fetal spine. **B** Sagittal scan of hydronephrotic fetal kidney (between crosses). Hyperechoic parenchyma with macrocysts suggestive of dysplasia.

Table 5.4.3   Ascites in the neonate

Urinary origin
  Obstruction
    Posterior urethral valves
    Pelviureteric junction
    Vesicoureteric junction
Gastrointestinal
  Perforation
  Appendicitis
  Imperforate anus
  Obstruction
Cardiac
  Cardiac malformations
  Heart failure
Hepatic
  Diffuse liver disease/hepatitis
  Meckel–Gruber
  Biliary atresia
  Common bile duct perforation
  Portal vein obstruction
Systemic infection
Obstruction thoracic duct
Hydrometrocolpos
Ruptured ovarian cysts

Antenatal and perinatal ultrasound may demonstrate ascites and perirenal urinomas in infants with posterior urethral valves. Urinary tract obstruction is an important cause of neonatal ascites (Table 5.4.3). A cystic pararenal mass compressing the kidney (Fig. 5.4.26) is seen in cases of antenatal urinoma. These are caused by leakage of urine, under pressure from the collecting system into the perinephric space, or the retroperitoneum or, as in ascites, the peritoneum. This is thought to be due to perforation of a calyceal fornix and accumulation of urine in a subcapsular or perirenal location with subsequent rupture or transudation across the peritoneum. Rarely perforation of the bladder may occur. This results in decompression of the urinary tract, so that the bladder may appear small and the kidneys may not be hydronephrotic. It is important that posterior urethral valves are excluded in cases of neonatal ascites and urinoma. Following relief of the primary obstruction most cases of urinoma will resolve spontaneously. Percutaneous drainage is indicated if there is infection or respiratory compromise secondary to the mass.

Following the findings of bladder outlet obstruction on antenatal US, decompresssion of the bladder in utero and the insertion of vesicoamniotic shunts have been performed. However, it is still unclear whether this results in consistent benefit to the fetus. After birth, the diagnosis of posterior urethral valves is confirmed by US and a micturating cystourethrogram. A thickened bladder wall, dilated posterior urethra and dilatation of the collecting systems is seen on US (Fig. 5.4.27). As described previously there may be ascites and/or a urinoma. The MCUG demonstrates a dilated posterior urethra and a thickened, trabeculated bladder wall (Fig. 5.4.28). There may be reflux into a dilated utricle, prostatic glands, urachus and commonly into the ureters. Bladder diverticula may be present. Functional studies with radioisotopes, preferentially MAG3, are necessary to assess parenchymal function and drainage but should be left for a month after primary treatment.

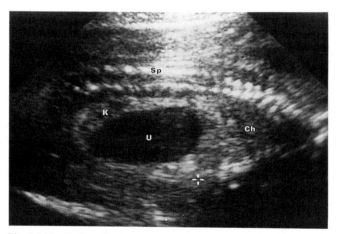

Fig. 5.4.26 Perirenal urinoma in posterior urethral valves. In utero. Sagittal scan of fetal trunk. Urinoma (U) in front of the kidney (K). Sp = spine, Ch = fetal chest.

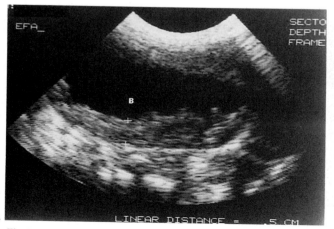

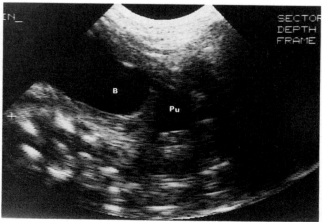

Fig. 5.4.27 Posterior urethral valves. Ultrasound of the bladder (B). **A** Thickened irregular bladder wall. **B** Dilated posterior urethra (Pu).

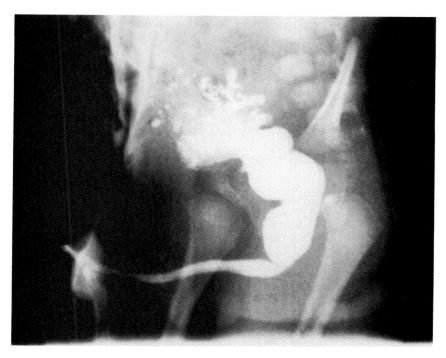

Fig. 5.4.28 Posterior urethral valves in a neonate. Note dilated posterior urethra with small grossly trabeculated bladder.

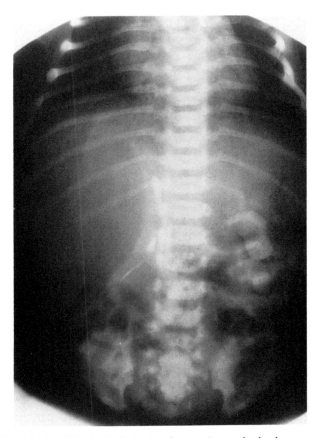

An IVU will demonstrate a urinoma (Fig. 5.4.29) and also the anatomy and function of the kidneys, but has now been superseded by US and radioisotope studies. In neonates with severe renal dysplasia in whom oligohydramnios has resulted in hypoplastic lungs, pneumothoraces may occur and may be a cause of death.

Fig. 5.4.29 IVU at birth. Patient with posterior urethral valves. Perirenal urinoma with displacement and compression of the right kidney. The urinoma is not opacified by the contrast medium.

Diagnosis in older children

In some patients posterior urethral valves are not diagnosed in the neonatal period. Clinical presentation is of a urinary tract infection, a renal mass or renal failure. The diagnosis is made with an MCUG (Figs 5.4.30). In these late cases the valve may result in a lesser degree of bladder outlet obstruction and the upper tract dilatation is variable. The classical bicuspid folds are not present, instead there is an incomplete diaphragm traversing the posterior urethra just distal to the verumontanum.

Incomplete non-obstructive folds are commonly seen in the posterior urethra of male children. These do not cause obstruction to urethral flow and are of no clinical significance.

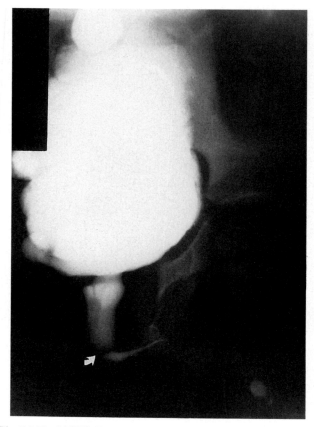

Fig. 5.4.30 MCUG. Two-year-old boy. Posterior urethral valves with trabeculated bladder wall, diverticula and typical comma-like appearance of the valves (arrow).

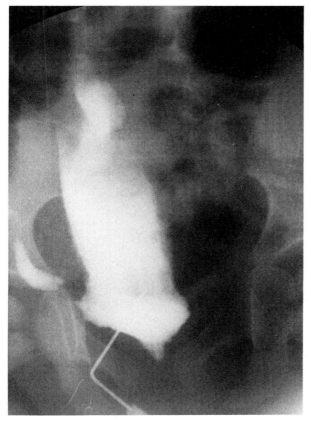

Fig. 5.4.31 Suprapubic MCUG. Prune belly syndrome with elongated bladder, urachal opacification and right vesicoureteric reflux.

REFERENCES

Callen P W, Bolding D, Filly R A, Harrisson M R 1983
Ultrasonographic evaluation of fetal paranephric pseudocysts.
Journal of Ultrasound in Medicine 2: 309–312

Cass A S, Stephen F D 1974 Posterior urethral valves: diagnosis and
treatment. Journal of Urology 112: 519–525

Cremin B, Aaronson I 1983 Ultrasonic diagnosis of posterior
urethral valves in neonates. British Journal of Radiology
56: 435–438

Chevalier R 1989 Obstructive nephropathy in early development.
Seminars in Nephrology 9: 5–9

Elder J S, Duckett J W, Snyder M M 1987 Intervention for fetal
obstructive uropathy: has it been effective? Lancet 1007–1010

Feinstein K A, Fernbach S K 1987 Septated urinomas in the neonate.
American Journal of Roentgenology 149: 997–1000

Glick P L, Harrisson M R, Golbus M S et al 1985 Management of the
fetus with congenital hydronephrosis II. Prognostic criteria and
selection for treatment. Journal of Pediatric Surgery 20: 376–387

Griscom N T, Colodny A H, Rosenberg H K, Fliegel C P, Hardy B E
1977 Diagnostic aspects of neonatal ascites: report of 27 cases.
American Journal of Roentgenology 128: 961–970

Heaton N D, Kadow C, Yates-Bell A J 1989 Late presentation of
congenital urethral valves. British Journal of Urology 64: 98

Kirchner S G, Braren V, Heller R M, Kirchner F K 1980 Uriniferous
perirenal pseudocysts: an unusual cause of calcified abdominal
mass in the newborn. Pediatric Radiology 9: 43–44

MacPherson R I, Gordon L, Bradford B L 1984 Neonatal urinomas:
imaging considerations. Pediatric Radiology 14: 396–399

MacPherson R I, Leithiser R E, Gordon L et al 1986 Posterior
urethral valves: an update and review. Radiographics 6: 753–791

Mahony B S, Callen P W, Filly R A 1985 Fetal urethral obstruction:
US evaluation. Radiology 157: 221–224

Mahony B S, Filly R A, Callen P W, Hricak H, Colbus M S,
Harrisson M R 1984 Fetal renal dysplasia: sonographic
evaluation. Radiology 152: 143–146

Reha W C, Gibbons M D 1989 Neonatal ascites and urethral valves.
Urology 33: 468–471

Reuss A, Wladimiroff J W, Stewart P A, Scholtmeiser R J 1988 Non-
invasive management of fetal obstructive uropathy. Lancet
949–951

Rittenberg M H, Hulbert W C, Snyder H M, Duckett J W 1988
Protective factors in posterior urethral valves. Journal of Urology
140: 993–996

Schultze L J, Blickman J G, Van Es A D, Hew J M 1984
Retroperitoneal reabsorption of extravasated urine in renal
transplant patients. Radiology 153: 625–626

Soulez G, Montagne J P H, Fauré C, Giruner M 1989 Urinome du
nouveau-né compliquant une uropathie congénitale. Journal de
Radiologie (Paris) 70: 471–476

Vintzileos A M, Campbell W A, Rodis J A, Nochinson D J, Pinette
R G, Retrikovsky B M 1989 Comparison of six different
ultrasonographic methods for predicting lethal fetal pulmonary
hypoplasia. American Journal of Obstetrics and Gynecology
161: 606–612

PRUNE BELLY SYNDROME

The prune belly syndrome occurs almost exclusively in males and consists of deficient abdominal musculature, undescended testes and a dilated, dysplastic urinary tract. Other associated abnormalities include, malrotation of bowel, congenital hip dislocation, Hirschsprungs' disease, and congenital heart disease.

On US dilated and tortuous ureters with bilateral hydronephrosis are seen. An MCUG demonstrates an elongated, large bladder with an irregular contour, and bilateral vesicoureteric reflux (Fig. 5.4.31). The urethra is usually abnormal, the posterior urethra is typically dilated and the prostatic utricle is opacified (Fig. 5.4.32). Later utricular calculi may form. There may be a megalourethra or in severe cases urethral atresia. Dysmorphic kidneys with dilated, tortuous and laterally placed ureters and flared iliac wings with a wide interpubic distance are seen on IVU (Fig. 5.4.33).

REFERENCES

Berdon W E, Baker D H, Wigger H J et al 1977 Radiologic and pathologic spectrum of the prune-belly syndrome. Radiologic Clinics of North America 15: 83–92
Cremin B J 1971 The urinary tract anomalies associated with agenesis of the abdominal walls. British Journal of Radiology 44: 767–772
Christoffer C R, Spinelli A, Severt D 1982 Ultrasonic diagnosis of prune-belly syndrome. Obstetrics and Gynecology 59: 391
Greskovich F J, Nyberg L M 1988 The prune-belly syndrome: a review of its etiology, defects, treatment and prognosis. Journal of Urology 707–712

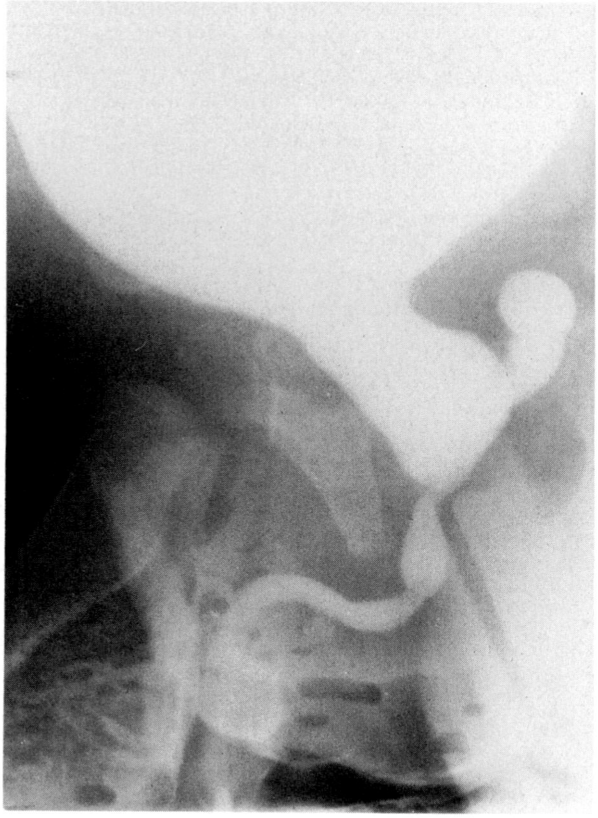

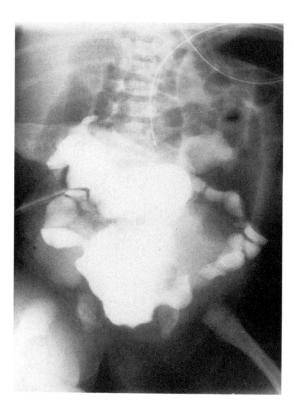

Fig. 5.4.32 MCUG. Prune belly syndrome during micturition. Dilatation of posterior urethra without obstruction. Opacification of a large utricle is seen posteriorly.

Fig. 5.4.33 IVU. Prune belly syndrome. Dysmorphic kidneys, ureters and bladder.

5.5 DUPLEX SYSTEMS, URETERIC ECTOPIA AND RELATED ANOMALIES

Duplication of the renal collecting system is a common anomaly and is the result of aberrant ureteral budding from the Wolffian duct at 5 weeks after conception. If the tip of the bud bifurcates before invading the metanephric stoma, a bifid pelvis results. If bifurcation from the Wolffian duct is more proximal, but the resultant ureters stay close together, the collecting system is duplex. Complete duplication involves the renal pelvis and whole length of ureter so that each division of the pelvis is drained by its own ureter opening separately into the bladder. The ureters cross in the abdomen or pelvis so that the ureter draining the upper renal segment always opens below and medial to the normally sited ureteric orifice for the lower renal segment (Table 5.5.1).

Table 5.5.1   Glossary of duplex systems, ectopic ureters and ureterocoeles

Duplex kidney	A kidney with two pelvicalyceal systems
Upper (lower) pole	One of the components of a duplex kidney
Duplex system	Duplex kidney with a single, a bifid or two ureters
Bifid system	Two pelvicalyceal systems that join before emptying in the bladder either at the pelviureteric junction (bifid pelvis) or at the vesicoureteric junction (bifid ureter)
Double ureter	Complete duplication. Separate openings into the urinary or genital tract
Upper (lower) pole ureter	Ureter that drains the upper pole of a duplex system
Upper (lower) pole orifice	Orifice associated with the ureter that drains the upper pole
Lateral ectopic	Orifice situated lateral to the normal position
Caudal or medial ectopic	Ureteral orifice situated at the proximal tip of the bladder neck or beyond.
Ectopic ureter	Ureter that drains to an abnormal site
Intravesical ureterocoele	Ureterocoele located entirely within the bladder (associated with single or duplex system)
Ectopic ureterocoele	Ureterocoele in which some portion of ureterocoele is situated permanently at the bladder neck or in the urethra. Ureterocoeles are stenotic, sphincteric or sphinctero-stenotic

UNCOMPLICATED DUPLEX SYSTEMS

The diagnosis of an uncomplicated duplex kidney is usually an incidental finding on US or IVU. The duplex kidney may be longer than the opposite normal kidney and a discrepancy of more than 1 cm in size should alert one to the diagnosis. US may demonstrate two distinct echogenic hilar complexes separated by a band of parenchyma (Fig. 5.5.1). However, diagnosis with US is unreliable and an IVU may be necessary to demonstrate the abnormal anatomy more clearly (Fig. 5.5.2). If the patient has presented with urinary tract infection an MCUG may be necessary as vesicoureteric reflux commonly occurs to the lower pole, even if there is no pelvicalyceal dilatation on US.

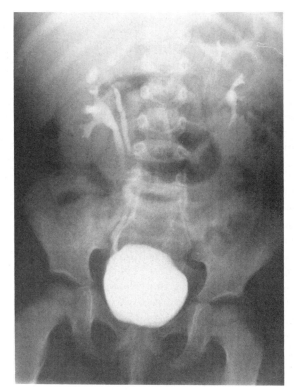

Fig. 5.5.2   IVU showing bilateral duplex systems.

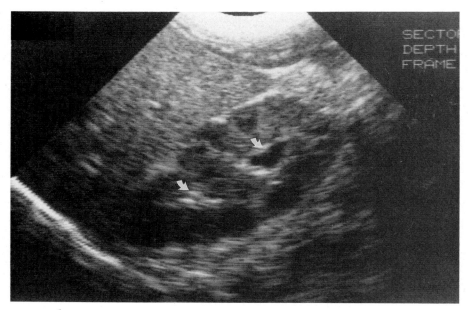

Fig. 5.5.1   US of duplex kidney with two collecting systems (arrows) separated by a central band of parenchyma.

COMPLICATED DUPLEX SYSTEMS

Ureteral duplication becomes clinically significant when it is associated with symptoms of infection of the urinary tract, vaginal discharge or wetting, abdominal mass or loin pain. The ureter draining the upper pole is the ectopic ureter and inserts medial to and below the orthotopic ureter. In females the insertion may be into the trigone, urethra, perineum, uterus or vagina. In males the ectopic ureter may insert into the trigone, the posterior urethra, an ejaculatory duct, seminal vesicle or vas deferens. Many ectopic ureters are associated with a stenotic orifice and a ureterocoele. Hydronephrosis of the upper pole of a duplex kidney results from obstruction and hydronephrosis, and scarring of the lower pole may be present secondary to vesicoureteric reflux.

Perinatal diagnosis

Dilatation of the pelvicalyceal system (usually the upper pole) and a single dilated ureter may be detected with antenatal US and suggests the presence of a duplex kidney (Fig. 5.5.3). If there is marked hydronephrosis, this may obscure the non-dilated lower pole and a wrong diagnosis of a single system will be made. Ureterocoeles are rarely demonstrated antenatally.

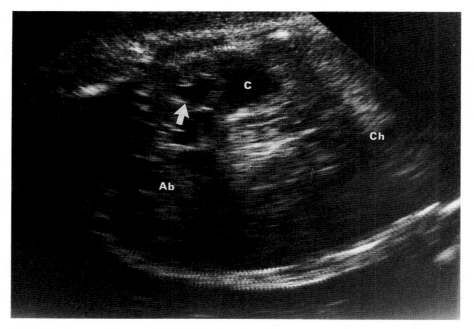

Fig. 5.5.3 Antenatal ultrasound with dilated renal pelvis (arrow).

After birth, US will more clearly demonstrate the abnormal duplex system (Fig. 5.5.4). The hydronephrotic upper pole appears as a cystic mass which must be distinguished from other cystic masses (Table 5.5.2). The surrounding upper pole renal parenchyma may be dysplastic and appear thin and echogenic. It may be very small and dysplastic and completely missed on US. A dilated ureter with a ureterocoele in the bladder is seen (Fig. 5.5.5). Sometimes the ectopic insertion of the ureter is into the vagina and this may be seen on US (Fig. 5.5.6). An MCUG is essential and will demonstrate vesicoureteric reflux into the lower pole of the duplex system. During bladder filling a ureterocoele is seen as a filling defect (Fig. 5.5.7A). When the bladder is full, the ureterocoele may flatten and is less clearly seen,

therefore it is important to look at the bladder during the early part of bladder filling. A ureterocoele may prolapse into the urethra during micturition, resulting in bladder outlet obstruction (Fig. 5.5.7B). Antenatally acute obstruction with rupture of an upper pole fornix and urinoma formation has occurred in these cases.

Table 5.5.2 Cystic lesion at the upper pole of the kidney
Duplex obstructed system
Multicystic dysplastic kidney
Simple renal cyst
Adrenal haemorrhage
Cystic neuroblastoma
Cystic nephroblastoma
Retroperitoneal lymphangioma

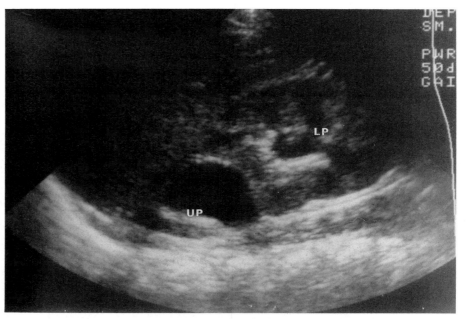

Fig. 5.5.4 Postnatal US showing duplex kidney with hydronephrotic upper pole (UP) and normal lower pole (LP).

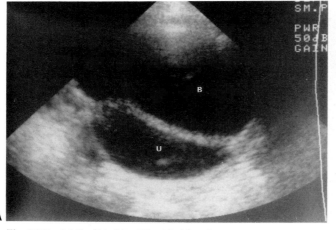

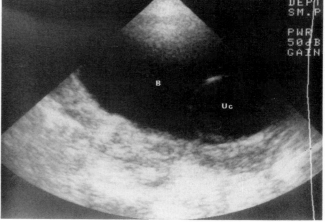

Fig. 5.5.5 **A** US of bladder (B) with dilated ureter (U) behind it. **B** US of bladder (B) with ureterocoele (Uc) within it.

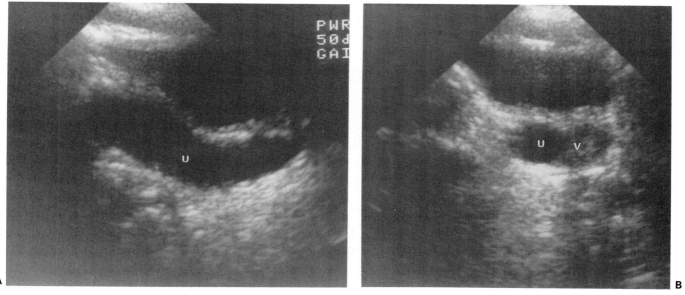

Fig. 5.5.6 **A** US showing ureter (U) inserting below the bladder. **B** Ureter (U) inserting into the vagina (V).

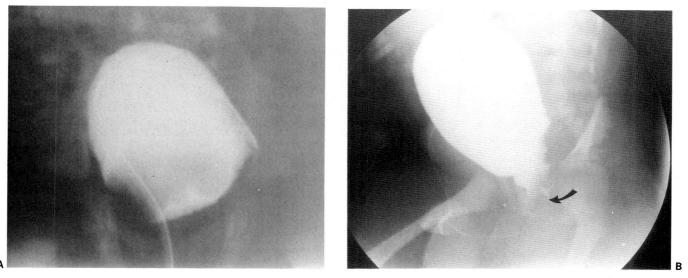

Fig. 5.5.7 **A** MCUG. During the filling phase, the ureterocoele is seen as a filling defect. **B** Ureterocoele (arrow) prolapsing into urethra during micturition.

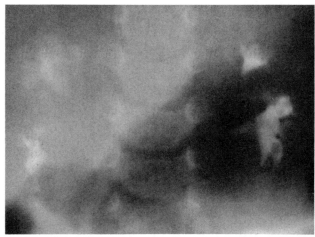

Fig. 5.5.8 Bilateral duplex systems with dysplastic right upper moiety.

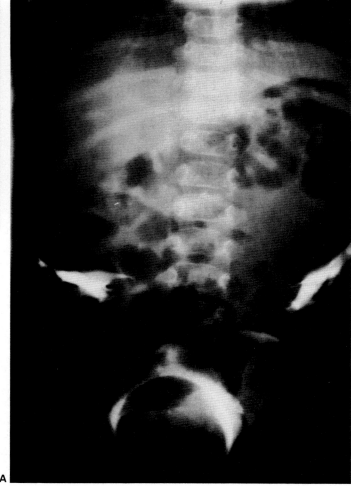

A

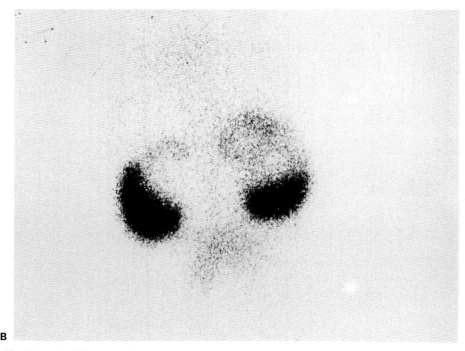

B

Fig. 5.5.9 **A** IVU in an infant with bilateral duplex kidneys with hydronephrotic upper moieties displacing the functioning lower moieties laterally. Note large ureterocoele in bladder. **B** DMSA scan of same infant. There is very poor function in the upper poles.

This may contribute to dysplasia and poor function of the renal parenchyma (Fig. 5.5.8). In some ectopic ureters, inserting outside the bladder, reflux is occasionally visualized during micturition.

An IVU may show the upper pole, depending on its function, and delayed films will be necessary (Figs 5.5.9, 5.5.10). The anatomy of the ureters is clearly seen.

Radioisotope studies with DMSA are required to assess the function of the kidney and in particular the upper pole.

Older children

Constant wetting and vaginal discharge is the typical presenting symptom in girls with a duplex system and ectopic ureter. Other presentations include an inter-labial mass in girls or infection. An IVU may demonstrate the dilated upper pole and ectopic ureter. If upper pole function is poor and it does not opacify, a duplex system should be strongly suspected if there is an increased distance between the top of the renal outline and the collecting system, an abnormal axis of the collecting system, fewer calyces compared to the

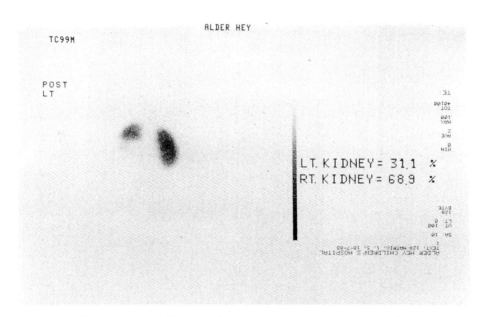

LT. KIDNEY = 31.1 %
RT. KIDNEY = 68.9 %

Fig. 5.5.10 DMSA scan in a child with right duplex kidney. Non-function of the lower moiety is due to reflux damage.

opposite, normal side, lateral displacement of the kidney and a ureter with a spiral course (Fig. 5.5.11). These appearances have been described as the 'drooping flower' (Fig. 5.5.9A).

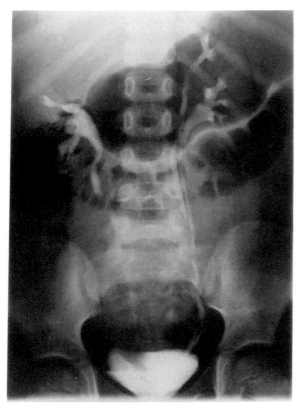

Fig. 5.5.11 IVU. Bilateral duplex systems, with lateral displacement of right lower pole collecting system.

Ureterocoeles: diagnostic difficulties

Ureterocoeles represent a congenital cystic dilatation of the terminal ureter. They are classified as simple or ectopic. Simple ureterocoeles are relatively rare in children and have been described (Fig. 5.5.12) (see '5.4 Urinary tract dilatation'). Ectopic ureterocoeles are more common and are associated with the upper pole of a duplex system in 85–90% of cases. The sonographic appearance of a cystic structure in the bladder is typical. However, in certain situations a ureterocoele is not visualized and can be missed. If the bladder is full it may collapse and 'disappear' (Fig. 5.5.13). Similarly during bladder filling in an MCUG or IVU ureterocoeles may efface and 'disappear' (Fig. 5.5.14A, B). When the bladder is full the ureterocoele may herniate into its own ureter and resemble a diverticulum (Fig. 5.5.14C).

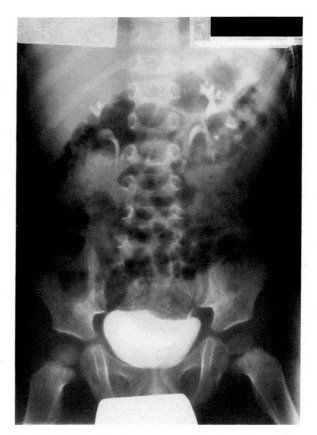

Fig. 5.5.12 Cobra head appearance of simple ureterocoele in the left side of the bladder.

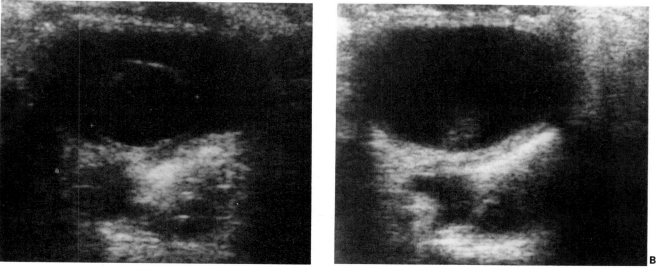

Fig. 5.5.13 **A** US of bladder with large ureterocoele. **B** Collapse of the large ureterocoele within the bladder.

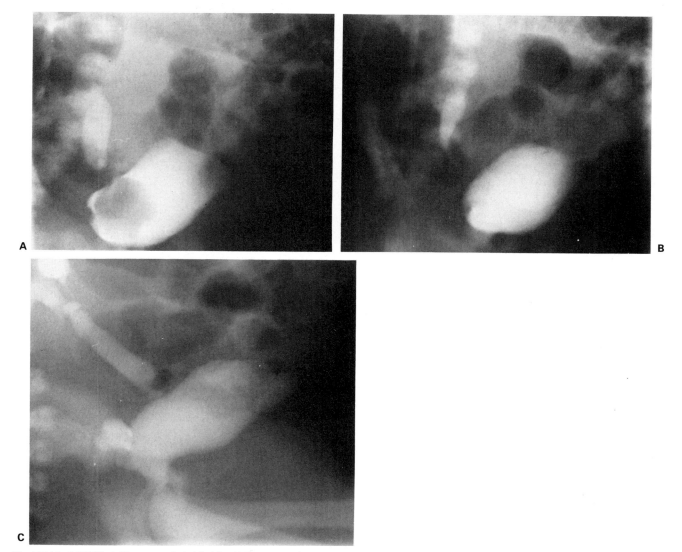

Fig. 5.5.14 MCUG. **A** Ureterocoele in bladder. **B** Ureterocoele not easily seen because of effacement during bladder filling. **C** Herniation of ureterocoele.

All causes of a filling defect in the bladder must be differentiated from a ureterocoele, especially a calculus, blood clots and air bubbles.

There may be a discrepancy between the size of the upper pole dilatation and the size of the ureterocoele, and the upper pole may be difficult to see even on US.

The upper pole connected to the ureterocoele may be a multicystic dysplastic moiety. Most ureterocoeles are separated into stenotic (orifice in the bladder and obstructed) or sphincteric (orifice in the urethra) or sphinctero-stenotic. An uncommon variety of ureterocoele may prolapse into the urethra, and in these cases the orifice of the ureterocoele is large and may be incompetent (Fig. 5.5.15). This type is associated with anomalies of the posterior musculature of the urethra.

Ectopic ureters: diagnostic difficulties

Ureteric orifices may present in any part of the developing Wolffian duct or urogenital sinus: vesical neck, prostatic urethra, seminal vesicle, vas deferens or ejaculation ducts in males; vesical neck, urethra in females. Therefore, opacification of any of these sites and ducts can occur during an MCUG.

Wolffian remnants or müllerian duct remnants in the girl may explain the ectopic insertion into vagina, uterus or Gartner duct leading to cystic masses in the vaginal wall (see 'Multicystic dysplastic kidney' in 5.3). A unilateral single ectopic ureter is a very rare entity. It is associated with a dysplastic poorly functioning kidney that may be demonstrated by US and isotopes (Fig. 5.5.16). It is more frequent in boys in which an MCUG may show reflux into an ectopic ureter, the ejaculatory duct or seminal vesicle. Another variant in boys is a vasoureteric connection in which an MCUG shows reflux into the ureter and vas deferens, both Wolffian duct remnants. This condition is often associated with anorectal malformations.

Lower pole anomalies

Vesicoureteric reflux

The commonest anomaly seen in the renal lower pole is reflux (Fig. 5.5.17). An MCUG or isotope cystogram should be performed in all children with complete duplication. Reflux into the upper pole is uncommon but possible. Reflux into both ureters occurs when both ureters open into a common bladder canal. US may show dilatation of the pelvicalyceal system and thinning of the renal parenchyma in cases of scarring and reflux nephropathy. These abnormalities are also demonstrated on an IVU (Fig. 5.5.18). Large and atonic ureters may be seen.

Pelviureteric junction obstruction

Pelviureteric junction obstruction may affect the lower part of a duplex system (Fig. 5.5.19). The appearances are characteristic of a simple pelviureteric junction obstruction and the diagnosis is made, with US, isotope studies and IVU. Tumours or cysts of the lower pole are easily differentiated.

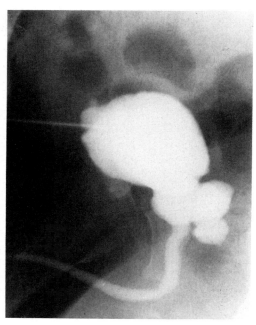

Fig. 5.5.15 Prolapse of part of a ureterocoele into the urethra. The orifice of the ureterocoele is large and incompetent.

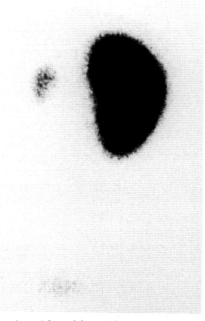

Fig. 5.5.16 DMSA scan in a girl aged five with constant wetting. IVU and US showed no right kidney. DMSA scan shows a tiny dysplastic right kidney whose ureter was found to have an ectopic insertion in the vagina. This was a single system.

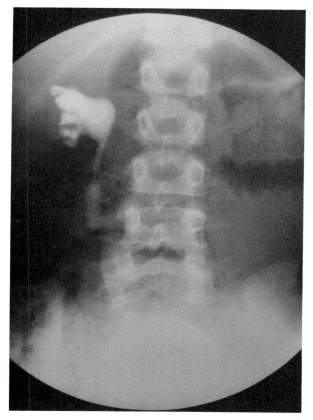

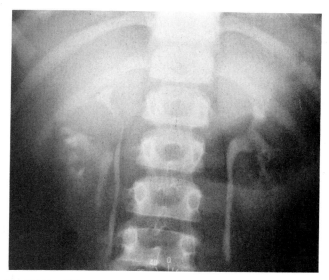

Fig. 5.5.17 MCUG. Vesicoureteric reflux into the lower moiety of a right duplex kidney.

Fig. 5.5.18 IVU. Right duplex kidney with parenchymal thinning and clubbing of calyces in the lower moiety.

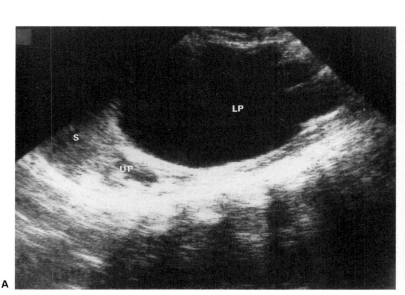

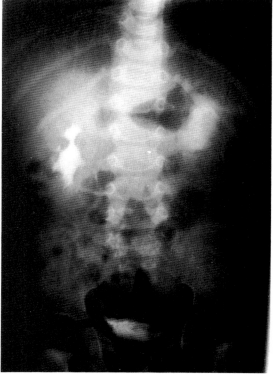

A

B

Fig. 5.5.19 **A** US. Pelviureteric junction obstruction with hydronephrotic lower moiety (LP). The spleen (S) and upper moiety (UP) are identified. **B** IVU. Same patient. Pelviureteric junction obstruction of the lower moiety of left duplex kidney.

Unusual variants of the duplex system

- Ureteral triplication
- Blind-ending ureter (see under ureteral diverticula)
- Yoyo reflux (occurring in incomplete duplications)
- Pyelopelvic or ureteroureteric reflux.

Postoperative studies

If a heminephrectomy with removal of the obstructed upper pole is performed, renal size is reduced. In the bladder, localized thickening of the posterior wall can be seen secondary to reimplantation.

If the ureterocoele is left in place and heminephrectomy and ureterectomy performed, the collapsed ureterocoele can be seen in the bladder (Fig. 5.5.20). When the ureterocoele is incised, as occurs more and more in newborns, reduction of the upper pole dilatation can be monitored by US.

In cases of ectopic ureter, the distal part is usually left and reflux may occur into the unused ureter (Fig. 5.5.21). Another potential complication is infection of this segment. Other postoperative complications include urine leakage or haemorrhage which can be detected and followed by US and IVU.

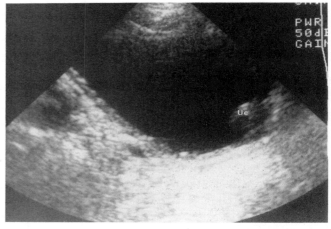

Fig. 5.5.20 US. Collapsed ureterocoele (Uc) in the bladder following heminephrectomy.

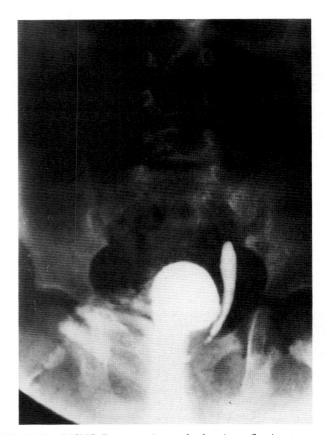

Fig. 5.5.21 MCUG. Postoperative study showing reflux into a residual distal ectopic ureter.

REFERENCES

Bauer S B, Retik A B 1978 The non-obstructive ectopic ureterocoele. Journal of Urology 119: 804–807

Balchick R J, Nasrallah P F 1987 Cecoureterocoele. Journal of Urology 137: 100–101

Caoine P, Zaccara A, Capozza N, De Gennaro M 1989 How prenatal ultrasound can effect the treatment of ureterocoele in neonates and children? European Urology 16: 357–364

Curarino G 1982 Single vaginal ectopic ureter and Gartner's duct cysts with ispilateral renal hypoplasia and dysplasia. Journal of Urology 128: 988–993

Dinkel E, Dittrich M, Peters H et al 1985 Sonographic biometry in obstructive uropathy in children: preoperative diagnosis and post-operative monitoring. Urologic Radiology 7: 1–7

Eklof O, Makinen E 1974 Ectopic ureterocoele: a radiological appraisal of 66 consecutive cases. Pediatric Radiology 11–120

Fitzsimons P J, Frost R A, Millward et al 1986 Prenatal and post natal US diagnosis of ureterocoele. Journal of Canadian Association of Radiology 37: 189

Gibbons M D, Cromie W J, Duckett J W 1978 Ectoptic vas deferens. Journal of Urology 120: 597–604

Glassberg K I, Braren V, Duckett J W et al 1984 Suggested terminology for duplex system, ectopic ureters and ureterocoeles. Journal of Urology 132: 1153–1154

Gomez F, Stephens F D 1983 Cecoureterocoele: morphology and clinical implications. Journal of Urology 129: 1017–1019

Hartman G W, Hodson C J 1969 Duplex kidneys and related abnormalities. Clinical Radiology 20: 387–400

Joseph D B, Bauer S B, Colodny A H, Mandell J, Lebowitz R L, Retik A B 1989 Lower pole ureteropelvic junction obstruction and incomplete renal duplication. Journal of Urology 141: 896–99

Lebowitz F L, Avni E F 1980 Misleading appearances in pediatric uroradiology. Pediatric Radiology 10: 15–31

Mandell J, Bauer S B, Colodny A H, Lebowitz R L, Retik A B 1981 Ureteral ectopia in infants and children. Journal of Urology 126: 219–222

Mezzacappa P M, Price A P, Kassner E G, Haller J O, Glassberg K I 1987 Cohen ureteral reimplantations – sonographic appearances. Radiology 165: 851–852

Nussbaum A R, Dorst J P, Jeffs R D, Gearhart J P, Sander R C 1986 Ectopic ureter and ureterocoele: their varied sonographic manifestations. Radiology 159: 227–235

Nussbaum A R, Lebowitz R L 1983 Interlabial masses in little girls review and imaging recommendations. American Journal of Roentgenology 141: 65–71

Perkins P J, Kroorand R L, Evans A T 1973 Ureteral triplication. Radiology 108: 533–538

Privett J T, Jean W D, Roylance J 1976 The incidence and importance of renal duplication. Clinical Radiology 27: 521–530

Schulman C C 1976 The single ectopic ureter. European Urology 2: 64–69

Share J C, Lebowitz R L 1988 Ectopic ureterocoele without ureteral and calyceal dilatation. Findings on urography and US. American Journal of Roentgenology 152: 567–571

Teele R L, Lebowitz R L, Colodny A H 1976 Reflux into the unused ureter. Journal of Urology 115: 310–313

Tressider G C, Blandy J P, Murray R S 1970 Pyelo-pelvic and uretero-ureteric reflux. British Journal of Urology 42: 728–735

Vodermark J S 1983 The persisting mesonephric duct syndrome: the description of a new syndrome. Journal of Urology 130: 958–961

5.6 INFECTIOUS DISEASES OF THE URINARY TRACT

IMAGING URINARY TRACT INFECTIONS

Urinary tract infection (UTI) is the most common non-epidemic bacterial infectious disease. During infancy and childhood, about 5% of girls and 0.5% of boys will be affected by at least one episode.

The role of imaging is to detect any predisposing underlying congenital abnormalities. These include vesicoureteric reflux, obstruction and other structural abnormalities. Imaging may also be important in the diagnosis and follow-up of severe and complicated infections such as renal abscesses, acute lobar nephronia, fungal diseases, tuberculosis and xanthogranulomatous pyelonephritis. Renal scarring and damage may be a consequence of an infection; imaging is used to detect scarring and to monitor any progressive damage.

REFERENCES

Avni E F, Van Sinoy M L, Hall M, Stallenberg B, Matos C 1989 Reduced renal mass with glomerular hyperfiltration: a cause of renal hyperechogenicity in children. Pediatric Radiology 19: 108–110

Capdeville R, Fortier Beaulieu M, Gauthier N, Mareschal J L 1973 Images striees du haut appareil urinaire. Journal de Radiologie (Paris) 54: 509–513

Dinkel E, Orth S, Dittrich M, Schulte Wisserman H 1986 Renal sonography in the differentiation of upper from lower urinary tract. American Journal of Roentgenology 146: 775–780

Galaknoff C, Hospitel S, Dana A, Michel J R 1986 Pyelo-ureterite cystique. Journal de Radiologie (Paris) 67: 463–468

Johnson C E, Debaz B P, Shurin P A, Debartholomeo R 1986 Renal US evaluation of UTI in children. Pediatrics 78: 871–878

Levin R, Burbridge K A, Abramson S, Berdon W E, Hensle T W 1984 The diagnosis and management of renal inflammatory processes in children. Journal of Urology 132: 718–721

Montgomery P, Kuhn J P, Afshani E 1987 CT evaluation of severe renal inflammatory disease in children. Pediatric Radiology 17: 216–222.

Morehouse H T, Weiner S N, Hoffman J C 1984 Imaging in inflammatory disease of the kidney. American Journal of Roentgenology 143: 135–141

Padovani J, Grangier M L, Faure F, Devred P H, Panuel M 1983 Les varices essentielles chez l'enfant. Annales de Radiologie (Paris) 27: 482–486

Paltiel H, Lebowitz R L 1989 Neonatal hydronephrosis due to primary reflux: changing patterns in diagnosis and treatment. Radiology 170: 787–789

Picirillo M, Rigsby C M, Rosenfield A T 1987 Sonography of renal inflammatory disease. Urologic Radiology 9: 66–78

CONGENITAL ABNORMALITIES

- Vesicoureteric reflux
- Obstruction
    pelviureteric junction obstruction
    megaureter
    posterior urethral valves
    duplex kidney and ectopic ureterocoele
- Structural abnormalities:
    bladder diverticula.

VESICOURETERIC REFLUX

The detection of vesicoureteric reflux and its role in the aetiology of urinary tract infection and reflux nephropathy, originally known as chronic pyelonephritis, has been the subject of considerable work over the last two decades.

In primary reflux there is abnormal function of the vesicoureteric junction secondary to a short distal ureteric submucosal tunnel in the bladder and an incompetent orifice.

Reflux is most frequently detected after a urinary tract infection. Between 1% and 2% of prepubertal children have asymptomatic bacteriuria, 14–33% of these children have vesicoureteric reflux. If the infection is symptomatic, the percentage of children with reflux rises to 18–50%. Up to one-third of children with reflux will develop reflux nephropathy. Vesicoureteric reflux and infection are therefore important complementary factors in the aetiology of reflux nephropathy. Reflux nephropathy is also an important cause of renal failure. Between 0.4% and 18% of normal children, including 10% of newborns, have been shown to have reflux. It is therefore important to detect reflux as early as possible in order to be able to institute prophylactic antibiotic treatment and hopefully reduce the risk of scarring and reflux nephropathy. Vesicoureteric reflux is also associated with renal dysplasia, which may be an untreatable contributory factor to reflux nephropathy.

Methods of detection

Detection of vesicoureteric reflux in the young infant is with an MCUG. It should be performed after the first well-documented urinary tract infection in both boys and girls. The examination is usually delayed for approximately 6 weeks during which a 15-day course of antibiotics is administered. While MCUG has been considered to be the 'gold standard' for the detection of vesicoureteric reflux, it has certain disadvantages.

The bladder is filled in a non-physiological manner, the examination is of limited duration so that intermittent reflux may be missed and it involves the use of radiation. During the MCUG, not only should the presence of reflux be documented, but also the grade of reflux, whether it occurs during micturition alone or also during filling, and the degree of bladder emptying. Grading of reflux is important for follow-up because higher grades of reflux are less likely to disappear spontaneously (Fig. 5.6.1). Grading of reflux is based on the International Reflux Committee Study (I–V) (Fig. 5.6.2).

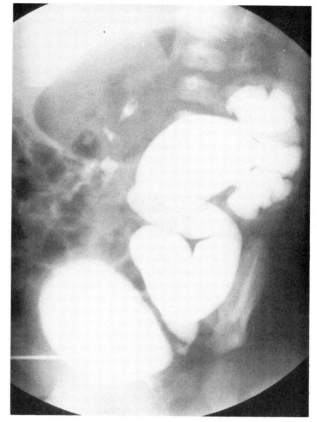

Fig. 5.6.1 Grading reflux. MCUG Left grade 5, right grade 2 reflux.

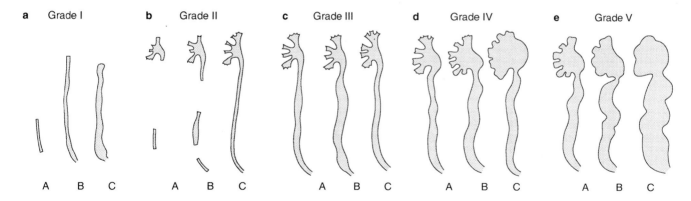

Fig. 5.6.2 Grades of reflux. Diagrams illustrating variations within grades I – V vesicoureteric reflux. **a** *Grade I*: vesicoureteric reflux does not reach the renal pelvis, with A, B, C: different degrees of ureteral dilatation. **b**. *Grade II*: vesicoureteric reflux extending up to the renal pelvis without dilatation, with A and B: filling of the ureter and calyces incomplete. C: filling of the ureter and calyces complete. **c** *Grade III*: vesicoureteric reflux extending up to the kidney, with A: mild dilatation of the ureter, renal pelvis and calyces, no blunting of the calyceal fornices B: moderate dilatation of the ureter and renal pelvis and mild ureteral tortuosity, no blunting of the calyceal fornices. C: mild dilatation of the ureter, moderate dilatation of the renal pelvis, slight blunting of the calyceal fornices. **d** *Grade IV*: moderate dilatation of the ureter with complete obliteration of the sharp angles of the calyceal fornices, but the papillary impressions visible, with A: moderate dilatation of the renal pelvis and calyces, complete obliteration of the sharp angles in majority of fornices. B: moderate tortuosity of the ureter and moderate dilatation of the renal pelvis. Complete obliteration of the sharp angles of all fornices. C: moderate tortuosity of the ureter, extensive dilatation of the renal pelvis, though papillary impressions are visible in the majority of calyces. **e** *Grade V* with A: moderate dilatation of the tortuous ureter, moderate dilatation of the renal pelvis, a papillary impression visible in only one of the calyces. B: gross dilatation of a tortuous ureter, renal pelvis and calyces; no papillary impressions visible. C: extreme dilatation of the whole upper urinary tract. (Reproduced with permission from Lebowitz R L et al 1985 International system of radiographic grading of vesicoureteric reflux. Pediatric Radiology 15: 105–109.)

Intrarenal reflux occurs in 5–15% of children with vesicoureteric reflux (Fig. 5.6.3). It is more likely to occur at the upper and lower poles of the kidneys because of the particular orientation of the precalyceal tubules at these sites. Intrarenal reflux with infected urine is thought to be an important cause of renal scarring.

Vesicoureteric reflux may also be detected with radionuclide studies, the direct and indirect isotope cystogram (Fig. 5.1.27). The technique of direct isotope cystography (DIC) is similar to MCUG. The advantages are the high sensitivity of the technique and the low radiation exposure compared with a conventional MCUG, the dose being reduced by a factor of 20. However, like MCUG, the child has to be catheterized (Fig. 5.6.4).

In the toilet-trained child, the indirect radionuclide cystogram (IRC) can be performed with ^{99m}Tc-DTPA or ^{99m}Tc-MAG3. The sensitivity of IRC is approximately equal to MCUG when ^{99m}Tc-DTPA is used, and may be higher with ^{99m}Tc-MAG3. Not only does this technique have a low radiation exposure but also does not require bladder catheterization. Vesicoureteric reflux during the filling phase of the IRC cannot be demonstrated, but it has been demonstrated that only 3% of all refluxing kidneys reflux only during filling. Both DIC and IRC are therefore useful in the diagnosis and follow-up of children with vesicoureteric reflux.

US is unable at present to demonstrate vesicoureteric reflux reliably. Recent work with colour flow has attempted to look at the jet phenomenon and urine flow into the bladder and reflux, without any useful conclusion. The development of ultrasound contrast media may enable a cystogram to be performed with ultrasound imaging.

When small, scarred kidneys are seen with US the presence of vesicoureteric reflux must be excluded, either in association with renal dysplasia or reflux nephropathy. An irregular renal outline with focal parenchymal loss is characteristic of the scarring seen in reflux. Hydronephrosis and ureteric dilatation may be seen in reflux, but ureteric dilatation behind the bladder may be intermittent. However, in the minor grades of reflux, particularly if scarring is subtle or absent, the renal ultrasound may be completely normal.

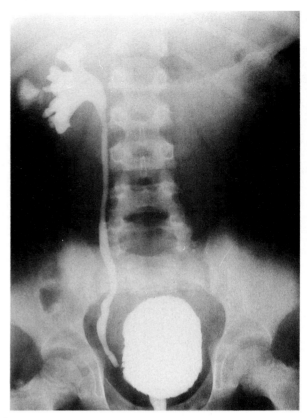

Fig. 5.6.3 Intrarenal reflux. MCUG. Right grade 3 reflux with intrarenal reflux.

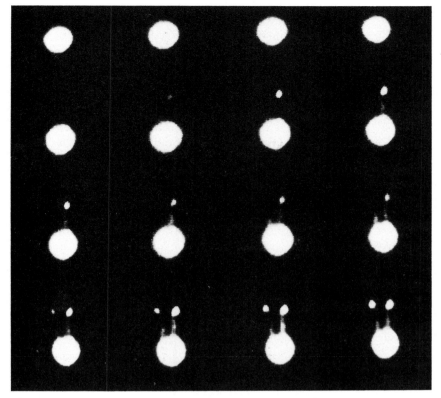

Fig. 5.6.4 Radionuclide cystography. Progressive appearance of bilateral reflux.

Intravenous urography has little value in the detection of vesicoureteric reflux. The examination may be normal in cases of mild reflux and may underestimate the severity of reflux. Dilatation developing during an IVU is indicative of reflux. In more severe reflux, dilated ureters with striations are suggestive (Fig. 5.6.5), and if there is evidence of renal scarring with associated calyceal clubbing, then reflux nephropathy is likely to be present. Vesicoureteric reflux may also result in an appearance on IVU which is the same as an obstructive uropathy, with dilated collecting systems, diffuse cortical loss and failure of renal growth. In very severe reflux, the IVU should be performed with a catheter in the bladder to prevent reflux during the examination as this may mimic function.

Vesicoureteric reflux is associated with numerous congenital urinary tract abnormalities. These include:

- Posterior urethral valves
- Multicystic kidney
- Megaureters
- Ectopic ureters, single and duplex (Fig. 5.6.6) (in the duplex kidney, reflux is typically into the lower moiety ureter) (see 5.5)
- Hutch diverticulum
- Prune belly syndrome
- Pelviureteric junction obstruction (see 5.4 'Urinary tract dilatation').

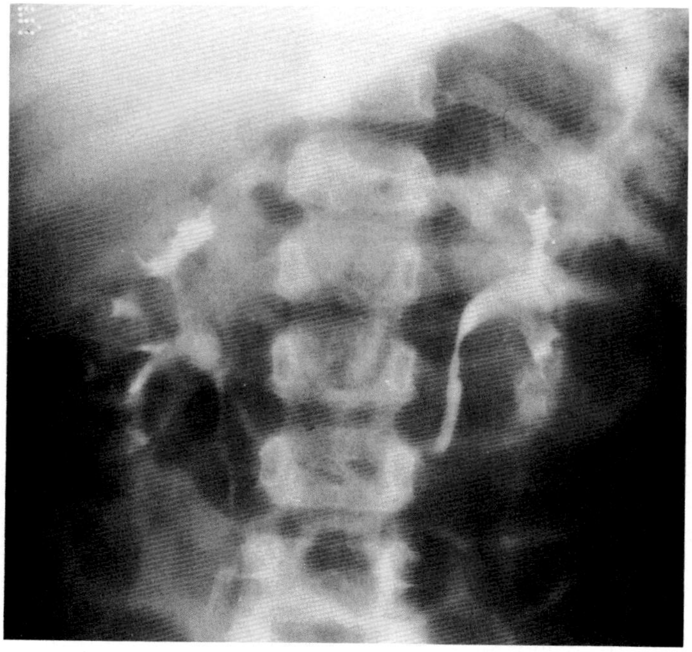

Reflux in the neonate

With antenatal US the presence of vesicoureteric reflux in the fetus may be demonstrated. Reflux detected in utero corresponds to Grade III–V and is more frequent in boys. Dilated pelvicalyceal systems are seen, and causes other than reflux such as obstruction must be excluded. Variation in the size of the pelvicalyceal dilatation during the ultrasound scan is more likely to be due to reflux than obstruction (Fig. 5.6.7). Dysplasia of the renal parenchyma may be an associated finding.

Fig. 5.6.5 IVU: Note striated right renal pelvis. This is a manifestation of reflux which was later proven on MCUG.

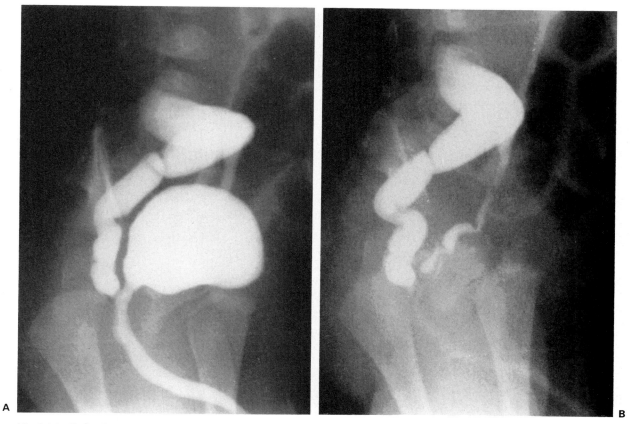

Fig. 5.6.6 Reflux in ectopic ureters. Case of fused pelvic kidneys. **A** Right reflux in ectopic ureter inserting just above the verumontanum. **B** At left, reflux occurs in vas deferens wherein the ureter connects.

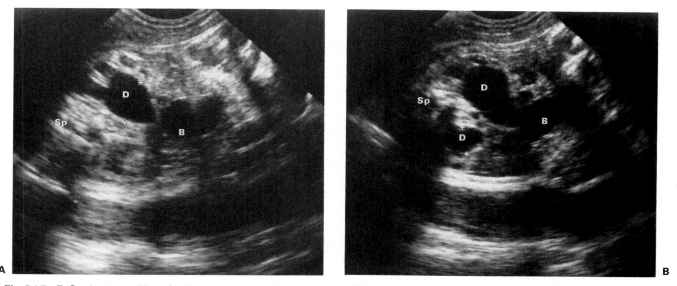

Fig. 5.6.7 Reflux in utero – 32 weeks. Transverse scans of fetal abdomen. Dilated (D) systems varying in size during different moments (**A, B**) of same examination. At birth, bilateral grade IV reflux was present. B = fetal bladder, Sp = fetal spine.

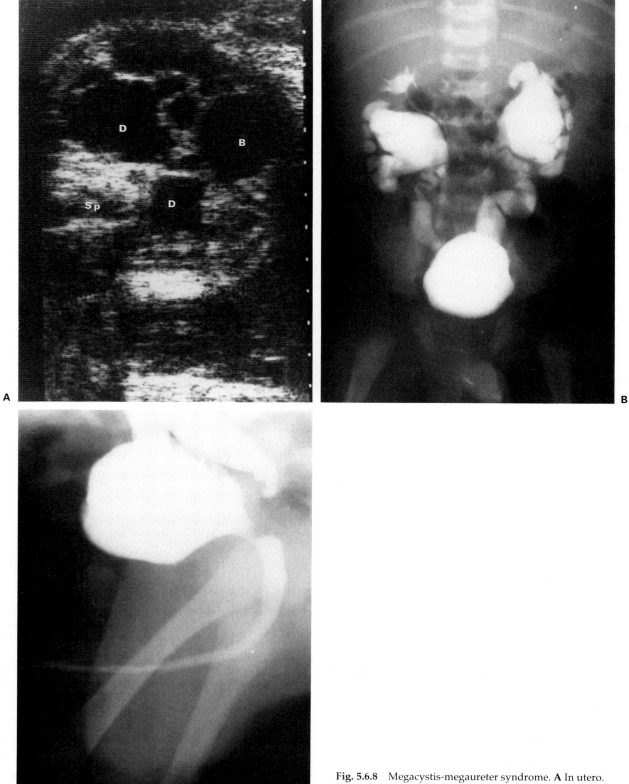

Fig. 5.6.8 Megacystis-megaureter syndrome. **A** In utero. Transverse scan of fetal abdomen. D = dilated systems, B = fetal bladder, sp = fetal spine. **B** MCUG at birth. Bilateral grade 4/5 reflux. **C** MCUG. Normal urethra.

A particular form of reflux detected in utero or directly after birth is the 'megacystis megaureter syndrome' in which the pelvicalyceal system, and the ureters and bladder are grossly dilated. Abnormal micturition results in marked vesicoureteric reflux, refilling of the bladder with refluxed urine and eventual incompetence of the detrusor muscle (Fig. 5.6.8). Antenatally this condition is associated with a normal amount of amniotic fluid and normal lung development, and is therefore distinguished from posterior urethral valves in which oligohydramnios is present.

Another very rare condition in which there is a dilated bladder, ureters and pelvicalyceal system and vesicoureteric reflux is the 'megacystis-microcolon hypoperistalsis syndrome'. In this condition severe abnormalities of the urinary tract are associated with abnormal function of the bowel.

All neonates with an antenatal diagnosis of an abnormal urinary tract including those with suspected reflux should have an ultrasound and MCUG soon after birth to confirm the diagnosis.

Familial reflux

Vesicoureteric reflux is a familial condition and therefore it has been suggested that all siblings of a child with vesicoureteric reflux and reflux nephropathy should be investigated with an ultrasound scan and a radionuclide cystogram, either indirect with MAG3 or a direct cystogram depending on the child's age.

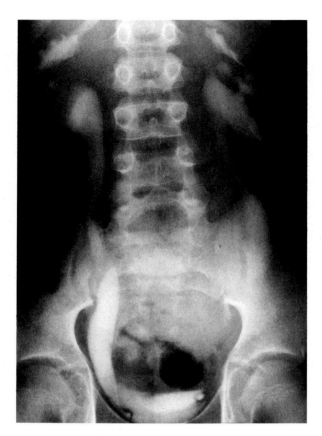

Fig. 5.6.9 Post reimplantation IVU. Typical deformity of the vesicoureteric junctions.

Treatment and postoperative studies

In most cases, vesicoureteric reflux resolves spontaneously and the risk of further scarring is low if infection does not occur. In these children, medical treatment with prophylactic antibiotics is sufficient and follow-up is with ultrasound and radionuclide cystography.

Other treatments may be necessary in cases in which there is failure of medical treatment for clinical or social reasons, in high grade reflux and in cases with severe reflux persisting after 2 years.

The aim of surgery is to elongate the submucosal ureteric tunnel, with reimplantation of the ureter. The success rate is 90%. Ultrasound demonstrates localized thickening of the bladder wall secondary to reimplantation, and a characteristic appearance is seen on IVU (Fig. 5.6.9), depending on the type of surgery.

Subureteric injection of Teflon paste or collagen may also prevent reflux, with a success rate of 80–85%. This is seen on US as an echogenic area with acoustic shadowing at the vesicoureteric junction (Fig. 5.6.10). Complications such as urinary tract dilatation are monitored with US.

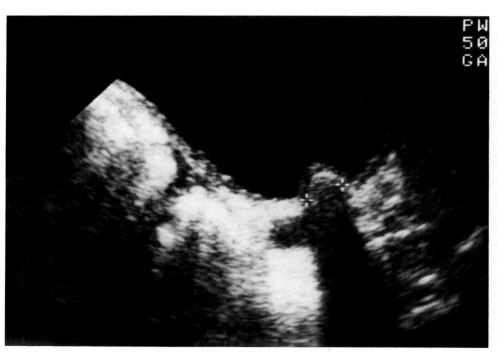

Fig. 5.6.10 Subureteric Teflon injection. US. Sagittal scan of the bladder. Teflon is seen as a hyperechoic focus with acoustic shadowing (between crosses).

REFERENCES

Becu L, Quesada E M, Medel R et al 1988 Small kidneys associated with primary reflux in children. A pathological overhand. European Urology 14: 127–140

Bellinger M F 1985 Management of vesicoureteric reflux. Urologic Clinics of North American 12: 23–29

Berdon W E, Baker D H, Blanc W A 1976. Megacystis microcolon intestinal hypoperistalsis syndrome: new case of intestinal obstruction in the newborn. Report of the radiological findings in five girls. American Journal of Roentgenology 126: 957–964

Ginalski J M, Michaud A, Genton N 1985 Renal growth retardation in children: sign suggestive of vesicoureteral reflux? American Journal of Roentgenology 145: 617–619

Gore M D, Fernbach S K, Donaldson J S, Shkdink A, Zaontz M R, Kaplan W E 1989 Radiographic evalution of subureteric injection of Teflon to correct vesicoureteral reflux. American Journal of Roentgenology 152: 115–119

Guignard J P 1989 Reflux vesico-ureteral. Archives Francaises de Pediatrie 46: 477–479

Hollowel J G, Altman H G, Mac Snyder H, Duckett J W 1989 Coexisting ureteropelvic junction obstruction and VUR: diagnostic and therapeutic implications. Journal of Urology 142: 490–493

International Reflux Study Committee 1981 Medical versus surgical treatment of primary vesico-ureteral reflux: a prospective international study in children. Journal of Urology 125: 277–283

International Collaborative Reflux Study in Children 1984 Clinical trial versus surgical treatment of VUR. Pediatric Research 18: 373A

Lebowitz R L 1986 The detection of VUR in the child. Investigative Radiology 519–531

Lebowitz R L, Olbing H, Parkkulaien K V, Smellie J M, Tammuren-Mobius T E 1985 International system of radiographic grading of VUR. Pediatric Radiology 15: 105–109

Maizels M, Smith C K, Firlit C F 1984 Management of children with VUR and UPJ obstruction. Journal of Urology 131: 722–727

O'Donnell B, Puri P 1984 Treatment of VU reflux by endoscopic injection of Teflon. British Medical Journal 289: 7–9

Roberts J P, Atwell J D 1989 Vesico-ureteral and urinary calculi in children. British Journal of Urology 64: 10–12

Schulman C C, Simon J, Pamart D, Avni E F 1987 Endoscopic treatment of VU reflux in children. Journal of Urology 138: 950–951

Seruca H 1989 Vesicoureteral reflux and voiding dysfunction: a prospective study. Journal of Urology Part 2, 142: 494–498

Shimada K, Matsin T, Ogino T, Arima M, Mori Y, Ikoma F 1988 Renal growth and progression of reflux nephropathy in children with VU reflux. Journal of Urology 140: 1097–1100

Sirota L, Herz M, Langer J, Jonas P, Boichis H 1986 Familial VU reflux: a study of 16 families. Urologic Radiology 8: 22–24

Tones V E, Velosa J A, Holley K E, Kelali P P, Stickler G B, Kurz S B 1980 The progression of vesicoureteral reflux nephropathy. Annals of Internal Medicine 92: 776–784

Whitaker R H, Fowler C D 1979 Ureters that show both reflux and obstruction. British Journal of Urology 51: 471–474

White R H R 1989 VU reflux and renal scarring. Archives of Diseases in Childhood 64: 407–412

Willi U, Lebowitz R L 1979 The so-called megaureter-megacystis syndrome. American Journal of Roentgenology 133: 409–416

Williamson B, Hartman G W, Hattery R R 1986 Multiple and diffuse ureteral filling defects. Seminars in Roentgenology 21: 214–223

REFLUX NEPHROPATHY

Reflux nephropathy describes the characteristic findings of cortical atrophy, calyceal dilatation and thinning of papillae, which represent the renal scars appearing after a urinary tract infection. These changes are irreversible and the complications and consequences of reflux nephropathy are hypertension and renal failure. Fifteen per cent of patients with chronic renal failure have reflux nephropathy, and the percentage ranges from 8.1% to 24.7% under 15 years. It is therefore mandatory to follow up all patients with reflux, both clinically and radiologically.

Progressive reflux nephropathy is demonstrated by further renal scarring, loss of renal volume and renal function. Compensatory hypertrophy of remaining renal parenchyma may occur. Assessment of renal growth is important.

Anatomically renal growth is best followed by US. Areas of cortical irregularity and thinning represent scars (Fig. 5.6.11). A localized hyperechoic area (Fig. 5.6.12), or diffuse hyperechogenicity of the kidney is seen if hyperfiltration is associated with reflux nephropathy.

An irregular renal outline with thinning of the renal cortex and clubbed calyces, affecting the upper and lower poles, are the diagnostic changes of reflux nephropathy shown on an IVU (Fig. 5.6.13).

Renal function is best evaluated with radionuclide studies, DMSA for structure and DTPA or MAG3 for function (Figs. 5.6.13, 5.6.14, 5.6.15). Regular isotope studies are important for follow-up.

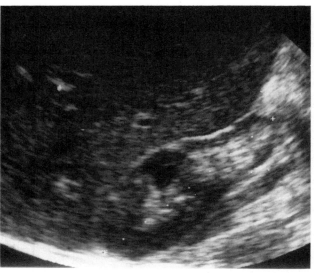

Fig. 5.6.11 Reflux nephropathy. US (sagittal scan of right kidney – between crosses.) Duplex system. Thinned cortex in the lower pole related to reflux nephropathy. Reflux into the lower pole was present on MCUG.

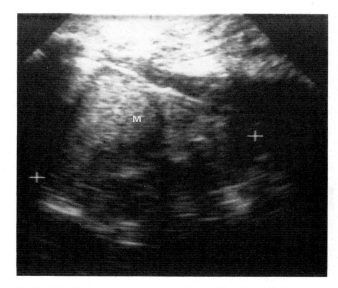

Fig. 5.6.12 Reflux nephropathy and hyperfiltration. US. Prone sagittal scan of left kidney (between crosses). A hyperechoic pseudo-mass (M) is seen; it corresponds to a focus of hyperfiltration (confirmed by isotopes).

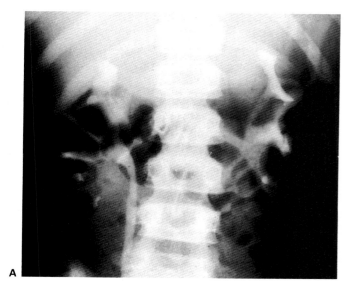

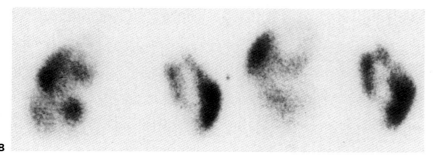

Fig. 5.6.13 **A** IVU. **B** DMSA scan , two views. Reflux nephropathy due to chronic pyelonephritis. Note clubbed calyces with loss of adjacent cortex in both kidneys. The extent of damage is better appreciated on DMSA.

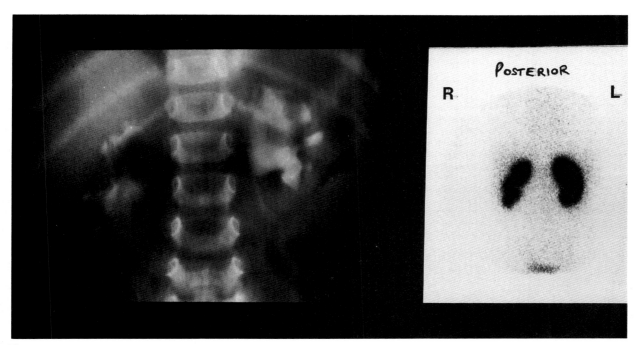

Fig. 5.6.14 IVU and DMSA scan in a child with reflux nephropathy. Uptake on the right is 38%; 62% on the left.

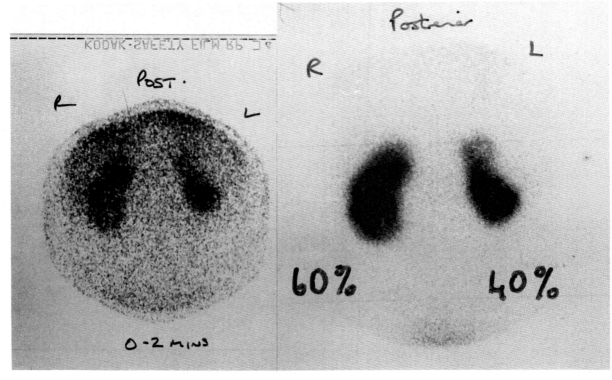

Fig. 5.6.15 Comparison of first two minutes of Mag 3 renogram with static DMSA scan. DMSA gives better anatomical definition of left upper pole scarring.

REFERENCES

Diard F, Nicolau A, Bernard S 1987 Intrarenal reflux: a new cause of medullary hyperechogenicity? Pediatric Radiology 17: 154–155

Habib R, Terdjman S 1985 Pathologie de la nephropathie de reflux. Journal d'Urologie 91: 104–106

Jacquier S, Jacquier J C 1989 Reliability of voiding cystourethrography to detect reflux. American Journal of Roentgenology 153: 807–810

Letner G R, Fleishmann L E, Pelmutter A D 1987 Reflux nephropathy. Pediatric Clinics of North America 34: 747–770

Mannhardt W, Schofer O, Schulte Wisserman H 1986 Pathogenic factors in recurrent UTI and renal scar formation in children. European Journal Pediatrics 145: 330–336

Matsumoto J S 1986 Acquired lesions involving the ureter in childhood. Seminars in Roentgenology 21: 166–167

Ransley P G, Risdon R A 1978 Reflux and renal scarring. British Journal of Radiology Suppl 14: 1–35

Ransley P G, Risdon R A 1981 Reflux nephropathy. Kidney International 20: 733–742

Rolleston G L, Maling T M Y, Hodson C J 1974 Intrarenal reflux and the scarred kidney. Archives of Disease in Childhood 49: 531–539

Scott J E 1987 Fetal ureteric reflux. British Journal of Urology 59: 291–296

Steele B T, Robitaille P, De Maria J, Grignon A 1989 Follow-up evaluation of prenatally recognized VU reflux. Journal of Pediatrics 115: 95–96

Tammimen T E, Kapiro E A 1977 The relation of the shape of renal papillae and of collecting duct opening to intrarenal reflux. British Journal of Urology 49: 345–354

Thomsen H S 1985 VU reflux and reflux nephropathy. Acta Radiologica Diagnostica 26: 3–13

INFECTIVE CONDITIONS OF THE KIDNEY

Acute pyelonephritis

Acute pyelonephritis describes diffuse haematogenous infection of the kidney. *E. coli* is the commonest infecting organism. US may be normal or demonstrate enlargement of the kidney due to inflammation and oedema (Fig. 5.16.16). Localized areas of infection may occur and are sometimes referred to as acute lobar nephronia. A hypoechoic area is seen within renal parenchyma, unless haemorrhage has occurred when a hyperechogenic segment is seen (Fig. 5.6.17). If a CT scan is performed, localized areas of decreased contrast enhancement corresponding to oedema and

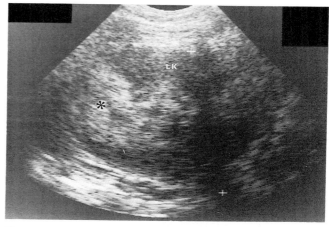

Fig. 5.6.17 Haemorrhagic acute lobar nephronia. US. Transverse scan of left kidney (LK). Hyperechoic area corresponding to the acute lobar nephronia (*).

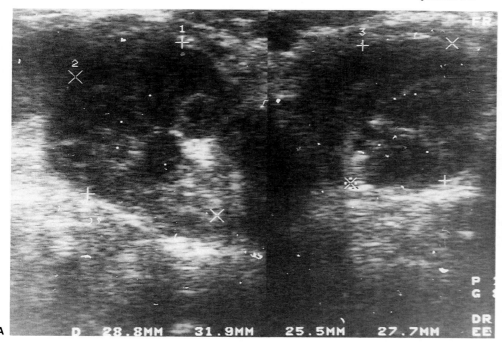

Fig. 5.6.16 Acute pyelonephritis. US. **A** Enlarged left kidney as compared to right on the transverse scans. **B** Left renal pelvis wall is thickened (arrows) on the sagittal scan.

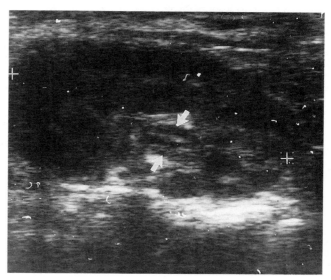

ischaemia are demonstrated (Fig. 5.6.18). Isotope scans with DMSA are a very sensitive method for the detection of acute parenchymal inflammation and renal scars (Figs 5.6.19, 5.6.20). Solitary or multiple focal defects or asymmetry in total uptake are seen (Fig. 5.6.19). These lesions may rapidly improve after adequate antibiotic therapy or remain unchanged if scar formation occurs (Fig. 5.6.20). There is little role for intravenous urography in the diagnosis of acute pyelonephritis, as other methods are less invasive and more sensitive. If performed, a persistent dense nephrogram or increased renal volume and scars may be seen (Fig. 5.6.21). Focal areas of poor contrast medium excretion may also be seen (Fig. 5.6.22).

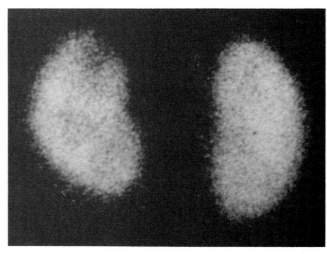

Fig. 5.6.19 Acute pyelenophritis. DMSA. Post view. Acute involvement. Typical ill-defined focal defect at the upper pole of left kidney.

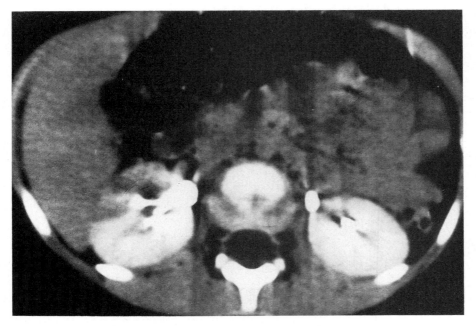

Fig. 5.6.18 Acute pyelonephritis. CT. Contrast-enhanced scan. The right kidney is swollen. There are areas of hypodensities corresponding to ischaemic or oedematous changes. (Courtesy of Dr P. Le Dosseur.)

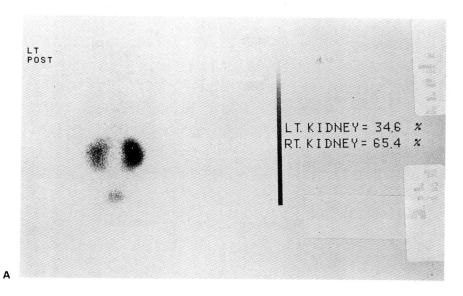

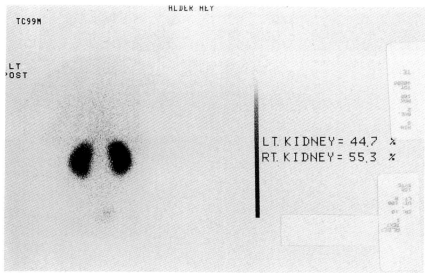

Fig. 5.6.20 DMSA scan in acute urinary infection. **A** During first 72 hours. There is diminished uptake on the left due to acute nephronia. **B** Six months later. There has been considerable improvement in function as oedema resolves.

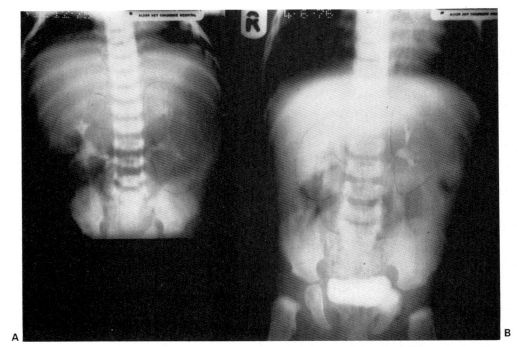

Fig. 5.6.21 **A** IVU during acute infection. **B** 6 months later. Note swelling of both kidneys in **A** with return to normal size in **B**.

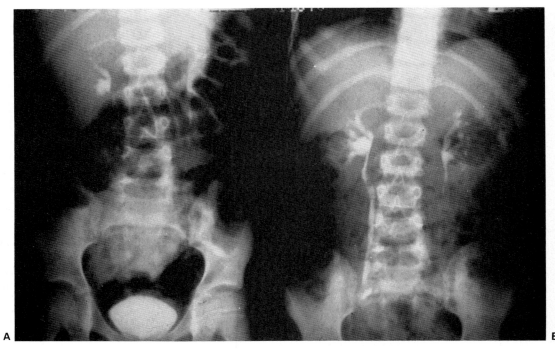

Fig. 5.6.22 **A** IVU during acute infection. **B** 6 months later following recovery. Note non-filling of the right middle and lower pole calyces during acute infection.

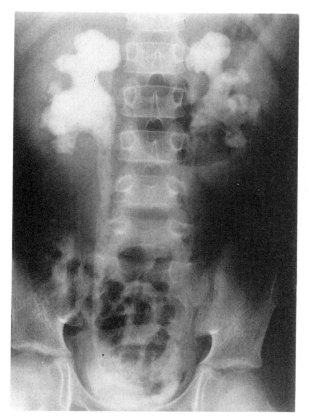

Fig 5.6.23 Pyelitis and ureteritis cystica. IVU. Multiple filling defects in the pelvis and ureters. Dilatation is also present as well as cortical thinning (upper poles).

Radiolucent folds at the level of the collecting system or in the ureter may represent pyelitis (Fig. 5.6.5) and ureteritis or reflux; diffuse filling defects are seen in pyelitis and ureteritis cystica (Fig. 5.6.23). There are various other causes of ureteral filling defects described in Table 5.4.2.

Renal abscess

Acute pyelonephritis may, if inadequately treated, progress to renal abscess or renal carbuncle formation. It is important to follow up acute pyelonephritis with US in order to detect this complication. A renal abscess can have various patterns on ultrasound examination. There is usually a mass with a complex echopattern and areas of necrosis (Fig. 5.6.24). Extrarenal extension can be demonstrated. CT is also useful in cases when abscess formation is suspected, a circumscribed mass with a low attenuation centre and perirenal inflammatory changes is seen (Fig. 5.6.25). CT is the most useful method for demonstrating extrarenal extension of an abscess.

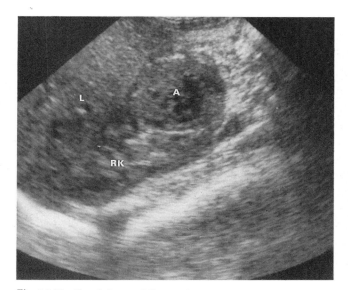

Fig. 5.6.24 Renal abscess (A) extending into the liver. US. Sagittal scan of the right kidney (RK). The echogenicity of the abscess is heterogeneous, probably corresponding to central necrosis. L = Liver.

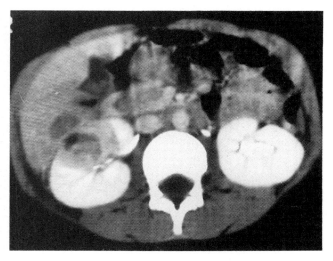

Fig. 5.6.25 Renal abscess with liver involvement. CT. Contrast-enhanced scan. Heterogeneous solid mass in the right kidney corresponding to the abscess. Hypodense area in the liver.

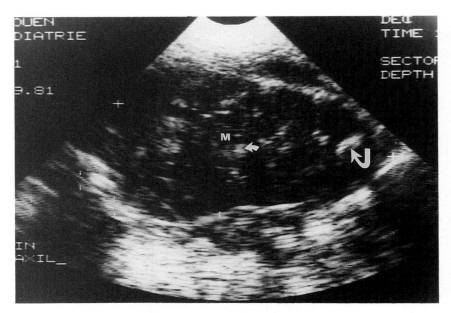

Fig. 5.6.26 Xanthogranulomatous pyelonephritis. US. Complex mass (M) at the lower pole of the left kidney. Calcifications are present (arrows) (Courtesy of Dr P. Le Dosseur.)

The differential diagnosis includes renal tumours, but the associated clinical findings and the presence of perirenal and extrarenal inflammatory changes should suggest an infective aetiology.

If calcification is present within the mass, xanthogranulomatous pyelonephritis should be suspected (Fig. 5.6.26).

Xanthogranulomatous pyelonephritis

This condition is rare in children and is associated with renal calculi. The ultrasound and CT appearances are of a renal mass, with multiple anechoic or non-enhancing areas. Calyceal dilatation with deposition of granulomatous material occurs. Occasionally fat may be seen within the mass on the plain film. The fat deposition may cause increase of echoic areas without acoustic shadows (Fig. 5.6.27).

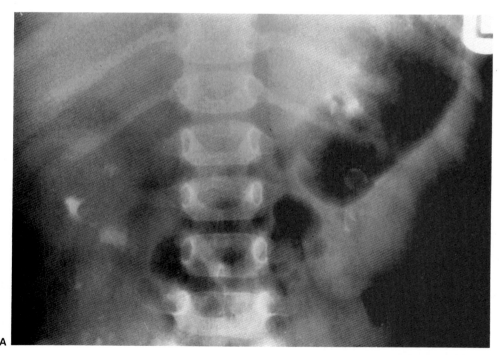

A

Fig. 5.6.27 Xanthogranulomatous pyelonephritis: **A** IVU **B** US. Note large nonfunctioning right kidney with calculi and surrounding perinephric low density area due to fat. **B** complex renal mass, with central bright echoes due to fat and calculi.

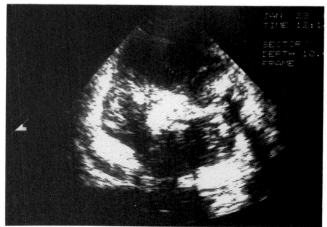

B

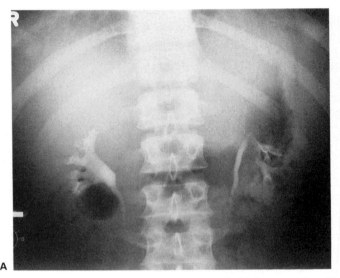
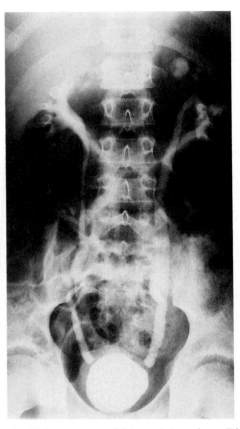

Fig. 5.6.28 Tuberculosis. IVU. **A** Early film. Non-opacified left upper calyx. 'Drooping lily' appearance of the remaining calyces. **B** late film. Opacified left hydrocalyx. Dilatation of both (mainly left) ureters. Thickened bladder wall. Calcifications were present on the radiograph of the abdomen.

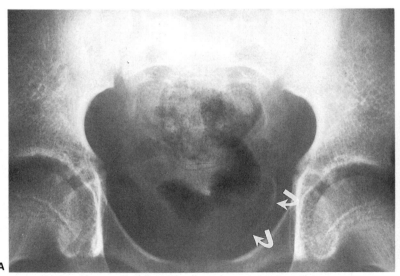
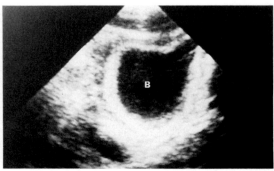

Fig. 5.6.29 Schistosomiasis. **A** Plain film of the abdomen. Fine calcification of the bladder wall (arrows). **B** US. Small bladder (B) with thickened hyperechoic wall.

Tuberculosis

Tuberculosis of the urinary tract, while uncommon in the western world, is still an important cause of renal disease in the developing world. Intravenous urography demonstrates the diagnostic features of a poorly functioning kidney with curvilinear calcification, hydrocalyx, ureteric strictures and a reduced bladder capacity (Fig. 5.6.28). US may show a thickened bladder wall, renal calcification and dilatation of the urinary tract. Similarly, CT demonstrates renal calcification and loss of volume.

Schistosomiasis

Calcification of the bladder wall and ureter, and mucosal irregularity are the typical findings (Fig. 5.6.29). Bladder capacity is markedly reduced.

Hydatid disease

Cystic lesions may be seen in renal hydatid disease; when present they are diagnostic and there may be irregular thickening of the cyst wall and echogenic debris within the cyst due to daughter cysts.

Fungal diseases

Renal candidiasis is a typical complication of acutely ill and ventilated newborns. It also occurs in immunocompromised patients. US is the most useful examination and demonstrates diffuse parenchymal hyperechogenicity with dilatation of the pelvicalyceal system and echogenic fungus balls within the collecting system (Fig. 5.6.30). Secondary obstruction may occur. The appearances on IVU and CT are the same with round filling defects, although these investigations are rarely necessary as the diagnosis should be made on US.

REFERENCES

Avni E F, Vandermerckt C, Braude P, Van Gansbeke D, Schulman C C 1988 Sonographic evaluation of renal inflammatory diseases in children. World Journal of Urology 6: 18–21

Avni E F, Van Gansbeke D, Thoua Y et al 1988 Ultrasonic demonstration of pyelitis and ureteritis in children. Pediatric Radiology 18: 134–139

Berliner L, Bosniak M A 1982 The striated nephrogram in acute pyelonephritis. Urologic Radiology 4: 41–44

Brettman L R 1988. Pathogenesis of UTI: host susceptibility and bacterial virulence factors. Urology 82: 9–11

Chaovachi B, Bensalah S, Lakhova R, Hammou A, Gharbi H A, Saied H 1989 Kystes hydatiques chez l'enfant. Aspects diagnostiques et therapeutiques. Annales de Pediatric (Paris) 36: 441–449

Cohen H L, Haller J O, Schechter S, Slovis T, Merola R, Eaton D K 1986 Renal candidiasis in the infant: US evaluation. Urologic Radiology 8: 17–21

Greenfield S P, Montgomery P 1987 CT and acute pyelonephritis in children. Urology 291: 137–140

Kangarloo H, Gold R H, Fine R N, Diament M J, Boechat M I 1985 UTI in infants and children evaluated by US. Radiology 154: 367–373

Kierce F, Carroll R, Guiney E J 1985 Xanthogranulomatous pyelonephritis in children. British Journal of Urology 57: 261–264

Kincaid Smith P 1975 Glomerular lesions in atrophic pyelonephritis and reflux nephropathy. Kidney International 8: 75–81

Lebowitz R L, Mandell J 1987 UTI in children putting radiology in its place. Radiology 165: 1–9

Rigsby C M, Rosenfield A T, Glickman M G, Hodson J 1986 Hemorrhagic focal bacterial nephritis: findings on sonography and CT. American Journal of Roentgenology 146: 1173–1177

Vankirk O G, Go R T, Wedel V J 1980 Sonographic features of XPN. American Journal of Roentgenology 134: 1035–1038

Yadin O, Benezer G, Golan A, Sober I, Barki Y, Carmi R 1900 Survival of a premature neonate with obstructive anuria due to candida. European Journal of Pediatrics 147: 653–655

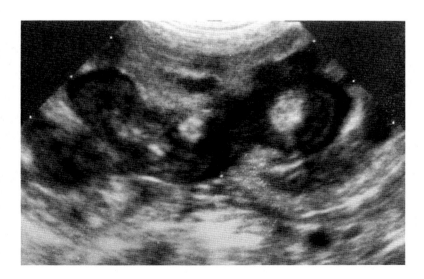

Fig. 5.6.30 Renal candidiasis. US. Sagittal scan of left kidney (between crosses). Filling of renal cavities with echogenic material (arrows).

5.7 TUMOURS OF THE URINARY TRACT *S. Neuenschwander*

RENAL NEOPLASMS

Approximately 55% of abdominal masses in childhood are of renal origin. In the neonate, the majority of these renal masses are benign and are due to a congenital abnormality. In older children, the incidence of neoplasia increases, with a decrease in congenital abnormalities.

Wilms' tumour

Wilms' tumour is the most common renal tumour in childhood and accounts for about 12% of all cancers occurring in children. The peak incidence is between 30 months and 3 years of age. The incidence is approximately 8 in 1 million children each year.

The most common presentation is with an asymptomatic abdominal mass. Pain, haematuria, fever or hypertension are less common presenting features.

One per cent of Wilms' tumours are familial and present at a younger age than the more common sporadic group.

Associated congenital abnormalities occur in approximately 15% of all children with Wilms' tumour. These primarily involve the genitourinary tract such as in cryptorchidism, hypospadias, horseshoe kidney and cystic renal disease. Specific associated malformations include hemihypertrophy, Beckwith–Wiedemann syndrome, cerebral gigantism (Soto's syndrome), neurofibromatosis, pseudohermaphroditism (Drash's syndrome), Perlman's syndrome and sporadic aniridia. Ninety per cent of Wilms' tumours occurring in Beckwith–Wiedemann syndrome, Drash's syndrome and hemihypertrophy will appear by 6 years of age. Wilms' tumour is associated with chromosomal abnormalities, the best known being deletion of the short arm of chromosome 11, a consistent finding in sporadic congenital aniridia. Wilm's tumour will develop in approximately 30% of children with aniridia, usually during the first 3 years of life. Other chromosomal abnormalities associated with Wilms' tumour include certain trisomies, 45X and various translocations.

Scanning of patients with congenital malformations associated with Wilms' tumour is recommended in some centres. This consists of repeated clinical examinations and ultrasound scanning, two or three times a year for the first 4 years of life. However, it is known that Wilms' tumour may grow very quickly, arising between screening ultrasound scans, and also that repeated scanning may impose considerable psychological stress on the family.

Wilms' tumour is bilateral in approximately 5% of patients, two-thirds of which are synchronous and one-third metachronous. Bilateral tumours present at a younger age than unilateral tumours, and are often associated with congenital anomalies, and familial cases. Nephroblastomatosis is commonly found in bilateral tumours.

Wilms' tumour may arise in any portion of the kidney, and is usually solid with a fibrous pseudocapsule that separates it from normal renal parenchyma. There may be areas of haemorrhage, necrosis and calcification. Wilms' tumour may infiltrate the capsule or invade the renal vein and inferior vena cava; enlargement of local lymph nodes may be due to metastases or reactive changes. Distant metastases most commonly involve the lungs; the liver is the next most frequent site.

Stage and histology are the most important prognostic factors. Two histological classifications are in current use, the predominantly American (NTWS) and European (SIOP) classifications. Classically the histology of Wilms' tumour is described as 'triphasic' and made up of primitive blastemal cells and their more differentiated derivatives, i.e. tubular, epithelial and mesenchymal elements. In some cases the histology may consist predominantly or exclusively of one component, e.g. monomorphous epithelial tumour, cystic partially differentiated nephroblastoma and rhabdomyomatous nephroblastoma. Both classifications consider these different forms as 'favourable' histology. 'Unfavourable' histological forms include anaplastic tumours. The NTWS classification also includes sarcomatous tumours whereas the SIOP classification excludes them from the 'unfavourable' histology. The cure rate for Stage 1 Wilms' tumour with favourable histology is greater than 90%. Unfavourable histology constitutes only 10% of cases but accounts for at least 60% of deaths.

Two further variants of histology are described. These are the rhabdoid type, which occurs in older children and metastasizes to the CNS and liver and the clear cell, sarcomatous type which frequently metastasizes to bone. In many centres these renal tumours are not included in the spectrum of Wilms' tumours. Although some radiological features suggestive of the different histologies have been described, such as marked necrosis in the rhabdoid type, histology cannot be predicted reliably from imaging and the diagnosis has to be made following surgery or biopsy.

The characteristic radiological findings of Wilms' tumour are a solid intrarenal mass and the first and often diagnostic examination is an abdominal ultrasound scan.

This will demonstrate a mass of uniform echogenicity equal to or slightly less than liver. Anechoic areas representing haemorrhage, necrosis or cystic components may be present. Large tumours are more often heterogeneous than small tumours (Fig. 5.7.1). In most cases ultrasound will demonstrate the tumour clearly, particularly if it arises from one of the poles of the kidney (Fig. 5.7.2). Rarely it arises in the subcapsular area resulting in a predominantly extrarenal mass. True extrarenal tumours have been described.

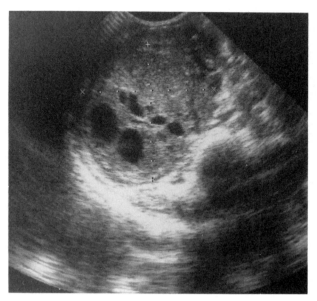

Fig. 5.7.1 Wilms' tumour: transverse ultrasound scan. A heterogenous, large, central intrarenal mass is present. CT scanning is required to delineate this more clearly.

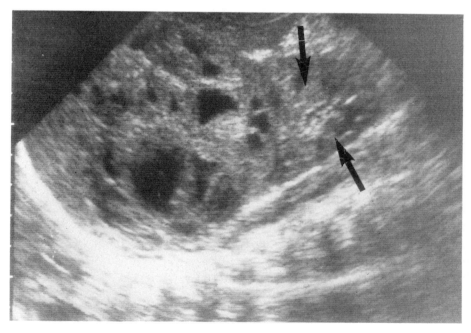

Fig. 5.7.2 Wilms' tumour of the upper pole of the kidney. The crescent-shaped renal parenchyma (arrows) is identified at the periphery of the tumoral mass.

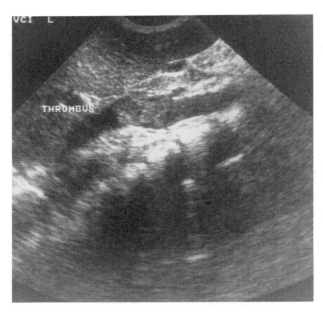

Fig. 5.7.3 Wilms' tumour. Tumoral thrombus within the inferior vena cava (ultrasound longitudinal scan). The upper limit of the thrombus is important to locate.

Ultrasound scanning is an excellent method for demonstrating the presence of tumour thrombosis in the inferior vena cava and right atrium. Thrombus is visualized as echogenic material within an expanded inferior vena cava, with loss of the normal change in calibre with respiration (Fig. 5.7.3). Renal vein thrombosis may also be seen (Fig. 5.7.4). With very large tumours, evaluation of the inferior vena cava may be difficult because of extrinsic displacement and compression. Contrast medium studies with CT, MRI and Colour Flow Doppler ultrasound are useful, although all may result in false negatives. Plain radiographs and intravenous urography (IVU) now have a minor role in the assessment of Wilms' tumour with current imaging techniques. When performed, a mass with displacement of adjacent bowel loops is seen; calcification is rare (about 5%). Following contrast medium, stretching, distortion and amputation of the pelvicalyceal system by the mass is seen. Prior to surgery, an IVU may be helpful in the demonstration of ureteric anatomy, particularly in patients with congenital abnormalities such as duplex or horseshoe kidneys.

CT is used to clarify the sonographic findings and confirms the intrarenal location of the mass, its extent, and morphological characteristics. CT is particularly useful in very large or central intrarenal tumours, when ultrasound alone may have difficulty in making the diagnosis of a Wilms' tumour. Abdominal lymph node enlargement is best appreciated at CT, as are small foci of tumour in the contralateral kidney.

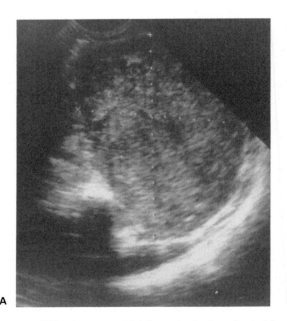

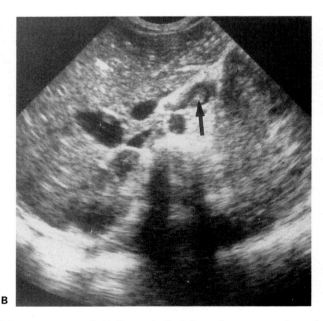

Fig. 5.7.4 Wilms' tumour with left renal vein thrombosis. Ultrasound, transverse scans. **A** At diagnosis, the left renal mass was so huge that the renal vein could not be identified. **B** After 2 weeks of chemotherapy, the tumour has shrunk, the left renal vein is well seen, with a dilated proximal lumen and a thrombus within it (arrow).

The tumour mass has a rounded, well-defined contour and is of low attenuation with little contrast enhancement. The normal compressed renal parenchyma is clearly seen following IV contrast medium (Fig. 5.7.5). The mass is usually solid with cystic areas due to haemorrhage and necrosis. Recent haemorrhage within the mass gives rise to areas of increased attenuation. Calcification is seen more frequently on CT than with plain films. Unlike neuroblastoma, the major vessels are displaced and not encased by the mass. Evaluation of the renal arteries, veins and inferior vena cava is possible following IV contrast.

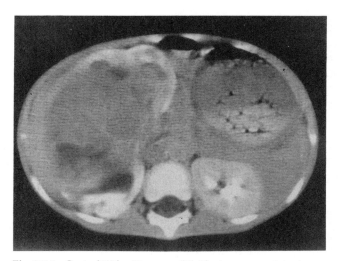

Fig. 5.7.5 Central Wilms' tumour. CT. The tumour contains low attenuation areas. A rim of functioning renal parenchyma is splayed out by the intrarenal tumour. The tumour abuts a dilated calyx. (Courtesy Pr. Kalifa.)

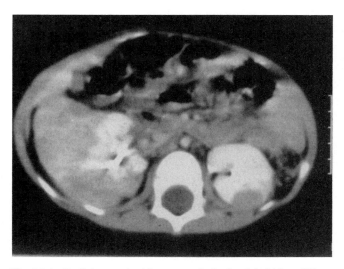

Fig. 5.7.6 Perilobar nephroblastomatosis. In the right kidney CT shows confluent peripheral non-enhanced soft tissue masses. They are sharply demarcated from normal enhanced parenchyma. In the left kidney, the posterior nodule does not distort the pelvicalyceal system: no normal renal outline.

The contralateral kidney is best assessed for bilateral lesions by CT (Fig. 5.7.6). Assessment of the liver, regional lymph nodes and the chest for metastases is also possible with CT. At the time of diagnosis, pulmonary metastases are present in over 10% of patients and 10% of these are only visible on CT.

MRI has been evaluated in the diagnosis of Wilms' tumour. The tumour has prolonged T_1 and T_2 relaxation times, but the signal intensity is variable due to areas of haemorrhage and necrosis. The extent of the mass, its renal origin and the inferior vena cava and other vessels are clearly seen. MRI is able to demonstrate tumour thrombus without the use of IV contrast. At present, MRI provides the same information as US and CT, but in the future, because of the lack of radiation in young children, it may prove to be the favoured imaging technique (Fig. 5.7.7).

Radionuclide scanning has been used in cases of bilateral Wilms' tumour to assess the amount of functioning renal tissue before conservative surgery with partial nephrectomy. The tumour tissue does not take up the isotope. Isotope scanning with ^{99m}Tc-DMSA has little role in the routine evaluation of Wilms' tumour.

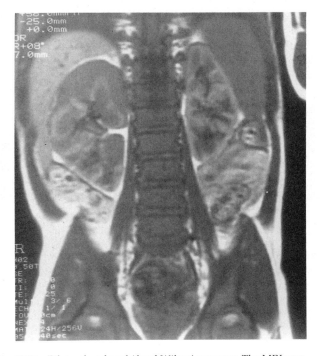

Fig. 5.7.7 Bilateral and multifocal Wilms' tumours. The MRI was performed preoperatively after 1 month of chemotherapy, resulting in dramatic debulking of tumours. The right kidney is enlarged, with a rather irregular outline. Tumours appear on this sequence (SE: 380/25) as hypointense areas compressing the renal parenchyma at the upper pole and in the inferior margin of the sinus (the left renal lesion is not illustrated in this section). This appearance is quite similar to nephroblastomatosis.

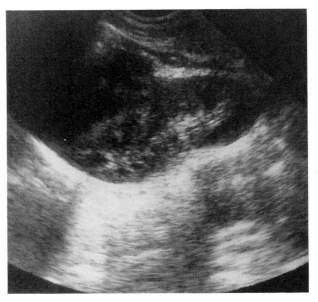

Fig. 5.7.8 Abscess of the upper pole of the kidney. There is an apparantly solid heterogeneous intrarenal mass. Pain, fever and elevated WBC in a 9-year-old child led to doubt in the diagnosis of Wilms' tumour. Abscess was confirmed by a posterior percutaneous puncture.

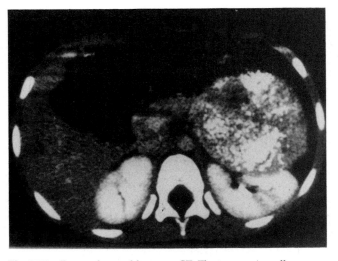

Fig. 5.7.9 Prerenal neuroblastoma. CT. The tumour is well delineated but is strongly calcified which is quite unusual in Wilms' tumour. Compressed renal parenchyma is seen between tumour and pelvis. The diagnosis of neuroblastoma was confirmed by the specific biochemical markers.

Arteriography is performed infrequently, most surgeons relying on US and CT, but may occasionally be used when partial nephrectomy is contemplated in cases of Wilms' tumour associated with congenital renal anomalies such as horseshoe kidney, or if bench dissection is needed.

The differential diagnosis of Wilms' tumour includes inflammatory lesions such as xanthogranulomatous pyelonephritis, renal abscess (Fig. 5.7.8) and lobar nephronia. It also includes haematoma following trauma and other neoplastic conditions such as renal cell carcinoma, mesoblastic nephroma, tuberous sclerosis and intrarenal neuroblastoma (Fig. 5.7.9).

The differential diagnosis of bilateral Wilms' tumour includes nephroblastomatosis, renal lymphoma and multiple renal abscesses.

Radiologically detectable complications of Wilms' tumour treatment include a severe rickets in children treated with Ifosfomide. Irradiation of the renal bed is no longer practised, so the complications of scoliosis, skeletal and muscle atrophy and post irradiation osteochondromata should no longer be encountered.

REFERENCES

Beckwith J B 1983 Wilms' tumour and other renal tumours of childhood. A selective review from the NWTS Pathology Centre. Human Pathology 14: 481–492

Beckwith J B, Kiviat N B 1981 Multilocular renal cysts and cystic renal tumours. American Journal of Roentgenology 136: 435–436

Bonnin J M, Rubinstein L J, Palmer N F et al 1984 The association of embryonal tumour originating in the kidney and in the brain. Cancer 54: 2137–2146

Cohen M D, Siddiqui A, Weetman R et al 1982 A rational approach to the radiologic evaluation of children with Wilms' tumour. Cancer 50: 887–892

De Campo J F 1986 Ultrasound of Wilms' tumour. Pediatric Radiology 16: 21–24

Gay B B, Dawes R K, Atkinson G O et al 1983 Wilms' tumour in horseshoe kidneys. Radiology 146: 693–697

Gibson J M, Hall-Craggs M A, Dicks-Mireaux C, Finn J P 1990 Intracardiac extension of Wilms' tumour: demonstration by magnetic resonance. British Journal of Radiology 63: 566–569

Montgomery P, Kuhn J P, Berger P R 1985 Rhabdoid tumour of the kidney: a case report. Urologic Radiology 7: 42–44

Reiman T A H, Siegel M J, Shackelford G D 1986 Wilms' tumour in children: abdominal CT and US evaluation. Radiology 160: 501–505

Nephroblastomatosis

Nephroblastomatosis represents a spectrum of congenital lesions of renal parenchyma. Primitive renal tissue is normally present until 36 weeks' gestation. The presence of this tissue postnatally is abnormal. Lesions may consist of rests of renal blastema, nodular renal blastema and confluent nephroblastomatosis. Rests of renal blastema are found in most cases of bilateral Wilms' tumour but are also found in approximately 1% of autopsies of all patients under 3 months of age. These lesions, sometimes called 'Wilms' tumour-in-situ', may be perilobar, intralobar or panlobar. They may occur singly or multiply, with or without Wilms' tumour, and in both kidneys or the ipsilateral or contralateral kidney in Wilms' tumour. Nodular renal blastema resembles Wilms' tumour but has no excess mitosis. Renal blastema and nodular renal blastema are visualized with US and may be hyperechoic or anechoic. They are more easily demonstrated by CT as non-enhancing nodules or cortical plaques of tissue sharply demarcated from normal renal parenchyma (Fig. 5.7.6). They are usually small with a diameter of less than 4 cm.

Massive or confluent nephroblastomatosis (Fig. 5.7.10) results in enlarged kidneys with calyceal distortion on intravenous urography. US may demonstrate hyperechoic or hypoechoic nodules. CT with IV contrast medium shows gross renal enlargement with low attenuation, non-enhancing peripheral tumour nodules and compression of central normal renal tissue.

It is believed that rests of renal blastema represent precursors of Wilms' tumour. The level of risk for developing a Wilms' tumour is not known, nor is the natural history clearly understood, but there is a definite increased incidence of Wilms' tumour in children with nephroblastomatosis.

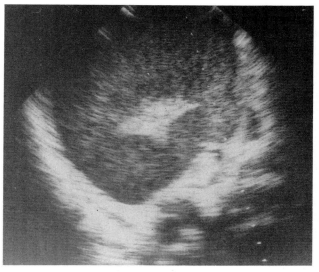

Fig. 5.7.10 Perilobar nephroblastomatosis. Diffuse form. US (transverse scan). The kidney is huge. A central echo is identifiable, but the normal corticomedullary differentiation is replaced by a thick homogeneous hypoechoic rim, with scalloped inner margins.

REFERENCES

Fernbach S K, Feinstein K A, Donaldson J S et al 1988 Nephroblastomatosis: comparison of CT with US and urography. Radiology 166: 153–156

Hennigar R A, Othersen H B, Garvin A J 1989 Clinico-pathologic features of nephroblastomatosis. Urology 33: 259–270

Machin G A 1980 Persistent renal blastema (nephroblastomatosis) as a frequent precursor of Wilms' tumour: a pathological and clinical review. 1 et 2. American Journal of Pediatric Hematology and Oncology 2: 165–172, 253–261

Machin G A, McCaughey W T E 1984 A new precursor lesion of Wilms' tumor (nephroblastoma): intralobar multifocal nephroblastomatosis. Histopathology 8: 35–53

Sebag A, Garel L, Pariente D, Sauvegrain J 1984 Nephromegalies bilaterales neonatales: interet de l'echographie. Annales de Radiologie 27: 580–588

Mesoblastic nephroma

Mesoblastic nephroma is a benign tumour and the most common neonatal renal neoplasm. It is almost always discovered in the first few months of life, although rarely it is detected in older children. It has also been detected antenatally (Fig. 5.7.11). The neonate usually presents with a large non-tender abdominal mass, and, occasionally, hypertension. The tumour may occur in the fetus and be detected on prenatal US. The typical tumour is a solid, unencapsulated mass arising from the medulla, and measures up to 30 cm in diameter. It may penetrate the renal capsule and extend into the perinephric space or retroperitoneum but does not metastasize. Local recurrence may result from capsular penetration or incomplete resection. Haemorrhage and necrosis are uncommon, but the neoplasm may show degenerative changes (Fig. 5.7.12). Microscopically, mesoblastic nephroma consists of spindle cells, which grow in sheets between intact nephrons at the interface with normal kidney. Mature nephrons can occur within the tumour.

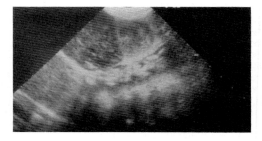

Fig. 5.7.11 Ultrasound. A mass in the upper pole of the right kidney was noted on antenatal ultrasound. Post delivery ultrasound shows the mass, which in this child is sharply demarcated from normal renal tissue.

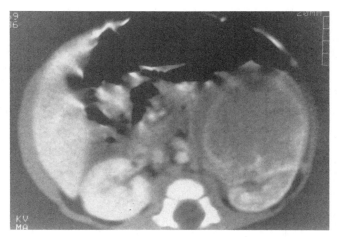

Fig. 5.7.12 Mesoblastic nephroma. CT shows an intrarenal mass. In this case, the outline of the tumour is not as well demarcated as observed in Wilms' tumour (Courtesy Pr. Diard.)

Ultrasound examination demonstrates a solid intrarenal mass of mixed echogenicity. The mass resembles a Wilms' tumour radiologically but does not always have a clearly defined capsule, the diagnosis being confirmed histologically following surgical excision. Wilms' tumour, although much less common than mesoblastic nephroma in this age group, does occur. CT is rarely necessary. When performed it demonstrates a solid intrarenal mass with minimal contrast enhancement. Although seldom performed, the tumour shows uptake of radionuclides such as ^{99m}Tc-DMSA during isotope scanning. This is thought to be due to the presence of nephrons within the tumour.

Malignant mesoblastic nephroma

Also known as malignant mesenchymal sarcoma, an unusual malignant form of mesoblastic nephroma exists which shows abundant mitotic activity and large areas of necrosis. This is reflected in the appearances on imaging with irregular hyperechoic and low attenuation areas within the tumour.

The differential diagnosis of mesoblastic nephroma and its malignant form includes Wilms' tumour, intrarenal neuroblastoma, nephroblastomatosis, renal vein thrombosis and infantile polycystic kidney disease.

REFERENCES

Hartman D S, Lesar M S L, Madewell J E et al 1981 Mesoblastic nephroma: radiologic–pathologic correlation of 20 cases. American Journal of Roentgenology 135: 69–74
Slasky B S, Penkrot R L, Bron K M 1982 Cystic mesoblastic nephroma. Urology 19: 220–223

Multilocular cystic nephroma

Multilocular cystic nephroma is an uncommon benign renal neoplasm that is characterized by a well-circumscribed encapsulated mass with numerous septae and fluid-filled locules. The lesion mainly affects young children (boys more than girls) and adults (predominantly young women).

Children normally present with a palpable abdominal mass. Imaging with US and CT demonstrates a well-circumscribed mass which is cystic with numerous locules and septae (Fig. 5.3.16). No discrete solid tissue is seen and the cysts do not enhance with IV contrast medium. There are a number of multilocular cystic masses in the kidney which cannot be distinguished from one another. These include a benign multilocular renal cyst, a well-differentiated cystic Wilms' tumour and a multilocular cystic nephroma which may contain foci of renal blastema, Wilms' tumour or renal cell carcinoma. The treatment, therefore, is nephrectomy with careful histological examination of the specimen.

REFERENCES

Garrett A, Carty H, Pilling D 1987 Multilocular cystic nephroma: report of three cases. Clinical Radiology 38: 55–57
Madewell J E, Goldman S M, Davis C J, Hardman D S, Fergin D S, Lichenstein J E 1983 Multilocular cystic nephroma: a radiographic–pathologic correlation of 58 patients. Radiology 146: 309–321

Renal cell carcinoma

Renal cell carcinoma rarely presents in childhood. The mean age in paediatric patients is 12 years. Presenting symptoms include a palpable mass, abdominal flank pain and haematuria. US and CT demonstrate a solid renal mass which may be calcified. Treatment is surgical and the prognosis is poor.

REFERENCE

Chan H S L, Daneman A, Gribbin M, Martin D J 1983 Renal cell carcinoma in the first two decades of life. Pediatric Radiology 3: 324–328

Renal lymphoma and leukaemia

Metastatic lymphoma frequently presents in the kidney. Primary lymphoma is rare in the kidney but renal involvement is seen in non-Hodgkin's lymphoma and most commonly in B-cell Burkitt lymphoma. Imaging demonstrates renal enlargement with discrete renal masses which may be multiple and occur in both kidneys. These are anechoic on US and do not enhance on CT with IV contrast medium. CT is thought to be more sensitive than US in the detection of renal lymphoma. When seen on IVU, the kidneys are enlarged and have an appearance resembling polycystic kidneys (5.7.13). Prior to commencement of chemotherapy, all children should have ultrasound of the kidneys performed to ensure normality. If there is ultrasonic evidence of renal involvement, chemotherapy may have to be adjusted, as affected kidneys may not be able to excrete tumour metabolites and renal failure may be precipitated.

Leukaemic infiltration of the kidney is common at autopsy but rarely detected clinically or radiologically. Renal involvement is diffuse, presenting with renal enlargement and hypoechoic or hyperechogenic masses on US (Fig. 5.7.14).

REFERENCES

Andre C, Garel L, Sauvegrain J 1982 Ultrasound of kidney lymphoma in children. Annales de Radiologie 25: 385–394
Araki T 1982 Leukemic involvement of the kidney in children: CT features. Journal of Computed and Assisted Tomography 6: 781–784
Hartman D S, Davis C J Jr, Goldman S M et al 1982 Renal lymphoma. Radiologic–pathologic correlation of 21 cases. Radiology 144: 759–766

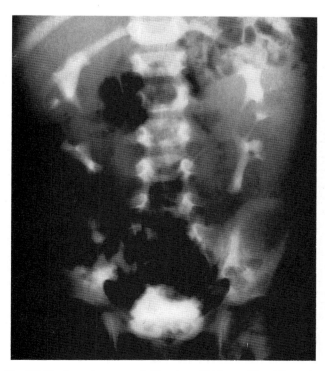

Fig. 5.7.13 Lymphomatous infiltration of kidneys. Note bilateral enlarged kidneys with splaying of the calyces.

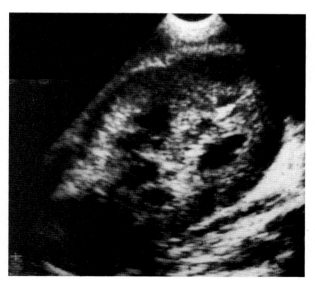

Fig. 5.7.14 Leukaemic infiltration of the kidneys. Note renal enlargement and diffuse hyperechogenicity.

Angiomyolipoma

Angiomyolipoma is a benign lesion seen in up to 50% of patients with tuberous sclerosis. It is uncommon in childhood, and the renal lesions in early childhood are often multiple and entirely cystic. Solid tumours are seen in children 6 years and older, however, the typical mixed lesion containing fat is not seen until late childhood or early adulthood (Fig. 5.7.15).

REFERENCE

Avni F E, Szliwowski H, Spehl M 1984 L'atteinte renale dans la sclerose tubereuse de Bourneville. Annales de Radiologie 27: 207–214

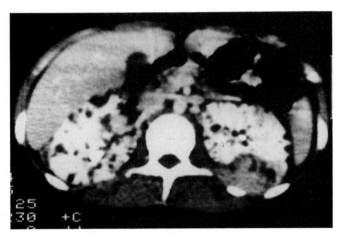

Fig. 5.7.15 Angiomyolipoma. CT. Bilateral fatty tumour involvement. Large angiomyolipoma is present in the posterior part of the left kidney. Case of tuberous sclerosis.

NEOPLASMS OF THE PELVIS AND URETER

Primary neoplasms of the collecting system are very rare in children. Involvement of the pelvicalyceal system may occur in Wilms' tumour and renal cell carcinoma, resulting in haematuria. Benign fibro-epithelial polyps occur, presenting with intermittent abdominal pain and haematuria. They are more common in boys. Detection with imaging is best with IVU or US, when minimal dilatation of the pelvi-calyceal system without obstruction and smooth filling defects or echogenic lesions in the pelvis and ureter are seen.

REFERENCE

Tschappeler H, Fischedick A R 1983 Benign pelvic ureteral tumors in children. Annales de Radiologie 26: 199–202

NEOPLASMS OF THE BLADDER AND URETHRA

Neoplasms of the bladder and urethra are uncommon in children.

The following lesions have been described:

- Rhabdomyosarcoma
- Neurofibroma
- Haemangioma
- Papillary neoplasm
- Benign epithelial polyp.

Rhabdomyosarcoma

Rhabdomyosarcoma is the most common neoplasm of the bladder in childhood. The age at presentation is 2–3 years and presenting features include an abdominal mass, haematuria and acute urinary retention.

The tumour often arises in the area of the trigone, extending into the bladder lumen with a polypoid botryoid configuration (Fig. 5.7.16). Extension through the wall of the bladder and into the perivesical tissues may occur (Fig. 5.7.17). The tumour may arise at the bladder base, in the region of the prostate in boys, presenting with a large pelvic mass behind the bladder which may extend into the bladder. In girls the tumour often arises in the vagina. Three histological subtypes are described, embryonal, alveolar and undifferentiated. Distant metastases arise in lung and bone. Following treatment with surgery, chemotherapy and radiotherapy local recurrence may still occur. Prognosis is related to the site of origin of the tumour and histology, with endophytic polypoid bladder tumours and alveolar type histology having a better outcome.

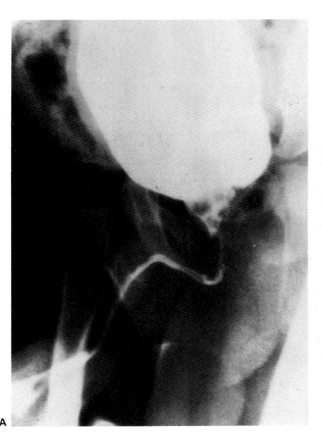

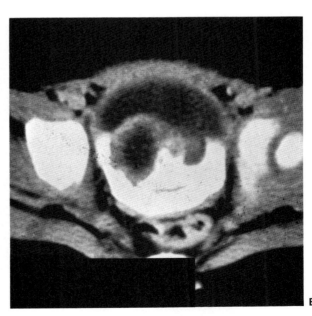

Fig. 5.7.16 2 year old boy presenting with stranguria. **A** Cystogram showing botryoid tumour projecting into the bladder base. Note poor urinary stream. **B** CT. Note the tumour projecting into the bladder lumen.

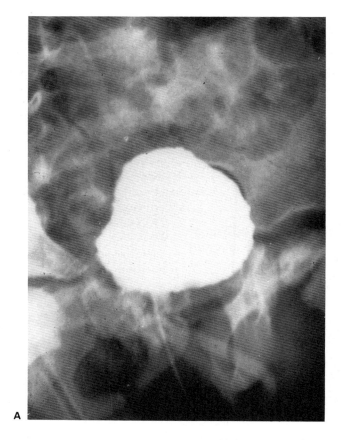

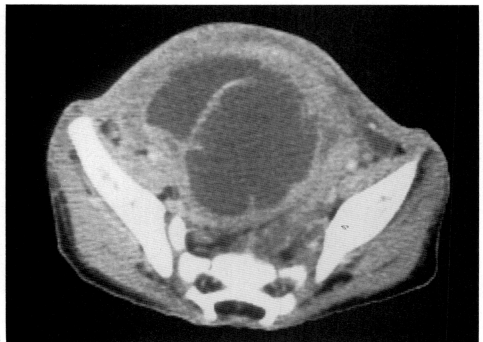

Fig. 5.7.17 **A** Cystogram. **B** CT of a child with a rhabdosarcoma. Note the small capacity bladder, the irregular bladder wall due to infiltration by tumour, on the cystogram, and the thickened bladder wall with intraluminal tumour on CT.

The diagnosis is made with a combination of imaging, cystoscopy and biopsy. Ultrasound examination demonstrates a polypoid echogenic mass within the bladder or a large solid homogeneously echogenic mass behind the bladder, often compressing and displacing the bladder anteriorly and out of the pelvis (Fig. 5.7.18). The same features are seen on CT, with enhancement of the mass initially during injection of IV contrast medium, but little enhancement during later scans. Prolapse or extension of the mass into the urethra or ureters will result in urinary retention, a large bladder and dilatation of the ureters and pelvicalyceal systems. Bilateral hydronephrosis may also be seen if there is compression and displacement of the ureters by a large pelvic mass.

CT demonstrates extension into perivesical tissues, both into soft tissue, regional lymph nodes, bone and large bowel. Oral contrast to opacify the colon is useful in these instances.

MRI is also able to demonstrate rhabdomyosarcoma which has a high signal intensity on T_2-weighted images and high or low signal on T_1-weighted images. Multiplanar imaging with MRI is very useful in the assessment of spread of the tumour into perivesical tissues.

At present, endoluminal tumours are most easily visualized with US, while bladder base tumours and perivesical extensions are best assessed with CT and MRI.

Distant metastases to the lungs are imaged with CT and skeletal lesions with radioisotope studies.

During treatment with chemotherapy and following surgery, frequent US, CT and MRI may be necessary to assess tumour shrinkage and recurrence. MRI with intravenous gadolinium is particularly useful in the assessment of response to treatment and the detection of recurrence.

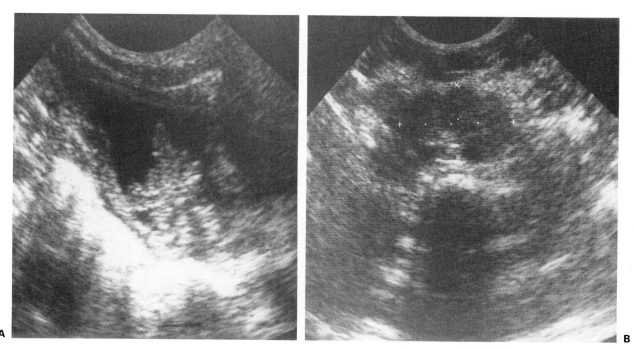

Fig. 5.7.18 Rhabdomyosarcoma of the bladder. **A** US shows a lobulated solid mass within the bladder. **B** Nodal involvement around the aorta and inferior vena cava is demonstrated.

The differential diagnosis of rhabdomyosarcoma includes plexiform neurofibromas, and pseudotumoral eosinophilic cystitis which is a benign inflammatory lesion. Children with these conditions present with frequency and sometimes haematuria. Bladder outlet obstruction will lead to obstructive uropathy and may progress to renal failure.

Benign epithelial polyps in the bladder are extremely rare in childhood and usually present with haematuria (Fig. 5.7.19).

REFERENCE

Geoffray A, Couanet D, Montagne J P H et al 1987 Ultrasonography and computed tomography for diagnosis and follow-up of pelvic rhabdomyosarcoma in children. Pediatric Radiology 17: 132–136

NEUROBLASTOMA

Background

Neuroblastoma is the second most common solid tumour of childhood. It arises from cells of neural crest origin in the adrenal medulla and sympathetic ganglia and has the potential to mature into ganglioneuroma (benign) or to regress spontaneously. Approximately 60% of neuroblastoma present in the abdomen, and two-thirds of these are adrenal in origin. The next most common site is the chest. Most cases (75%) are diagnosed by 4 years of age. The aetiology is unknown and familial cases occur.

The clinical picture at diagnosis varies greatly, because of the various sites of the primary tumour and the different patterns of dissemination. An apparently healthy child may present with an asymptomatic, paraspinal localized intrathoracic mass, with an excellent prognosis. At the other extreme is the pale, anxious child with periorbital ecchymoses, scalp nodules, a large abdominal mass, bone pain from widespread metastases and a poor prognosis. Other less common symptoms and signs of neuroblastoma include Horner's syndrome, sweating, diarrhoea (Fig. 5.7.20), hypertension and cerebellar encephalopathy, typically opsomyoclonus (dancing eyes), attributable to metabolic and immunological disturbances associated with the tumour.

The prognosis depends on the stage of the disease at diagnosis. Localized disease is defined as Stage I, II or III depending on the presence of disease across the midline and lymphadenopathy. Five-year survival in these cases varies from 40% to 90%. Stage IV disease includes patients with evidence of distant metastases; 5-year survival is about 10% to 60%. Metastases, present in 60–70% of children at the time of diagnosis, are usually to the skeleton, bone marrow and lymph nodes. Stage IVS is found in neonates and infants and is described below.

Neuroblastoma tumours excrete catecholamines and the detection of raised levels of vanillylmandelic acid (VMA) and homovanillic acid (HVA) in the urine is important in establishing the diagnosis.

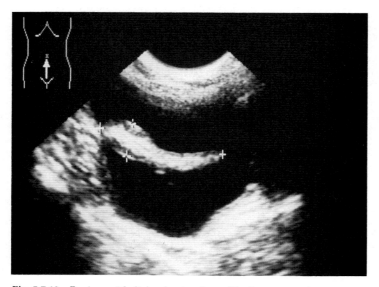

Fig. 5.7.19 Benign epithelial polyp in a boy of 9 who presented with haematuria.

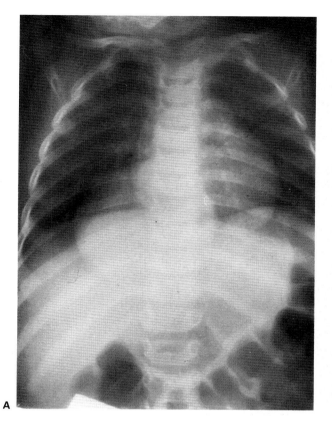

A

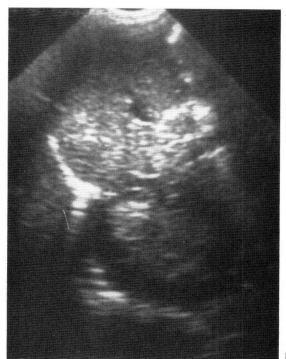

B

Fig. 5.7.20 **A** Chest radiograph. **B** Ultrasound and **C** MDP bone scan in a child with a neuroblastoma. This child presented with profuse watery diarrhoea, which was due to vasoactive intestinal polypeptide (VIP) excretion by the tumour. Following excision, the clinical symptoms, resolved. The child is well 12 years post treatment. The bone scan shows tumour uptake.

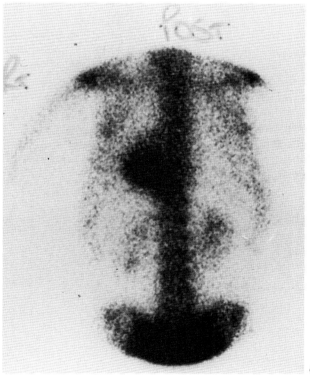

C

Imaging

Imaging has a crucial role in both making the diagnosis and also in detecting the extent of the tumour and the presence of metastases.

Plain radiographs

Plain radiographs of the abdomen may demonstrate a large abdominal mass, with irregular calcification (Fig. 5.7.21). Displacement of the paravertebral stripe secondary to retrocrural and para-aortic lymphadenopathy is often present (Fig. 5.7.22). Metastatic spread to the bones and bone marrow results in characteristic changes of osteoporosis, diffuse abnormal bony trabecular pattern, lytic bone lesions, pathological fractures and sutural diastasis with sutural irregularity (Fig. 5.7.23). Paraspinal masses with widening of the spinal canal and intervertebral foramina are seen. Irregularity of the posterior ends of the ribs indicate the posterior mediastinal location of these lesions. Collapse of vertebral bodies and occasionally acute spinal cord block may be present.

An IVU is now rarely performed, but if intravenous contrast medium is given displacement of the kidney inferiorly and laterally by a suprarenal mass is seen.

Ultrasound

Abdominal ultrasound is the first examination performed in a child presenting with an abdominal mass. The features of neuroblastoma are of an ill-defined echogenic mass, often containing calcification, displacing the ipsilateral kidney and extending across the midline, encasing and displacing the aorta and inferior vena cava (Fig. 5.7.24). Involvement of lymph nodes and the liver is also seen. Biopsy of the mass is possible with ultrasound guidance but must avoid areas of necrotic tumour.

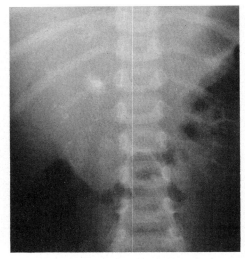

Fig. 5.7.21   Plain film showing irregular calcification in a large abdominal neuroblastoma.

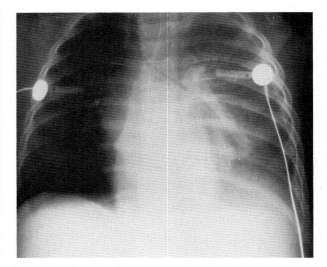

Fig. 5.7.22   There is widening of the paravertebral tissues due to tumour extension from an abdominal neuroblastoma.

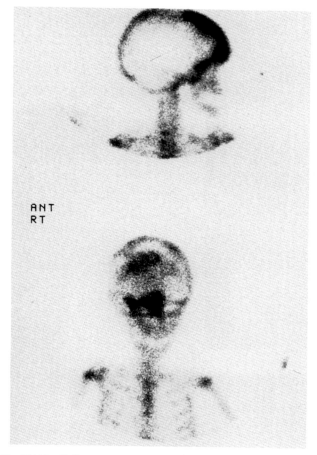

Fig. 5.7.23 Different child showing typical distribution of skull bony metastases from neuroblastoma.

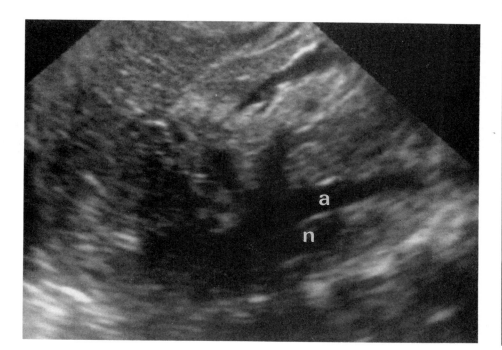

Fig. 5.7.24 Longitudinal ultrasound scan of abdomen showing tumour behind and displacing the abdominal aorta. n = neuroblastoma, a = aorta.

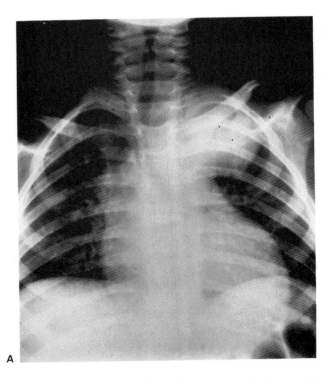

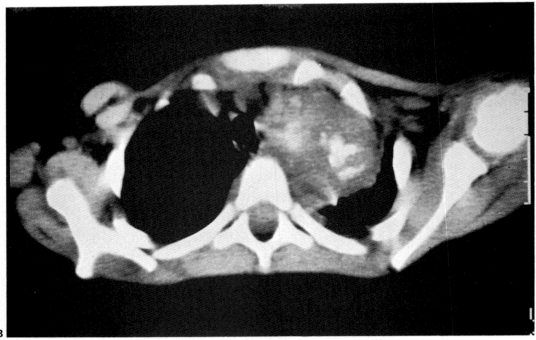

Fig. 5.7.25 **A** Chest radiograph and **B** CT of a child with a thoracic neuroblastoma.

CT

CT is used to demonstrate the presence and extent of neuroblastoma in the chest, abdomen and pelvis. In thoracic neuroblastoma a posterior mediastinal mass is seen (Fig. 5.7.25). The mass may be small and well defined, or extensive with displacement of the aorta and extension across the midline. Erosion of the posterior ribs and spine with disease in the spinal canal may be present. The presence of disease in the spinal canal is usually clearly seen following the administration of intravenous contrast medium (Fig. 5.7.26). Retrocrural nodes may be present in the lower part of the chest in association with an abdominal neuroblastoma.

CT scanning of the abdomen demonstrates an abdominal mass which may be confined to the suprarenal area, but is more usually poorly defined and extensive, occupying most of the central abdomen. The mass may displace the kidneys, extend into the renal hilum resulting in obstruction and hydronephrosis, and extend into the kidney itself (Fig. 5.7.27). Using intravenous contrast medium, encasement and displacement of the aorta, inferior vena cava and aortic branches is seen, and is a characteristic feature of neuroblastoma (Fig. 5.7.28). Neuroblastoma tissue itself does not enhance following intravenous contrast. Extensive paraaortic lymphadenopathy is common. Calcification within neuroblastoma on CT is common (70%). Extension into the spinal canal, erosion of vertebral bodies and metastatic disease in the liver may be demonstrated. Neuroblastoma may also occur in the pelvis. A mass is seen displacing the bladder anteriorly, and extension into the sacrum and sacral foramina may occur. If the mass is large, acute urinary retention with bladder outlet obstruction may occur.

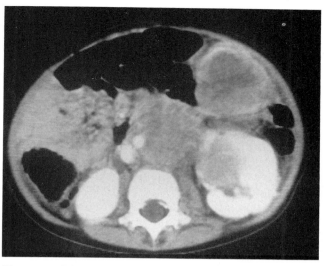

Fig. 5.7.27 CT scan with central neuroblastoma extending into the hilum of the left kidney. The aorta and inferior vena cava are displaced to the right.

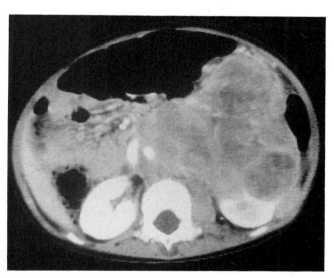

Fig. 5.7.28 CT scan. Large left-sided abdominal neuroblastoma displacing and encasing the aorta and inferior vena cava.

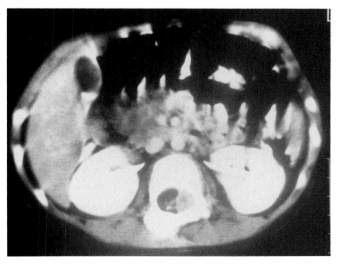

Fig. 5.7.26 CT scan with small right paravertebral neuroblastoma and enhancing mass in the spinal canal.

MRI

MRI is as good as CT or US in demonstrating neuro-blastoma in the abdomen or pelvis and has advantages. The mass demonstrates medium signal intensity on T_1-weighted images and high signal intensity on T_2-weighted images. MRI is able to identify the organ of origin of the neuroblastoma, define the extent and its characteristic relationship to adjacent vessels (Fig. 5.7.29). MRI is easily able to demonstrate extension of neuroblastoma into the spinal canal, without the need for contrast medium. In thoracic neuroblastoma it is the imaging method of choice. Neurological signs and symptoms are often absent and therefore it is important to look for disease in the spinal canal in all cases.

MRI is also able to image bone marrow and to demonstrate metastatic disease, which is seen as foci of low signal intensity on T_1-weighted images (Fig. 5.7.30).

Radionuclide imaging

Bone scanning with ^{99m}Tc-MDP is a sensitive method for the detection of metastatic disease to the skeleton. Multiple 'hot spots' of increased uptake of radioisotope are seen throughout the skeleton, particularly in the spine, skull and the proximal metaphyses of the limbs (Fig. 5.7.23). Characteristic symmetrical lesions around the knee are found (Fig. 5.7.31). Good technique is essential in order to be able to evaluate the metaphyses, as increased uptake in the epiphyses is normal at this age and may make assessment of the images difficult. The primary is often imaged on ^{99m}Tc-MDP scans, as uptake of the isotope is common (Fig. 5.7.20).

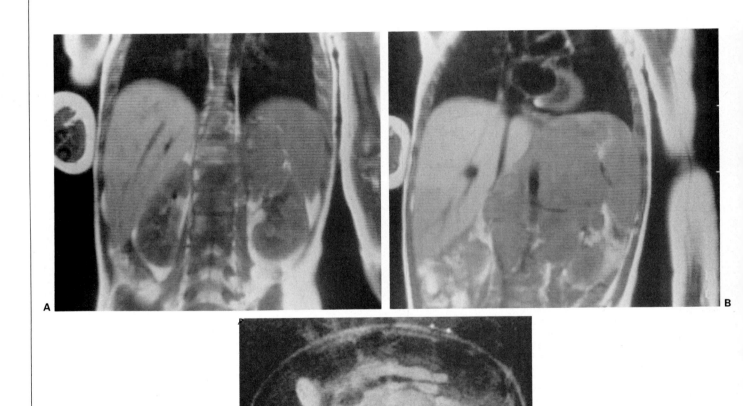

Fig. 5.7.29 **A** MRI coronal T_1-weighted image of left suprarenal neuroblastoma. **B** MRI coronal T_1-weighted image of central abdominal neuroblastoma encasing the aorta and left renal artery. **C** MRI transverse STIR image with high signal central abdominal neuroblastoma encasing the aorta and inferior vena cava. The left kidney is displaced.

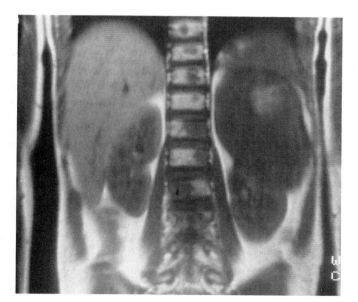

Fig. 5.7.30 MRI coronal T_1-weighted image. Left suprarenal neuroblastoma and metastases (low signal lesions) in the spine.

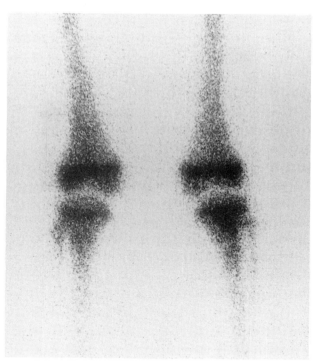

Fig. 5.7.31 ^{99m}Tc-MDP isotope scan of both knees. Symmetrical abnormal increased uptake in the metaphyses with blurring of the epiphyses.

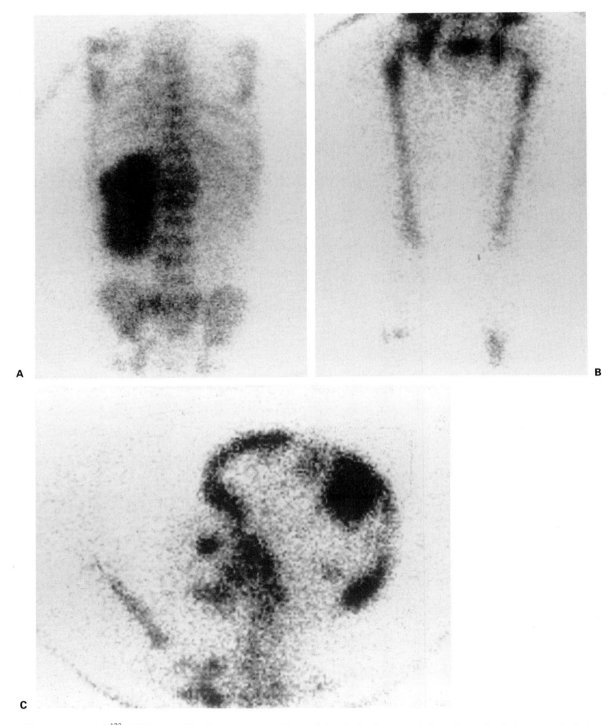

A

B

C

Fig. 5.7.32 **A – C** ^{123}I-MIBG scan. Uptake is seen in the large abdominal primary and throughout the skeleton particularly in the marrow cavities in the shafts of the long bones.

A catecholamine derivative, metaiodobenzylguanidine (MIBG), is also used in the detection of metastatic disease in neuroblastoma. MIBG is taken up by neurosecretory granules and when labelled with ^{123}I behaves as a specific radionuclide agent, which is taken up by neuroblast cells. Multiple 'hot spots' are seen throughout the bone marrow, in lymph nodes and in the primary lesion (Fig. 5.7.32). Uptake in the salivary glands, heart and adrenal glands is normal. All other sites represent disease. A small proportion of neuroblastoma cells do not take up MIBG and therefore in many institutions both bone scans with ^{99m}Tc-MDP and MIBG scans are used in the detection of metastases.

When labelled with a long-acting isotope [(131)]I), MIBG may be used as a form of targeted radiotherapy.

There is considerable research interest in the development of monoclonal antibodies which can be labelled with isotopes and act as specific radionuclides for diagnosis and therapy.

Neuroblastoma 4S

Neuroblastoma 4S occurs in infants less than 12 months of age. In this variant of neuroblastoma a particular pattern of metastatic spread to the skin, liver and bone marrow, but not to bone, is seen. Spontaneous recovery may occur, and if treatment is required, it is often far less than in standard Stage IV neuroblastoma, with more than 80% of patients surviving 5 years. Patients may present antenatally or in the early neonatal period, with hepatomegaly and characteristic bluish skin lesions. Respiratory difficulty due to massive hepatomegaly may require ventilation, and treatment with chemotherapy or radiotherapy to shrink the liver. Imaging with ultrasound is diagnostic and demonstrates hepatomegaly with an abnormal heterogeneous echopattern throughout the liver (Fig. 5.7.33). Primary suprarenal masses are often small, may be bilateral or even absent. The diagnosis of neuroblastoma 4S is confirmed with radioisotope scanning of the skeleton with ^{99m}Tc-MDP, when the absence of bony metastases is demonstrated. Following resolution of disease, the liver reduces in size, but the abnormal echogenicity persists for some time.

Follow-up

Chemotherapy is used in the treatment of all patients with metastatic disease and with inoperable tumours. Follow-up with radioisotope scans, both MIBG and ^{99m}Tc-MDP, is required to establish resolution of metastases. Persistent abnormalities, following treatment, on isotope bone scans do not necessarily indicate residual metastases, and may represent a non-specific bone response following healing. Residual abnormalities on MIBG scans are more worrying and probably require further treatment. Shrinkage of the primary tumour is seen following chemotherapy; both CT and ultrasound will demonstrate a small, residual calcified mass which is often confined to the para-aortic area. Surgical removal of the residual mass may be important in establishing a cure.

Differential diagnosis

The diagnosis of neuroblastoma is confirmed histologically and is usually straightforward in a patient with raised urinary catecholamines and characteristic radiology. The differential diagnosis of a large abdominal neuroblastoma includes a Wilms' tumour, teratoma, rhabdomyosarcoma and lymphoma. Displacement of the aorta anteriorly from the spine is a diagnostic feature of neuroblastoma and is not found in the above conditions; in these cases the mass usually extends across the aorta anteriorly. Neurenteric cysts present as posterior mediastinal masses and may be of soft tissue attenuation on CT, and should be distinguished from a thoracic neuroblastoma. They do not cause bone destruction, and are not metabolically active.

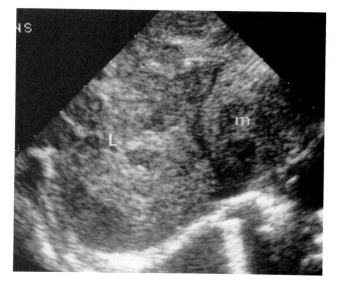

Fig. 5.7.33 Abdominal ultrasound scan. Enlarged liver with abnormal heterogeneous echogenicity and right suprarenal mass, in patient with 4S neuroblastoma. L = liver, M = mass.

GANGLIONEUROMA

Ganglioneuroma is a benign tumour of neural crest origin that can arise anywhere in the sympathetic chain or rarely in the adrenal gland, mesentery, alimentary tract, genitourinary system or nasopharynx. Ganglioneuroma and neuroblastoma represent mature and highly malignant extremes, respectively, of the same kind of tumours. Ganglioneuromas are frequently discovered as an incidental finding on clinical examination or a radiograph. When large they may spread through the neural foramina into the spinal canal, producing pain, alteration of gait or paraplegia. Plain radiography demonstrates a soft tissue mass with widening of the intervertebral foraminae and destruction of vertebral bodies. These findings are more clearly demonstrated with CT and MRI (Fig. 5.7.34).

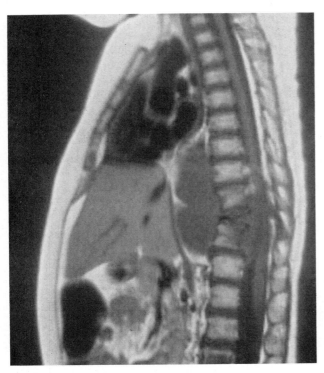

Fig. 5.7.34 MRI scan. Sagittal T_1-weighted images. Ganglioneuroma with retroperitoneal mass, collapse of upper lumbar vertebrae and extension into the spinal canal.

REFERENCES

Neuroblastoma and ganglioneuroma

Baker M E, Kirks D R, Korobkin M et al 1985 The association of neuroblastoma and myoclonic encephalopathy: an imaging approach. Paediatric Radiology 15: 185–189

Brodeur A M, Seeger R C, Barrett A et al 1988 International criteria for diagnosis staging and response to treatment in patients with neuroblastoma. Journal of Clinical Oncology 6: 1874–1881

Cohen M D, Klatte E C, Baehner R et al 1984 Magnetic resonance imaging of bone marrow disease in children. Radiology 151: 715–718

Cohen M D, Weetman R, Provisor A et al 1984 Magnetic resonance imaging of neuroblastoma with a 0.15T magnet. American Journal of Roentgenology 143: 1241–1248

Dietrich R B, Kangarloo H, Lenarsky C et al 1987 Neuroblastoma: the role of MR imaging. American Journal of Roentgenology 148: 937–942

Gordon I, Peters A M, Gutman A et al 1990 Skeletal assessment in neuroblastoma – the pitfalls of ^{123}I MIBG scans. Journal of Nuclear Medicine 31: 129–134

Hoefnagel C A, Voute O A, de Kraker J, Maraise H E 1987 Radionuclide diagnosis and treatment of neural crest tumours using iodine-131-meta-iodobenzyl guanidine. Journal of Nuclear Medicine 28: 308–314

Hownaan-Giles R B, Gilday D A, Ash J M 1979 Radionuclide skeletal survey in neuroblastoma. Radiology 131: 497–502

Ng Y Y, Kingston J E 1993 The role of radiology in the staging of neuroblastoma. Clinical Radiology 47: 226–235

Novak-Hofer I et al 1992 Radioimmuno localization of neuroblastoma xenografts with chimeric antibody [chCE]. Journal of Nuclear Medicine 33: 231–236

Peretz G S, Lam A 1985 Distinguishing neuroblastoma from Wilms' tumor by computed tomography. Journal of Computer Assisted Tomography 9: 889–893

Podrasky A E, Stark D O, Hattner R I et al 1983 Radionuclide bone scanning in neuroblastoma: skeletal metastasis and primary tumor localization of Tc [99m] MOP. American Journal of Roentgenology 141: 469–472

Rosenfield N S, Leonidas J C, Barwick K W 1988 Aggressive neuroblastoma simulating Wilms tumor. Radiology 166: 165–167

Stark D D, Moss A A, Brasch R C et al 1983 Neuroblastoma: diagnostic imaging and staging. Radiology 148: 101–105

5.8 RENAL HYPERTENSION

The exact incidence of hypertension in children is unknown; neither are there adequate figures to determine what proportion is essential hypertension and what is secondary. The lack of specific signs and symptoms in children emphasizes the need to measure blood pressure routinely as part of the clinical examination.

There are many causes of sustained hypertension in children. Excluding cardiac disease, renal pathology is the cause in 90% of children over 1 year of age (Table 5.8.1). Renal or abdominal tumours may also cause hypertension. Investigating the cause of hypertension requires clinical examination, biochemical tests and imaging. Initially an ultrasound and radioisotope scan of the kidneys should be performed. Ultrasound will detect significant hydronephrosis, a small or scarred kidney, due to dysplasia or reflux nephropathy, and tumours of the kidney and adrenal gland (Fig. 5.8.1).

Table 5.8.1   Abdominal causes of hypertension
Congenital renal disease – cystic dysplasia Polycystic disease: autosomal dominant Polycystic disease: autosomal recessive
Renal parenchymal disease Scarring after infection (reflux nephropathy) Nephritis Collagen vascular disorder
Obstruction – pelviureteric junction obstruction
Renovascular disease Renal vein thrombosis Fibromuscular hyperplasia Neurofibromatosis Middle aortic syndrome Takayasu's disease
Tumours Wilms' tumour Neuroblastoma Phaeochromocytoma

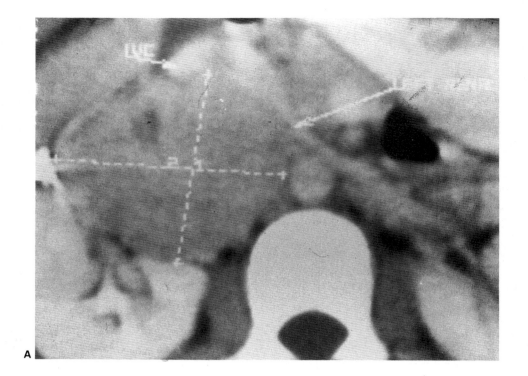

A

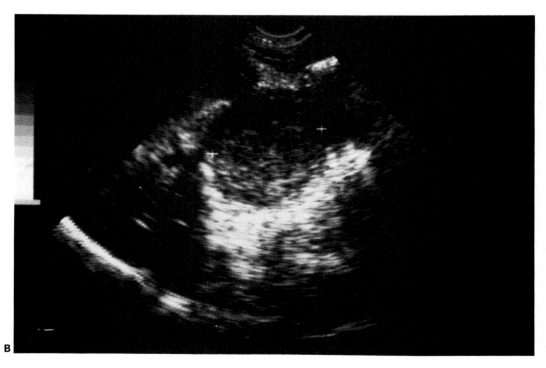

B

Fig. 5.8.1 Boy of 12 who presented with hypertensive encephalopathy. **A** CT of abdomen. A tumour of the right adrenal gland is present. This was a phaeochromocytoma. **B** Inferior venocavogram. The tumour is infiltrating the cava. **C** [123]I MIGB scan: Extensive uptake in the tumour.

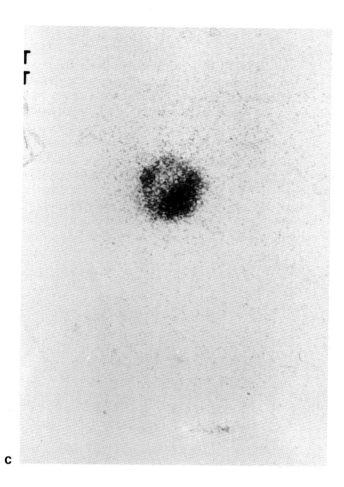

c

In the neonate, ultrasound may demonstrate renal vein thrombosis, and vascular complications such as renal artery spasm or clot, in patients with umbilical artery catheters. Duplex Doppler imaging, although difficult in neonates, may be helpful; colour Doppler clearly demonstrates blood flow to and from the kidney. Abdominal ultrasound may, however, fail to detect subtle renal scarring, vesicoureteric reflux, renovascular disease and phaeochromocytoma.

Isotope scanning with ^{99m}Tc-DMSA is the most sensitive technique for demonstrating a focal scar. ^{99m}Tc-DTPA or preferably Mag 3 is used to demonstrate renal function, obstruction of the collecting system and also the presence of vesicoureteric reflux by direct or indirect radionuclide cystogram. Intravenous urography is little used now in the assessment of the hypertensive child. It may be useful to demonstrate calyceal anatomy in a small kidney in which reflux has been excluded.

If both the ultrasound and a ^{99m}Tc-DMSA scan are normal, the cause of hypertension may be renovascular disease or a phaeochromocytoma. The presence of a phaeochromocytoma should be indicated by raised urinary catecholamine levels. If the lesion is not found in the adrenal glands by ultrasound then an ^{123}I-MIBG isotope scan will localize the tumour or tumours, and these can be further imaged with CT.

Renovascular hypertension

The diagnosis of renovascular hypertension is based on imaging. Plasma renin levels, as measured from a peripheral vein, are elevated in only 77% of patients.

The diagnosis of renovascular disease is not made by renal ultrasound alone. The specificity and sensitivity of imaging of the renal arteries with duplex and colour Doppler has not been fully evaluated in a large study yet. Nevertheless, these may be useful non-invasive techniques in the future. Isotope scanning with ^{99m}Tc-DTPA may demonstrate asymmetry of renal perfusion. Combined with an angiotensin-converting enzyme (ACE) inhibitor such as captopril, a ^{99m}Tc-DMSA or -DTPA scan may have an 85% sensi-

tivity in the diagnosis of renovascular hypertension (Fig. 5.8.2).

In all cases with hypertension in whom renovascular disease is suspected, angiography is required to confirm the diagnosis and demonstrate the site of the abnormality. Renal vein sampling for renin levels can also be performed at the same examination. The commonest causes of renovascular hypertension in children are fibromuscular hyperplasia, the middle aortic syndrome and William's syndrome. The classical appearance of the renal artery in fibromuscular hyperplasia is an irregular 'beaded' appearance with multiple stenoses. Segmental narrowing of the abdominal aorta and narrowing of the renal arteries is seen in both William's syndrome and the middle aortic

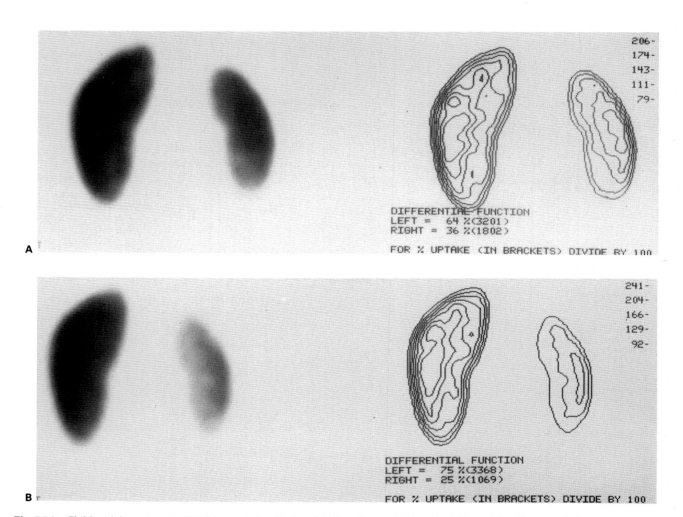

Fig. 5.8.2   Child with hypertension. DMSA scan **A** Pre Captopril. **B** Post Captopril. Note the failure of the affected right kidney to respond to Captopril, indicating a significant renal artery stenosis.

syndrome. Isolated renal artery stenosis may be idiopathic but is also a complication of renal transplantation.

Magnetic resonance imaging with magnetic resonance angiography is now able to demonstrate stenoses of the abdominal aorta and its branches. Cooperation of the patient is necessary at present and therefore precludes this imaging from many paediatric patients. In the future, however, magnetic resonance angiography may become the most useful screening and diagnostic technique.

Treatment

Percutaneous angioplasty may be a useful treatment in selected patients. A good response to dilatation of a renal artery stenosis with a balloon catheter is seen in fibromuscular hyperplasia and in postsurgical stenoses, e.g. renal transplantation. If angioplasty fails or is impossible, surgery may also correct renal artery stenosis. In some inflammatory conditions, e.g. Takayasu's arteritis, and in patients with extensive vessel involvement, e.g. the middle aortic syndrome, neither angioplasty nor surgery are successful and medical treatment alone may be the most useful.

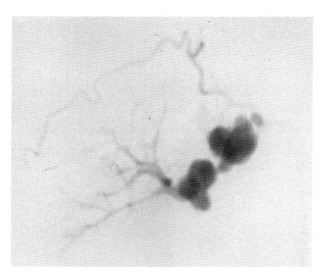

Fig. 5.8.3 Selective right renal angiogram in the same child. The renal artery contains multiple aneurysms due to a congenital vasculopathy. Note the collateral circulation.

REFERENCES

Aliabadi H, McLorie G S, Churchill B A, McMullin N 1991 Percutaneous dilatation for transplant renal artery stenosis in children. Journal of Urology 143: 569–573

Balfe J W, Levin L, Tzuru N, Chan J C 1989 Hypertension in childhood. Advances in Pediatrics 36: 201–246

Barth M O, Gagnadoux M F, Mareschal J L, Garel L, Mamou Mani T, Brunelle F O 1989 Angioplasty of renal transplant artery stenosis in children. Pediatric Radiology 19: 383–387

Chevalier R L, Tegtmeyer C J, Gomez R A 1987 Percutaneous transluminal angioplasty for renovascular hypertension in children. Pediatric Nephrology 1: 89–98

Diament M J, Stanley P, Boechat M I, Kangarloo H, Gilsanz V, Lieberman E R 1986 Pediatric hypertension: an approach to imaging. Pediatric Radiology 16: 461–467

Daniels S R, Loggie J M H, McEnery P T, Towbin R B 1987 Clinical spectrum of renovascular hypertension in children. Pediatrics 80: 689–784

Guzzetta P C, Potter B M, Ruley E J, Majd M, Bock G H 1989 Renovascular hypertension in children: current concepts in evaluation and treatment. Journal of Pediatric Surgery 24: 1236–1240

Ino T, Nishimoto K, Iwahara M et al 1988 Progressive vascular lesions in Williams–Beuren syndrome. Pediatric Cardiology 9: 55–58

Makker J P, Moorthy B 1979 Fibromuscular dysplasia of renal arteries as an important cause of renovascular hypertension in children. Journal of Pediatrics 95: 940–945

Merguerian P A, McLorie A G, Balfe J W, Khoury A E, Churchill B M 1990 Renal autotransplantation in children: a successful treatment for renovascular hypertension. Journal of Urology 144: 1443–1445

Novick A C 1991 Management of renovascular disease: a surgical perspective. Circulation 83 (suppl I, I): 167–171

Robinson L, Gedroyc W, Reidy J, Saxton H M 1991 Renal artery stenosis in children. Clinical Radiology 44: 376–382

Seibert J J, Northington F J, Miers J F, Taylor B J 1991 Aortic thrombosis after umbilical artery catheterization in neonates: prevalence of complications on long-term follow-up. American Journal of Roentgenology 156: 567–569

Siegel M J, St Amour T E, Siegel B A 1987 Imaging techniques in the evaluation of pediatric hypertension. Pediatric Nephrology 1: 76–88

Tonkin I L, Stapleton F B, Roy S 1988 Digital subtraction angiography in the evaluation of renal vascular hypertension in children. Pediatrics 81: 150–158

Wilson D I, Appleton R E, Coulthard M G, Lee R E J, Wren C, Bain H H 1990 Fetal and infantile hypertension caused by unilateral renal arterial disease. Archives of Disease in Childhood 65: 881–884

5.9   URINARY TRACT LITHIASIS

Urolithiasis is less common in children than in adults but is not infrequent. Calculi occur more often in infants (20% before 1 year, 34% before 2 years) than in older children and are more frequent in boys (2 : 1).

Presentation is by urinary tract infection (55%), haematuria (23%), pain (20%), micturition problems (12%) or proteinuria (10%). Underlying causes are multiple (Table 5.9.1). Proteus is the most common pathogen (30%), while *E. coli* (15%), enterococcus, pseudomonas, staphylococcus and klebsiella are other pathogens.

Stone composition is mainly calcium phosphate in North America, whereas struvite 'infection' stones are more common in Europe (Table 5.9.1).

The role of imaging is to diagnose lithiasis, to detect any underlying anatomical abnormality and to demonstrate the effect on the urinary tract so that treatment can be appropriate. Skeletal changes secondary to calculous disease can be monitored.

Table 5.9.1   Composition and aetiology of urolithiasis in North America and Europe

	North America %	Europe %
Oxalate calcium phosphate	58	37
Struvite (infectious stones)	25	54
Uric acid	8	1
Cystine	6	3
Abnormal metabolism	33	12
Anatomical anomaly	33	3
Infection	4	43
Unknown	28	30

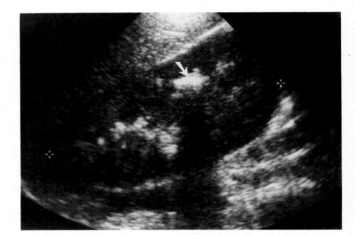

Fig. 5.9.1   Renal lithiasis. US. Typical appearance: hyperechoic focus (arrow) with acoustic shadowing. Left kidney between crosses.

IMAGING KIDNEY AND URETERIC STONES

Ultrasound

A calculus shows as a hyperechoic area with acoustic shadowing located within the pelvicalyceal system or ureter (Fig. 5.9.1). US can demonstrate the development of calculous disease as postulated by the Anderson–Carr theory of stone formation (Fig. 5.9.2).

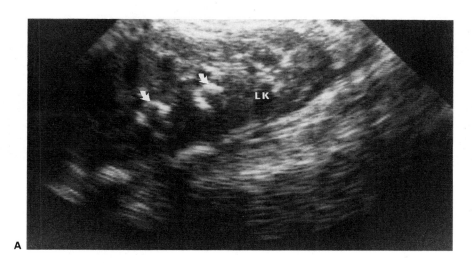

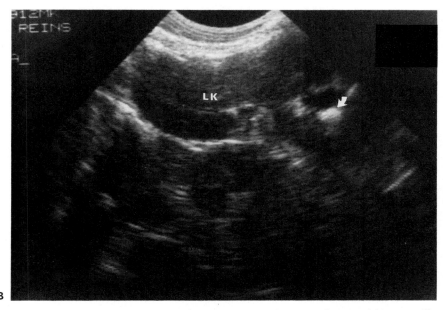

Fig. 5.9.2 Anderson–Carr theory. US. **A** Stage one. Hyperechoic encirclement of the pyramids tips (arrows). **B** Lithiasis. Same patient 2 months later. A stone is present (arrow) within a dilated system. LK = left kidney

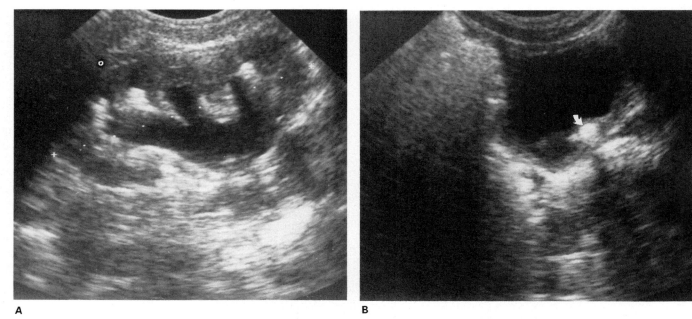

A   **B**

Fig. 5.9.3   Obstructing ureteral stone. US. **A** Sagittal scan of the kidney (between crosses). Pyelocalyceal dilatation. **B** Left sagittal scan of the bladder. The obstructive stone can be seen at the vesicoureteric junction (arrow).

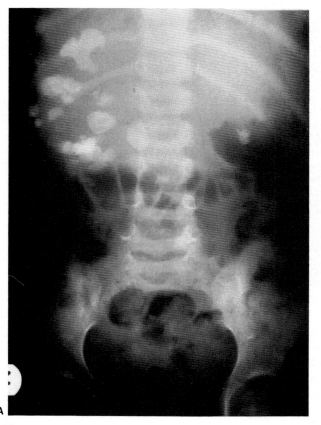

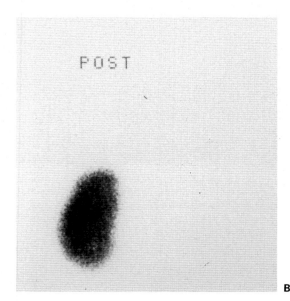

A   **B**

Fig. 5.9.4   **A** Multiple calculi are present in a dilated right kidney with a solitary left calculus. **B** DMSA scan. No right renal function but the left kidney is normal.

In suspected obstruction by a calculus, ultrasound examination should include the kidneys, ureters and bladder to determine the level of obstruction. The bladder should be filled prior to examination so that dilated ureters can be visualized (Fig. 5.9.3).

Radiography

On a scout film of the abdomen, calculi are seen as radiopacities in the renal areas, the line of the ureters or the bladder region (Fig. 5.9.4). Tomography may better delineate the number and size of stones prior to treatment. Differential diagnosis of a ureteric stone includes appendicolith, intracolic foreign body, calcified ovarian mass or adenopathy. An IVU is useful to localize ureteric stones (Fig. 5.9.5), and to characterize an underlying anomaly (Fig. 5.9.6).

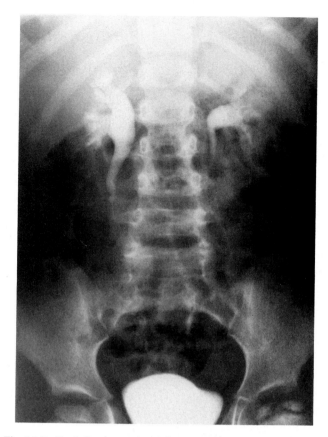

Fig. 5.9.5 Partially obstructive right ureteral stone. IVU. Dilated upper urinary tract secondary to a stone in a child who also has Legg–Perthes disease (left hip). The stone lies between the transverse processes of L3 and L4.

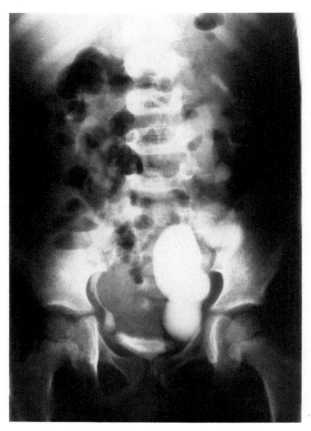

Fig. 5.9.6A Primary megaureter and lithiasis. IVU. Same patient as in Figure 5.9.7 with left ureteral and vesical lithiasis.

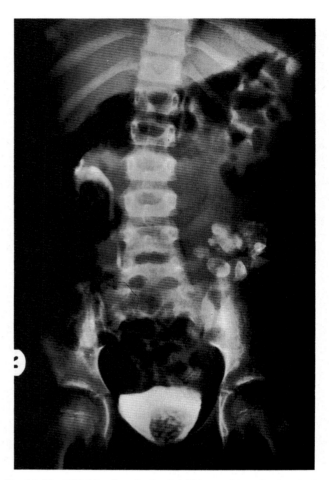

Fig. 5.9.6B IVU. Non functioning left kidney with multiple calculi contained in a ureterocoele in the bladder, and calculi in the left lower pole due to reflux.

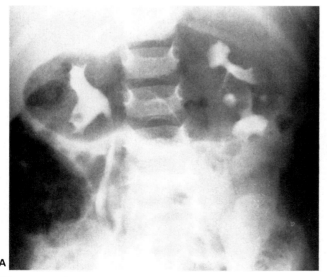

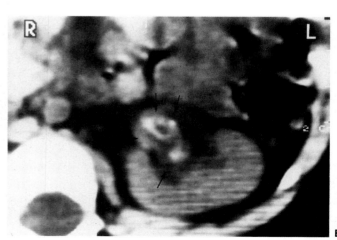

Fig. 5.9.7 Infectious stone. **A** IVU. Radiolucent left kidney lithiasis in a case with infected megaureter. **B** CT. Non-enhanced scan. Multilayered partially hyperdense lithiasis.

Rarely, retrograde urography may be necessary to visualize the level of obstruction.

Oxalic stones are densely radiopaque and may be associated with nephrocalcinosis. Associated skeletal anomalies are frequent in oxalosis.

Calcium magnesium-phosphate stones are also radiopaque. Non-opaque stones are usually composed of uric acid, with xanthine and mucoid matrix stones occurring less commonly. Cystine stones are usually multiple, may be voluminous and are of low radiopacity—often outlined by deposition of calcium salts. A voiding contrast or isotope cystogram is mandatory in such patients to detect associated reflux. The relation between coexisting reflux and lithiasis is unclear in cystine stone formation but reflux is almost always present with infective stones.

CT

Because of the greater density discrimination of CT, the detection of calculi is not so dependent on calcium content. CT is important in visualizing non- or poorly radiopaque stones (Fig. 5.9.7). Uric acid and cystine calculi can be identified by their low densities. Other types of calcium-containing stones cannot be distinguished reliably. CT also helps to determine the exact extent of calculi, especially in bilateral diffuse involvement.

CHARACTERISTICS OF BLADDER AND URETHRAL STONES

The urinary bladder is a typical location of 'endemic' stones related to ethnic, nutritional and climatic factors. On the contrary, in western countries, bladder stones are most frequently secondary to stasis, infection and foreign body, and are also associated with repair of extrophy, and after ileal surgery.

US is diagnostic showing a mobile echogenic zone with acoustic shadowing within the bladder (Fig. 5.9.8A). Calcified stones are easily detected on plain KUB radiographs. In contrast medium studies, a calculus appears as a round filling defect to be differentiated from a ureterocoele or blood clot (Fig. 5.9.8B).

Urethral lithiasis is rare. Suprapubic MCUG is diagnostic showing a urethral defect during micturition. A urethral polyp can give a similar appearance.

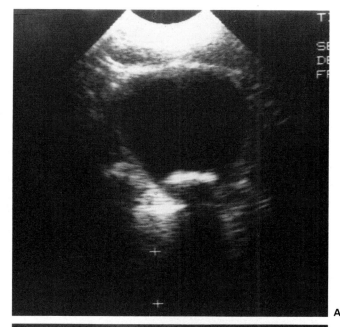

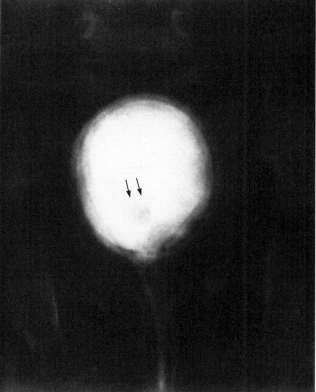

Fig. 5.9.8 Bladder stone (postureteral reimplantation). **A** US. Transverse scan of the bladder (mobile) hyperechoic focus with acoustic shadowing. **B** MCUG. Radiolucent filling defect.

NEPHROCALCINOSIS AND RELATED CONDITIONS

Nephrocalcinosis is the localized or diffuse deposition of calcium compounds within the renal parenchyma (Table 5.9.2).

Table 5.9.2   Cause of nephrocalcinosis
Renal tubular acidosis
Oxalosis
Primary hyperparathyroidism
Sarcoid
Hypervitaminosis D
Milk-alkali syndrome
Williams' syndrome
Medullary sponge kidney
Frusemide therapy
Post-tubular necrosis
Hyperthyroidism
Tumours
Tuberculosis
Hydatid disease

Medullary nephrocalcinosis (90% of cases)

When bilateral, there is typically an underlying metabolic disturbance inducing stone formation.

In neonates, prematurity, low birthweight and frusemide (Fig. 5.9.9) therapy are predisposing conditions. Gentamicin and theophylline have also been implicated. Although a plain radiograph may demonstrate these calcifications and suggest the condition (Fig. 5.9.10A), US is the most sensitive method. As described in 'Imaging kidney and ureteric stones' above, the appearances are of a gradual progression to a more diffuse hyperechoic medulla and reversed corticomedullary differentiation (Fig. 5.9.10B).

Cortical nephrocalcinosis

Sonographically, hyperechoic linear cortical areas are demonstrated which correspond to linear calcifications seen by urography.

Cortical nephrocalcinosis is usually a sequel of cortical ischaemia, cortical necrosis or renal vein thrombosis (see 5.16 'Renal transplant').

Localized nephrocalcinosis

Localized nephrocalcinosis is usually the consequence of chronic inflammatory disease but is occasionally seen in tumours or with a localised vascular lesion. Calcification also occurs in renal tumours. Localized medullary nephrocalcinosis may be seen in neonates, premature infants and neonates on frusemide therapy and is best appreciated on ultrasound examination.

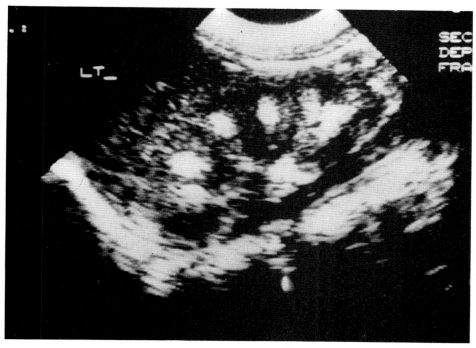

Fig. 5.9.9 Premature infant with prolonged frusemide therapy. Note nephrocalcinosis.

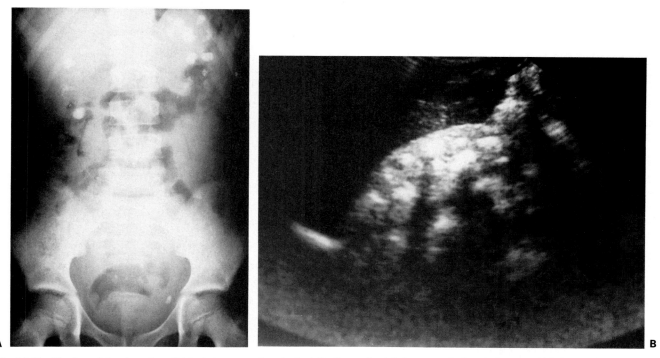

A   B

Fig. 5.9.10 Nephrocalcinosis and urolithiasis in a case of oxalosis. **A** Radiograph of abdomen including kidneys and bladder. Bilateral renal calcifications. A left ureteral stone is also present. **B** US. Sagittal scan of right kidney. Reversed corticomedullary differentiation with hyperechoic medulla. The cortex is quite hyperechoic. Associated nephrocalcinosis with acoustic shadowing.

THERAPY AND FOLLOW-UP

US is the best modality to follow cases after medical or surgical treatment.

In extracorporeal shock short wave lithotripsy (ESWL), US and a plain radiograph before treatment are necessary as a baseline study. Following ESWL, US may show residual hydronephrosis and radiography will demonstrate progressive disappearance of the fragments from the ureter (the so-called 'Steinstrasse') and thereafter from the bladder (Fig. 5.9.11). Perirenal haematoma and pulmonary oedema are rare complications of ESWL.

Surgery is now reserved for cases that cannot be managed by ESWL, particularly those with stones in difficult locations, or an underlying anatomical anomaly. Percutaneous lithotripsy has also been used as an alternative to surgery when ESWL is not possible; this procedure is monitored by fluoroscopy after IV opacification of the urinary tract with contrast medium. Whatever the treatment, follow-up US and radiographs are necessary to exclude recurrence (approximately 10%).

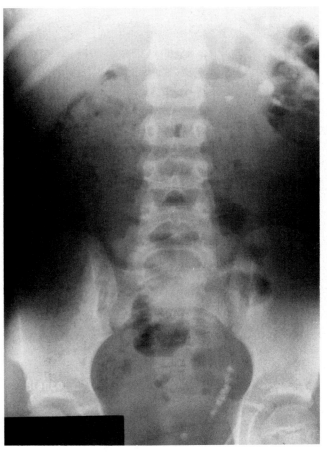

Fig. 5.9.11 Radiograph of abdomen including kidneys and bladder post ESWL. Reduced number and size of lithiasis. Some fragments can be seen in the left ureter (Steinstrasse). Same patient as Fig. 5.9.10.

REFERENCES

Androulakalis P A, Barratt T M, Ransley P G, Innes Williams D 1982 Urinary calculi in children. A 5 to 15-years follow-up with particular reference to recurrent and residual stones. British Journal of Urology 54: 176–180

Bettex M, Oetliker O, Zimmerman A, Kehrer B 1987 Urinary calculi in association with glomerular immaturity. European Urology 13: 182–185

Breatnach E, Smith S E W 1983 The radiology of renal stones in children. Clinical Radiology 34: 59–64

Clark J H, Fitzgerald J F, Bergstein J M 1985 Nephrolithiasis in childhood inflammatory bowel disease. Journal of Pediatric Gastroenterology and Nutrition 4: 829–834

Das G, Dick J, Bailey M J et al 1988 1500 cases of renal and ureteric calculi treated in an integrated stone centre. British Journal of Urology 62: 301–305

Dean T E, Harrison N W, Bishop N L 1988 CT scanning in the diagnosis and management of radiolucent urinary calculi. British Journal of Urology 62: 405–408

Jacinto J S, Madanlou H D, Grade M, Strauss A A, Bosu S K 1988 Renal calcification: incidence in very low birth weight infants. Pediatrics 81: 31–35

Laudone S M, Jenkins A D, Howards S S, Riehle R, Keating M A, Walker R D 1987 Initial experience with extracorporeal shock wave lithotripsy in children. Journal of Urology 183: 830–841

Lebowitz R, Vargas B 1987 Stones in the urinary bladder in children and young adults. American Journal of Roentgenology 148: 491–495

Lingeman J E, Smith L H, Woods J R, Newman D M 1989 Urinary calculi. Lea & Febiger, Philadelphia, pp 238–247

Myracle M R, McGahan J P, Goetzman B W, Adelman R D 1986 US diagnosis of renal calcification in infants on chronic frusemide therapy. Journal of Clinical Ultrasound 14: 281–287

Newhouse J H, Prien E L, Amis E S, Dietler S P, Pfister R C 1984 CT analysis of urinary calculi. American Journal of Roentgenology 142: 545–548

Papanicolaou N, Pfister R C, Young H H, Yoder I C, Herrin J T 1986 Percutaneous US lithotripsy of symptomatic renal calculi in children. Pediatric Radiology 16: 13–16

Patriquin H, Lafortune M, Filiatrault D 1985 Urinary milk of calcium in children and adults. American Journal of Roentgenology 144: 407–413

Patriquin H, Rotibaille P 1986 Renal calcium deposition in children: sonographic demonstration of the Anderson–Carr progression. American Journal of Roentgenology 146: 1253–1256

Pavanello L, Rizzoni G, Dussini N et al 1981 Cystinuria in children. European Urology 7: 139–143

Pearse D H, Kaude J V, Williams J L, Bush D, Wright P G 1984 Sonographic diagnosis of frusemide-induced nephrocalcinosis in newborn infants. Journal of Ultrasound in Medicine 3: 553–556

Polinsky M S, Kaiser B A, Balvarte H J 1987 Urolithiasis in childhood. Pediatric Clinics of North America 34: 683–710

Turnock R R, Rangecroft L 1989 Ureteral calculi in children: review of 50 consecutive cases. Urology 33: 211–214

Wilbert D H, Schofer O, Riedmiller H 1988 Treatment of pediatric urolithiasis by extracorporeal shock-wave lithotripsy. European Journal of Pediatrics 147: 579–581

5.10 BLADDER AND URACHUS

EXSTROPHY–EPISPADIAS COMPLEX AND ASSOCIATED ANOMALIES

Cloacal exstrophy

Incidence (1 : 200 000)/OEIS complex: OEIS complex is the association of Omphalocele, cloacal Exstrophy, Imperforate anus and Sacral meningocoele, and can be detected with antenatal US at 20–22 weeks.

Cloacal anomaly

In cloacal anomalies, there is confluence of the intestinal, genital and urinary tract with a single perineal orifice. The exact relationship of the different components is demonstrated with a lateral 'cloacogram' and an MCUG which demonstrates the bladder neck and its competence. Any associated hydrocolpos is seen on US.

Persistent urogenital sinus

In a persistent urogenital sinus, the rectum and anus are normal but the vagina and urethra are confluent. Female hypospadias is a variant of the condition. The urethral orifice opens into the anterior wall of the vagina and may be difficult to catheterize. Vesicoureteral reflux is common.

Bladder exstrophy (1 : 10 000 live births)

Plain radiographs of the abdomen show wide separation of the pubic bones (Fig. 5.10.1). The upper urinary tract is usually normal at birth. US will detect and monitor urinary tract dilatation, which may follow bladder reconstruction, and which may be complicated by calculous formation.

Epispadias

There is an incidence of 1 : 50 000 in the population. In epispadias there is an abnormal dorsal opening of the urethra. The bladder neck is poorly developed and urinary incontinence frequent. Plain radiographs of the pelvis in boys and girls show separation of the pubic symphysis greater than 1 cm.

An MCUG is necessary to determine bladder neck competence.

REFERENCES

Bockrath J M, Maizels M, Firlit C F 1982 Benign bladder polyp causing tandem obstruction of the UT in a patient with Beckwith–Wiedman S. Journal of Urology 128: 1309–1312

Escobar L E, Weaver D D, Bixler D, Hodes M E, Mitchell M 1987 Urorectal septum malformation sequence. American Journal of Diseases in Children 141: 1021–1024

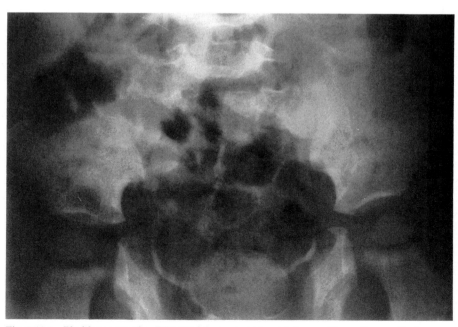

Fig. 5.10.1 Bladder exstrophy. IVU. Widely separated pubic bones. Normally opacified ureters enter into the open bladder.

Friedman A P, Haller J O , Schultze G, Schaffer R 1983 Sonography of vesical and perivesical abnormalities in children. Journal of Ultrasound in Medicine 2: 285–290

Gillerot Y, Koulisher L 1988 Major malformations of the UT. Anatomic and genetic aspects. Perinatal Nephrology and Biology of the Neonate 53: 186–196

Hendren W H 1980 Urogenital sinus and anorectal malformation: experience with 22 cases. Journal of Pediatric Surgery 15: 628–641

Hendren W H 1988 Urological aspects of cloacal malformations. Journal of Urology 140: 1207–1213

Hurwitz R S, Manzoni G A M, Ransley P G, Stephens D F 1987 Cloacal exstrophy: a report of 34 cases. Journal of Urology 138: 1060–1064

Jacquier S, Rousseau O 1987 Sonographic measurements of the normal bladder wall in children. American Journal of Roentgenology 149: 563–566

Marshall F F, Jeffs R D, Serafyan W K 1979 Urogenital sinus abnormalities in the female patient. Journal of Urology 122: 568–572

Marshall F F, Muecke E C 1968 Variations in exstrophy of the bladder. Journal of Urology 88: 766–796

Mirk P, Calisti A, Fileni A 1986 Prenatal sonographic diagnosis of bladder exstrophy. Journal of Ultrasound in Medicine 5: 291–293

Muecke E C, Curranino G 1968 Congenital widening of the pubic symphysis. Associated clinical disorders and roentgen anatomy of the affected bony pelvis. American Journal of Roentgenology 107: 179–185

Parott T S 1985 Urologic implications of ano-rectal malformations. Urologic Clinics of North America 12: 13–21

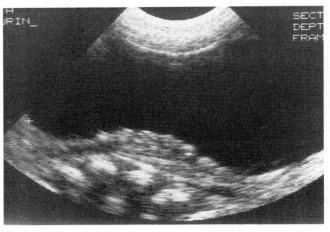

Fig. 5.10.2 Megabladder in a case of a neonate with posterior urethral valves. US. Sagittal scan of the huge bladder (12 cm).

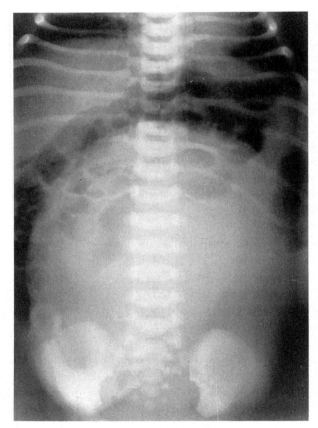

Fig. 5.10.3 Asphyxiated neonatal bladder. KUB. A pelvic 'mass' displaces the intestine upward and laterally. No bladder outlet obstruction was found; it resolved spontaneously.(Courtesy of Dr. F. Diard.)

LARGE BLADDERS (TABLE 5.10.1)

Table 5.10.1 Large bladder
Neurogenic bladder
Bladder outlet obstruction
Primary megacystis of childhood
'Asphyxiated' neonatal bladder
Megacystis megaureter (reflux)
Megacystis microcolon hypoperistalsis

Large bladders are relatively common findings in children. On US, a bladder should be considered large if its upper limit lies above the umbilicus and if emptying is never visualized. Antenatally or in the neonatal period, bladder outlet obstruction (from urethral valves) (Fig. 5.10.2) and massive reflux, leading to the so-called 'megacystis-megaureter syndrome' are the usual causes of large bladders (see 5.4 'Urinary tract dilatation'). 'Megacystis microcolon hypoperistalsis' is an uncommon cause and can also be detected in utero. US shows a large bladder and permanently dilated intestinal loops.

A particular type of large bladder that is seen in the last weeks of pregnancy and in the neonatal period is the so-called 'asphyxiated bladder'. The bladder is large but no obstructive aetiology is found and the condition resolves spontaneously (Fig. 5.10.3).

In older children, primary vesical gigantism is an uncommon but well-documented condition of unknown cause.

Bladder enlargement from obstruction may result from a prolapsed polyp, tumour (Fig. 5.10.4), uretero-coele or diverticulum protruding into the bladder neck.

Large bladders are also associated with neurogenic abnormalities.

REFERENCES

Inamdar S, Mallough C, Ganguly R 1984 Vesical gigantism or congenital megacystis. Urology 24: 601–603

Ivey H H 1978 Asphyxiated bladder as a cause of delayed micturition in the newborn. Journal of Urology 120: 498–499

Koefott R B, Websher G D, Anderson E E, Glenn J F 1981 Primary megacystis syndrome. Journal of Urology 125: 232–234

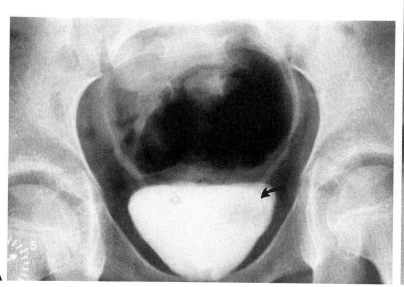
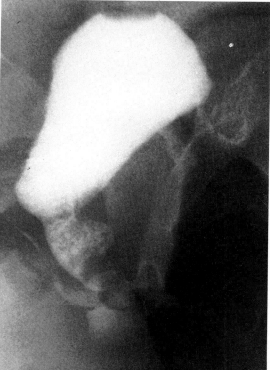

Fig. 5.10.4 Bladder tumour protruding into the urethra. **A** IVU. Inhomogenous aspect of the left vesicoureteric junction due to the tumour (arrow). **B** MCUG (micturition phase). Inhomogeneous mass within the urethra (arrow) corresponding to the bladder transitional cell tumour (8-year-old girl).

THICKENED BLADDER WALL (Table 5.10.2)

Table 5.10.2 Thickened bladder wall
Neurogenic bladder and voiding dysfunction Infection Tumoral, neurofibromatosis Haemorrhagic Bladder outlet obstruction (posterior urethral valves) Eosinophilic cystitis Post chemotherapy.

On sonography, bladder wall thickness above 4 mm is considered abnormal when the bladder is full. This thickness is a common finding especially in girls. It may or may not be associated with infection (Fig. 5.10.5).

Neurogenic bladder and micturition dysfunction

A neurogenic bladder is usually associated with neurological disorders; spinal dysraphism is a common cause. Spinal injury, spinal infection or tumour are less frequent. In dysraphism, either in utero or directly after birth, the urinary tract will appear normal and US is sufficient as a baseline examination.

Later, when 'dynamic' voiding starts, the bladder size increases, the wall thickens and becomes irregular and multiple diverticula may develop due to the dyssynergic contractions (Fig. 5.10.6). This is well seen on US, as can the dilatation of the upper urinary tract secondary to reflux. MCUG typically shows a large trabeculated bladder with spontaneous filling of the urethra due to an incompetent bladder neck (Fig. 5.10.7).

A milder form of neurogenic bladder is associated with vesicosphincteric dysynergia and with detrusor instability typically in young girls with urge micturition. The bladder capacity is small and the urethra appears narrow on MCUG (Fig. 5.10.8) and is best evaluated by combining this examination with urodynamic studies.

Infection and inflammatory cystitis

This is a common cause of thickening of the bladder. *E coli* is the commonest pathogen.

Eosinophilic cystitis is an uncommon inflammatory process. The bladder wall appears thickened. Vesicoureteric reflux may be present. The condition resolves spontaneously.

Haemorrhagic cystitis typically affects boys (Fig. 5.10.9) and is usually associated with *E. coli* or adenovirus. The bladder wall is thickened and the urine may appear echogenic on US due to blood.

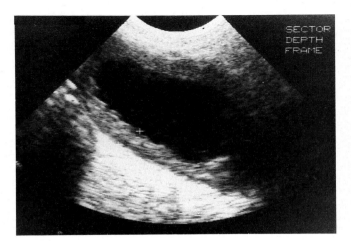

Fig. 5.10.5 Thickened bladder wall. US. Bladder wall thickness 6 mm in a non-infected asymptomatic baby boy.

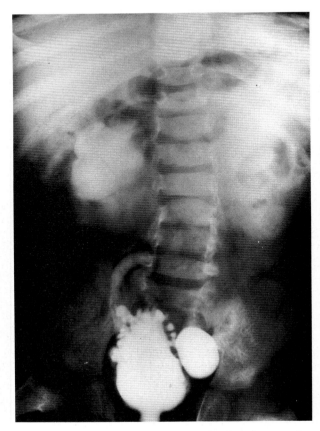

Fig. 5.10.6 Spinal dysraphism. MCUG. Dilated upper tracts due to reflux. Note multiple bladder diverticula and open posterior urethra.

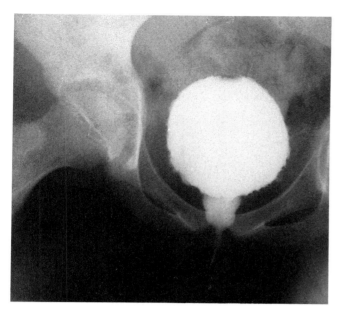

Fig. 5.10.7 Neurogenic bladder. MCUG. Filling phase. Irregular elongated bladder with incompetent neck in a case of operated myelomeningocoele.

Neoplastic involvement of the bladder

Involvement of the bladder with rhabdomyosarcoma or with neurofibromatosis may be localized or diffuse (see 5.7 'Tumours of the urinary tract').

US demonstrates the abnormal thickening of the bladder wall secondary to tumour. CT or MRI are necessary to determine the full extent of disease, particularly extravesically.

REFERENCES

Aaronson I, Cremin B J 1984 Neuropathic bladder. In : Aarnson I, Cremin B J (eds) Clinical pediatric uroradiology. Churchill Livingstone, Edinburgh, pp 266–285

Bartholomew T H 1985 Neurogenic voiding: function and dysfunction. Urologic Clinics of North America 12: 67–73

Lalmand B, Avni E F, Simon J, Verhest A, Schulman C C, Struyven J 1987 Transitional cell papillary carcinoma of the bladder in a child. Pediatric Radiology 17: 77–79

Sutphin M, Middleton A W 1984 Eosinophilic cystitis in children: a self limited process. Journal of Urology 132: 117–119

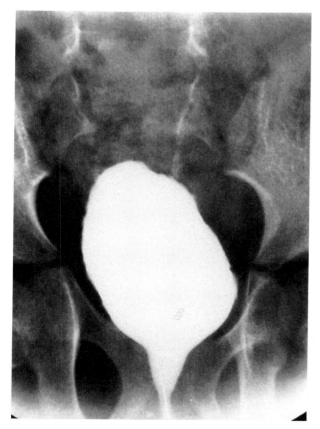

Fig. 5.10.8 Vesicosphincteric dyssynergia. MCUG. During micturition there is a thickened irregular bladder wall in a non-infected girl with urge micturition. Spastic urethra.

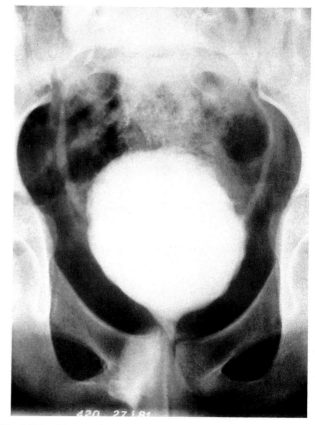

Fig. 5.10.9 Haemorrhagic cystitis. IVU. Irregular thickened bladder in a 10-year-old boy with haematuria.

BLADDER DUPLICATION

The usual form of bladder duplication is in the sagittal plane. Duplication may be partial or complete. The abnormality is demonstrated with an IVU and MCUG (Fig. 5.10.10). One part of the abnormal bladder may be obstructed, and US will demonstrate this.

REFERENCE

Abrahamson J 1961 Double bladder and related anomalies. British Journal of Urology 33: 195–214

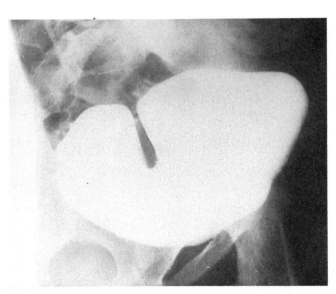

Fig. 5.10.10   Bifid bladder. MCUG.

BLADDER DIVERTICULA (Table 5.10.3)

Table 5.10.3   Bladder diverticula
Primary
Hutch (Vesicoureteric junction)
Neurogenic bladder
Post-reimplantation
Prune belly syndrome
Kinky hair syndrome
Williams' syndrome
Ehlers–Danlos syndrome
Cutis laxa syndrome
Fetal alcohol syndrome

The commonest type of bladder diverticulum is the so-called Hutch diverticulum at the vesicoureteric junction (Fig. 5.10.11). It may be associated with reflux; when prolapsed, it may also cause ureteric or bladder outlet obstruction.

Radiographically, the IVU typically underestimates the size and type of the diverticulum. It may be seen with US but an MCUG most accurately demonstrates the size and location of these diverticula which may become very large (Fig. 5.10.12). Multiple bladder diverticula may be part of a syndrome (Fig. 5.10.13; Table 5.10.3). Finally, diverticula may be secondary to surgery on the vesicoureteric junction.

REFERENCES

Boechat M I, Lebowitz R L 1978 Diverticula of the bladder in children. Pediatric Radiology 7: 22–28

Verghese H, Belman A B 1984 Urinary retention secondary to congenital bladder diverticula in infants. Journal of Urology 132: 1186–1188

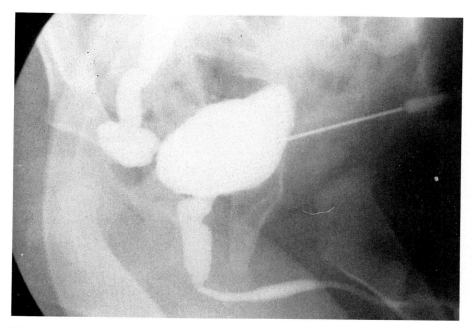

Fig. 5.10.11 Bladder diverticulum with vesicoureteral reflux. MCUG.

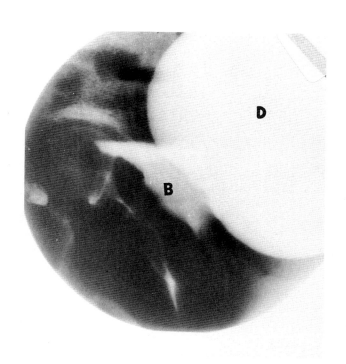

Fig. 5.10.12 Voiding cystogram in a boy with a huge solitary bladder diverticulum (D). Note size of diverticulum relative to the empty bladder (B).

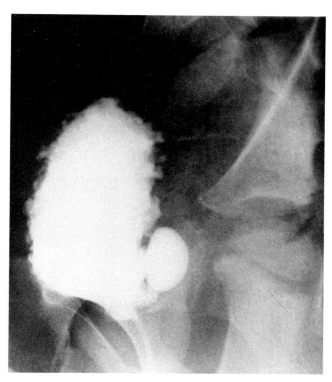

Fig. 5.10.13 Multiple bladder diverticula. MCUG. Case of fetal alcohol syndrome.

713

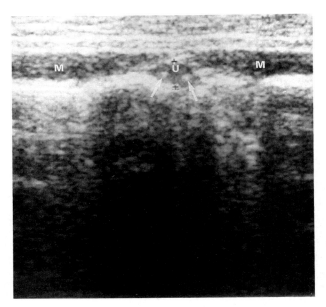

Fig. 5.10.14 Normal urachus. US. Supravesical transverse scan of the abdomen. The normal urachus (U) appears as a 3 mm oval area between the rectus muscles (M). Arrows point to the umbilical artery remnants.

URACHUS AND MIDLINE OMPHALOVESICAL ANOMALIES

Omphalovesical midline anomalies are unusual congenital malformations. Among them, patent anomalies are the most common. Some patency is found in 1 : 1000 autopsies. Symptomatic patency is rare. A patent urachus may be diagnosed in utero and associated with posterior urethral valves. Because of the easy demonstration of the anatomy, US is the best imaging method.

The urachus represents the fibrosed allantoic stalk connecting the umbilicus and bladder, and lies in the space of Retzius between the peritoneum and fascia transversalis. The umbilicovesical fascia surrounds the urachus. The fascia inludes both umbilical arteries. On a transverse scan, the urachus measures approximately 3 mm in diameter (Fig. 5.10.14).

Urachal anomalies have been classified into four groups: the completely patent urachus; urachal sinus (opening to the umbilicus); the urachal diverticulum (opening to the bladder), and urachal cysts.

Sonographically, the cystic type of anomaly presents as a mass. The contents of the cystic mass may be echogenic due to infection (Fig. 5.10.15). The sinus type of anomaly presents as a thick cord-like appearance. MCUG most clearly demonstrates the diverticulum type of anomaly (Fig. 5.10.16) and the completely patent urachus; the latter is seen in the prune belly sequence (Fig. 5.10.17).

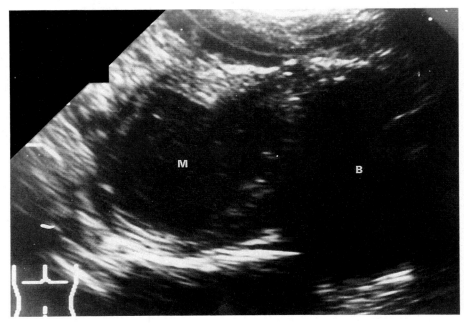

Fig. 5.10.15 Infected urachus (cystic type). US. Sagittal midline scan of the bladder (B). An echogenic mass (M) is seen above the bladder. (Courtesy of Dr M. Le Dosseur.)

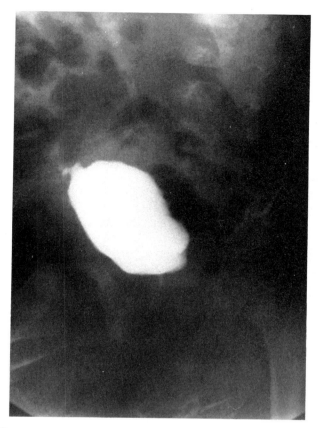

The differential diagnosis includes a rare urachal carcinoma in which CT will demonstrate the extent of the solid mass. It also includes other cystic lesions of the abdomen (mainly mesenteric cysts and ovarian cysts). Dystrophic calcifications of umbilical arteries' remnants can also be demonstrated within the umbilicovesical fascia by US and plain radiography.

REFERENCES

Avni E F, Diard D, Schulman C C 1988 Midline omphalo-vesical anomalies in children. Contribution of US imaging. Urologic Radiology 10: 189–194

Avni E F, Matos C, Van Regemorter G, Goolaerts J P, Diard F 1987 Symptomatic patent urachus in children. Contribution of US. Annales de Radiologie (Paris) 30: 482–485

Ney C, Friedenberg R H 1968 Radiographic findings in anomalies of the urachus. Journal of Urology 99: 288–291

Persutte W Y, Lenke R R, Kropp K, Ghareeb C 1988 Antenatal diagnosis of fetal patent urachus. Journal of Ultrasound in Medicine 7: 399–403

Srano R C, Klauber G, Carter B L 1983 CT of urachal abnormalities. Journal of Computer Assisted Tomography 7: 674–676

Thomas A J, Pollack M S, Libshitz H I 1986 Urachal carcinoma: evaluation with CT. Urologic Radiology 8: 194–198

Valla J S, Mollard P 1981 Pathologie de l'Ouraque chez l'enfant. Chirurgie Pédiatrique 22: 17–23

Fig. 5.10.16 Diverticulum type urachus. MCUG. A diverticulum is seen at the top of the bladder.

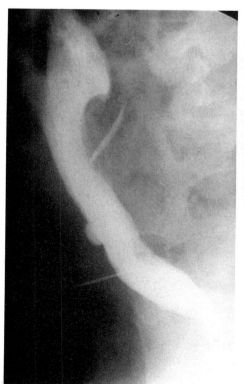

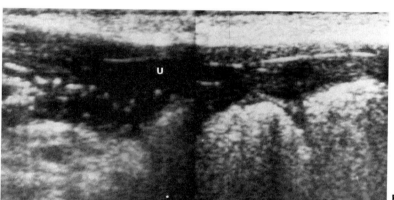

Fig. 5.10.17 Completely patent urachus. Case of prune belly syndrome. **A** MCUG. Suprapubic approach. Lateral view. Opacification of the bladder and the omphalovesical channel. Ureteral reflux is present. **B** US. Midabdominal sagittal scan. The patent urachus (U), a tubular structure, joins the umbilicus to the top of the bladder. It is partially cystic.

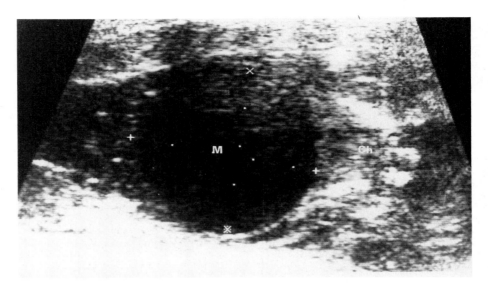

Fig. 5.11.1   Urethral atresia. In utero, 16 weeks. Sagittal scan of fetal trunk. A cystic mass (M) occupies the entire abdomen (4 × 3 cm) and corresponds to the extremely distended bladder. Ch = fetal chest.

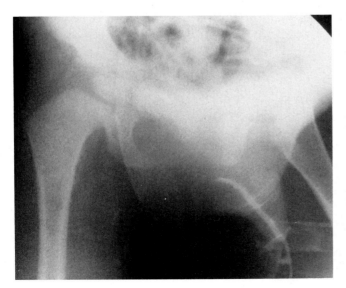

Fig. 5.11.2   Urethral atresia. Retrograde urethrogram. Case of prune belly syndrome.

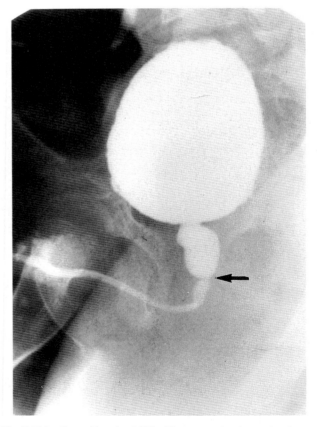

Fig. 5.11.3   Boy with spina bifida. The narrowing (arrow) is due to spasm of the external sphincter and is not a valve.

THE MALE URETHRA

Urethral atresia

Urethral atresia is a cause of early urinary tract obstruction in utero (Fig. 5.11.1), and is associated with poor outcome. It may be associated with the prune belly syndrome (Fig. 5.11.2).

Valves and strictures

Posterior urethral valve (PUV) is the commonest cause of urethral obstruction in boys and has been discussed in 5.4 under bladder outlet obstruction. MCUG is diagnostic in showing the valve and any associated reflux. US visualizes the upper urinary tract.

Functional radionuclide studies are performed when the child recovers from treatment, and are subsequently used to monitor renal function. PUV should be differentiated from external sphincter spasm as may be seen in children with neurogenic bladders (Fig. 5.11.3) and from physiological indentation and tortuosity of the posterior urethra.

Another common type of congenital stenosis is diaphragmatic obstruction of the bulbomembranous region. Other types of congenital stenosis are rare and may occur at any level of the penile and bulbous urethra (Fig. 5.11.4). Urethral stenosis and angular deformity may also be associated with rectourethral fistula, in association with anorectal atresia (Fig. 5.11.5).

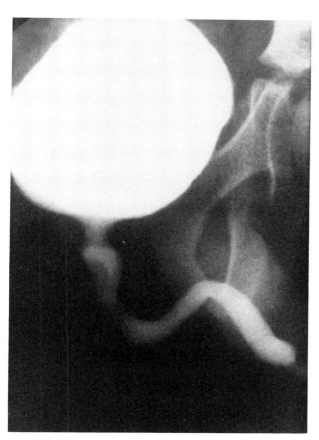

Fig. 5.11.4 Anterior urethral stenosis. MCUG. Dilatation of the urethra up to the stenosis of possibly congenital origin.

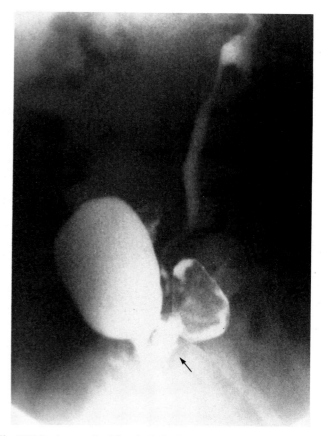

Fig. 5.11.5 Anourethral fistula. MCUG. Case of imperforate rectoanus. The fistula opacifies during micturition. Vesicoureteric reflux is also present.

Acquired urethral strictures secondary to catheterization or surgery usually occur in the anterior urethra. Strictures secondary to trauma may occur anywhere. MCUG (Fig. 5.11.6) or retrograde urethrography will define the stenosis. Retrograde urethrography may be performed by the insertion of an appropriately sized Foley catheter into the anterior urethra, or by using a simple catheter and occluding the distal urethra with fingers or a bandage.

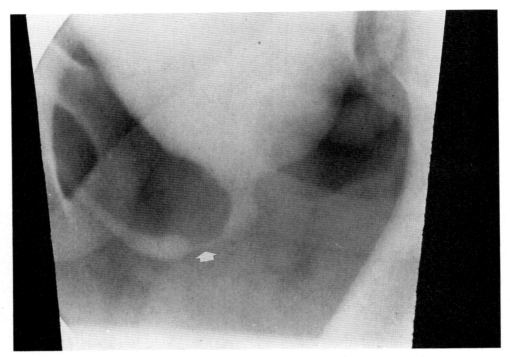

Fig. 5.11.6   Stricture of the posterior urethra (arrow) secondary to an old straddle injury.

Diverticula

The prostatic utricle is the commonest type of posterior urethral diverticulum. Opacifying during micturition (Fig. 5.11.7), it may be small or large, isolated or associated with other urogenital anomalies particularly the prune belly syndrome.

Anterior urethral diverticula are rare but may cause urinary tract obstruction (Fig. 5.11.8). Megalourethra is, in a sense, a large urethral diverticulum but corresponds to dilatation of the urethra due to corpus spongiosum deficiency (Fig. 5.11.9).

A lacuna magna is a dorsal urethral diverticulum of the fossa navicularis, which may cause pain and haematuria. A distal urethrogram is necessary to opacify the lesion with a catheter inserted directly into the diverticulum.

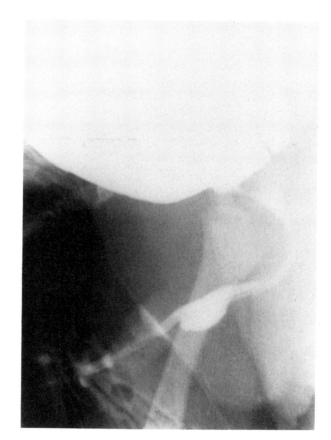

Fig. 5.11.8 Anterior diverticulum. MCUG (with catheter).

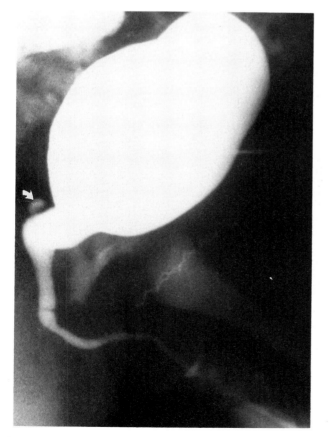

Fig. 5.11.7 Utricle. MCUG. A small utricle (arrow) opacifies during micturition. Partially obstructive posterior urethral valves are also present.

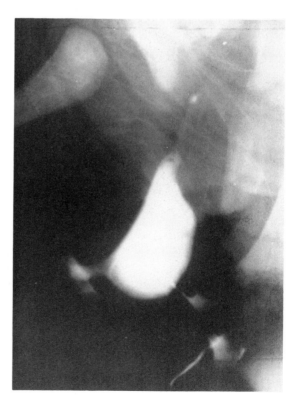

Fig. 5.11.9 Megalourethra. MCUG.

Cowper's ducts cyst and diverticulum

A retention cyst of Cowper's duct is seen as a filling defect on the floor of the bulbous urethra during voiding urethrography (Fig. 5.11.10). The duct and gland itself may opacify from reflux and appear as a tubular channel parallel to the urethra at the level of the posterior urethra. After fulguration of a retention cyst, massive reflux into the duct may occur resembling a diverticulum (Fig. 5.11.11).

Hypospadias

Hypospadias refers to abnormal location of the meatus somewhere between the normal site (glandular type) and the perineum (perineoscrotal type) (Fig. 5.11.12). Imaging of the upper urinary tract by US should be performed to exclude associated anomalies. After surgery, an MCUG is necessary to exclude acquired urethral stricture (Fig. 5.11.13).

Meatal stenosis and phimosis

These are rare causes of urinary tract obstruction. A small urinary jet is typical of meatal stenosis on voiding films (Fig. 5.11.12). In cases of phimosis, the prepuce opacifies and distends. In some severe cases secondary to meatal stenosis, there is dilatation of the entire urethra with retrograde opacification of the vas deferens and prostatic glands (Fig. 5.11.14). Ritual circumcision in poor hygienic conditions is an important cause of meatal stenosis.

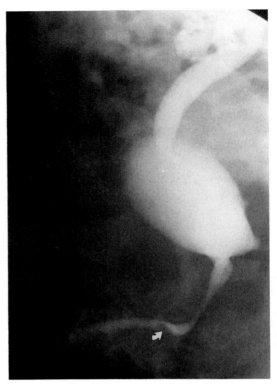

Fig. 5.11.10 Cowper's duct cyst. MCUG. A filling defect is seen at the base of the bulbous urethra (arrow).

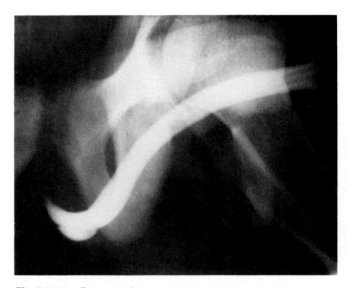

Fig. 5.11.11 Cowper's duct post fulguration of a cyst. The duct is partially opacified.

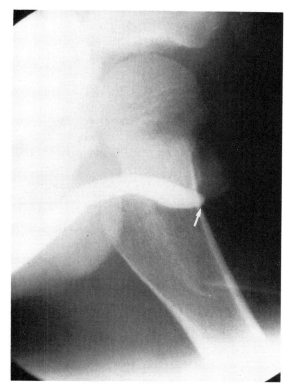

Fig. 5.11.12 Hypospadias with meatal stenosis. MCUG. Ventral opening of the urethra. Dilatation of the urethra up to the stenosed meatal opening (arrow). The urine jet is distal markedly small.

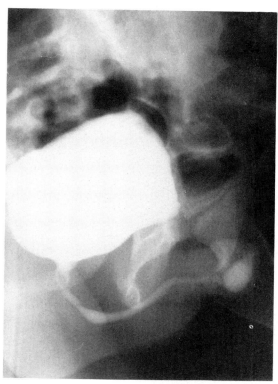

Fig. 5.11.13 Post hypospadias repair. MCUG. No significant stenosis is seen.

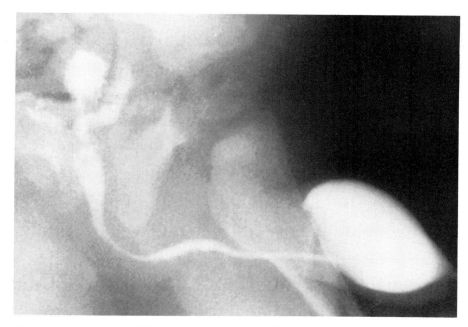

Fig. 5.11.14 Phimosis. MCUG. End of voiding phase. Distended opacified prepuce. Note reflux into the vas deferens.

Urethral polyps

Urethral polyps are uncommon causes of urinary tract obstruction and may be in the anterior or posterior urethra. MCUG is diagnostic (Fig. 5.11.15).

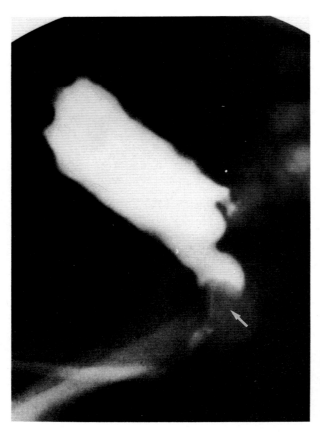

Fig. 5.11.15 Poor urinary stream and haematuria were the presenting complaints. The filling defect (arrow) in the posterior urethra is due to a polyp.

Urethral duplications

Urethral duplications occur almost always in the sagittal plane and may be complete or partial. If the two channels join above the sphincter, there is no incontinence and the lesion is discovered incidentally. When the ectopic channel communicates directly with the bladder, the child often presents with wetting. An MCUG may opacify both channels, or only one, in which case retrograde opacification may be necessary (Fig. 5.11.16).

THE FEMALE URETHRA

Congenital diverticulum of the female urethra is rare and will opacify on MCUG. An ectopic ureter may resemble a diverticulum if reflux occurs into the end of it.

Urethral duplication is usually associated with other caudal anomalies or bladder duplication. In girls, meatal stenosis is exceptional; urethral 'masses' may be a prolapsed ureterocoele or urethral polyp.

In the adrenogenital syndrome, there is 'masculinization' of the urethra which will appear longer and narrower than normal (Fig. 5.11.17), but without the verumontanum or morphology typical of the male urethra.

REFERENCES

Cambell J, Beasley S, McMullin N, Hutson J M 1987 Congenital prepubic sinus: a possible variant of dorsal urethral duplication. Journal of Urology 137: 505–506

Colodny A H, Lebowitz R L 1978 Lesion of Cowper's duct and glands in infants and children. Urology 11: 321–325

Effman E L, Lebowitz R, Colodny A H 1976 Duplication of the urethra. Radiology 119: 179–185

Gaisie G, Mandell J, Scatliff J H 1984 Congenital stenosis of the male urethra. American Journal of Roentgenology 142: 1269–1271

Kelly D, Harte F B, Roe P 1984 Urinary tract anomalies in patients with hypospadias. British Journal of Urology 56: 316–318

Kennedy H A, Steidle C P, Mitchell M E, Rink R C 1988 Collateral urethral duplication in the frontal plane. A spectrum of cases. Journal of Urology 139: 332–334

Madden N P, Turnock R R, Rickwood A M K 1986 Congenital polyps of the posterior urethra in neonates. Journal of Paediatric Surgery 21: 193–194

Madgar I, Ora H B Herz M, Mari H, Goldwasser B, Jonas P 1987 Urethral strictures in boys. Urology 30: 46–49

Morgan R J, Williams D I, Prior J P 1979 Mullerian duct remnants in the male. British Journal of Urology 51: 488–492

Moskowitz P S, Newton N A, Lebowitz R L 1976 Retention cysts of Cowper's duct. Radiology 120: 377–380

Parott T S 1985 Urologic implications of ano-rectal malformations. Urologic Clinics of North America 12: 13–21

Sommer J T, Stephens F D 1980 Dorsal urethral diverticulum of the fossa navicularis: symptoms, diagnosis and treatment. Journal of Urology 124: 94–97

Williams D I, Retik A B 1968 Congenital valves and diverticula of the anterior urethra. British Journal of Urology 41: 228–234

Woodhouse C R, Flym J T, Molland E A, Blandy J P 1980 Urethral diverticulum in females. British Journal of Urology 52: 305–310

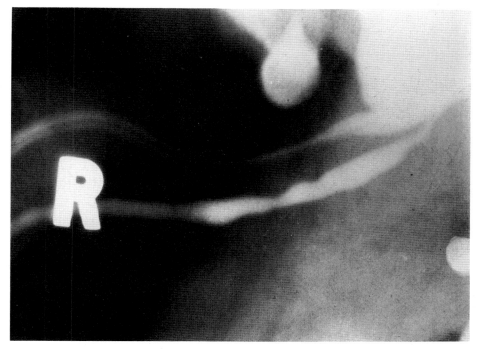

Fig. 5.11.16 Urethral duplication. MCUG. A catheter is in the accessory upper channel and enters the bladder separately.

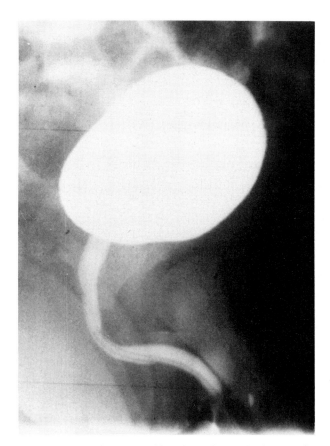

Fig. 5.11.17 Masculinization of female urethra. MCUG. Case of adrenogenital syndrome. There is an abnormally long tubular urethra.

5.12   SCROTUM

US is currently the best method to visualize the testis, the scrotum and the inguinal areas.

NORMAL SONOGRAPHIC ANATOMY

The testis appears as an ovoid echogenic mass measuring about 10–12 mm in length at birth and $40 \times 30 \times 25$ mm at puberty (Fig. 5.12.1). It is uniformly echogenic apart from the central hyperechoic area of the testicular hilum.

The head of the epididymus can be seen as a 5–10 mm solid mass above the testis (Fig. 5.12.1). A small amount of fluid around the testis is physiological, especially in the neonate.

Testicular and peritesticular vessels can be visualized with colour Doppler imaging. The tunica vaginalis around the testis can be traced up to the inguinal area.

UNDESCENDED TESTIS

The incidence in the male population is 1% at 1 year. US is effective in the preoperative assessment of an inguinal testis (Fig. 5.12.2). Intra-abdominal ectopic testes are difficult to find by US, although CT and MRI may prove helpful. If the ipsilateral kidney is absent in a child with an undescended testis, then the testis will also be absent, and searching is unfruitful. A frequent differential diagnosis of inguinal testis is inguinal lymphadenopathy.

The problem of the undescended testis is also discussed in Chapter 7.

HYDROCOELE

Hydrocoele is the most common cause of scrotal enlargement and results from late closure of the

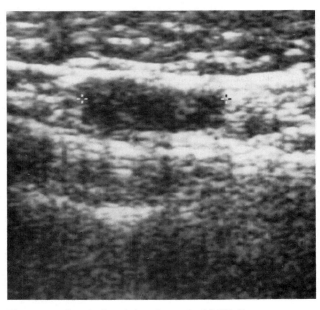

Fig. 5.12.2   Inguinal testis in a 6-month-old. US. Transverse scan of the left inguinal canal. The testis has normal shape and size (17 mm). It is surrounded by fat and muscles.

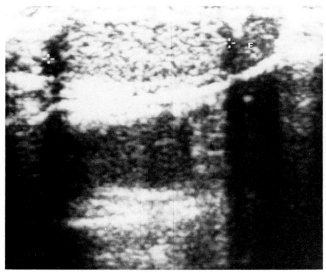

Fig. 5.12.1   Normal testis. US. Ovoid homogeneous solid appearance. Testis of a 3-year-old-child. 25 mm between crosses. E = head of epididymis.

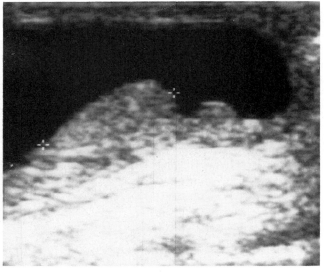

Fig. 5.12.3   Communicating hydrocoele in a newborn. US. Large fluid collection around a normal testis (between crosses).

processus vaginalis. It is a frequent finding in utero. The fluid tends to resolve by the age of 9 months. If the closure is incomplete, the hydrocoele is termed communicating and is abnormally persistent.

Hydrocoele appears as an echo-free collection around the normal testis (Figs 5.12.3, 5.12.4). An inguinal hernia may be associated (Fig. 5.12.4). In meconium peritonitis, the fluid appears echogenic and the scrotum shows calcifications (Fig. 5.12.5).

A hydrocoele may be a reaction to trauma, infection or torsion.

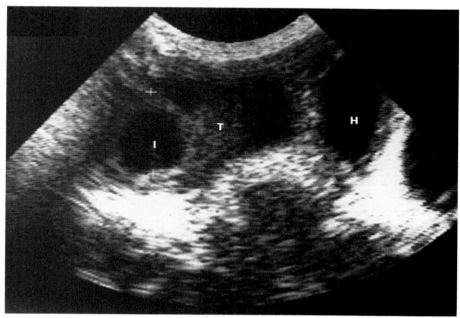

Fig. 5.12.4 Associated hydrocoele and inguinal hernia. US. Transverse scan of the scrotum. Fluid is seen around the testis (T). Peristalsis of the herniated intestine (I) was seen during ultrasound examination. A contralateral hydrocoele (H) is also present.

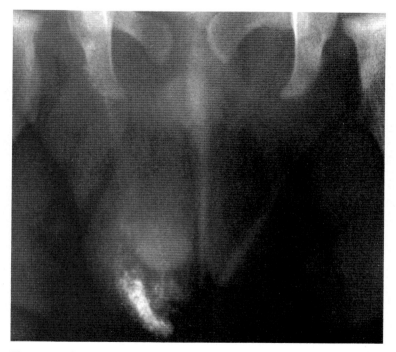

Fig. 5.12.5 Calcified meconium in the scrotum due to old meconium peritonitis.

THE ACUTE AND SUBACUTE SCROTUM

The causes of 'acute' and 'subacute' scrotum are various and include infection, trauma and torsion. Extrascrotal causes for 'acute scrotum', such as inguinal hernia, appendicitis, adrenal haemorrhage or spontaneous rupture of the common bile duct, should not be forgotten (Table 5.12.1).

Table 5.12.1   Acute and subacute scrotum (US)
Hydrocoele
Hernia
Trauma
Torsion of testis and testicular appendages
Epididymo-orchitis
Tumour
Leukaemia
Varicocoele
Adrenal haemorrhage
Appendicitis
Common bile duct perforation
Meconium peritonitis

Epididymo-orchitis

Inflammatory changes will increase the volume of the testis and epididymus. The tunica vaginalis around the testis is thickened and a hydrocoele may be present. Echogenicity is variable (Fig. 5.12.6).

In epididymo-orchitis an MCUG should be performed to exclude obstruction or reflux into the vas deferens, or any other unusual type of reflux, or anatomical variation.

Trauma

Trauma may induce a haematocoele (Fig. 5.12.7) or testicular haematoma that will appear as a hyperechoic focus. Complete testicular rupture may occur. Subsequent infarcts within the testis will appear as hypoechoic areas.

Torsion

Torsion of the testis may occur at any age and even in utero. In the perinatal period, the condition results from intravaginal torsion of the spermatic cord and tunica vaginalis. In the acute stage there is swelling of the testicular and paratesticular structures; at a later stage there may be only a small dysplastic calcified nubbin of tissue. Torsion is extravaginal and more frequent about the age of 12–15 years. Sonographically, both hyperechoic and hypoechoic patterns are found. The testis is enlarged (Fig. 5.12.8) in the acute phase.

Colour Doppler imaging has proved useful, with absence of vascular signals (Fig. 5.12.9). In the testis a technetium[99m] study is also a good imaging procedure when a cold area is consistent with lack of vascular flow in acute torsion.

The differential diagnosis includes infection which will show hyperaemia, and torsion of testicular appendages, in which the enlarged twisted adnexa appears as an echogenic paratesticular mass.

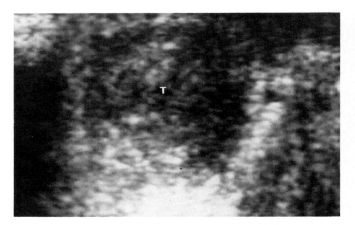

Fig. 5.12.6   Epididymo-orchitis. US. Four-year-old-boy with acquired urethral stenosis and vas deferens reflux. Swollen heterogeneous testis (T). The limits between testis and surrounding tunica vaginalis are ill defined.

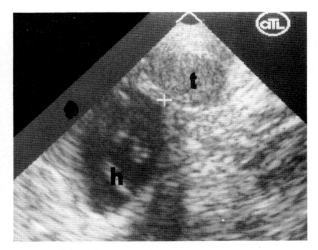

Fig. 5.12.7   Scrotal haematocoele (H), displacing a normal testis (T).

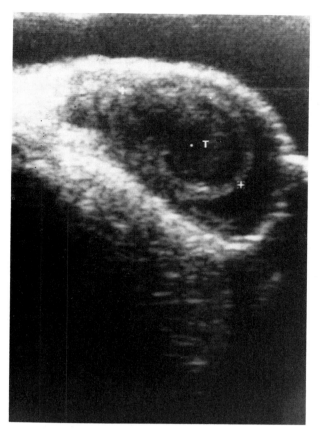

Fig. 5.12.8 Perinatal testicular torsion. Enlarged hypoechoic testis (T). A secondary hydrocoele is present.

VARICOCOELE

Varicocoeles are usually confined to the left side. Sonographically, the diagnosis is easily made by colour Doppler imaging, a method also useful in postoperative assessment. Embolization of the veins by selective catheterization has proved therapeutic. Varicocoele, especially in young children, may be a presenting feature of upper urinary tract tumour and abdominal ultrasound examination should be routinely undertaken.

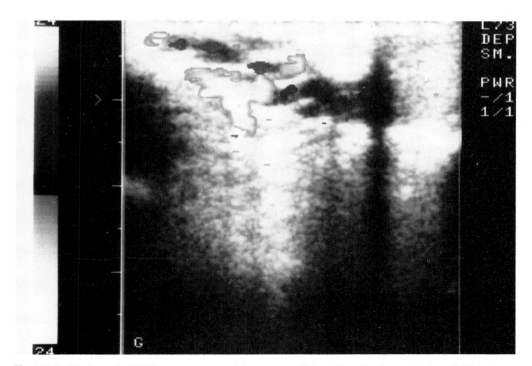

Fig. 5.12.9 Varicocoele. US. Transverse scan of the scrotum. Colour Doppler demonstration of dilated vessels above and around the testis (T).

REFERENCES

Audry G, Tazi M, Brueziere J 1987 Varicocecle chez l'enfant et l'adolescent. Annales de Pediatries 24: 625–628

Bird K, Rosenfield A T 1984 Testicular infarction secondary to acute inflammatory disease: demonstration by B. Scan US. Radiology 152: 785–788

Cunningham J J 1989 Unusual lesions imaged with scrotal US pictorial essay. Urology 34: 316–324

Finkelstein M S, Rosenberg H K, Snyder H M, Duckett J W 1986 US evaluation of scrotum in pediatrics. Urology 27: 1–9

Fritzche P J, Hricak H, Kogan B A et al 1987 Undescended testis: value of MR imaging. Radiology 164: 169–173

Han B K 1986 Uncommon causes of scrotal and inguinal swelling in children: sonographic appearance. Journal of Clinical Ultrasound 14: 421–427

Karp B, Nybonde T 1989 Adnexal hemorrhage versus testicular torsion: a diagnostic dilemma in the neonate. Pediatric Surgery International 4: 337–340

Kenney P J, Spirt B A, Ellis D A, Patil U 1985 Scrotal masses caused by meconium peritonitis: prenatal US diagnosis. Radiology 154: 362

Kogan S J, Gill B, Bennett B, Smey P, Reda E F, Levitt S B 1985 Human normochism: a clinicopathological study of unilateral absent testis in 65 boys. Journal of Urology 135: 758–761

Lupetin A R, King W, Rich P J et al 1983 The traumatized scrotum: US evaluation. Radiology 148: 203–207

Madrazzo B L, Klugo R C, Parts J R et al 1979 US demonstration of undescended testes. Radiology 133: 181–183

Martin B, Tubiana J M 1988 Aspects normaux et pathologiques de la sereuse vaginale en echographie. Annales de Radiologie (Paris) 31: 410–417

Meizner I, Katz M, Zmora E, Insler V 1983 In utero diagnosis of congenital hydrocele. Journal of Clinical Ultrasound 11: 449–450

Mendel J B, Taylor C A, Treves S et al 1985 Testicular torsion in children: scintigraphic assessment. Pediatric Radiology 15: 110–115

Mueller D L, Amundson G M, Rubin S Z, Wesenberg R L 1988 Acute scrotal abnormalities in children: diagnosis by combined sonography and scintigraphy. American Journal of Roentgenology 150: 643–646

Orazi C, Fariello G, Malena S, Caterino S, Ferro F 1989 Torsion of pardidymis of Giraldes Organ: an uncommon cause of acute scrotum in pediatric age group. Journal of Clinical Ultrasound 17: 598–601

Rifkin M D, Kurz A B, Goldberg B B 1984 Epididymitis examined by US. Correlation with pathology. Radiology 151: 187–190

Ring K S, Axelrod S L, Burbige K A, Hensle T W 1989 Meconium hydrocele: an unusual etiology of a scrotal mass in the newborn. Journal of Urology 141: 1172–1173

Rohnik D, Kawanoue S, Szarito P et al 1968 Anatomical incidence of testicular appendages. Journal of Urology 100: 755–756

Schaffer R M 1985 US of scrotal trauma. Urologic Radiology 7: 245–249

Teele R L, Share J C 1981 Scrotal ultrasonography. In Teele R L, Share J C (eds) Ultrasonography of infants and children. Saunders W B, Philadelphia

Thon W F, Gall H, Danz B, Bahren W, Sigmund G 1989 Percutaneous sclerotherapy of idiopathic varicocele in childhood: a preliminary report. Journal of Urology 141: 913–915

5.13   TRAUMA TO THE URINARY TRACT

Road traffic accidents are the commonest cause of urinary tract trauma in children. Iatrogenic damage and sexual abuse are other causes of traumatic haematuria.

The care of children following traffic accidents is initially directed towards stabilizing cardiorespiratory and haemodynamic functions. Imaging procedures should be performed only if the child is clinically stable, and then only when properly monitored in the radiology department.

UPPER URINARY TRACT TRAUMA

Renal injuries occur in 10% of patients who sustain blunt abdominal trauma; 75–80% of these lesions are minor and treated non-surgically. Careful evaluation is of paramount importance and the traumatized urinary tract as well as other organ involvement are best shown by CT.

To save time, the examination is initially performed with IV contrast medium enhancement. A haematoma is the most frequently encountered lesion. Intrarenal haematoma and contusions will appear as hypodense areas with irregular margins (Fig. 5.13.1). These have to be differentiated from a segmental infarct that results from occlusion or laceration of an intrarenal artery; an infarct would have a sharply marginated wedge-shaped appearance. Both lesions may coexist (Fig. 5.13.1).

Perirenal subcapsular haematoma results from haemorrhage confined to the immediate extrarenal space. The fluid collection flattens and displaces the kidney, and appears hypodense after contrast injection (Fig. 5.13.2, Fig. 5.13.3). On unenhanced scans it is hyperdense as compared with normal renal parenchyma. If postcontrast enhancement occurs (on early or late scans), persistent haemorrhage or pelvicalyceal system laceration with urine leakage should be suspected (Fig. 5.13.4).

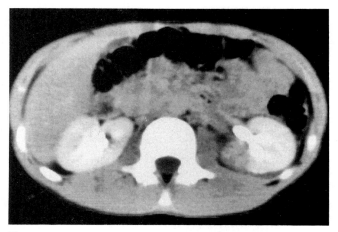

Fig. 5.13.1   Renal contusion and ischaemic lesions. Contrast-enhanced CT. Posterior hypodense parenchyma in the left kidney.

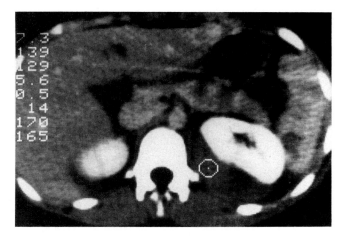

Fig. 5.13.2   Perirenal haematoma. Contrast-enhanced CT. The perirenal collection displaces and flattens the left kidney.

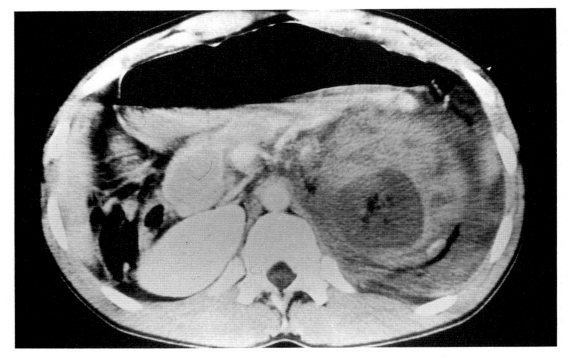

Fig. 5.13.3   Contrast enhanced CT: Note non-function of the left kidney, hyperdense perirenal collection relative to the non-functioning kidney due to persisting haemorrhage and subcapsular splenic haematoma.

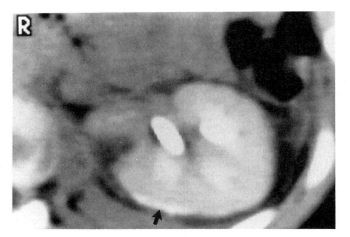

Fig. 5.13.4   Urine leakage in case of renal fracture/laceration. Contrast-enhanced CT. Fracture of renal parenchyma probably extending into the pyelocalyceal system and leading to urine leakage; contrast can be seen posteriorly (arrow).

Large haematomas may become infected or markedly compress the kidney and should be evacuated. Laceration or fracture of the kidney corresponds to more extensive damage (Fig. 5.13.4, Fig. 5.13.5). For a shattered kidney with multiple disrupted fragments and with frequent complications, nephrectomy is preferred but this must not be done until function of the contralateral kidney is confirmed. Ultrasound is not sufficient for this. The question of operative intervention arises also in cases of persistent urine leakage and in cases of serious vascular compromise leading to extensive ischaemic lesions. On enhanced CT, the ischaemic kidney fails to opacify and vascular thrombosis or laceration must be suspected when a rim of perfused parenchyma is seen around a hypodense non-perfused kidney.

Conservative treatment is now preferred in children with minor or moderate trauma. In most cases, there is progressive resolution of a haematoma, although calcification and scars may occur. Evolution is monitored both clinically and with follow-up CT.

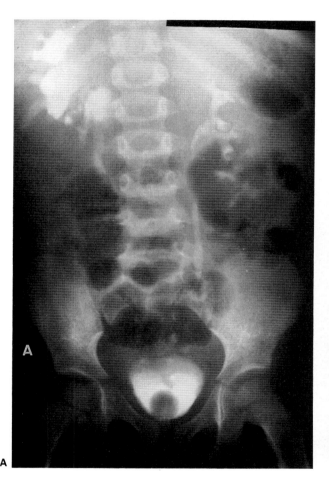

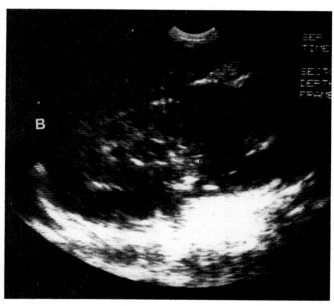

Fig. 5.13.5 A IVU. Note extravasation of contrast around the right kidney and in particular the renal pelvis. **B** Ultrasound. The echofree collection is due to a peripelvic urinoma, due to pelvic laceration.

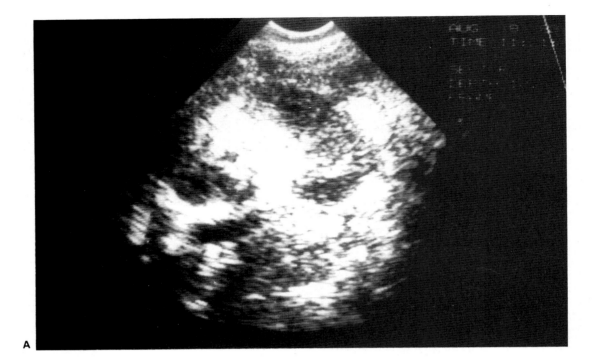

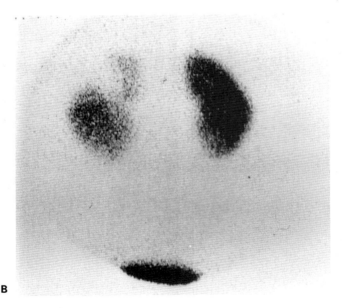

Fig. 5.13.6 US and DMSA scan in a boy with renal contusions. The bright echoes in the kidney indicate an area of haemorrhage. Note the severe impairment of function of the middle and upper pole of the kidney on a DMSA scan, 3 months later.

US may show a renal haematoma and can be performed if CT is not available. However, US underestimates lesions (Fig. 5.13.6) and may be almost normal even in cases of kidney laceration; furthermore, the examination may be difficult because of paralytic ileus and patient discomfort. On US, fresh haematoma appears as an echogenic area within or around the kidney (Fig. 5.13.6, Fig. 5.13.7A).

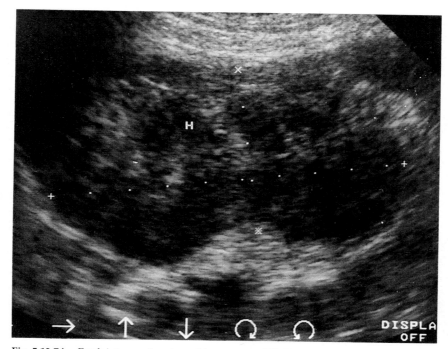

Fig. 5.13.7A Fresh intra- and peri-renal haematoma. US. Prone sagittal scan of the left kidney. Heterogeneous haemorrhage (H) is seen around the kidney (between crosses).

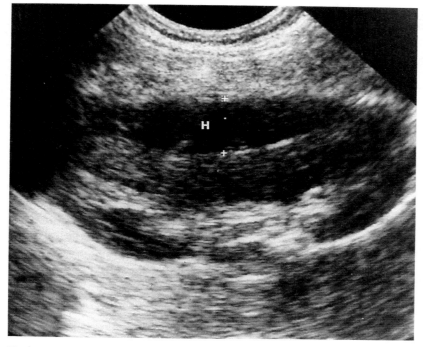

Fig. 5.13.7B Perirenal haematoma. US. Prone sagittal scan of left kidney. Fibrinolysed haematoma (H). Same case as in Figure 5.13.4, 1 month later.

The echogenicity of a haematoma decreases with fibrinolysis (Fig. 5.13.5). US is a useful follow-up technique. An IVU is generally inadequate to evaluate renal trauma but may demonstrate blood clot in the renal pelvis or extravasation (Fig. 5.13.5 and 5.13.8). Function must be confirmed by radionuclide imaging.

About 5% of children admitted to hospital with renal trauma will be found to have underlying renal pathology. CT will demonstrate the pathology along with the haematoma; plain radiographs of the abdomen after contrast medium enhanced CT will provide a urogram and delineate pelvicalyceal anomalies.

Birth trauma is a rare cause of haematuria and an encapsulated perirenal haematoma is best demonstrated with US. It should be differentiated from other neonatal tumours and other causes of haematuria such as renal vein thrombosis.

LOWER URINARY TRACT TRAUMA

To evaluate a patient with lower urinary tract injury associated with skeletal trauma, a plain film of the abdomen including the pelvic girdle should first be obtained. If CT is available this is the preferred next imaging procedure.

Thereafter, a retrograde urethrogram is performed to detect urethral or bladder neck tears. Contrast medium is introduced into the urethra carefully and cautiously under sterile conditions with fluoroscopic control. The bladder and damage to surrounding structures are best visualized with CT, when IV contrast medium and good distension of the bladder are helpful. Extravesical haematoma and pelvic fractures can be evaluated. A plain radiograph of the abdomen following contrast-enhanced CT will help evaluation of the ureters and will show the typical appearance of the compressed bladder, surrounded by the perivesical haematoma and urine leak (Fig. 5.13.9). Urethral strictures are common following complete or partial rupture and are shown on urethrograms, which can be conveniently performed if a suprapubic bladder catheter has been introduced.

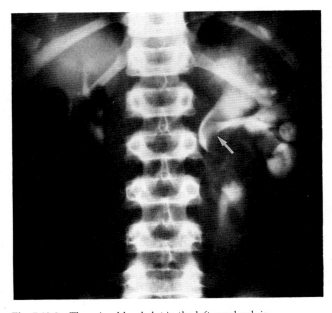

Fig. 5.13.8   There is a blood clot in the left renal pelvis.

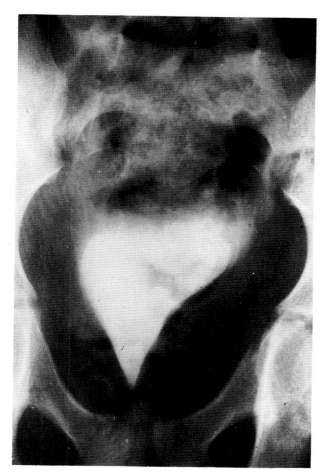

Fig. 5.13.9 Typical appearance of compressed bladder, caused by urine leak from a ruptured bladder neck.

REFERENCES

Eichelberger M R, Randolph J G 1985 Progress in pediatric trauma. World Journal of Surgery 9: 222–235

Fanney D R, Casillas J, Murphy B J 1990 CT in the diagnosis of renal trauma. Radiographics 10: 29–40

Furtzchegger A, Egender G, Jakse G 1988 The value of sonography in the diagnosis and follow-up of patients with blunt renal trauma. British Journal of Urology 62: 110–116

Haller J O, Bass I S, Sclafani S J A 1985 Imaging evaluation of traumatic hematuria in children. Urologic Radiology 7: 211–218

Karp M P, Jewett T C, Kuhn J P et al 1986 The impact of CT on the child with renal trauma. Journal of Pediatric Surgery 21: 617–625

Kaufman R A, Towbin R, Babcock D S et al 1984 Upper abdominal trauma in children. Imaging evaluation. American Journal of Roentgenology 142: 449–460

Merchant W C, Gibbons M D, Gonzales E T 1984 Trauma to the bladder neck, trigone and vagina in children. Journal of Urology 131: 747–750

Newman B, Smith S 1987 Unusual renal mass in a newborn infant. Radiology 163: 193–194

Siegel H J, Balfe D M Blunt renal and ureteral trauma in childhood. CT patterns of fluid collections. American Journal of Roentgenology 152: 1043–1047

5.14 RENAL PARENCHYMAL DISEASE: SYSTEMIC DISEASES WITH RENAL INVOLVEMENT

The role of imaging is to demonstrate the presence and extent of renal involvement. US is the most useful investigation. In many cases, the sonographic appearances are non-specific (Figs 5.14.1, 5.14.2); occasionally the features are characteristic and diagnostic (e.g. recessive polycystic kidney disease).

The abnormalities demonstrated on US are increased echogenicity of the cortex and/or medulla. There may be alteration of corticomedullary differentiation and also abnormalities in renal size.

Hyperechogenicity of the kidneys is assessed by comparison with the adjacent liver and spleen, and may occur in utero (Fig. 5.14.3). It is physiological in premature babies, but abnormal in older children in whom there is a wide differential diagnosis (Table 5.14.1).

The cause of increased echogenicity of the kidneys is multifactorial and includes oedema, inflammation, infection, fibrosis, glomerulosclerosis and hyperfiltration, nephrocalcinosis and cystic tubular dilatation. Hyperechogenicity is usually diffuse but may be localized as in reflux nephropathy. In most cases there is no correlation between the severity of the disease and the level of hyperechogenicity. Alteration of corticomedullary differentiation (Table 5.14.1), age of patient and size of kidneys are also important factors in reaching a differential diagnosis (see Chapter 5.3).

As hyperechogenicity and alteration in corticomedullary differentiation are non-specific features in renal parenchymal disease, the most useful added information is the size of the kidneys. Small, echogenic kidneys indicate chronic disease.

The diagnosis is made on histological examination of a renal biopsy which should be performed with ultrasonic guidance.

Table 5.14.1 Cortical hyperechogenicity

	Corticomedullary differentiation
Normal: newborns and prematures	Present
Glomerular disease	
Nephrotic syndrome	± Present
Glomerulosclerosis and hyperfiltration	Usually present
Haemolytic uraemic syndrome	Present
Acute glomerulonephritis	Present
Tubulointestinal disease	
Acute tubular necrosis	
Toxic	Present
Anoxic/shock kidney	Present
Tamm–Horsfall proteinuria	Reversed
Myoglobinuria	Present
Polycystic kidney disease	
Recessive	
Newborn	Absent
Infantile	Reversed
Dominant (adult)	Variable
Glomerulocystic disease	Absent
Nephronophthisis	Absent
Dysplasia	Present/variable
Storage disease	Present
Sickle cell disease	Present
Biliary atresia	Present
Renal vein thrombosis	
Acute	Absent
Chronic/sequelae	Present
Kawasaki disease	Present
Uric acid deposition	Absent

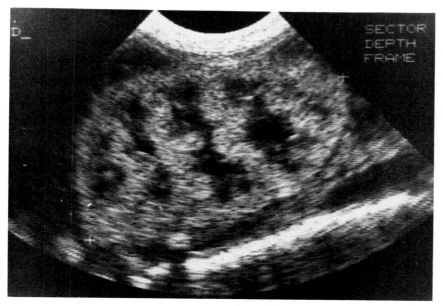

Fig. 5.14.1 Unclassified tubulopathy in a newborn. Sagittal scan of right kidney (between crosses). Increased cortical echogenicity with preserved corticomedullary differentiation. (The parents refused biopsy.)

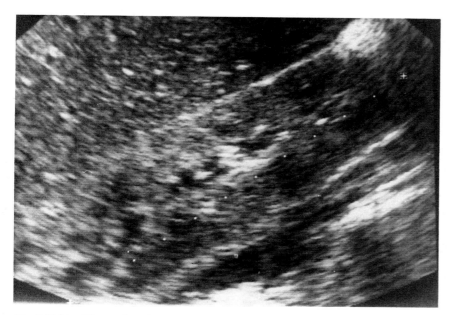

Fig. 5.14.2A Glomerulopathy in a 10-year-old girl. Sagittal scan of right kidney. Sonographic discovery of abnormal kidneys. Hyperechoic cortex – corticomedullary differentiation is partially preserved.

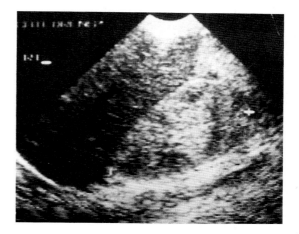

Fig. 5.14.2B Different child with more advanced change. The kidney is now more echogenic than liver and corticomedullary differentiation has disappeared.

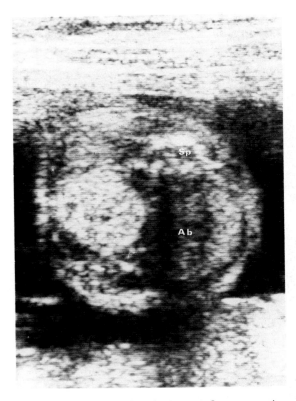

Fig. 5.14.3 Unclassified tubulopathy in utero. Same case as in Figure 5.14.1. Transverse scan of fetal abdomen (Ab). Hyperechogenicity of the kidney is striking. The other kidney was ectopic and pelvic. Sp = fetal spine.

GLOMERULAR DISEASE

Glomerulonephritis

This group of conditions may be primary or associated with Henoch–Schönlein purpura, systemic lupus erythematosis, polyarteritis nodosa or found in syndromes such as Goodpasture's syndrome and Wegener's granulomatosis. The ultrasound findings of renal hyperechogenicity are non-specific.

Nephrotic syndrome

Both kidneys are enlarged, with increased echogenicity and preservation of corticomedullary differentiation. This appearance may be seen in utero. The condition is characterized by marked albuminuria, a low plasma albumin and a high platelet count. Pleural effusions and ascites are common. Renal vein thrombosis secondary to the coagulopathy may occur.

The congenital nephrotic syndrome (Finnish type) also presents with similar sonographic appearances.

Haemolytic uraemic syndrome (HUS)

This condition, which is often preceded by an acute viral or enteropathic bacteria infection and diarrhoea, represents a group of entities in which there is a direct toxic injury to the glomerular capillaries with an associated micro-angiopathy, haemolytic anaemia, thrombocytopenia and acute renal insufficiency.

The kidney may be normal or increased in size. The cortex is hyperechoic with preserved corticomedullary differentiation (Fig. 5.14.4). This is related to calcium and collagen deposition and to some degree of cortical necrosis. As the clinical condition improves, the appearance of the kidney returns to normal. It has been suggested that examination of the kidneys with Doppler US is able to follow improvement in renal function and may be able to distinguish patients with a poor prognosis who will develop chronic renal failure. In the acute phase of the disease, there may be absent or reversed diastolic flow, which returns to normal as the acute vascular lesions heal.

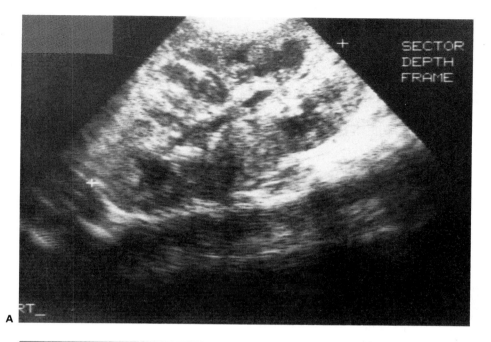

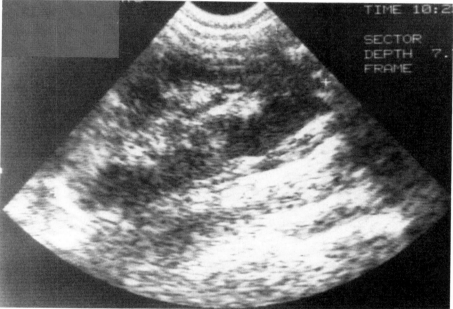

Fig. 5.14.4   Haemolytic uraemic syndrome. Sagittal scans of the kidneys. **A** Acute phase. Cortical hyperechogenicity with increased corticomedullary differentiation. **B** Improvement phase. Normalization of kidney appearance.

Hyperfiltration and glomerulosclerosis

Any condition leading to chronic renal hyperfiltration may induce glomerulosclerosis which will result in parenchymal hyperechogenicity due to dilated tubules with increased interfaces and fibrosis. These changes are seen in patients with decreased amount of renal tissue, whether congenital (as in multicystic dysplastic kidney) or acquired (as in reflux nephropathy or post-nephrectomy). Hyperechogenicity is either diffuse (post-nephrectomy or the contralateral kidney of multicystic kidney, see 5.3 'Cystic disease of the kidney' and 5.4 'Urinary tract dilatation') or localized (as in reflux nephropathy) with a pseudotumoral appearance (Fig. 5.14.5). These changes correspond to what used to be called compensatory hypertrophy.

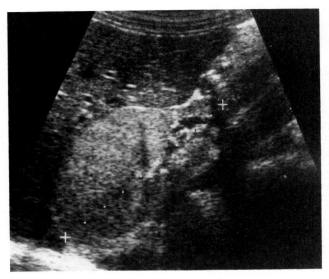

Fig. 5.14.5 Hyperfiltration and glomerulosclerosis. Sagittal scan of the right kidney in a 15-year-old girl with reflux nephropathy. Pseudotumoral appearance of the upper pole – hyperechoic cortex. Corticomedullary differentiation is not well preserved.

TUBULOINTERSTITIAL DISEASES

Tubulointerstitial nephritis

Tubulointerstitial nephritis is a pathological term used to describe an inflammatory process with involvement of the renal tubules and few glomerular alterations. Acute tubulointerstitial nephritis may be due to infections such as streptococcus, but the importance of drugs in the aetiology is being increasingly recognized. These include non-steroidal anti-inflammatory agents, antibiotics and some anticonvulsants. The sonographic changes include increased cortical echogenicity with normal corticomedullary differentiation.

Acute tubular necrosis

Acute ischaemia of the kidney from arterial occlusion may demonstrate a swollen kidney with a blurred corticomedullary junction on US. Doppler examination may be useful in demonstrating absence of flow. Drugs such as aminoglycosides may also result in acute tubular necrosis in which US demonstrates increased cortical echogenicity and normal corticomedullary differentiation.

Acute tubular obstruction due to precipitation of Tamm–Horsfall proteins leads to echogenic pyramids with normal cortex (see 5.17 'Urinary tract diversion and reconstruction').

Sickle cell disease

Renal hyperechogenicity is often seen as an incidental finding in patients with sickle cell disease. Repeated sickling in the papillary blood vessels results in areas of papillary necrosis which may calcify.

Uric acid nephropathy

Crystals of uric acid are deposited in distal tubules and collecting ducts in this condition. Children who are receiving chemotherapy for malignant disease, especially leukaemia and lymphoma, are at risk of uric acid nephropathy. US demonstrates increased parenchymal echogenicity with no distension of the collecting systems.

Hyperechogenicity associated with neoplasia

Hyperechogenicity may be associated with diffuse infiltration of the kidneys with leukaemia and lymphoma. Complications of therapy may also result in hyperechogenicity.

Biliary atresia

Hyperechogenicity in biliary atresia is related to accumulation of biliary salts and dilatation of renal tubules.

Renal cystic diseases

See 5.4 'Urinary tract dilatation'.

Renal shock

See 5.17 'Urinary tract diversion and reconstruction'.

REFERENCES

Alkrinawi S, Gradus D B, Goldstein J, Barki Y 1989 US pattern of congenital nephrotic syndrome of Finnish type. Journal of Clinical Ultrasound 17: 434–444

Avni E F, Van Sinoy H L, Hall M 1989 Hypothesis: reduced renal mass with glomerular hyperfiltration. A cause of renal hyperechogenicity in children. Pediatric Radiology 19: 108–110

Boechat M I, Quesfeld U, Dietrich R B, Cohen A, Kangarloo H, Vargas J 1986 Large echogenic kidneys in biliary atresia. Annales de Radiologie 29: 660–662

Choyke P L, Grant E G, Hoffer F A, Tina L, Korec S 1988 Cortical echogenicity in the hemolytic uremic syndrome: clinical correlation. Journal of Ultrasound in Medicine 7: 439–442

Evans J B, Shapeero L G, Roscelli J D 1988 Infantile glomerulonephritis mimicking polycystic kidney disease. Journal of Ultrasound in Medicine 7: 29–32

Garel L, Habib, Babin C, Lallemand D, Sauvegrain J, Broyer M 1982. Hemolytic uremic syndrome. Diagnostic and prognostic value of US. Annales de Radiologie 26: 169–174

Hayden K C, Santa Cruz F R, Amparo E G, Brouhard B, Swischuk L E, Arendt D K 1984 US evaluation of the renal parenchyma in infancy and childhood. Radiology 152: 413–417

Krensky A M, Reddisch J M, Teele R L 1983 Causes of increased renal echogenicity in pediatric patients. Pediatrics 72: 840–846

Patriquin H B, O'Regan S, Robitaille P, Paltiel H 1989 Haemolytic-uremic syndrome: intrarenal arterial doppler patterns as a useful guide to therapy. Radiology 172: 625–628

5.15   OLIGOANURIA IN THE NEWBORN

Understanding the radiological appearances of the normal and poorly functioning neonatal kidney requires some appreciation of transitional nephrology. This refers both to the adaptation of the fetus to the external environment and the maturation of the kidney. In the infant there is a relatively large extravascular space so that many injected substances which are freely diffusible, such as DTPA, will have a low plasma concentration. The glomerular filtration rate (GFR) is very low at birth (20–40 ml/min/1.73 m^2) and the tubules are even more immature than the glomeruli. These physiological factors explain why intravenous urography in the normal neonate is characterized by poor visualization of the kidneys.

Failure of micturition in the neonate may have prerenal, renal or postrenal causes. Hypoperfusion of the kidneys results in prerenal failure and may be secondary to dehydration, shock, respiratory distress syndrome or chronic heart failure.

Primary renal causes may be congenital, such as renovascular anomalies or absent kidneys. Postrenal failure is commonly caused by obstructive abnormalities. In all cases of renal failure in the newborn, US is the imaging modality of choice, and is particularly useful in distinguishing obstructive from non-obstructive causes.

ISCHAEMIC KIDNEYS, ACUTE TUBULAR NECROSIS

Anoxic damage of the kidneys varies in severity, as do the appearances on ultrasound scanning. Acute tubular necrosis occurs with oedema of the renal tubules and results in increased echogenicity of the renal parenchyma, particularly the medullae, or in milder forms, normal renal echogenicity. In some patients (usually dehydrated or asphyxiated newborns), acute tubular obstruction is due to precipitation of Tamm–Horsfall protein. This results in oliguria and a characteristic sonographic pattern with hyperechoic medullae and reversal of corticomedullary differentiation (Fig. 5.15.1). Depending on the time of the examination, hyperechogenicity of the medullae, may be partial or complete. Tamm–Horsfall proteinuria produces a characteristic persistent nephrogram on an IVU (Fig. 5.15.2). The condition is transitory and the ultrasound appearances and clinical condition return to normal within 1 or 2 days.

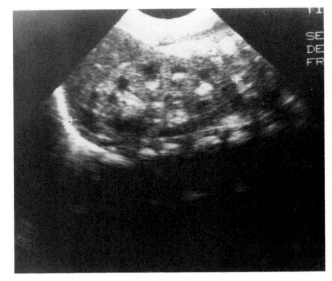

Fig. 5.15.1   Tamm–Horsfall proteinuria in a newborn. US. Sagittal scan of left kidney. Partially hyperechoic medulla with reversed corticomedullary differentiation.

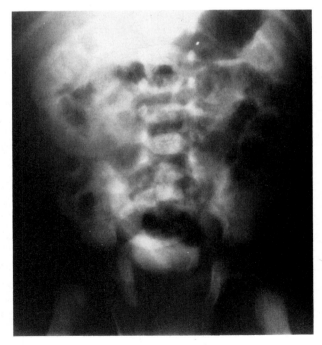

Fig. 5.15.2   Tamm–Horsfall proteinuria. IVU. Delayed nephrogram 2 hours post injection.

If medullary hyperechogenicity persists, other diagnoses should be considered (Table 5.15.1) and other investigations may be helpful.

Table 5.15.1   Hyperechoic medulla

Tamm–Horsfall proteinuria
Nephrocalcinosis
Vesicoureteric reflux
Autosomal recessive polycystic kidney disease
Cacchi–Richi syndrome — medullary sponge kidneys
Beckwith–Wiedemann syndrome
Bartter's syndrome

With more severe ischaemia, acute medullary and acute cortical necrosis may occur. In cortical necrosis, US demonstrates striking hyperechogenicity of the cortex (Fig. 5.15.3A) which, in favourable cases, may be transitory. In severe cases, the changes are irreversible and follow-up sonographic examinations demonstrate a small, shrunken kidney with diffuse, dystrophic cortical calcification (Fig. 5.15.3B). These appearances may also be visible on a plain abdominal radiograph.

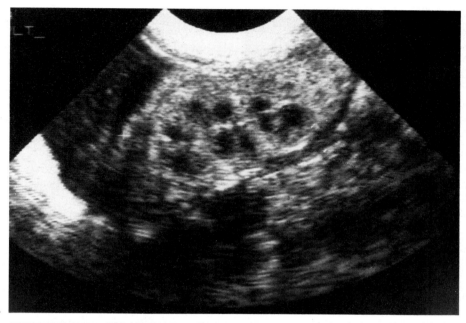

A

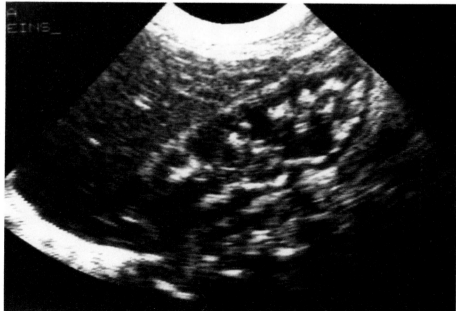

B

Fig. 5.15.3   Shock kidney. Cortical necrosis. US. Premature baby with hyaline membrane disease. Sagittal scan of right kidney. **A** Acute episode. Hyperechoic cortex with preserved corticomedullary differentiation. **B** Follow-up. Shrunken cortex with dystrophic diffuse calcifications.

In acute medullary necrosis, the sonographic changes are non-specific. However, an IVU will demonstrate characteristic changes with contrast-filled cavities in the precalyceal areas (Fig. 5.15.4).

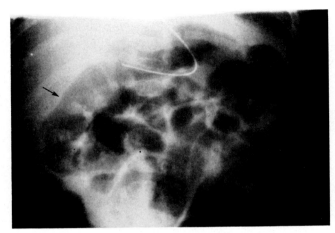

Fig. 5.15.4 Medullary necrosis. IVU. Streaks of contrast within precalyceal areas in the right kidney.

RENOVASCULAR LESIONS

Renal vein thrombosis

Neonatal renal vein thrombosis was thought to be a serious and rare condition, but examination of autopsy material demonstrates an incidence varying from 1 : 150 to 1 : 250. Clinical presentation is variable; classically there is renal insufficiency, a painful flank mass and haematuria. However, the condition may be asymptomatic. This is related to the extent and rapidity of thrombus formation and the development of collateral circulation. In the neonate the aetiology is multifactorial and includes dehydration, decreased renal perfusion and a high haematocrit. Renal vein thrombosis may occur in utero, may be unilateral or bilateral, and is more common in infants of diabetic mothers. It is often associated with adrenal haemorrhage.

The sonographic appearances are variable and reflect the presence of haemorrhage, oedema and ischaemia. Hyperechoic perilobar and interlobar streaks are said to be specific. In the acute phase these changes are associated with swelling of the kidney and loss of corticomedullary differentiation, and probably correspond to oedema and haemorrhage at the level of the interlobar vessels (Fig. 5.15.5). These changes are transitory and reversible, and follow-up US will demonstrate a return to normal appearances.

The chronic changes seen if the kidneys do not return to normal also include characteristic hyperechoic streaks, typically around the pyramids, which represent dystrophic calcification secondary to haemorrhage (Fig. 5.15.6). This is not associated with renal enlargement and corticomedullary differentiation is preserved. These changes are permanent and may be seen on a plain abdominal radiograph as patchy calcification.

Sometimes thrombus can be demonstrated in the inferior vena cava. Colour flow Doppler imaging is potentially helpful in demonstrating abnormal renal blood flow. Duplex Doppler is technically difficult in neonates but may demonstrate increased vascular resistance with a raised resistive index in renal vein thrombosis.

Intravenous urography is unhelpful, as the affected kidney is often non-functioning. In cases of chronic sequelae following renal vein thrombosis, DMSA scans are useful in demonstrating loss of renal function.

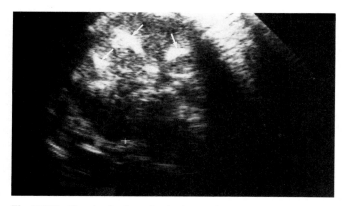

Fig. 5.15.5 Renal vein thrombosis. Acute phase. Newborn baby boy. Transverse scan of right kidney. Massively swollen kidney; corticomedullary differentiation is lost. Hyperechoic streaks (arrows) probably corresponding to haemorrhage around the interlobar vessels.

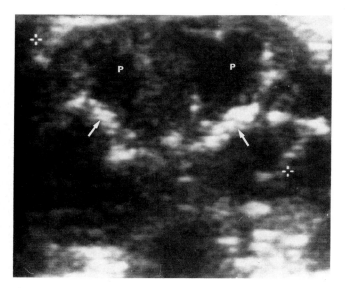

Fig. 5.15.6 Renal vein thrombosis. Sequelae of a perinatal episode. Sagittal scan of left kidney. Dystrophic hyperechogenicity (calcifications) in the interlobar areas (arrows). Asymptomatic newborn baby boy. A calcified thrombosis was also present in the inferior vena cava. P = pyramids.

Renal artery thrombosis

Aortic thrombosis and renal artery thrombosis may occur in the neonate and are related to aortic and umbilical artery catheterization. Unexplained hypertension with normal renal appearances on US should suggest renal artery thrombosis. Doppler US will demonstrate absence of arterial flow in the kidney. Rarely, echogenic blood clot is seen. The diagnosis may be confirmed with a DTPA or MAG3 isotope scan, and angiography. MR scanning may be able to demonstrate the occluded vessel and the absence of blood flow.

REFERENCES

Avni E F, Spehl M, Lebrun D, Gomes H, Garel L 1983 Transient acute tubular disease in the newborn characteristic US pattern. Annales de Radiologie (Paris) 26: 175–182

Chevalier R L, Campbell F, Brenbridge A N A G 1984 Prognostic factors in neonatal acute renal failure. Pediatrics 74: 265–272

Clark R L, Klein S 1983 Renal arcuate veins: new microangiographic observations. American Journal of Roentgenology 141: 755–759

Feld L G, Springate J E, Fildes R D 1986 Acute renal failure: pathophysiology and diagnosis. Journal of Pediatrics 109: 401–408

Keating M A, Althausen F F 1985 The clinical spectrum of renal vein thrombosis. Journal of Urology 133: 945–988

Koch K J, Cory D A 1986 Simultaneous RVT and bilateral adrenal hemorrhage MR demonstration. Journal of Computer Assisted Tomography 10: 681–683

Kozlowski K, Brown R W 1978 Renal medullary necrosis in infants and children. Pediatric Radiology 7: 85–89

Lalmand B, Avni E F, Nasr A, Ketelbant P, Struyven J 1993 Perinatal renal vein thrombosis: US demonstration. Journal of Ultrasound in Medicine (in press)

Marchal G, Verbeken E, Oyen R, Noeman F, Baert A L, Lauwerijns J 1986 US of the normal kidney. Ultrasound in Medicine and Biology 12: 999–1009

McDonald P, Tarar R, Gilday D, Reilly B J 1974 Some radiologic observations in renal vein thrombosis. Radiology 120: 369–387

Metreweli C, Pearson R 1984 Echographic diagnosis of renal vein thrombosis. Pediatric Radiology 14: 105–108

Paling M R, Wakefield J A, Watson L R 1985 Sonography of experimental acute renal vein occlusion. Journal of Clinical Ultrasound 13: 647–653

Sanders L D, Jacquier S 1989 Ultrasound demonstration of prenatal renal vein thrombosis. Pediatric Radiology 19: 133–135

Seibert J J, Lindley S G, Corbitt S S, Seibert R W, Arnold W C 1986 Clot formation in the renal artery in the neonate demonstrated by US. Journal of Clinical Ultrasound 14: 470–473

Spies J B, Hricak H, Stemmer T M et al 1984 Sonographic evaluation of experimental acute renal arterial occlusion in dogs. American Journal of Roentgenology 142: 341–346

Sty J R, Starshak R J, Hubbard A M 1983 Acute renal cortical necrosis in hemolytic uremic syndrome. Journal of Clinical Ultrasound 11: 175–178

As more children with chronic renal disease are surviving, renal transplantation is becoming increasingly common in infants and young children.

Imaging forms part of the pretransplantation investigation and is also important in the diagnosis of rejection and other complications following the transplant.

Pre-transplant imaging

In most cases imaging of the kidney prior to transplantation consists of a follow-up ultrasound of chronic renal parenchymal disease. Rarely a patient presents in renal failure, and imaging is required to establish the cause of the renal failure. It is important to image the diseased, native kidneys for a number of reasons. In some cases such as hydronephrosis, previous chronic infection, hypertension and massive proteinuria, nephrectomy prior to transplantation is performed. Some renal diseases may recur in transplanted kidneys; these include oxalosis, Henoch–Schönlein purpura and some of the glomerulonephritides.

Imaging is also required to evaluate the patient's bladder and urethra, and is particularly important when the cause of renal failure is associated with a neuropathic bladder and an MCUG and videourodynamics may be required.

Post-transplant imaging

An important role of imaging the renal transplant is to determine the cause of malfunction of the transplant kidney and assess which cases need further investigation with a renal biopsy. Radionuclide imaging with flow studies and US with Doppler are the most frequently performed and most useful studies in the follow-up of renal transplants.

An early baseline study should be performed after surgery and subsequent imaging should follow an established protocol with consistency of technique so that studies may be compared, enabling small changes to be detected. Blood flow studies with ^{99m}Tc-DTPA or MAG3 enable assessment of perfusion and function of the transplant. Sonographically, changes in renal volume, corticomedullary differentiation, hydronephrosis and the Doppler characteristics of blood flow are important indicators of pathology (Fig. 5.16.1). More specific complications of transplantation such as renal artery stenosis and unusual fluid collections may require angiography and CT scanning.

EARLY POST-TRANSPLANT STUDIES (less than 15 days postoperatively)

In cases of deterioration in renal function or clinical condition of the patient, US is initially important to differentiate obstructive from non-obstructive causes. When hydronephrosis is present further investigation of the pelvicalyceal system and ureter is necessary (see 'Urological complications' below).

In other cases, acute rejection of the transplant should be considered and must be distinguished from other causes of transplant dysfunction. Rejection may be primarily vascular, cellular (interstitial) or commonly mixed, both vascular and cellular. Sonographic examination may demonstrate an increase in renal volume due to oedema, reduction or absence of echoes from the central sinus fat and altered echogenicity (increased or mottled) of the parenchyma (Fig. 5.16.2). However, it is recognized that the sonographic appearance of the kidney can be normal in the presence of proven rejection. The role of Doppler US is important in the diagnosis, particularly in the presence of predominantly vascular rejection. Colour Doppler is used to demonstrate arterial and venous flow and also to point to specific vessels for sampling with duplex sonography. Examination of the waveform of the intrarenal arteries in rejection will demonstrate decreased forward velocity of diastolic flow, and measurements such as the resistive index (RI) or Pourcelot index (PI) may be used to detect subtle changes indicating early rejection. The patient is his or her best control subject and a sudden or sustained gradual change in measurements is suggestive of rejection. The normal RI is approximately 0.50, and the upper limit of normal is 0.75 (or 75%), the upper limit of normal for the pulsatility index is 1.8; any measurements above these indicate pathology. A high RI is not specific for acute rejection and is also found in renal vein obstruction and acute tubular necrosis.

Doppler sonography is also useful in the examination of the blood supply to the transplant and in the diagnosis of acute renal artery or vein thrombosis. Digital angiography may be needed to confirm these findings or to demonstrate the extent of renal infarction.

Radionuclide imaging allows quantitative assessment of the perfusion and the function of the transplanted kidney. This allows early detection of failure of graft perfusion rejection and recovery from acute tubular necrosis. In acute rejection the features on the ^{99m}Tc-DTPA scan are deterioration in renal perfusion,

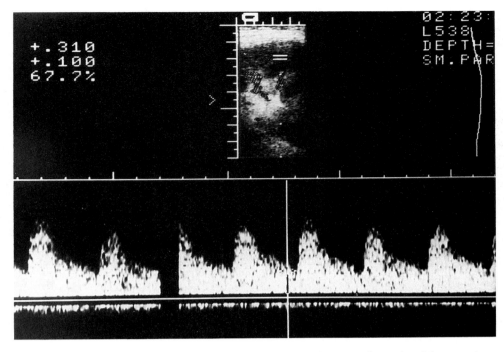

Fig. 5.16.1 Normal Doppler study. The sample volume analysed is situated in an interlobar vessel. RI is 68%.

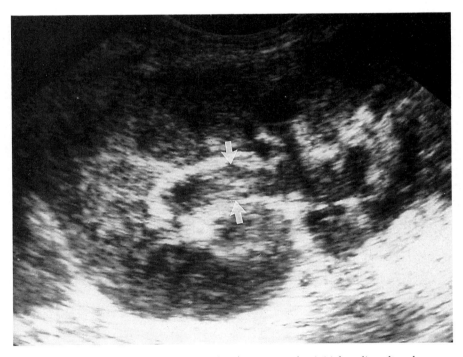

Fig. 5.16.2 Acute rejection. US. Swollen kidney as compared to initial studies; altered echogenicity. Thickened renal pelvis wall (arrows).

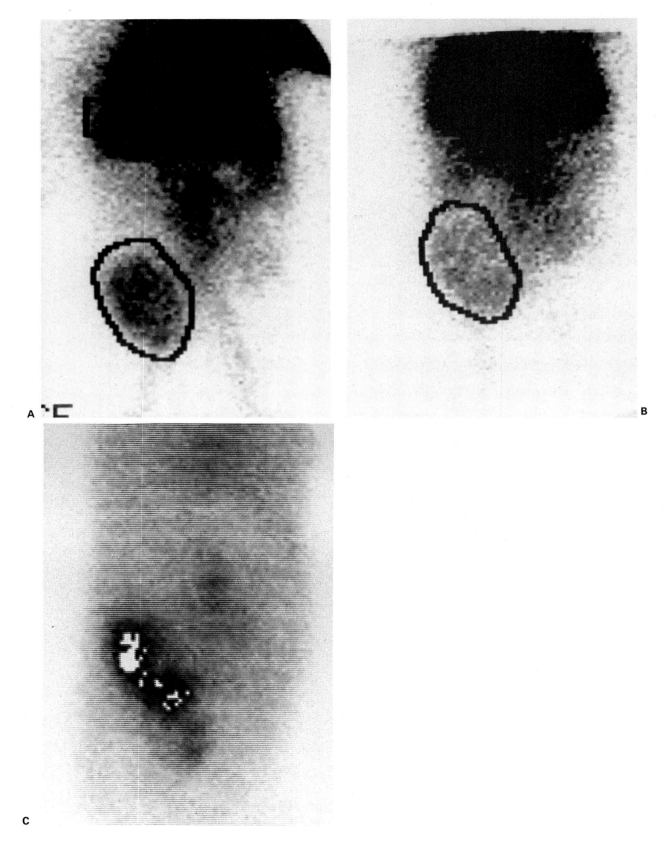

Fig. 5.16.3 DTPA scan in a patient. **A** Day 1 postoperatively showing good perfusion of the transplant kidney. **B** Day 5 postoperatively showing markedly reduced perfusion of the transplant kidney. **C** Day 5 postoperatively, 20-minute images showing very poor excretion of isotope.

decreased uptake of DTPA and decreased excretion of tracer (Fig. 5.16.3). In acute tubular necrosis, perfusion is maintained although excretion of tracer and decreased uptake of DTPA is seen. Serial nuclear medicine studies are probably the best method for distinguishing acute rejection from acute tubular necrosis.

Recently, MRI has been shown to demonstrate specific features of acute rejection on T_1-weighted images with disappearace of corticomedullary differentiation. However, it is not a first line investigation in the early post-transplant period.

Renal biopsy and cytology are still important in difficult cases, and remain the definitive standard.

LATE POST-TRANSPLANT STUDIES (more than 15 days postoperatively)

Obstruction must be excluded as a cause of deteriorating renal function and an ultrasound examination is essential.

Acute rejection can occur and must be differentiated from cyclosporin toxicity and unusual infections. Using Doppler US and isotope studies it is difficult to distinguish rejection from cyclosporin toxicity, although the deterioration in renal perfusion may be more marked in the former.

There is a high incidence of renal artery stenosis following transplantation in children. Doppler imaging may demonstrate arterial narrowing, but the findings are confirmed by angiography. Angioplasty may be successful in widening the stenosis. Pseudoaneurysms may occur within the kidney following biopsy and are seen as an echolucent area with abnormal Doppler signal within the kidney.

UROLOGICAL COMPLICATIONS

The rate of complications is greater in children than in adults. The main complication is obstruction. Hydronephrosis may be secondary to an abnormal surgical anastomosis or oedema of the transplant compressing the ureter in the early postoperative period. Later, ischaemia and rejection with fibrosis at the anastomosis may occur. An initial US, followed by an antegrade study, will demonstrate the abnormality (Fig. 5.16.4A). Percutaneous nephrostomy and balloon dilatation of any stricture under US and fluoroscopic guidance may treat this complication (Fig. 5.16.4B).

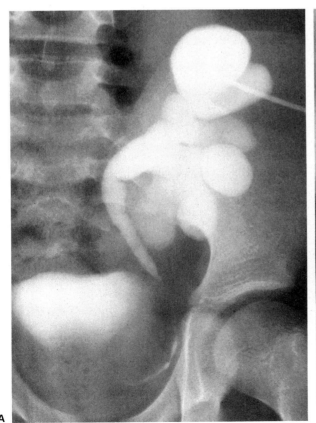
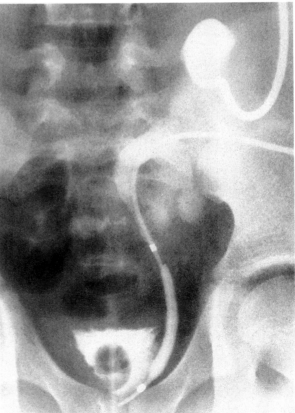

A   **B**

Fig. 5.16.4 Ureteral stenosis. **A** Diagnostic procedure. Opacification through nephrostomy tube. Stenosis of lower ureter. **B** Therapeutic procedure. Balloon dilatation.

Urinomas secondary to leakage at the anastomosis or to obstruction may occur.

Lymphocoele, haemorrhage (sometimes post biopsy) and abscess formation also occur and are detected with US. CT may also be useful in delineating complicated collections of lymph. These can be treated with percutaneous drainage with ultrasound guidance, and a nephrostomy may also be inserted in order to decrease pressure in the renal pelvis.

REFERENCES

Allen K S, Jorkasky D K, Arger P H et al 1988 Renal allografts: prospective analysis of Doppler sonography. Radiology 169: 371–376

Argyropoulou M, Brunelle F 1990 Apport du Doppler pulse dans la transplantation renale. Annales de Pediatrie 37: 177–119

Birnholz J C, Merkel F K 1985 Fibromucosal edema of the collecting system: a new ultrasonic sign of severe, acute renal allograft rejection. Radiology 154: 190

Brunelle F, Gagnadoux M F 1990 Traitement par angioplastie transluminale des stenoses arterielles du rein transplante chez l'enfant. Annales de Pediatrie 37: 99–102

Cochlin D L, Wake A, Salaman J R, Griffin P J A 1988 US changes in the transplant kidney. Clinical Radiology 39: 373–376

Dubosky E V, Russel C D 1988 Radionuclide evaluation of renal transplants. Seminars in Nuclear Medicine 18: 181–198

Genkins S M, Ganfihippö F P, Caroll B A 1989 Duplex doppler sonography of renal transplants: lack of sensitivity and specificity in establishing pathologic diagnosis. American Journal of Roentgenology 152: 535–540

Haddick W, Filly R A, Backman U et al 1986 Renal allograft rejection: US evaluation. Radiology 161: 469–473

Hall J R, Kim E E, Pjura G A, Maklad N F, Sandler C M, Verati R 1988 Correlation of radionuclide and US studies with biopsy findings for diagnosis of renal transplant rejection. Urology 32: 172–179

Lear J R, Raff U, Jain R, Horgan J G 1988 Quantitative measurement of renal perfusion following transplant surgery. Journal of Nuclear Medicine 29: 1656–1661

Letourneau J G, Day D L, Ascher N L, Castaneda Zuniga W R 1988 Imaging of renal transplants (perspective). American Journal of Roentgenology 150: 833–838

Pollak R, Verenis S A, Maddux M S, Mozes M F 1988 The natural history of and therapy for perirenal fluid collections following renal transplantation. Journal of Urology 140: 716–720

Renther G, Waujusra D, Bauer H 1989 Acute renal vein thrombosis in renal allografts: detection with duplex doppler US. Radiology 70: 557–558

Slovis T L, Babcock D S, Hricak H et al 1984 Renal transplantation rejection: sonographic evaluation in children. Radiology 153: 659–665

Smith T P, Hunter D W, Letourneau G G et al 1988 Urine leaks after renal transplantation: value of percutaneous pyelography and drainage for diagnosis and treatment. American Journal of Roentgenology 151: 511–514

Thomsen H S, Nielsen S L 1989 Imaging in renal transplantation. Current Opinion in Radiology 1: 297–305

Wrisett H, Amparo E G, Fawcett H D et al 1988 Renal transplant dysfunction MR evaluation. American Journal of Roentgenology 150: 319–323

5.17 URINARY TRACT DIVERSION AND RECONSTRUCTION

URINARY TRACT DIVERSION

For many years (up to the early 1970s), an ileal conduit was the standard method of supravesical urinary diversion. With better methods for emptying the bladder and improved surgery for severe reflux and bladder exstrophy, this has become obsolete.

Nevertheless, those children with ileal conduit diversion need continuous follow-up studies. Yearly US preferably, or IVU, are necessary to detect secondary dilatation and calculus formation. Complications include obstruction (at the ileal stoma, within the ileal loop, at the ileo-ureteric anastomosis or at the level of passage through the mesentery of the ureter), urine leakage, and urine stasis with secondary infection or stones. Renal failure is uncommon.

Introduction of water-soluble contrast medium into the loop with a Foley ballon catheter within the stoma (loopogram) may be necessary to show the ileal loop and any stenosis (Fig. 5.17.1). Reflux is virtually always present and results in the presence of air bubbles within the pelvicalyceal system.

Colon conduit was an alternative to ileal conduit, with the advantage of a possible antireflux anastomosis.

Ureterosigmoidostomies were used in bladder exstrophy and more severe cloacal anomalies, when the ureters were connected to the sigmoid in an antireflux manner. Reflux and obstruction secondary to stricture or inflammatory polyps at the site of anastomosis are important complications, for the detection of which periodic US or IVU are necessary. Furthermore, young patients with ureterosigmoidostomy are at risk of developing adenocarcinoma of the sigmoid about 10 years after surgery. This has led to virtual abandonment of this operation. Cutaneous ureterostomies were once used to divert a markedly abnormal urinary tract (Fig. 5.17.2). Following reconstruction the ureters may run an unusual angulated lateral course which should not cause obstruction. Recently, percutaneous bladder catheterization through an appendicovesicostomy (Mitrofanoff) has been developed for neuropathic and other bladders with chronic outlet obstruction.

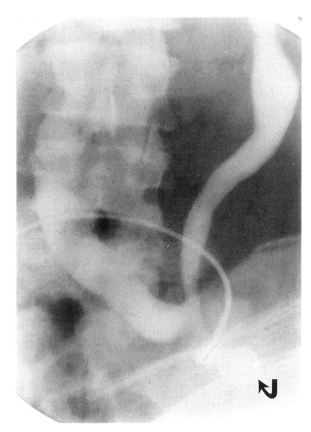

Fig. 5.17.1   Loopogram. Opacification of the ileal conduit and both ureters through the stoma (arrow).

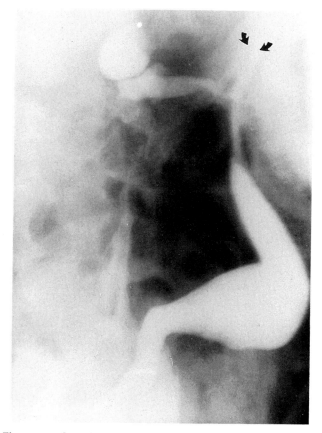

Fig. 5.17.2   Opacification through cutaneous ureterostomies (arrows). Case of prune belly syndrome.

URINARY TRACT RECONSTRUCTION

Reconstruction of the urinary tract may be achieved by ureter-to-ureter or ureter-to-bladder anastomosis. If necessary, the bladder can be brought closer to the ureter either by the Boari flap technique (a flap of the bladder is partially excised and interposed between the bladder and ureter) or by the psoas hitch technique (the elongated bladder is attached to psoas). Reflux is a possible complication of the technique.

BLADDER AUGMENTATION

Bladder augmentation may be necessary in patients requiring urinary tract diversion or reconstruction, and in those with small and non-compliant bladders, e.g. bladder exstrophy, neuropathic bladder. A segment of ileum, colon or stomach may be used (Fig. 5.17.3), or the bladder may be opened and refashioned to form a cystoplasty. The augmented bladder has a characteristic shape on MCUG and US. Following augmentation, intermittent catheterization may be required to empty the bladder; the efficacy of this technique can be monitored with pre- and post-catheterization ultrasound examinations. With colonic augmentations echogenic debris, corresponding to mucus secreted by the bowel, is seen in the bladder (Fig. 5.17.4).

Artificial sphincters may also be required in children with neurogenic bladders, to control wetting. Each sphincter has a different appearance. The reservoirs are filled with contrast when inserted so that any disruption is easily detected with plain radiographs.

REFERENCES

Aaronson I A, Morgan T C 1979 Ureterosigmoidostomy in childhood: the quality of life. Journal of Pediatric Surgery 14: 74–76

Amis E S, Pfister R C, Hendren W H 1981 The radiology of undiversion. Urologic Radiology 3: 161–169

Hanna M K, Shoengold S, Vy C, Heiliczer J D, Arboit J, Fine B P 1983 The results of urinary undiversion in children. Urology 21: 123–126

Lebowitz R L 1981 Post-operative uroradiology. Appleton-Century-Crofts, New York

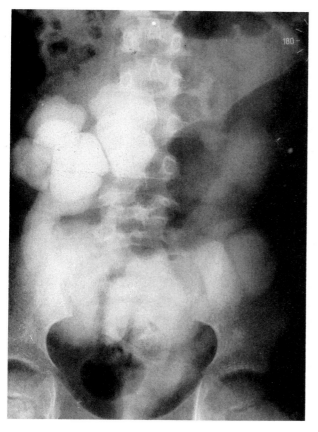

Fig. 5.17.3 Bladder augmentation with segment of colon. IVU.
Case of pelvic fused kidneys in an 8-year-old child. Multiple
previous surgical procedures.

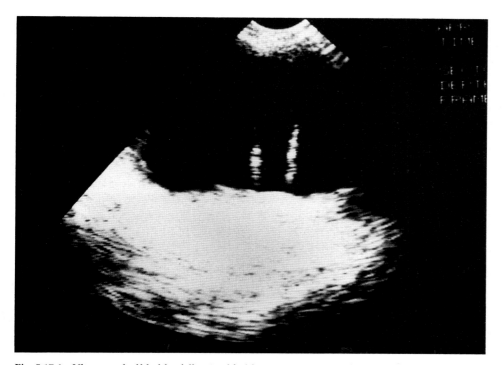

Fig. 5.17.4 Ultrasound of bladder following bladder augmentation with bowel. Note echogenic mucus
streaks.

Gynaecology and intersex

E. Phelan

INTRODUCTION

Imaging of the paediatric genital tract has been revolutionized by ultrasound (US) which is the most sensitive and non-invasive means of assessing the female pelvis. After a plain abdominal and chest radiograph when indicated, US is the first and often the only imaging carried out. US also makes an excellent assessment of the upper urinary tracts for dilatation and congenital anomalies, obviating the need for urography. Studies should be of high quality and performed by a radiologist familiar with paediatric pathology.

The indications for US are, abdominal pain, an abdominal mass, precocious puberty or amenorrhoea. In the infant and child high frequency 5 MHz and 7.5 MHz transducers are required for good quality imaging.

US should always be performed prior to any planned invasive study, e.g. MCU. In children under 3 years a 3 hour fast is recommended. The child may then be fed during the examination. Sedation is rarely required but where necessary the fasting patient may be given chloral hydrate, 50 mg/kg, orally. Examination of the abdomen is best carried out by examining the pelvis first, particularly in an infant, and by exposing only that part of the abdomen required for imaging. If the bladder is not full pelvic ultrasound may be difficult. However, the bladder will fill in the course of an examination and catheterization using a 5 or 6 F (neonate) or 8 F feeding tube is rarely required.

The ovary in the prepubertal female is ovoid in shape. At least one ovary can be visualized in 80% of females under 5 years and in 95% over 5 years. Normal ovarian volume is less than 1 cm^3 in prepubertal children and no larger than 6 cm^3 in the postpubertal child. The volume (V) is calculated using the formula for a modified prolate ellipse, $L \times W \times D/2$, where the length (L) and thickness (D) are measured in the sagittal section, the lines intersecting at 90 degrees to each other. The width (W) of the ovary is measured in transverse plane.

The uterus can be visualized in 90% of female neonates and has a mean length of 3.4 cm. In the neonatal period small amounts of fluid may be seen in the uterine cavity due to maternal stimulation with oestrogen. This should not be confused with larger collections of fluid due to hydrocolpos. After 1 month the uterus is 2.6–2.8 cm long. The cervix is large relative to the uterus representing two-thirds of the total uterine length. The uterus does not alter in size until age 6–8 years when it undergoes a gradual increase in size until puberty when it reaches 5–8 cm in length, 1.5–3 cm in AP diameter and 3–5 cm in width.

Other methods of investigation may be required for specific abnormalities, e.g. MCU and genitography in patients with cloacal or urogenital sinus anomalies, or intersex disorders. Computed tomography (CT) is also employed in the assessment of abdominal masses, although the same information can be obtained with a careful ultrasound study without the need for intravenous and oral contrast and ionizing radiation and, occasionally, general anaesthesia. Magnetic resonance imaging (MRI) provides excellent cross-sectional anatomical images of the abdomen. It has the advantage of being non-irradiating, and the ability to present images in several planes and in three dimensions will be valuable particularly for surgical planning.

REFERENCES

Nussbaum A R, Sanders R C, Jones M D 1986 Neonatal uterine morphology as seen on real-time US. Radiology 160: 641–643

Salardi S, Orsini L F, Cacciari E, Bovicelli L, Tassoni P, Reggiani A 1985 Pelvic ultrasonography in premenarchal girls: relation to puberty and sex hormone concentrations. Archives of Disease in Childhood 60: 120–125

CONGENITAL ANOMALIES

Congenital anomalies of the female genital tract result from müllerian duct abnormalities and/or abnormalities of the urogenital sinus or cloaca. Failure of fusion of the müllerian ducts results in a wide variety of fusion abnormalities of the uterus, cervix and upper vagina, ranging from bicornuate uterus to complete duplication of the uterus, cervix and vagina (Fig. 6.1). Müllerian duct abnormalities may occur alone or in association with urogenital sinus or cloacal abnormali-ties. Persistence of the cloaca results from failure of the urorectal septum (which divides into the dorsal anal membrane and ventral urogenital membrane) to fuse with the cloacal membrane at the end of the sixth gestational week. When fusion fails there is a common opening onto the perineum which serves as the outlet for urine, genital secretions and for faeces and meconium. Cloacal anomalies are seen in 1 in 40 000 to 50 000 newborns and are seen exclusively in pheno-typic females.

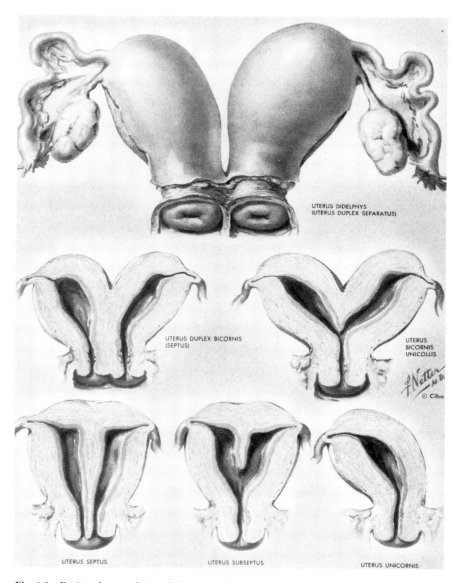

Fig. 6.1 Fusion abnormalities of the uterus. (With permission CIBA collection).

Persistence of the urogenital sinus (Fig. 6.2) results from incomplete development of the lower vagina resulting in drainage of urine and vaginal secretions into a common perineal orifice. It is seen alone, in association with a cloacal defect, and may also be seen in patients with intersex disorders. A fistula may be present between the rectum and the genital tract, usually communicating with the vagina or vestibule. The configuration of the types of urogenital sinus and cloacal anomalies and their development are shown in Figure 6.3.

Jaramillo classifies cloacal abnormalities on imaging studies according to the cloacal configuration (urethral, vaginal), the type of urinary–cloacal communication (urethral, vesical), and the level of rectal communication (vaginal, cloacal, vesical or other). The cloacal configuration is catagorized as urethral when there is a narrow, long and curved cloaca which tends to be a continuation of the urethra. The cloacal orifice is usually small. The vaginal configuration tends to have a wider more straight cloaca which is usually a continuation of the vagina. These two configurations have an approximately equal incidence. The urinary–cloacal communication is urethral in the majority of patients (77%). These patients have a well-formed urethra with a good sphincter. In patients with a vesical–cloacal communication the urethra is absent and there is direct communication between the bladder and the cloaca.

The level of rectal communication is at the vagina in most patients (68%). In the remaining patients it may be at the level of the cloaca. When the rectum communicates with the vagina it is at the level of the lower vagina, or, when there is vaginal duplication, at the level of the vaginal septum. Rarely the rectum may communicate higher in the vagina or with the anterior wall. The rectum may also open directly onto the perineum through an anteriorly placed anus.

The radiological investigation of urogenital sinus and cloacal anomalies centres on the accurate delineation of the anatomy of the anomaly for surgical planning, and also on the demonstration of associated anomalies, both genitourinary and of other organ systems. Associated anomalies of particular importance are anomalies of the uterus which include duplication of the uterus, vagina or both, uterine aplasia or vaginal atresia or stenosis. All patients with a cloacal anomaly will have some form of uterine or vaginal anomaly.

Contrast studies of the urogenital sinus and cloaca are best performed by placing the patient in the lateral or steep oblique position. An inflated balloon catheter is placed at the opening of the perineal orifice with the ballon resting on the perineal surface providing a seal for the injection of water-soluble contrast into the orifice. Using this technique the whole urogenital sinus or cloaca can be opacified often with retrograde

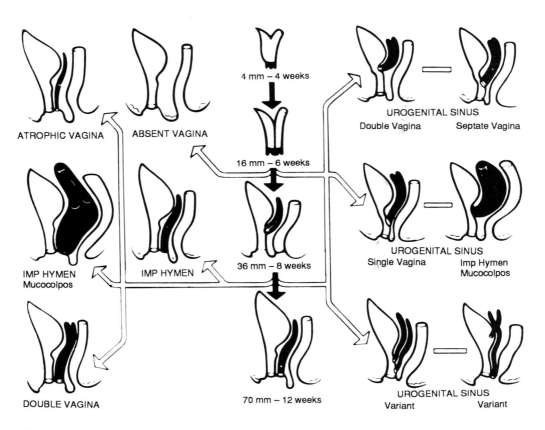

Fig. 6.2 Various configurations of the urogenital sinus.

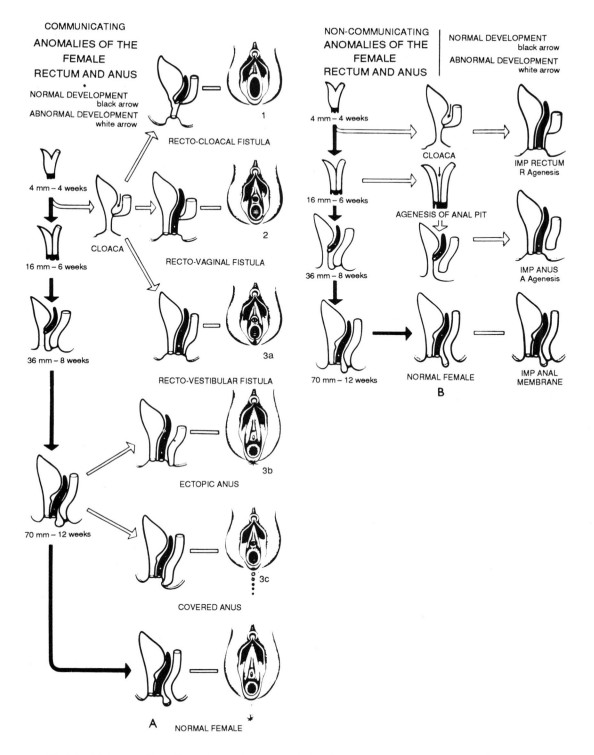

Fig. 6.3 Various configurations of cloacal anomalies in females.
(With permission Lippincott Co.).

filling of the vagina and uterus and in the case of cloacal anomalies, the rectum. Depending on the configuration of the bladder it may fill using this technique; however separate catheterization and filming during micturition will often provide additional information on the level of communication of the bladder, vagina and rectum. It is also important to obtain micturating films, as 60% of patients with cloacal abnormalities have vesicoureteric reflux. A catheter may preferentially pass into the rectum through a rectovaginal, rectocloacal or rectovesical fistula, in which case the lower rectum will be opacified and the communication with the cloaca shown. If the communication with the rectum is small it may not fill retrogradely and the only means of demonstrating a fistula from the rectum may be from filling of the rectum from above if a defunctioning colostomy has been performed.

MRI elegantly displays the anatomy of the urogenital and cloacal anomalies, particularly using sagittal T_1-weighted images. In addition to demonstrating the uterus and vagina it also demonstrates any congenital anomalies such as vaginal obstruction. The gonads can also be imaged in the pelvis or inguinal canal. This may be particularly useful for the location of intra-abdominal gonads, as these are usually too small to be loated by US in the neonatal period. Streak gonads have been successfully imaged in this way with MRI. Gradual enlargement of the gonads, or the presence of a mass in a patient in whom streak gonads would be expected such as gonadal dysgenesis should raise the possibility of malignancy.

The upper urinary tract should be examined using US for congenital renal anomalies such as horseshoe kidney, renal dysplasia, unilateral renal agenesis and ectopic ureters. Non-genitourinary anomalies include oesophageal atresia, congenital heart disease and vertebral anomalies. The high incidence of spinal cord abnormalities in infants with imperforate anus and cloacal anomalies has led to the recommendation that all infants should have spine US in the neonatal period to look for cord tethering and other dysraphic abnormalities. The presence of a spinal cord abnormality does not correlate with the presence of vertebral anomalies on plain film. Older children should be examined with MRI.

Genital tract obstruction

Two-thirds of patients with genital tract obstruction have an imperforate hymen. Until late fetal life the lumen of the vagina is separated from the cavity of the urogenital sinus by the hymen which forms the junction between the müllerian duct-derived upper vagina and the lower vagina derived from the urogenital sinus. The hymen usually ruptures in the perinatal period and remains as a thin fold around the vaginal orifice. Imperforate hymen is not associated with an increased incidence of müllerian duct abnormalities, however vaginal stenosis, vaginal atresia or a vaginal membrane are associated with an increased incidence of fusion abnormalities of the uterus, cervical and uterine stenosis, and hypoplasia or absence of the uterus, fallopian tubes and cervix.

Genital tract obstruction may present in the neonate or at puberty. The neonate presents with a pelvic mass due to hydrocolpos or hydrometrocolpos. Retrograde reflux of uterine contents into the peritoneal cavity may produce calcification similar to that due to meconium peritonitis. In adolescents, obstruction produces haematocolpos or haematometrocolpos accompanied by cyclical pain and amenorrhoea. When cyclical pain is not a feature in an adolescent with amenorrhoea then vaginal stenosis and absence of the uterus and other müllerian structures is likely.

Rokitansky–Mayer–Küster–Hauser syndrome is the association of congenital absence of the vagina, absence or abnormalities of the uterus, together with renal anomalies, particularly unilateral renal agenesis or ectopy. The uterus may be normal except for the lack of a conduit to the introitus, or be a rudimentary bipartite uterus as originally described by Rokitansky, or have any of the fusion abnormalities. Skeletal abnormalities, particularly vertebral anomalies, are seen in 12% of patients. The ovaries are normal in all

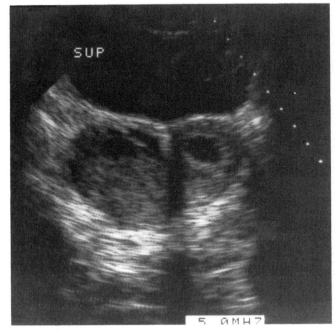

Fig. 6.4 Rokitansky–Meyer–Küster–Hauser syndrome. Fourteen-year-old girl with right iliac fossa pain. Longitudinal scan demonstrating two masses in the pelvis. At surgery the superior homogeneous mass was a haemorrhagic ovarian cyst with a fluid-debris level and the lowermost mass with a fluid centre the obstructed left uterine horn. The left kidney was absent. No skeletal anomalies were seen in this patient.

patients. Congenital absence of the vagina is also associated with Klippel–Feil anomaly. These patients present either as neonates or in adolescence in the same manner as those with imperforate hymen. A second mass, the unobstructed portion of a duplicated uterus, may be seen on US in addition to an obstructed uterine horn (Fig. 6.4). If there is cervical or high vaginal stenosis there will be fluid and echoic material in the uterus only.

ABNORMALITIES OF SEXUAL DIFFERENTIATION

Intersex disorders are abnormalities of non-accord of chromosomal, gonadal and genital sex. Their classification is based on gonadal and genital anatomy, chromosomal findings and specific genetic or metabolic abnormalities. Intersex abnormalities are divided into those associated with apparently normal chromosome constitutions, e.g. female and male pseudohermaphroditism, most of which are associated with ambiguous genitalia, and those associated with abnormal chromosomal constitutions which may, or may not, be associated with sexual ambiguity (Table 6.1).

The sex of the patient is uncertain in all patients with ambiguous genitalia. This in itself constitutes a medical emergency and early assessment, including radiological investigation, must be made to determine the sex of rearing. Delay in establishing gender may give rise to ambivalent feelings on the part of the parents and jeopardize their relationship with their child.

In addition to radiological investigation immediate biochemical assessment should be made to exclude adrenogenital syndrome, particularly the salt-losing form which is life-threatening if untreated. Buccal smear followed by full chromosomal analysis will determine the karyotype, 46XX, 46XY or mosaic. Gender is often assigned before the results of karyotyping are known. Regardless of karyotype the assignment of gender depends on the anatomy of the external genitalia. If the diagnosis of ambiguous

Table 6.1 Classification of intersex (with permission of S. J. Robboy and Haines & Taylor)

Category	Aetiology
Normal chromosome constitutions	
Female pseudohermaphroditism	Adrenogenital syndrome:
	Enzyme deficiencies
	21-hydroxylase – 95%
	11-hydroxylase
	3-beta-hydroxysteroid dehydrogenase
	Maternal androgen ingestion
	Maternal virilizing tumour
Male pseudohermaphroditism	**Primary gonadal defect**
	Testicular regression syndrome (gonadal destruction)*
	Leydig cell agenesis
	Defect in testosterone synthesis:
	Enzyme deficiencies
	20,22-desmolase
	3-beta hydroxysteroid dehydrogenase
	17 alpha-hydroxylase
	17,20-desmolase
	17 beta-ketosteroid reductase
	End-organ defect
	Disordered androgen action
	Androgen insensitivity
	syndrome (testicular feminization)
	Incomplete androgen insensitivity syndrome (e.g. Reifenstein's syndrome)
	Disorder of testosterone metabolism
	5α-reductase deficiency
Abnormal sex chromosomal constitutions	
Sexual ambiguity frequent:	
Mixed gonadal dysgenesis, including:	
Pure gonadal dysgenesis (some forms)	
Dysgenetic male	
Pseudohermaphroditism	
True hermaphrodite	
Sexual ambiguity infrequent	
Klinefelter's syndrome	
Turner's syndrome	
XX male	
Pure gonadal dysgenesis (some forms)	

* May appear phenotypically male.

genitalia is made in the neonatal period prior to the acceptance of the child as belonging to one or other sex, most will be raised as female, particularly if the phallus is thought to be too small for adequate function as a male. This provides the most satisfactory functional result because it is almost impossible to construct a penis that is sexually functional whereas a vagina suitable for coitus and normally appearing female external genitalia are more easily created surgically.

Embryology

Sexual differentiation of the gonads, internal and external genitalia, occurs in the first half of fetal life. At 6 weeks' gestation the müllerian ducts develop lateral to the wolffian ducts. The fallopian tubes, uterus, cervix and upper vagina are derived from the müllerian ducts, and the wolffian system gives rise to the epididymis, vas deferens and seminal vesicle.

The sex chromosomes determine whether the indifferent gonad (urogenital ridge) will develop into a testis or ovary. Differentiation of the male internal and external genitalia is an active process which requires H-Y antigen. This was thought to be located on the Y chromosome, however it may be autosomal and genes on the X and Y chromosomes may regulate its expression. Müllerian inhibiting substance produced by testicular Sertoli cells causes regression of the müllerian ducts. In the absence of this substance the fallopian tubes, uterus and upper vagina develop passively from the müllerian ducts. Müllerian inhibiting substance has a local action which inhibits the development of the ipsilateral fallopian tube. However to prevent development of the uterus and vagina both testes must secrete adequate amounts of müllerian inhibiting substance. This explains why patients with a testis and contralateral streak ovary or ovotestis generally have a uterus and single fallopian tube on the side of the streak ovary or ovotestis.

Testosterone, produced by fetal Leydig cells, is required for the development of the wolffian ducts into the epididymes, vas deferens and seminal vesicle. Testosterone acts locally on the ipsilateral wolffian duct. In the absence of testosterone, or the inability of the testis to produce testosterone, or insensitivity of the wolffian duct to testosterone, differentiation into the epididymes, vas deferens and seminal vesicle does not occur.

Development of the male external genitalia into the penis and scrotum and prostate is mediated by dihydroxytestosterone which is produced from testosterone by the action of the enzyme 5α-reductase. The absence of male development in the presence of a testis may be due to a lack of adequate testosterone secretion, deficient enzyme (5α-reductase) at end-organ level to convert testosterone to dihydroxytestoserone, or complete end-organ insensitivity (testicular feminization) to testosterone. Lesser degrees of deficiency or end-organ insensitivity may result in partial male development characterized by small penis, hypospadias, deficient formation of the scrotum, or persistent urogenital sinus.

Ovarian differentiation is a passive process which occurs in the absence of H-Y antigen activity. In the absence of müllerian inhibiting substance the uterus, fallopian tubes and upper vagina develop by 17 weeks' gestation. The lower vagina develops from the urogenital sinus.

Female pseudohermaphroditism

Female pseudohermaphroditism is the most common cause of ambiguous genitalia. It is due to excessive exposure of genetic (46XX) females to androgens in utero (Table 6.1). This results from deficiencies in adrenal enzymes for cortisol synthesis. Ninety per cent of patients have 21-hydroxylase deficiency, an autosomal recessive condition which may be familial. The remaining patients are deficient in 11-hydroxylase or 3β-hydroxylase. The intermediary metabolites formed result in virilization of the female genitalia. The uterus, ovaries and vagina are normal in these children and all should be raised as females regardless of the degree of virilization of the external genitalia. Perineal reconstruction of the external structures provides normal appearing female external genitalia.

When androgen excess is present prior to 16 weeks' gestation the vagina and urethra may open into a common urogenital sinus. If virilization is severe the vagina may open into the urogenital sinus above the external urethral sphincter. This requires an altered surgical approach necessitating a vaginal pullthrough at about 2 years of age in additional to genital reconstruction in the neonatal period. Marked clitoral enlargement and an opening of the urogenital sinus at the clitoral base may mimic penile hypospadias.

Maternal virilizing tumours such as luteoma of pregnancy, most often seen in multiparous women, may also produce female pseudohermaphroditism. Female pseudohermaphroditism may also be caused by excessive maternal ingestion of androgens. This was common practice in the late 1950s for treatment of habitual or threatened abortion.

The role of the radiologist is to demonstrate the anatomy of internal genitalia, particularly the presence of a uterus, cervix and vagina.

The degree of masculinization of the external genitalia determines the configuration of the urogenital sinus (Fig. 6.2). The level of communication between the vagina and the urethra determines the surgical approach. If the vagina enters the urethra below the external sphincter then a cutback or flap vaginoplasty can be performed in the neonatal period at the time of genital reconstruction, or at 3–6 months of age. If the vagina enters the urethra above the external sphincter, e.g. at the level of the posterior urethra, then reconstruction of the external genitalia is performed in the neonatal period but vaginal pullthrough is deferred until approximately 2 years of age.

Contrast studies require the catheterization of the urethra and/or urogenital sinus. Barium paste or other opaque material should mark the external orifice on the perineum. If the catheter enters the bladder an MCU should be performed with the patient in the lateral position. A vagina or utriculus may fill in the course of micturition. A cervical impression indicates the presence of a cervix (Fig. 6.5). A uterine cavity and fallopian tubes may also be outlined (Fig. 6.6). If the vagina is outlined without contrast entering the bladder the vaginal catheter may be left in place and a second catheter passed anteriorly into the urogenital sinus in an attempt to catheterize the urethra. The relative position of the vaginal orifice both to the urethra and the exterior can also be demonstrated in this manner. If no vaginal filling occurs on MCU and no other orifice is catheterized, US is valuable in demonstrating a uterus and endoscopy may demonstrate a vaginal orifice arising from the posterior urethra at the level of the verumontanum above the external urethral sphincter.

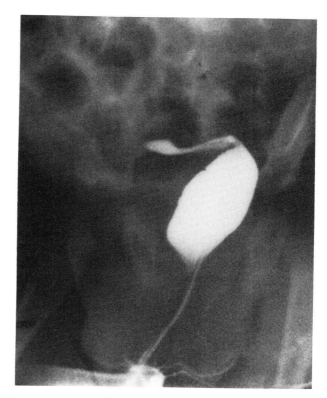

Fig. 6.6 Female pseudohermaphrodite with congenital adrenal hyperplasia. Sinogram demonstrates the vagina and also the uterine cavity and fallopian tubes.

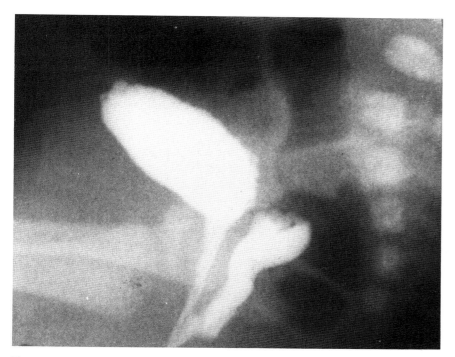

Fig. 6.5 46XX female pseudohermaphrodite with congenital adrenal hyperplasia and ambiguous genitalia. Sinogram demonstrates the vagina arising from the inferoposterior aspect of the urogenital sinus. The cervical impression is seen at the apex of the vagina.

Table 6.2 Intersex clinical features

Category	Aetiology	Müllerian structures*	Wolffian structures†	External genitalia	Malignant potential
Normal chromosome constitutions					
Female pseudohermaphroditism 46XX	Adrenogenital syndrome, maternal androgen ingestion, maternal virilizing tumour	Normal	Absent	Ambiguous	None
Male pseudohermaphroditism 46XY	**Primary gonadal defect** Testicular regression syndrome				None
	Early	Absent	Absent	Female	
	Intermediate	Rudimentary	Variable	Ambiguous	
	Late	Absent	Normal	Male	
	Leydig cell agenesis	Absent	Variable		None
	Defect in testosterone synthesis – enzyme deficiencies	Absent	Variable	Ambiguous or female	None
	End-organ defect Disordered androgen action				
	Androgen insensitivity syndrome (testicular feminization)	Absent	Absent	Female or ambiguous	4% by age 25 yr, 33% by 50 yr
	Disorder of testosterone metabolism 5α-reductase deficiency	Absent	Normal	Female or ambiguous	None
Abnormal sex chromosomal constitutions					
Sexual ambiguity frequent					
Mixed gonadal dysgenesis, 45X/46XY		Present (95%)	Variable	Ambiguous	33% gonadoblastoma
Other mosaics True hermaphrodite, 46XX (50%), 46XY(20%)		Present	Present	Ambiguous	2.6% germ cell tumours

* Uterus, fallopian tubes, upper vagina.
† epididymis, vas deferens, seminal vesicle.

If a cervical impression or uterus are demonstrated using contrast studies then male pseudohermaphroditism is unlikely (Table 6.2).

Male pseudohermaphroditism

Patients with male pseudohermaphroditism have a 46 XY karyotype but have deficient external genitalia due to relative or absolute androgen deficiency which is due to primary gonadal or end-organ defects (Table 6.1). The external genitalia are usually feminine or ambiguous.

The end-organ defect, androgen insensitivity (testicular feminization), is the most common form of male pseudohermaphroditism. The external genitalia are usually female and the diagnosis rarely made before puberty when the patient presents with primary amenorrhoea. The vagina is short and the uterus and cervix absent. The testes are cryptorchid and located in the inguinal canal, the pelvis or rarely the labia. The incidence of malignancy in the gonads is 4% by 25 years and 33% by 50 years, of which the most common is seminoma. Because malignancy is rare before puberty the gonads are usually not removed until after

adolescence to allow the patient the normal pubertal growth spurt and to develop feminine secondary sexual characteristics.

About 10% of patients in this group have partial androgen insensitivity (incomplete testicular feminization), also known as Reifenstein's syndrome.

The other end-organ defect, 5α-reductase deficiency, is an autosomal recessive familial condition. Affected males are either phenotypically female or have ambiguous genitalia at birth. In most patients the urogenital sinus has an anterior orifice which is the urethra and a posterior orifice which ends in a blind vaginal pouch.

Primary gonadal disorders include testicular regression syndrome, Leydig cell agenesis, defects in testosterone synthesis and defects in the müllerian system. A broad spectrum of abnormalities may be seen, ranging at one end from feminine external genitalia with absent internal genitalia, to an intermediate spectrum with sexual ambiguity and various combinations of wolffian and/or müllerian development (Table 6.2). At the other end of the spectrum patients appear phenotypically male with infantile or nearly normal male external genitalia, normally differentiated wolffian structures and inhibited müllerian structures. Some patients in this group may be raised as males; however, if they present as neonates and have a small phallus it is preferable to raise them as females.

The radiological investigation of male pseudohermaphroditism depends on the time of presentation. Patients presenting in the neonatal period should have contrast studies in the same way as female pseudohermaphrodites. In this situation a male urethra and utriculus arising from the posterior urethra may be demonstrated (Fig. 6.7). No cervical impression is seen as the uterus is almost always absent. Pelvic US will confirm the absence of müllerian structures.

Phenotypic females may present with amenorrhoea after the onset of secondary sexual characteristics. Pelvic US may show absent or rudimentary müllerian structures (Table 6.2). Pelvic US may also be useful in assessing impalpable gonads for malignancy in postpubertal patients. Asymmetry or enlargement of the gonads is suspicious of malignant change.

True hermaphroditism

True hermaphroditism is defined by the presence of well-developed testicular and ovarian tissues in the same patient. Sixty per cent of true hermaphrodites have a 46XX karyotype. The remainder are 46XY or mosaics. All have both well-developed male and female gonadal tissue in various morphological combinations, i.e. a testis on one side and an ovary on the other, two ovotestes, or a normal gonad on one side and an ovotestis on the other. Only 10% of uteri are normal, the abnormalities encountered include uterine hypoplasia (50%), and a 10–15% incidence of each of the following, unicornuate uterus, absent cervix or absent uterus.

In the past many hermaphrodites were not diagnosed until adolescence when males were investigated for gynaecomastia and females for amenorrhoea. The condition is now recognized more often in the neonate because of greater awareness of ambiguous genitalia. Germ cell tumours, including gonadoblastoma, develop in 2.6% of gonads.

Radiological investigation of true hermaphroditism centres around the investigation of primary amenorrhoea and of possible malignancy if the gonads have not been removed. In the neonatal period contrast studies and US may establish the presence of uterus and vagina.

Mixed gonadal dysgenesis

Mixed gonadal dysgenesis is characterized in most patients by a mosaic 45X/46XY karyotype, persistent müllerian structures (95%), asymmetry of the gonads with an abnormal testis and a contralateral streak gonad. There is poor development of the testis and

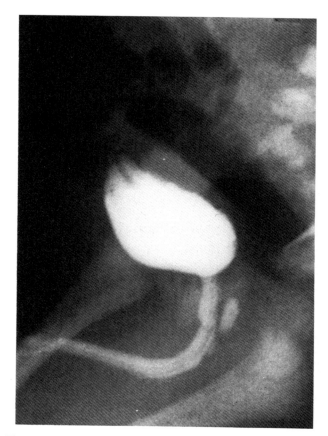

Fig. 6.7 46XY male pseudohermaphrodite with ambiguous genitalia. Male type urethra with a utriculus filling from the posterior urethra. No cervical impression is present. The phallus was inadequate and the child reared as a female with genital reconstruction and removal of the gonads.

deficient masculinization of the external genitalia. These patients should be raised as females with perineal reconstruction and removal of the gonads. Ninety-five per cent of patients have müllerian duct remnants. The uterus is usually infantile or rudimentary.

Approximately one-third of patients will develop gonadoblastoma. The likely time of development of gonadoblastoma is 3% by 10 years, 10% by 13 years, 20% by 15 years and 75% by 26 years. Gonadoblastoma may be seen in the neonatal period. The development of virilization or breast development other than at puberty in a patient with mixed gonadal dysgenesis usually indicates the presence of tumour.

Imaging of the gonads in intersex disorders

Removal of the gonads is required in all patients with male pseudohermaphroditism, mixed gonadal dysgenesis and true hermaphroditism because of their malignant potential. When the gonads are present in the inguinal canal or in the labia or scrotum they are palpable and do not require imaging. The location of the gonads in the pelvis at surgery is usually easy and so imaging prior to laparotomy is usually not required.

MRI with its superior resolution in demonstrating pelvic anatomy may identify intra-abdominal gonads, either ovaries or testes or streak gonads, with greater accuracy than US or CT, and may find a role in surgical planning. However, when the gonads are very small they are not distinguishable using any imaging method. Asymmetric enlargement of a gonad should raise the possibility of malignancy. Malignant change however may be found only on microscopic examination.

Abnormalities without ambiguous genitalia

These disorders include a variety of syndromes in which there is usually no sexual ambiguity but there is a discrepancy between the external and internal genitalia.

Turner's syndrome

Turner's syndrome, XO gonadal dysgenesis, is the most common disorder in this group. The gonads are streaks of connective tissue at the site of the ovaries. The fallopian tubes, uterus and vagina are present and the external genitalia are female. No secondary sexual characteristics develop at puberty and the genitalia remain infantile. The physical signs of Turner's syndrome are well described. Horseshoe kidney and coarctation of the aorta are associated.

A rare chromatin-positive form of Turner's syndrome occurs, karyotype XO/XX or other mosaic, e.g. XO/XXX or XX with an abnormal second X chromosome. The gonads range from streaks to dysplastic to hypoplastic. The somatic features of Turner's syndrome are present and secondary sex characteristics including menstruation may occur at puberty.

Klinefelter's syndrome

Klinefelter's syndrome affects 1 in 750 males. The most common karyotype is 47XXY. Other karyotypes include two or more X plus two or more Y chromosomes. The diagnosis is usually made at or after puberty. These males are often tall with small external genitalia, especially the testes. Twenty-five per cent of patients are mentally retarded. Fifty per cent of adults have gynaecomastia, and azoospermia and infertility are usual.

Klinefelter's syndrome with the karyotype 49XXXXY may be recognized before puberty because of associated severe mental retardation, hypotonia, abnormal facies, short neck, radioulnar synostosis, elongated radius and coxa valga.

Pure gonadal dysgenesis

Patients with pure gonadal dysgenesis have a 46XX or 46XY karyotype and are phenotypic females with streak gonads and normal müllerian structures usually without sexual ambiguity. The name Swyer's syndrome is also given to those with the 46XY karyotype.

Sex reversal syndrome – XX male

This syndrome is extremely rare. These patients have a 46XX karyotype but male phenotype and male internal and external genitalia. In contrast to true hermaphroditism there are no internal müllerian duct remnants. The disorder is similar to Klinefelter's syndrome with the exception of hypospadias which occurs in 50% but is uncommon in Klinefelter's syndrome.

REFERENCES

Cremin B J 1974 Intersex states in young children: the importance of radiology in making a correct diagnosis. Clinical Radiology 25: 63–73

Currarino G 1984 Caffey's pediatric X-ray diagnosis: the genitourinary tract. Year Book Publishers, Chicago, pp 1719–1732

Donahoe P K, Crawford J D 1986 Ambiguous genitalia in the newborn. In: Pediatric surgery. Year Book, Chicago, pp 1363–1382

Gambino J, Caldwell B, Dietrich R, Walot I, Kangarloo H 1992 Congenital disorders of sexual differentiation: MR findings. American Journal of Roentgenology 158: 363–367

Grimes C K, Rosenbaum D M, Kirkpatrick J A 1982 Pediatric gynecologic radiology. Seminars in Roengtenology 17: 284–301

Jaramillo D, Lebowitz R L, Hendren W H 1990 The cloacal malformation: radiological findings and imaging recommendations. Radiology 177: 363–367

Jeffs R D 1987 Exstrophy, epispadias, and cloacal and urogenital sinus abnormalities. Pediatric Clinics of North America 34: 1233–1257

Josso N 1981 Normal sexual differentiation. In: The intersex child. Karger, Basel, pp 1–13

Kogan B A, Hricak H, Tanagho E A 1987 Magnetic resonance imaging in genital anomalies. Journal of Urology 138: 1028–1030

Robboy S J, Welch W R, Cunha G R (Eds) The pathological basis of intersex. Obstetric and gynaecological pathology. 3 Edn, Churchill Livingstone, Edinburgh, pp 928–943

Wood B P 1990 Cloacal malformations and extrophy syndromes. Radiology 177: 326–327

Sober I, Bar-Ziv Y, Lieberman E 1980 The radiological evaluation of intersex: technique of demonstrating müllerian duct remnants in difficult cases. Journal of Urology 123: 439–440

INFLAMMATORY DISEASE

Pelvic inflammatory disease (PID) is becoming increasingly common in adolescents. The appearances and differential diagnosis of PID are the same for adolescents as in adults. There may be unilateral or bilateral complex adnexal masses (Fig. 6.8) which may be associated with fluid in the pouch of Douglas. If PID is suspected in a prepubertal female the possibility of sexual abuse should be considered.

Endometriosis is a laparoscopic diagnosis more common in the adolescent postpubertal female than previously recognized. There is no racial predilection. The principle presenting features are increasing dysmenorrhoea, often acquired, chronic pelvic pain of a cyclic or acyclic nature and menorrhagia. In one group of patients studied biopsy-proven endometriosis was found in 53% of 43 adolescents investigated by laparoscopy. The average interval between menarche and the onset of symptoms is 4.5 years.

The differential diagnosis of endometriosis in adolescents is the same as for adults.

VAGINAL DISCHARGE

Vaginal discharge in a child is an unusual complaint. Bloody vaginal discharge may be the first manifestation of precocious puberty and the child may require investigation for true precocious puberty or precocious pseudopuberty. In assessing the cause of vaginal discharge, bleeding or vulval injury, the differential diagnosis includes foreign body, infection, urethral prolapse and unintentional straddle injury in addition to sexual trauma. If signs of trauma to the vulva or vagina are evident on physical examination unintentional straddle injury may be the cause but sexual abuse should be considered.

Pelvic US may be very helpful in the investigation of vaginal discharge in children. In the presence of a full bladder the normal contour of the vaginal walls is well seen and the presence of local causes of vaginal discharge such as foreign body, or vaginal neoplasm such as rhabdomyosarcoma or endodermal sinus tumour are readily detected as a mass within the vagina. US signs of PID may be detected in sexually abused children. In postmenarchal females pregnancy may also be excluded.

TRAUMA

Major perineal injury may occur in children as a result of road trauma, falling astride or impalement. These injuries result in rupture of the urethra, bladder, vagina or rectum, or a combination of any of the above. In most instances the perineal signs do not reflect the severity of the lesion. Patients with bladder or urethral rupture may have minimal symptoms.

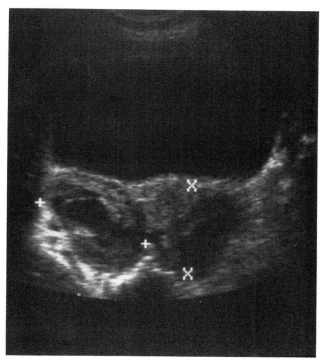

Fig. 6.8 Pelvic inflammatory disease. Transverse scan of the pelvis showing bilateral tubo-ovarian masses in a sexually active 15 year old.

Urethral bleeding may be absent in up to 70% of patients. They may present with macroscopic haematuria, inability to void or with peritoneal irritation or ileus. Most urethral ruptures are associated with pelvic fracture (70%). Urethral rupture may be isolated or more often occurs in association with bladder rupture. The tears may be continuous or separate. Retrograde urethrography may demonstrate urethral tear directly, or indirectly if extravasation of contrast is seen. Urethral catheterization should be avoided as it provides minimal information and may aggravate the injury. Indirect evidence of bladder or urethral tear may also be seen with extravasation of contrast into the pelvis after IV contrast injection either for urography or abdominal CT.

Rectal trauma is usually the result of impalement. Though signs of perineal injury or rectal bleeding are usual, up to one-third of patients will not have perineal signs and may present with an acute abdomen only. Most diagnoses of rectal tear are made by direct endoscopic visualization of the rectum. The outcome of rectal laceration is more favourable in children than in adults.

Perineal injury from sexual abuse is uncommon and a substantial number of sexually abused children do not experience injury because the offenders wish to avoid detection. Abuse by a relative or aquaintance is less likely to produce trauma than assault by a stranger. Coexistence of sexual abuse and physical abuse is uncommon.

REFERENCES

Paradise J 1990 The medical evaluation of the sexually abused child. Pediatric Clinics of North America 37: 839–862

Reinberg O, Yazbeck S 1989 Major perineal trauma in children. Journal of Pediatric Surgery 24: 982–984

OVARIAN CYSTS

Ovarian cysts, single or multiple, account for 70% of masses in the female pelvis. The ovaries of normal prepubertal females contain multiple tiny cysts due to unstimulated (primordial) follicles which measure up to 9 mm in diameter. At puberty, ova-containing (non-primordial) follicles are present under the surface of the ovary. Late developing primordial follicles may also be present up to age 14 years giving the ovary a polycystic appearance, which may give rise to difficulty in distinguishing between this and poly-cystic ovaries in postpubertal girls.

Follicular and lutein cysts measuring up to 3 cm in diameter are common in the neonatal period and at puberty and are regarded as physiological. They may also be found in young children but with lesser frequency. These lesions originate from unruptured graafian follicles or follicles which have ruptured and immediately resealed. These uncomplicated cysts are unilocular and transonic with good through transmission on US. There are no US criteria which distinguish between the various cyst types.

Follicular cysts

Cysts up to 3 cm in diameter are generally asymptomatic and resolve spontaneously over a period of days to several weeks (Fig. 6.9A). Fluid may be noted in the pouch of Douglas on resolution of the cyst (Fig. 6.9B). Large follicular cysts are found most often in post-pubertal girls but they occasionally present in younger children with torsion or haemorrhage. Rarely these cysts may secrete oestrogen, resulting in isosexual precocious puberty. The endocrine changes resolve with resolution of the cyst on serial US examination.

Cysts of the corpus luteum and theca lutein cysts

Cysts of the corpus luteum (Fig. 6.10) do not generally occur before ovulation and so are rare prior to puberty. They are generally asymptomatic in the adolescent, however instead of undergoing involution in the latter part of the menstrual cycle they may continue to produce oestrogen and progesterone resulting in dysfunctional uterine bleeding.

Theca lutein cysts result from unruptured follicles rather than corpora lutea. They are approximately the same size as follicular cysts. These are more numerous in peripubertal and postpubertal girls but have also been described in neonates and young infants.

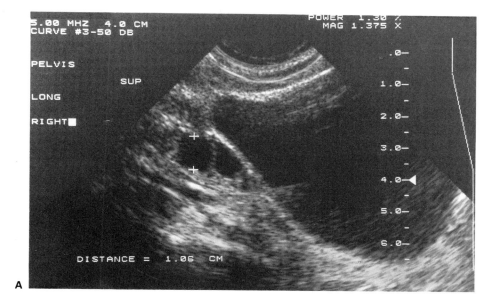

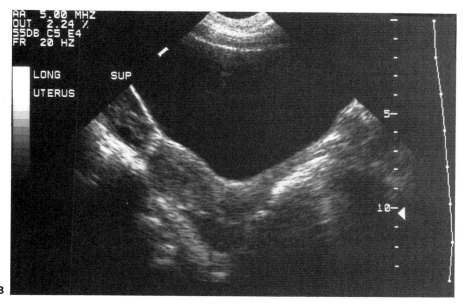

Fig. 6.9 **A** Follicular cyst in an 8-year-old girl. **B** Fluid in the pouch of Douglas following resolution of the cyst.

Simple cysts

These are regarded as follicular cysts whose lining has been destroyed by hydrostatic pressure and are similar in appearance to follicular and lutein cysts.

Paraovarian cysts

Paraovarian cysts are derived from the organ of Rosenmüller or epoophoron which is a remnant of the wolffian system and consists of Gartner's duct and many tubules. Cysts may arise in the main duct or in the tubules and lie in the mesosalpynx between the ovary and tube. These cysts are indistinguishable from other adnexal cysts.

Neonatal cysts

Very large cysts are occasionally seen in neonates, either diagnosed antenatally or in the immediate postnatal period when they present as an abdominal mass. These cysts may be so large as to produce dystocia at delivery. Most are follicular or luteinizing cysts and they are thought to be due to stimulation by maternal chorionic gonadotrophin during pregnancy. An increased incidence of luteinizing cysts is seen in infants of diabetic mothers, or in infants whose mothers have had toxaemia of pregnancy or maternal isoimmunization. These conditions are associated with raised levels of human chorionic gonadotrophin. There is also an increasing incidence of ovarian cysts in premature infants because of their increased sensitivity to human chorionic gonadotrophin.

Large uncomplicated cysts are unilocular, without septation and show through transmission on sonography. If they bleed or undergo torsion they develop internal fine echoes and may exhibit a fluid/fluid level. They may be aspirated under US control with surgery reserved for complicated or recurrent cysts. Spontaneous regression of cysts under 5 cm diameter may occur. Rupture of large neonatal cysts is a rare event and an unusual cause of neonatal ascites.

The differential diagnosis of neonatal ovarian cysts is:

— hydronephrosis
— enteric duplication
— hydrocolpos
— urachal cyst.

After hydronephrosis and hydrocolpos, ovarian cysts are the next most common cause of a neonatal cystic mass. When examining the child with a cystic intra-abdominal mass it is important to locate both ovaries as the presence of a normal ovary on the side of the cyst makes an ovarian origin for the cyst very unlikely. Duplication cysts may be distinguishable by the presence of a thin hypoechoic rim of smooth muscle under the capsule of the cyst.

Management of uncomplicated ovarian cysts

The management of uncomplicated ovarian cysts has become increasingly conservative. Serial US examinations show resolution of most cysts, particularly those up to 5.5 cm in diameter, over a 6 week period. Repeated aspiration of uncomplicated cysts has been described in the neonate and in adult women but not in children. It may have a role in the management of simple cysts in adolescents in whom a cyst persists with symptoms insufficient to require surgical intervention.

The child presenting with abdominal pain and found to have a simple follicular cyst should be managed conservatively. If the clinical course is benign, i.e. there is no deterioration or development of peritonitis or signs of perforation, the patient may be followed up with US after an interval of 2–3 weeks. By examining the pelvis at a different time of the menstrual cycle the cyst usually resolves or shows a reduction in size. If the clinical condition of the child deteriorates a repeat US may show development of fine echoes within the cyst suggesting haemorrhage and/or torsion. Absence of the cyst and free fluid in the pouch of Douglas indicates cyst rupture.

Torsion and haemorrhage

The adnexae in children are very mobile and lie in the abdomen descending into the pelvis at puberty. Torsion of a normal ovary and fallopian tube may present as an acute abdomen. The ovary is enlarged having the appearance of a complex mass. Distended follicles may be seen in the periphery of the torted ovary. Rarely, massive ovarian oedema, either unilateral or bilateral, may occur following torsion and may simulate tumour. Torsion may also result in amputation of the ovary which may then calcify and form a freely mobile mass within the abdomen.

Torsion or haemorrhage into an ovarian cyst results in a complex mass in the adnexal region. The mass may appear completely solid, however though transmission is usually present posteriorly (Fig. 6.11). The differential diagnosis includes ovarian tumour, appendiceal abscess, PID and ectopic pregnancy. The presence of persistent pyrexia makes appendiceal or other abscess more likely. Torsion and haemorrhage may not be distinguishable on US. Both produce increased echogenicity within the cyst with or without fluid in the pouch of Douglas. Serial US, if the patient's clinical status allows, may show gradual change in an haemorrhagic cyst as the haemorrhage lyses whereas torsion of a cyst alone or of the uterine adnexa may show an unchanging appearance over a period of days.

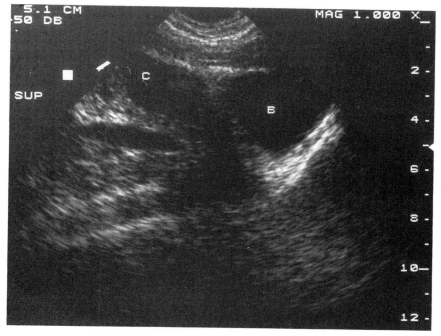

Fig. 6.10 Corpus luteum cyst in a 14-year-old girl.

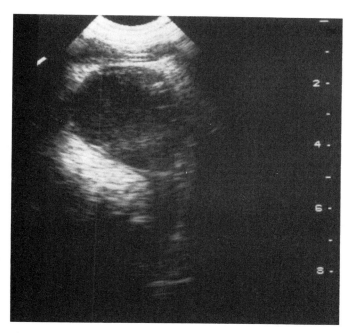

Fig. 6.11 Haemorrhagic ovarian cyst. Note the homogeneous appearance with through transmission posteriorly. At surgery a cystectomy was performed with preservation of the ovary.

Polycystic ovaries

Single or multiple cysts are a common finding in normal females both pre and postpubertal. Polycystic ovaries (Stein–Leventhal syndrome) is very rare in adolescents and this diagnosis should be made with caution in this group. The syndrome classically consists of amenorrhoea, hirsutism and polycystic ovaries. The ovaries are typically enlarged, pale and thick walled. The US criteria for the diagnosis of polycystic ovaries are the presence of 10 or more cysts 2–8 mm in diameter associated with increased ovarian stroma. The diagnosis may be made on clinical and biochemical grounds in the presence of ovaries appearing normal on US.

Other associations

Multiple ovarian cysts measuring up to 6 cm in diameter have been described in untreated juvenile hypothyroidism. The ovaries in these patients return to normal after treatment with thyroxine. Cysts have also been described in patients with cystic fibrosis.

REFERENCES

Farrell T P, Boal D K, Teele R L, Ballantine T V 1982 Acute torsion of normal uterine adnexa in children: sonographic demonstration. American Journal of Roentgenology 139: 1223–1225
Graif M, Shalev J, Strauss S, Engelberg S, Mashiach S, Itzchak Y 1984 Torsion of the ovary: sonographic features. American Journal of Roentgenology 143: 1331–1334
Han B K, Babcock D S 1983 Ultrasonography of torsion of normal uterine adnexa. Journal of Ultrasound in Medicine 2: 321–323
Kennedy L A, Pinckney L E, Currarino G, Votteler T P 1981 Amputated calcified ovaries in children. Radiology 141: 83–86
Thind D R, Carty H M L, Pilling D W 1989 The role of ultrasound in the management of ovarian masses in children. Clinical Radiology 40: 180–182
Warner M A, Fleischer A C, Edell S L, Thieme G A, Bundy A L, Kurtz A B, James Jr A E 1985 Uterine adnexal torsion: sonographic findings. Radiology 154: 773–775

OVARIAN NEOPLASMS

Ovarian neoplasms account for 30% of ovarian masses in children and 1–1.6% of all paediatric tumours. These tumours can be divided into germ cell and non-germ cell tumours (Table 6.3). Germ cell tumours predominate in children, accounting for 70–80% of all ovarian neoplasms in girls under 20 years, the largest proportion of which, 60%, are mature benign teratomas. In contrast, epithelial neoplasms account for 80% of ovarian neoplasms in adults.

Between 15 and 35% of all ovarian tumours are malignant, with a peak incidence after puberty at about 13 years. Benign tumours are seen in all ages but occur predominantly in prepubertal children.

The most common presenting complaint is abdominal pain (70% of patients), and most common physical sign an abdominal mass. Other modes of presentation include increasing abdominal distension, constipation, or genitourinary symptoms. Thirty per cent of teratomas present with torsion. Hormonally active tumours (7% of all ovarian tumours) usually present with isosexual precocious puberty. Masculinizing ovarian tumours are extremely rare.

The differential diagnosis of ovarian tumours is listed on Table 6.4. The distinction between benign and malignant tumours and occasionally complicated ovarian cysts cannot be made reliably using US or other imaging methods. All such lesions may present as complex masses of varying echogenicity with cystic and solid components. It must be borne in mind,

Table 6.3 Classification of ovarian masses		
	% Pelvic masses	% Ovarian tumours
Cysts	70	
Follicular		
Lutein		
Simple		
Paraovarian		
Neoplasms	30	
1. Primary neoplasms		60
Germ cell tumours		
Teratoma		36
Mature (benign)		
Immature		
Malignant		
Germinoma		
Embryonal carcinoma		
Endodermal sinus tumour		
Choriocarcinoma		
Gonadoblastoma		
Polyembryoma		
Non-germ cell tumours	10	30
Epithelial		
Serous cystadenoma		
Mucinous cystadenoma		
Serous cystadenocarcinoma		
Mucinous cystadenocarcinoma		
Clear cell carcinoma		
Endometrioid		
Sex cord tumours		<10
Fibroma		
Sertoli–Leydig		
Granulosa theca		
2. Secondary neoplasms		<10
Lymphoma		
Leukaemia		

Table 6.4 Ovarian masses: differential diagnosis
Appendicitis
Torsion of ovary +/− cyst
Haemorrhagic cyst
Ectopic pregnancy
Pelvic inflammatory disease
Duplication cyst

however, that malignant ovarian neoplasms are very rare and most complex cystic masses in childhood will be cysts which have undergone torsion or haemorrhage and more rarely a benign dermoid which may also have undergone torsion. However in the presence of a complex mass the liver, para-aortic region and peritoneum should be examined for metastatic disease and ascites and a chest radiograph should be done for metastases.

Germ cell tumours

Mature (benign) teratoma, also called benign cystic teratoma, is the commonest ovarian tumour, seen in children of all ages with a peak at 15 years. They are predominantly multicystic but may be solid or contain mixed echoes (Fig. 6.12). Posterior acoustic shadowing results from the presence of calcification or fat. A fat/fluid level may be visible within the cyst and hair or sebaceous material which may be mobile may be visible as areas of intermediate or increased echoes within the cyst. Fifty per cent show calcification on plain abdominal radiograph (Fig. 6.13). Up to 9% are bilateral.

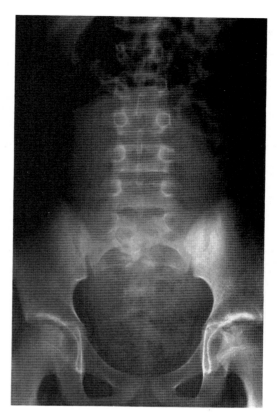

Fig. 6.13 Calcification overlying the sacrum in a benign cystic teratoma (same patient as in Fig. 6.12).

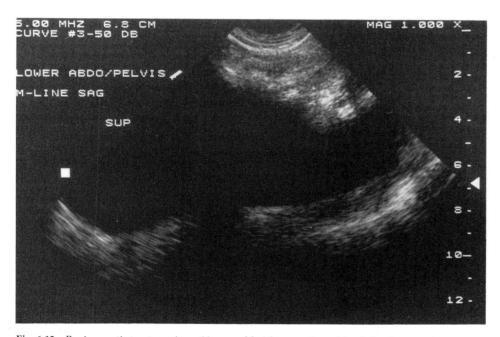

Fig. 6.12 Benign cystic teratoma in an 11-year-old girl presenting with a 2-day history of abdominal pain. Note the large cystic component with echogenic material anteriorly which is fat within the teratoma.

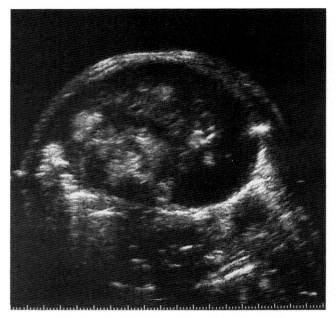

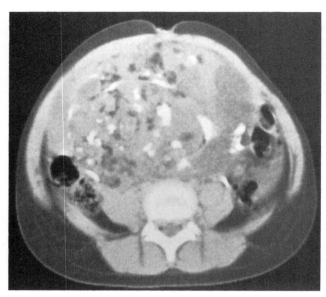

Fig. 6.14 Immature teratoma in a 23-month-old girl presenting with a 3 week history of lethargy, poor appetite and increasing abdominal distension. Neuroglial implants were present in the peritoneum at surgery.

Fig. 6.15 CT scan of the lower abdomen in an 8-year-old girl with a 4 week history of increasing abdominal pain. Calcification in a malignant teratoma with yolk sac elements. Serum AFP was elevated. (With acknowledgements to Dr J.G. Stuckey).

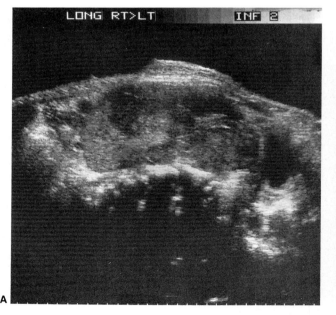

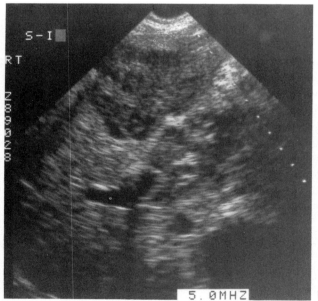

Fig. 6.16 **A** Germinoma in a 12-year-old girl presenting with abdominal distension for 2 years with increasing distension for 6 months. Longitudinal scan shows a large predominantly solid mass occupying the whole abdomen. Torsion and also lymph node involvement were present at initial surgery. **B** The patient was lost to follow-up and re-presented 10 months later with a further mass. Longitudinal scan showed metastases in the liver and also in the para-aortic regions.

Immature teratomas account for 11% of germ cell tumours. These lesions are not frankly malignant but contain embryonic neuroglial or neuroepithelial elements as well as mature elements. They are associated with an increased incidence of malignancy but appear to have a better prognosis in children than in adults. Neuroglial implants in the peritoneum are described in these tumours but with a relatively benign course. They may have both cystic and solid components and are found in all age groups, average age 11 years (Fig. 6.14).

Up to 30% of teratomas in childhood are malignant. These tumours, also known as teratocarcinomas, contain one or more of the components of malignant germ cell tumours (Fig. 6.15). The prognosis is dependent on the most malignant component of the tumour.

Germinoma

Germinomas comprise 16% of all germ cell tumours. This is the single most common malignant ovarian tumour. There are no US criteria which distinguish these from other ovarian neoplasms (Fig. 6.16A). Between 5 and 20% are bilateral. Metastatic disease occurs to regional lymph nodes and liver (Fig. 6.16B).

Other germ cell tumours

The remaining malignant germ cell tumours, embryonal carcinoma (yolk-sac tumour), endodermal sinus tumour, choriocarcinoma and gonadoblastoma are seen solely or in combination with other tumours of germ cell origin, e.g. teratoma, and are very rare.

Choriocarcinoma may present in the neonate with disseminated metastatic disease. It may be seen as a gestational tumour. Gonadoblastoma occurs almost exclusively in the dysgenetic gonads in patients with intersex disorders. The most frequent karyotypes are 46XY and 45XO/XY. Calcification is characteristic.

Biochemical markers in germ cell tumours

Table 6.5 shows the tumours for which biochemical markers may be identified. Alpha-fetoprotein (AFP) is the marker for malignant germ cell and embryonal cell tumours. Other conditions in which AFP may be raised include hepatic malignancy, hepatitis, some gastrointestinal tract malignancies and hereditary tyrosinaemia.

Beta HCG (human chorionic gonadotropin) will be raised in any tumour which contains trophoblastic elements, i.e. choriocarcinoma, embryonal carcinoma and polyembryoma. Beta HCG is also elevated in pregnancy and in the presence of an hydatidiform mole.

Table 6.5   Germ cell tumours: tumour markers

	AFP	HCG
i. Teratoma		
Mature (benign)	–	–
Immature	–(+)	–
Tumours containing other malignant germ cell components*	+	(+)
ii. Germinoma*	–	–(+)
iii. Embryonal carcinoma*	+	–(+)
iv. Endodermal sinus tumour*	+	–
v. Choriocarcinoma*	–	+
vi. Gonadoblastoma	–	–
vii. Polyembryoma		

* Tumours containing other malignant germ cell components ii – v.

Non-germ cell tumours

Non-germ cell tumours comprise 30% of all ovarian tumours. This group includes stromal tumours, i.e. sex-cord tumours and ovarian fibromas, epithelial tumours, and also metastatic lesions.

Epithelial tumours represent 17% of ovarian tumours in the paediatric age group. These tumours are found almost exclusively in postpubertal females, most commonly 18–19 year olds.

The frequency of occurrence of the individual epithelial tumours is: serous cystadenoma, 52%; mucinous cystadenoma, 32%; serous cystadenocarcinoma, 8%; mucinous cystadenocarcinoma, 5%; clear cell carcinoma, 2%. The malignant potential of these tumours is less than that in adults, e.g. 7–13% for cystadenoma.

Stromal tumours comprise 12% of ovarian tumours. These tumours include fibromas and sex-cord tumours such as granulosa-theca and luteal tumours and Sertoli–Leydig tumours. The latter are referred to as arrhenoblastoma and androblastoma when hormonally active.

The remaining stromal tumours are rare, particularly in the prepubertal child. Thecomas constitute 5% of stromal tumours and 0.6% of all ovarian tumours. All thecomas are endocrinologically active, and 1% exhibit calcification.

Sertoli–Leydig tumours (androblastoma, arrhenoblastoma) constitute 15% of stromal tumours in children. Less than 15% are malignant. Fibroma, oat cell carcinoma, endometroid carcinoma of the ovary have been reported.

Seven per cent of all ovarian tumours are endocrinologically active. Granulosa-theca cell tumours are the most common ovarian tumour to produce gonadal isosexual precocious puberty. Forty per cent of these tumours produce precocious puberty. They occur mostly in the second decade. The postpubertal child may manifest hypermenorrhoea, amenorrhoea, ascites or abdominal fullness. The tumours are usually well encapsulated and contain areas of cystic degeneration and haemorrhage; 2.5% are bilateral.

Metastatic disease

Metastatic involvement of the ovaries in Burkitt's lymphoma and leukaemia (Fig. 6.17) is well described in childhood. Like lymphoma and leukaemia elsewhere, these tumours may be mistaken for cysts due to their decreased echogenicity. The presence of bilateral lesions should alert the examiner to the possibility of metastatic infiltration.

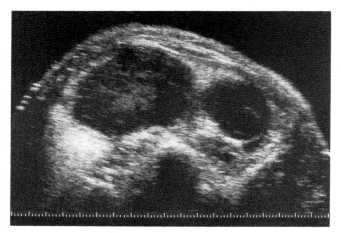

Fig. 6.17 Transverse scan of the abdomen showing bilateral hypoechoic masses due to ovarian infiltration in acute lymphoblastic leukaemia.

OTHER GENITAL TUMOURS

Tumours of the genital tract other than ovarian tumours are rare.

Embryonal rhabdomyosarcoma of the vagina (botryoid type) is almost exclusively seen in young girls (Fig. 6.18). Ninety per cent occur before the age of 5 years, with two-thirds appearing before 3 years. These tumours arise from the anterior vaginal wall and may invade the vesicovaginal septum or bladder wall. They commonly present with haemorrhagic vaginal discharge and less commonly by extrusion of the mass from the vagina, urethral obstruction or a palpable abdominal mass. Metastases may occur to regional lymph nodes, lungs or bone. The differential diagnosis includes endodermal sinus tumour, embryonal carcinoma of the vagina, Gartner's duct cysts, and benign vaginal or hymenal polyp. Rhabdomyosarcoma of the vulva is less common than vaginal rhabdomyosarcoma and may be mistaken for infection of Bartholin's gland prior to biopsy. The mean age at presentation of these tumours is 8 years as opposed to the younger age at presentation for vaginal rhabdomyosarcoma. The uterus is an unusual site for rhabdomyosarcoma and when seen it occurs in older females, mean age 14 years.

Clear cell adenocarcinoma of the vagina and cervix is described in females aged 7 years to adulthood. These tumours arise from the anterior vaginal wall. In 65% of patients there is a history of maternal exposure to diethylstilboestrol and other non-steroidal oestrogens prior to the 18th week of pregnancy. Ninety per cent of these tumours occur after 12 years. The most common symptom is vaginal discharge or bleeding.

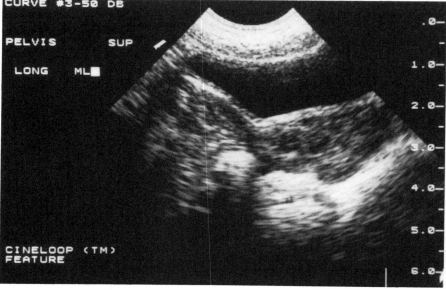

Fig. 6.18 Rhabdomyosarcoma of the vagina.

REFERENCES

Athey P A, Malone R S 1987 Sonography of ovarian fibroma/thecomas. Journal of Ultrasound in Medicine 6: 431–436

Barr L L, Swischuk L E, Hayden C K 1988 Muscular rim sign in enteric duplication cysts. Radiology 169 (suppl): 463

Bickers G H, Siebert J J, Anderson J C, Golladay S, Berry D L 1981 Sonography of ovarian involvement in childhood acute lymphocytic leukaemia. American Journal of Roentgenology 137: 399–401

Breen J L, Maxson W S 1977 Ovarian tumors in children and adolescents. Clinical Obstetrics & Gynecology 20: 607–623

Ehren I M, Mahour G H, Isaacs Jr H 1984 Benign and malignant ovarian tumors in childhood and adolescents. American Journal of Surgery 147: 339–344

Ein S H 1973 Malignant ovarian tumors in children. Journal of Pediatric Surgery 8: 539–542

Ein S H, Darte J M M, Stephens C A 1970 Cystic and solid ovarian tumors in children: a 44-year review. Journal of Pediatric Surgery 5: 148–156

Favara B E, Franciosi R A 1972 Ovarian teratoma and neuroglial implants on the peritoneum. Cancer 31: 678–681

Goldsmith C I, Hart W R 1975 Ataxia-telangiectasia with ovarian gonadoblastoma and contralateral dysgerminoma. Cancer 36: 1838–1842

Golladay E S, Mollitt D L 1983 Ovarian masses in the child and adolescent. Southern Medical Journal 76: 954–957

Hays D M, Shimada H, Raney Jr R B, Tefft M, Newton W, Christ W M, Lawrence Jr W, Ragab A, Beltangady M, Maurer H M 1988 Clinical staging and treatment results in rhabdomyosarcoma of the female genital tract among children and adolescents. Cancer 61: 1893–1903

Herbst A I, Robboy S J, Scilly R E, Poskanzer D C 1974 Clear-cell carcinoma of the vagina and cervix in girls: analysis of 170 registry cases. American Journal of Obstetrics and Gynecology 119: 713–724

Hilgers R D, Malkasion Jr G D, Soule E H 1970 Embryonal rhabdomyosarcoma (botryoid type) of the vagina; a clinicopathological review. American Journal of Obstetrics and Gynecology 107: 484–502

Lucraft H H 1979 Ovarian tumours in children – a review of 40 cases. Clinical Radiology 30: 279–285

Mahour G H, Woolley M M, Landing B H 1976 Ovarian teratoma in children. American Journal of Surgery 132: 587–589

Maurer H M, Ruymann F B, Pochedly C (eds) 1991 Rhabdomyosarcoma and related tumors in children and adolescents. CRC Press, Boca Raton, Florida, pp 355–362

Towne B, Mahour G H, Woolley M M, Isaacs Jr H 1975 Ovarian cysts and tumours in infancy and childhood. Journal of Pediatric Surgery 10: 311–320

ENDOCRINE

Precocious puberty

Sexual precocity is the development of secondary sexual characteristics before the normal age; in females there is breast enlargement, or pubic or axillary hair before 8 years, or onset of menarche before 9 years.

Isosexual precocious puberty is always appropriate for the patient's phenotype. Heterosexual precocity is at variance with the patient's phenotype, i.e. virilization in the female or feminization in the male. True precocious puberty is present when all secondary sexual characteristics have developed and is always appropriate for the gender of the child, i.e. isosexual, and has an endocrine profile similar to normal puberty. Ovulation occurs and the ovaries and uterus are increased in size (Table 6.6). It occurs with premature maturation of the hypothalamus and is idiopathic in 85% of females and 66% of males. It may also be associated with a variety of central nervous system disorders (Table 6.7).

Pseudoprecocious puberty is present when only some of the secondary sexual characteristics have developed and may be isosexual, i.e. appropriate for the child's gender, or heterosexual, i.e. male characteristics appearing in female or vice versa. The endocrine pattern of isosexual pseudoprecocious puberty in the female is more varied but is generally associated with elevated oestrogen and androgen levels and low gonadotrophin levels. The gonads remain small and ovulation does not occur. The cause is peripheral rather than a central lesion, such as granulosa-theca cell tumours of the ovary (Table 6.7). Pseudoprecocious puberty producing heterosexual (male) secondary characteristics is seen in adrenal hyperplasia and tumours where there are adrenal rests in the ovary or cysts.

Heterosexual precocious puberty in the female is caused by ovarian tumours such as arrhenoblastoma in patients with dysgenetic gonads, adrenal hyperplasia, virilizing adrenal adenoma or carcinoma, androgen-producing teratomas or by the administration of androgens.

The approach to the patient presenting with precocious puberty is simplified if it can be divided into true precocious puberty or pseudoprecocious puberty. However it is not always possible to distinguish between these entities and premature thelarche or premature adrenarche. Isolated premature thelarche and adrenarche are benign conditions and are not associated with neoplasma, either central or peripheral, or with premature epiphyseal closure. Premature thelarche (premature breast development) and adrenarche (premature development of pubic or axillary hair) can cause confusion because they may be the first signs of precocious or pseudoprecocious puberty. These patients should be closely followed to ensure that further signs of puberty, either true precocious puberty or precocious pseudopuberty, do not develop.

In patients with isolated premature thelarche or adrenarche pelvic US will demonstrate a normal premenarchal uterus and ovaries. In precocious pseudopuberty the appearance of the pelvic organs varies according to the underlying cause such as the presence of an autonomously functioning ovarian cyst. Most autonomously functioning cysts involute without the need for surgery. Large ovarian cysts have also been documented in McCune–Albright syndrome, neurofibromatosis and congenital hypothyroidism. Rarely the cause of precocious pseudopuberty may be a granulosa-theca or granulosa cell tumour of the ovary. Although adrenal lesions are more likely to cause heterosexual precocious pseudopuberty, the adrenals should be examined in all patients as congenital adrenal hyperplasia has been reported to cause isosexual precocious puberty. An intermediate or postmenarchal uterus and adult size ovaries are seen in patients with true precocious puberty. Both true precocious puberty and pseudopuberty have been documented in McCune–Albright syndrome.

US should be the first method of investigation of a patient with premature thelarche, adrenarche, true precocious puberty or precocious pseudopuberty. Although true precocious puberty is usually idiopathic, a central cause should be sought (Table 6.7). MRI is the most sensitive method of assessing the pituitary and hypothalamic regions for neoplasm. Imaging of the CNS in the early investigation of premature thelarche or adrenarche is not necessary. However should other signs of true precocious puberty develop the patient should be investigated for a central cause.

Amenorrhoea

Primary amenorrhoea exists when menarche is delayed beyond 16 years. The causes of primary amenorrhoea are listed in Table 6.8. Amenorrhoea before 16 years may be constitutional and a family history of late onset menarche is often elicited. Investigation should not be delayed after 16 years however.

In primary amenorrhoea physical examination should establish whether the external genitalia are normal and if there is imperforate hymen. Pregnancy should be excluded by pregnancy test and pelvic US. US will establish whether the uterus and ovaries are present, their degree of maturity and will also exclude haematometrocolpos. Careful examination of the

Table 6.6 Precocious puberty: clinical features

True precocious puberty (complete)	Pseudoprecocious puberty (incomplete)
Isosexual	Isosexual or heterosexual
Increased gonadotrophins	Decreased gonadotrophins
Exaggerated gonadotrophin response to GHRH	Elevated oestrogens
Ovulation	No ovulation
Adult/intermediate uterus and ovaries	Infantile uterus and ovaries

Table 6.7 Causes of isosexual precocious puberty in females

I Central
A Idiopathic
B Congenital
    Hydrocephalus
    Arachnoid cyst
C Inflammatory
    Encephalitis
    Meningitis
    Cerebral abscess
D Tumour
    Optic glioma
    Hypothalamic
    Pineal
E Trauma
F Miscellaneous
    Neurofibromatosis
    McCune–Albright syndrome
    Tuberous sclerosis
    Hypothyroidism
      Primary
      Iatrogenic
    Silver's syndrome

II Gonadotrophin-secreting tumours
A Chorioepithelioma
B Teratoma
C Hepatoblastoma

III Gonads
A Ovarian tumours
    Granulosa theca cell tumour
    Luteal cyst

IV Adrenal
A Tumours
    Adenoma
    Carcinoma

V Miscellaneous
A Premature thelarche
B Premature adrenarche
C Ingestion of oestrogens
D Iatrogenic administration of human
    chorionic gonadotrophin
E Vaginitis, vaginal tumour, foreign body or
    trauma presenting with vaginal bleeding

Table 6.8 Causes of primary amenorrhoea

Congenital
    Imperforate hymen
    Vaginal atresia
    Uterine aplasia
Endocrine
    Stein–Leventhal syndrome
    Hypopituitarism
    Adrenal hyperplasia
    Hypothyroidism
Intersex disorders*
    Testicular feminisation (androgen insensitivity syndrome)
    17α-hydroxylase deficiency (defect in testosterone synthesis)
    Pure gonadal dysgenesis
    True hermaphroditism
Chromosomal
    Turner's syndrome
Other
    Pregnancy
    Anorexia nervosa
    Radiation therapy
Neoplasm
    Craniopharyngioma
    Masculinizing tumours
      Adrenal tumour
      Hilus cell
      Arrhenoblastoma
    Granulosa theca cell tumour
Drugs
    Androgen ingestion

* May not be detected until puberty.

ovaries should be performed to exclude neoplasm. The US examination should also include the adrenals as they may be a source of tumour. The uterus of patients with anorexia nervosa may remain premenarchal in size and shape. The ovaries show no evidence of follicles and once treated adequately ovarian follicles will appear. If no pelvic or intra-abdominal cause of amenorrhoea can be found a central cause should be sought such as pituitary tumour or hypopituitarism. Chromosomal analysis should be performed if the external genitalia are abnormal or if the uterus is absent or hypoplastic or if the ovaries cannot be located or if gonads are found in the inguinal canal or labia. The adrenals may be assessed by US or CT if the biochemical assay suggests a tumour rather than adrenal hyperplasia.

Stein–Leventhal syndrome may present with primary amenorrhoea. The ovaries may appear morphologically normal on US, however the superior resolution of MRI may demonstrate an increase in the number of follicles or ovarian stroma in patients hitherto thought to have normal ovaries on pelvic sonography. Vaginal sonography may also demonstrate the ovaries with greater resolution.

REFERENCES

Cohen H L, Heller J O 1989 Paediatric and adolescent genital abnormalities in neonatal and paediatric ultrasound. Clinics in Diagnostic Ultrasound 24: 187–251

Faure N, Prat X, Bastide A, Lemay A 1989 Assessment of ovaries by magnetic resonance imaging in patients presenting with polycystic ovarian syndrome. Human Reproduction 4: 468–472

Haller J O, Bass I S, Nardi P M, Novogroder M 1985 A problem oriented approach to the imaging of pediatric endocrine disorders. Seminars in Ultrasound, CT and MR 6: 321–336

Root A W 1973 Endocrinology of puberty, part II: aberrations of sexual maturation. Journal of Pediatrics 83: 187–200

Shawker T H, Comite F, Rieth K G, Dwyer A J, Cutler G B, Loriaux L 1984 Ultrasound evaluation of isosexual precocious puberty. Journal of Ultrasound in Medicine 3: 309–316

SACROCOCCYGEAL GERM CELL TUMOURS

Sacrococcygeal germ cell tumours are the commonest solid tumour in neonates occurring in approximately 1 in 35–40 000 live births. Between 50 and 70% of these tumours present in the first few days of life, with less than 10% presenting after 2 years of age. They show varying degrees of differentiation from embryonal carcinoma to mature teratoma. The incidence is two to four times higher in females than in males; however malignancy is more common in boys. Malignancy is also more common if diagnosed after 2 months of age. These tumours arise in totipotential cells within the anterior portion of the coccyx and usually grow posteriorly and inferiorly below the coccyx. They may also grow anteriorly and superiorly, giving rise to an intrapelvic presacral tumour. These tumours are classified by the American Association of Pediatrics, Surgical Section, according to location: type I, predominantly external with minimal presacral component; type II, tumours presenting externally but with a significant presacral component; type III, tumours presenting externally but with predominant presacral component; type IV, presacral tumour with no external presentation. The majority of lesions are types I and II.

The differential diagnosis of type I and II tumours includes myelomeningocoele, lipoma, lymphangioma and haemangioma. Type IV tumours may mimic neuroblastoma, anterior meningocoele, rectal abscess or duplication, or chordoma. Treatment consists of surgical removal of the tumour and the coccyx and is usually curative. Recurrence may be seen if removal is incomplete. Malignancy has been documented in previously benign tumours.

The imaging of sacrococcygeal germ cell tumours centres around the demonstration of the anatomical extent of the lesion, particularly the presacral intrapelvic portion. They may be cystic, partly cystic and solid, or solid. Teratomatous components such as fat, sebaceous material and hair may be present and 30–50% of these tumours contain calcification. Plain radiography (Fig. 6.19A) of these masses should include the pelvis, lumbar spine and sacrum to exclude a dysraphic abnormality or sacral defect. If a sacral defect is seen the possibility of the Currarino triad should be considered (see below). Cross-sectional imaging using US, CT (Fig. 6.19B) and MRI will demonstrate the extent of the tumour, its characteristics and its relationship to the rectum, adnexa and bladder, all of which will be displaced anteriorly by any intrapelvic, presacral portion of the mass. The anterior relationship of the rectum to the mass is important in distinguishing a germ cell tumour from masses arising from the uterus or bladder, such as hydrocolpos or rhabdomyosarcoma. It is useful to place an uninflated Foley catheter in the rectum to mark its position in relation to the mass, particularly when

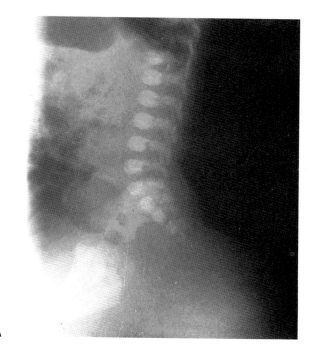

A

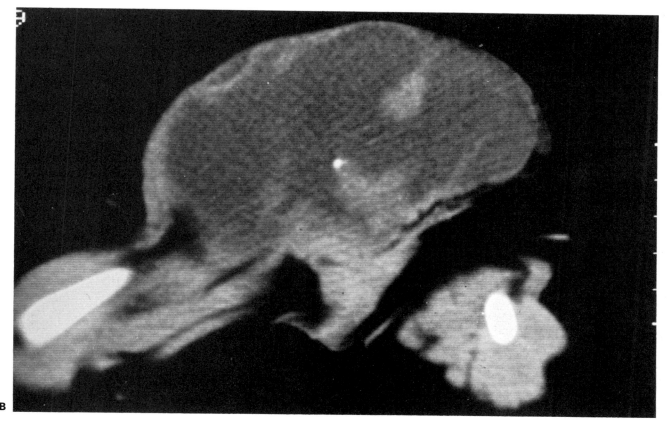

B

Fig. 6.19 Sacrococcygeal teratoma. **A** Plain film. **B** CT.

using US. The US, CT and MRI appearances of these lesions varies according to the amounts of fat, calcification, and cystic and solid components of the lesion. Fat-fluid levels may be seen on all three imaging modalities. The presence of cystic components and calcification is more common in benign teratomas; however this is not specific for benign disease. The presence of local invasion or necrosis in a predominantly solid mass suggests malignancy. The presence of raised serum AFP is also specific for malignancy. The upper urinary tract should be imaged in all patients as urinary obstruction may be present, particularly if there is a large presacral component to the mass.

The Currarino triad malformation complex consists of three main features: (1) a congenital anorectal stenosis or other low anorectal malformation; (2) an anterior sacral defect of the type seen in anterior sacral meningocele (scimitar, crescent or sickle deformity of the sacrum); and (3) a presacral mass which may be a meningocele, a teratoma or occasionally an enteric cyst or a combination of these. This triad has been described in families and also in unrelated patients. In members of the same family one or two features may be lacking, suggesting an incomplete form of the syndrome.

Fetal bowel perforation with a fluid collection in the coccygeal region has also been reported to mimic sacrococcygeal teratoma on antenatal US and also postnatally.

REFERENCES

Altman R P, Randolph J G, Lilly J R 1974 Sacrococcygeal teratoma: American academy of pediatrics surgical section survey – 1973. Journal of Pediatric Surgery 9: 398
Bale P 1984 Sacrococcygeal developmental abnormalities and tumors in children. Prospectives in Pediatric Pathology 1: 9–56
Currarino G, Coln D, Votteler T 1981 Triad of anorectal, sacral and presacral anomalies. American Journal of Roentgenology 137: 395–398
Lockwood C, Ghidini A, Romero R, Hobbins J C 1988 Fetal bowel perforation simulating sacrococcygeal teratoma. Journal of Ultrasound in Medicine 7: 227–229
Shey W L, Shkolnik A, White H 1977 Clinical and radiographic considerations of sacrococcygeal teratomas: an analysis of 26 new cases and review of the literature. Pediatric Radiology 125: 189–195
Wells R G, Sty J 1990 Imaging of sacrococcygeal germ cell tumours. Radiographics 10: 701–713

PAEDIATRIC BREAST DISEASE

Breast disease is rare in children and when encountered is usually seen in adolescents, both male and female. Approximately 90% of all breast disease is benign, and malignancy either primary or secondary is extremely rare (2–10% of all paediatric breast lesions). The onset of breast development (thelarche) usually begins at age 11–11.5 years, range 8–15 years. Development of one breast may begin before the other. The discoid subareolar tissue may be confused with pathology and excised, resulting in poor or absent breast development. Significant breast asymmetry may occur in early adolescence. Catch-up usually occurs by late adolescence, though asymmetry may persist into adulthood. Pseudoasymmetry of the breasts may occur if there is rib cage deformity or scoliosis or Poland syndrome. At thelarche, idiopathic breast hypertrophy may occur with explosive development of breast tissue either unilateral or bilateral. This may be confused with tumour such as giant fibroadenoma.

Breast asymmetry or the presence of a palpable mass is the most common reason for investigation of the breast in childhood and adolescence. An initial conservative approach to management of breast masses is justified in most patients because of the extremely low incidence of malignancy in this age group. The initial assessment of a breast mass should be with US. Although US will not reliably distinguish between benign and malignant disease it will, however, characterize cystic and solid masses and may act as a guide for aspiration or biopsy. Mammography is not recommended in the assessment of the adolescent with breast disease because of the sensitivity of the growing breast to irradiation and the extremely low incidence of malignancy in patients under 20 years.

The most common breast mass encountered in adolescent females is the classic fibroadenoma. This accounts for 70% of all lesions in this age group. The peak age of incidence is 17–20 years but they have been described in patients up to 2 years before menarche. Fibroadenomas may reach 10–15 cm in size. Fibroadenomatosis, multiple and or bilateral fibroadenomas, is seen in up to 25% of patients. Giant fibroadenoma (Fig. 6.20) is by definition at least 5 cm in size and is less common than classic fibroadenoma. These lesions may enlarge rapidly over a 3–6 month period, may be single or multiple and are said to occur earlier in adolescence than classic fibroadenoma. The typical US appearance of giant fibroadenoma and classic fibroadenoma is a smooth round or oval mass with homogeneous internal echoes, however this is not specific and there is considerable variation in their appearances. The differential diagnosis should include other benign lesions such as abscess, haematoma, papillary duct hyperplasia or juvenile papillomatosis, or much less likely, a malignant lesion such as

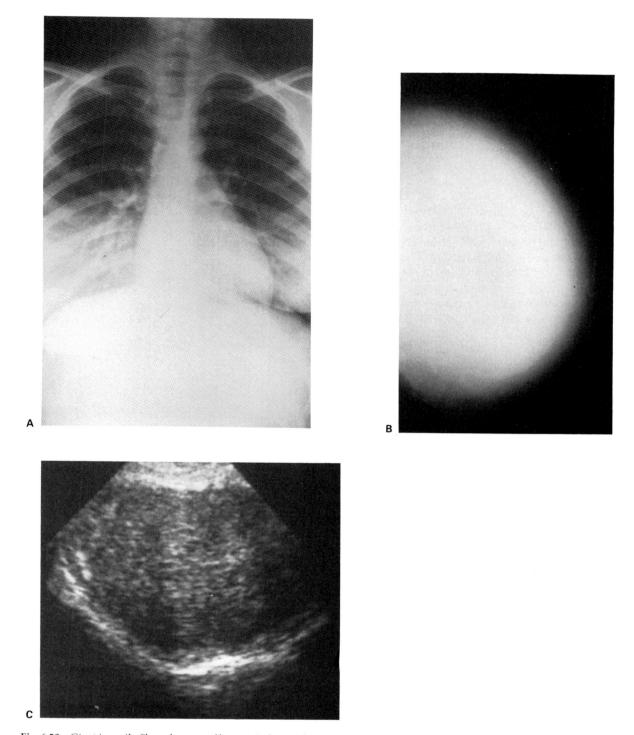

Fig. 6.20 Giant juvenile fibroadenoma of breast. **A** chest radiograph. **B** Mammogram. **C** US.

cystosarcoma phalloides, carcinoma or metastatic disease. Other less common lesions encountered include lipoma and haemangioma. Papillary duct hyperplasia includes the entities papilloma, papillomatosis and sclerosing papillomatosis. Juvenile papillomatosis is now regarded as a separate entity. A family history of carcinoma is reported in 28% of patients with juvenile papillomatosis and 5% have associated carcinoma. The earliest age at diagnosis of concurrent carcinoma is 17 years. Thirteen per cent of patients with papillary duct hyperplasia have a family history of carcinoma. Both conditions may present with a mass and may be confused with fibroadenoma.

Primary malignancy of the breast is rare. Cystosarcoma phalloides (also known as phalloides tumour) is the commonest malignant breast lesion in adolescents. Most are seen in the 16–19 year age group. The majority of these tumours are benign; however, fatal cases with metastatic disease have been reported. The diagnosis may be suggested by the presence of fluid-filled spaces or clefts in a solid mass on US but the lesion may not be distinguishable from fibroadenoma.

Less than 1% of breast carcinoma is seen in patients under 20 years. However, it has been reported in children, both male and female, as young as 3 years. Radiation as for scoliosis radiography may predispose to increased malignancy. Metastatic disease to the breast is more common than primary malignancy and may be seen in lymphoma (Fig. 6.21), both Hodgkin's and non-Hodgkin's type, leukaemia, rhabdomyosarcoma and neuroblastoma. Primary lymphoma and rhabdomyosarcoma of the breast are rare.

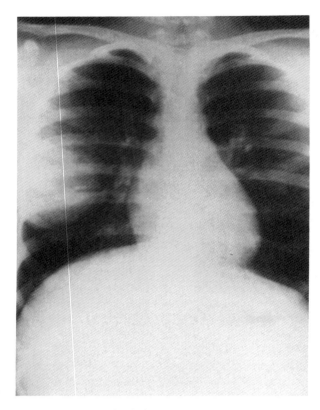

Fig. 6.21 Lymphoma of right breast.

REFERENCES

Feig S A 1992 Breast masses. Mammographic and sonographic evaluation. Radiologic Clinics of North America 30: 67–92

Feig S A, Ehrlich S M 1990 Estimation of radiation risk from screening mammography: recent trends and comparison with expected benefits. Radiology 174: 638–647

Greydanus D E, Parks D S, Farrell E G 1989 Breast disorders in children and adolescents. Pediatric Clinics of North America 36: 601–638

Pettinato G, Manivel J C, Kelly D R, Wold L E, Dehner L P 1989 Lesions of the breast in children exclusive of typical fibroadenoma and gynaecomastia: a clinicopathologic study of 113 cases. Pathology Annual 24: 296–328

Rosen P P 1984 Papillary duct hyperplasia of the breast in children and young adults. Cancer 56: 1611–1617

Endocrine Disease

U. Willi   D. Shaw   H. Carty

INTRODUCTION

Disorders of the endocrine organs include abnormalities of the hypothalamus and the pituitary gland, the thyroid and parathyroid glands, the adrenals, the pancreas and the gonads. There are conditions in which more than one endocrine organ is involved, and also disease of organs outside the endocrine system which may cause endocrine disturbances.

The purpose of this chapter is to describe and discuss abnormalities of the endocrine organs and associated lesions with or without functional endocrine impact as far as these lesions can be demonstrated by imaging means. Therefore, the endocrine system will not be reviewed encyclopaedically, but rather from a clinical and imaging standpoint. Also, due to the organization of this book, the chapter on endocrine disease is incomplete in itself and reference is made to other parts of the book, in particular Chapter 10 on imaging the central nervous system, in which the hypothalamus and pituitary gland are discussed. Abnormalities involving the endocrine aspects of the ovaries are primarily included in Chapter 6 on imaging paediatric gynaecology. Some aspects of testicular and adrenal imaging are dealt with in Chapter 5 on the genitourinary tract. Finally, there are multiple syndromes associated with hypogonadism or hypergonadism, including precocious puberty, with direct or indirect impact upon endocrinological function. The more common syndromes are included in the appropriate section of this chapter; others are included in the tables.

The chapter is divided into seven sections:

7.1 Thyroid
7.2 Parathyroid
7.3 Adrenals
7.4 Pancreas
7.5 Gonads
7.6 Precocious and delayed puberty
7.7 Complex cases (diseases originating outside the endocrine organ system).

The sections are introduced by a brief assessment of the embryology, anatomy and function of the respective organ(s). Some technical notes on the approach to diagnostic imaging then precede the description and discussion of the pathological conditions. An attempt to arrange the pathological conditions according to clinical categories such as malformation, neoplasm, infection, trauma, etc. is made as far as it seemed appropriate for the different sections.

Current technology includes conventional and digital radiographic procedures, high resolution computed tomography (CT), ultrasonography (US), scintigraphy, magnetic resonance imaging (MRI) and magnetic resonance angiography, as well as interventional procedures. US is the most versatile and useful tool in the initial imaging approach to paediatric endocrine disease outside the central nervous system. This procedure is supplemented, as indicated, by the other imaging modalities according to the needs of the individual case.

7.1 THYROID

EMBRYOLOGY, ANATOMY, FUNCTION

The thyroid gland originates predominantly from the endodermal primitive pharynx at about $3\frac{1}{2}$ weeks of gestation, primarily as a diverticulum and is connected with the tongue by the thyroglossal duct. It divides into two lobes joined by the isthmus and reaches its definitive location by the end of the 7th week. The migration of the thyroid gland during its development may be disturbed so that the gland may lie in ectopic sites such as the base of the tongue, the tracheal wall, the superior retrosternal area and others.

The thyroglossal duct becomes solid and atrophic and, in about half the population, its lower part develops into a pyramidal lobe in continuity with the isthmus.

The lateral portions of the thyroid gland originate from neurodermal material, i.e. the ultimobranchial bodies. This part of the gland will become the parafollicular cell-line of which C-cells will secrete calcitonin. Along the dorsolateral border of the thyroid lobes run the carotid arteries, paralleled laterally by the internal jugular veins.

The size of the thyroid gland is highly variable with geographical differences. According to a German study of 1080 children, the mean thyroid volume was 4.3 ml at 7 years of age and 13.6 ml at 16 years, while in a study from Sweden a mean thyroid volume of 4.1 ml was found at the age of 13 years.

Within the thyroid gland the synthesis of the hormones tri-iodothyronine (T3) and thyroxine (T4) takes place under the effect of iodine. T3 is also produced within the liver and kidney as well as elsewhere in the body by deiodination of T4. These substances have an essential effect upon growth and metabolism. The thyroid stimulating hormone (TSH) produced by the anterior part of the pituitary gland regulates the function of the thyroid. Its synthesis and release is governed by the thyroid releasing hormone (TRH) produced within the hypothalamus. Overproduction of TSH or TRH will result in hypertrophy or hyperplasia of thyroid tissue and overproduction of thyroid hormones; while an increased synthesis or intake of thyroid hormones will decrease the production of TSH.

IMAGING APPROACH AND TECHNIQUE

US has become the primary modality for imaging the thyroid gland following physical examination. Scintigraphy is an established and often useful tool for topographic functional evaluation of the thyroid. It should be performed after morphological assessment when necessary. A special scintigraphic technique with functional suppression of normal thyroid tissue allows visualization of an autonomous thyroid adenoma.

Colour Doppler US may yield information about abnormal blood flow to the thyroid and is increased in hyperthyroidism. MRI and CT may be indicated in imaging ectopic thyroid tissue or some related pathological process, especially in the mediastinum. Occasionally, calcification in the thyroid gland may be apparent on a plain film.

Due to its anterior and superfical location, the thyroid gland, along with the normal parathyroid glands, is easily accessible to ultrasonographic examination. This is best done with the child in the supine position with the head tilted slightly downwards and the neck supported by a shaped pad. If needed, the parent or nurse may help by holding the child's head, sitting either alongside the examination table or at the end of the table on the headside of the child. In small children with a relatively short neck access to the anterior neck region by the linear probe may be difficult but usually possible. A linear 7.5- or 10-MHz probe is recommended, supplemented by a transsonic pad at times, but this is usually not needed for nearfield definition with modern 10-MHz transducers. If the thyroid gland is normally located, its size, shape, echogenicity and echo pattern should be evaluated in longitudinal and transverse planes. A volumetric assessment is most useful in assessing mass lesions. There is considerable geographical variability in thyroid size. A relatively large isthmus, asymmetry and other morphological variations as well as operator dependence, limit the usefulness of thyroid volume in assessing normality. Patience and calm combined with experience or skill will allow a successful examination in most children.

PATHOLOGY

Hypothyroidism

Hypothyroidism is a common endocrine disorder in paediatrics, while hyperthyroidism is less frequent. In the majority of cases, hypothyroidism is due to an anatomical defect, usually aplasia, hypoplasia or dysplasia of the thyroid gland. This may or may not be associated with thyroid ectopia. (Fig. 7.1.1). A lingual or oesophageal thyroid may cause dysphagia or bleeding. Tracheal wall or laryngeal ectopia may present with respiratory disturbance. Thyroid ectopia does not necessarily imply hypothyroidism but this

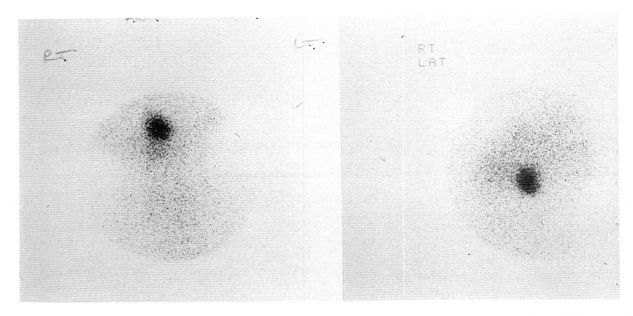

Fig. 7.1.1 Technetium thyroid scan in a neonate with hypothyroidism diagnosed on routine screening. Anterior and lateral view. There is a lingual thyroid.

may be a complication of partial or total surgical removal of the ectopic thyroid tissue.

Hypothyroidism may be congenital or acquired, anatomical or functional. It may be permanent ('intrinsic') or transitory ('extrinsic') as a consequence of prematurity or by transplacental influence of a substance ingested by the pregnant mother or by placental transmission of inhibitory immunoglobulins from a mother with autoimmune thyroiditis. Whether any imaging procedure is necessary in an infant with clinically known hypothyroidism and no anterior neck mass is questionable, since it will not affect the management by replacement therapy.

Clinical manifestations of infants with hypothyroidism are sleepiness, sluggishness, low temperature, cold extremities, muscular hypotonia, low heart rate, anaemia, little crying, poor appetite, choking at feeding, large tongue, short neck, constipation, myxoedema

of scalp, eyelids, hands, feet and external genitalia, cardiomegaly, distended abdomen often associated with an umbilical hernia and a wide fontanelle.

Hypothyroidism may be acquired as a consequence of partial or complete removal of an ectopic thyroid gland or follow radiation therapy of the neck for Hodgkin's disease. Nephropathic cystinosis as well as lymphocytic thyroiditis and Hashimoto's disease, are other possible aetiologies of acquired hypothyroidism.

Hashimoto's thyroiditis is the most frequent cause of goitre in this age group as well as the most common overall cause of thyroid disease in paediatrics. There is diffuse infiltration of the thyroid gland causing a heterogeneous scintigraphic pattern with areas of decreased and increased uptake. Ultrasonographically, the gland has a homogeneously reduced echogenicity with symmetrical enlargement of the thyroid (Fig. 7.1.2) and may appear similar to Graves' disease.

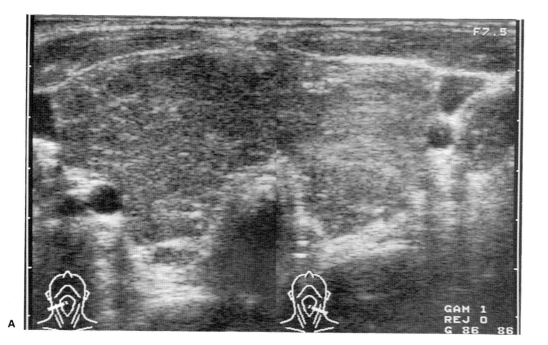

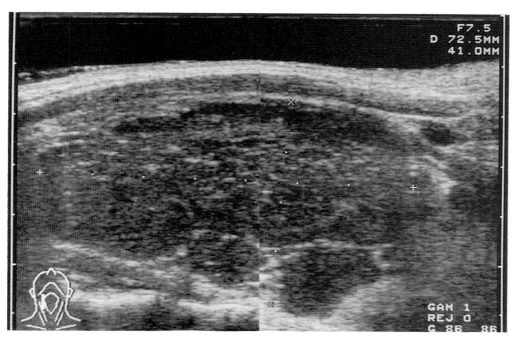

Fig. 7.1.2 Fifteen-year-old hypothyroid boy with Hashimoto's disease. Transverse (**A**) and longitudinal (**B**) ultrasonographic scans show slightly asymmetrical enlargement of thyroid with homogeneous echogenicity. Due to an irregular surface, dorsoinferior portions of the right lobe (**B**) fail to show continuity with the gland. This should not be mistaken for local adenopathy. Also, note the similarity with Graves' disease (Fig. 7.1.4)

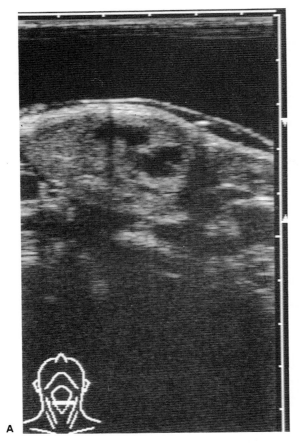

Pendred's syndrome, also referred to as deaf-mutism-goitre-euthyroidism syndrome, may cause hypothyroidism as well as presenting at an early stage without enlargement of the thyroid gland (Fig. 7.1.3).

The commonest cause of hypothyroidism in school-age children is Hashimoto's thyroiditis which is an autoimmune disorder. Initially the children present with an enlarged thyroid and are commonly euthyroid at presentation but occasionally there is initial hyperthyroidism which may lead to a mistaken diagnosis of Graves' disease.

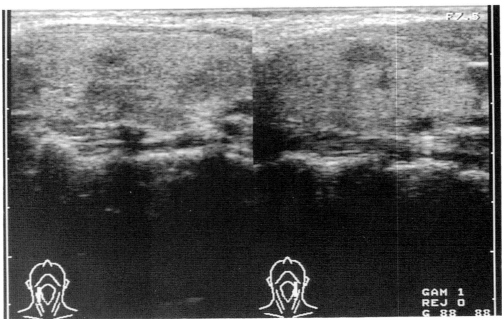

Fig. 7.1.3 Eleven and a half-year-old girl with Pendred's syndrome and primary hypothyroidism. Two years earlier normal size thyroid. Transverse ultrasonographic scans through caudal portions (**A**) of thyroid now show mild to moderate enlargement of gland in the left inferior region with cystic degenerative components as proven by fine needle biopsy. At 15 years, right and left longitudinal scans (**B**) show progression of enlargement and multiple hypoechoic foci bilaterally.

Hyperthyroidism

Graves' disease, although not frequent in paediatrics, is the most common cause of hyperthyroidism in children. The patients will present clinically with goitre, tachycardia, exophthalmus and restlessness. Commonly associated symptoms in Graves' disease are local and diffuse lymphadenopathy, inflammatory infiltrates of the retro-ocular space and splenomegaly. Adrenal insufficiency, myasthenia gravis and pernicious anaemia are recognized associations. Graves' disease may coexist with chronic lymphocytic thyroiditis. While Graves' disease (Fig. 7.1.4) has an ultrasonographic appearance similar to chronic lymphocytic thyroiditis, Hashimoto's disease, it differs from the latter scintigraphically by a homogeneous high photon activity throughout the gland with rapid acquisition of counts. Scintigraphy is not indicated as a routine procedure in these patients because of their characteristic clinical presentation. Graves' disease occurs mainly in girls in adolescence.

Congenital hyperthyroidism is usually transient, lasting weeks to months, and may be seen in children of mothers with active or treated Graves' disease or chronic lymphocytic thyroiditis. Most of these newborns present with goitre, restlessness, tachycardia, respiratory distress and fever. The characteristic radiographic signs are cranial synostosis, frontal bossing and advanced osseous maturation.

The autonomous thyroid adenoma is a rare benign cause of hyperthyroidism in a child (Fig. 7.1.5). It is solid ultrasonographically and shows normal or high photon uptake on scintigraphy.

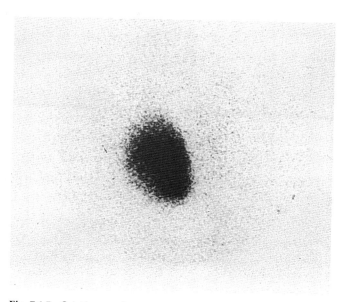

Fig. 7.1.5 Scintigram of autonomous functioning adenoma. This is suppressing all activity from the rest of the gland.

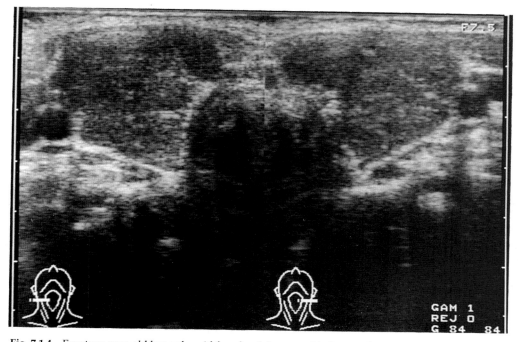

Fig. 7.1.4 Fourteen-year-old hyperthyroid female adolescent with Graves' disease. Transverse ultrasound scan through midportion of thyroid. Symmetrical enlargement of lobes; lobular appearance; homogeneous echo-quality. Note similarity with Hashimoto's disease (Fig. 7.1.2).

Goitre

Goitre is most commonly due to benign enlargement of the thyroid gland, the children being euthyroid. In some cases, it may be associated with hypothyroidism or hyperthyroidism. It may be congenital or acquired, resulting from some hormonal disturbance, or be due to an inflammatory infiltration. Neoplasms will also produce thyroid enlargement, these children also being euthyroid.

In a newborn infant, goitre is often induced by antithyroid drugs or iodide intake during pregnancy. In congenital hyperthyroidism, a goitre is usually present. A thyroid teratoma may mimic goitre, and may contain calcification.

Endemic goitre is due to iodine deficiency and its resulting hyperactivity of the thyroid gland leads to hyperplasia.

Chronic lymphocytic thyroiditis (Hashimoto's thyroiditis), also mentioned under 'Hypothyroidism' above (Fig. 7.1.2), is the most common cause of sporadic goitre. Although it occurs below school age and even in infancy, its frequency is highest in adolescent girls who are euthyroid in most cases. Its course varies from case to case, resolving spontaneously after weeks to months or persisting for years. A common aetiological and genetic basis with Graves' disease has been hypothesized. Goitrous enlargement of the thyroid may occasionally occur in other causes of thyroiditis such as mumps and tuberculosis. Sporadic goitre may be induced by medications containing iodide or a competitive substance such as lithium.

A patient with a colloid goitre, irrespective of size, is typically euthyroid. Its aetiology is not understood. An autoimmune aetiology has been suggested but is unproven. To differentiate it from lymphocytic thyroiditis requires a biopsy. In a multinodular goitre, US may show cystic or solid areas or both, each area being homogeneous or heterogeneous in echo quality.

With time, a solid colloid goitre may become increasingly heterogeneously nodular or cystic by US (Figs. 7.1.6–7.1.8). There may even be calcification from necrosis. Regressive, i.e. cystic, changes may be altered by haemorrhage. However, differentiation ultrasonographically between adenomatous nodular hyperplasia and epithelial neoplasia, i.e. between macro- and micro-follicular adenoma, both being benign, is not possible. Even the hypodense rim of a solid lesion, a frequent ultrasonographic sign of a benign adenoma, is no guarantee of the absence of malignancy (Fig. 7.1.9).

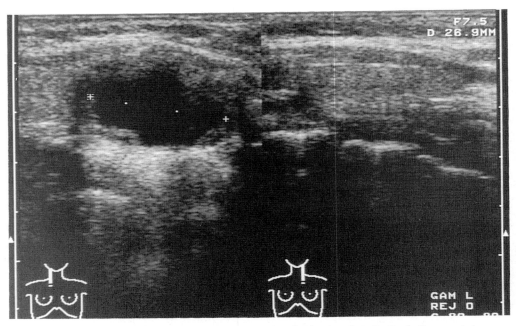

Fig. 7.1.6 Eleven and a half-year-old euthyroid girl with colloid goitre. Longitudinal ultrasound scans through normal left and enlarged right lobes. Purely cystic lesion on the right with irregular hypoechoic rim. Biopsy yielded chronic inflammatory changes with fibrosis; no malignancy.

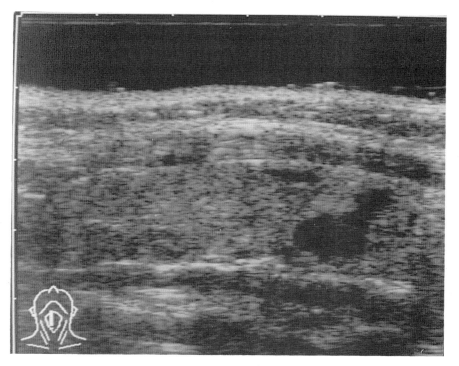

Fig. 7.1.7 Fourteen and a half-year-old euthyroid girl with mild goitre. She has pituitary insufficiency with hypogonadotropic hypogonadism and delayed puberty. Longitudinal ultrasound scan through the right thyroid lobe shows mild nodular heterogenicity with degenerative cystic alterations, with photon-deficient areas on scintigraphy. Fine needle biopsy showed no malignancy.

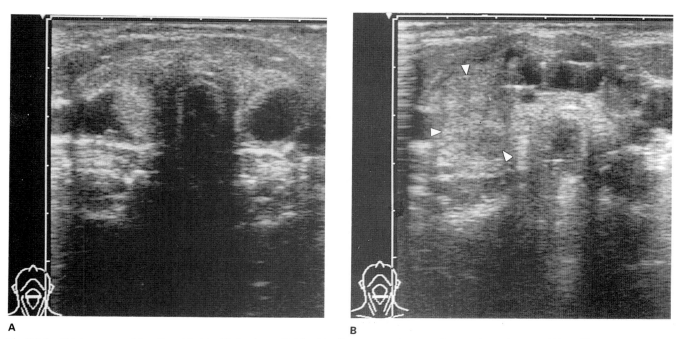

A **B**

Fig. 7.1.8 Thirteen-year-old euthyroid girl with benign colloid goitre. Transverse ultrasound scans through upper (**A**) and lower (**B**) portions of the thyroid gland: hyperplasia confirmed histologically.

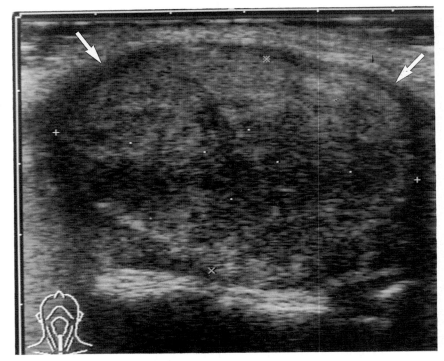

Fig. 7.1.9 Sixteen-year-old euthyroid adolescent girl with benign thyroid adenoma. Longitudinal ultrasound scan shows gross solid enlargement of the entire left lobe with a hypoechoic rim (arrows). Because of complete photon deficiency on scintigraphy, a left hemithyroidectomy with partial resection of the isthmus was performed, which histologically proved to be a follicular adenoma without malignancy.

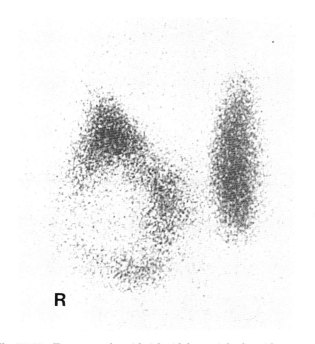

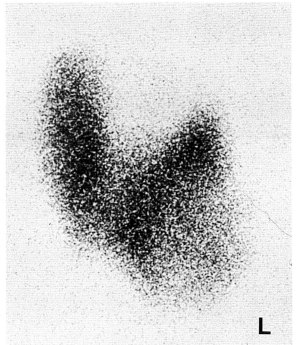

Ultrasonic cystic lesions are photon deficient at scintigraphy. Benign solid ultrasonographic lesions may show normal, deficient or increased photon activity. Scintigraphy cannot differentiate benign and malignant lesions (Figs. 7.1.10, 7.1.11).

US and scintigraphy are complementary and indispensable in the evaluation of a goitre.

Helpful distinguishing features of benign and malignant disease are:

- A normal scintigram does not exclude malignancy while a normal ultrasound examination does with a high degree of confidence.
- A hypoechoic nodular lesion with proven endocrine activity and photon uptake on scintigraphy is very likely to be benign.
- A diffusely hypoechoic nodular lesion with complete photon deficiency at scintigraphy is suspicious of malignancy.

Biopsy is then indicated before partial or total thyroidectomy is performed. Percutaneous needle biopsy is about 90% accurate.

Fig. 7.1.10 Teenage euthyroid girl with large right thyroid mass. Scintigraphy shows a large photopenic area within the lower part of enlarged right thyroid lobe. US (not shown) demonstrated a heterogeneous mass with multiple cystic components in the corresponding location. Right hemithyroidectomy yielded non-functioning benign adenoma.

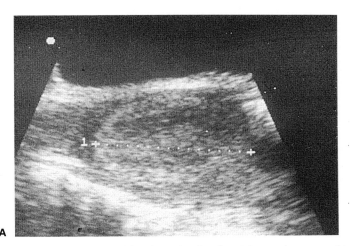

Fig. 7.1.11 Twelve-year-old euthyroid girl with painless neck mass on the left. **A** Longitudinal ultrasound scan of left thyroid lobe shows solid, well-defined mass. **B** Scintigraphy shows left thyroid enlargement by a photopenic mass. A total thyroidectomy was performed. Histology yielded papillary carcinoma.

Thyroid carcinoma

Carcinoma of the thyroid is a rare disease in children. Its clinical manifestation is usually a painless solitary nodule or mass. Associated bilateral cervical lymphadenopathy is common. Metastases occur mainly within the lungs, skeleton and lymphatic system; sites of predilection are the lung bases, skull, long bones as well as cervical, axillary and mediastinal lymph nodes. Pulmonary metastases may have a small, nodular appearance with a miliary distribution.

Most thyroid carcinomas in children are of the papillary type histologically (Figs. 7.1.11, 7.1.12). Less frequent and more aggressive are the follicular or mixed papillary/follicular type carcinomas. A thyroid carcinoma may be associated with benign goitrous abnormalities including thyroiditis. The medullary type of thyroid carcinoma arises from the parafollicular cells (C-cells) which secrete calcitonin, serum levels of which are used in diagnosis and follow-up. This type of carcinoma may occur sporadically, but is also part of the genetic disorder known as multiple endocrine neoplasia syndrome and is associated with phaeochromocytoma, parathyroid hyperplasia and neuromatosis of the intestinal tract including the lips, tongue and buccal mucosa. This type of carcinoma may appear in early childhood and is prone to metastasize early, therefore complete thyroid resection is advocated.

Irradiation to the head and neck is a major aetiological factor in the occurrence of thyroid carcinoma, although the latent period may be in the order of decades. Whether combined radiation and chemotherapy increases the risk of developing malignancy is questionable.

Other anterior neck masses

When an 'anterior neck mass' is observed by the referring clinician, diagnostic imaging is required to identify the site of origin and the kind of 'mass'.

A thyroglossal duct cyst is due to the persistence of the thyroglossal duct, possibly associated with locally developing glandular tissue. Thyroglossal duct cysts may appear at any site along the descent of the thyroid gland from the base of the tongue to the cranial border of the isthmus of the thyroid gland. These cysts are non-tender midline lesions. They may become infected and perforate and, thus, be associated with a thyroglossal duct sinus. A paramedial or anterolateral cystic mass is more likely to be a branchial cleft cyst. If infected, the cyst is tender and should be differentiated from cervical lymphadenopathy, which is much more common, as well as from thyroiditis, although some infected branchial arch cysts especially arising from the pyriform fossae may cause local thyroiditis with decreased isotope uptake. A single medial thyroid or an ectopic thyroid may both present as

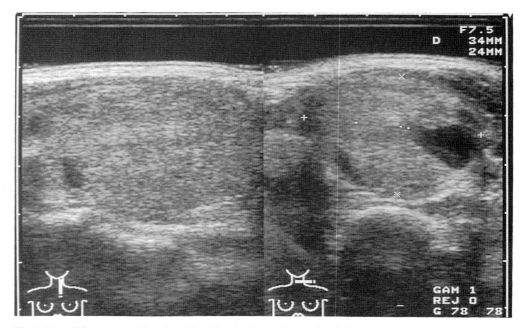

Fig. 7.1.12 Fifteen-year-old euthyroid adolescent boy with painless left thyroid mass. Longitudinal and transverse ultrasound scans through the left thyroid lobe show moderate enlargement with a heterogeneous hyperechoic mass with a few cystic components, which was photon deficient at scintigraphy. A left hemithyroidectomy was performed for a papillary carcinoma.

midline neck masses, the latter also as a paramedian mass.

Cystic lymphangiomas are usually large and multi-loculated ultrasonographically.

Rarely a jugular venous varix may present as a soft cystic swelling in the lateral aspect of the neck. Doppler US examination should be combined with conventional grey-scale imaging in all neck masses to exclude a vascular lesion.

REFERENCES

Bamforth J S, Hughes I, Lazarus J, John R 1986 Congenital anomalies associated with hypothyroidism. Archives of Disease in Childhood 61: 608–609

Bonakdarpour A, Kirkpatrick J A, Renzi A, Kendall N 1972 Skeletal changes in neonatal thyrotoxicosis. Radiology 102: 149–150

Brooks P T, Archard N D, Carty H M L 1988 Thyroid screening in congenital hypothyroidism: a review of 41 cases. Nuclear Medicine Communications 9: 613–617

Connors M A, Styne D M 1986 Transient neonatal 'athyreosis' resulting from thyrotropin binding inhibiting immunoglobulins. Pediatrics 70: 287–290

Gerald B 1968 Cardiac failure in infancy secondary to thyrotoxicosis. Radiology 91: 59–60

Hempelmann L H, Hall W J, Phillips M et al 1975 Neoplasms in persons treated with X-rays in infancy: fourth survey in 20 years. Journal of the National Cancer Institute 555: 519–530

Hernandez R J, Poznanski A K 1979 Distinctive appearance of the distal phalanges in children with primary hypothyroidism Radiology 132: 83–84

Lecklitner M I 1992 Neonatal and pediatric thyroid imaging. In: Sandler M P, Patton J A, Gross M D, Shapiro B, Falke T H M (eds) Endocrine imaging. Appleton & Lange, New York

Lindsay A N, Voorhess M L, MacGillivray M H 1980 Multicystic ovaries detected by sonography in children with hypothyroidism. American Journal of Diseases in Children 134: 588

Lucaya J, Berdon W, Enriques G, Regas J, Carrero J 1990 Congenital pyriform sinus fistula: a cause of acute left sided suppurative thyroiditis and neck abscess in children. Pediatric Radiology 21: 27–30

Muller-Leise C, Troger J, Khabirpour F, Pockler C 1988 Schilddrusenvolumen-Normunerte. Deutsche Medizinische Wochenschrift 113: 1872–1875

Nelson W E 1992 The endocrine system. In: Behrman R E, Kliegman R M, Nelson W E, Vaghan V C (eds) Textbook of pediatrics, 14th ed. W B Saunders, Philadelphia

Refetoff S, Harrison J, Karanifilski B T et al 1975 Continuing occurrence of thyroid carcinoma after irradiation to the neck in infancy and childhood. New England Journal of Medicine 292: 171–175

Rezvani I, DiGeorge A M, Cote M L 1977 Primary hypothyroidism in cystinosis. Journal of Pediatrics 91: 340–341

Riggs W Jr, Wilroy R S Jr, Etteldorf J N 1972 Neonatal hyperthyroidism with accelerated skeletal maturation, craniosynostosis, and brachydactyly. Radiology 105: 621–625

Stewart R R, David C L, Eftedhari F, Ried H L, Fuller L M, Fornage B D 1989 Thyroid gland: US in patients with Hodgkin disease treated with radiation therapy in childhood. Radiology 172: 159–163

Swischuk L E 1970 The beaked, notched, or hooked vertebra; its significance in infants and young children. Radiology 95: 661–664

Vane D, King D R, Dales C T Jr 1984 Secondary thyroid neoplasm in pediatric cancer patients: increased risk with improved survival. Journal of Pediatric Surgery 19: 855–859

7.2 PARATHYROID

EMBRYOLOGY, ANATOMY, FUNCTION

The superior parathyroid glands originate from the fourth branchial pouch. They descend with the thyroid gland to their final correct location adjacent dorsally to the superior parts of the thyroid lobes. The inferior parathyroid glands originating from the third branchial pouch migrate caudally with the thymic gland, sometimes into the superior mediastinum. One-third of inferior parathyroid glands are located within the cervical lobes of the thymus or adjacent to the cricoid cartilage.

Aberrant locations of the superior parathyroid glands may be at various levels between the thyroid and the oesophagus, in close vicinity to the carotid arteries or within the mediastinum. The inferior parathyroid glands are more likely to be aberrant; their ectopic position is variable and includes upper thyroid, intrathyroid or mediastinal location. Figure 7.2.1 shows the distribution of aberrant locations of the parathyroid glands.

Various types of cells comprise the parathyroid glands: chief cells develop after childhood and adolescence into light and dark cells with distinct functions of parathyroid hormone secretion and production; oxyphil and water clear cells become active also after puberty as sites of hormone secretion.

The functional aspects of parathyroid hormone are the absorption of calcium from the gastrointestinal tract, the stimulation of osteoclasts to mobilize calcium and phosphate for resorption, and the inhibition of phosphate resorption and stimulation of calcium resorption in the kidneys.

IMAGING APPROACH AND TECHNIQUES

The object is the detection of the parathyroid glands. Successful localization of an adenoma or hyperplasia of the glands depends largely on whether the glands are in normal or aberrant position. Although US might be the overall initial imaging modality (Fig. 7.2.2), it has become complementary to MRI, if available. The same is true for CT. MRI, because of its sensitivity for tissue differentiation and high degree of specificity for a parathyroid adenoma, is increasingly used for anatomical definition and localization of the glands. Thallium-technetium isotope subtraction scintigraphy is a practical non-invasive method to establish the diagnosis of a functionally active parathyroid adenoma (Fig. 7.2.3), although there is a spectrum of false-positive results. If available, the combination of MRI and dual isotope subtraction scintigraphy seems the best approach for imaging parathyroid-related hyperparathyroidism.

US may be used to guide percutaneous fine needle biopsy for a histological diagnosis of parathyroid adenoma. Digital selective angiography may be used for diagnosis also.

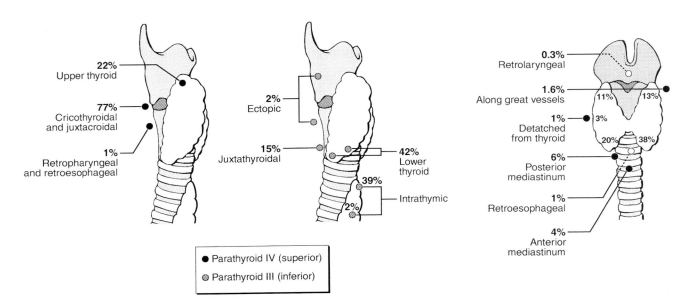

Fig. 7.2.1 Showing position of normal and ectopic location of the parathyroids. (Reproduced with permission from Sacks B A et al 1980 Parathyroid adenomas: cinearteriography. American Journal of Roentgenology 135: 535–538)

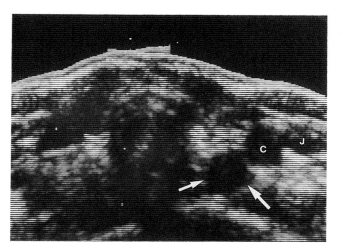

Fig. 7.2.2 Fifteen-year-old girl with primary hyperparathyroidism. Evaluation for recurrent urinary tract infection led to a diagnosis of nephrolithiasis. Because of hypercalcaemia and normal serum phosphorus, the diagnosis was suspected. Transverse compound ultrasound scan just below the thymic isthmus showed a cyst-like mass on the left (arrows). C = Carotid, J = jugular vein. At surgery, the mass proved to be a 10 × 8 × 20 mm solitary adenoma from the aberrantly located left upper parathyroid gland. Both right and lower left parathyroid glands were normal.

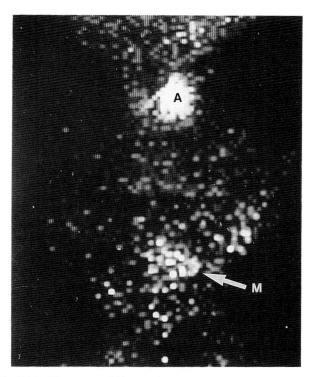

Fig. 7.2.3 Three-year-old boy with polyostotic fibrous dysplasia. Presented as a newborn with rickets and jaundice, multiple rib fractures and, at 6 weeks, with a femoral fracture. Thallium-technetium subtraction scintigraphy shows high photon intensity in the left aspect of the neck due to a functioning solitary parathyroid adenoma (A). Note, less well defined area of activity in the chest due to thallium uptake by the myocardium (M).

PATHOLOGY

Hypoparathyroidism/pseudohypoparathyroidism

Hypoparathyroidism and pseudohyparathyroidism are diagnosed by clinical and laboratory means. Radiographic findings include thickening of the vault and base of the skull, widening of the sutures (from increased intracranial pressure), widespread intracranial calcification, especially in the basal ganglia, choroid plexus and cerebellum, soft tissue calcification and areas of increased bone density.

In pseudohypoparathyroidism (Albright's hereditary osteodystrophy), shortening of the metacarpals, metatarsals and phalanges is a prominent additional feature, as are a relatively narrow lumbar spinal canal, para-articular ossification and calcification and short stature.

Hyperparathyroidism

The most common clinical manifestations of hyperparathyroidism are nephrolithiasis and skeletal abnormalities, i.e. subperiosteal bone resorption, resorption of the lamina dura, general loss of bone density along with a 'ground glass' appearance of the bone, and focal osteoclastic bone lesions (so-called brown tumours associated with haemorrhage in the bone). Primary hyperparathyroidism occurs uncommonly in children, with the most likely cause being a solitary adenoma (Fig. 7.2.3). It may be suspected in the presence of hypercalcaemia or in the absence of a reason for secondary hyperparathyroidism (Figs. 7.2.2, 7.2.3). Investigations may be delayed due to unexplained clinical abnormalities. Parathyroid hyperplasia as a cause for primary hyperparathyroidism and carcinoma is rare.

More common than primary is the occurrence of secondary hyperparathyroidism in children. Its anatomopathological correlate is usually hyperplasia of all parathyroid glands.

Chronic or end-stage glomerular renal disease leading to hyperphosphataemia and hypocalcaemia is the most common cause of secondary hyperparathyroidism in the young patient (Figs. 7.2.4, 7.2.5).

Although osteomalacia and secondary rickets are part of this condition, the primary pathology is ostiitis fibrosa.

Any type of longstanding hypocalcaemia, except for hypoparathyroidism, can induce secondary hyperparathyroidism, e.g. rickets.

Hyperparathyroidism may be associated with abnormalities of other endocrine organs, i.e. the adrenals, pancreas and pituitary gland in the multiple endocrine neoplasia (MEN) syndromes.

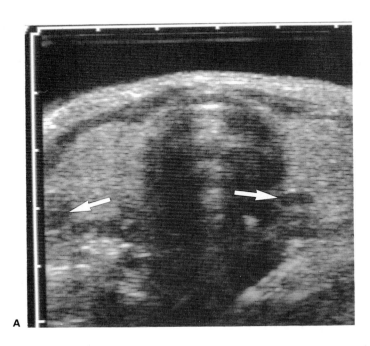

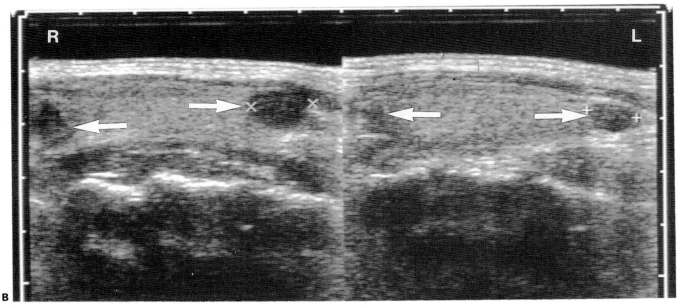

Fig. 7.2.4 Eighteen-year-old female with chronic glomerulonephritis, renal insufficiency and secondary hyperparathyroidism. Transverse ultrasound scan through cranial third of thyroid lobes (**A**) and bilateral longitudinal sections (**B**) show hyperplasia of all four normally located parathyroid glands (arrows). R = Right, L = left.

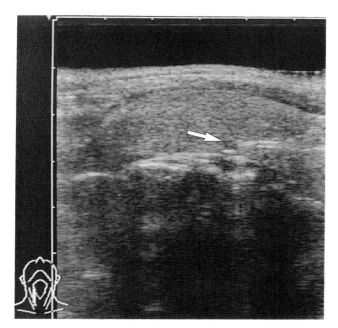

Fig. 7.2.5 Twelve and a half-year-old girl with end-stage renal disease from congenital hypoplastic kidneys and secondary hyperparathyroidism. Longitudinal ultrasound scan through the right thyroid lobe shows the right inferior parathyroid gland (arrow) presumed due to mild hyperplasia with 3.2 mm diameter. The other parathyroid glands were not detectable.

REFERENCES

Auffermann W, Gooding G A W, Okerlund M D, Clark O H, Turner S, Levin K E, Higgins C B 1988 Diagnosis of recurrent hyperparathyroidism: comparison of MR imaging and other imaging techniques. American Journal of Roentgenology 150: 1027–1033

Eftekhari F, Yusefzadeh D K 1982 Primary infantile hyperparathyroidism: clinical, laboratory and radiographic features in 21 cases. Skeletal Radiology 8: 201–208

Erman W A, Breslau N A, Weinreb J C et al 1989 Non-invasive localization of parathyroid adenomas: a comparison of X-ray, computerized tomography, ultrasound, scintigraphy and MRI. Magnetic Resonance Imaging 7: 187–194

Falke T H M, Schipper J, Patton J A, Sandler M P 1992 Parathyroid glands. In: Sandler M P, Patton J A, Gross M D, Shapiro B, Falke T H M (eds) Endocrine imaging. Appleton & Lange, New York

Glass E J, Barr D G D 1981 Transient neonatal hyperparathyroidism secondary to maternal pseudohypoparathyroidism. Archives of Disease in Childhood 56: 565–568

Gooding G A W, Okerlund M D, Stark D D, Clark O H 1986 Parathyroid imaging: comparison of double-tracer (T1-201, Tc-99m) scintigraphy and high-resolution US. Radiology 161: 57–64

Grantmyre E B 1973 Roentgenographic features of 'primary' hyperparathyroidism in infancy. Journal of the Canadian Association of Radiology 24: 257–260

Higgins C B, Aufferman W 1988 MR imaging of thyroid and parathyroid glands: a review of current status. American Journal of Roentgenology 161: 1096–1106

Maltby C, Russell C F, Laird J D et al 1989 Thallium-technetium isotope subtraction scanning in primary hyperparathyroidism. Journal of the Royal College of Surgeons of Edinburgh 34: 40

Sacks B A, Eisenberg H, Pallotta J 1980 Parathyroid adenomas: cinearteriography. American Journal of Roentgenology 135: 535–538

Spritzer C E, Gefter W B, Hamilton R, Greenberg R M, Axel I, Kressel H Y 1987 Abnormal parathyroid glands. High resolution MR imaging. Radiology 162: 487–491

Young A E, Gaunt J T, Croft D N et al 1983 Localisation of parathyroid adenomas by thallium-201 and technetium-99m subtraction scanning. British Medical Journal 286: 1384–1385

7.3 ADRENALS

EMBRYOLOGY, ANATOMY, FUNCTION

The adrenal glands arise from two sites, the mesoderm and the neuroectoderm. The cortical primordium arises from coelomic epithelial cells of the posterior abdominal wall, forming the fetal adrenal cortex around the 6th week of gestation. The medullary primordium derives from sympatic ganglion cells of the neural crest. At 8 weeks' gestation, the medullary primordium 'intrudes' into the cortical primordium and becomes surrounded by the fetal cortex over the following weeks, while the primordium of the permanent cortex differentiates from further mesenchymal cells originating in the coelomic epithelium. From the primordium of the permanent cortex, the zona glomerulosa and the zona fasciculata begin to evolve and differentiate at about the 12th week of gestation. Throughout the intrauterine period the fetal cortex forms the bulk of the adrenal gland. At birth, the fetal cortex accounts for 80% of the size of the gland, the permanent cortex for 20% of the adrenal cortex, while the adrenal medulla consists of a few clusters of chromaffin cells. Involution of the fetal cortex then occurs in the first 4 weeks of life with a corresponding decrease in size of the adrenal gland. By 2–4 months of age no fetal cortex remains. The fetal adrenal gland is 10–20 times larger than the adult gland relative to body size. The third zone of the permanent cortex appears by the age of four. The fetal adrenal medulla consists of a cluster of chromaffin cells and can usually not be appreciated macroscopically at birth. It is only after birth, and somewhat synchronously with the involution of the fetal cortex, that the adrenal medulla will grow to an ultrasonographically recognizable structure.

The adrenal glands are supplied by multiple arteries, arising from the inferior phrenic artery, the aorta, and the renal artery. Venous drainage is by a single cortical vein on the right side which directly enters the inferior vena cava. On the left, after joining the inferior phrenic vein, the adrenal vein enters the renal vein.

The two adrenal glands are not symmetrical. On the right side, the gland assumes a suprarenal dorsomedial position in continuity with the long renal axis. On the left side, the gland lies medially adjacent to the renal upper pole and is slightly anteverted with respect to the kidney. The shape of the adrenal glands is determined by the neighbouring anatomical structures. On the right side, these are the renal upper pole, the posterior segment of the right hepatic lobe, the crus of the diaphragm and, possibly, the inferior vena cava; on the left, the medial aspect of the renal upper pole, the spleen, the crus of the diaphragm and the pancreatic tail.

Epinephrine and norepinephrine are the important hormones produced and secreted by the chromaffin tissue of the adrenal medulla. The sympathetic ganglia and other extra-adrenal chromaffin tissues also secrete norepinephrine. Control of this function is by the splanchnic nerves and acetyl choline released by the central nervous system. The adrenal medulla may be stimulated by stress, both somatic and psychological.

The adrenal cortex produces and secretes different steroid hormones within each of its three zones. Aldosterone secretion occurs in the zona glomerulosa – the outer part of the adrenal cortex – and acts upon the distal nephron to maintain the salt water balance. Cortisol production occurs in the midportion of the adrenal cortex, the zona fasciculata. Androgens are secreted in the zona reticularis, the inner layer of the adrenal cortex adjacent to the adrenal medulla. The hypothalamic–pituitary–adrenal axis consists of a complex control and feedback system controlling production of adrenal cortical hormones, especially cortisol. The renin–angiotensin–aldosterone axis is also a control and feedback system including the juxtaglomerular apparatus for salt water balance.

IMAGING APPROACH AND TECHNIQUES

US is the first imaging technique in the evaluation of suspected adrenal abnormality in a child. Due to the large size of the adrenal glands in the newborn, they are easily seen by US, but ease of visualization decreases rapidly with age. Longitudinal coronal sections with the transducer in the longitudinal renal axis using the kidneys, liver or spleen as an ultrasonographic window are the optimal ultrasonic approach. In case of a mass lesion, a plain abdominal radiographic film supplements the ultrasound examination, recommended for the appreciation of associated calcifications, mass effect and the abdominal gas pattern.

Further imaging of the glands usually by CT, but increasingly by MRI, is indicated in mass lesions. Contrast enhancement of the gastrointestinal tract, dynamic IV contrast enhancement and targetted, narrow contiguous slices are required for CT examination of small adrenal lesions. The child's normal adrenal gland is difficult to see by CT due to lack of body fat and requires meticulous attention to technique. The right adrenal has a bilobed appearance and lies close to the inferior vena cava and liver. The left is more triangular in shape and lies under the tail of the pancreas and the spleen. It is easier to distinguish the adrenals from the surrounding tissues by MR than CT, but movement artefacts arise from bowel movement and respiration and young children will need sedation.

Gross et al have published an excellent review of the different imaging techniques for specific pathological conditions. Both the cortex and medulla may be functionally imaged by scintigraphy – [75]selenocholesterol being used for the adrenal cortex. In paediatrics, adrenal scintigraphy is almost exclusively used for the demonstration of functional activity of a sympathico-adrenergic tumour in the form of ^{123}I-labelled meta-iodobenzylguanidine (MIBG).

More invasive diagnostic procedures such as venous blood sampling and percutaneous biopsy are sometimes of use for diagnosis.

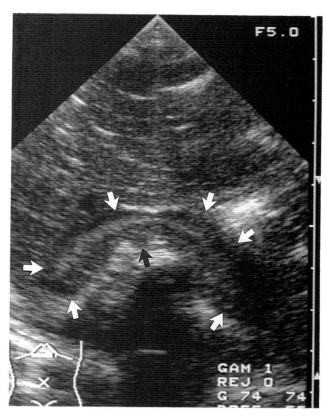

Fig. 7.3.1 Newborn girl on day 1. Asplenia syndrome with right-sided aorta (black arrow) immediately behind 'isthmus', i.e. fusion of adrenals (white arrows) on transverse abdominal US. Child died at 26 hours of life. Autopsy confirmed presence of 'horseshoe adrenal'.

PATHOLOGY

Neuroblastoma is described in Chapter 5.

Most adrenal tumours, except neuroblastoma, in children have clinical endocrine manifestations so that the organ of origin of a mass discovered by imaging is not in doubt. Occasionally lesions arising in structures adjacent to the adrenal glands cause confusion. On the right side, lesions of the kidney, liver, inferior vena cava and gallbladder may mimic adrenal lesions. On the left side, these may originate in the kidney, tail of the pancreas, spleen or accessory spleen and their vessels, stomach, and occasionally a pulmonary sequestration.

Morphological and structural abnormalities

Absence of the adrenal glands has been reported rarely in association with multiple congenital abnormalities and in complex hydrocephalus, possibly as part of a syndrome. Severe hypoplasia or underdevelopment is known to occur in conjunction with anencephaly. Maldevelopment of the fetal adrenal cortex seems to correlate with the structural abnormality of the hypothalamic–pituitary axis, with disturbance of ACTH production or stimulation. Severe hydrocephalus and pituitary lesions may lead to adrenal underdevelopment. In congenital cytomegaly, there may be associated hypoplasia of the adrenal glands with absence or maldevelopment of the permanent fetal cortex leading to adrenal insufficiency. Fusion of the adrenal glands, 'horseshoe' adrenals, is known to be associated with the asplenia syndrome (Fig. 7.3.1), and has also been reported in Cornelia de Lange syndrome and some other rare conditions. Ectopic adrenal cortical tissue has been described in various locations in the abdomen as well as in the thoracic para-aortic regions, the coeliac plexus, broad ligament, epididymis and hilum of the ovary.

Adrenogenital syndrome

21-Hydroxylase deficiency and 11-beta-hydroxylase deficiency account for the vast majority of the adrenal manifestations of this syndrome, also known as congenital adrenal hyperplasia, although adrenal enlargement may be difficult to demonstrate in the individual patient beyond infancy. However, in the newborn, the adrenal glands seem to be larger than average, and a characteristic 'cerebriform morphology' has been described by Wigglesworth (Fig. 7.3.2). Imaging is not routinely indicated.

The more severe form of 21-hydroxylase deficiency characteristically presents with life-threatening salt loss and ambiguous genitalia at birth or in the first few weeks of life. In these patients, adrenal-like tissue has been consistently found within the testes (Fig. 7.3.3).

Adrenoleukodystrophy is characterized by various hypofunctional states of the adrenal cortex associated with a demyelinating disorder of the central nervous system. Its neonatal form presents with seizures and hypotonia at birth and has an especially severe course leading to death within the first 5 years of life. Occasionally associated degenerative hepatic changes in leukodystrophy can lead to a mistaken diagnosis of Zellweger's syndrome, cerebrohepatorenal syndrome, in which the adrenals are normal but there are abnormal cartilaginous calcifications in the epiphyseal regions of hip and knee, and renal cortical cysts.

Wolman's disease is a rare, severe lysosomal disease due to a deficiency of lysosomal acid lipase. Life expectancy is only a few months. The adrenal glands are symmetrically large and heavily calcified and are easily imaged. The inner portion of the zona fasciculata, the zona reticularis and the fetal cortex are involved.

Genetic abnormalities of the adrenal glands leading to disturbance of aldosterone secretion are hypoaldosteronism and hyperaldosteronism. Conn's syndrome, hyperaldosteronism, is rarely found as part of MEN syndromes. The adenoma, which may be very small, may be seen occasionally by US but is best imaged by CT. It appears as a smooth solid low density lesion within the gland. Presentation is with hypertension. In Bartter's syndrome, hyperplasia of the juxtaglomerular apparatus with high renin and angiotension secretion and subsequent hypokalemic alkalosis, moderate adrenal enlargement affecting the zona glomerulosa is usually present. Transient pseudohypoaldosteronism with salt wasting occurs in neonates due to aldosterone-receptor deficiency as well as in conjunction with sepsis in obstructive uropathy.

Adrenal insufficiency, i.e. Addison's disease, occurs in a large number of adrenal developmental disorders, i.e. adrenal hypoplasia, some forms of congenital adrenal hyperplasia, congenital adrenoleukodystrophy and Wolman's disease, but also transiently in newborns. The most frequent abnormality leading to adrenal insufficiency is cytotoxic autoimmune atrophy of the adrenal gland. Imaging is not indicated. A radiographically small heart has been described in some children. Occasional complications of treatment, mainly steroid related, such as moniliasis of the oesophagus may be encountered.

Infection

Various infective agents may affect the adrenal glands. Tuberculosis may cause granulomatous change and even abscess formation (Fig. 7.3.4). The adrenal gland will calcify following treatment. Most calcified adrenal

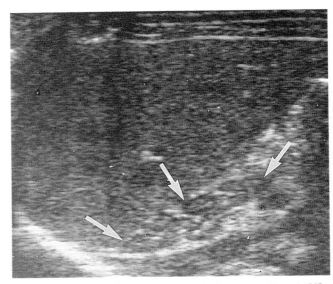

Fig. 7.3.2 Seven-week-old boy. Failure to thrive, vomiting. At US no evidence of hypertrophic pyloric stenosis, but relatively large adrenal glands with convoluted 'cerebriform' arrangement (arrows); right longitudinal US view.

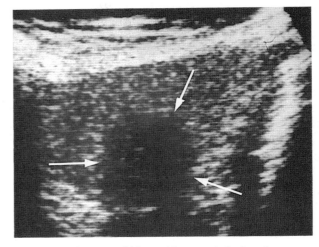

Fig. 7.3.3 Twelve-year-old boy with congenital adrenal hyperplasia, diagnosed at 6 weeks of age with salt loss. Longitudinal ultrasound scan of right testis showed well-defined hypoechoic intrinsic lesion, 'testicular adrenal-like tissue' (arrows).

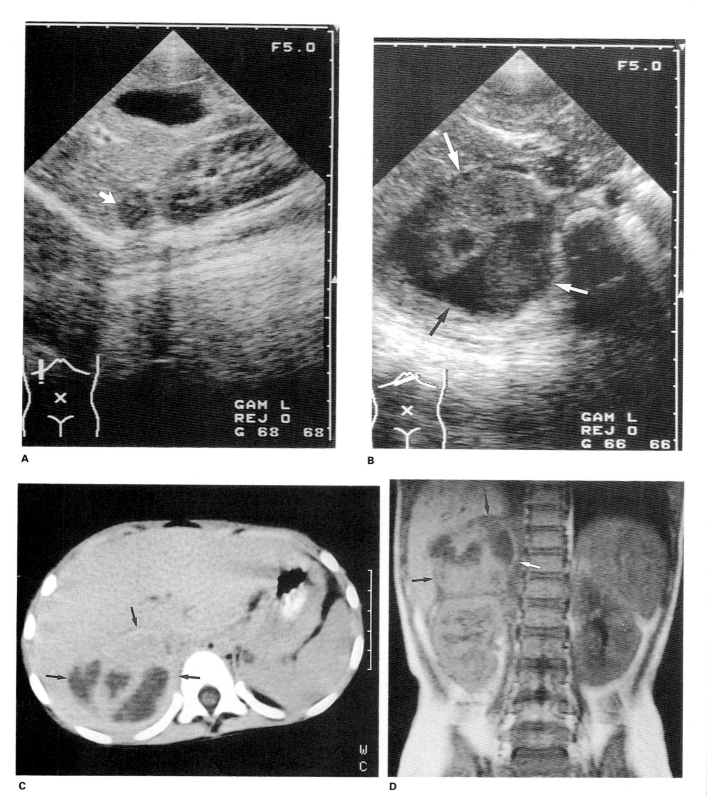

A

B

C

D

Fig. 7.3.4   Almost 3-year-old girl. BCG-vaccination at 5 months of age into left deltoid region. Subsequently a local solitary ulcerative lymph node was removed as well as a secondary solitary right inguinal lymph node abscess. **A** Longitudinal ultrasound scan through the right abdomen 4 months later showed mild adrenal enlargement (arrow), while the child was well. Eight months later, the child became very sick. **B** Transverse ultrasound scan through right upper abdominal quadrant showed a huge heterogenic adrenal mass (arrows), confirmed by CT without intravenous contrast (**C**) and MRI (**D**) and impinging on the kidney. At operation a tuberculous abscess was evacuated.

glands discovered on abdominal radiography in the western world are the result of adrenal haemorrhage and not tuberculosis. This is of no clinical consequence and is not associated with adrenal insufficiency. Acute infectious involvement may also be caused by a variety of viruses, such as cytomegalovirus, herpes simplex virus, enterovirus and echovirus.

Meningococcal septicaemia may be associated with acute adrenal insufficiency and hypotensive collapse – the Waterhouse-Friderichsen syndrome – due to haemorrhagic necrosis of the adrenal glands. At ultrasound examination the adrenal haemorrhage is usually easy to see. If the child recovers, adrenal calcification usually follows. Pneumococcal and streptococcal septicaemia may also occasionally involve the adrenal glands. Fungal agents, candida and aspergillus, may colonize the adrenal glands as opportunistic infection.

Cushing's syndrome

Cushing's syndrome, rare below 7 years, may be caused by bilateral hyperplasia of the adrenal cortex, usually due to a primary pituitary tumour or a disruption of the hypothalamic–pituitary–adrenal regulating mechanism, or by a primary adrenal tumour. Clinical, endocrine and radiological investigation is directed towards identifying the source of the endocrine malfunction. US of the abdomen is the first imaging procedure, followed by CT if a tumour is located. In suspected adrenal hyperplasia, imaging of the brain and pituitary gland is indicated. Other radiological manifestations of Cushing's disease include osteoporosis with vertebral compression fractures and increased fat deposition in the subcutaneous tissues, mediastinum and abdomen. Tumours of the adrenal cortex may be adenomas (Fig. 7.3.5) or carcinomas (Fig. 7.3.6). Both may calcify and undergo central necrosis. Carcinomas may metastasize to the lungs. The radiological differentiation of carcinoma and adenoma is based on the size of the tumour rather than imaging characteristics. Tumours over 6 cm in size are usually carcinomas. Bilateral tumours may occur. Regression of symptoms follows resection of the primary tumour.

Cushing's syndrome may be produced by primary adrenocortical nodular hyperplasia as an autosomal dominant disease with associated myxoma formation within various parts of the body including the skin and heart. Other primary lesions such as neuroblastoma and islet cell adenoma of the pancreas may occasionally lead to adrenocortical hyperplasia and Cushing's syndrome. Exogenous administration of glucocorticoids or ACTH as well as endogenous overproduction of ACTH mediated by some hypothalamic/pituitary process are further causes of Cushing's syndrome. Virilization may be an associated sign in an adrenal adenoma or carcinoma, in the child presenting with 'precocious puberty'.

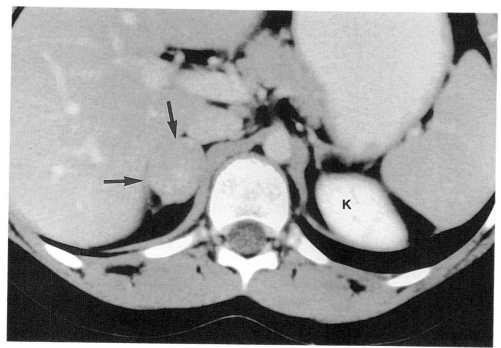

Fig. 7.3.5 Nine and a half-year-old girl with Cushing's syndrome. A suspicion of an adrenal tumour was confirmed by CT. Transverse scan with intravenous contrast demonstrates a right suprarenal, solid mass (arrows). Histology after resection was consistent with an adrenal adenoma. K = left renal upper pole, contrast enhanced.

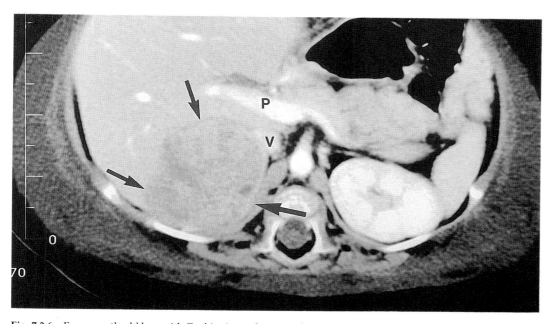

Fig. 7.3.6 Four-month-old boy with Cushing's syndrome and suspicion of adrenal tumour. US confirmed right suprarenal mass. CT with intravenous contrast showed mild heterogenic enhancement of a moderately large tumour mass (arrows), displacing the inferior vena cava (V). Histology after resection of tumour yielded evidence of malignancy, although there were no metastases. P = portal vein.

Phaeochromocytoma

Children with a phaeochromocytoma present with hypertension. The tumour is rare in childhood, occasionally familial with an autosomal dominant inheritance, and may be found as part of the MEN syndromes. It is also rarely found in association with the phakomatoses. The tumour mostly occurs in the adrenal medulla, but common extra-adrenal sites are the retroperitoneum, and mediastinum and the urinary bladder. Acute hypertensive crises may occur during micturition in children with tumours located in the bladder. Although the tumours may be multiple, they are usually benign. Malignant tumours may metastasize to bone, liver and lungs. Histologically benign phaeochromocytomas may be locally aggressive and invasive, making resection difficult or impossible if they involve major vessels.

The clinical diagnosis is based on the discovery of raised urinary catecholamines. Imaging is then directed to locating the tumour. US of the adrenal glands is the primary imaging technique, followed by CT (Fig. 7.3.7). Scintigraphy with ^{123}I-MIGB will help determine if the tumour is unilateral or bilateral (Fig. 7.3.7). Doppler US and CT will confirm that the major vessels are not involved. If the adrenal glands are normal, further imaging should be deferred until after ^{123}I-MIGB scanning to locate the tumour. Imaging of the abnormal focus of uptake by CT or MRI is then required for surgical planning and may be supplemented by venous sampling for hormonal assay using percutaneous catheterization techniques.

A phaeochromocytoma is usually of homogeneous echo texture and on CT is also of uniform density, seldom with central necrosis. In endocrinely active but non-resectable tumours, therapy with ^{131}I-MIBG may be successful.

Primitive neuroectodermal tumour (PNET)

PNET, more common in the central than in the peripheral nervous system, is related to neuroblastoma and Askin's tumour and is similar in many respects although cytogenetically different.

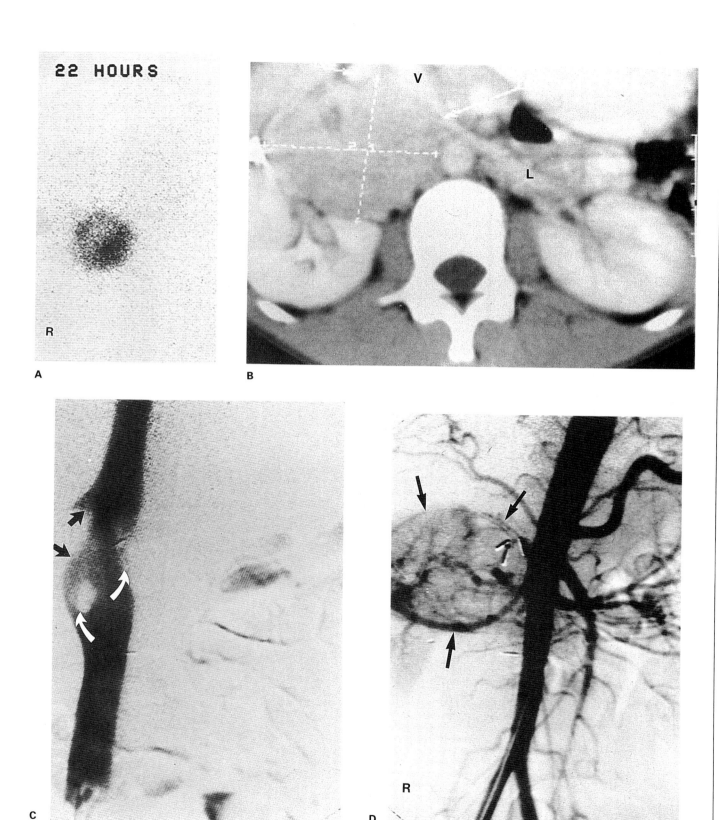

Fig. 7.3.7 Twelve-year-old boy with hypertension. US showed solid mass in right adrenal region, thought to be a phaeochromocytoma. Catecholames were high. **A** ^{123}I-MIBG scintigraphy showed intensive uptake by tumour at 22 hours. **B** CT with intravenous contrast showed the lesion impinging on the right kidney and displacing the inferior vena cava (V). L = left renal vein. There were two attempts at surgery. Only partial resection was possible due to invasion of the inferior vena cava. **C** Digital subtraction cavography showed a distorted right contour by tumour invasion (black arrows). Flow defects from renal veins (curved arrows). Histology yielded paraganglioma. The child was treated with ^{131}I-MIBG. Tumour size remained stable, but tumour activity decreased. **D** Digital subtraction arteriography by aortic injection showed the vascular supply of the tumour (arrows).

Adrenal haemorrhage

Adrenal haemorrhage occurs almost exclusively in newborns in association with perinatal asphyxia or trauma but also may occur with bacterial septicaemia. Acute or late adrenal insufficiency is rare, even in bilateral and gross adrenal haemorrhage. The haemorrhagic process may involve both (Fig. 7.3.8) or one (Figs. 7.3.9, 7.3.10) of the adrenal glands or only one part of a gland (Fig. 7.3.11). In a moderate or massive degree of adrenal haemorrhage, there is clinically a palpable flank mass due to the mass effect of the haemorrhage with caudal displacement of the kidney. However, renal vein thrombosis is a common association and may cause true renal enlargement. The mass is usually not palpable at birth and develops over the subsequent 24 hours. The child will often become jaundiced and present with vomiting. The mass usually regresses rapidly with resorption of the clot. Posthaemorrhagic calcification subsequently occurs and is the commonest cause of adrenal calcification seen on abdominal radiographs.

US demonstrates these morphological changes along with the changes of the echo quality due to clot formation and involution (Fig. 7.3.8).

If there is no ultrasonographic resolution after several days, other diagnoses, including neuroblastoma and its variants, but also benign conditions such as an adrenal cyst or extra-adrenal abnormalities from a surrounding organ including an enteric duplication cyst, need to be considered.

Post-traumatic adrenal haemorrhage has been described in blunt abdominal injury in some 3% of cases mostly associated with liver, spleen or kidney trauma. This usually occurs on the right but without evidence of subsequent adrenocortical insufficiency.

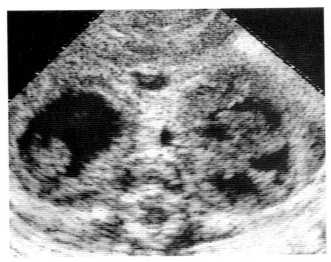

Fig. 7.3.8 Newborn with bilateral adrenal haemorrhage. Transverse ultrasound scan through the upper abdomen at 7 days. There is bilateral heterogeneity due to the coagulation process within initially completely 'cystic' adrenal glands. Ten weeks later there was complete resolution of the haemorrhages without calcification.

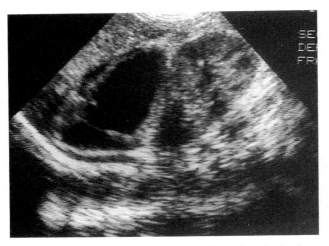

Fig. 7.3.9 Newborn with adrenal haemorrhage. Longitudinal ultrasound scan through the right abdomen showed massive enlargement of the adrenal gland from haemorrhage. Note adrenal mass effect upon kidney with flattening and caudal displacement.

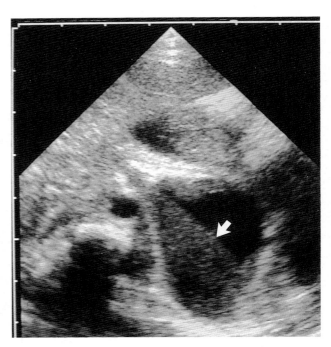

Fig. 7.3.10 Newborn with left-sided adrenal haemorrhage in conjunction with ipsilateral renal vein thrombosis. Initially completely cystic appearance. Transverse ultrasound scan at 3 days of age showed fluid–fluid level (arrow) from sedimentation. (Oblique position of transducer.)

REFERENCES

Armanini D, Kuhnle U et al 1985 Aldosterone-receptor deficiency in pseudohypoaldosteronism. New England Journal of Medicine 313: 1178–1181

Burke B A 1992 The pituitary, pineal, adrenal, thyroid, and parathyroid glands. In: Stocker J T, Dehner L P (eds) Pediatric pathology. Lippincott, Philadelphia

Carty A, Stanley P 1974 Bilateral adrenal abscesses in a neonate. Pediatric Radiology 1: 63–64

Cohen E K, Daneman A, Stringer D A, Soto G, Thorner P 1986 Focal adrenal hemorrhage: a new US appearance. Radiology 161: 631–633

deSa D D 1991 The adrenal glands. In: Wigglesworth J S, Singer D B (eds) Textbook of fetal and perinatal pathology. Blackwell Scientific Publications, Oxford

Evans A E, D'Angio G J, Randolph J 1971 A proposed staging for children with neuroblastomas. Children's Cancer Study Group A. Cancer 27: 374–378

Gross M D, Falke T H M, Shapiro B, Sandler M P 1992 Adrenal glands. In: Sandler M P, Patton J A, Gross M D, Shapiro B, Falke T H M (eds) Endocrine imaging. Appleton & Lange, New York

Harrison R B, Francke P Jr 1977 Radiographic exhibit; radiographic findings in Wolman's disease. Radiology 124: 188

Kelley R I, Datta N S, et al 1986 Neonatal adrenoleukodystrophy: new cases, biochemical studies, and differentiation from Zellweger and related peroxisomal polydystrophy syndromes. American Journal of Medical Genetics 23: 896–901

Lough J, Fawcett J, Wiegensberg B 1970 Wolman's disease. An electron microscopic, histochemical, and biochemical study. Archives of Pathology 89: 103–110

McCauley R G K, Beckwith J B, Elias E R, Faerber E N, Prewitt L H Jr, Berdon W E 1991 Benign hemorrhagic adrenocortical macrocysts in Beckwith–Wiedemann syndrome. American Journal of Roentgenology 157: 549–552

Moore K L 1988 The urogenital system. In: Moore K L (ed) The developing human, 4th edn. W B Saunders, Philadelphia

Neville A M, O'Hare M J 1982 The human adrenal cortex. Springer, Berlin

Page D L, DeLellis R A, Hough A J 1986 Neuroblastoma. In: Hartman W N, Gobin L H (eds) Tumors of the adrenal. Washington, D C, Armed Forces Institute of Pathology

Rodriguez-Soriano J, Vallo A, Oliveros R, Castillo G 1983 Transient pseudohypoaldosteronism secondary to obstructive uropathy in infancy. Journal of Pediatrics 103: 375–380

Sivit C J, Hung W, Taylor G A, Catena L M, Brown-Jones C, Kushner D C 1991 Sonography in neonatal congenital adrenal hyperplasia. American Journal of Roentgenology 156: 141–143

Sivit C J, Ingram J D, Taylor G A, Bulas D I, Kushner D C, Eichelberger M R 1992 Post-traumatic adrenal hemorrhage in children: CT findings in 34 patients. American Journal of Roentgenology 158: 1299–1302

Symington T 1982 The adrenal cortex. In: Bloodworth J M B (ed) Endocrine pathology, general and surgical, 2nd edn. Williams & Wilkins, Baltimore

Willi U, Atares M, Prader A, Zachmann M 1991 Testicular adrenal-like tissue (TALT) in congenital adrenal hyperplasia: detection by ultrasonography. Pediatric Radiology 21: 284–287

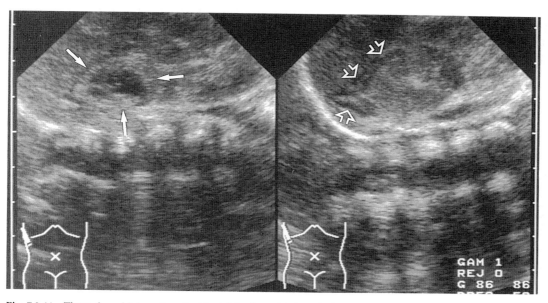

Fig. 7.3.11 Three-day-old, term boy. Incidental finding of right-sided partial adrenal haemorrhage. Coronal ultrasound scans showed mild to moderate cystic enlargement of the medial part of the adrenal gland (arrows) and normal lateral aspect (open arrows). Complete spontaneous resolution 2 weeks later with no calcification. Note the difficulty in differentiating the permanent from the fetal cortex in the haemorrhagic part of the gland.

7.4 PANCREAS

EMBRYOLOGY, ANATOMY, FUNCTION

The pancreas forms from a dorsal and ventral primordium, arising in the 5th gestational week from the ventral foregut. The ventral bud consists of a right and a left portion. Only the right one persists, rotating dorsally along the duodenum and fusing with the dorsal primordium at 7 weeks of gestation, while the left portion regresses (Fig. 7.4.1). The dorsal primordium forms the body and tail of the pancreas and variably the duct of Santorini; the persisting part of the ventral primordium forms the pancreatic head and uncinate process as well as the duct of Wirsung. Exocrine or acinar differentiation becomes apparent at 10 weeks of gestation but further development is slow until birth. After birth, it develops rapidly. The endocrine islet cells differentiate from the ductular system of the pancreas. The distribution of islet cells varies between fetal, neonatal and later life. The relative mass of endocrine pancreatic tissue is greatest during the third trimester of gestation, decreasing rapidly in relation to the developing exocrine tissue after birth. The alpha-cells are the first to appear at 9 weeks of gestation, producing glucagon. D-cells generate somatostatin, beta-cells insulin and PP-cells the pancreatic peptides. There is controversy about the origin of the pancreatic islets of Langerhans and it is unclear whether the cells originate from the same endodermal source as the exocrine acini, or whether there are different types of endoderm for the two different tissues, or whether the two types of cells may react differently according to their respective functional demands. Exocrine enzyme secretion, trypsin, chymotrypsin and lipase, begins shortly before the third trimester of pregnancy. Secretion of amylase occurs only after birth. There is wide interaction of the pancreatic exocrine secretion with cholecystokinin, pancreozymin and secretin. The endocrine secretion is controlled by neural elements and by endocrine 'signals' from the intestine to the islets.

IMAGING APPROACH AND TECHNIQUE

The pancreas can be well demonstrated by US, which is the first imaging procedure, but also by CT or MRI. Proportionately, the AP dimensions of the pancreas are greater than in the adult; consequently, if the body of the pancreas measures more than 1.5 cm at any age, enlargement is present. Ultrasound echogenicity is variable and low echogenicity in the very young can be normal and not indicative of pancreatitis. Two main ultrasonographic approaches are used, the oblique transverse ventral view using the liver as an acoustic window or, in a thin patient with no air in the stomach, the direct view through the abdominal wall. The normal duct of Wirsung will only be appreciable longitudinally as a fine linear echostructure running through the central part of the pancreas. A second plane from the left flank is longitudinal-coronal, using the spleen as the acoustic window and angling the transducer ventrally, and may show the tail. Alternatively, a longitudinal-oblique ventral scanning plane with angulation of the transducer from its midline position to the left side toward the spleen may permit visualization of the pancreatic tail.

Oral contrast is essential in CT evaluation, particularly to assess the head. If the lumen of the duct is clearly delineated, it is likely to be enlarged. Axial slices should be 5 mm or less. A first pass should be

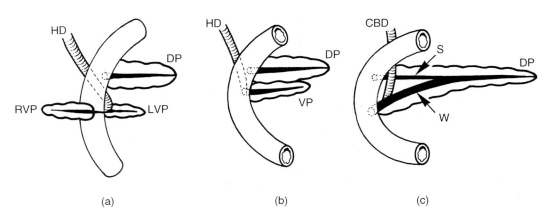

(a)   (b)   (c)

Fig. 7.4.1 Developmental anatomy of the pancreas. HD, hepatic duct; DP, dorsal pancreas; RVP, right ventral pancreas; LVP, left ventral pancreas; CBD, common bile duct; S, duct of Santorini; W, Wirsung.

done without intravenous contrast. A rapid sequence should then follow with bolus injection of intravenous contrast.

MRI may demonstrate tumours on the basis of their contrast properties in the different sequences. Angiography may be necessary in the context of a gastroenteropancreatic tumour for localization of the tumour as well as transhepatic portal vein catheterization and blood sampling for quantitative hormone assay.

PATHOLOGY

Annular pancreas

Failure of posterior migration of the ventral primordium as well as premature fixation of the latter to the duodenum prior to its dorsal rotation both result in a ring-like morphology of the pancreatic head area. Annular pancreas is known to be associated with trisomy 21, tracheoesophageal fistula, intrinsic duodenal obstruction and rotation anomalies of the gastrointestinal tract. The fusion of the two primordia may be incomplete or absent. In the latter case, a relative stenosis of the duct of Santorini may occur as the child grows, leading to obstructive pancreatitis. Any congenital maldevelopment may be associated with pancreatitis.

Ectopic pancreatic tissue has been described in the wall of the proximal gastrointestinal tract, including stomach, duodenum and jejunum, but also in the liver, the porta hepatis and the mesentery as well as in association with enteric duplication anomalies. The ectopic tissue may consist of both exocrine and endocrine components, contain only exocrine tissue, or be just adenomatous proliferation of ducts.

Pancreatic aplasia

Incomplete development of the pancreas may occur. This may be limited to exocrine aplasia, or complete agenesis with absence of both the exocrine and the endocrine part of the organ may occur. Incomplete formation may involve a specific anatomical area of the pancreas.

Other associations

Polycystic renal disease and various syndromes, such as Saldino–Noonan, Jeune's, Meckel–Gruber and the trisomies 13, 18 and 21 may characteristically involve the pancreas by various degrees of cystic changes.

Exocrine abnormalities

Hypoglycaemia, hyperinsulinaemia

Hypoglycaemia in infants is frequently a transitory phenomenon, related to intrauterine growth retardation, maternal drug ingestion particularly of hypoglycaemic agents. If persisting into infancy and childhood, hypoglycaemia may be caused by hyperinsulinism, various enzyme deficiencies, other endocrine insufficiencies such as panhypopituitarism, congenital heart disease, or be due to drugs such as ethyl alcohol or salicylates.

Excess insulin secretion should be considered when hypoglycaemia is unaccompanied by enlargement of the liver or in the presence of excess ketones in the blood or urine.

Hyperinsulinism can result from beta cell pancreatic adenoma, or hyperplasia, but localized benign or malignant endocrinely active tumours of the pancreas are rare in infants or children. More common in children under 1 year is the condition of nesidioblastosis, in which there are increased numbers of beta cells in the exocrine portion of the pancreas.

Because of the diffuse involvement of the pancreas, imaging procedures such as US or CT generally have little to offer in the evaluation of these infants before they undergo the usual treatment of subtotal pancreatectomy. Increased echogenicity has been described with US but the specificity of this technique is too low. In the older child, where more discrete lesions may occasionally be found in the form of an adenoma, pancreatic US and CT may demonstrate the lesion. Such insulinomas are poorly reflective. In older children, retrograde percutaneous catheterization of the pancreatic branches of the splenic vein may allow not only confirmation of the diagnosis of hyperinsulinism but also some degree of localization. Similarly, intraoperative US has proved a useful diagnostic technique.

Should an islet cell adenoma be diagnosed, particularly in later childhood, hyperparathyroidism, excess gastrin secretion and pituitary tumours may be associated, sometimes familially, in the MEN syndromes, MEN type I.

True endocrine hyperplasia has been demonstrated in infants of diabetic mothers, in adenomatosis of the pancreas, and in Beckwith–Wiedemann syndrome. In children of diabetic mothers, there is hypertrophy of the islets as well as increase of the individual islet cell volume, pleomorphism of the B-cell nuclei, eosinophil infiltration and peri- as well as intra-insular fibrosis.

Diabetes mellitus

The idiopathic forms, either insulin dependent or non-insulin dependent, are much the commonest cause of this condition. Insulin insufficiency, however, may be due to localized pancreatic disease such as congenital hypoplasia, following surgery or pancreatitis, associated with some other endocrine conditions such as Cushing's syndrome, acromegaly, associated with drug ingestion and, rarely, as part of genetically determined syndromes such as hyperlipidaemia, the

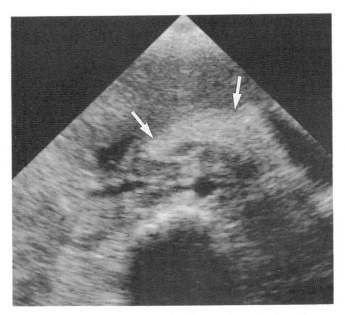

Fig. 7.4.2 Mitochondrial cytopathy (Kearns–Sayre syndrome). Fibrolipomatous atrophy of the pancreas with exocrine and endocrine insufficiency with diabetes mellitus.

Prader–Willi syndrome, and myotonic dystrophy. Diabetes mellitus with fatty infiltration of the pancreas is a feature of mitochondrial cytopathy (Kearns–Sayre syndrome); also associated are progressive external ophthalmoplegia, retinitis pigmentosa, cardiac conduction defects, delayed sexual maturation and hypoparathyroidism (Fig. 7.4.2).

Children with diabetes mellitus are at increased risk of chest disease, particularly pulmonary tuberculosis, and this is one of the rare occasions in childhood where routine chest radiography is indicated. Radiological features of the disease otherwise in childhood are not prominent, although there is a generalized increased risk of infections. Abnormal motility in the gastrointestinal tract is a recognized complication, as is renal enlargement, which may be associated with the nephrotic syndrome.

Pancreatitis, trauma and pseudocyst

Pancreatitis is uncommon in childhood and rare in the infant and newborn. Most pancreatitis is associated with trauma, and the position of the pancreas draped over the vertebral bodies and close to the child's anterior abdominal wall is a predisposing factor in blunt blows to the abdomen. Many such injuries are accidental but traumatic pancreatitis is a feature of the physically abused child.

There are a variety of other causes of pancreatitis which include viruses such as infectious mononucleosis and mumps, steroids, L-asparaginase, biochemical abnormalities (such as hyperparathyroidism, hypercalcaemia and hyperlipidaemia), anaphylactoid purpura and hereditary pancreatitis, which is often calcific.

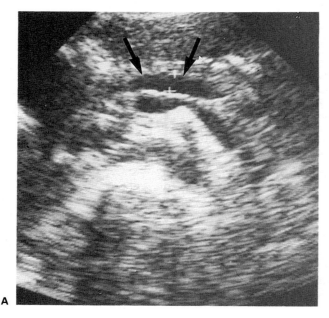

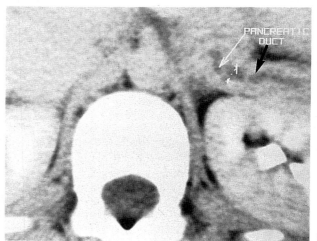

Fig. 7.4.3 Pancreatitis with enlargement of the duct. (**A**) US. (**B**) CT.

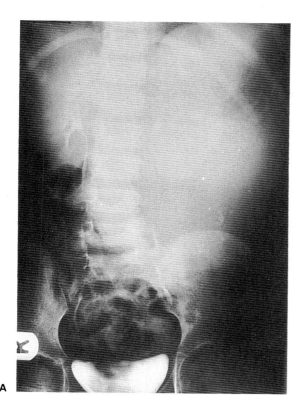

Radiographic examination is usually by plain abdominal radiographs and US. Enlargement and increased sonolucency of the pancreas with dilatation of the pancreatic duct are features (Fig. 7.4.3). The necrosis associated with release of pancreatic enzymes can produce large cystic areas in the region of the pancreas itself and in the retroperitoneum, and such collections can extend up into the pleural cavities, mediastinum and pericardial sac. Ascites is common (Fig. 7.4.4). An upper gastrointestinal study frequently reveals oedematous thickening of the mucosal pattern of the duodenum and upper small bowel, with displacement of the bowel from the mass effect of any pseudocyst. In cases of blunt trauma, it is important to remember the possible coincidence of transection of the duodenal loop in addition to traumatic pancreatitis. US is of particular value in the monitoring of resolution of pancreatic inflammation and pseudocysts which are usually treated conservatively, although percutaneous drainage may be undertaken, but CT is better in initial evaluation, particularly of trauma.

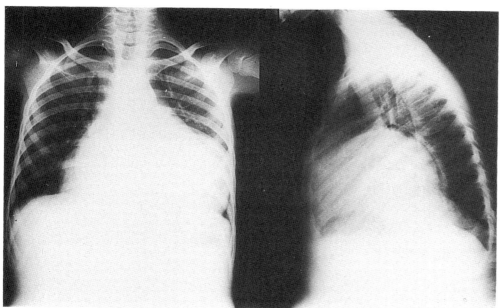

Fig. 7.4.4 Pancreatic pseudocyst with abdominal calcification shown on urography (**A**) extending into the thorax (**B**).

As most pancreatitis in childhood is not recurrent, calcification is not a prominent feature, but may be marked in the recurrent hereditary pancreatitis (Fig. 7.4.5). Recurrent, unexplained pancreatitis may also arise in association with abnormalities of the ducts of Santorini and Wirsung, particularly in the presence of pancreas divisum. Choledochal cysts and biliary calculi should be excluded. Pancreatitis may be associated with duplications of the stomach and duodenum. Ascaris is a bile-loving nematode and an occasional cause of pancreatitis.

The enlargement of the pancreatic head can cause obstructive jaundice (Fig. 7.4.6).

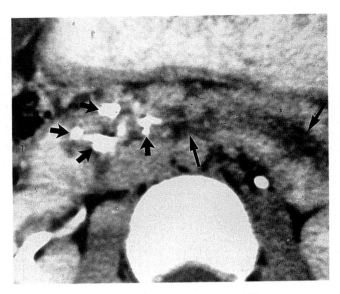

Fig. 7.4.5 Hereditary pancreatitis in an 8-year-old boy. Calcification (short arrows) and dilated pancreatic duct (long arrows).

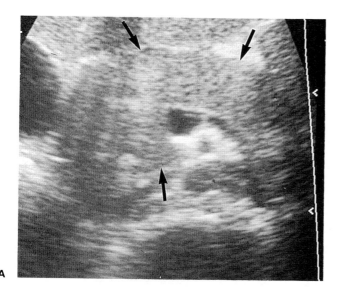

A

Fig. 7.4.6 Pancreatitis, simple chronic. Presentation with abdominal pain and jaundice. US (**A**) shows pancreatic enlargement, confirmed by CT (**B, C**). **D** Percutaneous cholangiogram shows narrowing of distal common bile duct in pancreatic head.

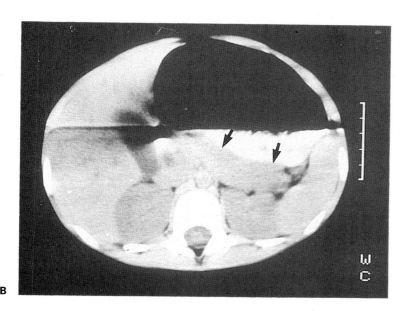

B

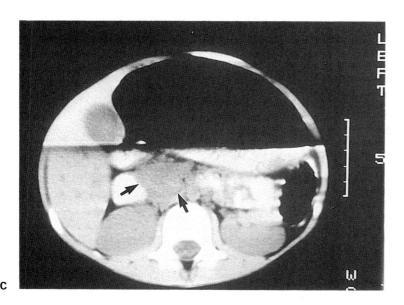

C

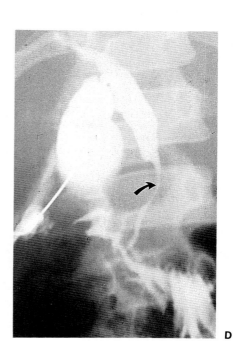

D

In mucoviscidosis (cystic fibrosis of the pancreas) exocrine pancreatic function is typically deficient. Fatty replacement of the pancreas is easily perceived on CT and revealed by increased echogenicity via US (Fig. 7.4.7). In later childhood, punctate calcifications may be seen on plain abdominal radiography and ectasia of the pancreatic duct is seen on US. The advent of paediatric endoscopes has facilitated delineation of the pancreatic and biliary duct systems in greater detail than can be achieved by US.

Inspissation of pancreatic secretions may also occur in various states of dehydration, acidosis or with hyperalimentation.

The Pearson syndrome consists of refractory sideroblastic anaemia with iron deposition, and is associated with pancreatic fibrosis and insufficiency. The pancreas is highly echogenic as in cystic fibrosis (Fig. 7.4.8). The same can be found in neonatal haemochromatosis which may involve the entire pancreas in addition to the liver and heart.

Shwachman's syndrome in which pancreatic insufficiency is associated with cyclical neutropenia and metaphyseal chondrodysplasia shows fatty replacement of the pancreas with high echogenicity (Fig. 7.4.8). High echogenicity is a feature of thalassaemia and haemosiderosis (Fig. 7.4.9).

True cysts of the pancreas are a well-recognized feature of polycystic disease of the kidney (autosomal dominant type) in later life. Von Hippel–Lindau disease may include true pancreatic cysts as well as solid tumours. Pancreaticoblastomas often seen in Beckwith–Wiedemann syndrome can similarly present as solid or cystic lesions. Other primary tumours are rare but secondary retroperitoneal lymphoma and neuroblastoma are the most common. Benign teratoma, haemangioendothelioma and hamartoma have all been described.

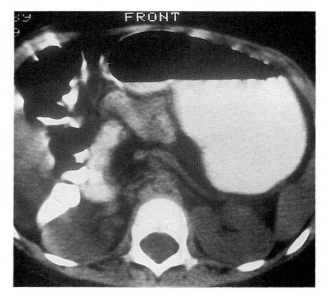

Fig. 7.4.8 Shwachmann's syndrome. CT. Fatty atrophy of pancreas.

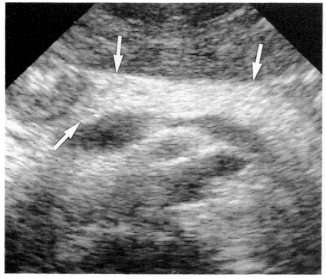

Fig. 7.4.7 Cystic fibrosis of the pancreas (mucoviscidosis). Fatty echogenic pancreas.

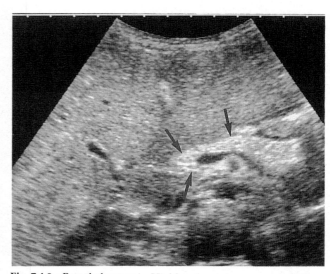

Fig. 7.4.9 Beta thalassaemia. Highly echogenic pancreas on US (arrows).

REFERENCES

Atkinson G, Wyly J, Gay B, Ball T, Winn K 1988 Idiopathic fibrosing pancreatitis: a cause of obstructive jaundice in childhood. Pediatric Radiology 18: 28–32

Aynsley-Green A, Polak J M, Bloom S R et al 1981 Nesidioblastosis of the pancreas: definition of the syndrome and the management of the severe neonatal hyperinsulinaemic hypoglycaemia. Archives of Disease in Childhood 56: 496–508

Bruncton J N, Drouillard J, Balu-Maesturo C, Francois E, Normand F, Tiran A 1988 Lymphoma of the pancreas. Journal of Medical Imaging 2: 137–143

Burt T B, Condon V R, Matlak M E 1983 Fetal pancreatic hamartoma. Pediatric Radiology 13: 287–290

Choyke P L, Glenn G M, Walther M M et al 1992 The natural history of renal lesions in von Hippel–Lindau disease: a serial CT study in 28 patients. American Journal of Roentgenology 159: 1229–1234

Fleischer A C, Parker P, Kirchner S G, James A E Jr 1983 Sonographic findings of pancreatitis in children. Radiology 146: 151–155

Forbes A, Leung J W C, Cotton P B 1984 Relapsing acute and chronic pancreatitis. Archives of Disease in Childhood 59: 927–935

Franken E A, Chin L C, Smith W L, Lu C H 1984 Hereditary pancreatitis in children. Annales de Radiologie 27: 130–137

Garel L, Brunelle F, Lallemand D, Sauvegrain J 1983 Pseudocysts of the pancreas in children. Which cases require surgery? Pediatric Radiology 13: 120–123

Herman T E, Siegel M J 1991 Pictorial essay: CT of the pancreas in children. American Journal of Roentgenology 157: 375–383

Jaffe R 1991 The pancreas. In: Wigglesworth J S, Singer D B (eds) Textbook of fetal and perinatal pathology. Blackwell Scientific Publications, Oxford, pp 1021–1055

Kloppel G, Lenzen S 1984 Anatomy and physiology of the endocrine pancreas. In: Kloppel G, Heitz P U (eds) Pancreatic pathology. Churchill Livingstone, Edinburgh, pp 133–153

Koh T H H G, Cooper J E, Newman C L, Walker T M, Kiely E M, Hoffman E B 1986 Pancreatoblastoma in a neonate with Wiedemann–Beckwith syndrome. European Journal of Pediatrics 145: 435–438

Lucas A, Sarson D L, Bloom S R, Aynsley-Green A 1980 Developmental aspects of gastric inhibitory polypeptide (GIP) and its possible role in the enteroinsular axis in neonates. Acta Paediatrica Scandinavica 69: 321–325

McHugo J M, McKeown C, Brown M T et al 1987 Ultrasound findings in children with cystic fibrosis. British Journal of Radiology 60: 137–141

McLean J M 1979 Embryology of the pancreas. In Howat H T, Sarles H (eds) the endocrine pancreas. Saunders, Philadelphia, pp 3–13

Merril J R, Raffensberger J G 1976 Pediatric annular pancreas: twenty years experience. Journal of Pediatric Surgery 11: 921–925

Nicholson R L 1981 Abnormalities of the perinephric fascia and fat in pancreatitis. Radiology 139: 125–127

Pearson H A, Lobel J S, Kocoshis S A et al 1979 A new syndrome of refractory sideroblastic anemia with vacuolisation of marrow precursors and exocrine pancreatic dysfunction. Journal of Pediatrics 95: 976–984

Suarez F, Bernard O, Gauthier F et al 1987 Bilio-pancreatic common channel in children: clinical, biological and radiological findings in 12 children. Pediatric Radiology 17: 206–211

Taussig L M 1984 Cystic fibrosis. Thieme-Stratton

Robey G, Daneman A, Martin D J 1983 Pancreatic carcinoma in a neonate. Pediatric Radiology 13: 284–287

Seifert G 1984 Congenital anomalies. In: Kloppel G, Heitz P U (eds) Pancreatic pathology. Churchill Livingstone, Edinburgh, pp 22–26

Sharma S, Puri S, Chaturvedi P, Kulssgrishtha R, Baijar V 1988 Mediastinal pancreatic pseudocyst following traumatic rupture of diaphragm. Pediatric Radiology 18: 337

Willi U V, Reddish J M, Littlewood-Teele R 1980 Cystic fibrosis: its characteristic apppearance on abdominal sonography. American Journal of Roentgenology 134: 1005–1010

Wong K C, Lister J 1981 Human fetal development of the hepato-pancreatic duct junction – a possible explanation of congenital dilatation of the biliary tract. Journal of Pediatric Surgery 16: 139–145

7.5 GONADS

EMBRYOLOGY, ANATOMY, PHYSIOLOGY

The development of both the male and female gonads is common for the first 2 weeks of gestation. At about 5 weeks of gestation, germ cells migrate from the yolk sac to the gonadal ridges of the mesonephros. The sex cords originating from the mesothelium project into the gonadal ridges. As disorders of intersex and testicular disease occur in association with both gynaecological problems and genitourinary problems, there is some repeat discussion of aspects of these lesions in Chapter 6. Testicular development begins around 7 weeks of gestation due to the effect of the HY-antigen on gonad-specific receptors of the gonadal cell membrane.

The seminiferous tubules begin to form around 7 weeks of gestation, the interstitial cells at about 8 weeks, and, at the same time, the genital tract is being masculinized. Prespermatogonia and Sertoli cells are components of the seminiferous tubules. Testosterone synthesis by the interstitial Leydig cells of the testis initiates virilization. Internal and external genital structures develop under the action of testosterone and dehydrotestosterone. The latter is essential for normal development of the external genitalia. The müllerian structures normally regress completely in the male, under the influence of a müllerian inhibiting substance produced by testicular Sertoli cells.

A prostatic utricle which is a normal anatomical variant is formed by the fused caudal ends of the müllerian ducts. Occasionally this can form a cyst.

The wolffian system gives rise to the epididymis, vasa deferentia and seminal vesicles.

The ovarian germ cells are surrounded by granulosa cells originating from the sex cords and by mesenchymal theca cells developing from the genital ridge. At 6 weeks of gestation, the müllerian ducts appear and develop in conjunction with the mesonephric ducts. They fuse at about 7 weeks of gestation to a single tube anterior to the mesonephric ducts and give rise to the uterus including the cervix and proximal part of the future vagina. At 8 weeks of gestation, the canalicular structure resulting from the fused müllerian ducts reaches the urogenital sinus at the müllerian tubercle. At the same time, the vaginal plate develops distally. It advances cranially toward the proximal region of the future vagina, obliterating its lumen. Recanalization then develops from its distal part up to the cervix. This process may be incomplete or disrupted and thus lead to various degrees of vaginal obstruction, i.e. imperforate hymen, vaginal stenosis or atresia. In late pregnancy, the vaginal epithelium becomes prominent due to glycogen accumulation but gradually regresses after birth as the effect of maternal oestrogens decreases. In contrast to the male development, the mesonephric ducts regress in the female. Persistence may lead to Gartner's duct cysts in the lateral aspects of the vagina.

At 3½ weeks of gestation, the genital tubercle forms above the cloacal membrane giving rise to an internal urogenital and external labioscrotal pair of folds. At 7 weeks of gestation, at the same time as fusion of the müllerian ducts, the cloaca is separated into the anterior urogenital sinus and the posterior anorectal canal by the urorectal membrane. Between 8½ and 9 weeks of gestation, the external genitalia differentiate to male or female phenotype. In the male, the phallus, having formed from the former genital tubercle, grows in length and produces the corpus spongiosum and the corpora cavernosa from its own mesenchymal substance. The urogenital folds develop into the urethra. Its urothelium is of endodermal origin from the urogenital sinus except for its most distal portion which is lined by ectodermal epithelium. The labioscrotal folds fuse and form the scrotum.

In the female, the phallus remains small and becomes the clitoris. The urogenital folds develop into the labia minora. The labioscrotal folds remain unfused and become the labia majora. The urogenital sinus forms the vaginal vestibule containing the vestibular glands, the vaginal opening and the urethral orifice.

For the general pathophysiology of the female genitalia, reference is made to Chapter 6 on paediatric gynaecology.

Endocrinological manifestation of maternal oestrogens are the relatively large size of the neonatal uterus and its prominent endometrial echo on US.

At birth, the uterus measures 2.3–4.6 cm in length (mean 3.4 cm) and 0.8–2.2 cm in width (mean 1.3 cm). As maternal oestrogen effect diminishes the length reduces to 2–3 cm and width to 0.5–1.0 cm, and adopts an infantile configuration with the width of the cervix being the same as the body. Adult configuration develops at puberty. The width of the cervix is then smaller than the body.

While the effects of maternal oestrogens gradually decrease and disappear, this physiological behaviour may be disturbed in very premature infants of 26 weeks or so. Immaturity of the negative feedback mechanism in very premature girls may lead to the development of large ovarian cysts when they reach the postconceptional age of their calculated term.

IMAGING APPROACH AND TECHNIQUE

Initial imaging of genitalia in both sexes is by US, although it is likely that MRI will play an increasing role in determining the presence of genital organs in cases of doubtful sex with ambiguous genitalia.

The urinary bladder should be moderately full in order to serve as a convenient ultrasonographic 'window'. Too little as well as too much urine in the bladder may preclude good visualization. If the bladder is too full, not only will the uterus be flattened but also the ovaries may become indistinct from neighbouring structures and even ascites may be pushed out of the cul-de-sac and pelvis. Also, such a patient will not be comfortable for investigation and cooperation is limited. Lifting the upper part of the patient's body may facilitate the examination by relieving the abdominal strain.

To examine the scrotum by US, a boy should keep his legs straight and close to each other. A towel supporting the scrotum and surrounding it from both sides may be used to immobilize it. A cooperative patient best does this himself; a smaller child can be helped by his nurse or parent. With the penis positioned upwards, the ultrasonographic access to the scrotum is ideal. A linear high-resolution transducer of 7.5 MHz or 10 MHz is recommended for scrotal and testicular evaluation, while a sector or curved transducer of 5 MHz is usually adequate for the investigation of the inner genitalia in older children. In fat girls 3.5 MHz probes may be needed. Higher MHz linear transducers may be advantageous in babies. Some advocate the use of transvaginal US in young adults who have been sexually active. With the development of smaller probes, this technique may become applicable also for younger girls.

Colour Doppler US supplementing the two-dimensional grey-scale morphology is useful in expert hands for the evaluation of gonadal perfusion and its impairment. In testicular torsion, pertechnetate perfusion scintigraphy is also a reliable technique for differentiating torsion from epididymo-orchitis.

For CT examination of the pelvis, it is essential that the bowel is fully opacified with contrast, and IV contrast used to opacify vessels, in an attempt to distinguish them from lymph nodes. MRI will increasingly replace CT in the assessment of the paediatric pelvis and its content.

REFERENCES

Coffin C M, Dehner L P 1992 The male reproductive system. In: Stocker J T, Dehner L P (eds) Pediatric pathology. J.B. Lippincott, Philadelphia

Gilsanz V, Cleveland R H, Reid B S 1982 Duplication of the müllerian ducts and genitourinary malformations. Part 1: the value of excretory urography. Radiology 144: 793–796

Gilsanz V, Cleveland R H, Reid B S 1982 Duplication of the müllerian ducts and genitourinary malformations. Part 2: analysis of malformations. Radiology 144: 797–801

Golimbu M 1984 HY antigen: genetic control and role in testicular differentiation. Urology 24: 115–121.

Ivarsson S A, Nilsson K O, Persson P H 1983 Ultrasonography of pelvic organs in prepubertal and post pubertal girls. Archives of Disease in Childhood 58: 352–354

Jost A 1972 A new look at the mechanisms controlling sex differentiation in mammals. Johns Hopkins Medical Journal 130: 38–53

Nussbaum A R, Sanders R C, Jones M D 1986 Neonatal uterine morphology as seen on real-time US. Radiology 160: 641–643

Sedin G, Bergquist C, Lindgren P G 1985 Ovarian hyperstimulation syndrome in preterm infants. Pediatric Research 19: 548–552

Table 7.5.1   Abnormal sexual development

Abnormality of sex chromatin
Monosomy Y (lethal)
Monosomy X (e.g. Turner's syndrome)
Polysomy Y (XYY karyotype)
Polysomy X (XXX and XXY karyotype)

Abnormality of gonads
Abnormal germ cell migration (e.g. agonadism)
Hermaphroditism
Testicular regression (failure of testicular function with sequelae according to time of occurrence)
Leydig cell agenesis

Endocine abnormality
Persistent müllerian duct syndrome (i.e absent müllerian inhibiting factor)
Abnormality of central nervous system (i.e. absent or abnormal production/release of gonadotropin)
Abnormal synthesis/function of sex steroids: e.g. 21-alpha-hydroxylase or 11-beta-hydroxylase deficiency; androgen resistance (5-alpha reductase deficiency; testicular feminization)

Maternal endocrine disturbance
Virilization during pregnancy
Effect of exogenous hormones (i.e. contraceptives)
Diethylstilboestrol

Abnormality of müllerian ducts
Imperforate hymen
Atresia/agenesis of vagina, uterine cervix or fundus
Failure of fusion of müllerian ducts (uterus didelphys, bicornuate/septate uterus)
Unilateral absence of müllerian duct (unicornuate uterus)

Agenesis of cloacal membrane
Absent anal, genital, urinary orifice(s)

Hypospadias/epispadias

Agenesis of penis/micropenis

Adapted from Lauchlan.

PATHOLOGY

The spectrum of congenital abnormalities of the gonads and sexual development is listed in Table 7.5.1. These disorders may be divided into those of sex differentiation without ambiguous genitalia and those with ambiguous external genitalia (Tables 7.5.2, 7.5.3).

REFERENCES

Conte F, Grumbach M M 1988 Pathogenesis, classification and treatment of anomalies of sex. In : DeGroot L J (ed) Endocrinology. W B Saunders, Philadelphia
Lauchlan S C 1991 The reproductive system. In Wigglesworth J S, Single D B (eds) Textbook of fetal and perinatal pathology. Blackwell Scientific Publications, Oxford

Table 7.5.2   Differentiation disorders with normal external genitalia

Chromosome abnormalities
1. Classic Turner's syndrome X0 gonadal dysgenesis
2. Chromatin-positive variants of Turner's: including mosaics X0/XX, X0/XXX, X0/XX/XXX or 46XX with an abnormal X
3. Klinefelter's syndrome: commonly 47XXY but many mosaics
4. XX male: (X-reversal syndrome)
5. Persistent müllerian duct syndrome
6. Some male pseudohermaphrodites

In 1, 2 and 6 the external appearance is female and in 3, 4 and 5 the external appearance is male

Table 7.5.3   Sex differentiation disorders with ambiguous genitalia

	Gonads	Chromosomes	Urerus

1. *Female pseudohermaphroditism*
   Congenital adrenal hyperplasia
   Maternal androgen effect
	Ovary	46XX	+

2. *Male pseudohermaphroditism*
   Decreased testosterone synthesis
   Dihydrotestosterol deficiency
   Testicular feminization
   Male hypospadias
	Testes	46XY	−

3. *Dysgenetic male pseudohermaphroditism and XY gonadal agenesis* Mixed gonadal dysgenesis	Testis and streak testis	X0/XY or Y line mosaics	+/−
Familial XY gonadal dysgenesis	Bilateral streak	46XY	+/−
Drash syndrome	Testes	46XY	−
XY gonadal dysgenesis	Absent testes	46XY	+/−
4. *True hermaphroditism*	Testicular and ovarian tissue	46XX + mosaics 46XY with Y line	+

DISORDERS OF SEXUAL DIFFERENTIATION WITH NORMAL EXTERNAL GENITALIA

Turner's syndrome

This is a relatively common non-familial disorder in which in addition to the chromosomal abnormality, there are numerous somatic associations.

In males, the 'Turner phenotype' with normal karyotype is also known as 'male Turner syndrome' or Noonan syndrome with multiple related anomalies.

On fetal ultrasound, Turner's syndrome may present with hydrops, ascites and cystic hygroma.

The skeletal abnormalities include a short fourth metacarpal, osteoporosis, a V-shaped distal radio-ulnar joint and a slightly decreased bone age, particularly as the child approaches maturity (Fig. 7.5.1). Clinically the children have a characteristic facies, broad chest, widely spaced nipples and neck webbing with a low hairline. Lymphoedema of hands and feet is common. Coarctation of the aorta is the main cardiac abnormality and is present commonly in those with a webbed neck. Renal anomalies including horseshoe kidney are present in about 30% of patients. Hypertension is common. There is an increased incidence of autoimmune disorders. Secondary signs of sexual development fail to develop at puberty. Menstruation is usually absent, though there are rare reports of successful pregnancy. In most children with Turner's syndrome the fallopian tubes, uterus and vagina are present but ovaries are absent or streak like.

In the mosaic forms of Turner's syndrome, somatic abnormalities are less frequent.

REFERENCE

Hall J G, Gilchrist D M 1990 Turner syndrome and its variants. Pediatric Clinics of North America 37: 1421–1440

46XX gonadal dysgenesis

This may be sporadic or inherited with an autosomal recessive pattern. Sensineuronal deafness may occur in the familial variety. The ovaries are either streaks, absent or hypoplastic. Other organs are normal. The patients are phenotypically female.

Klinefelter's syndrome

Patients have a male external appearance but the testes are small and cryptorchidism and hypospadias are common. The carrier type is typically 47XXY but numerous mosaics have been described. The patients are generally sterile. Mental retardation is present in 25% of patients. Gynaecomastia develops in almost half of the older patients. Azoospermia and infertility are usual. Diagnosis is usually made around puberty. Patients with the 47XXY carrier type have an increased risk of developing breast cancer after puberty.

A variant of Klinefelter's syndrome with a 49XXXXY carrier type has been described. This has associated radioulnar synostosis, coxa valga, abnormal facies, decreased bone age and hypotonia with severe mental retardation.

XX male or sex reversal syndrome

This is a rare disorder of sex differentiation in which the external appearances and internal genitalia are those of a male but the chromosomal type is 46XX. Fifty per cent of patients have hypospadias. The clinical appearances are similar to Klinefelter's syndrome and the testicular histology is the same. Gynaecomastia is common at puberty.

Persistent müllerian duct syndrome

This is also known as uterine hernia syndrome. This is a very rare type of male sexual differentiation. The testicular hormone responsible for normal regression of the müllerian ducts in the male fetus is deficient. Patients have an external male appearance with the normal 46XY carrier type but have a small uterus and fallopian tubes and a small vagina connected with the posterior urethra at the level of the verumontanum. Cryptorchidism is common. Inguinal hernias are common. The uterus, tubes and sometimes the testes may be found in the hernias.

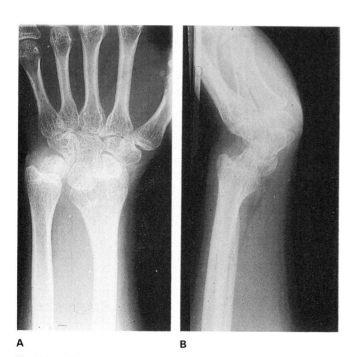

A　　　**B**

Fig. 7.5.1 Typical features on the hand and wrist radiographs (**A**, **B**) in Turner's syndrome. Note short metacarpal, osteoporosis and abnormal radioulnar articulation.

REFERENCE

Fernandes E T, Hollabraugh R S, Young J A, Wilroy SR, Schriocki
E A 1990 Peristent müllerian duct syndrome. Urology
36: 516–518

Male pseudohermaphroditism – testicular feminization syndrome

Male pseudohermaphroditism associated with the testicular feminization syndrome is due to an inherited defect of androgen receptors. It is inherited as an X-linked recessive trait and affects 50% of males in the family. Affected females are carriers. Patients have a normal female habitus and a blind-ending vagina (Fig. 7.5.2). A diagnosis is usually made at puberty when menstruation fails. Breast development is normal but axillary and pubic hair scanty. The diagnosis is now made increasingly early as chromosome tests on an unborn infant are now quite common, following antenatal US. In this situation the infant has been shown to have a normal 46XY chromosome karyotype, but when the infant is born it appears entirely female. It is important that testicular tissue is identified and removed as, with all abnormally located testicular tissue, there is an increased incidence of neoplasia, which approaches 50% by 50 years. The testes, which are small, may be in the inguinal canal or abdomen.

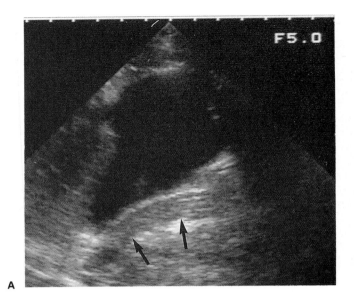

A

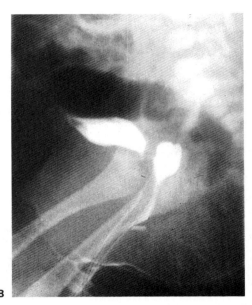

B

Fig. 7.5.2 A Testicular feminization syndrome in a 17 year old. The patient is phenotypically female but has 46XY karyotype. US shows a vagina but no uterus. **B** Infant with 46XY karyotype on amniotic fluid; although infant born phenotypically female, karyotype confirmed post delivery. Genitogram shows a normal bladder and vagina, with separate orifices.

SEX DIFFERENTIATION WITH AMBIGUOUS EXTERNAL GENITALIA

These conditions are briefly summarized in Table 7.5.3.

Female pseudohermaphroditism

These patients have ambiguous external genitalia, usually with a prominent phallus and sometimes partially fused labial scrotal folds. The patients are a female 46XX carrier type and have normal ovaries, fallopian tubes and uterus but the patients are subjected to androgens in utero. There is no testicular tissue. The urethra is usually connected to the vagina posteriorly and forms a urogenital sinus. The orifice is usually at the base of the phallus (Fig. 7.5.3).

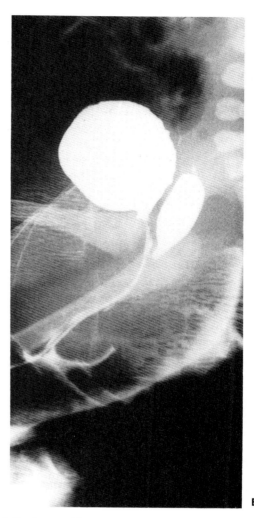

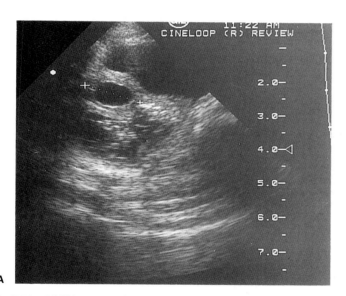

Fig. 7.5.3 46XXY mosaic infant with ambiguous external genitalia – an enlarged clitoris resembling severe hypospadias, and enlarged labia resembling a bifid scrotum. **A** US shows an enlarged vagina. Also seen were an ovary with two follicles and a bicornuate uterus. **B** Genitogram. Note an elongated urethra, filling of a normal vagina and the distal end of the cervical canal. This child subsequently developed a hernia and an ovotestis was removed from the right inguinal canal.

Congenital adrenal hyperplasia

This is the commonest cause of ambiguous genitalia in females. There is an inherited defect of enzymes involved in hormone synthesis by the adrenal cortex. This results in a decrease in hydrocortisone production with an increase in ACTH production by the pituitary. The ACTH increase causes overstimulation of the adrenal cortex with hyperplasia of it. The commonest enzyme defect is 21-hydroxylase deficiency which is inherited as an autosomal recessive condition. The condition in these patients is severe and is usually complicated by salt wasting. A less frequent defect is 11-beta-hydroxylase deficiency. This is associated with systemic arterial hypertension.

The degree of ambiguity of the external genitalia is variable. Imaging generally demonstrates an enlarged, elongated male type posterior urethra which is fairly featureless (Figs. 7.5.4, 7.5.5). Excess maternal androgens may also produce ambiguous genitalia.

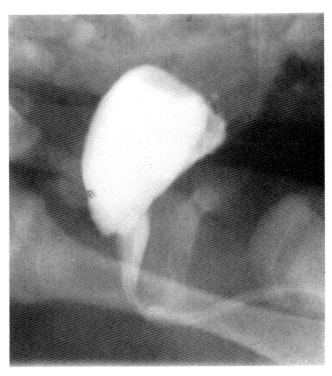

Fig. 7.5.4 Congenital adrenal hyperplasia. The patient, a 46XX karyotype, has an elongated featureless urethra.

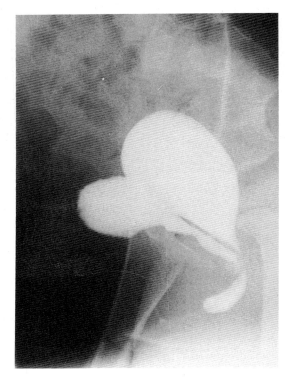

Fig. 7.5.5 Congenital adrenal hyperplasia in an infant with urogenital sinus.

Male pseudohermaphroditism

These patients have varying degrees of ambiguous external genitalia commonly with undescended or absent testes. They have a normal 46XY carrier type. There are no müllerian derivatives. Relative or absolute androgen deficiency due to primary gonadal or end-organ defects causes the failure of development of the external genitalia.

5-Alpha reductase deficiency – dehydrotestosterone deficiency

This form of male pseudohermaphroditism used to be referred to as pseudovaginal perineal hypospadias. These patients have normal testosterone. Testes are well developed, but they are often located intra-abdominally or in the inguinal canal (Fig. 7.5.6b). The hallmark of the disease clinically is that there is poor masculinization of the external genitalia. The vagina is blind ending (Fig. 7.5.6a) but there is no uterus or fallopian tubes. Some patients at puberty develop improved masculinization.

Testicular feminization

These patients have end-organ failure of response to the action of the normal androgen. The defect may be complete or incomplete (Fig. 7.5.2). When complete the patients appear female. The incomplete form depends on the degree of end-organ failure and may variably appear either as males or females.

Mixed gonadal dysgenesis

A variety of carrier types is seen in this condition. The commonest varieties are 45X/46XY karyotype or 45X0 or 46XX. Varying mosaics are also described. The external appearance varies from a virtually normal female to a male with severe hypospadias. In most cases, however, there is frank ambiguity of external genitalia. The testis is usually intra-abdominal but may be in the inguinal canal. As with most other forms of abnormally located testis in intersex situations, the testis should be removed for fear of neoplasia. Gonadoblastoma occurs in 75% of patients by 26 years. The development of secondary sexual characteristics, other than at puberty, in these patients indicates development of a tumour.

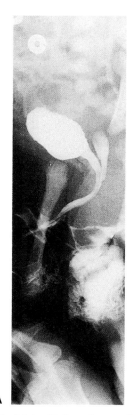

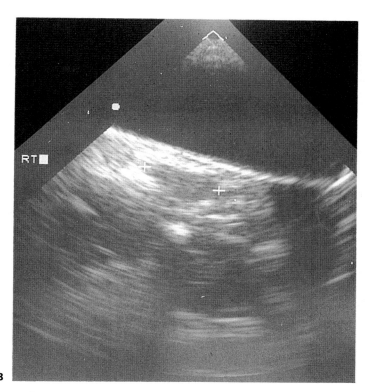

A   **B**

Fig. 7.5.6   Alpha reductase deficiency. **A** Genitogram in a child with severe perineal hypospadias. Note filling of blind vagina. **B** US showing testis behind the bladder.

Familial 46XY gonadal dysgenesis

This condition is inherited as an X-linked autosomal dominant trait most commonly. Sporadic cases are known. The carrier type is 46XY. There may be associated campomelic dwarfism. The gonads vary from being streak testes to dysgenetic and undescended testes. Patients with streak gonads have a female phenotype, most commonly with normal tubes, uterus and vagina. Amenorrhoea occurs at puberty. Those patients with dysgenetic testes have incompletely masculinized external genitalia. Some virilization usually takes place at puberty but is incomplete. The risk of neoplasm in the abnormal gonads exists.

Drash syndrome

This condition encompasses male pseudohermaphroditism, gonadal dysgenesis, nephropathy and Wilms' tumour. The patients have a 46XY carrier type, gonadal dysgenesis with variable histology, ambiguous external genitalia but intra-abdominal testes, chronic glomerulonephritis and the development of Wilms' tumour in more than 50% of the patients. If the gonads are left behind, neoplasia in these organs is also common.

46XY gonadal agenesis

This is also known as the vanishing testis syndrome. Although the patients are of a 46XY carrier type there are no gonads present and there is incomplete male sex differentiation, probably due to testicular resorption in early fetal life. External genitalia are ambiguous.

True hermaphroditism

These patients have characteristically both testicular and ovarian tissue. The most common sex carrier type is 46XX but many mosaics with a Y line are also known (Fig. 7.5.3). These patients usually have a testis or an ovary on one side and an ovo-testis on the other. The testis or the ovo-testis may be within the abdomen or in the groin, scrotum or labia. The testis or the ovo-testis is usually dysgenetic. There is usually a vas on the side of the testis and a fallopian tube on the side of the ovary. Most patients have a uterus but it is often hypoplastic or bicornuate. External genitalia are almost always ambiguous but have a tendency towards male phenotypes. A urogenital sinus may be present.

REFERENCES

Cremin B J 1974 Intersex states in young children: the importance of radiology in making a correct diagnosis. Clinical Radiology 25: 63–73

Eddy A A, Mauer S M 1985 Pseudohermaphroditism, glomerulopathy, and Wilms tumour (Drash syndrome): frequency in end-stage renal failure. Journal of Pediatrics 106: 584–587
White P C, New M I, Dupont B 1987 Congenital adrenal hyperplasia (1). New England Journal of Medicine 316: 1519–1524

IMAGING

Imaging in intersex disorders is concerned with the demonstration of what gonads and internal organs are present. The first approach is US. The varying internal organs may be small or rudimentary and may be missed on US even in expert hands. For further identification of these organs by radiological techniques, two other procedures are helpful. One is MRI which is increasingly being shown to have exquisite sensitivity in the demonstration of the pelvic organs, particularly when used with appropriate surface and body coils. The other is genitography. This is fully described in Chapter 6 on gynaecology. The basic principle of all genitography is to opacify all orifices presenting on the perineum following careful catheterization of these orifices and identifying their communication (Fig. 7.5.7).

REFERENCE

Kogan B A, Hricak H, Tanagho E A 1987 Magnetic resonance imaging in genital anomalies. Journal of Urology 138: 1028–1030

TUMOUR ASSOCIATED WITH DISORDERS OF SEX DIFFERENTIATION

The increased risk of neoplasia in patients who have abnormally located gonads, particularly testes, is well known. The neoplasms are usually of the germ cell type, and will therefore include seminoma, dysgerminoma, gonadoblastoma, teratocarcinoma and yolk sac tumour. Embryonal carcinoma and choriocarcinoma have also been described. The tumours are more common in those patients with a Y chromosome and, in fact, are rare in patients who have not got this chromosome.

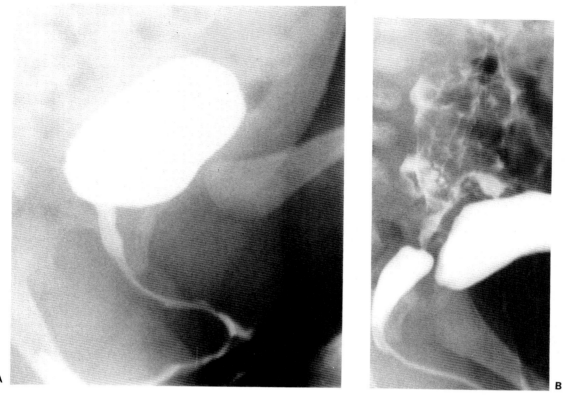

Fig. 7.5.7 **A** 46XX infant with enlarged clitoris. Cystogram showing elongated urethra and normal bladder. **B** Catheter in vagina. A normal vagina is demonstrated with reflux of contrast through the uterus into the peritoneum.

7.6 PRECOCIOUS AND DELAYED PUBERTY

Puberty occurs at different ages in males and females. In females, puberty begins between the ages of 8 and 13 years and, in males, 9 and 14 years. Generally speaking, the clinical appearances are earlier in girls than in boys. Puberty is due to the effect of the hypothalamus–pituitary complex becoming activated and resulting in maturation of the gonads, with increased production of the sex hormones and the development of secondary sex characteristics, a growth spurt and the development of reproductive capabilities. Precocious puberty is defined as the appearance of external signs of adolescence before expected. This is generally accepted as being before the age of 8 in girls or 9 in boys, although if signs of puberty develop this early in either sex, children will often be brought to the hospital for investigation as both of these are at the extremes of normal. Precocious puberty is far commoner in girls than in boys and may be complete or incomplete. In the complete forms, there is a normal appearance of iso-sexual characteristics. In the incomplete forms, the clinical appearances may be either iso-sexual or heterosexual. In girls, heterosexual precocious puberty is manifest by virilization and in boys by gynaecomastia.

COMPLETE PRECOCIOUS PUBERTY

In complete precocious puberty there is an increased production of gonadotrophic and sex hormones with an early onset of ovulation, or in boys spermatogenesis. This is due to premature activation of the hypothalamus–pituitary–gonadal complex. The causes are detailed in Table 7.6.1. Most commonly, complete precocious puberty is idiopathic but occasionally it can be secondary to an organic CNS lesion, particularly tumours of the hypothalamus or pituitary gland, and clinical investigation is directed towards excluding these.

Table 7.6.1 True precocious puberty (gonadotrophin dependent)
Idiopathic, i.e. constitutional
Lesion of the central nervous system (indirect or direct involvement of the hypothalamo-pituitary system) Hydrocephalus (primary or secondary) Sequelae of meningoencephalitis, meningitis or trauma Tumour, malignant or benign (including tuberous sclerosis and neurofibromatosis
Gonadotrophin-producing tumours of the central nervous system, mediastinum (association: Klinefelter's syndrome), liver or gonads
Effect of exogenous gonadotrophin
McCune–Albright syndrome
Prolonged untreated hypothyroidism
Adapted from DiGeorge.

CNS abnormality

The most frequent cause of abnormal precocious puberty is a CNS tumour and, as previously stated, it is most commonly in the hypothalamus or in the pituitary fossa. This tumour is more common in boys than in girls. The tumours are generally benign but because of the location are seldom resectable. The tumours are usually hamartomas and are either in the hypothalamus or in the tuber cinereum. The tumour exerts its effect by releasing gonadotrophin-releasing hormone. When these tumours are present, the presentation of precocious puberty is usually at a very young age. Other tumours that have been described as causing precocious puberty will be those located near the hypothalamus and include gliomas, often in patients with neurofibromatosis, astrocytomas and dysgerminomas. Precocious puberty is also associated with hydrocephalus or occasionally with the sequelae of previous infection and abscess.

Precocious puberty is a manifestation of McCune–Albright syndrome, in patients with polyostotic fibrous dysplasia. It can also occur following chronic exposure to either endogenous or exogenous androgens or oestrogens.

PRECOCIOUS PSEUDOPUBERTY

Children may present with some features of precocious puberty, though seldom with a complete manifestation. The causes are many and are listed in Table 7.6.2.

Table 7.6.2 Precocious pseudopuberty (gonadotrophin independent)

Girls
Isosexual precocity (feminization)
Autonomous functional ovarian cyst
Effect of exogenous oestrogen
McCune–Albright syndrome
Adrenocortical tumour (oestrogen producing)
Ovarian tumour
 Germ cell teratoma, chorionepithelioma
 Sex cord stroma: granulosa-theca cell (association: Ollier's disease); with annular tubules (association: Peutz–Jeghers syndrome)

Heterosexual precocity (virilization)
Congenital adrenal hyperplasia
Adrenocortical tumour (testosterone producing)
Ovarian germ cell tumour (androgen producing)
Extraovarian teratoma (androgen producing)
Androblastoma (arrhenoblastoma)
Effect of exogenous androgen

Boys
Isosexual precocity (masculinization)
Congenital adrenal hyperplasia
Adrenocortical tumour (testosterone producing)
Leydig cell hyperplasia, primary
Testicular Leydig cell tumour
Extratesticular teratoma (androgen producing)
Effect of exogenous androgen

Heterosexual precocity (feminization)
Effect of exogenous oestrogen
Adrenocortical tumour (oestrogen producing)
Testicular and extratesticular sex cord stroma tumour:
 Sertoli tumour
 With annular tubules (association: Peutz–Jeghers syndrome)

Adapted from DiGeorge.

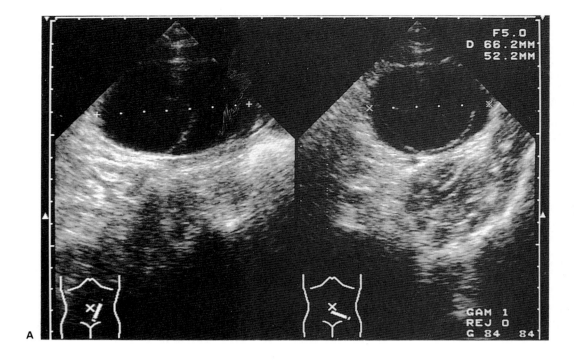

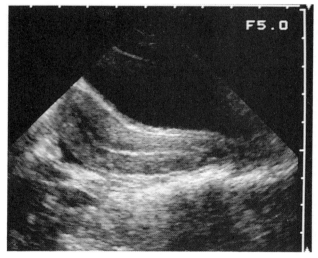

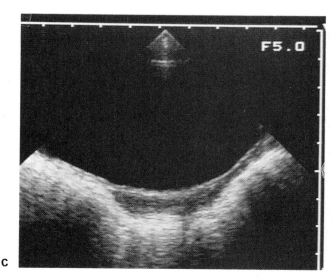

Fig. 7.6.1 Isosexual precocious puberty. Nine-year-old girl with delayed bone age 8, trisomy 21, who presented with vaginal bleeding. **A** US of pelvis. There is a large ovarian cyst. **B** The uterus is 5.6 cm long with a prominent midline endometrial echo and enlarged fundus, both features of a postmenarchal uterus. Hypothyroidism was also present and the presumed cause of the uterine and ovarian change was overstimulation of the pituitary gland due to excess TSH production. Spontaneous resolution occurred following treatment of hypothyroidism. **C** Normal infantile uterus, length 3.4 cm, following treatment.

Incomplete iso-sexual precocious puberty in girls

These children will present usually with the effects of excess oestrogen production, of which the commonest clinical presentation is vaginal bleeding. Secondary sex characteristics are not usually prominent. Investigation is directed at identifying any underlying ovarian neoplasm that may be causing this lesion (Fig. 7.6.1). The most commonly discovered lesion is granulosa thecal cell cyst of the ovary, but true, malignant neoplasms also occur (Fig. 7.6.2). Initial radiological investigation is by US in an effort to identify an ovarian cyst. The cyst may be easily identified but the uterus and vagina usually remain immature.

Premature breast development or premature development of pubic and axillary hair are relatively common, self-limited variants of pubertal development in girls. Premature breast development is defined as enlargement of the breasts without other signs of precocious puberty in children less than 8 years of age. This commonly occurs between 1 and 4 years of age and may affect only one breast. This is known as premature thelarche.

The early appearance of pubic or axillary hair without other signs of sexual maturity in girls under the age of 8 is referred to as premature adrenarche.

Premature breast development may resolve spontaneously. When puberty occurs, it usually proceeds normally. Biochemical investigation in these children is normal.

Heterosexual precocious puberty – virilizing disorders in girls

These children present with the appearance of male secondary sex characteristics and include excessive body and facial hair, acne, increased muscle mass, deepening of the voice and cliteromegaly. In the girl who is already menstruating, menstrual abnormalities are common and may revert to amenorrhoea. Breast size may also decrease and vaginal atrophy may occur. The commonest cause of this is congenital adrenal hyperplasia, but other causes of excess circulating androgen or androgen-like substances will also produce the same effects.

Radiological investigation is directed towards excluding an underlying adrenal neoplasm. The commonest lesion will be a carcinoma of the adrenal gland. Occasionally, ovarian neoplasms, in particular arrhenoblastoma, thecoma and some of the gonadal blastomas, will also produce virilization.

Polycystic ovarian disorder may also result in idiopathic hirsutism and will be identified by ultrasound examination. In this condition, there is an increase in the body and facial hair but there are no other signs of virilization. The trait is often familial.

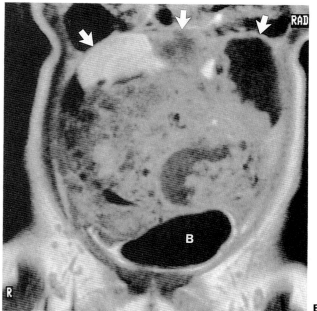

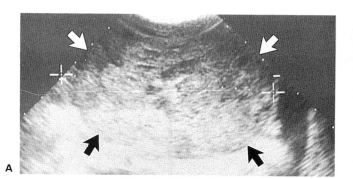

Fig. 7.6.2 Four-year-old girl presenting with vaginal bleeding and breast development. Ultrasound examination demonstrated a 5 cm solid ovarian neoplasm (arrows), which histologically was a malignant granulosa cell tumour. **B** Nine-year-old girl with huge abdominal mass (arrows) and precocious puberty due to malignant teratoma of ovary. B = bladder.

Precocious puberty in males

Iso-sexual precocious puberty in boys is due to an increase in circulating androgen or androgen-like substances produced by the adrenal glands or testes (Figs 7.6.3, 7.6.4). Occasionally it can occur from an exogenous source. As with females, congenital adrenal hyperplasia is the most common cause. A rare form of iso-sexual precocious puberty in boys is caused by an extrapituitary tumour releasing human chorionic gonadotrophic (HCG) hormone which has an effect on stimulating testosterone production. Tumours that have been thus described include hepatomas, hepatoblastomas and teratomas (Fig. 7.6.5). A suprasellar germinoma or pinealoma may also produce a similar effect.

The premature appearance of pubic and axillary hair in boys without the appearance of secondary sexual characteristics is relatively common. These children will often have a slightly advanced bone age and an increase in growth rate. Gynaecomastia may occur as a transient abnormality in adolescent boys. It can be pronounced but generally spontaneously regresses. The regression, however, may take 2–3 years. In some patients it persists into adult life. Gynaecomastia may also be associated with other signs of feminization as a result of exposure to oestrogen, which may occur from oestrogen-secreting neoplasms of the testis or adrenal cortex or a prolactin-secreting tumour of the pituitary gland. Gynaecomastia is a clinical feature of Klinefelter's syndrome but has no underlying endocrine abnormality.

Radiological investigation of precocious puberty

Most of the investigation is clinical and biochemical. The initial radiological investigations include the hand and wrist for bone age, together with an ultrasound examination of the abdomen and internal genitalia, and of external genitalia in boys. When carrying out the ultrasound examination of the pelvis, attention should be focused on the shape and development of the uterus, i.e. is it infantile or menarchal? The finding of an adult-type uterus in an infant below the age of 8 indicates underlying oestrogen stimulation. If these are all normal and there is no clinical suspicion of intracranial lesion, then further investigation is not warranted. If there is clinical or biochemical suspicion of an underlying tumour and it cannot be found within the abdomen or within the reproductive organs, then an MR scan of the brain is warranted to exclude a hypothalamic or pituitary lesion. In all patients with neurofibromatosis presenting with precocious puberty, an MR scan of the brain is indicated.

Monitoring of the effects of precocious puberty is by regular assessment of bone age.

REFERENCES

Arisaka O, Shimura N, Nakayama Y et al 1989 Ovarian cysts in precocious puberty. Clinical Pediatrics 28: 44–47

Burton E M, Ball Jr W S, Crone K, Dolan L M 1989 Hamartoma of the tuber cinereum: a comparison of MR and CT findings in four cases. American Journal of Neuroradiology 10: 497–501

Clarke C F, Piesowicz A T, Edmonds K, Grant D 1989 Polycystic ovary syndrome in a virilized premenarcheal girl. Archives of Disease in Childhood 64: 1307–1309

DiGeorge A M 1992 The endocrine system. In: Berrman R E, Kliegman R M, Nelson W E, Vaughan III V C (eds) Nelson textbook of pediatrics, 14th edn.

Hahn F J, Leibrock L G, Huseman C A, Makos M M 1988 The MR appearance of hypothalamic hamartoma. Neuroradiology 30: 65–68

Lee P A, O'Dea L S 1990 Primary and secondary testicular insufficiency. Pediatric Clinics of North America 37: 1359–1387

Lyon A J, De Bruyn R, Grant D B 1985 Transient sexual precocity and ovarian cysts. Archives of Disease in Childhood 60: 819–822

Lyon A J, De Bruyn R, Grant D B 1985 Isosexual precocious puberty in girls. Acta Paediatrica Scandinavica 74: 950–955

Mahoney C P 1990 Adolescent gynecomastia. Differential diagnosis and management. Pediatric Clinics of North America 37: 1389–1404

Nakagawara A, Ikeda K, Tsuneyoshi M et al 1985 Hepatoblastoma producing alpha-fetoprotein and human chorionic gonadotropin. Cancer 56: 1636–1642

Pasquino A M, Tebaldi L, Cives C, Maciocci M, Boscherini B 1987 Precocious puberty in McCune–Albright syndrome. Progression from gonadotropin-independent and gonadotropin-dependent puberty in a girl. Acta Paediatrica Scandinavica 76: 841

Rieth K G, Comite F, Shawker T H, Culter G B 1984 Pituitary and ovarian abnormalities demonstrated by CT and ultrasound in children with features of McCune–Albright syndrome. Radiology 153: 389–393

Rieth K G, Comite F, Dwyer A J et al 1987 CT of cerebral anomalies in precocious puberty. American Journal of Roentgenology 148: 1231–1238

Wheeler M D, Styne D M 1990 Diagnosis and management of precocious puberty. Pediatrics Clinics of North America 37: 1255–1271

DELAYED PUBERTY

The time of onset of puberty is variable. It is considered to be delayed in girls when there are no secondary sex characteristics by about the age of 13 or menstruation has not begun by the age of 16, and in boys when there is no sign of enlargement of testis and penis by about the age of 14. Delayed puberty may be constitutional and related to severe illness. It is also frequent in disorders of the hypothalamus–pituitary complex, causing decreased gonadotrophin secretion, or in primary disorders of the gonads. The commonest cause, however, is idiopathic constitutional pubertal delay.

Delayed puberty in chronic systemic disorders

Delayed puberty in chronic systemic disorders is relatively common. It is seen with chronic inflammatory bowel disease, malabsorption, chronic renal, cardiac or pulmonary disease, such as one will find in patients with cystic fibrosis, and in any longstanding debilitation, i.e. children on treatment for tumours.

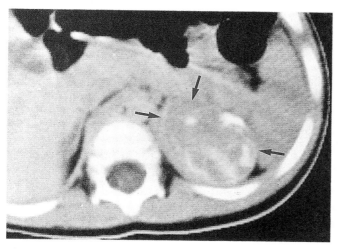

Fig. 7.6.3 Four-month-old male child with penile enlargement. CT of upper abdomen revealed a well-encapsulated partially calcified left adrenal tumour (arrows) which histologically was a benign adrenocortical adenoma.

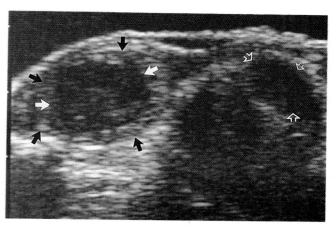

Fig. 7.6.4 Four-year-old boy with precocious puberty and enlargement of the right testis, and advanced bone age. Scrotal US showed a normal left testis (open white arrows) and a right intratesticular tumour (closed white arrows) surrounded by hyperechogenic normal testicular tissue (black arrows). Histology revealed a Leydig cell tumour. Serum testosterone fell to normal in 24 hours following tumour excision.

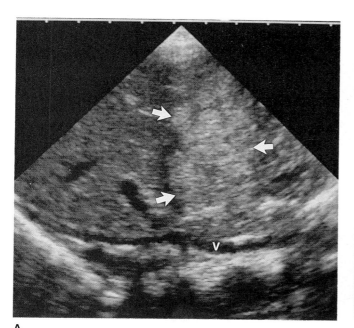

A

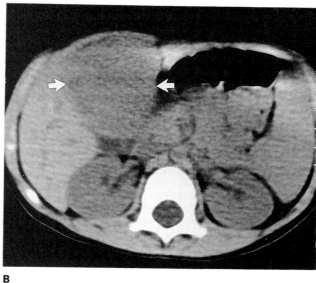

B

Fig. 7.6.5 Sixteen-month-old boy with precocious puberty and hepatomegaly. Ultrasound (**A**) and CT (**B**) show a hepatic tumour (arrows), which histologically was a hepatoblastoma. V = vein.

Delayed puberty is a feature of children with severe psychological disorders and anorexia nervosa. It is also a feature of intensive athletic training and is very commonly delayed in children undergoing international training for gymnastics or swimming.

Constitutional delay is well recognized. In these children the onset of puberty and menstruation may be delayed for several years but once it commences it occurs normally. There may be a genetic predisposition. Investigation is directed at excluding an underlying cause requiring treatment but apart from this the children will develop normally and observation is all that is required.

Hypothalamic pituitary disorders may result in delayed puberty. The lesion leads to a decreased gonadotrophin production with a decrease in the development of the normal gonadal sex steroids as a result. Gonads, therefore, fail to develop normally. Secondary sexual characteristics also are delayed or absent. There is often a delay in skeletal maturation with persistent failure of epiphyseal closure. The organic lesions include cerebral tumours such as craniopharyngioma, hypothalamic and optic glioma, or a variety of other tumours in the region of the pituitary gland or hypothalamus. Dysgerminoma is a relatively common one. Histiocytosis X may also destroy the normal pituitary function. Congenital lesions such as septo-optic dysplasia and holoprosencephaly are often associated with maldevelopment of the hypothalamus and pituitary gland and may result in hypogonadism with failure of development of puberty.

Idiopathic hypopituitarism, isolated gonadotrophin deficiency and a variety of familial causes of failure of normal pituitary development also will lead to delayed or absent puberty.

Delayed puberty and hypogonadism is a feature of the Prader–Willi syndrome, Laurence–Moon–Biedl syndrome and Klinefelter's syndrome.

Hypogonadism from any cause may lead to failure of pubertal development. Congenital absence of the ovaries or testes, Turner's syndrome and many of the other chromosomal abnormalities, are well known to be associated with delayed puberty. A tragic consequence of bilateral testicular torsion is testicular atrophy with pubertal failure.

Investigation

As with precocious puberty, radiological investigation is directed to identifying the degree of delay (by bone age assessment), and identifying the presence of the uterus, vagina and testes initially by ultrasound examination, and excluding a congenital anomaly or a tumour of the CNS, adrenal or gonad, although tumours of these last two rarely result in delayed puberty.

REFERENCE

Rosenfield R L 1990 Clinical review 6: diagnosis and management of delayed puberty. Journal of Clinical Endocrinology and Metabolism 70: 559–562

7.7 COMPLEX CASES

UNDESCENDED TESTIS – CRYPTORCHIDISM

Failure of descent of the testis into the scrotum is a relatively uncommon occurrence. There is an incidence of about 1% at 1 year of age. Failure of descent on the right is far more frequent than that on the left, though 30% of patients have bilateral cryptorchidism. An associated inguinal hernia is common on the affected side and the testis may lie in the inguinal canal. Urinary tract anomalies are said to be present in 10–20% of patients. These include the whole range of urinary tract anomalies found congenitally. If there is failure of development of the kidney, then the testis on that side will not have developed and searching for it is not fruitful. The undescended testis lies in the inguinal canal in between 60% and 70% of patients and is frequently palpable there. In fat children, it may not be palpable and it is in these patients that US is extremely helpful. The undescended testis is more prone to undergo torsion than a normal testis because of poor fixation. If left in the ectopic position it has a 20–40% increased risk of neoplasia and this risk rises if the testis is within the abdomen. Hence the importance of identifying the location of an undescended testis. A neoplasm usually develops in the third decade of life and is usually of a germ cell type tumour.

The cause of idiopathic cryptorchidism is unknown. It is, of course, seen in patients with forms of hermaphroditism and is common in association with hypospadias.

Imaging approaches

It is often not possible to locate an undescended testis by imaging. The initial imaging approach should be an ultrasound examination of the kidneys to establish the presence of an ipsilateral kidney. If this is absent, then there is no point in proceeding further. If this is present then one should ultrasound the inguinal canals and pelvis, looking particularly behind the bladder. It is rare to find a testis on US within the abdominal cavity, but it is quite common to find them within the inguinal canal. Testicular venography and spermatic arteriography have been carried out on older patients but they are technically difficult to perform in young children and are therefore not commonly utilized or indicated. On occasion, CT may demonstrate a testis, particularly within the abdomen, but this is a relatively rare occurrence and the radiation dose is not warranted. Recent reports of MRI suggest that this will be the method of choice for locating an undescended testis non-invasively. In most units, however, the initial imaging approach, if US cannot locate the testis within the inguinal canal, is by laparoscopic imaging and all radiological procedures are used as a secondary approach.

On MRI, a normal testis has a high signal on intermediate and T2-weighted images which is homogeneous. With fat suppression techniques, the testis can often be demonstrated in the inguinal canal very clearly.

REFERENCES

Benson C B, Doubilet P M, Richie J P 1989 Sonography of the male genital tract. American Journal of Roentgenology 153: 705–713

Friedland G W, Chang P 1988 The role of imaging in the management of the impalpable undescended testis. American Journal of Roentgenology 151: 1107–1111

Fritzsche P J, Hricak H, Kogan B A, Winkler M L, Tanagho E A 1987 Undescended testis: value of MR imaging. Radiology 164: 169–173

Guiney E J, Corbally M, Malone P S 1989 Laparoscopy and the management of the impalpable testis. British Journal of Urology 63: 313–316

Kier R, McCarthy S, Rosenfield A T, Rosenfield N S, Rapoport S, Weiss R M 1988 Nonpalpable testes in young boys: Evaluation by MR imaging. Radiology 169: 429–433

Lee P A, O'Dea L S 1990 Primary and secondary testicular insufficiency. Pediatric Clinics of North America 37: 1359–1387

Pappis C H, Argianas S A, Bousgas D, Athanasiades E 1988 Unsuspected urological anomalies in asymptomatic cryptorchid boys. Pediatric Radiology 18: 51–53

Troughton A H, Waring J, Langstaff A, Goddard P R 1990 The role of magnetic resonance imaging in the investigation of undescended testes. Clinical Radiology 41: 178–181

TESTICULAR TUMOURS

Testicular neoplasms are listed in Table 7.7.1.

Testicular neoplasms are a relatively uncommon tumour in childhood, constituting only about 2% of all solid tumours. The peak incidence is at 2 years of age. Clinical presentation is with a firm, painless swelling of the scrotum, but if torsion supervenes then the child may present with a painful swelling, making the diagnosis increasingly difficult. The lump may be present for weeks to months. Rarely, tumours are associated with secondary sexual characteristics. The commonest tumour is a yolk sac tumour and most testicular tumours have a tumour marker, commonly alpha-feto protein or occasionally HCG (human chorionic gonadotrophin).

Table 7.7.1 Testicular neoplasms
Germ cell neoplasia
Endodermal sinus tumour (i.e. yolk sac tumour)
Teratoma
– Mature (20% metastasize)
– Immature
Embryonal carcinoma
Teratocarcinoma
Seminoma
Intratubular germ cell neoplasia
Epidermoid cyst
Sex cord-stroma tumour
Leydig cell tumour
Leydig cell hyperplasia
Sertoli cell tumour
Juvenile granulosa cell tumour
Gonadoblastoma
Others
Rhabdomyosarcoma
Secondary/metastatic tumour
Leukaemia
Lymphoma
Neuroblastoma
Wilms' tumour
Langerhan's cell histiocytosis
Haemangioma
Juvenile xanthogranuloma etc.

Imaging approach

Initial imaging is by ultrasound examination of the testis and inguinal canal. The ultrasound should include Doppler assessment of tumour vascularity. The ultrasound examination must include a review of the whole abdomen looking for intra-abdominal nodes or hepatic metastases. This is accompanied by a chest radiograph. Further investigation is by CT. This is not required for assessment of the primary tumour but assessment of nodal or pulmonary spread.

On ultrasound examinations, most testicular neoplasms are of mixed echogenicity but are mainly hypoechoic. Areas of necrosis will show up as very low echo lesions. Areas of calcification have an increased echogenicity. Many of the tumours are associated with a small hydrocele, even in very young children. In the adolescent, a hydrocele may surround a tumour in the child presenting ostensibly with the clinical problem of hydrocele. Continuation of tumour into the groin is rare with the primary neoplasms but does occur with secondary neoplasms. At US, an attempt should be made to see whether the tumour is entirely limited to the testis or has broken through its capsule.

Follow-up examination while the child is on treatment is usually by US of the abdomen, and chest radiograph. CT is indicated if there is a rise in a tumour marker and the tumour cannot be identified with US. MRI will increasingly play a part in the detection of intra-abdominal pathology.

Yolk sac tumour

Also known as endodermal sinus tumour, orchidoblastoma and embryonal carcinoma of infancy, this is the commonest germ cell testicular tumour in childhood. It produces raised levels of serum alpha-feto protein, thus tumour activity can be monitored by biochemistry. At US the tumour is usually of mildly raised echogenicity and is seldom calcified (Fig. 7.7.1).

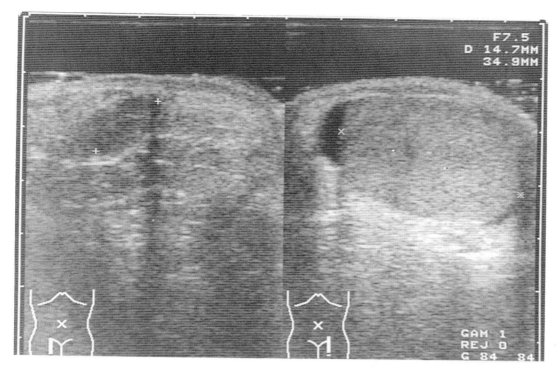

Fig. 7.7.1 Testicular US. One-year-old male child with painless swelling of the left testis. The left testis is enlarged with homogeneous increased enchodensity relative to the right. Histologically this was an endodermal sinus tumour.

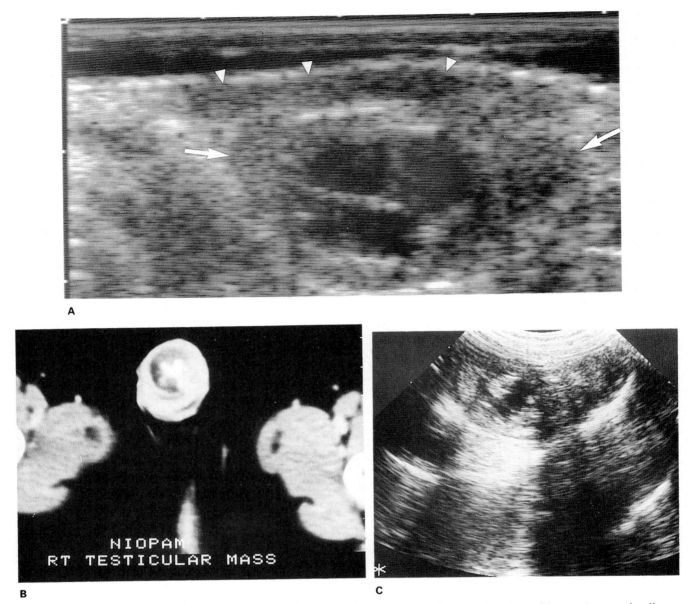

Fig. 7.7.2 **A** Benign intratesticular teratoma in an 18-month-old boy. The arrowheads indicate local swelling of the anterior scrotal wall. The mass itself (arrows) is mainly cystic. **B** Another boy with a testicular teratoma which is partially calcified. CT shows well-encapsulated tumour. **C** US of testis: heterogeneous mass.

Testicular teratoma

Testicular teratoma is the next most common tumour in childhood. This tumour has an increased incidence of calcification and this may well be palpable clinically as a hard, craggy mass. When a teratoma develops in the postpubertal age group there is an increased incidence of malignant potential, but in the prepubertal age group they are usually benign (Fig. 7.7.2). Radiological investigation is as for all other testicular tumours.

Other testicular tumours

Seminoma or choriocarcinoma are very rare during childhood, as is gonadoblastoma. Most sex cord-stroma tumours present in infancy. The Leydig cell tumour is the most common one and iso-sexual precocious pseudopuberty is a frequent feature. Leydig cell hyperplasia is bilateral and characteristically occurs in neonates of diabetic mothers or in association with Beckwith–Wiedemann syndrome and chromosomal abnormalities. Testicular Sertoli cell tumour is rare. There is a large cell type, calcifying Sertoli cell-like tumour known to occur bilaterally, multifocally and in association with complex endocrine abnormalities, Peutz–Jeghers syndrome, tuberous sclerosis and cardiac myxoma. Juvenile granulosa cell tumour of the testis occurs in babies under 6 months of age and has no endocrine features as opposed to its female counterpart.

Benign testicular lesions such as leiomyoma, fibromas and haemangiomas have all been described.

The testis is often affected by secondary neoplasm, most commonly leukaemia. Once infiltration takes place it is usually bilateral. The testis may be normal in size or enlarged and may well have a normal echodensity. Diagnosis is often by testicular biopsy. Leukaemic infiltration of the testis, though common during treatment, also occurs following treatment or during bone marrow remission. When it occurs following bone marrow transplant, there is often a very rapid relapse. Other secondary tumours in the testis are very rare but include Wilms' tumour, lymphoma, neuroblastoma and Langerhan's cell histiocytosis.

A rhabdomyosarcoma (Fig. 7.7.3) may arise anywhere within the perineum and has been described arising from the spermatic cord, the testicular appendages and the tunica. It has no characteristic radiological features. These tumours tend to grow rapidly and metastasize early to regional and retroperitoneal lymph nodes.

The differential diagnosis of all testicular masses must include a diagnosis of chronic torsion, and Doppler US is most effective in resolving the clinical problem.

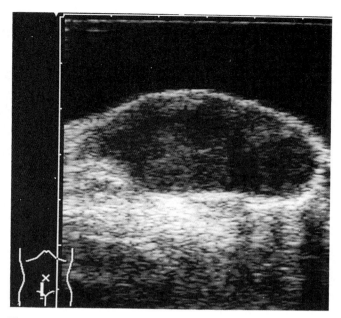

Fig. 7.7.3 Longitudinal scan of enlarged right testis containing an embryonal rhabdosarcoma in a $3\frac{1}{2}$-year-old boy with painless enlargement of the testis.

Torsion and testicular atrophy may result in absent puberty. Bilateral testicular damage from any cause, surgery, radiation or tumour, will have the same effect. Toxic injury may also result from chemotherapy.

REFERENCES

Dehner I P 1986 Gonadal and extragonadal germ cell neoplasms – teratomas in childhood. In: Finegold M (ed.) Pathology of neoplasia in children and adolescents. W B Saunders, Philadelphia, p 282

Heaney J A, Klauber G T, Conley G R 1983 Acute leukemia: diagnosis and management of testicular involvement. Urology 21: 573–577

Lorigan J G, Shirkhoda A, Dexeus F H 1989 CT and MR imaging of malignant tumor of the undescended testis. Urologic Radiology 11: 113–117

Lupetin A R, King W, Rich P, Lederman R B 1983 Ultrasound diagnosis of testicular leukemia. Radiology 146: 171–172

Pritchard J, Mitchell C D 1988 Testicular tumors in children. In: Broecker B H, Kelin F A (eds) Pediatric tumors of the genitourinary tract. Alan R Liss, New York, p 187

Raney R B Jr, Duckett J W, Donaldson M R 1984 Malignant genitourinary tumors. In: Sutow W W, Fernback D J, Vietti T J (eds) Clinical pediatric oncology, 3rd edn. Mosby-Year Book, St Louis, p 734

MULTIPLE ENDOCRINE NEOPLASIA SYNDROMES

At least three different forms of multiple endocrine neoplasia (MEN) syndromes are described and are detailed in Table 7.7.2.

Table 7.7.2   Multiple endocrine neoplasia syndrome
Type I Werner's syndrome Parathyroid adenoma or hyperplasia Islet tumours of the pancreas Pituitary tumours Adrenal cortical adenomas Thyroid adenomas
Type II (or IIA) Sipple's syndrome Medullary thyroid carcinoma Phaeochromocytoma Parathyroid adenoma or hyperplasia
Type III (or IIb) mucosal neuroma syndrome or Gorlin's syndrome *(Fig. 7.7.6)* Medullary thyroid carcinoma Phaeochromocytoma Parathyroid adenoma or hyperplasia Neuromas of the tongue, salivary glands, pancreas, gallbladder and gastrointestinal ganglia

Werner's syndrome

The pituitary tumours are mostly benign. Islet cell tumours of the pancreas include nesidioblastomas. In addition to the adenoma of the thyroid and adrenal glands, carcinoid tumours of the bronchus and of the intestinal tract have been described.

The adrenal lesions in the MEN II A and B syndromes tend to be bilateral and multiple as opposed to the sporadic form of phaeochromocytoma.

There are, in addition, unclassified manifestations of multiple or complex endocrine neoplasias including pituitary adenoma, multiple medullary thyroid carcinoma, parathyroid hyperplasia, extra-adrenal paraganglioma, gastric leiomyoma, phaeochromocytoma, islet cell tumour of the pancreas, associated with Maffucci's syndrome and phakomatosis. Unusual pathophysiological phenomena and disease courses may also suggest a multiple endocrine syndrome on initial presentation (Figs 7.7.4, 7.7.5). Endocrine disease may be associated with or complicated by some systemic infectious disease, immunodeficiency, metabolic disorder and others.

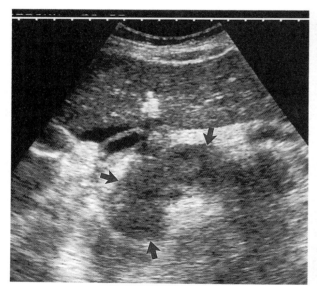

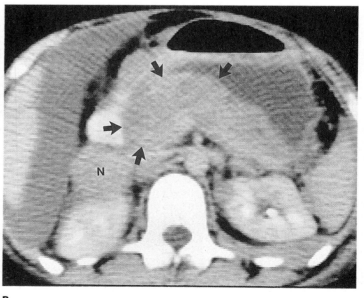

A **B**

Fig 7.7.4   Twelve-year-old girl presenting with massive ascites, pleural effusion, hilar and mesenterial lymphadenopathy as well as bilateral huge ovarian tumours. US (**A**) as well as CT (**B**) showed an enlarged pancreas (arrows) with mild structural irregularities. CT also shows ascites and tumour nodule (N) in front of right renal upper pole. Patient died after rapid deterioration over 6 weeks. Autopsy revealed extensive diffuse metastases of all organ systems including brain, heart, skeleton and soft tissues. The final diagnosis was malignant neuroendocrine tumour of ovaries.

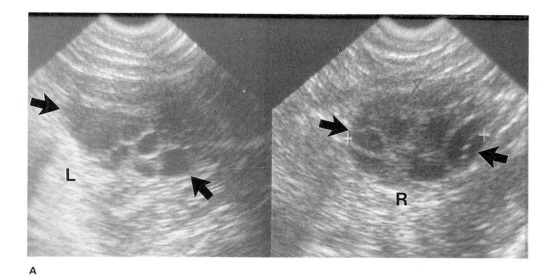

A

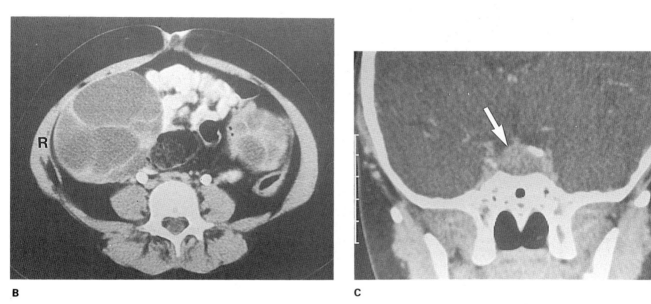

B   **C**

Fig. 7.7.5 A 13-year-old girl presenting with an adbominal mass. **A** US shows multiple cysts within enlarged ovaries (arrows). **B** CT confirms the finding. Further investigation revealed low-grade chronic hypothyroidism. **C** Cranial CT demonstrates hyperplasia of the pituitary gland (arrow) secondary to chronic hypothyroidism.

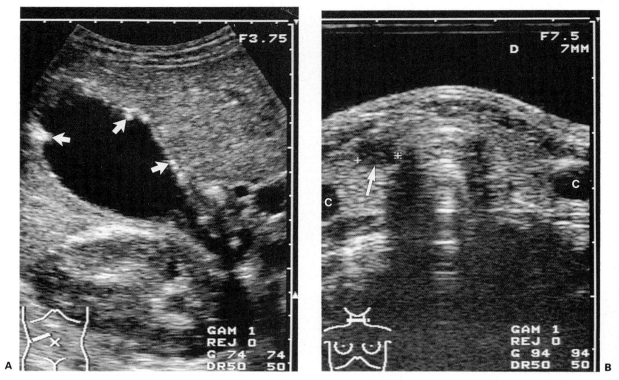

Fig. 7.7.6 Twelve-year-old boy with abdominal pain. **A** US shows multiple echogenic nodules (arrows) in the gallbladder wall. Histologically these were multiple neuromas of the gallbladder wall and suggested diagnosis of multiple endocrine neoplasia (MEN II syndrome). **B** Follow-up US of the neck demonstrated a hypoechoic right thyroid mass (arrow). Partial thyroidectomy and histology revealed thyroid carcinoma. C = carotid artery.

REFERENCES

Amano S, Hazama F et al 1978 Ectopic ACTH-MSH producing carcinoid tumor with multiple endocrine hyperplasia in a child. Acta Pathologica Japonica 28: 721

Brandi M L, Marx S H, Aurbach G D, Fitzpatrick L A 1987 Familial multiple endocrine neoplasia type I: a new look at pathophysiology.

Burke B A 1992 The pituitary, pineal, adrenal, thyroid, and parathyroid glands. In: Stocker J T, Dehner L P (eds) Pediatric pathology. JP Lippincott, Philadelphia, pp 941–1001

Carney J A, Sizemore G W, Hayles A B 1978 Multiple endocrine neoplasia, type IIB. In: Ioachim H L (ed) Pathobiol annual, vol 8. Raven, New York, p 105

Leshin M 1985 Multiple endocrine neoplasia. In: Wilson J D, Foster D W (eds) W.B. Saunders, Philadelphia, p 1274

Rabin D, McKenna T J 1982 Polyendocrine syndrome and parendocrine diseases. In: Dietchy J M (ed) Clinical endocrinology and metabolism. Principles and practice, vol 9, Grune and Stratton, New York, p 614

Webb T A, Sheps S G, Carney J A 1980 Differences between sporadic pheochromocytoma and pheochromocytoma in multiple endocrine neoplasia type II. American Journal of Surgical Pathology 4: 121

Index

N.B. The 'cele' ending has been used throughout the Index to incorporate both 'coele' and 'cele'.